PLEASE STAMP DATE DUE, BOTH BELOW AND ON CARD

DATE DUE	DATE DUE	DATE DUE	DATE DUE
OCT 8 1988	5/31/98		
OCT 2 0 1988	JUN 1 1 1990		
NOV 0 1988	SEP 2 5 2000		
NOV 1988	SEP 3 0 2002		
MAY 2 1 1990	4-30-03		
JUN 1 5 1990			
APR 0 1 1991			
MAR 2 2 1993			
APR 0 8 1993			
JUN 0 1 1994			
AUG 0 3 1996			
SEP 3 0 1996			
DEC 2 9 1996			

GL-15(3/71)

The
Bacteriophages
Volume 2

THE VIRUSES

Series Editors
HEINZ FRAENKEL-CONRAT, *University of California*
Berkeley, California

ROBERT R. WAGNER, *University of Virginia School of Medicine*
Charlottesville, Virginia

THE VIRUSES: Catalogue, Characterization, and Classification
Heinz Fraenkel-Conrat

THE ADENOVIRUSES
Edited by Harold S. Ginsberg

THE BACTERIOPHAGES
Volumes 1 and 2 • Edited by Richard Calendar

THE HERPESVIRUSES
Volumes 1–3 • Edited by Bernard Roizman
Volume 4 • Edited by Bernard Roizman and Carlos Lopez

THE PAPOVAVIRIDAE
Volume 1 • Edited by Norman P. Salzman
Volume 2 • Edited by Norman P. Salzman and Peter M. Howley

THE PARVOVIRUSES
Edited by Kenneth I. Berns

THE PLANT VIRUSES
Volume 1 • Edited by R. I. B. Francki
Volume 2 • Edited by M. H. V. Van Regenmortel and Heinz Fraenkel-Conrat
Volume 3 • Edited by Renate Koenig
Volume 4 • Edited by R. G. Milne

THE REOVIRIDAE
Edited by Wolfgang K. Joklik

THE RHABDOVIRUSES
Edited by Robert R. Wagner

THE TOGAVIRIDAE AND FLAVIVIRIDAE
Edited by Sondra Schlesinger and Milton J. Schlesinger

THE VIROIDS
Edited by T. O. Diener

The Bacteriophages
Volume 2

Edited by
RICHARD CALENDAR
University of California, Berkeley
Berkeley, California

PLENUM PRESS • NEW YORK AND LONDON

Library of Congress Cataloging in Publication Data

(Revised for vol. 2)

The Bacteriophages.

  (The Viruses)
  Includes bibliographies and index.
  1. Bacteriophages. I. Calendar, Richard. II. Series.
QR342.C35   1988   576′.6482   88-9770
ISBN 0-306-42853-9 (v. 2)

© 1988 Plenum Press, New York
A Division of Plenum Publishing Corporation
233 Spring Street, New York, N.Y. 10013

Printed in the United States of America

Contributors

Akira Aoyama, Department of Biology, University of California at San Diego, La Jolla, California 92093

Dennis H. Bamford, Department of Genetics, University of Helsinki, Helsinki SF-00100, Finland

Randall Benson, Department of Biological Sciences, University of Nebraska, Lincoln, Nebraska 68588-0118

L. Elizabeth Bertani, Biology Division, California Institute of Technology, Pasadena, California 91125

William R. Bishai, Evans Department of Medicine and Clinical Research, Boston University Medical Center, and Department of Microbiology and Molecular Genetics, Harvard Medical School, Boston, Massachusetts 02115

Lindsay W. Black, Department of Biological Chemistry, University of Maryland Medical School, Baltimore, Maryland 21201

Fred Eiserling, Department of Microbiology, University of California, Los Angeles, California 90024

Olivier Fayet, Centre de Recherche de Biochimie et de Genetique Cellulaires du CNRS, Toulouse, France 31062

David I. Friedman, Department of Microbiology and Immunology, University of Michigan Medical School, Ann Arbor, Michigan 48109-0620

Costa Georgopoulos, Department of Cellular, Viral, and Molecular Biology, University of Utah School of Medicine, Salt Lake City, Utah 84132

Marie N. Hayashi, Department of Biology, University of California at San Diego, La Jolla, California 92093

Masaki Hayashi, Department of Biology, University of California at San Diego, La Jolla, California 92093

Yen Sen Ho, Department of Molecular Genetics, Research and Development Division, Smith Kline and French Laboratories, King of Prussia, Pennsylvania 19406-0939

France Keppel, Department of Molecular Biology, University of Geneva, Geneva 1211, Switzerland

Diane R. Kiino, Departments of Biochemistry and Molecular Biology, and Molecular Genetics and Cell Biology, University of Chicago, Chicago, Illinois 60637

Eugene Martin, Department of Biological Sciences, University of Nebraska, Lincoln, Nebraska 68588-0118

Leonard Mindich, Department of Microbiology, Public Health Research Institute, New York, New York 10016

Peter Model, The Rockefeller University, New York, New York 10021

Gisela Mosig, Department of Molecular Biology, Vanderbilt University, Nashville, Tennessee 37235

John R. Murphy, Evans Department of Medicine and Clinical Research, Boston University Medical Center, Boston, Massachusetts 02118

Anthony R. Poteete, Department of Molecular Genetics and Microbiology, University of Massachusetts Medical School, Worcester, Massachusetts 01605

Delwood L. Richardson, Jr., Department of Chemistry, University of California at San Diego, La Jolla, California 92093

Martin Rosenberg, Department of Molecular Genetics, Research and Development Division, Smith Kline and French Laboratories, King of Prussia, Pennsylvania 19406-0939

Lucia B. Rothman-Denes, Departments of Biochemistry and Molecular Biology, and Molecular Genetics and Cell Biology, University of Chicago, Chicago, Illinois 60637

Marjorie Russel, The Rockefeller University, New York, New York 10021

Erich W. Six, Department of Microbiology, University of Iowa, Iowa City, Iowa 52242

Preface

It has been 10 years since the Plenum Publishing Corporation printed a series of review articles on bacteriophages in *Comprehensive Virology*. Articles in that series contained physical–genetic maps but very little DNA sequence information. Now the complete DNA sequence is known for some phages, and others will soon follow. During the past 10 years, two phages have come into common use as reagents: λ phage for cloning single copies of genes, and M13 for cloning and DNA sequencing by the dideoxy termination method. Also during this period the use of alternative sigma factors by RNA polymerase has become established for SPO1 and T4. This seems to be a widely used mechanism in bacteria, since it has been implicated in sporulation, heat shock response, and regulation of nitrogen metabolism. The control of transcription by the binding of λ phage CII protein to the −35 region of the promoter is a recent finding, and it is not known how widespread this mechanism may be. This rapid progress made me eager to solicit a new series of reviews. These chapters are of two types: each of the first type deals with an issue that is exemplified by many kinds of phages. Chapters of this type should be useful in teaching advanced courses. Chapters of the second type provide comprehensive pictures of individual phage families and should provide valuable information for use in planning experiments. During the next 10 years, at least, phages will still be attractive model systems for studies of the interactions between DNA, RNA, and proteins, since they are so easy to handle and since so much is already known about them.

These volumes are dedicated to Arthur Kornberg on the occasion of his 70th birthday. When I was a graduate student in his department, Arthur was always available, and his advice had enormous value. Recently, the success of my research on P4 phage DNA replication has depended upon generous gifts of purified proteins from Arthur's laboratory. In facing life's predictable crises, I invariably find the path to humility by asking myself "how did Arthur handle this?"

Richard Calendar

Berkeley, California

Contents

Chapter 1

Biology of the Bacteriophage φX174

*Masaki Hayashi, Akira Aoyama, Delwood L. Richardson Jr., and
Marie N. Hayashi*

Chapter 2

The P2-like Phages and Their Parasite, P4

L. Elizabeth Bertani and Erich W. Six

Chapter 3

Strategies of Bacteriophage DNA Replication

France Keppel, Olivier Fayet, and Costa Georgopoulos

Chapter 4

Regulation of Phage Gene Expression by Termination and Antitermination of Transcription

David I. Friedman

Chapter 5

DNA Packaging in dsDNA Bacteriophages

Lindsay W. Black

Chapter 6

Filamentous Bacteriophage

Peter Model and Marjorie Russel

Chapter 7

Bacteriophage N4

Diane R. Kiino and Lucia B. Rothman-Denes

Chapter 8

Lipid-Containing Bacteriophages

Leonard Mindich and Dennis H. Bamford

Chapter 9

Phage T4 Structure and Metabolism

Gisela Mosig and Fred Eiserling

Chapter 12

Bacteriophage Gene Products That Cause Human Disease

William R. Bishai and John R. Murphy

Chapter 13

Structure and Function of the Transcription Activator Protein cII and Its Regulatory Signals

Yen Sen Ho and Martin Rosenberg

CHAPTER 1

Biology of the Bacteriophage φX174

MASAKI HAYASHI, AKIRA AOYAMA, DELWOOD L.
RICHARDSON, JR., AND MARIE N. HAYASHI

I. INTRODUCTION

φX174 is a small, icosahedral, bacteriophage consisting of circular, single-stranded DNA and a protein capsid (Sinsheimer, 1959a,b). Because φX174 has a small genome and the structure of the mature phage is relatively simple, it has been an attractive system for investigating DNA replication, gene expression, DNA-protein and protein-protein interactions, and morphogenesis.

This review is divided into two sections. In the first section, some pertinent results are described as background material. Denhardt (1977) and Denhardt et al. (1978) have published extensive reviews covering most aspects of the isometric phages. Therefore, the background material will summarize the progress made up to the time of their reviews, and the references will not be exhaustive. Since then, there have been a large number of publications. We review these in more detail later. A few areas not covered in the later sections were brought up to date with new references. General references on related areas are available; Casjens (1985) for virus structure and assembly, Kornberg (1980, 1982, 1983) for DNA replication, Baas (1985) for DNA replication of single-stranded DNA phages, Geider and Hoffmann-Berling (1981) for proteins controlling DNA helical

MASAKI HAYASHI, AKIRA AOYAMA, AND MARIE N. HAYASHI • Department of
Biology, University of California at San Diego, La Jolla, California 92093.   DELWOOD L.
RICHARDSON, JR. • Department of Chemistry, University of California at San Diego,
La Jolla, California 92093.

structure, McHenry (1985) for structure and function of DNA polymerase III holoenzyme, and Hubscher and Spadari (1984) for enzymes involved in DNA replication.

II. BACKGROUND

A. The Genomes

The group of isometric, single-stranded (SS) DNA phages consists of about 15 members (see Godson, 1978, for review). Among them, φX174, S13, and G4 have been extensively studied. Sanger *et al.* (1977, 1978) sequenced all 5386 nucleotides of the φX174 genome. This was the first sequencing of the entire genome of a DNA-containing organism. Subsequently, G4 (Godson *et al.*, 1978a) and S13 (Lau and Spencer, 1985) sequences were determined. Although the gene orientations on the genome are identical in these phages, the DNA sequences are significantly different. The S13 genome contains 5386 nucleotides (identical to φX174) and differs from φX174 by 87 transitions and 24 transversions. The G4 genome consists of 5577 nucleotides and has 67% homology with the φX174 genome (Godson *et al.*, 1978b).

Recently, various mutants of alpha3 (α3), an isometric SS DNA phage, have been isolated. Complementation tests and partial DNA sequences indicated that α3 is very similar to φX174 in gene orientations, but there are significant differences in nucleotide sequences (Kodaira and Taketo, 1984a,b; Kodaira *et al.*, 1985).

B. The Genes

The φX174 genome encodes nine essential genes: A, B, C, D, E, F, G, H, and J (see Tessman and Tessman, 1979; Hayashi, 1978, for reviews). Protein capsids of mature phages consist of gpF (major capsid protein), gpG (major spike protein), gpH (minor spike protein), and gpJ (internal protein). A protein capsid precursor (prohead) is composed of gpF, gpG, gpH, and nonphage structural proteins gpB and gpD. gpA is a site-specific, strand-specific endonuclease (Section V.B). gpE is not required for intracellular phage development, but controls lysis of host cells. The 10th gene, A*, was found encoded within gene A (Linney *et al.*, 1972; Linney and Hayashi, 1973). gpA* is responsible for shutting off host DNA replication (Funk and Snover, 1976; Martin and Godson, 1975; Colasanti and Denhardt, 1985). The 11th gene, K, was proposed by Tessman *et al.* (1980). gpK is apparently not needed for phage synthesis, but it seems to stimulate phage production (Tessman *et al.*, 1980; Gillam *et al.*, 1985). The function(s) of gpK remain(s) unknown. Table I lists the φX174 genes and their functions.

TABLE I. Genes of øX174

Gene	Gene function	DNA replication stages[a] blocked by mutation	Mol. wt. of gp in PAGE[a]	Mol. wt. of gp from sequence
A	Stg. II, stg. III	RF→RF, RF→SS	60,000	58,650
A*	Shut off host DNA repl.	Unknown (see text)	37,000	38,700
B	Morphogenesis, Ω[b]	RF→SS	20,000	13,830
C	Switch stg. II to stg. III	RF→SS[c]	5,800[d]	10,050
D	Morphogenesis, Ω,[b] 132S comp.	RF→SS	14,000	16,920
E	Lysis	None	10,000[e]	10,370
F	Major capsid protein, Ω[b]	RF→SS	50,000	48,440
G	Major spike protein, Ω[b]	RF→SS	20,000	19,020
H	Minor spike protein, Ω,[b] adsorption	RF→stable SS	37,000	34,370
J	Phage internal protein, stg. III	RF→stable SS[f]	4,050[g]	4,220
K	Stimulation of phage synthesis	None	8,000[h]	6,380

[a] See Denhardt (1977) for A, A*, B, D, F, G, and H.
[b] Ω Prohead component.
[c] Aoyama and Hayashi (1985).
[d] Aoyama et al. (1983).
[e] Pollock et al. (1978).
[f] Hamatake et al. (1985).
[g] Freymeyer et al. (1977).
[h] Tessman et al. (1980).
Abbreviations: comp., component; repl., replication; stg. II and stg. III, stage II and stage III DNA replication.

C. Genetic Map

The nine essential genes were mapped by standard crosses of mutants (Baker and Tessman, 1967; Benbow *et al.*, 1974) or heteroduplex transfection methods (Hayashi and Hayashi, 1974; Weisbeek *et al.*, 1976) and were arranged along the circular genome, except for gene J (mutants have not been found). The presence of K (Tessman *et al.*, 1980) and J (Burgess and Denhardt, 1969; Gelfand and Hayashi, 1969) were deduced by gel electrophoresis. Gene A* was predicted by gel analysis of a series of A mutant proteins and by fingerprinting of gpA and gpA* (Linney *et al.*, 1972; Linney and Hayashi, 1973). The exact positions of these genes were determined from the Sanger sequence.

The protein products of most of these genes had been identified by polyacrylamide gel electrophoresis (PAGE) by 1977 (see Denhardt, 1977, for review). The sum of the estimated molecular weights is about 2.7×10^5 daltons. This corresponds to a coding capacity of about 6800 nucleotides, which is far more than the 5500 nucleotides estimated at the time (Sinsheimer, 1959a). This was interpreted either by anomaly of protein migrations in PAGE gels or by the existence of some unknown, peculiar orientation of genes in the genome. An early study by Linney *et al.* (1972) showed that gene A region codes two genes, A and A*. Translation of gene A region was initiated at two different sites in the same reading frame. The larger protein is A, and the smaller one is A*. Two overlapping genes that were read in different reading frames were subsequently discovered. Weisbeek *et al.* (1977) have shown, by genetic evi-

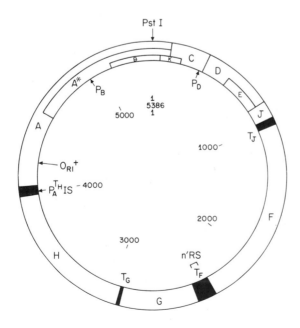

FIGURE 1. Genetic map of φX174. This map is constructed according to the Sanger *et al.* (1978) sequence data. A unique PST 1 site is the reference point (nucleotide 1). $O_{RI}{}^+$ is the origin of the (+) strand DNA synthesis. P_A, P_B, and P_D are promoters, and T_J, T_F, T_G, and T_H are transcription terminators (Hayashi *et al.*, 1986). IS is the incompatibility sequence (Van der Avoort *et al.*, 1982, 1984). n'RS is the n' protein recognition site (Shlomai and Kornberg 1980a).

dence, that gene B is encoded completely within gene A. They proposed that the overlap region can be translated in two ways with different reading frames: one frame for the synthesis of the A and A* proteins, another for the synthesis of B protein. Sanger *et al.* (1977) confirmed these results by DNA sequence analysis. Barrell *et al.* (1976) found that gene E lies within the gene D coding sequence. Gene K was deduced from the Sanger sequence to overlap genes A and C. These frugal uses of DNA sequence to code for multiple genes triggered the numerous findings of overlapping genes in other organisms (see Normark *et al.*, 1983; Kozak, 1986, for review). The genetic map of φX174 is shown in Fig. 1.

D. Outline of the Infection Process

The morphogenesis was outlined in several reviews (Dressler *et al.*, 1978; Hayashi, 1978) and is outlined in Fig. 2. The infection of *E. coli* by φX174 involves three steps: adsorption to lipopolysaccharide receptors on the cell surface, eclipse of the capsid with the ejection of the DNA, and DNA penetration into the host cell (see Incardona, 1978, for review). gpH (pilot protein) is transferred into the cell with the viral DNA and is thought to direct binding to a specific membrane site. During the life cycle in host cell, the viral genome undergoes three stages of DNA replication. Stage I DNA replication is the conversion of SS DNA to RF DNA at this specific membrane site and requires at least 13 host-originated proteins but no phage-encoded proteins. Stage II is semiconservative replication of RF DNA and is carried out by the proteins involved in stage I plus two additional proteins, *E. coli rep* protein and φX174 gpA. gpA cleaves at the *ori*$^+$ site of the viral strand [(+) strand] and binds at the 5' end. This allows further replication of RF. Stage III is the synthesis of viral circular DNA from RF-gpA complex. This process is tightly coupled to the formation of mature phage and requires the φX174-coded proteins gpA, gpB, gpC, gpD, gpF, gpG, gpH, and gpJ as well as host proteins, DNA polymerase III holoenzyme, and *rep* protein. Prohead is a capsid precursor that is assembled from gpF, gpH, gpG, gpB, and gpD. The RF-gpA complex associates with prohead to form a replication assembly (50S complex). gpC controls conversion from stage II replication to DNA packaging into prohead (Aoyama and Hayashi, 1986). The viral DNA synthesis proceeds in the 50S complex by a rolling circle mechanism with the displaced viral strand packaged into prohead. gpJ is incorporated into prohead along with the displaced viral strand, and gpB is removed from the replication complex by an unknown mechanism. When one round of replication is completed, gpA cleaves the viral strand at *ori*$^+$ and joins the two ends to form a packaged circular genome. The products of this stage are RF-gpA complex and a 132S particle, which is infectious. When gpD is eliminated from the 132S particle, stable, mature φX174 (114S) is made. These stages are shown schematically in Fig. 2.

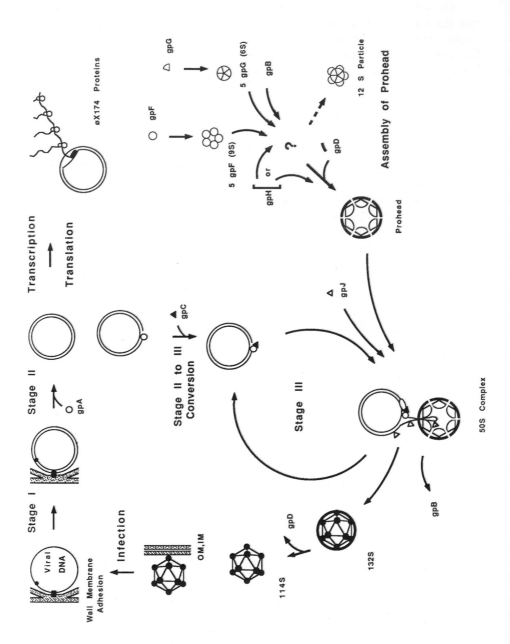

E. Gene Expression

In the φX174 system, transcription and consequently translation occur throughout the phage infection period. There is no temporal switch from one class of genes to another, as has been observed in more complex bacteriophages. No evidence exists for alteration or modification of the host transcriptional and translational apparatus due to φX174 infection. Host transcription is not shut off and seems to proceed after infection, although the host system tends to be inhibited as the phage development progresses.

An early work showed that φX174 mRNA *in vivo* is exclusively transcribed from the complementary strand [(−) strand of RF]; thus, the sequence of mRNA is identical to that of viral DNA [(+) strand] (Hayashi et al., 1963). No antimessages were found. These observations were also reproduced in an *in vitro* transcription system that consisted of RF DNA and purified RNA polymerase (Hayashi et al., 1964).

Smith and Sinsheimer (1976a,b,c) and Axelrod (1976a,b) found that promoters are located near the beginnings of gene A (P_A), gene B (P_B), and gene D (P_D) in *in vitro* transcription systems. Grohman et al. (1975) determined the nucleotide sequences of the 5′ termini of the *in virto* transcripts initiated at these sites. Sanger et al. (1977) have determined the entire genome sequence of φX174, and with the information from Grohman et al. (1975), Smith and Sinsheimer (1976a,b,c), and Axelrod (1976a,b), they were able to locate the exact position of P_A, P_B, and P_D.

Axelrod's results (1976a,b) suggested the presence of four possible termination sites on φX174 RF DNA. Two of these sites (T_1 and T_3) function only in the presence of the termination factor *rho*. Termination *in vitro* at the other two sites was *rho*-independent. Smith and Sin-

---

FIGURE 2. Model of overall morphogenesis of φX174. The infection of the host cell by φX174 results in the viral SS DNA attached to a bacterial membrane site (the black rectangle) at a wall membrane adhesion region. gpH (the minor spike protein; small black circle) is transferred along with the DNA and remains associated with the DNA. DNA replication proceeds by three discrete stages. Stage I (SS → DS) requires 13 host proteins. Stage II (DS → DS) requires gpA and host proteins. DNA replicating by stage II is converted to stage III by the binding of gpC. Stage III (DS → packaged SS) also requires prohead (see below) and gpJ and proceeds via the 50S complex to yield phage particles. The 132S phage particle is converted to the 114S phage upon exposure to divalent cations in a maturation process that results in the release of gpD. Transcription and translation occur throughout infection. Five molecules of gpF (major capsid protein) associate to form the 9S particle, and five molecules of gpG (major spike protein) associate to form the 6S particle. gpB is required along with the 6S and 9S to form a prohead precursor which is inferred but has not been identified. Attempts to isolate this particle have yielded the 12S particle, which contains 5 gpF and 5 gpG. The prohead precursor combines with gpD to form the prohead structure, which contains gpF, gpG, gpB, gpD, and optimally gpH. The timing of the incorporation of gpH during prohead morphogenesis is unclear. OM, outer membrane; IM, inner membrane; outer circle of DNA is the viral (+) strand; inner is the (−) strand. Adapted from Fujisawa and Hayashi (1977c).

sheimer (1976b) observed only one *in vitro* termination site that was independent of *rho*. Kapitza *et al.* (1979) found in an *in vitro* system three *rho*-dependent sites. These promoter and termination sites are shown in Fig. 3.

Because of the complexity of the termination events *in vitro* (as observed in differences among *in vitro* systems), the termination sites have not been sequenced. Several papers attempted to deduce possible termination sites from the known DNA sequences using computer programs based on duplex stability (McMahon and Tinoco, 1978), G + C–rich palindromes followed by poly T or A sequences (Otsuka and Kunisawa, 1982), and

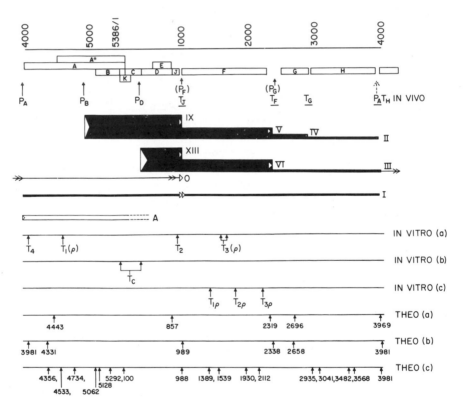

FIGURE 3. Transcription map of φX174. Black bars represent transcripts of φX174 *in vivo* (Hayashi *et al.*, 1976). Thickness of the bars is proportional to the amount of the RNA. 0 and Roman numerals I to XIII represent major RNA species in infected cells. Species 0 starts at P_D and terminates at T_J after one round of transcription. Species I is the whole genome transcript which may be initiated at P_F (a rare initiation site; Van der Avoort *et al.*, 1983) and terminated at T_J. A is unstable functional gene A mRNA; termination site is unknown. Termination sites deduced from *in vivo* systems (a) Axelrod (1976a), (b) Smith and Sinsheimer (1976a), (c) Kapitza *et al.* (1979). Termination sites deduced from the sequence analysis THEO (a) McMahon and Tinoco (1978), (b) Otsuka and Kunisawa (1982), (c) Brendel (1985).

normalization of known terminator sequences (Brendel, 1985). These sites are also shown in Fig. 3.

Hayashi and Hayashi (1970) and Clements and Sinsheimer (1975) found that most φX174 mRNAs *in vivo* were stable and could be separated as discrete size species in a gel electrophoresis. These mRNAs were mapped by hybridization to the restricted RF DNA fragments (Hayashi *et al.*, 1976) (Fig. 3). This map indicates that promoters exist before genes B and D (P_B and P_D). Transcription terminators are found after genes J, F, G, and H (T_J, T_F, T_G, and T_H). As shown previously by Linney and Hayashi (1974) and Puga *et al.* (1973), Hayashi *et al.* (1976) found that functional gene A mRNA was unstable, and it was therefore not possible to determine the transcription unit of gene A mRNA. The functional, unstable gene A mRNA may start at P_A. Promoters and *in vivo* terminators are also shown in Fig. 3.

φX174 apparently lacks any sophisticated regulation mechanism, such as positive or negative regulation systems. However, the arrangement of promoters and termination sites along the genome, and the efficiencies of termination events, may serve as a simple control mechanism (Fig. 3). The dosage of message for each φX174 gene can be estimated, because the molecular weight and relative amount of each RNA species and the cistrons encoded in each RNA species are known (Fig. 3). A comparison between each protein synthesized in infected cells and its RNA dosage shows a positive relationship between the amount of mRNA and the amount of protein. Promoters P_B and P_D are located at positions such that the most abundantly expressed genes (probably the most needed proteins), such as B and D, are most frequently transcribed. Alternatively, gpH is synthesized in the smallest amount (probably a less needed protein), because the gene is located at the distal ends of the promoters, and mRNA passing through gene H has escaped three termination events. Amounts of gpC, gpF, and gpG are roughly proportional to the amount of mRNA. Thus, this type of regulation of gene expression may be regarded as a primitive attenuation system (see Yanofsky, 1981, for review). The affinity of ribosome-binding sites (RBS) will further control the gene expression more delicately. One exception from these regulation mechanisms is gpE. Since gene E overlaps gene D, translation of gene E is tightly regulated by gene D expression (Section VI.F).

III. PHAGE STRUCTURE

A. The 114S Particle

The φX174 capsid is icosahedral in shape, with prominent spikes, and measures 25 nm in diameter. There are 60 gpF, 60 gpG, 12 gpH, and

60 gpJ per phage (Burgess, 1969). The viral DNA is circular, single-stranded (SS), and 5386 bases long (Sanger *et al.*, 1977, 1978).

The spikes were removed from the capsid by treatment with 4M urea (Edgell *et al.*, 1969). The capsid contained gpF, gpJ, and the viral DNA, and the spikes contained gpG and gpH (Shank *et al.*, 1977). Additionally, a precipitate was formed upon urea treatment that contains a significant amount of gpF and gpG. It has been postulated that gpJ binds to and condenses the viral DNA inside the capsid (Freymeyer *et al.*, 1977; Hamatake *et al.*, 1985). gpJ binds both SS and DS DNA, although there is a slight preference for SS DNA in competitive binding experiments (Hamatake, 1983; Hamatake *et al.*, 1985).

Yazaki (1981) observed that the spike is pentagonal and frustum-shaped by electron microscopy using a combination of staining with uranyl acetate and shadowing with platinum-palladium. The spikes measure 9 nm at the base and 6 nm high (Fig. 4). The phage capsid was 25 nm in diameter.

The basic model of ϕX174 structure (see Fig. 5) is a capsid of 60 gpF arranged with icosahedral symmetry (12 pentamers of F) containing SS DNA and 60 gpJ. It is proposed that the 12 prominent spikes, arranged at the vertices of an icosahedron, are composed of pentamers of gpG and a single gpH (Shank *et al.*, 1977). Dunker (1974) suggests that ϕX174 is a T=1 icosahedron, since is contains 60 each of gpF and gpG. This would correspond to a regular icosahedron made of 12 pentameric assemblies, capped with a gpH, distributed at the vertices of the icosahedron.

The laser Raman spectrum of the phage capsid was used to study the structure of the DNA and the proteins in the capsid (Incardona *et al.*, 1987). The Raman profile of the encapsidated DNA indicates the nucleosides have *C2'-endo* sugar pucker and *anti* glycosidic bond orientation as would be true of B-form DNA, but the nucleic acid backbone does not have the geometry characteristic of the B-form DS DNA. Instead, the Raman profile indicates that the backbone is in a conformation more characteristic of a heat-denatured form rather than a B form (Incardona *et al.*, 1987). Their finding suggests limited interbase interactions in the capsid, in contrast to the observed (Edlind and Ihler, 1980) and predicted (Nussinov and Pieczenik, 1984) long-range base pairing of SS ϕX174 DNA. The limited interbase interactions of encapsidated ϕX174 DNA contrasts with the DS A-form RNA secondary structure observed in SS RNA plant viruses and bacteriophages by laser Raman spectroscopy (Thomas, 1986). Incardona *et al.* (1987) suggest that the lack of interbase interactions is the result of constraints imposed by the viral capsid, and suggest the possibility of DNA-protein interactions in the phage structure. Fourier deconvolution of the Raman amide I band provide an estimate of 60% total β-sheet secondary structure in all proteins of the virion. The amide III region of the spectrum confirms that β-sheet and irregular domains are the predominant protein secondary structures.

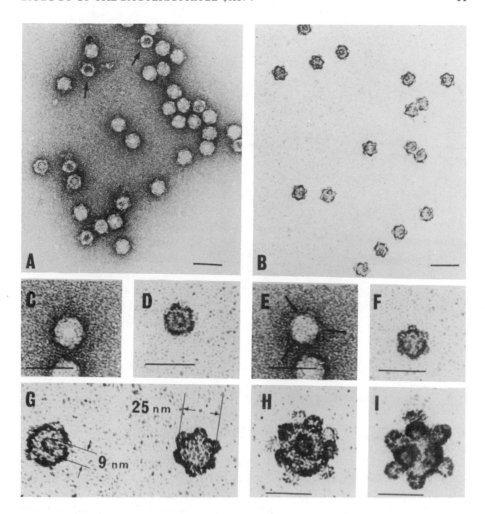

FIGURE 4. Electron micrographs of phage. (A) Negatively stained φX174 particles with 2.5% uranyl acetate. Arrows indicate empty particles. Some particles have electron-transparent (white) spots on the particle. (B) φX174 visualized by the staining and shadowing method. Spikes of the particle are clearly observed. (C) Negatively stained φX174 particle having one spot at the uppermost part of the particle. (D) φX174 particle having the same positioning on the support film as the particle of C, visualized by the staining and shadowing method. (E) Negatively stained φX174 particle with three spots on the particle (arrows). (F) φX174 particle positioned in a similar manner to that of E, visualized with the staining and shadowing method. (G) Sizes of the φX174 particle, 25 nm in diameter for the icosahedral capsid and 9 nm in diameter for the base part of the pentagonal frustum-shaped spike. (H, I) CPV (cytoplasmic-polyhedrosis virus from silkworm) particles visualized with the staining and shadowing method. The particle in H is in the same spatial orientation as the φX174 particle in D, and that in I is similar to that in F. All bars indicate 50 nm. C–F, H, and I are shown under the same magnification. Note the difference in size of these two kinds of viruses. Electron micrographs were kindly provided by Dr. K. Yazaki. Figure from Yazaki (1981).

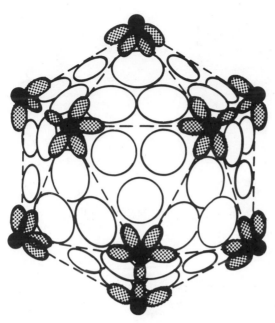

FIGURE 5. Model of phage structure. Sixty molecules of gpF (large white circles) are distributed with icosahedral symmetry. The spikes at the vertices of the icosahedron are composed of pentamers of gpG (cross-hatched) and a single gpH (black circle). Model from Hayashi (1978), adapted from Shank *et al.* (1977).

B. The 132S Particle

The 132S particle, which is also infectious, is made up of the proteins gpF, gpG, gpH, gpJ, and gpD and the viral DNA (140S particle of Weisbeek and Sinsheimer, 1974; Fujisawa and Hayashi, 1977a,b). The relative amounts of gpF, gpH, gpG, and gpJ in this particle are similar to that of phage (Weisbeek and Sinsheimer, 1974). It appeared spherical with a diameter of 40 nm in electron micrographs when stained by neutral sodium phosphotungstate (Fujisawa and Hayashi, 1977b). The phage had prominent spikes and measured 32 nm in the same conditions (Fujisawa and Hayashi, 1977b). Fujisawa and Hayashi (1977a) found that the presence of gpD protects the 132S particle from inactivation by antiphage sera (under conditions that would inactivate mature phage) and proposed that gpD was in the external layer of the particle.

The 132S particle can be converted to the 114S particle *in vitro* (Weisbeek and Sinsheimer, 1974; Fujisawa and Hayashi, 1977b). However, pulse and pulse-chase experiments indicated no clear precursor-product relationship between the 132S and 114S phage particles *in vivo* (Fujisawa and Hayashi, 1977b). Exposure of the 132S particle to Mg^{2+}, Ca^{2+}, or Mn^{2+} results in release of gpD, leaving infectious phage (114S particle). When gpD is removed by exposure to Zn^{2+} or dilution in 20 mM TRIS buffer (pH 7.4), the resultant particles are uninfectious (Fujisawa and Hayashi, 1977b). The conversion is probably not reversible, since the 114S particle cannot be converted to the 132S particle by incubating with an extract containing gpD (Weisbeek and Sinsheimer, 1974). Fujisawa and

Hayashi (1977b) suggested that the 132S might be the result of stage III DNA synthesis and packaging *in vivo*, which is subsequently converted to 114S upon lysis. Alternatively, some intercellular conversion of 132S to 114S may occur depending on the intracellular concentration of divalent cations. At this time it is impossible to distinguish these possibilities.

IV. INFECTION

A. Host Requirements

φX174 binds to lipopolysacharide (LPS) in the outer membrane of rough strains of *E. coli* and *Salmonella typhimurium*. The binding site is in the core polysaccharide of the LPS in *S. typhimurium* (Jazwinski *et al.*, 1975a) and *E. coli* (Incardona and Selvidge, 1973). The specificity for phage binding in the core polysaccharide of the LPS was studied using a series of *S. typhimurium* mutants that make defective LPS. An N-acetyl-glucosamine at the nonreducing end of the core polysaccharide is required for optimal binding of φX174 but no S13 (Jazwinski *et al.*, 1975a). Both phages absolutely required the terminal glucose and side chain galactose (underlined in Fig. 6A) for binding.

The core polysaccharide of LPS from φX174-sensitive *E. coli* C strain has a different structure from that of *S. typhimurium* (Fig. 6B) (Feige and

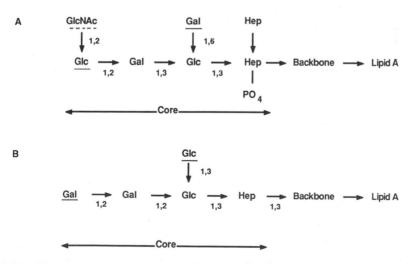

FIGURE 6. Structure of LPS core required for phage binding. (A) The core oligosaccharide from *Salmonella typhimurium* (Jazwinski *et al.*, 1975a; Luderitz *et al.*, 1971). (B) The core oligosaccharide from *E. coli* C (Feige and Stirm, 1976). GlcNAc, N-acetylglucosamine; Hep, heptose; P, phosphate.

Stirm, 1976). It was proposed that the (1→2)-linkage is important for φX174 binding (Feige and Stirm, 1976; Ohkawa, 1980). Testing phage sensitivity of various mutants with altered LPS core structures showed that the heptose region was not required for binding, loss of the branch (1→3)-linked glc reduced binding by 50%, and loss of the terminal (1→2)-linked gal reduced binding by greater than 99% (Feige and Stirm, 1976). The *E. coli* K-12 strain is resistant to φX174, but a mutant of *E. coli* K-12 with an altered LPS core was sensitive to φX174 (Ohkawa, 1980). Feige and Stirm (1976) reported that the altered LPS core had the same structure as that of the φX174-sensitive *E. coli* C strain; however, their *E. coli* C LPS core structure differed from that previously reported.

Phage binding requires the genes *rfa* and *phxB* in *E. coli* (Bachmann, 1983). *rfa* is a cluster of genes at 81 min, including *phx*, *con*, and *lpsA*, that code for LPS biosynthesis (Schmidt, 1973; McFadden and Denhardt, 1974; Havekes *et al.*, 1977). The *phx* gene is required for φX174 sensitivity and is present in *E. coli* C strain but not K-12 strain (McFadden and Denhardt, 1974). The gene *phxB* is required for φX174 adsorption (Munekiyo *et al.*, 1979) and is present in *E. coli* C and K-12 strains. It is located between *gal* and *aroG* at 17 min on the *E. coli* genetic map.

Host range mutants of φX174 map in genes G, F, and H. Newbold and Sinsheimer (1970a) have isolated temperature-sensitive gene G mutants that affected host range, and Weisbeek *et al.* (1973) mapped three host range mutants of φX174 to gene G by marker rescue of DNA restriction fragments. Dowell *et al.* (1981) reported isolation of host range mutants of φX174 capable of infecting some K-12 strains that mapped in gene F. One mutant had a wide range that included *E. coli* C and B and *Shigella* YbR. Host range mutants of gene H were located by Sinsheimer (1968). In S13, gene F mutants affected host range and adsorption (Tessman, 1965).

B. Attachment

Attachment (or adsorption) is the reversible binding of φX174 to LPS receptors. There are two forms of phage, one of which will bind to the cell or LPS at low temperatures (Bleichrodt and Van Abkoude, 1967; Incardona, 1981). The nonbinding form is more stable to heat denaturation (Bleichrodt and Van Abkoude, 1967). There is an equilibrium between the two forms that is shifted toward the binding form by exposure to pH above 7 or phosphate greater than 25 mM. Phage isolated by lysis of the infected cells at low temperature are of the nonbinding form and can be converted to the binding form by incubation at 37°C (Incardona, 1981).

Kinetics of phage binding, when observed at temperatures low enough to avoid eclipse, are first order in the presence of excess bacteria (Newbold and Sinsheimer, 1970b; Bayer and Starkey, 1972). Diffusion limits the attachment of phages to cells, as shown by close agreement of the experimentally determined binding constant and that calculated from the diffusion constant (Bayer and Starkey, 1972; Incardona, 1983a). A review of theoretical papers (Incardona, 1983a) indicates that there is a hyperbolic relationship between the per-cell binding constant and the receptor density; the binding constant (per receptor) is essentially independent of receptor density when the density is above 1000 sites per cell.

Incardona (1983b) has proposed a kinetic model for the attachment process (see Fig. 7) that includes reversible binding to free (SF) and cell-bound (S) LPS and shedding of LPS with or without bound phages from cells. This model takes into account the dynamic state of the bacterial membrane which includes the continual shedding of LPS-containing membrane fragments (Rothfield and Pearlman-Kothencz, 1969). Three variations of this model with different sets of rate constants were shown to fit the experimental binding data (Incardona, 1983b); however, in each case the binding to cell-bound receptors is irreversible (i.e., k_{-1} is zero). Incardona *et al.* (1985) have proposed that binding to cell-bound LPS is essentially irreversible owing to cooperative binding to multiple adjacent LPS on the cell. They postulate that a single φX174 vertex binds to the LPS receptor, but dissocation from the cell is prevented by the subsequent interaction of adjacent receptor molecules with additional vertices. The release (shedding) of virus receptor complexes from infected cells and the dissociation of these complexes were confirmed by electron microscopy. The binding data were shown to fit the theoretical model (Incardona *et al.*, 1985) for wild-type virus at 15°C and account for the non-linearity observed at 37°C in the kinetics for mutant and wild-type virus.

Brown *et al.* (1971) and Bayer and Starkey (1972) observed that usually 2–3 spikes become imbedded in cell wall. The phage becomes submerged in the cell wall to one-half of its diameter. Bayer and Starkey (1972) observed that approximately 70% of the adsorbed particles were found at the points of adhesion between the cell wall and the inner membrane (Section IV.D).

Binding of negatively charged phages and anionic LPS requires cations to neutralize the repulsive charges. Comparison of the relative ef-

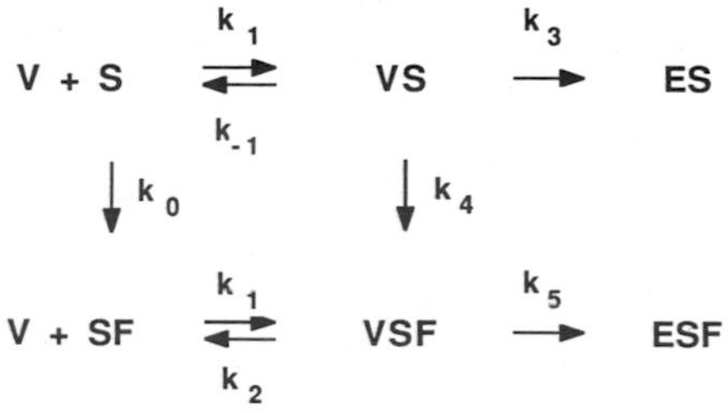

FIGURE 7. Kinetic model for phage binding and eclipse. Virus (V) binds reversibly to LPS, which is either attached to the cell (S) or free (SF; recently shed from the cell), to give a virus-LPS complex (VS, attached to cell; VSF, free). This virus-LPS complex can undergo eclipse (release of the viral DNA) on attached (ES) or free (ESF) LPS. This

$$V + S \underset{k_{-1}}{\overset{k_1}{\rightleftarrows}} VS \xrightarrow{k_3} ES$$

$$\downarrow k_0 \qquad\qquad \downarrow k_4$$

$$V + SF \underset{k_2}{\overset{k_1}{\rightleftarrows}} VSF \xrightarrow{k_5} ESF$$

model also depicts the shedding of LPS receptors, with (VSF) or without (SF) virus bound, from the cell. Model adapted from Incardona (1983b).

fects of different concentrations of uni- and multivalent ions on the inactivation of phage by LPS show that Na^+ neutralizes electrostatic repulsion by an ionic strength effect while binding is also involved for bi- and trivalent ions (Rowatt, 1984). For inactivation by different types of multivalent metal ions and polyamines, the concentration required for 50% inactivation varies inversely with the charge on the cation (Rowatt and Williams, 1985). The increase in activity as the charge rises suggests that electrostatic binding is overwhelmingly important.

C. Eclipse

The eclipse is an irreversible reaction in which the DNA is ejected from the capsid. Binding to the LPS isolated from phage-sensitive cells, which requires 1 mM Ca^{2+} or Mg^{2+}, was sufficient for eclipse when the temperature is above 20°C (Incardona and Selvidge, 1973). The lipid A portion of the LPS was required for eclipse but not for adsorption (Jazwinski *et al.*, 1975a). Alternatively, phages can be eclipsed by exposure to high concentrations of $CaCl_2$ (100 mM) at temperatures above 20°C (Incardona, 1974), with kinetics similar to that of phage bound to intact host cells. The eclipse rate approaches zero at 15°C owing to the high (approximately 35 kcal/mole) energy of activation (Newbold and Sinsheimer, 1970b; Incardona, 1974, 1981).

Incardona (1981) designed a novel selection protocol to enrich for cold-sensitive eclipse mutants by the application of Arrhenius kinetic theory. He found that mutants could be isolated with altered eclipse rates due to structural changes affecting two parameters, the entropy and enthalpy of activation. Enrichment of a mutagenized virus population for mutants that failed to eclipse after a short period at 37°C gave an increase for the cs (cold-sensitive) phenotype from 0.2% to 2–4%, while the frequency of the ts (temperature-sensitive) phenotype remained unchanged (less than 0.2%). As predicted, the cs mutants characterized had either a higher enthalpy of activation or a lower entropy of activation.

Further investigations have attempted to use the physical parameters indicated by the eclipse rate to detect and characterize altered quaternary structures (Incardona and Müller, 1985). The eclipse kinetics of Fcs70 (a previously characterized cs mutant in gpF) have shown that the enthalpy of activation is equal to wild type, whereas the entropy of activation is reduced (Incardona, 1974). Later experiments on the eclipse kinetics of Fcs70 over a wider range of temperatures showed that the enthalpy of activation is also larger (Incardona and Müller, 1985). The deletion of 27 bases in the J–H intercistronic region caused a small (approximately 50%) increase in the eclipse rate, whereas the insertion of 163 bases or deletion of seven bases did not effect the eclipse rate (Incardona and Müller, 1985). They propose that the increased eclipse rate is specific to this sequence, but an alternative explanation is that a deletion of seven bases does not alter the structure enough to increase the rate, but a deletion of 27 does.

Although isolated LPS is sufficient for the eclipse reaction, there is evidence that other host factors may be involved for eclipse associated with the cell. The membrane associated *dnaP* gene product, which initiates DNA replication in *E. coli*, was found to participate in the eclipse and DNA penetration by Mano *et al.* (1979). The rate of eclipse and DNA penetration were reduced in *dnaP* mutants at the restrictive temperature.

Cell envelopes were treated with heat and detergent to look for factors involved in the eclipse reaction. Isolated cell envelope fraction had a higher eclipsing activity than isolated LPS (Mano *et al.*, 1982b). The eclipsing activity of the cell envelope fraction was heat-labile, but that of the LPS was not (Mano *et al.*, 1982b). The activity necessary to convert phages to eclipsed particles was removed by the ionic detergents cetyltrimethylammonium bromide (CTAB) and N-laurylsarcosine sodium salt (Sarkosyl) but was not removed by many nonionic detergents (Mano *et al.*, 1982a). A moderate loss of eclipsing activity by treatment with the nonionic detergent Span80 was reduced by a higher concentration of divalent cations. Mano *et al.* (1982b) proposed that a membrane-bound protein component that is heat-labile and susceptible to removal by ionic detergents is essential for the eclipse and subsequent DNA penetration.

The isolated eclipsed particle sediments at 70S, and the DNA has become sensitive to nucleases (Newbold and Sinsheimer, 1970a). Electron microscopy of eclipsed particles has been made possible by a combination of negative staining and shadowing techniques (Yazaki, 1981). The eclipse of phage immobilized on electron microscopy grids with 100 mM Ca^{2+} showed the genome extruding from the spike, and in one-third of the cases the genome extruded from two or more spikes. Some deformation of the capsid around this spike was observed (Yazaki, 1981). Phages eclipsed with LPS or cell envelope fractions and then visualized using Yazaki's (1981) negative staining and shadowing technique showed somewhat different structures (Mano *et al.*, 1982b). Eclipse with LPS gave one sort of particle where the phage DNA was extruded as a short, thick bundle.

Eclipse with the cell envelope fraction gave two types of particles. In one of them phage DNA was extruded as a short, thick bundle, and in the other more than 95% of the phage DNA was extruded from the phage particle, associated with a membrane fragment (Mano *et al.*, 1982b). For eclipse by both LPS and the cell envelope fraction, the DNA was extruded through only one spike (Mano *et al.*, 1982b). The DNA in the particles eclipsed by high Ca^{2+} formed various thicknesses and shapes such as bending, looping, or branching, which were thought to reflect the compact form of the DNA in the virus particle (Yazaki, 1981). The DNA in the particle eclipsed by the cell envelope fraction was the thickness of two strands of SS DNA and existed in a highly extended, unknotted configuration (Mano *et al.*, 1982b).

D. DNA Penetration

The eclipsed viral DNA penetrates the cell by an unknown mechanism. The process requires active metabolism by the cell and the function of gpH as a pilot protein. The DNA becomes attached to the bacterial outer membrane, where it is replicated to form RF DNA (Section V.A).

Infection of starved cells results in eclipsed phage which can be removed by buffer containing EDTA. The DNA does not penetrate the cell (Francke and Ray, 1971; Knippers *et al.*, 1969). Addition of nutrients results in rapid resumption of normal infection. Knippers *et al.* (1969) observed that the role of the host seemed to be related to some favorable condition of the cell wall or membrane instead of an active metabolism. Francke and Ray (1971) proposed that the penetration required DNA replication—that is, that penetration was somehow linked to Stage I DNA synthesis.

Involvement of and requirement for gpH in DNA penetration led Jazwinski *et al.* (1975b,c) to postulate that gpH acted as a pilot protein to guide the DNA into the cell and direct stage I DNA synthesis. gpH enhanced viral SS DNA transformation of *E. coli* spheroplasts (Jazwinski *et al.*, 1975b). gpH is transferred into the cell with the phage DNA and can be isolated on the resultant RF DNA after infection (Jazwinski *et al.*, 1975c).

The DNA is inserted and transferred to the outer membrane (Jazwinski *et al.*, 1975a). The outer membrane fraction, which contained ϕX174 DNA, was contaminated with a significant fraction of DPNH oxidase, which was used as a marker for the inner membrane. Jazwinski *et al.* (1975a) suggested that the contamination might be indicative of attachment to the wall membrane adhesion regions, which were identified as the predominate sites of phage binding by Bayer and Starkey (1972).

Van der Avoort *et al.* (1982) found that cells containing plasmids with the cloned H–A intercistronic sequence had a reduced ability to propagate ϕX174. The reduction was due to lower burst size, with only 10% of viral DNA converted to RF, and fewer progeny RF DNA synthesized. The H–A intercistronic sequence of G4 on a plasmid acts as an incompatibility sequence for both ϕX174 and G4, but that of ϕX174 only affects ϕX174 (Van der Avoort *et al.*, 1984). There is an equivalent sequence in M13, but it acts completely independent of ϕX174 and G4. It is suggested that the sequence interacts with a limiting host component, probably a specific membrane site, that the phage DNA is associated with during replication (Section V.A).

The relation of DNA penetration to stage I DNA synthesis (Section V.A) is unclear. Intact ϕX174 (Jazwinski and Kornberg, 1975) and S13 (Watabe *et al.*, 1981) are converted to RF DNA by crude extracts of *E. coli*. In the case of ϕX174, a membrane fraction was necessary that included LPS and some other, unidentified factor (Jazwinski and Kornberg, 1975).

Watabe *et al.* (1981) reported that the extract they used for S13 did not require a membrane fraction; however, Brij 58 (a detergent that may have solubilized some membrane proteins) was used to prepare the crude extract.

The φX174 DNA-membrane complex was isolated and purified by isopycnic sucrose gradient sedimentation and zone electrophoresis by Azuma *et al.* (1980). Labeled viral DNA was associated with the intermediate density membrane fraction (wall membrane adhesion region) and the cytoplasmic membrane in cells that were blocked for protein synthesis (no stage II DNA synthesis could occur). DNA in the form of RF I is chased from the wall membrane adhesion region to the cytoplasmic membrane. Azuma *et al.* (1980) suggested that the viral DNA was converted to RF I DNA on the wall membrane adhesion region. Proteins of 80,000 and 13,000 daltons were enriched in the DNA-membrane complex (Azuma *et al.*, 1980), and there is circumstantial evidence that the larger peptide may be identical to a polypeptide that is enriched in the host cell-chromosomal membrane complex.

V. DNA SYNTHESIS AND PACKAGING

A. Stage I (SS→RF)

The first stage of φX174 DNA replication is the conversion of the viral circular SS DNA to the covalently closed, supertwisted duplex form (RF I) DNA. Although this conversion takes place in the membrane fraction of the host cell and requires gpH (Section IV.D), it can be reconstituted in an *in vitro* soluble system without the membrane fraction or gpH. This *in vitro* process is entirely dependent on host enzymes and can be subdivided into six stages: prepriming (assembly of primosome), priming (formation of RNA primer), elongation (synthesis of viral DNA strand), gap filling (eliminating of RNA primer and formation of RF II DNA), ligation (formation of a covalently closed RF IV DNA), and supercoiling (formation of RF I DNA). In the prepriming stage, a group of proteins—the prepriming proteins (n', n, n", i, *dnaC*, and *dnaB*) and primase—are assembled at a specific region of the viral DNA to form a primosome. The primosome is mobile machinery for synthesizing the RNA primer along the viral DNA. The resultant RNA primer provides the initiation site for DNA polymerase III holoenzyme to synthesize the complementary strand on the template viral DNA by extending the 3' end of the RNA primer. The product of this reaction is an open circular duplex DNA with a 5' terminal RNA primer. DNA polymerase I fills the nick or the gap after its 5'→3' exonucleolytic removal of the 5' terminal RNA. A covalently closed duplex DNA (RF IV) is formed by DNA ligase, and negative twists are introduced by DNA gyrase to form RF I DNA. Reconstitution of this pathway was achieved from purified components in the laboratories of Kornberg and Hurwitz

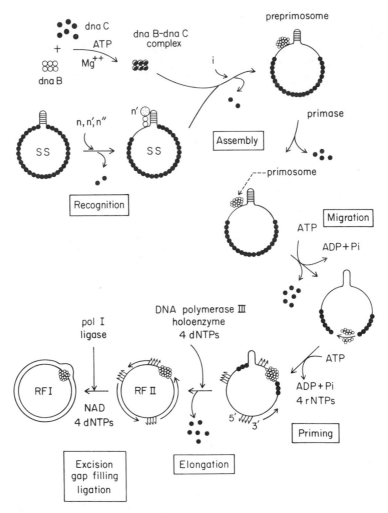

FIGURE 8. A model for stage I DNA replication. Adapted from Kobori and Kornberg (1982c).

(Shlomai *et al.*, 1981; Kornberg, 1980, 1982). The enzymology of the pathway has been elucidated in detail using these *in vitro* systems. The model of the pathway of stage I DNA replication is summarized in Fig. 8.

1. Single-Stranded DNA Binding Protein

Single-stranded DNA binding protein (SSB) of *E. coli* (Sigal *et al.*, 1972) is the first protein that interacts with the viral SS DNA. SSB is a tetrameric protein of 18,500-dalton protomers, which coats the viral DNA in a cooperative manner and destabilizes most hairpin structures (Molineux *et al.*, 1974; Molineux and Gefter, 1975; Weiner *et al.*, 1975). Chrysogelos and Griffith (1982) showed with electron microscopy that the complexes of SSB and fd SS DNA appear as beaded fiber loops similar to a nucleosome. Binding of SSB determines the specificity of the RNA priming system in E. coli cells infected by SS DNA phages (Kornberg, 1980, 1982). Three distinct priming systems have been observed in E. coli: the φX174 type, the G4 type, and the M13 type. These require for priming the primosome, primase, and RNA polymerase, respectively. A specific hairpin structure that is not destabilized by SSB provides a key signal for the initiation of priming in all cases (Kornberg, 1980, 1982).

2. Assembly of Primosome at a Specific Site on the Viral DNA

The primosome contains one molecule each of protein n', n, a hexameric dnaB protein, six molecules of dnaC protein, protein n", protein i, and primase (Arai et al., 1981c,d; Kobori and Kornberg, 1982a,b,c). The assembly of the primosome (Fig. 8) is initiated by the recognition of the specific site of the viral DNA by protein n' (Shlomai and Kornberg, 1980a). Protein n' (factor Y of Wickner and Hurwitz, 1975; a monomer of 75,000 daltons; Shlomai and Kornberg, 1980b) binds to the unique hairpin structure which is not destablized by SSB (see below). The binding of the protein n' enhances the affinity of protein n for the protein n' recognition site (Low et al., 1982). Although the purified protein n is a dimer of 13,000-dalton subunits, a monomer of protein n is incorporated into the protein n' recognition site. The binding of protein n is dependent upon SSB; direct interaction between protein n and SSB may be involved in this reaction. The formation of a complex with one protein n per one tetrameric SSB is observed in the absence of DNA (Low et al., 1982). The binding of protein n to the protein n' recognition site facilitates the binding of the protein n", which is required for the successive binding of the protein i, dnaC protein, and dnaB protein (Arai et al., 1981c,d; Low et al., 1982). Six molecules of dnaC protein (29,000 daltons; Kobori and Kornberg, 1982a,b) forms a tight complex with one molecule of hexameric dnaB protein (Kobori and Kornberg, 1982c) in the presence of ATP (Wickner and Hurwitz, 1975) and introduce dnaB protein to the preprimosome. Protein i (trimer of 22,000-dalton subunits) is required for the incorporation of the dnaB–dnaC protein complex into the preprimosome complex (Arai et al., 1981d). the dnaC proteins associate stably in the primosome during the DNA synthesis. However, the association of the dnaC proteins with the newly replicated DNA is unstable, and additional dnaC proteins may be required for the efficient further rounds of φX174 replication (Low et al., 1981). The assembly of the primosome is completed at or near the recognition site of the protein n' by the binding of primase (Arai and Kornberg, 1981a).

3. Assembly Site for Primosome

The target for binding the protein n' (factor Y) was localized to a 55-nucleotide fragment (2301–2354 of φX174 DNA sequence) that contains the potential for a 44-nucleotide hairpin structure (Fig. 9) between the

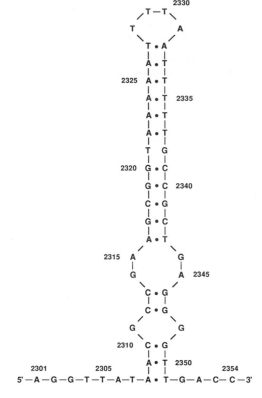

FIGURE 9. Possible secondary structure of DNA sequence at the recognition site of protein n′ (factor Y). Positions on the φX174 DNA sequence are indicated. Adapted from Shlomai and Kornberg (1980a).

genes F and G of φX174 (Shlomai and Kornberg, 1980a). The mechanism of the protein n′ recognition of the assembly site is not clear. The secondary structure may not be sufficient for the recognition of the protein n′, because the complementary strand, which can be folded into the same secondary structure, does not bind the protein n′ (Ray *et al.*, 1981). The primosome assembly sites of pBR322 (Zipursky and Marians, 1980), Col E1 (Zipursky and Marians, 1980; Nomura *et al.*, 1982), and mini F (Imber *et al.*, 1983) have been also identified on the specific hairpin structures. However, there is no apparent sequence homology between these protein n′ assembly sites (Marians *et al.*, 1982) except the stretch of seven nucleotides: G(orT)AAGCGG (Van der Ende *et al.*, 1983a). This sequence may be important for the protein n′ recognition. DNase footprinting and methylation protection experiments indicate that factor Y (protein n′) binds to the entire length of the effector site of pBR322 (Greenbaum and Marians, 1984). Since one molecule of factor Y cannot cover the entire length (if it is a globular protein as assumed), involvement of a specific tertiary interaction of DNA in the factor Y recognition was suggested (Greenbaum and Marians, 1984). Marians and his co-workers have proposed that the interaction between two hairpin structures in the factor Y recognition sites may be involved in the recognition event (Abarzua *et* al., 1984; Soeller et al., 1984; Greenbaum and Marians, 1985). However, the factor Y recognition sites of pBR322 are not essential for pBR322 replication in vivo (Van der Ende et al., 1983b), although they do support DNA synthesis in vitro (Zipursky and Marians, 1981). Therefore, the physiological roles of the target sequences for factor Y (protein n') in these plasmids are unclear.

4. Priming by Primosome

The primosome migrates along the SS DNA in a 5'→3' direction (opposite to the direction of primer synthesis and DNA elongation) (Arai and Kornberg, 1981a). The protein n', which has DNA-dependent ATPase and dATPase activities (Shlomai and Kornberg, 1980a,b), probably catalyzes the translocation of the primosome utilizing the energy of ATP or dATP hydrolysis (Arai et al., 1981a). The protein n' also destabilizes the SSB bound to the DNA during the translocation of the primosome (Shlomai and Kornberg, 1980b,c).

RNA primers are synthesized at many regions on the viral DNA when the DNA synthesis is not coupled. The distribution of the RNA primers on the DNA shows a distinct pattern, which suggests preferential transcription of certain regions. The dnaB protein of the primosome serves as a "replication promoter" that recognizes the regions where primase initiates RNA synthesis (McMacken et al., 1977; McMacken and Kornberg, 1978; Arai et al., 1981a; Arai and Kornberg, 1981c). Ogawa et al. (1983) reported that pppA-Pu is the preferred initiation sequence. When the priming reaction is coupled to the DNA synthesis, deoxyribonucleoside triphosphates are incorporated to form ribonucleotide-deoxyribonucleotide hybrids (Arai and Kornberg, 1981d). The average number of the primers on the viral DNA is approximately one primer per DNA with 1–10 ribonucleotides in each primer.

Primase (dnaG protein, a monomer of 60,000 daltons; Bouche et al., 1975; Rowen and Kornberg, 1978) requires the dnaB protein of the primosome as a replication promotor for its RNA priming of the φX174 SS DNA. The dnaB protein (a hexamer of a 50,000-dalton protomer; Reha-Krantz and Hurwitz, 1978a; Arai et al., 1981b) is an SS and DS DNA-dependent ATPase (Ueda et al., 1978; Lanka et al., 1978; Reha-Krantz and Hurwitz, 1978a,b; Arai and Kornberg, 1981b) and has distinct binding sites for ATP (or other ribonucleoside triphosphates), SS DNA, DS DNA, primase, and other proteins in its two domains (Nakayama et al., 1984). In the absence of SSB, the dnaB protein can bind to the SS DNA and promote RNA synthesis by primase (a general priming system; Arai and Kornberg, 1979). Experiments using DNA intercalating agents, such as ethidium bromide, indicate that the DNA domain inside the hexameric dnaB protein has a specific secondary structure (Arai and Kornberg, 1981c). Therefore dnaB protein may produce a structure that can be recognized by primase, within its domain by "wrapping the DNA around its surface." However, when the SS DNA is coated by SSB, the *dnaB* protein cannot bind; it can function only when it becomes one of the components of the primosome.

5. DNA Chain Elongation

The association of the holoenzyme with the primer on the SS DNA requires ATP (Burgers and Kornberg, 1982a,b; Johanson and McHenry, 1984; Biswas and Kornberg, 1984). The ATP-activated holoenzyme stays on the DNA stably during the DNA elongation.

O'Donnell and Kornberg (1985a) studied the movement of the holoenzyme at the end of the DNA elongation using a multiprimed DNA as a template. When the ATP-activated holoenzyme reaches at the 5' end of the primer, it can stop DNA synthesis, move to the 3' end of the next primer, and reinitiate the DNA synthesis without requiring energy from ATP hydrolysis. Since the holoenzyme cannot travel along the SS region of the DNA, it may bind to the duplex region rather than the 3' terminus at the replication fork.

6. Termination and Maturation

The termination of the DNA synthesis by the holoenzyme was studied using the SS DNA primed by either DNA or RNA as template (O'Donnell and Kornberg, 1985b). Virtually all (90%) of the RF II DNA synthesized by the holoenzyme had a nicked (not gapped) structure that can be sealed by ligase when the DNA-primed SS DNA was used as a template. The rest (10%) had one nucleotide beyond the 5' terminus displacing the annealed 5' terminus. When the template DNA was primed by RNA, the 5' terminus of the majority (85%) of the RF II was displaced by 1–5 nucleotides. Dissociation of the holoenzyme from the RF II DNA is a slow reaction and requires ATP hydrolysis (Burgers and Kornberg, 1983).

DNA polymerase I is required for removing the RNA primer and for sealing the RF II DNA. Since the RNA primer of the 5' terminus of the RF II DNA is displaced by DNA polymerase III holoenzyme (O'Donnell and Kornberg, 1985b), DNA polymerase I may be required only to remove the RNA and seal the RF II DNA.

In vitro studies have shown that once assembled on the viral strand, the primosome remains bound even after the viral SS DNA has become a covalently closed, supercoiled duplex form (RF IV or I DNA) (Arai *et al.*, 1980, 1981e; Low *et al.*, 1981; Kornberg, 1982). The primosome-associated RF I or RF IV DNA is a much better substrate for cleavage with gpA than supercoiled RF I DNA (Low *et al.*, 1981).

7. Incompatibility Sequence

Although stage I DNA synthesis can be reconstituted in an *in vitro* soluble system, it has been shown that stage I DNA synthesis occurs at a specific intracellular "essential bacterial site" (Knippers and Sinsheimer, 1968; Yarus and Sinsheimer, 1971). The association of parental RF DNA with the cell membrane has also been evident (Jazwinski *et al.*, 1975a; Azuma *et al.*, 1980). However, this aspect of DNA replication has not been well studied. The recent discovery of the incompatibility sequence of φX174 by Van der Avoort *et al.* (1982, 1984) is an important step toward solving this problem. They found that the intracellular presence of recombinant plasmids containing the Hind II restriction fragment 4 of φX174 greatly reduces the ability of E. *coli* cells to propagate φX174 (Van der Avoort *et al.*, 1982). This "reduction sequence" is located between nucleotides 3904 and 3989 of the φX174 DNA sequence and contains the intercistronic region between genes H and A as well as small portions of these genes (Fig. 3). Interference of phage propagation with the reduction sequence has the following characteristics: (1) Adsorption of phage to the cells is normal; (2) only 10% of infecting viral DNA is converted to RF DNA; (3) less progeny RF is synthesized; (4) the interference is φX174-specific and (5) independent of de novo protein or RNA synthesis. Therefore, the effect of the recombinant plasmids with the reduction sequence on infecting DNA is similar to the process of superinfection exclusion: the alteration of an infecting cell in such a way that superinfecting phages cannot initiate an infection (Hutchison and Sinsheimer, 1971; Tessman *et al.*, 1971). Van der Avoort *et al.* (1982) proposed that interaction between the φX174 reduction sequence and the intracellular component (membrane or protein) that is present in limited amounts. This intracellular component might be the "essential bacterial site" at which the parental RF DNA is thought to be replicated.

In a more recent study, Van der Avoort *et al.* (1984) tested the effects of the reduction sequence on the transduction of φX174-sensitive cells by chimeric phage. These chimeric phage consisted of plasmid DNA containing the φX174 origin with or without the reduction sequence packaged in the φX174 capsid. They showed that the reduction sequence inhibited the transduction when the recombinant plasmids with φX174 *ori*+ also contain the functional protein n' recognition site of φX174. Therefore, the interference also involves competition for the primosome. However, when the same recombinant plasmids were packaged into phage G4 capsid, the transduction was not affected by the φX174 reduction sequence. They proposed that the membrane sites for φX174 stage I and stage II DNAs syntheses are spatially connected to the adsorption sites for φX174 at which the infecting DNA enters the cell. The recombinant DNA packaged in a G4 particle may adsorb to a G4-specific receptor that is not connected to the φX174 replication site. Therefore, the function of the reduction sequence may be to bind the φX174 parental RF DNA to a limited number of specific sites where the replicative enzymes are present. In such a case the reduction sequence functions as a viral incompatibility element in a similar way as that proposed for plasmid incompatibility (Hakkaart *et al.*, 1982; Jacob *et al.*, 1963). Similar reduction sequences were also identified in G4 (Van der Avoort *et al.*, 1984) and M13 (Cleary and Ray, 1980, 1981;

Johnston and Ray, 1984). The G4 reduction sequence is not specific to G4, and it interferes with φX174 propagation. It may interact with the φX174-specific replication site (or component), although G4 and φX174 may have different entry sites. The M13 reduction sequence called "replication enhancer sequence" is suggested to interact with gpII, which is functionally equivalent to gpA of φX174. Therefore, it is independent of G4 or φX174 reduction sequence (Johnston and Ray, 1984).

B. Stage II (RF→RF)

The second stage of φX174 DNA replication is semiconservative replication of supercoiled RF I DNA. *In vitro* studies indicate that RF replication can be divided into viral and complementary strand synthesis (Eisenberg *et al.*, 1976b, 1978; Reinberg *et al.*, 1981). The viral strand synthesis proceeds through a rolling circle mechanism (Eisenberg *et al.*, 1976b, 1978). The complementary strand synthesis occurs in a mechanism that is essentially the same as that of the stage I DNA synthesis. These two pathways were reconstituted in a separate or a combined *in vitro* system from purified components (Shlomai and Kornberg, 1978; Arai *et al.*, 1980, 1981e; Brown *et al.*, 1983c). The mechanism of stage II DNA replication proposed from *in vitro* experiments is in good agreement with *in vivo* observations (Baas *et al.*, 1978, 1980a; Keegstra *et al.*, 1979). Figure 10 summarizes the model for stage II DNA replication.

1. Viral Strand Replication

In vitro studies show that viral strand replication requires supercoiled RF I DNA, φX174 gpA, *E. coli rep* protein, SSB, DNA polymerase III holoenzyme, ATP, deoxyribonucleoside triphosphates, and Mg^{2+} (Eisenberg *et al.*, 1976a). gpA initiates the viral strand synthesis (Eisenberg *et al.*, 1976a; Sumida-Yasumoto *et al.*, 1976) by introducing a nick on the viral strand of the supercoiled RF I DNA at the origin of the viral strand replication (ori^+) (Francke and Ray, 1972; Henry and Knippers, 1974; Van Mansfeld *et al.*, 1978). gpA then binds covalently to the newly generated 5' end of the viral strand and forms a relaxed open circular RF II DNA (RF II–gpA complex) (Ikeda *et al.*, 1979; Eisenberg and Kornberg, 1979). *rep* protein binds to the gpA of the RF II–gpA complex at the origin and unwinds the DNA strands (Scott *et al.*, 1977). Strand separation is maintained by SSB, which binds to the separated DNA strands (Scott *et al.*, 1977; Eisenberg *et al.*, 1977). DNA polymerase III holoenzyme associates the RF II–gpA–*rep* protein complex at the replication fork and extends the 3' end of the viral DNA while the 5' end of the viral strand is being displaced. The 5' end of the displaced viral strand, which is covalently attached to gpA, travels along with the replication fork in a looped rolling circle (Eisenberg *et al.*, 1977). When one round of the

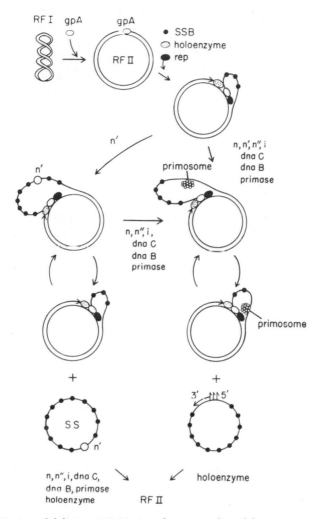

FIGURE 10. A model for stage II DNA replication. Adapted from Arai et al. (1981e).

looped rolling-circle synthesis of the viral strand is completed, the gpA bound at the 5' end of the parental viral strand cuts the viral strand at the newly synthesized origin and rejoins the two ends of the parental strand to generate circular viral DNA coated by SSB (Eisenberg et al., 1977). The gpA is transferred to the newly generated 5' end of the RF DNA and reforms the RF II–gpA–rep protein complex, which serves as template for further rounds of viral strand synthesis.

Matthes et al. (1980, 1982a,b) proposed from in vivo pulse-chase experiments that viral strand synthesis may also occur by a discontinuous process with initiations at other than the gpA nicking site. Three such sites that have some homology to the protein n' recognition site were indicated on the complementary strand. However, no functional protein n' recognition sites were detected on the complementary strand *in vivo* (Strathearn *et al.*, 1984) when the φX174 RF DNA restriction fragments were cloned into an M13 deletion mutant (Ray *et al.*, 1982). The possibility of discontinuous synthesis of the viral strand is therefore unclear.

2. Origin of DNA Replication

ori[+] is located inside of gene A between nucleotides 4305 and 4306 of the φX174 DNA sequence where gpA introduces an endonucleolytic cleavage (Langeveld *et al.*, 1978). A 30-nucleotide sequence surrounding the origin is conserved among the isomeric SS DNA phages (Fiddes *et al.*, 1978; Van Mansfeld *et al.*, 1978, 1980; Heidekamp *et al.*, 1980, 1982). This 30-nucleotide sequence is required for viral strand synthesis and has three functional domains: the recognition sequence for gpA, an AT-rich spacer sequence, and the key (binding) sequence of gpA (Fig. 11) (Baas *et al.*, 1981b). gpA has a SS DNA-specific endonuclease activity (Henry and Knippers, 1974; Van Mansfeld *et al.*, 1980; Baas *et al.*, 1980b; Eisenberg, 1980) and cleaves the SS DNA containing a consensus eight-nucleotide sequence of A(orT)ACTC(orT)GAT(orG) between the G and A residue (Van Mansfeld *et al.*, 1984a). Although the recognition sequence for gpA (between nucleotides 1 and 10 of the 30-nucleotide sequence) contains the consensus sequence that can be cut by gpA, it is not sufficient for the nicking action of gpA on the duplex DNA (Heidekamp *et al.*, 1981). The key (binding) sequence for gpA (between nucleotides 18 and 27) and the spacer sequence between the recognition sequence and the key (binding) sequence are also required (Fluit *et al.*, 1984a,b). Since the spacer sequence is AT-rich, this sequence may provide a starting point for the melting of the DS DNA. These results suggest that gpA first binds to the key (binding) sequence, which induces melting of the DS region containing the AT-rich spacer sequence and then the recognition sequence. The bound gpA recognizes the consensus sequence in the melted recognition sequence and cuts the viral strand at the origin.

The first nucleotide and the last three nucleotides of the 30-nucleotide sequence are not involved in the nicking action of the gpA; however, these nucleotides may be important to support subsequent stages of DNA replication (Section V.C). A recombinant plasmid containing the φX174 origin with a C→G substitution at the first position is

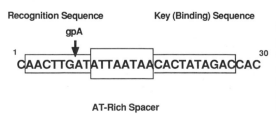

Recognition Sequence   **Key (Binding) Sequence**

gpA

1   30
CAACTTGATATTAATAACACTATAGACCAC

AT-Rich Spacer

FIGURE 11. The *ori*[+] region. The 30-nucleotide sequence (nucleotides 4299–4328 of the φX174 DNA sequence) with its three functional domains is shown. The arrow indicates the gpA cleavage site. Adapted from Baas *et al.* (1981b) and Baas (1985).

cleaved by gpA but is a poor template in the *in vitro* stage II DNA replication system (Brown *et al.*, 1983a,b).

3. Covalent Ester Bond between gpA and Viral Strand

gpA forms a covalent ester bond with the newly created 5' end of the
viral strand of the RF DNA (Ikeda *et al.*, 1979; Eisenberg and Kornberg,
1979). This linkage conserves the energy of the cleaved phosphodiester
bond, which is later used to rejoin the viral strands upon termination
(Eisenberg *et al.*, 1977; Brown *et al.*, 1984). The ester bond is formed
between a tyrosine-hydroxyl residue in gpA and the phosphate group of
the adenosine residue on the position 4306 (Van Mansfeld *et al.*, 1984a,b;
Roth *et al.*, 1984; Sanhueza and Eisenberg, 1985). After one round of viral
strand synthesis, gpA cleaves the regenerated origin, establishing a new
covalent bond with the new 5' end. During the second cleavage, the 3'
and 5' ends of the parental viral strands are ligated to form a circular
DNA (Eisenberg *et al.*, 1977; Brown *et al.*, 1984). Two catalytic groups
(tyrosine residues) are present in one gpA molecule to exert alternately
the successive cleavage steps (Roth *et al.*, 1984; Sanhueza and Eisenberg,
1985; Van Mansfeld *et al.*, 1986b). These two tyrosine residues are located in the repeating sequence: *tyr*-val-ala-lys-*tyr*-val-asn-lys (between
343 and 347 of the 513 residues of gpA;) Van Mansfeld *et al.*, 1986b). The
side chains of these tyrosine residues are in juxtaposition in an alpha-
helix, and either can function as the acceptor of the DNA chain. The
hydroxyl groups of the two tyrosyl side-chains in such a conformation
can occupy a symmetrical position toward the phosphorus atom. The
nicking-closing reaction of topoisomerases and gyrases proceeds via a
covalent DNA-protein complex (Champoux, 1977; Depew *et al.*, 1978;
Sugino *et al.*, 1977), and the bond in the intermediate structure is a
tyrosylphosphate ester (Tse *et al.*, 1980; Champoux, 1981).

4. *rep* Protein as a Helicase

E. coli rep protein (a monomer of 66,000 daltons) is a single-stranded,
DNA-dependent ATPase (Scott and Kornberg, 1978; Kornberg *et al.*,
1978; Arai *et al.*, 1981f). The protein has two distinct sites for the binding
of ATP and SS DNA (Arai *et al.*, 1981f). Binding of ATP to *rep* protein
increases the affinity of the protein to SS DNA, whereas the subsequent
hydrolysis of the ATP decreases affinity of the protein for SS DNA. Binding of SS DNA to *rep* protein is thus turned on and off by the binding and
hydrolysis of ATP.

rep protein functions as a helicase when a SS region is available in DS
DNA (Yarranton and Gefter, 1979; Baumel *et al.*, 1984). During stage II
DNA replication, the *rep* protein functions as a helicase by binding to the
RF II–gpA complex in a 1 : 1 ratio probably through the interaction with
the gpA (Scott *et al.*, 1977; Kornberg *et al.*, 1978; Arai and Kornberg,

1981). With the action of SSB, the *rep* protein separates the strands of duplex RF DNA and can thereby generate and advance a replication fork. Catalytic separation by *rep* protein of the strands of the duplex RF DNA requires ATP. Two molecules of ATP are hydrolized for every base pair melted (Kornberg *et al.*, 1978; N. Arai and Kornberg, 1981). Based on these results, the reaction sequence for unwinding the RF II–gpA complex has been summarized as follows (N. Arai and Kornberg, 1981): (1) recognition of gpA at the origin by *rep* protein to form a RF II–gpA–*rep* protein complex; (2) ATP binding to induce a conformational change of *rep* protein in the complex; (3) melting of a nucleotide base pair by the tightly bound gpA–*rep* protein–ATP complex; (4) ATP hydrolysis to promote displacement of the gpA–*rep* protein–ADP complex from the single-stranded region; (5) regeneration of a gpA–*rep* protein–ATP complex and its translocation to a base-paired region; and (6) binding of SSB to stabilize the newly created single-stranded region. Repetition of this sequence enables a single *rep* protein molecule to move unidirectionally and processively to separate the strands in advance of the replication fork.

When coupled to replication in the viral DNA synthesis, a "looped" rolling-circle intermediate is formed. DNA polymerase III holoenzyme does not bind tightly to the RF II–gpA complex, despite the available 3' hydroxyl terminus. The holoenzyme becomes stably complexed when the looped rolling-circle intermediate is formed (N. Arai and Kornberg, 1981). Presumably an association with the replication fork structure that is produced by helicase activity of the *rep* protein is essential for stable binding.

5. Termination and Reinitiation of Viral Strand Synthesis

In the termination stage of the viral strand synthesis, cleavage of the newly formed viral strand and ligation of the parental viral strand occur to form a circular parental viral strand. The gpA that is bound to the 5' end of the parental strand is transferred to the 5' end of the newly generated viral strand (Reinberg *et al.*, 1983; Brown *et al.*, 1984). This termination and reinitiation reaction requires more than the recognition sequence of the gpA. Studies with plasmids containing a functional origin and a part of the origin in the same orientation showed that the first 16 nucleotides do not function as a terminator signal either *in vivo* (Baas *et al.*, 1981a) or *in vitro* (Reinberg *et al.*, 1983). The presence of a second cleavage sequence on SS DNA for gpA, TTACTTGAGG (984–993), also implies that the recognition sequence itself is not sufficient for a termination event, because the second cleavage sequences does not function as a terminator (Van Mansfeld *et al.*, 1984a).

Brown *et al.* (1984) demonstrated that the gpA is transferred from the parental strand to the newly synthesized strand upon termination. They used 2',3'-dideoxyribonucleoside triphosphates to stop the viral strand synthesis at certain points within the 30-nucleotide origin sequence in the *in vitro* stage II DNA synthesizing system. When DNA synthesis was stopped 25 nucleotides into the origin sequence, gpA was transferred to the newly synthesized viral DNA fragment. However, when DNA synthesis was stopped 18 nucleotides into the origin sequence, no transfer of the gpA was observed.

Van Mansfeld *et al.* (1986a) reported that gpA does not cleave the SS restriction fragment containing the first 25 or 26 nucleotides of the 30-nucleotide sequence when SSB is present, whereas the SS DNA fragment containing the first 27 nucleotides of the origin region is cleaved by gpA *in vitro*. This result indicates a strict correlation between the nucleotide requirement for the gpA cleavage of the supercoiled RF I DNA and the SSB-coated SS DNA. Both DNAs require the key (binding) sequence as well as the recognition sequence of the gpA. The termination event may therefore require the same sequence of events as the initiation does: recognition of the key (binding) sequence by gpA, a proper arrangement of gpA so as to recognize the recognition sequence, and cleavage (Van Mansfeld *et al.*, 1986a). However, since these experiments were performed using free gpA, the relationship between the sequence requirement for the termination by free gpA and the gpA bound to the viral DNA is not clear.

Edlind and Ihler (1980) observed with electron microscopy that the 5' end and the 3' end of φX174 viral DNA cleaved at the origin of the viral DNA synthesis by gpA position closely each other owing to the long-range base-pairing. They proposed that such positioning of the ends of the viral DNA during the rolling-circle synthesis may also be important for gpA to recognize the ends for rejoining.

6. Complementary Strand Synthesis during RF DNA Replication

Complementary strand synthesis during RF replication follows the synthesis of the viral strand and requires the same proteins as for stage I DNA synthesis. The initiation mechanism of complementary strand synthesis during RF replication probably follows a pathway similar to that in the stage I replication (Section V.A). The question is how the complementary strand synthesis is coordinated with the viral strand synthesis during the RF replication. *In vitro* studies have shown that two paths of RF replication are possible (Fig. 10): one is discrete synthesis of RF→SS and SS→RF, and the other is a coupled synthesis of RF→SS and SS→RF in the rolling-circle structure containing gpA, *rep* protein, SSB, DNA polymerase III holoenzyme, and primosome (Arai *et al.*, 1981e). When the RF II–gpA complex is used as the template for the *in vitro* coupled stage II DNA replication system, the first reaction is the formation of the rolling-circle intermediate containing gpA, *rep* protein, DNA polymerase III holoenzyme, and SSB. This complex associates with protein n', which is the predominant intermediate in the initial stage of RF replication. During further replication, this complex produces a viral circular DNA containing protein n', which is converted to RF II DNA by the components needed for stage I DNA synthesis (discrete RF→SS and SS→RF stage). As assembly of the primosome on the viral strand progresses, the rolling-circle structure that has the primosome predominates (the coupled RF→SS and SS→RF stage).

Such a complex can initiate the complementary strand synthesis, in the presence of proteins i and *dnaC*, before the viral circular DNA has been completed. Since the primosome remains bound to the RF DNA, this complex synthesizes RF DNA with high efficiency, without the time-consuming prepriming stage of the primosome. These observations may indicate that viral strand synthesis during stage II replication occurs mainly in this primosome-associated complex. However, electron microscopic analysis of *in vivo* RF DNA showed that the majority (85%) of the rolling circles isolated during RF replication have single-stranded tails. This indicates that the greater part of the complementary strand synthesis is initiated after segregation of a circular SS viral DNA from the RF intermediate (Koths and Dressler, 1978; Keegstra *et al.*, 1979). The occurrence and the function of the primosome-associated complex *in vivo* are therefore unclear.

In the primosome-associated rolling-circle intermediate observed *in vitro*, the primosome might migrate processively along the viral strand coupled to movement of the replication fork generated by gpA and *rep* protein. The association of *rep* protein, the primosome, and DNA polymerase III holoenzyme in the intermediate structure suggests that these components interact with each other to form a replisomelike structure at the replication fork. This may be a useful model of the semidiscontinuous DNA replication of *E. coli* chromosome (Kornberg, 1983, 1984). However, recent studies on the *in vitro* replication of the host chromosomal *ori* C DNA indicate that only *dnaB* protein, *dnaC* protein, and primase are required for initiation of replication (Van der Ende *et al.*, 1985). No evidence for requirement of proteins n, n', n", or i for the host DNA replication has been reported. Moreover, LeBowitz and McMacken (1986) have recently demonstrated that *E. coli dnaB* protein has a DNA helicase action on duplex DNA, indicating that *dnaB* protein is solely involved in strand separation during the host chromosomal DNA replication.

Wang *et al.* (1984) studied the effects of DNA methylation on RF replication *in vivo*. They found that the replacement of all the cytosine residues in the complementary strand of RF DNA with 5-methylcytosine (m^{5}C) residues caused a 300- to 500-fold loss in its transfection activity. Replacing half of the cytosine residues on the complementary strand with m^{5}C residues gave a 20-fold decrease, whereas 10% replacement of C with m^{5}C resulted in a loss of only 60% of the transfecting activity. When only one-third of RF DNA is methylated and the remaining part, which includes gene A and origin of viral strand synthesis and possibly three promoter regions is not methylated, the transforming activity is about 2% of nonmethylated RF DNA. They concluded that gene A was not the main target for this inhibition by DNA methylation but that the loss of transfecting activity was caused by hemimethylation of the RF DNA, interfering with the processively catalyzed movement of the replication fork.

C. Stage III (RF→SS/Phage)

Asymmetric synthesis of the viral DNA during the third stage of φX174 DNA replication is tightly coupled to the morphogenetic pathway of φX174 phage (Hayashi, 1978). The DNA synthesis requires functions of the phage structural genes F, G, H, and J; the nonstructural but morphogenetic genes B, D, and C; and gene A. Packaging of the φX174 circular viral DNA into the phage capsid requires concomitant synthesis of viral DNA. Previous *in vivo* studies indicate that the coupling of DNA synthesis and the phage morphogenesis occurs in a specific intermediate structure in which a rolling-circle intermediate DNA is associated with phage capsid precursor (prohead; see Section V.E) (Koths and Dressler, 1980; Fujisawa and Hayashi, 1976a, 1977c). Establishment of an *in vitro* stage III system reconstituted from the purified components by Aoyama *et al.* (1981, 1983b) and Aoyama and Hayashi (1986) has clarified the mechanism of the stage III DNA replication. The *in vitro* stage III system is composed of φX174 RF I DNA, gpA, gpC, gpJ, prohead, *E. coli rep* protein, DNA polymerase III holoenzyme, dUTPase, SSB, ATP, deoxyribonucleside triphosphates, and Mg^{2+}. The asymmetric synthesis of the viral DNA and its concomitant packaging is initiated by the nicking action of gpA on the supercoiled RF I DNA and proceeds via rolling-circle mode similar to that described for the viral strand synthesis in the stage II replication. Synthesis of the viral strand occurs at the replication fork of the rolling-circle intermediate that is associated with prohead, in which the displaced viral strand is directly packaged during the viral strand DNA synthesis. gpC initiates the DNA synthesis and is thought to be required for the association of prohead to the template DNA. gpJ is required for condensing the viral strand DNA in the prohead (Aoyama *et al.*, 1981, 1983b; Hamatake *et al.*, 1985). After one round of rolling-circle synthesis, a circular viral DNA is formed within the prohead by the cutting-rejoining activity of the gpA (Fujisawa and Hayashi, 1976b). The product of this reaction is an infectious phage particle and RF II DNA containing the replicative enzymes, which is used for subsequent rounds of phage synthesis. Figure 12 summarizes the model for stage III DNA replication.

Studies using *in vitro* crude stage III systems or *in vivo* systems suggested the requirement for some other enzymes: DNA gyrase subunit A (Hamatake *et al.*, 1981), host factor(s) (Wolfson and Eisenberg, 1982), *dnaB* and *dnaC* proteins (Sumida-Yasumoto and Hurwitz, 1977, 1978),

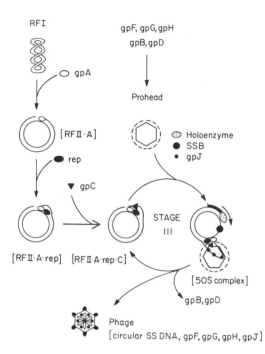

FIGURE 12. A model for stage III DNA replication and packaging. Adapted from Aoyama *et al.* (1983b).

and *dnaG* protein (Sumida-Yasumoto and Hurwitz, 1977, 1978; McFadden and Denhardt, 1974). These proteins are not required in the purified system (Aoyama *et al.*, 1983b). DNA gyrase subunit A and the unknown factor(s) (prepared by the method of Wolfson and Eisenberg) have no stimulating effects in the purified system (Hamatake and Aoyama, unpublished results). The requirement and the function of these proteins are unclear.

Stage III DNA synthesis and the concomitant synthesis of phage can occur in the absence of SSB in the *in vitro* system (Aoyama *et al.*, 1983b). However, the reaction is sensitive to salt. SSB is required for the stage III DNA synthesis at the physiological salt concentration (Aoyama and Hayashi, 1986). SSB may bind to the complementary strand to facilitate DNA elongation or to ensure the strand separation at the replication fork.

1. Initiation of Stage III DNA Synthesis

Although the same RF II–gpA–*rep* protein complex as that in the stage II replication is used as the intermediate structure for viral DNA synthesis in stage III replication, the initiation of viral strand synthesis requires additional enzymes (proteins): φX174 gpC and prohead. gpC is a SS DNA-specific binding protein with a molecular weight of approximately 8000 (Aoyama *et al.*, 1983a) and is required for the initiation of the stage III DNA synthesis. A dimer of this protein recognizes and binds specifically to the RF II–gpA–*rep* protein complex (initiation complex of RF replication) in the presence of ATP (Aoyama and Hayashi, 1986).

Hydrolysis of ATP, presumably by *rep* protein, is required for the binding of gpC, indicating that partial melting of the duplex DNA at the origin is required. The binding of the gpC is competitive with SSB, which also interacts with the RF II–gpA–*rep* protein complex. The RF II–gpA–*rep* protein–gpC complex (preinitiation complex for stage III) is inactive for DNA synthesis in the absence of prohead, even in the presence of SSB. These results indicate that the preinitiation complex for stage III has a specific structure with which only prohead can interact. When prohead is added to the preinitiation complex, a rolling-circle synthesis of the viral strand commences. These properties of gpC are important for the conversion of stage II DNA synthesis to stage III DNA synthesis (Section V.D).

Genetic studies indicate that gpF of the prohead, gpA, and *rep* protein interact directly with each other to achieve the association of prohead and RF II–gpA–*rep* protein–gpC complex at the replication fork (Tessman and Peterson, 1976). Furthermore, some mutations in *rep* protein abolish stage III replicative activity without affecting the stage II replication *in vivo* (Tessman and Peterson, 1976). Formation of a complex of prohead and the preinitiation complex specific for stage III replication is required for initiation of the rolling-circle synthesis in the stage III replication.

The molecular structure of the RF II–gpA–*rep* protein–gpC–prohead complex remains to be elucidated. Since gpC is an SS DNA-specific binding protein and requires ATP to bind to the RF II–gpA–*rep* protein complex, it might associate with the SS region of the RF II–gpA–*rep* protein complex created by partial unwinding reaction of the *rep* protein at the origin of replication. The approximate 1 : 1 stoichiometry of the gpC to RF II–gpA–*rep* protein complex in the preinitiation complex suggests a specific rather than a nonspecific interaction, such as is seen between SSB and SS DNA (Aoyama and Hayashi, 1986). Fluit *et al.* (1985) suggested the possibility that some of the viral components interact with a specific DNA sequence containing the last three nucleotides of the 30-nucleotide origin sequence that is not required for stage II replication (see below). gpC might recognize these last three nucleotides in the 30-nucleotide origin sequence. Alternatively, gpC might interact with the *rep* protein in the RF II–gpA–*rep* protein complex. Tessman and Peterson (1982) suggested an interaction between SSB and *rep* protein from *in vivo* experiments. Competition between gpC and SSB may occur by interacting with either the SS DNA region or the *rep* protein in the RF II–gpA–*rep* protein complex. The structure of the junction between the prohead and the RF II–gpA–*rep* protein–gpC complex remains unclear. No specific structure for the attachment site to the RF II–gpA–*rep* protein–gpC complex or for the entrance of DNA has been found. All available information indicates a symmetrical structure of prohead (Section V.E).

2. Origin of Stage III DNA Synthesis

Plasmid DNA containing the φX174 origin region of viral DNA replication can be packaged in the phage capsid either directly in the *in vitro* stage III replication system (Aoyama and Hayashi, 1982, 1985) or *in vivo* by superinfection with φX174 phage (Van der Ende *et al.*, 1982b; Fluit *et al.*, 1985). These experiments indicate that the 30-nucleotide origin sequence is necessary and sufficient for the stage III replication (Fluit *et al.*, 1985). This result contrasts to the requirement of the first 27 nucleotides of the 30-nucleotide sequence for the stage II replication (Baas *et al.*, 1981; Brown *et al.*, 1983a,b). Plasmid DNA containing the first 27 or the 28 nucleotides of the 30-nucleotide sequence are packaged 10- to 100-fold less efficiently than the plasmid DNA containing the complete 30-nucleotide sequence (Fluit *et al.*, 1985). The last three nucleotides of the 30-nucleotide sequence may be a part of the "φX174 morphogenetic signal" that overlaps the key (binding) sequence of gpA and may provide an additional and essential interaction site for gpF or gpC in the RF II–gpA–*rep* complex (Fluit *et al.*, 1985; Aoyama and Hayashi, 1986).

3. Synthesis and Packaging of Viral Strand

Packaging of the viral DNA into the prohead requires an additional viral encoded protein: gpJ (Aoyama *et al.*, 1981, 1983b; Hamatake *et al.*, 1985). In the absence of gpJ, a circular viral DNA is synthesized at essentially the same rate as that of the normal stage III replication both *in vivo* (Hamatake, 1983) and *in vitro* (Hamatake *et al.*, 1985). However, in the absence of gpJ, the viral DNA is not packaged correctly; the particles sediment heterogeneously in a sucrose gradient, suggesting that the DNA is exposed to the outside of the capsid to various extents (Hamatake *et al.*, 1985). These DNAs are digested by nucleases rapidly *in vivo* (Hamatake, 1983). Kodaira and Taketo (1984a) have isolated mutants in gene J of the isometric SS DNA phage α3. They observed no SS DNA synthesis (stage III) in gene J mutant-infected cells.

gpJ is a small basic protein with a molecular weight of 4000 (Freymeyer *et al.*, 1977). gpJ is a generalized nucleic acid binding protein and can bind to both DS and SS DNA (Hamatake *et al.*, 1985). Approximately 100 molecules of gpJ bind to one molecule of φX174 SS or DS DNA (Hamatake, 1983). This number is comparable to that found in a phage particle (60 gpJ per particle) (Burgess, 1969). Since a molecule of gpJ is too small to wrap a long stretch of DNA strand around it, a specific interaction among gpJ on the DNA might be occurring. Such an interaction may produce a nucleosomelike structure of the RF DNA and a compact, condensed structure of a SS DNA inside a phage particle.

Hamatake *et al.* (1985) proposed that gpJ binds first to the RF DNA template, then enters directly into the prohead along with the viral strand during the packaging. The binding of gpJ prevents SSB-dependent stage II viral DNA synthesis (Hamatake *et al.*, 1985). DNA synthesis resumes when prohead is added to this complex. These results suggest a direct interaction between gpJ and the prohead. Recently, Kodaira and Taketo (1984a) and Kodaira *et al.* (1985) reported that mutants isolated in gene J of the phage α3 always contained second mutations in gene H and formed minute plaques on suppressor-minus cells. Therefore, a direct interaction between gpJ and gpH in the prohead may be essential for the formation of infectious phage. Spindler and Hayashi (1979) showed that the viral DNA is not packaged correctly in the gene H mutant infected cells. These cells produce defective particles that contain various length of DNA. This result also supports the possibility of the direct interaction between gpJ and gpH during the phage formation. Kodaira and Taketo (1984b) also observed a similar phenomenon in mutants in gene C of α3, which were always accompanied by second mutations in gene H. Although such phenomena are not observed in φX174, gpH might have an important role at the replication fork of φX174, where both gpC and gpJ are located, for packaging SS DNA during stage III DNA synthesis.

The size of DNA that can be packaged into phage particles has been studied both *in vivo* (Müller and Wells, 1980a; Van der Ende *et al.*, 1982b; Russell and Müller, 1984) and *in vitro* (Aoyama and Hayashi, 1985) using plasmid DNA carrying the φX174 origin or φX174 DNA with insertions. The size of DNA that can produce transducing particles is between 74–82% and 102–106% of the length of φX174 DNA. The upper limit may be determined by the spatial capacity of the virion, because part of the DNA becomes sensitive to digestion by DNase when DNA larger than 101% of the unit length is packaged (Aoyama and Hayashi, 1985). Determinants of the lower limit are unclear. Phage particles that have DNA smaller than 75.8% of the unit length loses its ability to adsorb to the host cell. This may be caused by an abortive change of phage structure (Aoyama and Hayashi, 1985). Such defective phage particles show slower sedimentation than expected in sucrose gradient (Aoyama and Hayashi, 1985; Aoyama and Hayashi, unpublished results). Circularization of the synthesized DNA is independent from the size of DNA but is determined only by the φX174 origin sequence (Aoyama and Hayashi, 1985).

4. Termination of Viral Circle Synthesis and Maturation of Phage Particles

After one round of the rolling-circle synthesis, the gpA that is bound to the RF DNA terminates the replication in a similar way to that of stage II replication and regenerates the RF II–gpA complex for the next round of synthesis. gpC as well as *rep* protein and DNA polymerase III holoenzyme may remain on the RF II–gpA complex (Aoyama and Hayashi, 1986). The parental viral circular DNA that is produced by the cutting-rejoining activity of gpA is packaged with gpJ into the prohead. During or after the rolling-circle synthesis of the viral strand, the following changes to the prohead occur: (1) elimination of gpB; (2) elimination of gpD depending on the divalent cation concentration; and (3) rearrangement of the phage structural components (proteins gpF, gpG, and gpH) to yield mature phage particles (Section V.E). These changes also occur in the *in vitro* stage III system and do not require any additional components other than those for stage III DNA synthesis (Aoyama *et al.*, 1981, 1983b; Richardson, Aoyama, and Hayashi, unpublished observation). Mechanisms of these processes remain to be elucidated.

D. Mechanism of Conversion from Stage II Replication to Stage III Replication

In the late stage of infection, transition from stage II RF replication to stage III viral DNA replication occurs. This transition involves shutdown of stage II DNA synthesis and initiation of stage III DNA synthesis. The transition coincides with shutdown of host DNA synthesis and increase of the number of the replicating RF DNA molecules. During stage II DNA replication, the number of active RF DNA molecules is relatively small. Most of the RF molecules are inactive for DNA synthesis but presumably are active for transcription. After the transition to the stage III replication, the number of the active RF DNA molecules for the stage III DNA synthesis increases to around 30 per cell. Although the molecular mechanism of this transition is not yet completely clear, several advances have been achieved recently.

1. gpA*

A role of gpA* in the shutdown of both stage II and host chromosomal DNA synthesis has been suggested by several laboratories (Martin and Godson, 1975; Funk and Snover, 1976; Langeveld *et al.*, 1979, 1981; Van der Ende *et al.*, 1981, 1982a; Eisenberg and Ascarelli, 1981). gpA* is translated from an in-frame start codon within gene A of ϕX174 and hence is a C-terminal part of gpA with a molecular weight of approximately 37,000 (Linney and Hayashi, 1973). This protein binds to SS DNA and also to DS DNA with less affinity (Eisenberg and Ascarelli, 1981; Van der Ende *et al.*, 1982a) and has relatively unspecific SS nuclease activity, with preference on the origin of the viral DNA synthesis (Lagenveld *et al.*, 1979, 1981). gpA* binds covalently to the 5' end of SS DNA through tyrosyl-phosphate ester (Eisenberg and Finer, 1980; Sanhueza and Eisenberg, 1984; Zolotukhin *et al.*, 1984) after cutting and also can ligate the SS DNA (Eisenberg and Finer, 1980; Sanhueza and Eisenberg, 1984). Recently, the mechanism of the shutdown of the host chromosomal DNA synthesis has become clear. Colasanti and Denhardt (1985) demonstrated that expression of the cloned gpA* inhibits the host chromosomal replication and cell division (Section VIII.A). The shutdown of the host chromosomal DNA replication may release the host DNA replicative enzymes so that they may be used by ϕX174 RF DNA for stage III DNA replication (Section VIII.A).

The effect of gpA* on stage II DNA synthesis is not clear. Two models have been proposed, neither of which has direct evidence. Eisenberg and Ascarelli (1981) showed that gpA* covers RF II DNA and prevents stage II DNA synthesis by inhibiting strand separation by *rep* protein. They suggested that association of prohead with the RF DNA overcomes the inhibitory effects of the gpA* on the rolling-circle synthesis of viral strand, although no evidence has been provided. Van Mansfeld *et al.* (1982) reported that a part of the gpA* isolated from the infected cells carries an oligonucleotide AGGATAA, which is probably a part of a sequence of the second cleavage site of gpA: TTACTTGAG-GATAA (984–997 of the φX174 DNA sequence). gpA* can cleave the SS restriction fragment containing the second cleavage site of gpA in the presence or the absence of SSB (Van Mansfeld *et al.*, 1986a). Based on these results, Van Mansfeld *et al.* (1986a) proposed that stage II replication might be interrupted by the gpA* cleavage at the second cleavage site of gpA.

Dubeau and Denhardt (1981) and Dubeau *et al.* (1981) reported that gpA* can cut the duplex RF DNA and bind covalently to it in the presence of gpA. They suggested that gpA* might function in a gpA-gpA* complex during stage III DNA replication.

2. gpC

Recently, Aoyama and Hayashi (1986) showed a direct correlation between the shutdown of the stage II DNA replication and the initiation of the stage III DNA replication in the *in vitro* system. As already mentioned, gpC of φX174 recognizes the RF II–gpA–*rep* protein complex and binds specifically to this complex. This action of gpC causes the inhibition of the stage II DNA synthesis *in vitro*. The inhibition is competitive with SSB. A remarkable aspect of this gpC inhibition of stage II DNA synthesis is that the gpC can bind to the RF II–gpA–*rep* protein complex and inhibit the DNA synthesis only at the initiation or the reinitiation step after one round of the rolling-circle DNA synthesis. Hence, the replicating rolling-circle intermediate of the stage II DNA synthesis can complete the process even in the presence of gpC. Such action of gpC converts all replicating rolling-circle molecules of the stage II DNA synthesis into a specific preinitiation complex, the RF II–gpA–*rep* protein–gpC complex, which is recognized by prohead to begin stage III DNA replication. These results indicate that gpC has a central role in the conversion of stage II DNA replication to stage III DNA replication. Based on these results, Aoyama and Hayashi (1986) proposed a model of the mechanism by which stage II replication is switched to stage III replication (Fig. 13).

In this model, a competition between gpC and SSB for interaction with the RF II–gpA–*rep* protein complex determines the course of the φX174 morphogenesis. If SSB binds first to the SS region of the RF II–gpA–*rep* protein complex, the rolling-circle synthesis of the SSB-coated

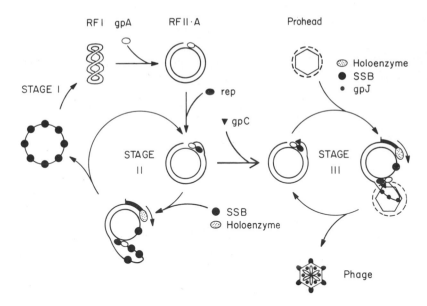

FIGURE 13. A model for stage II to stage III conversion. Adapted from Aoyama and Hayashi (1986).

viral strand occurs. gpC can interact with this replicating complex only after the completion of one round of DNA synthesis. However, if gpC binds first to the RF II–gpA–*rep* protein complex, the complex becomes accessible specifically to prohead and can serve as a DNA packaging apparatus. Since gpC stays on the complex to produce phage multiple times (Aoyama and Hayashi, 1986), all RF II–gpA–*rep* protein complexes are eventually converted to RF II–gpA–*rep* protein–gpC complexes. This model explains the early observation made *in vivo*. In the gene C mutant-infected cells, the newly synthesized RF II DNA is rapidly converted to RF I DNA (Fujisawa and Hayashi, 1977a). In the cells infected with a mutant in the gene F, G, B, or D, the newly synthesized RF II DNA maintains its open structure. Since the RF II–gpA–*rep* protein–gpC complex is inactive for the viral DNA synthesis of stage II, the RF II DNA remains as open structure in the absence of the competent prohead.

E. Structure and Morphogenesis of Prohead

Prohead is a 10-megadalton protein complex made up of five proteins; gpF, gpH, gpG, gpB, and gpD. The requirement for prohead in the reconstitution of stage III DNA synthesis and packaging *in vitro* supports the proposed role of prohead as a capsid precursor in φX174 morphogenesis. The structure of prohead is not well understood, although comparisons to other φX174 intermediates and precursors in the assembly pathway have revealed some information. A model for prohead morphogenesis was proposed by Fujisawa and Hayashi (1977c). The presence of gpB in the isolated prohead contradicts the proposal that gpB was catalytic in the formation of the 12S particle and forces us to reconsider the proposed morphogenesis pathway for prohead (Fig. 2).

1. Prohead Is Required for Stage III DNA Synthesis

Prohead was required for the synthesis of phage *in vitro* in the stage III DNA synthesizing system using both crude extracts of φX174-infected cells (Mukai *et al.*, 1979) and the pure system (Aoyama *et al.*, 1981, 1983b). Mukai *et al.* (1979) fractionated *ochre* C φX174-infected cell crude extract by sedimentation through sucrose gradients and tested fractions for complementation of *amber* B φX174-infected cell crude extract to make infectious phage *in vitro*. The 108S material (prohead) was active, whereas material from other parts of the gradient had little or no activity. The isolated prohead is required by the *in vitro* stage III system which utilizes purified phage and host components to make infectious phage (Aoyama *et al.*, 1981, 1983b).

2. Proposed Model of Prohead Structure

Prohead appeared in electron micrographs to be spherical, 40 nm in diameter, with a hollow core that was penetrated by the stain (Fujisawa and Hayashi, 1977c). The 132S particle appeared to be the same size and shape in electron micrographs when stained by the same procedure, but was not hollow (the 132S particle is described in Section III.B; briefly, it contains viral DNA and the proteins gpF, gpH, gpG, gpJ, and gpD). The phage appeared icosahedral, with prominent knobs in the same conditions, and it measured 32 nm from spike to spike. Fujisawa's prohead did not contain gpB, but the prohead isolated by Mukai *et al.* (1979) that was active in the *in vitro* stage III system does contain gpB. Hence, the structure of the Mukai's prohead may be slightly different from that of Fujisawa's prohead.

The relative amounts of gpF, gpH, and gpG are the same in prohead, phage, and the 132S particle (Fujisawa and Hayashi, 1977c). The relative amount of gpD is the same in prohead and the 132S particle. Mukai *et al.* (1979) estimated that prohead contains 60 gpF, 12 gpH, 60 gpG, 60 gpB, and 240 gpD. The capsid structural proteins gpF, gpG, and gpH are present in the same numbers as proposed for phage (see Section III). The only evidence for their conformation comes from the structures proposed for the phage and intermediates in the morphogenesis. gpB and gpD are not present in the mature phage. The arrangement or location of gpB is unknown. Mukai *et al.* (1979) proposed that gpB may be a scaffolding protein or involved in DNA packaging. gpD is thought to form an external scaffold.

The conformation of the capsid structural proteins may be different in prohead and in phage. Conformational changes probably do occur in the prohead to capsid transition of dsDNA phages without proteolysis (King, 1980), and they have been shown to occur in the polymerization of flagella (Uratani *et al.*, 1972). Fujisawa and Hayashi (1977b,c) suggested that a conformation change occurs in the capsid proteins when gpD is removed from the 132S particle. Additionally, the phage can exist in two forms which differ in their sensitivity to heat denaturation (Bleichrodt and Van Abkoude, 1967). The transition between the two forms probably involves a conformation change with the loss of one weak, noncovalent bond not located in the immediate vicinity of the adsorption site (Bleichrodt *et al.*, 1968; see Section IV.D).

3. Morphogenesis of Prohead

The morphogenesis of prohead has important implications for prohead structure. gpF and gpG form pentamers that sediment as 9S and 6S particles in sucrose gradients (Tonegawa and Hayashi, 1970). A 12S particle is formed during infection except with F, G, or B mutants (Tonegawa and Hayashi, 1970; Siden and Hayashi, 1974). It is chased into phage *in vivo* and contains pentamers of gpF and gpG (Siden and Hayashi, 1974). The observation that gpB was missing from the 12S particle, yet was required for 12S formation, was critical in Siden and Hayashi's (1974) conclusion that gpB was catalytic for the formation of the 12S particle. The presence of gpB in prohead (Mukai *et al.*, 1979) indicates that gpB is structural instead of catalytic; the requirement of gpB for the formation of 12S particles from 6S and 9S (Siden and Hayashi, 1974) suggests that it might hold gpF and gpG together. The 12S particle may be the result of dissociation or proteolysis of the prohead precursor, which might contain gpF, gpG, and gpB. It is interesting to note that there is a particle isolated from dissociated prohead which is similar in size to the 12S particle but contains gpF, gpG, gpH, and gpB (Richardson, Aoyama, and Hayashi, unpublished results). Fujisawa and Hayashi (1977c) proposed that twelve 12S particles aggregate in the presence of gpD to form the prohead structure. At this point it is unclear which particles do combine together to form the prohead. The lack of gpB in the prohead of Fujisawa and Hayashi (1977c) compared to the prohead isolated by Mukai *et al.* (1979) might be explained by comigration with gpG or gpD during gel electrophoresis, proteolysis during the isolation, or different lysis conditions.

Fujisawa and Hayashi (1977a,b,c) proposed that gpD acts as a scaffold for assembly of capsid proteins, since it was required for the accumulation of prohead and was present on the 132S, 50S, and 108S particles. That gpD protected the 132S particle from inactivation by antiphage antibodies further suggested that gpD was an external scaffold (Fujisawa and Hayashi, 1977a). Additionally, gpD is known to form a tetramer *in vitro* (Farber, 1976).

The timing and mode of the incorporation of gpH into prohead are not known. gpH is thought to be part of the phage spike (Edgell *et al.*, 1969) and has been named the pilot protein for its role in directing the DNA into the cell (Jazwinski *et al.*, 1975a,b,c). Infection with amber H mutants of φX174 does produce 12S particles (Tonegawa and Hayashi, 1970), proheadlike structures (unpublished observations cited by Mukai *et al.*, 1979), and small amounts of phagelike material (110S rather than 114S), which are not infectious but do contain complete circular viral DNA (Spindler and Hayashi, 1979). The absence of gpH in *amber* H mutants damages the packaging process in some way, as evidence by the increased amount of defective (70S) particles produced (Spindler and Hayashi, 1979; Siegel and Hayashi, 1969). The few 110S phagelike particles produced are uninfectious, but the DNAs isolated from these particles are infective to *E. coli* spheroplasts (Spindler and Hayashi, 1979).

The essential question is when the gpH needs to enter the prohead assembly pathway to enable efficient packaging to make infectious virus. Wild-type infections do not produce a large amount of defective particles (Siegel and Hayashi, 1969). There may be some kinetic control of assembly, such that proheads containing gpH are made preferentially. Alternatively, there may be enough gpH made during wild-type infections that a majority of the available binding sites are saturated with the protein.

Proheads are also utilized during the morphogenesis of the DS DNA bacteriophages, such as P22, T4, and T7 (Murialdo and Becker, 1978; Earnshaw and Casjens, 1980). Several patterns emerge in comparison of prohead morphogenesis among these different, related bacteriophages. Four of these are (1) core or scaffolding proteins utilized for prohead assembly, (2) proheads increase in size upon DNA packaging, (3) a primer protein that acts as a nucleus for prohead assembly (this protein is often not essential, but instead speeds up the assembly process), and (4) a specialized vertex for DNA insertion. Surprisingly, only the first has been shown to occur for φX174, and the proposed scaffold, gpD, is thought to be external instead of internal.

VI. GENE EXPRESSION

In this section recent papers on gene expression are collected.

A. RNA Polymerase-Binding Sites of RF DNA

Williams and Fisher (1980) examined RNA polymerase-binding sites of RF forms by an electron microscopy. RF I DNA-RNA polymerase binary complex cleaved with *Pst*I restriction enzyme or RF III–RNA polymerase complex were examined. A histogram constructed from the positions of 558 polymerase molecules bound to 181 DNA molecules showed three predominant peaks, at 3300, 3970, and 4900 of the Sanger sequence. These correspond to P_D, P_A, and P_B (see Fig. 3).

B. Minicells

Reeve (1981) investigated the process of ϕX174 development in minicells (anucleated cells). Infected minicells synthesized 11 ϕX174 coded proteins. Infecting SS DNA was converted to RFI. However, no further replication of RF took place, and no progeny SS DNA synthesis was detected. The lack of progeny RF and SS DNA was attributed to the small amount of ϕX174 proteins synthesized in minicells (particularly gpA) rather than deficiencies of the DNA synthesizing enzymes and precursors in minicells.

C. Mutation at Ribosome-Binding Site

Gillam *et al.* (1980) developed a method of inducing a mutation that is phenotypically silent. They chose the region containing the RBS of ϕX174 gene H.

```
16S rRNA 3' end:   3'HO-AUUC-CUCCACUA . . . 5'
φX RBS. . . CCAGCCACTTAAGTGAGGTGATTTATGTTT . . . 3'
                  |            |              |
                2910         2920           2930
Mutagenic oligo:    3'ACTCC-CTAAA 5'
```

A synthetic mutagenic oligodeoxynucleotide shown above was hybridized to wild-type ϕX174 SS DNA, and the heteroduplex was converted to RF using Klenow fragment and T4 ligase. The RF DNA was used to transfect *E. coli* spheroplasts and DNA isolated from the resultant mixture of wild-type and mutant phage. The DNA was used as a substrate for enrichment of mutant DNA by again using the same oligonucleotide as a primer for Klenow fragment. The principle of the method is that under limiting priming conditions (i.e., higher temperature and reduced concentration of the primer), mutant DNA will form more stable duplex with the primer than will wild-type DNA. After ligation, the residual SS DNA (mostly wild type) was inactivated with S1 endonuclease, and the mutant enriched DNA is used to infect *E. coli* spheroplasts.

After two cycles of enrichment, the isolated DNA contained approximately equal amounts of wild-type and mutant DNA (as determined by sequence analysis). After one more cycle of enrichment, four out of four plaques yielded mutant phages. The mutant phages were indistinguishable from the wild-type phages with respect to the plaque morphology, burst size, temperature dependency, and gene expression. Deletion of nucleotide 2925 has no major effect on the translation of gene H. This is an interesting result, because deletion of nucleotide 2925 interrupts the extended region of the mRNA that can complex with 16S RNA, and it may change the secondary structure involving the RBS of initiation codon. The absence of a significant effect as a consequence of this deletion indicates that some nucleotides at the RBS are more critical than others.

Gillam et al. (1984) mutated by site-specific mutagenesis using synthetic oligonucleotides the gene E ribosome-binding sequence GAGG to GAAG without affecting the amino acid glutamine, which is part of the overlapping gene D. This mutant does not lyse infected E. coli, but the infected cells accumulated a large number of intracellular mature phages. Thus, the mutation inactivates production of gene E lytic product, presumably by blocking translation of gene E, without affecting other phage functions. Similar mutations were found in the RBS of T7 gene 0.3 (GAG-GU→ GAAGU) (Dunn et al., 1978) and T4 gene rIIB (AGGA→ AGAA) (Singer et al., 1981). In both cases, these alterations in the RBS result in a 90% decrease in translation.

D. Transcription Termination

The peculiar features of φX174 transcription in vivo, such as the presence of a gene transcript in more than one message and the synthesis of mRNA larger than the entire genome, are the consequences of inefficient termination events (Fig. 3). In general, two types of transcription terminations are defined in prokaryotes: one is rho-dependent, the other independent (see Holmes et al., 1983; Von Hippel et al., 1984; Chamberlin et al., 1985; Platt, 1986; Imamoto and Nakamura, 1986, for reviews).

Most of the prokaryotic transcription termination signals (particularly rho-independent) contain a GC rich inverted repeat followed by a run of uridine (or adenine). The dyad symmetry forms a base-paired structure consisting of a stem and a loop in the DNA sequence and the transcribed RNA. Crucial signals reside in the RNA (see Platt, 1986, for review). Variations in the length of the stem, the sizes of the loop, and the run of uridines are assumed to determine the efficiency of termination.

It has been postulated that the six base-paired hairpin structures existing in the J-F intercistronic region may serve as the termination signal for T_J (Godson et al., 1978b). This hairpin is followed by only two sets of TT (TTACTT).

Hayashi et al. (1981) determined whether rho activity is involved in in vivo termination of φX174 transcription. A temperature-sensitive rho mutation was introduced into a φX174-sensitive cell. mRNAs synthesized with or without rho factor were analyzed in gels. The size distribution of φX174-specific mRNAs synthesized in rho⁻ cells is similar to that in wild-type cells, and no preferential synthesis of larger RNAs were

found in rho^- cells. With or without rho activity, transcription terminations at T_J, T_F, T_G and T_H were observed. Hayashi *et al.* (1981) concluded
that the transcription termination of φX174 is independent of rho factor
in vivo. However, rho factor was involved in premature termination
caused by nonsense mutations (Fassler and Tessman, 1981) or by chloramphenicol treatment of infected cells (see Adhya and Gottesman, 1978,
for review). With active rho factor, all messages treated with the drug
started at P_B and P_D and terminated at T_J. No elongation of mRNA beyond this point was observed. Gene F N-terminal polar mutants terminated mRNA at T_F, and gene G polar mutants at T_G. rho inactivation
partially suppressed these premature terminations of mRNA.

Patrushev *et al.* (1981) investigated the effects ot rho factor in an *in
vitro* transcription-translation-coupled system. In an S30 extract from the
wild-type cells, the predominant protein products from the template
φX174 RF DNA were gpA, gpB, and gpD. When rho activity was deficient
in the extract, additional synthesis of gpF, gpG, and gpH was observed.
Patrushev *et al.* (1981) proposed that the expression of these two classes
of genes was regulated by a termination and antitermination mechanism
occurring at one of the rho factor-dependent terminators located in gene F
(Fig. 3) (Kaptza *et al.*, 1979). Thus, the *in vitro* and *in vivo* termination
events are quite different with respect to the rho requirement.

E. Mutations around the T_J Site

Müller and Wells (1980a,b) and Müller (1983) constructed a series of
viable φX174 and G4 phage mutants, specifically altered in the hairpin
sequence of the J–F intercistronic region by deletions and insertions.
These mutants are very useful for determining the regulatory significance
of the J–F intercistronic region, including the terminator T_J.

Romantschuk and Müller (1983) measured phage-specific protein
synthesis in cells infected with mutants with these hairpin sequence
modifications. All mutants tested showed a relative decrease in the expression of upstream gene D as compared to downstream genes F, G, and
H. The mutations also appeared to affect the efficiency of the gene F
ribosome-binding site. Hayashi *et al.* (1983) compared φX174 mRNA size
species of infected cells with these mutants. The results showed that the
mutants could be grouped into two classes: (1) Cells infected with class 1
mutant (1 deletion and 3 insertions tested) contained all RNA species
found in wild-type infected cells, with a similar size distribution. Two
species of RNA—IX and XIII (Fig. 3)—of class 1 insertion mutants (+44,
+93, and +163 nucleotides) were shifted slightly to a higher-molecular-
weight region. This shift roughly corresponds to the size of DNA inserted
into these mutants. This indicated that the termination at T_J in class I
mutants occurs after the insertion sites. (2) In infected cells with class 2

mutants (2 deletions and 2 insertion mutants tested), no detectable RNA species IX and XIII were found.

The disappearance of T_J containing wild-type RNA species (IX and XIII) in class 2 mutants suggests two possibilities: (1) Because the mutations in the hairpin structure may disrupt the termination signal, the absence of these two RNA species may be due to read-through of transcription. RNA synthesis would continue until the termination signals located downstream of the J–F junction was reached (T_F, T_G, or T_H). This would result in an increased production of larger RNA species in the class 2 mutant infected cells. No such increase was seen in distributions of isolated mRNAs. The hybridization test showed that no increase in F and H messages were found in class 2 mutants. (2) The other possibility is that RNAs terminating at T_J of class 2 mutants became more unstable than class 1 or wild-type infected cells. To test this possibility, the stabilities of mRNA representing various regions of the genome were determined by hybridization of RNA with restricted RF DNA fragments. The messages covering gene F and gene H regions decay with very similar rates in class 1 and class 2 infected cells. A significant difference was observed in the decay curves of gene B and gene D regions. In class 2 mutants, these messages decayed rapidly (half-lives of 1–2 min). This fast decay was not observed in class 1 and wild types (half-lives of 6–8 min). Hayashi *et al.* (1983) concluded that the decay rate of mRNA containing T_J was controlled by the sequences between the J–F intercistronic region. They speculated that class 2 mutations produce an mRNA more susceptible to mRNA degrading nucleases (probably $3' \rightarrow 5'$ nuclease).

An apparent contradiction between Romantschuk and Müller's (1983) finding of a general decrease of gpD synthesis in these mutants, and the results of Hayashi *et al.* (1983) showing the presence of two distinct classes with respect to the stability of gene D and gene B messages, can be explained by the physiological differences of the host cell. gpD synthesis was measured in heavily UV-irradiated cells to reduce host-protein synthesis, whereas gene D mRNA decay was determined in normal cells.

F. Cloning of mRNA Stabilizing Sequences

Hayashi and Hayashi (1985) constructed pBR322 derivative plasmid-containing heat-labile lambda repressor and the lambda P_R promoter followed by gene B or gene D sequences lacking the φX174 promoters. They inserted the wild-type J–F intercistronic regions [*am*N11E, class 1, named (+) mutant] or of an insertion mutant [*ins*2, class 2, named (−) mutant] or of neither sequence [(0) mutant] immediately downstream of gene B or gene D.

Cells carrying these plasmids were grown at low temperatures, and the rates of synthesis of various mRNA species were determined with the active repressor. No messages corresponding to gene D or gene B were detected. On the other hand, RNAs from the pBR322 portion of the plasmids were detected in all cell species. When the repressor was heat-inactivated, synthesis of gene D or gene B mRNA was observed, indicating that P_R promoter controls synthesis of gpB or gpD. The decay rates of messages corresponding to gene D or gene B and the pBR322 portion of plasmids were determined at the high temperature. In all strains, pBR322-specific mRNA decayed with half-lives of 2 min. Decay rates of B or D messages with (+) sequence were 7 to 8 min; with (−) sequence, 2.2 min; and with (0) sequence, 2 min. These results showed that the cloned (+) sequence significantly increased half-lives of the preceding genes. The decay of the 5' or 3' portion of D message was also examined using the probes of covering these portions. The decay of these regions is very similar to the total decay of gene D message. The (+) sequence stabilized not only the total gene D mRNA decay but also the decay of the 5' and 3' terminal sequences of the message. This stabilizing effect disappeared when the (+) sequence was replaced with the (−) or (0) sequence.

When the rates of protein synthesis of these genes were compared in the cells carrying these plasmids, the ratios of the (+), (−), and (0) sequences were 3–8:~2:1. After rifampicin treatment, the ratio became 10–15:~2:1, indicating that stabilized gene D or gene B mRNA was functional.

These experiments indicate that (1) the degree of stability of gene D or gene B messages was mainly determined by the sequence at their 3' end; (2) the stability-controlling sequences do not function *in trans*; (3) stability of two ϕX174 mRNAs starting at P_B or P_D and terminating at T_J in infected cells is not due to physiological changes of the cells after infection; (4) none of the ϕX174-coded proteins were responsible for the stabilization; and (5) the stabilized mRNA is functional as well as structurally stable. These characteristic features of ϕX174 mRNA decay starting around T_J resemble the retroregulation system.

Retroregulation was first recognized in lambda phage. Schindler and Echols (1981) and Guarneros *et al.* (1982) found that the *sib* site, located distal to the *int* gene, functions in two ways in *int* mRNA decay. When mRNA initiates at the *int* promoter (P_I), RNA synthesis is terminated at the stem loop structure of the *sib* site. This transcript is stable. However, initiation at P_L promoter, modified by N protein, does not respond to the *sib* termination signal, and a longer read-through transcript results. This mRNA is unstable. The 3' end of P_I promoting mRNA serves as a barrier to 3'-exonuclease degradation. RNase III cleavage of the extended P_L transcript allows degradation of the longer transcript (Schmeissner *et al.*, 1984).

In the T_J terminater of ϕX174, transcription terminates downstream of the stabilizing sequences. Nucleases chew back to the sequence, probably in the 3'→5' direction. The class 1 sequence could potentially slow down the upstream procession of mRNA specific nucleases. When the (+) sequence was replaced by the (−) sequence to form class 2 mutants, the protecting effect of the sequence disappeared. Therefore, class 2 mRNA decays faster than class 1 mutant. The wild-type sequence (+) contains a six base-paired hairpin structure upstream of the termination sites. The hairpin structure was destroyed by the insertional mutation to create the (−) sequence. Thus, the hairpin structure would be a candidate for the barrier of 3'→5' hydrolysis of mRNA by nuclease(s). However, more detailed investigation involving eight different deletion or insertion mutants of φX174 or G4 revealed that the hairpin structure was not a primary requirement to form the (+) type sequence (Hayashi et al., 1983). For example, one deletion mutant, although it could stabilize gene B or gene D mRNA, as the wild-type phage does, does not contain a stable hairpin structure. Another insertion mutant has the potential for small perfectly base-paired secondary structure, but it is a (−)-type mutant. Thus, the distinction of (+) or (−) type sequence seems to demand more complicated structural requirements. φX174 mRNA synthesis and stabilities at T_J, T_F, T_G, or T_H terminators are identical in wild-type or in RNAase III–deficient cells (M. N. Hayashi, personal observation), implying that RNAase III may not be involved in gene B, gene D, or other φX174 mRNA species degradation.

Retroregulation also occurs at the termination sites of the tryptophane operon (Mott et al., 1985). Panavotatos and Truong (1985) found that a cloned T7 RNAase III site, upon cleavage, became a strong mRNA stabilization signal, relative to the full-length transcript. Wong and Chang (1986) reported that Bacillus thuringensis cry (an insecticidal paraporal crystal protein gene) contains a positive retroregulator that functions in both Bacillus subtilis and E. coli. These findings indicate that retroregulation mechanisms are probably widespread among prokaryotes, although detailed mechanisms, including the structure of stabilizers and enzymes involved in mRNA degradation, may differ.

G. Expression of Overlapping Genes

The most striking feature of φX174 gene arrangement on the genome is the presence of overlapping genes. Gene B overlaps gene A (Weisbeek et al., 1977; Sanger et al., 1977), gene E is included within gene D (Barrell et al., 1976), and gene K overlaps genes A and C (Sanger et al., 1977). These overlapping genes are read in different reading frames. An important problem in φX174 gene expression is how these genes are expressed. The transcription map, presented in Fig. 3, reveals that translation of gene B can be completely independent of gene A expression, because each gene is transcribed from a different promoter, P_A or P_B. Gene E expression, however, differs greatly from the situation of genes A and B. Because no promoter for gene E has been found, genes D and E must share the message starting at P_D for their expression.

Because D protein is the most abundant ϕX174 protein, the RBS of E gene would be covered by ribosomes translating the D gene. Thus, some positive measure may be necessary to ensure adequate synthesis of the lysis protein. One means of effecting this regulation, used by the expression of an overlapping lysis gene in the RNA phages MS2, R17, and f2 (Atkins *et al.*, 1979; Model *et al.*, 1979; Beremand and Blumenthal, 1979), is proposed by Kastelein *et al.* (1982). The model includes a frameshift in the upstream gene (in this case the coat protein gene) followed by termination of translation and reinitiation of translation by terminating ribosomes at RBS of the overlapping gene (lysis gene). Buckley (1985) and Buckley and Hayashi (1987) investigated whether or not a similar mechanism is involved in the expression of the ϕX174 lysis protein. They constructed a series of deletions in the upstream D gene region. These fragments were cloned into expression vectors with the regulatable lambda P_R promoter, heat-labile lambda repressor, and about 75 nucleotides of lambda *cro* 5' end. Sequences necessary for gpE synthesis were assayed either by comparing cell lysis in clones containing deletions in the D–E sequences to wild-type clones or by measuring β-galactosidase synthesis using ϕX174 gene E–*lac*Z gene fusions. There are two basic features of these gene fusion constructs. (1) The RBS and initiation codon of gene D were eliminated, and the first nine codons of *lac*Z were replaced by 20 nucleotides including the gene E RBS and initiation codon. Therefore, the expression of *lac*Z depended on the P_R promoter and RBS of *cro* and RBS of gene E—the situation identical to the original D–E overlap. (2) The *cro* part contained 76, 75, or 74 nucleotides of the 5' end of this gene so that the gene D part of the constructs can be read in three different reading frames—D(a), E(a+1), or 3rd(a-1)—by choosing appropriate *cro* clones. The reading frames E and 3rd create nonsense codons, whereas the reading frame D does not. The results from the gene fusion experiments are shown in Fig. 14.

When ribosomes enter into the D–E region with the reading frame D, β-galactosidese activity decreased if the deletion extended toward E_{RBS}. This decrease was not continuous, but there were two sites where the enzyme activity drastically reduced: one between nucleotides 456 and 489, the other between nucleotides 517 and 539 (Fig. 14a). When ribosomes read the E frame or the 3rd frame, there were two sites where the β-galactosidase activity changed discontinuously (Fig. 14b). One site is between 456 and 489, and the other between 517 and 539. The increase of the enzyme activity of deletion 456 (3rd reading frame) is probably due to the presence of a stop codon at 485, around where the reading frame may be changed. Similarly, the deletion 517(3rd) has a stop codon at 527, and deletions 539(3rd) and 541(3rd) have a stop codon at 554. These results indicated that there are two possible sites where the ribosomes change the

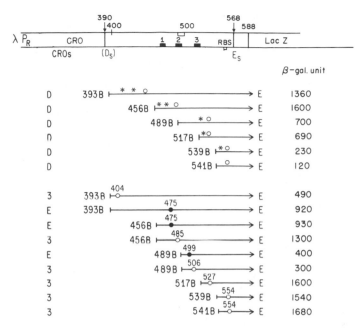

FIGURE 14. Gene fusion of lambda CRO φX174D-E and lacZ. Bars represent deleted region of the gene fusion construct (all start at 312). D, E, and (3) are three different reading frames: D (a); E (a+1); (3) (−1).

reading frame; one is somewhere between nucleotides 456 and 489, and the other between nucleotides 506 and 554.

The multiple alanine codons (GCN) in the φX174 D reading frame upstream of the E gene are potential cause of reading frame shifts. It has been shown that, in an *in vitro* system, *E. coli* tRNA$_{ser}^3$ is able to read an alanine codon as a doublet and as a consequence introduce a −1 reading frame shift (Bruce *et al.*, 1986; Dayhuff *et al.*, 1986; Atkins *et al.*, 1979). Of the 7 alanine codons upstream of the φX174 F gene region, 6 lie upstream of stop codons which lie in the −1 reading frame (shown with * in Fig. 14). A −1 frameshift at any of these sites would cause translational termination. From Fig. 14 deletion of 2 of these alanine codons, one at nuc. 456 and one at nuc. 462, caused a large drop in E expression as measured by β-galactosidase activity (compare X456B with X489B). A further drop in activity was not seen until a third alanine codon (at nuc. 522) was deleted (compare X489B or X517B with X539B). Deletion of the last alanine codon (at nuc. 540) lying upstream of a −1 reading frame stop codon, caused a further drop in activity (compare X539B with X541B).

Thus, the level of E expression may be the result of multiple frameshift-chain termination events. Chain termination at the stop codon at nuc. 485 appears to be the more favorable stopping point (in terms of allowing E gene expression). The presence of two alanine codons upstream of the stop codon at nucleotide 485, as opposed to one each for the other two stop codons, may be the reason.

Buckley and Hayashi (1987) proposed a model for φX174 E gene expressin. Due to misdecoding of a triplet as a doublet, ribosomes undergo a −1 reading frame shift. This decoding error may be a result of misreading alanine codons by tRNA$_{ser}$[3] in upstream of E gene. The shift of reading frame creates a termination codon where translation terminates. If the translation termination site is situated far upstream of the RBS of E gene, exposed mRNA would allow the entry of new ribosomes at RBS of E gene. If the termination occurs in the vicinity of the E gene RBS, then ribosomes reinitiate E gene translation. Both mechanisms result in synthesis of lysis protein, a protein needed by the phage to cause cell lysis.

There is another set of the overlapping gene in φX174. Gene K overlaps genes A and C. No reports have been found regarding regulation mechanisms in this set of the overlapping genes. One interesting aspect is from which promoter functional gene K mRNA is transcribed. If gene K is translated from the mRNA that begins at P_A, gene K overlaps gene A. If gene K is translated from the mRNA that begins at P_B, then gene C overlaps gene K. These situations may contain some controlling mechanisms different from those present in the D−E overlap.

VII. LYSIS

The φX174 E gene, part of the D−E overlapping gene system (Barrell et al., 1976), was first shown to encode a lysis protein by Hutchison and Sinsheimer (1966). Studies of φX174 mutants (Hutchison and Sinsheimer, 1966) and expression of the cloned φX174 E gene (Henrich et al., 1982; Young and Young, 1982; Bläsi et al., 1985) have demonstrated that of the φX174 coded proteins, only the E protein is necessary to cause cell lysis of E. coli. Most models for E protein action suggest a membrane insertion role for activity (Barrell et al., 1976; Young and Young, 1982), and recent works have shown that a functional, cellular, autolytic system is necessary for gpE-induced lysis (Lubitz et al., 1984a,b; Maratea et al., 1985).

Altman et al. (1985) and Bläsi et al. (1983) showed that gpE-induced lysis of E. coli is a result of its integration into the host cell inner membrane. In association with this membrane integration, a very limited degradiation of peptidoglycan occurs (Lubitz and Plapp, 1980). Hence, it is possible that gpE-induced autolysis of E. coli requires a specific interaction of the phage protein with enzymes that also represent targets for penicillin (Tomasz, 1979). However, Halfmann and Lubitz (1986) showed that cloned φX174 lysis gene is fully active in an E. coli temperature-sensitive, penicillin-tolerant mutant. This indicates that the modes of lysis induction by gpE and by penicillin differ and the trigger mechanism for autolysis depend on the specific inducer used. Lubitz and Pugsley (1985) pointed out that, as a consequence of membrane perturbation by gpE, a more indirect mechanism for the activation of peptidoglycan-synthesizing or degrading enzymes is possible.

Comparison of the E protein amino terminus with other membrane-spanning proteins, especially the lambda S (lysis) protein, shows several shared characteristics. Included is a potential membrane-spanning hydrophobic region terminated by positively charged amino acid residues (Young and Young, 1982). This further supports a membrane insertion role for the E protein. Recent work (Bläsi and Lubitz, 1985; Maratea et al., 1985) showed that lytic activity of E protein was localized to amino terminal section of the molecule at residues 51 to 59 (out of 91 total). Buckley and Hayashi (1986) found that this E gene activity has been further localized to the amino terminal 29 amino acids, a region of the protein that is thought to just span the cell membrane (Young and Young, 1982). The 29 amino acid region of gene E fused to both the lacZ gene and chloramphenicol acetyl transferase (CAT) gene resulted in fusion proteins with lytic activity. Fusion to a third protein, trpE, did not result in lytic activity. These results support a model of oligomerization of E protein for lytic activity (Struck et al., 1985), since both β-galactosidase and CAT exist as tetramers in their native state (Shaw, 1971; Zipser, 1963).

Gene E–containing plasmids can be used as cloning vehicles. Henrich and Plapp (1986) constructed a small positive selection vector (3.2 kb) containing modified gene E DNA downstream of the lac promoter (pUH84). The modified gene E DNA contains PstI, SalI, AccI, HincII, BamHI, and EcoRI sites. Plasmid pUH84 does not yield transformants after introduction into E. coli unless the lysis gene is inactivated by insertion of foreign DNA into one of the restriction sites in the modified gene E. Transcription of fragments cloned into pUH84 may be effectively regulated by the lac promoter, provided the host cells are cotransformed with the newly constructed plasmid, pUH7, which carries the I^Q allele of the lac repressor gene.

VIII. EFFECTS OF φX174 GENES ON HOST BACTERIAL CELLS

The most significant change in host cells after infection with φX174 is lysis of the cells. The mechanism of lysis is described in the preceding section.

A. Gene A*

Martin and Godson (1975) and Funk and Snover (1976) found that a product of gene A is responsible for shutoff of host DNA synthesis. However, these results did not reach a clear distinction between gpA and gpA*. Recently, Colasanti and Denhardt (1985) cloned gene A* in an expression vector carrying lambda ts repressor and lambda P_R promoter. Upon induction of expression of gpA*, DNA synthesis of a host carrying this plasmid was severely inhibited. However, the rate of β-galactosidase induction of the plasmid-containing cell was similar to that observed in control cells (no plasmid), indicating that gpA* had no effect on transcription and translation. Cells in which gpA* was expressed formed filaments and increased in mass for several hours after induction and were eventually killed. They also found that, upon induction of gpA*, the cell produced more recA protein, indicating a partial induction of the SOS response. However, gpA*-induced filamentation of host cells was also observed in recA56 and lexA3 (Ind⁻) strains in which the SOS response could not be induced. They proposed the following models: (1) gpA* may act specifically at single-stranded regions in the E. coli growing fork, breaking the DNA at the point and blocking further replication. It is known SS DNA has a greater sensitivity to cleavage by gpA* (section V.D); (2) gpA* makes a physical obstruction by binding to DNA or helicase; or (3) inhibition of cell division occurs as the result of an SOS-independent coupling of cell division to DNA replication (Burton and Holland, 1983).

Poddar's group published a series of papers on the effect of ϕX174 infection on the host cells. Host synthesis of β-galactosidase (Pal and Poddar, 1980), tryptophanase, D-serinedeaminase, and alkaline phosphatase (Ghosh et al., 1985) was reduced in ϕX174-infected cells. Pal and Poddar (1980) attributed the inhibition as due to the conformational change of the folded chromosome, the decrease of supercoiled regions, and the increase of relaxed regions. This change was the result of nicking of host DNA with gene A product, probably gpA* (Pal and Poddar, 1982).

B. Other Genes

Van der Avoort et al. (1983) cloned ϕX174 genes in pACYC177 and pBR322. The genes B, C, F, and G can be maintained stably in the cell with efficient expression of these genes. Genes D and E can only be maintained when the expression of these gene is completely blocked. Genes F and G are expressed even when they are not proceeded by promoters of ϕX174 or plasmid. This is due to the presence of two promoter-like sequences just in front of the two genes. Expression of complete A, H, or J genes could not be demonstrated. These experiments indicate that gpA or gpA*, gpH, and gpD may be lethal for cell growth, whereas gpB, gpC, gpF, and gpG proteins are nonlethal. The effect of gpJ is unknown.

IX. CONCLUDING REMARKS

An impressive number of isometric SS DNA phage papers have been accumulated in the past several years. This is an encouraging phenomenon for all SS DNA phage biologists, particularly in an apparently eukaryote-oriented era of molecular biology. ϕX174 is the first DNA-containing organism whose entire genome was sequenced. The sequence data have been invaluable for orienting genes and intercistronic regions, determining regulatory signals such as the origin of DNA replication, promoters, leaders, ribosome-binding sites, etc. Obviously, one can easily plan cloning strategies from the sequence. Exhaustive search for and extensive purification of the host factors and the availability of equally pure phage-encoded proteins have made it possible to advance our understanding of the biochemical processes involved in DNA replication and phage morphogenesis. Recent progress in gene manipulation techniques have been, and will continue to be, an enormous driving force in the exploration of unexpected profiles of isometric phages, as evidenced by many papers in this review. Simultaneously, we will be able to revisit the past descriptive or speculative results with new techniques. The interaction of the phage with the bacteria during adsorption, eclipse, and DNA penetration provides a unique opportunity to study the properties of the bacterial wall and membrane in conjunction with translocation of DNA and gpH. The lysis system also provides a way to probe wall and membrane structure of the host cells. We suspect that the phage will be an excellent vehicle with which to investigate the localization of the DNA replication at a membrane site. Continued dissection of the stage III DNA replication system will allow us to understand the molecular interactions in more detail and provide a wealth of new information on protein-protein and protein-DNA interactions. The molecular structures of prohead, phage, and the 50S complex remain to be elucidated. X-ray crystallography and laser Raman spectroscopy should provide useful information on the molecular structures. Chemical cross-linking as a structural probe may prove useful, as it has in other systems. The eclipse reaction provides a unique tool for probing the dynamic nature of DNA-protein and protein-protein interactions. The biology of the isometric SS DNA phages will, therefore, be significantly enriched in the coming years.

Acknowledgments. We thank our numerous colleagues who provided original figures, reprints, and preprints of their work for this review (concluded November 1986). We offer our apologies to anyone whose papers have been inadvertently neglected. We particularly thank Dr. Yazaki for providing original electron micrographs of φX174. We thank M. E. Dalphin for critically reading the manuscript. We thank E. Corets and S. Lindelsee for help in preparation of the manuscript. Our unpublished results are supported by grants NIH GM12934 and NSF 83-08385.

M.H. and M.N.H. dedicate their papers cited in this review, with affection and admiration, to the late professor Sol Spiegelman, at whose laboratory in Illinois it all started (M. Hayashi, M. N. Hayashi, and S. Spiegelman, 1963). They regret that their story has not yet been completed 25 years later.

REFERENCES

Abarzua, P., Soeller, W., and Marians, K. J., 1984, Mutational analysis of primosome assembly sites. I. Distinct classes of mutants in the pBR322 *Escherichia coli* factor Y DNA effector sequences, *J. Biol. Chem.* **259**:14287.

Adhya, S., and Gottesman, M., 1978, Control of transcription termination, *Annu. Rev. Biochem.* **48**:967.

Altman, E., Young, K., Garrett, J., Altman, R., and Young, R., 1985, Subcellular localization of lethal lysis proteins of bacteriophages λ and φX174, *J. Virol.* **53**:1008.

Aoyama, A., and Hayashi, M., 1982, *In vitro* packaging of plasmid DNAs into φX174 bacteriophage capsid, *Nature* **297**:704.

Aoyama, A., and Hayashi, M., 1985, Effects of genome size on bacteriophage φX174 DNA packaging *in vitro, J. Biol. Chem.* **160**:11033.

Aoyama, A., and Hayashi, M., 1986, Synthesis of bacteriophage φx174 *in vitro:* Mechanism of switch from DNA replication to DNA packaging, *Cell* **47**:99.

Aoyama, A., Hamatake, R. K., and Hayashi, M., 1981, Morphogenesis of φX174: *In vitro* synthesis of infectious phage from purified viral components, *Proc. Natl. Acad. Sci. USA* **78**:7285.

Aoyama, A., Hamatake, R. K., Mukai, R., and Hayashi, M., 1983a, Purification of φX174 gene C protein, *J. Biol. Chem.* **285**:5798.

Aoyama, A., Hamatake, R. K., and Hayashi, M., 1983b, *In vitro* synthesis of bacteriophage φX174 by purified components, *Proc. Natl. Acad. Sci. USA* **80**:4195.

Arai, K., and Kornberg, A., 1979, A general priming system employing only *dnaB* protein and primase for DNA replication, *Proc. Natl. Acad. Sci. USA* **76**:4308.

Arai, K., and Kornberg, A., 1981a, Unique primed start of phage φX174 DNA replication and mobility of the primosome in a direction opposite chain synthesis, *Proc. Natl. Acad. Sci. USA* **78**:69.

Arai, K., and Kornberg, A., 1981b, Mechanism of *dnaB* protein action. II. ATP hydrolysis by *dnaB* protein dependent on single- or double-stranded DNA, *J. Biol. Chem.* **256**:5253.

Arai, K., and Kornberg, A., 1981c, Mechanism of *dnaB* protein action. III. Allosteric role of ATP in the alteration of DNA structure by *dnaB* protein in priming replication, *J. Biol. Chem.* **256**:5260.

Arai, K., and Kornberg, A., 1981d, Mechanism of *dnaB* protein action. IV. General priming of DNA replication by *dnaB* protein and primase compared with RNA polymerase, *J. Biol. Chem.* **256**:5267.

Arai, K., Arai, N., Shlomai, J., and Kornberg, A., 1980, Replication of duplex DNA of phage φX174 reconstituted with purified enzymes, *Proc. Natl. Acad. Sci. USA* **77**:3322.

Arai, K., Low, R. L., and Kornberg, A., 1981a, Movement and site selection for priming by the primosome in phage φX174 DNA replication, *Proc. Natl. Acad. Sci. USA* **78**:707.

Arai, K., Yasuda, S., and Kornberg, A., 1981b, Mechanism of *dnaB* protein action. I. Crystallization and properties of *dnaB* protein, an essential replication protein in *Escherichia coli, J. Biol. Chem.* **256**:5247.

Arai, K., Low, R., Kobori, J., Shlomai, J., and Kornberg, A., 1981c, Mechanism of *dnaB* protein action. V. Association of *dnaB* protein, protein n', and other prepriming proteins in the primosome of DNA replication, *J. Biol. Chem.* **256**:5273.

Arai, K., McMacken, R., Yasuda, S., and Kornberg, A., 1981d, Purification and properties of *Escherichia coli* protein i, a prepriming protein in φX174 DNA replication, *J. Biol. Chem.* **256**:5281.

Arai, N., and Kornberg, A., 1981, Rep protein as a helicase in an active, isolatable replication fork of duplex φX174 DNA, *J. Biol. Chem.* **256**:5294.

Arai, N., Polder, L., Arai, K., and Kornberg, A., 1981e, Replication of φX174 DNA with purified enzymes. II. Multiplication of the duplex form by coupling of continuous and discontinuous synthetic pathways, *J. Biol. Chem.* **256**:5239.

Arai, N., Arai, K., and Kornberg, A., 1981f, Complexes of rep protein with ATP and DNA as a basis for helicase action, *J. Biol. Chem.* **256**:5287.

Atkins, J. F., Steiz, J. A., Anderson, C. W., and Model, P., 1979, Binding of mammalian ribosomes to MS2 phage RNA reveals an overlapping gene encoding a lysis function, *Cell* **18**:247.

Axelrod, N., 1976a, *In vitro* transcription of φX174: Selective initiation with oligonucleotides, *J. Mol. Biol.* **108**:753.

Axelrod, N., 1976b, *In vitro* transcription of φX174: Analysis with restriction enzymes, *J. Mol. Biol.* **108**:771.

Azuma, J., Morita, J., and Komano, T., 1980, Process of attachment of φX174 parental DNA to the host cell membrane, *J. Biochem.* **88**:525.

Baas, P. D., 1985, DNA replication of single-stranded *Escherichia coli* DNA phages, *Biochim. Biophys. Acta* **825**:111.

Baas, P. D., Teertstra, W. R., and Jansz, H. S., 1978, Bacteriophage φX174 RF DNA replication *in vivo*: A biochemical study, *J. Mol. Biol.* **125**:167.

Baas, P. D., Teertstra, W. R., Van der Ende, A., and Jansz, H. S., 1980a, Bacteriophage φX174 and G4 RF DNA replicative intermediates. A comparative study using different isolation procedures, *J. Mol. Biol.* **137**:283.

Baas, P. D., Heidekamp, F., Van Mansfeld, A. D. M., Jansz, H. S., Langeveld, S. A., Van der Martel, G. A., Veeneman, G. H., and Von Boom, J. H., 1980b, Studies on the φX RF DNA replication, in: *Mechanistic Studies of DNA Replication and Genetic Recombination* (B. Alberts and F. Fox, eds.), pp. 267–277, Academic Press, New York.

Baas, P. D., Teertstra, W. R., Van Mansfeld, A. D., Jansz, H. S., Van der Marel, G. A., Veeneman, G. H., and Van Boom, J. H., 1981a, Construction of viable and lethal mutations in the origin of bacteriophage φX174 using synthetic oligodeoxyribonucleotides, *J. Mol. Biol.* **152**:614.

Baas, P. D., Heidekamp, F., Van Mansfeld, A. D. M., Jansz, H. S., Langeveld, S. A., Van der Martel, G. A., Veeneman, G. H., and Von Boom, J. H., 1981b, Essential features of the origin of bacteriophage φX174 RF DNA replication: A recognition and a key sequence for φX gene A protein, in: *The Initiation of DNA Replication* (D. S. Ray, ed.), pp. 195–209, Academic Press, New York.

Bachmann, B. J., 1983, Linkage map of *Escherichia coli* K-12, edition 7, *Microbiol. Rev.* **47**:180.

Baker, R., and Tessman, I., 1967, The circular genetic map of phage S13, *Proc. Natl. Acad. Sci. USA* **58**:1438.

Barrell, B. G., Air, G. M., and Hutchinson, C. A. III, 1976, Overlapping genes in bacteriophage φX174, *Nature* **264**:34.

Baumel, I., Meyer, T. F., and Geider, K., 1984, Functional aspects of *Escherichia coli* rep helicase in unwinding and replication of DNA, *Eur. J. Biochem.* **138**:247.

Bayer, M. E., and Starkey, T. W., 1972, The adsorption of bacteriophage φX174 and its interaction with *Escherichia coli*: a kinetic and morphological study, *Virology* **49**:236.

Benbow, R. M., Zuccarelli, A. Z., Davis, G. C., and Sinsheimer, R. L., 1974, Genetic recombination in bacteriophage φX174, *J. Virol.* **13**:898.

Beremand, M. N., and Blumenthal, T., 1979, Overlapping genes in RNA phage: A new protein implicated in lysis, *Cell* **18**:257.

Biswas, S. B., and Kornberg, A., 1984, Nucleoside triphosphate binding to DNA polymerase III holoenzyme of *Escherichia coli*. A direct photoaffinity labeling study, *J. Biol. Chem.* **259**:7990.

Bläsi, V., and Lubitz, W., 1985, Influence of C-terminal modifications of φX174 lysis gene E on its lysis-inducing properties, *J. Gen. Virol.* **66**:1209.

Bläsi, V., Geisen, R., Lubitz, R., Henrick, B., and Plapp, R., 1983, Localization of bacteriophage φX174 lysis gene product in the cell envelope of *E. coli*, in: *The Target of Penicillin* (R. Hakenbeck, J. V. Holtje, and H. Labischiski, eds.), pp. 205–210, Walter de Gruyter, Berlin.

Bläsi, V., Henrich, B., and Lubitz, W., 1985, Lysis of *Escherichia coli* by cloned φX174 gene E depends on its expression., *J. Gen. Microbiol.* **131**:1107.

Bleichrodt, J. F., and Van Abkoude, E. R., 1967, The transition between two forms of bacteriophage φX174 differing in heat sensitivity and adsorption characteristics, *Virology* **32**:93.

Bleichrodt, J. F., Blok, J., and Berends–Van Abkoude, E. R., 1968, Thermal inactivation of bacteriophage φX174 and two of its mutants, *Virology* **36**:343.

Bouche, J.-P., Zechel, K., and Kornberg, A., 1975, *dna* G gene product, a rifampicin resistant

RNA polymerase, initiates the conversion of a single-stranded coliphage DNA to its duplex replicative form, *J. Biol. Chem.* **250**:5995.

Brendel, V., 1985, Mapping of transcription terminators of bacteriophages φX174 and G4 by sequence analysis, *J. Virol.* **53**:340.

Brown, D. R., Reinberg, D., Schmidt-Glenewinkel, T., Roth, M., Zipursky, S. L., and Hurwitz, J., 1983a, DNA structures required for φX174 A–protein–directed initiation and termination of DNA replication, *Cold Spring Harbor Symp. Quant. Biol.* **47**:701.

Brown, D. R., Schmidt-Glenewinkel, T., Reinberg, D., and Hurwitz, J., 1983b, DNA sequences which support activities of the bacteriophage φX174 gene A protein, *J. Biol. Chem.* **258**:8402.

Brown, D. R., Reinberg, D., Schmidt-Glenewinkel, T., Zipursky, S. L., and Hurwitz, J., 1983c, Analysis of the φX174 gene A protein using *in vitro* DNA replication systems, *Methods Enzymol.* **100**:21.

Brown, D. R., Roth, M. J., Reinberg, D., and Hurwitz, J., 1984, Analysis of bacteriophage φX174 gene A protein–mediated termination and reinitiation of φX DNA synthesis. I. Characterization of the termination and reinitiation reactions, *J. Biol. Chem.* **259**:10545.

Brown, D. T., MacKenzie, J. M., and Bayer, M. E., 1971, Mode of host cell penetration by bacteriophage φX174, *J. Virol.* **7**:836.

Bruce, A. G., Atkins, T. F., and Gestrand, R. F., 1986, tRNA anticodon replacement experiments show that ribosomal frame shifting can be caused by doublet decoding, *Proc. Natl. Acad. Sci. USA* **83**:5062.

Buckley, K. J., 1985, Ph.D. thesis, University of California at San Diego, La Jolla.

Buckley, K. J., and Hayashi, M., 1986, Lytic activity localized to membrane-spanning region of φX174 E protein, *Mol. Gen. Genet.* **204**:120.

Buckley, K. J., and Hayaski, M., 1987, The role of premature translational termination in the regulation of expression of the φX174 lysis gene, *J. Mol. Biol* **198**:599.

Burgers, P. M., and Kornberg, A., 1982a, ATP activation of DNA polymerase III holoenzyme of *Escherichia coli.* I. ATP-dependent formation of an initiation complex with a primed template, *J. Biol. Chem.* **257**:11468.

Burgers, P. M., and Kornberg, A., 1982b, ATP activation of DNA polymerase III holoenzyme from *Escherichia coli.* II. Initiation complex: Stoichiometry and reactivity, *J. Biol. Chem.* **257**:11474.

Burgers, P. M., and Kornberg, A., 1983, The cycling of *Escherichia coli* DNA polymerase III holoenzyme in replication, *J. Biol. Chem.* **258**:7669.

Burgess, A. B., 1969, Studies on the proteins of φX174. II. The protein composition of the φX coat, *Proc. Natl. Acad. Sci. USA* **64**:613.

Burgess, A. B., and Denhardt, D. T., 1969, Studies on φX174 proteins I. Phage specific proteins synthesized after infection of *E. coli, J. Mol. Biol.* **44**:377.

Burton, P., and Holland, I. B., 1983, Two pathways of division inhibition in UV-irradiated *E. coli, Mol. Gen. Genet.* **190**:309.

Casjens, S., 1985, *Virus Structure and Assembly,* Jones and Barlett, Boston.

Chamberlin, M. J., Briat, J.-F., Dedrick, R. L., Hanna, M., Kane, C. M., Levin, J., Reynolds, R., and Schmidt, M., 1985, Factors involved in elongation and termination of bacterial and mammalian transcription, in: *Genetics, Cell Differentiation, and Cancer* (P. A. Marks, ed.), pp. 47–73, Academic Press, New York.

Champoux, J. J., 1977, Strand breakage by the DNA untwisting enzyme results in covalent attachment of the enzyme to DNA, *Proc. Natl. Acad. Sci. USA* **74**:3800.

Champoux, J. J., 1981, DNA is linked to the rat liver DNA nicking-closing enzyme by a phosphodiester bond to tyrosine, *J. Biol. Chem.* **256**:4805.

Chrysogelos, S., and Griffith, J., 1982, *Escherichia coli* single-strand binding protein organizes single-stranded DNA in nucleosome-like units, *Proc. Natl. Acad. Sci. USA* **79**:5803.

Cleary, J. M., and Ray, D. S., 1980, Replication of the plasmid pBR322 under the control of a cloned replication origin from the single-stranded DNA phage M13, *Proc. Natl. Acad. Sci. USA* **77**:4638.

Cleary, J. M., and Ray, D. S., 1981, Deletion analysis of the cloned replication origin region from bacteriophage M13, *J. Virol.* **40:**197.

Clements, J. B., and Sinsheimer, R. L., 1975, Process of infection with bacteriophage φX174. XXXVII. RNA metabolism in φX174 infected cells, *J. Virol.* **15:**151.

Colasanti, J., and Denhardt, D. T., 1985, Expression of the cloned bacteriophage φX174 A* gene in *Escherichia coli* inhibits DNA replication and cell division, *J. Virol.* **53:**805.

Denhardt, D. T., 1977, The isometric single-stranded DNA phages, in: *Comprehensive Virology*, Vol. 7 (H. Fraenkel-Conrat and R. R. Wayner, eds.), pp. 1–104, Plenum, New York.

Denhardt, D. T., Dressler, D., and Ray, D. S., 1978, *The Single-Stranded DNA Phages*, Cold Spring Harbor Laboratory, Cold Spring Harbor, NY.

Depew, R. E., Liu, L. F., and Wang, J. C., 1978, Interaction between DNA and *Escherichia coli* protein ω: Formation of a complex between single-stranded DNA and ω protein, *J. Biol. Chem.* **253:**511.

Dowell, C. E., Jansz, H. S., and Zandberg, J., 1981, Infection of *Escherichia coli* K-12 by bacteriophage φX174, *Virology* **114:**252.

Dressler, D., Hourcade, D., Koths, K., and Sims, J., 1978, The DNA replication cycle of the isometric phages, in: *The Single-Stranded DNA Phages* (D. T. Denhardt, D. Dressler, and D. S. Ray, eds.), pp. 187–214, Cold Spring Harbor Laboratory, Cold Spring Harbor, NY.

Dubeau, L., and Denhardt, D. T., 1981, The mechanism of replication of φX174. XVIII. Gene A and A* proteins of φX174 bind tightly to φX174 replicative form DNA, *Biochim. Biophys. Acta* **653:**52.

Dubeau, L., Hours, C., and Denhardt, D. T., 1981, The mechanism of replication of φX174. XVII. Purification and partial characterization of the gene A and A* proteins, *Can. J. Biochem.* **59:**106.

Dunker, A. K., 1974, Structure of isometric viruses containing nonidentical polypeptide chains, *J. Virol.* **14:**878.

Dunn, J., Buzah-Pollert, E., and Studier, W., 1978, Mutations of bacteriophage T7 that affect initiation of synthesis of gene 0.3 protein, *Proc. Natl. Acad. Sci. USA* **75:**2741.

Earnshaw, W. C., and Casjens, S. R., 1980, DNA packaging by the double-stranded DNA bacteriophages. *Cell* **21:**319.

Edgell, M. H., Hutchison, C. A. III, and Sinsheimer, R. L., 1969, The process of infection with bacteriophage φX174. XXVIII. Removal of the spike proteins from the phage capsid, *J. Mol. Biol.* **42:**547.

Edlind, T. D., and Ihler, G. M., 1980, Long range base pairing in bacteriophage φX174 single-stranded DNA, *J. Mol. Biol.* **142:**131.

Eisenberg, S., 1980, Cleavage of φX174 single-stranded DNA by gene A protein and formation of a tight protein-DNA complex, *J. Virol.* **35:**409.

Eisenberg, S., and Ascarelli, R., 1981, The A* protein of φX174 is an inhibitor of DNA replication, *Nucleic Acids Res.* **9:**1991.

Eisenberg, S., and Finer, M., 1980, Cleavage and circularization of single-stranded DNA: A novel enzymatic activity of φX174 A* protein, *Nucleic Acids Res.* **8:**5305.

Eisenberg, S., and Kornberg, A., 1979, Purification and characterization of φX174 cistron A protein: A multifunctional enzyme of duplex DNA replication, *J. Biol. Chem.* **254:**5328.

Eisenberg, S., Scott, J. F., and Kornberg, A., 1976a, An enzyme system for replication of duplex circular DNA: The replicative form of phage φX174, *Proc. Natl. Acad. Sci. USA* **73:**1594.

Eisenberg, S., Scott, J. F., and Kornberg, A., 1976b, Enzymatic replication of viral and complementary strands of duplex DNA of phage φX174 proceeds by separate mechanisms, *Proc. Natl. Acad. Sci. USA* **73:**3151.

Eisenberg, S., Griffith, J., and Kornberg, A., 1977, φX174 cistron A protein is a multifunctional enzyme in DNA replication, *Proc. Natl. Acad. Sci. USA* **74:**3198.

Farber, M. B., 1976, Purification and properties of bacteriophage φX174 gene D product, *J. Virol.* **17:**1027.

Fassler, J. S., and Tessman, I., 1981, Relation between UV suppression of polarity in φX174 and UV sensitivity of *rho* mutants, *J. Virol.* **37:**955.

Feige, U., and Stirm, S., 1976, On the structure of the *Escherichia coli* C cell wall lipopolysaccharide core and on its φX174 receptor region, *Biochem. Biophys, Res. Commun.* **71**:566.

Fiddes, J. C., Barrell, B. G., and Godson, G. N., 1978, Nucleotide sequences of the separate origins of synthesis of bacteriophage G4 viral and complimentary DNA strands, *Proc. Natl. Acad. Sci. USA* **75**:1081.

Fluit, A. C., Baas, P. D., Van Boom, J. H., Veeneman, G. H., and Jansz, H. S., 1984a, Gene A protein cleavage of recombinant plasmids containing the φX174 replication origin, *Nucleic Acids Res.* **12**:64434.

Fluit, A. C., Baas, P. D., Jansz, H. S., Veeneman, G. H., and Van Boom, J. H., 1984b, Gene A protein interacting with recombinant plasmid DNAs containing 25-30 b.p. of the φX174 replication origin, *Adv. Exp. Med. Biol.* **179**:231.

Fluit, A. C., Baas, P. D., and Jansz, H. S., 1985, The complete 30-base-pair origin region of bacteriophage φX174 in a plasmid is both required and sufficient for *in vivo* rolling-circle DNA replication and packaging, *Eur. J. Biochem.* **149**:579.

Francke, B. R., and Ray, D. S., 1971, Fate of parental φX174-DNA upon infection of starved thymine-requiring host cells, *Virology* **44**:168.

Francke, B. R., and Ray, D. S., 1972, *cis*-limited action of the gene-A product of bacteriophage φX174 and the essential bacterial site, *Proc. Natl. Acad. Sci. USA* **69**:475.

Freymeyer, D. K. II, Shank, P. R., Edgell, M. H., Hutchinson, C. A. III, and Vanaman, T. C., 1977, Amino acid sequence of the small core protein from bacteriophage φX174, *Biochemistry* **16**:4550.

Fujimura, F. K., and Hayashi, M., 1978, Transcription of isometric single-stranded DNA phage, in: *The Single-Stranded DNA Phages* (D. T. Denhardt, D. Dressler, and D. S. Ray, eds.), pp. 485–505, Cold Spring Harbor Laboratory, Cold Spring Harbor, NY.

Fujisawa, H., and Hayashi, M., 1976a, Viral DNA synthesizing intermediate complex isolated during assembly of bacteriophage φX174, *J. Virol.* **19**:409.

Fujisawa, H., and Hayashi, M., 1976b, Gene A product of φX174 is required for site specific endonucleolytic cleavage during single-stranded DNA synthesis *in vivo*, *J. Virol.* **19**:416.

Fujisawa, H., and Hayashi, M., 1977a, Functions of gene C and gene D products of bacteriophage φX174, *J. Virol.* **21**:506.

Fujisawa, H., and Hayashi, M., 1977b, Two infectious forms of bacteriophage φX174, *J. Virol.* **23**:439.

Fujisawa, H., and Hayashi, M., 1977c, Assembly of bacteriophage φX174: Identification of a virion capsid precursor and proposal of a model for the functions of bacteriophage gene products during morphogenesis, *J. Virol.* **24**:303.

Funk, F. D., and Snover, D., 1976, Pleiotropic effects of mutants in gene A of bacteriophage φX174, *J. Virol.* **18**:141.

Geider, K., and Hoffmann-Berling, H., 1981, Proteins controlling the helical structure of DNA, *Annu. Rev. Biochem.* **50**:233.

Gelfand, D. H., and Hayashi, M., 1969, Electrophoretic characterization of φX174-specific proteins, *J. Mol. Biol.* **44**:501.

Ghosh, A., Pal, S. K., and Poddar, R. K., 1985, Modulation of gene expression in *Escherichia coli* infected with single-stranded bacteriophage φX174, *Mol. Gen. Genet.* **198**:304.

Gillam, S., Astell, C. S., and Smith, M., 1980, Site-specific mutagenesis using oligodeoxyribonucleotides: Isolation of a phenotypically silent φX174 mutant, with a specific nucleotide deletion, at very high efficiency, *Gene* **12**:129.

Gillam, S., Astell, C. R., Jahnke, P., Hutchison, C. A. III, and Smith, M., 1984, Construction and properties of a ribosome-binding site mutation in gene E of φX174 bacteriophage, *J. Virol.* **52**:892.

Gillam, S., Atkinson, T., Markham, A., and Smith, M., 1985, Gene K of bacteriophage φX174 codes for a protein which affects the burst size of phage production, *J. Virol.* **53**:708.

Godson, G. N., 1978, The other isometric phages, in: *The Single-Stranded DNA Phages* (D. T. Denhardt, D. Dressler, and D. S. Ray, eds.), pp. 103–112, Cold Spring Harbor Laboratory, Cold Spring Harbor, NY.

Godson, G. N., Barrell, B. C., Staden, R., and Fiddes, J. C., 1978a, Nucleotide sequence of bacteriophage G4 DNA, *Nature* **276**:236.

Godson, G. N., Fiddes, J. C., Barrell, B. G., and Sanger, F., 1978b, Comparative DNA sequence analysis of the G4 and φX174 genomes, in: *The Single-Stranded DNA Phages* (D. T. Denhardt, D. Dressler, and D. S. Ray, eds.), pp. 51–86, Cold Spring Harbor Laboratory, Cold Spring Harbor, NY.

Greenbaum, J. H., and Marians, K. J., 1984, The interaction of *Escherichia coli* replication factory Y with complementary strand origins of DNA replication. Contact points revealed by DNase footprinting and protection from methylation, *J. Biol. Chem.* **259**:2594.

Greenbaum, J. H., and Marians, K. J., 1985, Mutational analysis of primosome assembly sites. Evidence for alternative DNA structures, *J. Biol. Chem.* **260**:12266.

Grohman, K., Smith, L. H., and Sinsheimer, R. I., 1975, New method for isolation and sequence determination of 5' terminal region of bacteriophage φX174 *in vitro* mRNAs, *Biochemistry* **14**:1951.

Guarneros, G., Montanez, C., Hernandez, T., and Court, D., 1982, Post transcriptional control of bacteriophage in gene expression from a site distal to the gene, *Proc. Natl. Acad. Sci. USA* **79**:238.

Hakkaart, M. J. J., Wesseling, J. G., Veltkamp, E., and Nijkamp, H. J. J., 1982, Maintenance of bacteriocinogenic plasmid CloDF13 in *Escherichia coli* cells. I. Localization and mutual interactions of four CloDF13 incompatibility regions, *Mol. Gen. Genet.* **86**:531.

Halfmann, G., and Lubitz, W., 1986, Differential induction of *Escherichia coli* autolysis by penicillin and the bacteriophage φX174 gene E product, *J. Bacteriol.* **166**:683.

Hamatake, R. K., 1983, Ph.D. thesis, University of California at San Diego, La Jolla.

Hamatake, R. K., Mukai, R., and Hayashi, M., 1981, Role of DNA gyrase subunits in synthesis of bacteriophage φX174 viral DNA, *Proc. Natl. Acad. Sci. USA* **78**:1532.

Hamatake, R. K., Aoyama, A., and Hayashi, M., 1985, The J gene of bacteriophage φX174: *In vitro* analysis of J protein function, *J. Virol.* **54**:345.

Havekes, L., Tommassen, J., Hoekstra, W., and Lugtenberg, B., 1977, Isolation and characterization of *Escherichia coli* K-12 F⁻ mutants defective in conjugation with an I-type donor, *J. Bacteriol.* **129**:1.

Hayashi, M., 1978, Morphogenesis of the isometric phages, in: *The Single-Stranded DNA Phages* (D. T. Denhardt, D. Dressler, and D. S. Ray, eds.), pp. 531–547, Cold Spring Harbor Laboratory, Cold Spring Harbor, NY.

Hayashi, M., Hayashi, M. N., and Spiegelman, S., 1963, Restriction of *in vivo* genetic transcription to one of the complementary strand of DNA, *Proc. Natl. Acad. Sci. USA* **50**:664.

Hayashi, M., Hayashi, M. N., and Spiegelman, S., 1964, DNA circularity and mechanism of strand selection in the generation of genetic messages, *Proc. Natl. Acad. Sci. USA* **51**:351.

Hayashi, M., Fujimura, F. K., and Hayashi, M. N., 1976, Mapping of *in vivo* messenger RNAs for bacteriophage φX174, *Proc. Natl. Acad. Sci. USA* **73**:3519.

Hayashi, M. N., and Hayashi, M., 1974, Fragment maps of φX174 replicative DNA produced by restriction enzymes from *Haemophilus aphirophilus* and *Haemophilus influenzae* H-I, *J. Virol.* **11**:42.

Hayashi, M. N., and Hayashi, M., 1981, Stability of bacteriophage φX174-specific mRNA *in vivo*, *J. Virol.* **37**:506.

Hayashi, M. N., and Hayashi, M., 1985, Cloned DNA sequences that determine mRNA stability of bacteriophage φX174 *in vivo* are functional, *Nucleic Acids Res.* **13**:5937.

Hayashi, M. N., Hayashi, M., and Imai, M., 1981, Bacteriophage φX174-specific mRNA synthesis in cells deficient in termination factor *rho* activity, *J. Virol.* **38**:198.

Hayashi, M. N., Hayashi, M., and Müller, U. R., 1983, Role for the J–F intercistronic region of bacteriophages φX174 and G4 in stability of mRNA, *J. Virol.* **48**:186.

Hayashi, Y., and Hayashi, M., 1970, Fractionation of φX174 specific messenger RNA, *Cold Spring Harbor Symp. Quant. Biol.* **35**:17.

Heidekamp, F., Langeveld, S. A., Baas, P. D., and Jansz, H. S., 1980, Studies of the recognition sequence of φX174 gene A protein. Cleavage site of φX gene A protein in St-1 RFI DNA, *Nucleic Acids Res.* **8:**1009.

Heidekamp, F., Baas, P. D., Van Boom, J. H., Veeneman, G. H., Zipursky, S. L., and Jansz, H. S., 1981, Construction and characterization of recombinant plasmid DNAs containing sequences of the origin of bacteriophage φX174 DNA replication, *Nucleic Acids Res.* **9:**3335.

Heidekamp, F., Baas, P. D., and Jansz, H. S., 1982, Nucleotide sequences at the φX gene A protein cleavage site in replicative form I DNAs of bacteriophages U3, G14, and α3, *J. Virol.* **42:**91.

Henrich, B., and Plapp, R., 1986, Use of the lysis gene of bacteriophage φX174 for the construction of a positive selection vector, *Gene* **42:**345.

Henrich, B., Lubitz, W., and Plapp, R., 1982, Lysis of *Escherichia coli* by induction of cloned φX174 genes, *Mol. Gen. Genet.* **185:**493.

Henry, T. J., and Knippers, R., 1974, Isolation and function of the gene A initiator of bacteriophage φX174, a highly specific DNA endonuclease, *Proc. Natl. Acad. Sci. USA* **71:**1549.

Holmes, W. M., Platt, T., and Rosenberg, M., 1983, Termination of transcription in *E. coli*, *Cell* **32:**1029.

Hubscher, U., and Spadari, S., 1984, *Proteins Involved in DNA Replication*, Plenum Press, New York.

Hutchison, C. A. III, and Sinsheimer, R. L., 1966, The process of interaction with bacteriophage φX174. X. Mutations in φX lysis gene, *J. Mol. Biol.* **18:**429.

Hutchison, C. A. III, and Sinsheimer, R. L., 1971, Requirement of protein synthesis for bacteriophage φX174 superinfection exclusion, *J. Virol.* **8:**121.

Ikeda, J.-E., Yudelevich, A., Shimamoto, N., and Hurwitz, J., 1979, Role of polymeric forms of the bacteriophage φX174 coded gene A protein in φX RFI DNA cleavage, *J. Biol. Chem.* **254:**9416.

Imamoto, F., and Nakamura, Y., 1986, *Escherichia coli* proteins involved in regulation of transcription termination: Function, structure, and expression of the nusA and nusB genes, *Adv. Biophys.* **21:**175.

Imber, R., Low, R. L., and Ray, D. S., 1983, Identification of a primosome assembly site in the region of the ori 2 replication origin of the *Escherichia coli* mini-F plasmid, *Proc. Natl. Acad. Sci. USA* **80:**7132.

Incardona, N. L., 1974, Mechanism of adsorption and eclipse of bacteriophage φX174. III. Comparison of the activation parameters for the *in vitro* and *in vivo* eclipse reactions with mutant and wild-type virus, *J. Virol.* **14:**469.

Incardona, N. L., 1978, Adsorption and eclipse reactions of the isometric phages, in: *The Single-Stranded DNA Phages* (D. T. Denhardt, D. Dressler, and D. S. Ray, eds.), pp. 549–555, Cold Spring Harbor Laboratory, Cold Spring Harbor, NY.

Incardona, N. L., 1981, Application of Arrhenius kinetic theory to viral eclipse: Selection of bacteriophage φX174 mutants, *J. Virol.* **39:**510.

Incardona, N. L., 1983a, Binding of viruses and ligands to cells: Effect of receptor density, *J. Theor. Biol.* **104:**693.

Incardona, N. L., 1983b, A kinetic model for virus binding which involves release of cell-bound virus-receptor complexes, *J. Theor. Biol.* **105:**631.

Incardona, N. L., and Müller, U. R., 1985, Eclipse kinetics as a probe of quaternary structure in bacteriophage φX174, *J. Mol. Biol.* **181:**479.

Incardona, N. L., and Selvidge, L., 1973, Mechanism of adsorption and eclipse of bacteriophage φX174. II. Attachment and eclipse with isolated *Escherichia coli* cell wall lipopolysaccharide, *J. Virol.* **11:**775.

Incardona, N. L., Tuech, J. K., and Murti, G., 1985, Irreversible binding of phage φX174 to cell-bound lipopolysaccharide receptors and release of virus-receptor complexes, *Biochemistry* **24:**6439.

Incardona, N. L., Prescott, B., Sargent, D., Lambda, O. P., and Thomas, G. J. Jr., 1987, Phage φX174 probed by laser Raman spectroscopy: Evidence for capsid-imposed constraint on DNA secondary structure, *Biochemistry* **26:**1532.

Jacob, F., Brenner, S., and Cuzin, F., 1963, On the regulation of DNA replication in bacteria, *Cold Spring Harbor Symp. Quant. Biol.* **28:**329.

Jazwinski, S. M., and Kornberg, A., 1975, DNA replication *in vitro* starting with an intact φX174 phage, *Proc. Natl. Acad. Sci. USA* **72:**3863.

Jazwinski, S. M., Lindberg, A. A., and Kornberg, A., 1975a, The lipopolysaccharide receptor for bacteriophages φX174 and S13, *Virology* **66:**268.

Jazwinski, S. M., Lindberg, A. A., and Kornberg, A., 1975b, The gene H spike protein of bacteriophages φX174 and S13. I. Functions in phage-receptor recognition and in transfection, *Virology* **66:**283.

Jazwinski, S. M., Marco, R., and Kornberg, A., 1975c, The gene H spike protein of bacteriophages φX174 and S13. II. Relation to synthesis of the parental replicative form, *Virology* **66:**294.

Johanson, K. O., and McHenry, C. S., 1984, Adenosine 5′-0-(3-thiotriphosphate) can support the formation of an initiation complex between the DNA polymerase III holoenzyme and primed DNA, *J. Biol. Chem.* **259:**4589.

Johnston, S., and Ray, D. S., 1984, Interference between M13 and oriM13 plasmids is mediated by a replication enhancer sequence near the viral strand origin, *J. Mol. Biol.* **177:**685.

Kapitza, E. L., Stukacheva, E. A., and Shemyakin, 1979, Effect of *E. coli rho* factor and RNAase III on the formation of φX174 RNA *in vitro*, *FEBS Lett.* **98:**123.

Kastelein, R. A., Remaut, E., Ficro, W., and Van Duin, J., 1982, Lysis gene expression of RNA phage MS2 depends on a frame shift during translation of the overlapping coat protein gene, *Nature* **295:**35.

Kccgstra, W., Baas, P. D., and Jansz, H. S., 1979, Bacteriophage φX174 RF DNA replication *in vivo:* A study by electron microscopy, *J. Mol. Biol.* **135:**69.

King, J., 1980, Regulation of structural protein interactions as revealed in phage morphogenesis, in: *Biological Regulation and Development*, Vol. 2 (R. F. Goldberger, ed.), pp. 101–132, Plenum, New York.

Knippers, R., and Sinsheimer, R. L., 1968, Process of infection with bacteriophage φX174. XX. Attachment of the parental DNA of bacteriophage φX174 to a fast-sedimenting cell component, *J. Mol. Biol.* **34:**17.

Knippers, R., Salivar, W. O., Newbold, J. E., and Sinsheimer, R. L., 1969, Process of infection with bacteriophage φX174. XXVI. Transfer of the parental DNA of bacteriophage φX174 into progeny bacteriophage particles, *J. Mol. Biol.* **39:**641.

Kobori, J. A., and Kornberg, A., 1982a, The *Escherichia coli dnaC* gene product. I. Overlapping of the *dnaC* proteins of *Escherichia coli* and *Salmonella typhimurium* by cloning into a high copy number plasmid, *J. Biol. Chem.* **257:**13757.

Kobori, J. A., and Kornberg, A., 1982b, The *Escherichia coli dnaC* gene product. II. Purification, physical properties, and role in replication, *J. Biol. Chem.* **257:**13763.

Kobori, J. A., and Kornberg, A., 1982c, The *Escherichia coli dnaC* gene product. III. Properties of the *dnaB-dnaC* protein complex, *J. Biol. Chem.* **257:**13770.

Kodaira, K., and Taketo, A., 1984a, Isolation and some properties of bacteriophage α3 gene J mutants, *Mol. Gen. Genet.* **195:**541.

Kodaira, K., and Taketo, A., 1984b, Function and structure of microvirid phage α3 genome. II. Isolation and properties of various mutants of α3, *Biochim. Biophys. Acta* **783:**171.

Kodaira, K., Nakano, K., and Taketo, A., 1985, Function and structure of microvirid phage α3 genome. DNA sequence of H gene and properties of missense H mutant, *Biochim. Biophys. Acta* **825:**255.

Kornberg, A., 1980, *DNA Replication*, Freeman, San Francisco.

Kornberg, A., 1982, *Supplement to DNA Replication*, Freeman, San Francisco.

Kornberg, A., 1983, Mechanisms of replication of the *Escherichia coli* chromosome. 14th Sir Hans Krebs Lecture, *Eur. J. Biochem.* **137:**377.

Kornberg, A., 1984, Enzyme studies of replication of the *Escherichia coli* chromosome, *Adv. Exp. Med. Biol.* **179:**3.

Kornberg, A., Scott, J. F., and Bertsch, L. L., 1978, ATP utilization by *rep* protein in the catalytic separation of DNA strands at a replication fork. *J. Biol. Chem.* **253:**3298.

Koths, K., and Dressler, D., 1978, Analysis of the φX DNA replication cycle by electron microscopy, *Proc. Natl. Acad. Sci. USA* **75**:605.

Koths, K., and Dressler, D., 1980, The rolling circle–capsid complex as an intermediate in φX DNA replication and viral assembly, *J. Biol. Chem.* **255**:4328.

Kozak, M., 1986, Bifunctional messenger RNAs in eukaryotes, *Cell* **47**:481.

Langeveld, S. A., Van Mansfeld, A. D. M., Baas, P. D., Jansz, H. S., Van Arkel, G. A., and Weisbeek, P. J., 1978, Nucleotide sequence of the origin of replication in bacteriophage φX174 RF DNA, *Nature* **271**:417.

Langeveld, S. A., Van Mansfeld, A. D. M., De Winter, J. M., and Weisbeek, P. J., 1979, Cleavage of single-stranded DNA by the A and A* proteins of bacteriophage φX174, *Nucleic Acids Res.* **7**:2177.

Langeveld, S. A., Van Mansfeld, A. D., Van der Ende, A., Van de Pol, J. H., Van Arkel, G. A., and Weisbeek, P. J., 1981, The nuclease specificity of the bacteriophage φX174 A* protein, *Nucleic Acids Res.* **9**:545.

Lanka, E., Edelbluth, C., Schlicht, M., and Schuster, H., 1978, *Escherichia coli dnaB* protein: Affinity chromatography on immobilized nucleotides, *J. Biol. Chem.* **253**:5847.

Lau, P. C., and Spencer, J. H., 1985, Nucleotide sequence and genome organization of bacteriophage S13 DNA, *Gene* **40**:273.

LeBowitz, J. H., and McMacken, R., 1986, The *Escherichia coli dnaB* replication protein is a DNA helicase, *J. Biol. Chem.* **261**:4738.

Linney, E. A., and Hayashi, M., 1973, Two proteins of gene A of φX174, *Nature New Biol.* **245**:6.

Linney, E. A., and Hayashi, M., 1974, Intragenic regulation of the synthesis of φX174 gene A proteins, *Nature* **249**:345.

Linney, E. A., Hayashi, M. N., and Hayashi, M., 1972, Gene A of φX174, I. Isolation and identification of its products, *Virology* **50**:381.

Low, R. L., Arai, K., and Kornberg, A., 1981, Conservation of the primosome in successive stages of φX174 DNA replication, *Proc. Natl. Acad. Sci. USA* **78**:1436.

Low, R. L., Shlomai, J., and Kornberg, A., 1982, Protein n, a primosomal DNA replication protein of *Escherichia coli*. Purification and characterization, *J. Biol. Chem.* **257**:6242.

Lubitz, W., and Plapp, R., 1980, Murein degradation of *E. coli* infected with bacteriophage φX174, *Curr. Microbiol.* **8**:63.

Lubitz, W., and Pugsley, 1985, Changes in host cell phospholipid composition by φX174 gene E product, *EEMS Microbiol. Lett.* **30**:171.

Lubitz, W., Halfmann, G., and Plapp, R., 1984a, Lysis of *Escherichia coli* after infection with φX174 depends on the regulation of the cellular autolytic system, *J. Gen. Microbiol.* **130**:1079.

Lubitz, W., Harkness, R. E., and Ishiguro, E. E., 1984b, Requirement for a functional host cell autolytic enzyme system for lysis of *Escherichia coli* by bacteriophage φX174, *J. Bacteriol.* **159**:385.

Luderitz, O., Westphal, O., Staub, A. M., and Nikaido, H., 1971, Isolation and chemical and immunological characterization of bacterial lipopolysaccharides, in: *Microbial Toxins* (G. Weinbaum, S. Kadis, and S. J. Ajl, eds.), pp. 145–233, Academic Press, New York.

Mano, Y., Sakai, H., and Komano, T., 1979, Growth and DNA synthesis of bacteriophage φX174 in a *dnaP* mutant of *Escherichia coli*, *J. Virol.* **30**:650.

Mano, Y., Kawabe, T., Obata, K., Yoshimura, T., and Komano, T., 1982a, Effects of detergents and divalent cations on the functioning of cell envelopes of *Escherichia coli* in the early stages of infection with bacteriophage φX174, *Agric. Biol. Chem.* **46**:631.

Mano, Y., Kawabe, T., Komano, T., and Yazaki, K., 1982b, Involvement of a cell envelope component of *Escherichia coli* in the early stages of infection with bacteriophage φX174, *Agric. Biol. Chem.* **46**:2041.

Maratea, D., Young, K., and Young, R., 1985, Deletion and fusion analysis of the phage φX174 lysis gene E, *Gene* **40**:39.

Marians, K. J., Soeller, W., and Zipurski, S. L., 1982, Maximal limits of the *Escherichia coli* replication factor Y effector site sequences in pBR322 DNA, *J. Biol. Chem.* **257**:5656.

Martin, D. F., and Godson, G. N., 1975, Identification of a bacteriophage φX174 coded protein involved in the shut-off of host DNA replication, *Biochem. Biophys. Res. Commun.* **65**:323.

Matthes, M., and Denhardt, D. T., 1980, The mechanism of replication of φX174 DNA. XVI. Evidence that the φX174 viral strand is synthesized discontinuously, *J. Mol. Biol.* **136**:45.

Matthes, M., and Denhardt, D. T., 1982a, Mechanism of replication of bacteriophage φX174. XX. Sensitivity of nascent DNA to single-strand-specific nucleases, *J. Virol.* **42**: 12.

Matthes, M., Weisbeek, P. J., and Denhardt, D. T., 1982b, Mechanism of replication of bacteriophage φX174. XIX. Initiation of φX174 viral strand DNA synthesis at internal sites on the genome, *J. Virol.* **42**:301.

McFadden, G., and Denhardt, D. T., 1974, Mechanism of replication of φX174 single-stranded DNA. IX. Requirement for the *Escherichia coli dnaG* protein, *J. Virol.* **14**:1070.

McHenry, C. S., 1985, DNA polymerase III holoenzyme of *Escherichia coli:* Components and function of a true replicative complex, *Mol. Cell. Biochem.* **66**:71.

McMacken, R., and Kornberg, A., 1978, A multienzyme system for priming the replication of φX174 viral DNA, *J. Biol. Chem.* **253**:3313.

McMacken, R., Ueda, K., and Kornberg, A., 1977, Migration of *Escherichia coli dnaB* protein on the template DNA strand as a mechanism in initiating DNA replication, *Proc. Natl. Acad. Sci. USA* **74**:4190.

McMahon, J. E., and Tinoco, I. Jr., 1978, Sequences and efficiencies of proposed mRNA terminators, *Nature* **271**:275.

Model, P., Webster, R. E., and Zinder, N. D., 1979, Characterization of Op3, a lysis-defective mutant of bacteriophage f2, *Cell* **18**:235.

Molineux, I. J., and Gefter, M. L., 1975, Properties of the *Escherichia coli* DNA-binding (unwinding) protein interaction with nucleolytic enzymes and DNA, *J. Mol. Biol.* **98**:811.

Molineux, I. J., Friedman, S., and Gefter, M. L., 1974, Purification and properties of *Escherichia coli* deoxyribonucleic acid unwinding protein: Effects on deoxyribonucleic acid synthesis *in vitro*, *J. Biol. Chem.* **249**:6090.

Mott, J. E., Galloway, J. L., and Platt, T., 1985, Maturation of *Escherichia coli* tryptophan operon mRNA; evidence for 3' exonucleolytic processing after *rho*-dependent termination, *EMBO J.* **4**:1887.

Mukai, R., Hamatake, R. K., and Hayashi, M., 1979, Isolation and identification of bacteriophage φX174 prohead, *Proc. Natl. Acad. Sci. USA* **76**:4877.

Müller, U. R., 1983, Enzymatic construction and selection of bacteriophage G4 mutants with modifications of a DNA secondary structure in the J–F intercistronic region, *J. Virol.* **48**:170.

Müller, U. R., and Wells, R. D., 1980a, Intercistronic regions in φX174 DNA. I. Construction of mutants with altered intercistronic regions between genes J and F, *J. Mol. Biol.* **141**:1.

Müller, U. R., and Wells, R. D., 1980b, Intercistronic regions in φX174 DNA. II. Biochemical and biological analysis of mutants with altered intercistronic regions between genes J and F, *J. Mol. Biol.* **141**:25.

Munekiyo, R., Tsuzuki, T., and Sekiguchi, M., 1979, A new locus of *Escherichia coli* that determines sensitivity to bacteriophage φX174, *J. Bacteriol.* **138**:1038.

Murialdo, H., and Becker, A., 1978, Head morphogenesis of complex double-stranded deoxyribonucleic acid bacteriophages, *Microbiol. Rev.* **42**:529.

Nakayama, N., Arai, N., Kaziro, Y., and Arai, K., 1984, Structural and functional studies of the *dnaB* protein using limited proteolysis. Characterization of domains for DNA-dependent ATP hydrolysis and for protein association in the primosome, *J. Biol. Chem.* **259**:88.

Newbold, J. E., and Sinsheimer, R. L., 1970a, The process of infection with bacteriophage φX174. XXXII. Early steps in the infection process: Attachment, eclipse and DNA penetration, *J. Mol. Biol.* **49**:49.

Newbold, J. E., and Sinsheimer, R. L., 1970b, Process of infection with bacteriophage φX174. XXXIV. Kinetics of the attachment and eclipse steps of the infection, *J. Virol.* **5**:427.

Nomura, N., Low, R. L., and Ray, D. S., 1982, Selective cloning of Col/E1 DNA initiation sequences using the cloning vector M13 delta E101, *Gene* **18**:239.

Normark, S., Bërgstrom, S., Edlund, T., Grundström, T., Jaurin, B., Lindberg, F. P., and Olsson, O., 1983, Overlapping genes, *Annu. Rev. Genet.* **17**:499.

Nussinov, R., and Pieczenik, G., 1984, Folding of two large nucleotide chains, *J. Theor. Biol.* **106**:261.

O'Donnell, M. E., and Kornberg, A., 1985a, Dynamics of DNA polymerase III holoenzyme of *Escherichia coli* in replication of a multiprimed template, *J. Biol. Chem.* **260**:12875.

O'Donnell, M. E., and Kornberg, A., 1985b, Complete replication of templates by *Escherichia coli* DNA polymerase III holoenzyme, *J. Biol. Chem.* **260**:12884.

Ogawa, T., Arai, K., and Okazaki, T., 1983, Site selection and structure of DNA-linked RNA primers synthesized by the primosome in phage φX174 DNA replication *in vitro*, *J. Biol. Chem.* **258**:13353.

Ohkawa, T., 1980, On the structure of the lipopolysaccharide core in the cell wall of *Escherichia coli* K12 W2252-llu⁻ and its Ter-mutant cells, *Biochem. Biophys. Res. Commun.* **95**:938.

Otsuka, J., and Kunisawa, T., 1982, Characteristic base sequence patterns of promoter and terminator sites in φX174 and fd phage DNAs, *J. Theor. Biol.* **97**:415.

Pal, S. K., and Poddar, R. K., 1980, Identification of a φX174 coded protein involved in the inhibition of beta-galactosidase synthesis in *Escherichia coli*, *Biochem. Biophys. Res. Commun.* **95**:1341.

Pal, S. K., and Poddar, R. K., 1982, Effect of bacteriophage φX174 infection on the conformation of *Escherichia coli* DNA, *Mol. Gen. Genet.* **187**:162.

Panavotatos, N., and Truong, K., 1985, Cleavage within an RNAase III site can control mRNA stability and protein synthesis *in vitro*, *Nucleic Acids Res.* **13**:2227.

Patrushev, L. I., Kapitza, E. L., Stukacheva, E. A., and Shemyakin, M. F., 1981, Control of bacteriophage φX174 gene expression by the transcription termination factor *rho in vitro*, *Mol. Gen. Genet.* **182**:471.

Platt, T., 1986, Transcription termination and regulation of gene expression, *Annu. Rev. Biochem.* **55**:339.

Pollock, T. J., Tessman, E. S., and Tessman, I., 1978, Identification of lysis protein E of bacteriophage φX174, *J. Virol.* **28**:408.

Puga, A., Borrás, M.-T., Tessman, E. S., and Tessman, I., 1973, Difference between functional and structural integrity of messenger RNA, *Proc. Natl. Acad. Sci. USA* **70**:2171.

Ray, D. S., Cleary, J. M., Hines, J. C., Kim, M. H., Strathearn, M., Kaguni, L., and Roark, M., 1981, DNA initiation determinants of bacteriophage M13 and of chimeric derivatives carrying foreign replication determinants, in: *The Initiation of DNA Replication* (D. S. Ray, ed.), pp. 169–193, Academic Press, New York.

Ray, D. S., Hines, J. C., Kim, M. H., Imber, R., and Nomura, N., 1982, M13 vectors for selective cloning of sequences specifying initiation of DNA synthesis on single-stranded templates, *Gene* **18**:231.

Reeve, J. N., 1981, φX174-directed DNA and protein syntheses in infected minicells, *J. Virol.* **40**:396.

Reha-Krantz, L. J., and Hurwitz, J., 1978a, The *dnaB* gene product of *Escherichia coli*. I. Purification, homogeneity, and physical properties, *J. Biol. Chem.* **253**:4043.

Reha-Krantz, L. J., and Hurwitz, J., 1978b, The *dnaB* gene product of *Escherichia coli*. II. Single-stranded DNA–dependent ribonucleoside triphosphatase activity, *J. Biol. Chem.* **253**:4051.

Reinberg, D., Zipursky, S. L., and Hurwitz, J., 1981, Separate requirements for leading and lagging strand DNA synthesis during φX A protein-dependent RF→RF DNA replication *in vitro*, *J. Biol. Chem.* **256**:13143.

Reinberg, D., Zipursky, S. L., Weisbeek, P., Brown, D., and Hurwitz, J., 1983, Studies on the φX174 gene A protein-mediated termination of leading strand DNA synthesis, *J. Biol. Chem.* **258**:529.

Romantschuk, M. L., and Müller, U. R., 1983, Mutations in the J–F intercistronic region of bacteriophages φX174 and G4 affect the regulation of gene expression, *J. Virol.* **48**:180.

Roth, M. J., Brown, D. R., and Hurwitz, J., 1984, Analysis of bacteriophage φX174 gene A protein–mediated termination and reinitiation of φX DNA synthesis. II. Structural characterization of the covalent φX A protein–DNA complex, *J. Biol. Chem.* **259**:10556.

Rothfield, L., and Pearlman-Kothencz, M., 1969, Synthesis and assembly of bacterial membrane components: A lipopolysaccharide-phospholipid-protein complex excreted by living bacteria, *J. Mol. Biol.* **44**:477.

Rowatt, E., 1984, The role of bivalent ions in the inactivation of bacteriophage φX174 by lipopolysaccharide from *Escherichia coli* C, *Biochem. J.* **223**:23.

Rowatt, E., and Williams, R. J., 1985, The effect of multivalent ions on the inactivation of bacteriophage φX174 by lipopolysaccharide from *Escherichia coli* C, *Biochem. J.* **231**:765.

Rowen, L., and Kornberg, A., 1978, Primase, the *dnaG* protein of *Escherichia coli*: An enzyme which starts DNA chain, *J. Biol. Chem.* **253**:758.

Russell, P. W., and Müller, U. R., 1984, Construction of bacteriophage φX174 mutants with maximum genome sizes, *J. Virol.* **52**:822.

Sanger, F., Air, G. M., Barrell, B. G., Brown, N. L., Coulson, A. R., Fiddes, J. C., Hutchison, C. A. III, Slocombe, P. M., and Smith, M., 1977, Nucleotide sequence of bacteriophage φX174 DNA, *Nature* **265**:687.

Sanger, F., Coulson, A. R., Friedman, T., Air, G. M., Barrell, B. C., Brown, N. L., Fiddes, J. C., Hutchison, C. A. III, Slocombe, P. M., and Smith, M., 1978, The nucleotide sequence of bacteriophage φX174, *J. Mol. Biol.* **125**:225.

Sanhueza, S., and Eisenberg, S., 1984, Cleavage of single-stranded DNA by the φX174 A* protein: The A*-single-stranded DNA covalent linkage, *Proc. Natl. Acad. Sci. USA* **81**:4285.

Sanhueza, S., and Eisenberg, S., 1985, Bacteriophage φX174 A protein cleaves single-stranded DNA and binds to it covalently through a tyrosyl-dAMP phosphodiester bond, *J. Virol.* **53**:695.

Schindler, D., and Echols, H., 1981, Retroregulation of the int gene of bacteriophage λ. Control of translation completion, *Proc. Natl. Acad. Sci. USA* **78**:4475.

Schmeissner, V., McKenney, K., Rosenberg, M., and Court, D., 1984, Removal of terminator structure by RNA processing regulates in gene expression, *J. Mol. Biol.* **176**:39.

Schmidt, G., 1973, Genetical studies on the lipopolysaccharide structure of *Escherichia coli* K12, *J. Gen. Microbiol.* **77**:151.

Scott, J. F., and Kornberg, A., 1978, Purification of the rep protein of *Escherichia coli*: An ATPase which separates duplex DNA strands in advance of replication, *J. Biol. Chem.* **253**:3292.

Scott, J. F., Eisenberg, S., Bertsch, L. L., and Kornberg, A., 1977, Mechanism of duplex DNA replication revealed by enzymatic studies of phage φX174: Catalytic strand separation in advance of replication, *Proc. Natl. Acad. Sci. USA* **74**:193.

Shank, P. R., Hutchison, C. A. III, and Edgell, M. H., 1977, Isolation and characterization of the four major proteins in the virion of bacteriophage φX174, *Biochemistry* **16**:4545.

Shaw, W. V., 1971, Comparative enzymology of chloramphenicol resistance, *Ann. N.Y. Acad. Sci.* **182**:23.

Shlomai, J., and Kornberg, A., 1978, Deoxyuridine triphosphatase of *Escherichia coli*: Purification, properties, and use as a reagent to reduce uracil incorporation into DNA, *J. Biol. Chem.* **253**:3305.

Shlomai, J., and Kornberg, A., 1980a, An *Escherichia coli* replication protein that recognizes a unique sequence within a hairpin region in φX174 DNA, *Proc. Natl. Acad. Sci. USA* **77**:799.

Shlomai, J., and Kornberg, A., 1980b, A prepriming DNA replication enzyme of *Escherichia* coli. I. Purification of protein n': A sequence specific, DNA-dependent ATPase, J. Biol. Chem. **255**:6789.

Shlomai, J., and Kornberg, A., 1980c, A prepriming DNA replication enzyme of Escherichia coli. II. Actions of protein n': A sequence specific, DNA-dependent ATPase, J. Biol. Chem. **255**:6794.

Shlomai, J., Polder, L., Arai, K., and Kornberg, A., 1981, Replication of φX174 DNA with purified enzymes. I. Conversion of viral DNA to a supercoiled, biologically active duplex, J. Biol. Chem. **256**:5233.

Siden, E. J., and Hayashi, M., 1974, Role of the gene B product in bacteriophage φX174 development, J. Mol. Biol. **89**:1.

Siegel, J. E., and Hayashi, M., 1969, φX174 bacteriophage structural mutants which affect DNA synthesis, J. Virol. **4**:400.

Sigal, N., Delius, H., Kornberg, T., Gefter, M. L., and Alberts, B., 1972, A DNA-unwinding protein isolated from Escherichia coli: Its interaction with DNA and with DNA polymerases, Proc. Natl. Acad. Sci. USA **69**:3537.

Singer, B. S., Gold, L., Shinedling, S. T., Humnter, D., Pribnow, D., and Nelson, M. A., 1981, Analysis in vitro of translational mutants of the rIIB cistron of bacteriophage T4, J. Mol. Biol. **149**:405.

Sinsheimer, R. L., 1959a, Purification and properties of bacteriophage φX174, J. Mol. Biol. **1**:37.

Sinsheimer, R. L., 1959b, A single-stranded deoxyribonucleic acid from bacteriophage φX174, J. Mol. Biol. **1**:43.

Sinsheimer, R. L., 1968, Bacteriophage φX174 and related viruses, Prog. Nucleic Acid Res. Mol. Biol. **8**:115.

Smith, L. H., and Sinsheimer, R. L., 1976a, The in vitro transcription units of bacteriophage φX174. I. Characterization of synthetic parameters and measurement of transcript molecular weight, J. Mol. Biol. **103**:681.

Smith, L. H., and Sinsheimer, R. L., 1976b, The in vitro transcription units of bacteriophage φX174. II. In vitro initiation sites of φX174 transcription, J. Mol. Biol. **103**:699.

Smith, L. H., and Sinsheimer, R. L., 1976c, The in vitro transcription units of φX174. III. Initiation with specific 5' end oligonucleotides of in vitro φX174 RNA, J. Mol. Biol. **103**:711.

Soeller, W., Abarzua, P., and Marians, K. J., 1984, Mutational analysis of primosome assembly sites. II. Role of secondary structure in the formation of active sites, J. Biol. Chem. **259**:14293.

Spindler, K. R., and Hayashi, M., 1979, DNA synthesis in Escherichia coli cells infected with gene H mutants of bacteriophage φX174, J. Virol. **29**:973.

Strathearn, M. D., Low, R. L., and Ray, D. S., 1984, Selective cloning of a DNA single-strand initiation determinant from φX174 replicative-form DNA, J. Virol. **49**:178.

Struck, D. K., Maratea, D., and Young, R. 1985, Purification of hydrid beta-galactosidase proteins encoded by φX174 E phi lacZ and Escherichia coli prlA phi lacZ: A general method for the isolation of lacZ fusion polypeptides produced in low amounts, J. Mol. Appl. Genet. **3**:18.

Sugino, A., Peebles, C. L., Kreuger, K. N., and Kozzarelli, N. R., 1977, Mechanism of action of nalidixic acid: Purification of Escherichia coli nal A gene product and its relationship to DNA gyrase and a novel nicking-closing enzyme, Proc. Natl. Acad. Sci. USA **74**:4767.

Sumida-Yasumoto, C., and Hurwitz, J., 1977, Synthesis of φX174 viral DNA in vitro depends on φX replicative form DNA, Proc. Natl. Acad. Sci. USA **74**:4195.

Sumida-Yasumoto, C., Yudelevich, A., and Hurwitz, J., 1976, DNA synthesis in vitro dependent upon φX174 replicative form I DNA, Proc. Natl. Acad. Sci. USA **73**:1887.

Sumida-Yasumoto, C., Ikeda, J.-E., Benz, E., Marians, K. J., Vicuna, R., Sugrue, S., Zipursky, S. L., and Hurwitz, J., 1978, Replication of φX174 DNA: In vitro synthesis of φX174 RFI DNA and circular single-stranded DNA, Cold Spring Harbor Symp. Quant. Biol. **43**:311.

Tessman, E. S., 1965, Complementation groups in phage S13, Virology **25**:303.

Tessman, E. S., and Peterson, P. K., 1976, Bacterial *rep⁻* mutations that block development of small DNA bacteriophages late in infection, *J. Virol.* **20:**400.

Tessman, E. S., and Tessman, I., 1978, The genes of the isometric phages and their functions, in: *The Single-Stranded DNA Phages,* (D. T. Denhardt, D. Dressler, and D. S. Ray, eds.), pp. 9–29, Cold Spring Harbor Laboratory, Cold Spring Harbor, NY.

Tessman, E. S., and Peterson, P. K., 1982, Suppression of the ssb-1 and ssb-113 mutations of *Escherichia coli* by a wild-type *rep* gene, NaCl, and glucose, *J. Bacteriol.* **152:**572.

Tessman, E. S., Borras, M.-T., and Sun, I. L., 1971, Superinfection in bacteriophage S13 and determination of the number of bacteriophage particles which can function in an infected cell, *J. Virol.* **8:**111.

Tessman, E. S., Tessman, I., and Pollock, T. J., 1980, Gene K of bacteriophage φX174 codes for a nonessential protein, *J. Virol.* **33:**557.

Thomas, G. J. Jr., 1986, Applications of Raman spectroscopy in structural studies of viruses, nucleoproteins and their constituents, in: *Spectroscopy of Biological Systems* (R. J. H. Clark and R. E. Heston, eds.), pp. 233–309, Wiley, New York.

Tomasz, A., 1979, The mechanism of the irreversible antimicrobial effects of penicillins. How the beta-lactam antibiotics kill and lyse bacteria, *Annu. Rev. Microbiol.* **33:**113.

Tonegawa, S., and Hayashi, M., 1970, Intermediates in the assembly of φX174, *J. Mol. Biol.* **48:**219.

Tse, Y. C., Kirkegaard, K., and Wang, J. C., 1980, Covalent bonds between protein and DNA: Formation of phosphotyrosine linkage between certain DNA topoisomerases and DNA, *J. Biol. Chem.* **255:**5560.

Ueda, K., McMacken, R., and Kornberg, A., 1978, dnaB protein of *Escherichia coli:* Purification and role in the replication of φX174 DNA, *J. Biol. Chem.* **253:**261.

Uratani, Y., Asakura, S., and Imahori, K., 1972, A circular dichroism study of *Salmonella* flagellin: Evidence of conformational change on polymerization, *J. Mol. Biol.* **67:**85.

Van der Avoort, H. G., Van Arkel, G. A., and Weisbeek, P. J., 1982, Cloned bacteriophage φX174 DNA sequence interferes with synthesis of the complementary strand of infecting bacteriophage φX174, *J. Virol.* **42:**1.

Van der Avoort, H. G., Teertstra, R., Versteeg, R., and Weisbeek, P. J., 1983, Genes and regulatory sequences of bacteriophage φX174, *Biochim. Biophys. Acta* **741:**94.

Van der Avoort, H. G., Van der Ende, A., Van Arkel, G. A., and Weisbeek, P. J., 1984, Regions of incompatibility in single-stranded DNA bacteriophages φX174 and G4, *J. Virol.* **50:**533.

Van der Ende, A., Langeveld, S. A., Teertstra, R., Van Arkel, G. A., and Weisbeek, P. J., 1981, Enzymatic properties of the bacteriophage φX174 A protein on superhelical φX174 DNA: A model for the termination of the rolling circle DNA replication, *Nucleic Acids Res.* **9:**2037.

Van der Ende, A., Langeveld, S. A., Van Arkel, G. A., and Weisbeek, P. J., 1982a, The interaction of the A and A* proteins of bacteriophage φX174 with single-stranded φX DNA *in vitro, Eur. J. Biochem.* **124:**245.

Van der Ende, A., Teertstra, R., and Weisbeek, P. J., 1982b, Initiation and termination of the bacteriophage φX174 rolling circle DNA replication *in vivo:* Packaging of plasmid single-stranded DNA into bacteriophage φX174 coats, *Nucleic Acids Res.* **10:**6849.

Van der Ende, A., Teertstra, R., Van der Avoort, H. G., and Weisbeek, P. J., 1983a, Initiation signals for complementary strand DNA synthesis on single-stranded plasmid DNA, *Nucleic Acids Res.* **11:**4957.

Van der Ende, A., Teertstra, R., and Weisbeek, P. J., 1983b, n' Protein activator sites of plasmid pBR322 are not essential for its DNA replication, *J. Mol. Biol.* **167:**751.

Van der Ende, A., Baker, T. A., Ogawa, T., and Kornberg, A., 1985, Initiation of enzymatic replication at the origin of the *Escherichia coli* chromosome: Primase as the sole priming enzyme, *Proc. Natl. Acad. Sci. USA* **82:**3954.

Van Mansfeld, A. D., Langeveld, S. A., Weisbeek, P. J., Baas, P. D., Van Arkel, G. A., and Jansz, H. S., 1978, Cleavage site of φX174 gene A protein in φX and G4 RFI DNA, *Cold Spring Harbor Symp. Quant. Biol.* **43:**331.

Van Mansfeld, A. D., Langeveld, S. A., Baas, P. D., Jansz, H., S van der Marel, G. A., Veeneman,

G. H., and Van Boom, J. H., 1980, Recognition sequence of bacteriophage ϕX174 gene A protein—an initiator of DNA replication, *Nature* **288**:561.

Van Mansfeld, A. D., Van Teeffelen, H. A., Zandberg, J., Baas, P. D., Jansz, H. S., Veeneman, G. H., and Van Boom, J. H., 1982, A protein of bacteriophage ϕX174 carries an oligonucleotide which it can transfer to the 3′–OH of a DNA chain, *FEBS Lett.* **150**:103.

Van Mansfeld, A. D., Baas, P. D., and Jansz, H. S., 1984a, Gene A protein of bacteriophage ϕX174 is a highly specific single-strand nuclease and binds via a tyrosyl residue to DNA after cleavage, *Adv. Exp. Med. Biol.* **179**:221.

Van Mansfeld, A. D., Van Teeffelen, H. A., Baas, P. D., Veeneman, G. H., Van Boom, J. H., and Jansz, H. S., 1984b, The bond in the bacteriophage ϕX174 gene A protein–DNA complex is a tyrosyl-5′-phosphate ester, *FEBS Lett.* **173**:351.

Van Mansfeld, A. D., Van Teeffelen, H. A., Fluit, A. C., Baas, P. D., and Jansz, H. S., 1986a, Effect of SSB protein on cleavage of single-stranded DNA by ϕX gene A protein and A* protein, *Nucleic Acids Res.* **14**:1845.

Van Mansfeld, A. D., Van Teeffelen, H. A., Baas, P. D., and Jansz, H. S., 1986b, Two juxtaposed tyrosyl-OH groups participate in ϕX174 gene A protein catalysed cleavage and ligation of DNA, *Nucleic Acids Res.* **14**:4229.

Von Hippel, P., Bear, D. G., Morgan, W. D., and AcSwiggen, J. A., 1984, Protein–nucleic acid interaction in transcription: A molecular analysis, *Annu. Rev. Biochem.* **53**:389.

Wang, R. Y., Shenoy, S., and Ehrlich, M., 1984, DNA methylation inhibits the transfecting activity of replicative-form ϕX174 DNA, *J. Virol.* **49**:674.

Watabe, K., Kubota, M., Morita, J., and Komano, T., 1981, *In vitro* conversion of S13 viral DNA in phage particles to the double-stranded DNA, *Biochim. Biophys. Acta* **656**:189.

Weiner, J. H., Bertsch, L. L., and Kornberg, A., 1975, The deoxyribonucleic acid unwinding protein of *Escherichia coli:* Properties and functions in replication, *J. Biol. Chem.* **250**:1972.

Weisbeek, P. J., and Sinsheimer, R. L., 1974, A DNA-protein complex involved in bacteriophage ϕX174 particle formation, *Proc. Natl. Acad. Sci. USA* **71**:3054.

Weisbeek, P. J., Van de Pol, J. H., and Van Arkel, G. A., 1973, Mapping of host range mutants of bacteriophage ϕX174, *Virology* **52**:408.

Weisbeek, P. J., Vereijken, J. M., Baas, P. D., Janz, H. S., and Van Arkel, G. A., 1976, The genetic map of bacteriophage ϕX174 constructed with restriction fragments, *Virology* **72**:61.

Weisbeek, P. J., Borrias, W. E., Langeveld, S. A., Baas, P., and Van Arkel, G. A., 1977, Bacteriophage ϕX174: Gene A overlaps gene B, *Proc. Natl. Acad. Sci. USA* **74**:2504.

Wickner, S., and Hurwitz, J., 1975, Association of phage ϕX174 DNA dependent ATPase activity with an *Escherichia coli* protein replication factor Y required for *in vitro* synthesis of phage ϕX174 DNA, *Proc. Natl. Acad. Sci. USA* **72**:3342.

Williams, R. C., and Fisher, H. W., 1980, Electron microscopic determination of the preferential binding sites of *Escherichia coli* RNA polymerase to ϕX174 replicative form DNA, *J. Mol. Biol.* **140**:435.

Wolfson, R., and Eisenberg, S., 1982, *Escherichia coli* host factor required specifically for the ϕX174 stage III reaction: *In vitro* identification and partial purification, *Proc. Natl. Acad. Sci. USA* **79**:5768.

Wong, H. C., and Chang, S., 1986, Identification of a positive retroregulator that stabilizes mRNAs in bacteria, *Proc. Natl. Acad. Sci. USA* **83**:3233.

Yanofsky, C., 1981, Attenuation in the control of expression of bacterial operons, *Nature* **289**:751.

Yarranton, G. T., and Gefter, M. L., 1979, Enzyme-catalized DNA unwinding: Studies on *Escherichia coli rep* protein, *Proc. Natl. Acad. Sci. USA* **76**:1658.

Yarus, M. T., and Sinsheimer, R. L., 1971, The process of infection with bacteriophage ϕX174. XIII. Evidence for an essential bacterial site, *J. Virol.* **1**:135.

Yazaki, K., 1981, Electron microscopic studies of bacteriophage ϕX174 intact and "eclipsing" particles, and the genome by the staining and shadowing method, *J. Virol. Methods* **2**:159.

Young, K. D., and Young, R., 1982, Lytic action of cloned φX174 gene E, *J. Virol.* **44**:993.

Zipser, D., 1963, A study of the urea-produced subunits of β galactosidase, *J. Mol. Biol.* **7**:113.

Zipursky, S. L., and Marians, K. J., 1980, Identification of two *Escherichia coli* factor Y effector sites near the origins of replication of the plasmids ColE1 and pBR322, *Proc. Natl. Acad. Sci. USA* **77**:6521.

Zipursky, S. L., and Marians, K. J., 1981, *Escherichia coli* factor Y sites of plasmid pBR322 can function as origins of DNA replication, *Proc. Natl. Acad. Sci. USA* **78**:6111.

Zipursky, S. L., Reinberg, D., and Hurwitz, J., 1980, *In vitro* DNA replication of recombinant plasmid DNAs containing the origin or progeny replicative form DNA synthesis of phage φX174, *Proc. Natl. Acad. Sci. USA* **77**:5812.

Zolotukhin, A. S., Drygin, I. F., and Bogdanov, A. A., 1984, Bacteriophage φX174 A protein binds *in vitro* to the phage φX174 DNA by a phosphodiester bond via a tyrosine residue, *Biochem. Int.* **9**:799.

CHAPTER 2

The P2-like Phages and Their Parasite, P4

L. Elizabeth Bertani and Erich W. Six

I. INTRODUCTION

A. Origin and Distribution of the P2-like Phages

Three readily distinguishable phages—P1, P2, and P3—were isolated by
G. Bertani (1951) from a single source, the Lisbonne and Carrère strain of
Escherichia coli. All three cross-react serologically (Bertani and Bertani,
1971). P1, which differs from P2 in many respects, later found use as a
generalized transducing phage for *E. coli* (Lennox, 1955) and is reviewed
in a separate chapter in this volume. Another series of temperate phages,
isolated from strains of *E. coli* found in human feces, was characterized
by Jacob and Wollman (1961). The members were placed in a common
group on the basis of host range, noninducibility by ultraviolet light, and
inability to recombine with and serological unrelatedness to phage λ.
They included phages 186 and 299, although in the case of 186, induction
was not actually tested. Further historical details can be found in Bertani
(1958).

In addition to the above-mentioned phages, a number of others, including 18, PK, W-φ, and the φ-D series, were found to be serologically
related to P2 (Bertani and Bertani, 1971). Recent surveys of temperate
phages found in natural environments have turned up many new isolates
(Dhillon and Dhillon, 1972, 1973, 1981; Dhillon *et al.*, 1976; Poon and

L. ELIZABETH BERTANI • Biology Division, California Institute of Technology, Pasadena, California 91125. ERICH W. SIX • Department of Microbiology, University of
Iowa, Iowa City, Iowa 52242

Dhillon, 1986) and suggest that phages serologically related to P2 are quite numerous and widespread. Following a study of isolates active on enterobacteria, Dhillon *et al.* (1980) concluded that the P2-like phages are most frequently found as prophages, whereas λ-like phages are more frequently found as cell-free virions.

B. Phage P4

Six (1963) detected the defective phage P4 in a strain of *E. coli*, K-235, that also harbored the colicinogenic factor K and the P2-related phage PK. Although serologically cross-reacting with P2 (Bertani and Bertani, 1971), P4 might be more accurately described as an unrelated replicon that parasitizes the P2 family. P4 is lacking the genes that code for phage structural proteins and has acquired the ability to obtain these proteins from P2 or any of its relatives by activating their morphopoietic genes. As a consequence, P4 has the same virion proteins as P2 and is thus included in any screen for serological relatedness.

C. Special Features

In addition to serological cross-reactivity between members, the P2-like phages can be defined by a set of shared characteristics that include morphology—especially the contractile tail sheath—and unidirectional replication requiring a *cis*-acting phage protein and the bacterial *rep* function. Although one or another of these may be found in "unrelated" phages, the combination is unique to the P2 family. Phage P4, in comparison, is noticeably smaller and replicates bidirectionally and independently of *rep*.

More recently, the host–parasite relationship with the defective phage P4 has proved to be useful for taxonomic purposes because it requires that the P2-like phages have extensive similarity in the genes that code for and control the virion proteins, as well as nearly identical single-stranded DNA termini. It probably also includes another interesting feature of the P2 system: a mechanism for packaging phage DNA from covalently closed monomers. To date, this relationship has been found in all P2-like phages examined and not in any unrelated phages.

Still another property generally associated with the P2 group—non-inducibility by ultraviolet light—extends to all members tested with the exception of phage 186 (Woods and Egan, 1974).

Some minor differences may be host-related. Although *Shigella dysenteriae* was originally used to detect P2, *E. coli* C has been adopted as the laboratory host. In addition, the phage can multiply in most other strains of *E. coli* (K12, B) as well as in strains of *Serratia marcescens* and *Salmonella typhimurium* (Bertani and Bertani, 1971), *Klebsiella pneu-*

moniae (Streicher *et al.*, 1972; Ow and Ausubel, 1980), and *Yersinia* sp. (Camara and Kahn, personal communication). Phage 186 is unable to adsorb to *E. coli* C (Bradley *et al.*, 1975), so *E. coli* K12 is usually used as its host. Phage P3, on the other hand, does not plate on K12 (Six, unpublished). Phage P4 has the additional complication that it can only multiply in lysogens carrying a suitable helper phage (Six and Klug, 1973).

Studies on these phages have contributed substantially to our understanding of microbial genetics and basic regulatory mechanisms and to the current art of recombinant DNA technology. The exclusion of phage λ by prophage P2 forms the basis for a widely used cloning system (Section IV.D). The addition of a fragment of P2 DNA to the plasmid pBR322 results in a vector that can integrate very efficiently and stably into the host chromosome (Section III.C). P4, because of its small size, flexibility with respect to amount of packageable DNA, and ability to integrate or replicate as a plasmid, shows promise as a novel cloning vehicle (Section V.H).

D. Scope of This Review

The information concerning the phages P2, 186, and P4 that has accumulated during the past 15 years will be brought up to date and compared wherever possible. Unfortunately, little additional work has been done on the other members of the group, and only a few new facts concerning phages P3 and 299 can be provided. Additional background information and references to earlier work can be found in Bertani and Bertani (1971). With the exception of certain key references, those papers already cited there will not be referred to again here.

Detailed genetic and restriction maps of P2 (Bertani and Ljungquist, 1984) and P4 (Calendar *et al.*, 1984) are available elsewhere. Procedures for the preparation and purification of phage P2 can be found in Bertani and Bertani (1970) and a review of P2 integration in Calendar *et al.* (1977a). The interactions between P2 and P4 have been described in Calendar *et al.* (1977b) and more recently in Calendar *et al.* (1985). The ability of P4 to turn on the genes of P2 has been compared with similar activities in adenovirus and retrovirus (Calendar, 1986).

II. THE VIRIONS

A. Morphology

P2 and 186 are morphologically indistinguishable, each characterized by an icosahedral head of about 60 nm diameter and a straight tail of length 135 nm (Fig. 1). The head of P4 is only 45 nm in diameter, but the tail is of the same dimensions as that of P2 (Fig. 1). All P2-like phages

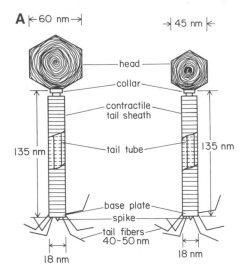

A

|← 60 nm →| →| 45 nm |←

head

collar

contractile
tail sheath

135 nm   tail tube   135 nm

base plate

spike

tail fibers
40-50 nm

18 nm   18 nm

P2 : DNA = 33 kb   P4 : DNA = 11.5 kb

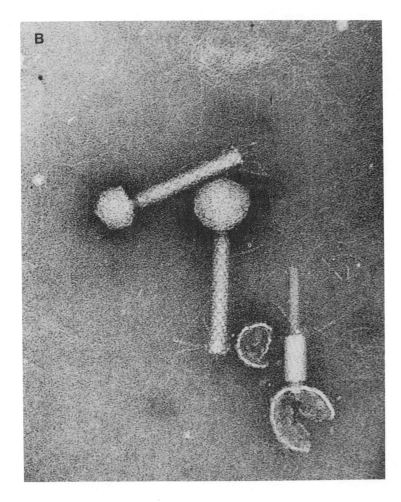

B

examined so far, as well as P4, have a contractile tail sheath. Because of the similarity in tail structure, these phages have been classified together with P1 and the T-even phages under the general heading of "myo-viridae" (Fraenkel-Conrat, 1985). It is doubtful, however, if there can be any functional interchangeability between the groups. Although the T-even tails are about the same size as those of the P2-like phages, they are more complex and require twice as many gene products to be synthesized (King and Laemmli, 1973). Interchangeability within the P2 group is more likely, especially as the extent of DNA sequence agreement in the late genes becomes more and more apparent (see Appendix B). Unfortunately, no heterologous *in vitro* reconstitution experiments involving the ex-change of whole heads and tails or gene complementation studies have been described, but viable P2-186 hybrids with tail genes derived from both phages have been reported (Hocking and Egan, 1982d).

B. Virion Proteins

The virion proteins of phages P2 and P4 have been resolved by SDS-PAGE (Lengyel *et al.*, 1973, 1974; Goldstein *et al.*, 1974) (Table I). Of the six proteins found in phage P2 heads, the four largest are all cleaved derivatives of the N gene product, and one of these, N^*, of molecular mass 36 kD, constitutes the major capsid component. As can be seen in Table I, P4 heads contain all of the proteins found in P2, but they have relatively less of the major N^* protein and relatively more of the minor components. The significance of a 20-kD protein found to be associated with P4 heads will be discussed in Section V.B. Triangulation numbers of 9 and 4 have been estimated for P2 and P4, respectively (Goldstein *et al.*, 1974; Geisselsoder *et al.*, 1982).

As anticipated, the tail proteins of P2 and P4, also listed in Table I, are not distinguishable. Details on the derivation of the P2 and P4 pro-teins will be discussed later (Sections IV.B and V.B). There is evidence that phage P2 attaches to the core region of the lipopolysaccharide of *E. coli* (Lindberg, 1973). Adsorption is greatly improved by the addition of calcium ion (Bertani and Bertani, 1970).

Although the virion proteins of phage 186 have not been studied extensively, its serological cross-reactivity with P2 suggests that the tail proteins must be similar, a conclusion supported by the sequences of the respective D genes (Kalionis *et al.*, 1986b; Appendix B). There are also important differences, however, as phage 186, unlike P2, does not adsorb

---

FIGURE 1. The morphology of P2 and P4 particles. (A) Schematic drawing of particles of P2 and P4, adapted from Goldstein *et al.* (1974). (B) Particles of P2 (larger heads) and P4 (smaller heads). A tail with contracted sheath is also visible. Electronmicrograph courtesy of R. Calendar.

TABLE I. Protein Composition of P2 and P4 Heads
and Tails[a]

| | | | Number of copies | |
Protein	Gene	Mol. wt. (kD)	P2	P4
h1	N	42	4 ± 2	23 ± 4
h2	N	41	10 ± 3	46 ± 7
h5 (N*)	N	36	484 ± 27	210 ± 19
h6	?	32	21 ± 5	21 ± 3
h7	?	18	95 ± 13	33 ± 6
#3	sid	27	0	8 ± 3
#4	psu	20	0	26 ± 16
t1	T	94	5 ± 2	6 ± 2
t2	H	71	18 ± 3	18 ± 3
t3	?	51	6	4 ± 1
t4	FI	46	181 ± 18	180
t5	?	31	22 ± 5	22 ± 3
t6	FII	20	273 ± 22	265 ± 52

[a]Data are taken from Lengyel et al. (1973, 1974) and Barrett et al.
(1976). P2 head proteins h3 and h4 have not been included, because they are difficult to resolve from the major head protein.

to *E. coli* C and does not require calcium ion for adsorption (Bradley *et al.*,
1975).

C. Structure of the DNA

The DNA found in particles of the P2-like phages or P4 is double-
stranded, linear, and nonpermuted and terminates in complementary single strands of 19 base pairs (Bertani and Bertani, 1971; Inman *et al.*, 1971;
Younghusband and Inman, 1974). The GC content of P2 DNA is 52%
(Skalka and Hanson, 1972), and no rare bases have been reported. P2 DNA
has a molecular mass of about 22×10^6 daltons or 33 kb (Bertani and
Bertani, 1971). The DNA molecule of phage 186 is slightly smaller, about
30 kb (Younghusband and Inman, 1974), whereas that of P4 is only 11.5
kb (Inman *et al.*, 1971).

Filter hybridization studies (Skalka and Hanson, 1972) and electron
microscope heteroduplex mapping (Younghusband and Inman, 1974) indicate about 50% sequence identity between P2 and 186. Although cross-
hybridization between P2 and P4 has been reported to be as little as 1%
(Lindqvist, 1974), there is some sequence identity between the P2 *ogr* and
P4 δ genes (Kalionis *et al.*, 1986b; Appendix B).

The single-stranded termini or cohesive ends of the DNA of all three
phages (Padmanabhan and Wu, 1972; Murray and Murray, 1973; Wang *et
al.*, 1973; Padmanabhan *et al.*, 1974; Murray *et al.*, 1977; Lindqvist,
1981a), as well as those of phage 299 (Murray and Murray, 1973; Murray
et al., 1977), have been sequenced (Appendix B). They are all of the same

length. P4 termini are indistinguishable from those of P2, whereas the termini of phage 299 differ in one base pair, and those of phage 186 differ in two (Appendix B). The first seven base pairs of double-stranded DNA at the left end are also identical for all four phages, except for one base pair in the case of P4 (Appendix B). The right end appears to be more divergent. The presence of cohesive ends permits both circularization of single molecules and the formation of hybrid dimers or multimers. Padmanabhan (1977) has synthesized chemically an octanucleotide complementary to a portion of one of the cohesive ends of P2 DNA and studied its interactions with the molecule.

D. Arrangement of DNA in the Particles

The DNA of P2 is arranged in the head in an orderly manner. In electron microscope pictures of flattened particles, the DNA appears as a series of concentric circles, as if wound into a ball or around a spool (Richards *et al.*, 1973). When the particles are ruptured by formaldehyde (Chattoraj and Inman, 1974a), a unique end of the DNA molecule, corresponding to the left cohesive end, remains attached to the tail. This result was obtained for phages 186 and P4 as well, and in all cases it is the same cohesive end that is involved (Chattoraj and Inman, 1974; Lindqvist, 1981a).

The fixation of one end of the DNA molecule to the tail may be necessary to maintain the linear configuration of the DNA in mature particles. P2 or P4 DNA, packaged into heads in the absence of tails (filled heads), appears "knotted" when extracted (Liu *et al.*, 1981a,b) owing to an interaction between the ends of the molecule. If P4 DNA is shortened by a deletion, the proportion of knotted molecules found even in whole, intact particles may increase to 80% (Wolfson *et al.*, 1985). It is not clear whether the knotting happens within the capsid itself or during the extraction of the DNA. The knots can be resolved either by heating the DNA to denature the hybridized termini or by treatment with a type II DNA topoisomerase (Liu *et al.*, 1981b). The resolution of knots in P4 DNA has been developed as a sensitive assay for this type of topoisomerase (Liu *et al.*, 1981b).

III. THE GENOMES

A. Deletions and Insertions

1. Phage P2

As in the case of other icosahedral phages, the heads of P2 particles are tightly packed with DNA (Earnshaw and Harrison, 1977). As a result, they may be damaged when exposed to increasing temperature in a medium such as standard saline citrate (Bertani, 1975). This has made possible the easy isolation of deletion mutants that have a higher probability of survival (Bertani and Chattoraj, 1980). A number of such mutants, isolated from P2 (Table II), have been very useful in correlating the physical and genetic maps.

One spontaneous duplication, *vir37* (Bertani and Bertani, 1974; Chattoraj and Inman, 1974), recognized by its virulent phenotype, has been obtained, and methods to select for phages containing more DNA than normal are available (Nicoletti and Bertani, 1983). An *IS2* insertion into the early region, producing the derivative *sig5* (Lindahl *et al.*, 1971; Saha and Haggård-Ljungquist, personal communication), may have been acquired as a result of using *E. coli* K12 as a host.

The upper and lower limits on the size of P2 DNA compatible with viability have not been established. Phages carrying both deletions *del1* and *del2* have lost 14% (4.5 kb) of their DNA but are still viable (Bertani and Chattoraj, 1980), as is the derivative P2 *sig5*, which carries a 3.7% (1.2 kb) insertion (Chattoraj *et al.*, 1975). In a more extreme case, P4 dimers, totaling only 23 kb of DNA, can be packaged into P2-size heads (Pruss *et al.*, 1974b; Goldstein *et al.*, 1974), whereas at the other end of

TABLE II. Deletions, Insertions, and Hybrids

A. Phage P2

Mutant[a]	Size (and position) of[b]		Phenotype[d]	Reference[e]
	Deletion	Insertion[c]		
del1	7.6% (92.1–99.7%)	—	Old⁻	(1)
del2	6.1% (45.5–51.6%)	—	Fun⁻	(2)
del3	3.6% (72.2–75.8%)	1.1%	Att⁻, Int⁻, C⁻ (Vir)	(3,4)
del4	7.0% (92.3–99.3%)	—	Old⁻	(2)
del5	3.3% (48.6–51.9%)	—	Fun⁻	(5)
del6	2.1% (72.2–74.3%)	—	Att⁻, Int⁻	(4)
del19	5.6% (72.9–78.5%)	—	Att⁻, Int⁻, C⁻	(9)
vir3	17 bp	—		(6)
vir6	1 bp	—		(6)
vir22	5.0% (72.2–77.2%)	0.5%		(1,4)
vir24	57 bp	—	Att⁻, Int⁻, C⁻	(6)
vir37	—	2.7% (77.2–79.9%)		(7)
vir40	75 bp	—		(8)
vir56b	4.1% (72.2–76.3%)	4.8%		(3,4)
vir65	17 bp	—	Att⁻, Int⁻, C⁻	(8)
vir79	1.1% (75.6–76.7%)	—	C⁻	(2)
vir94	5.9% (72.2–78.1%)	0.9%	Att⁻, Int⁻ C⁻, Cox⁻	(4)
sig5	—	3.7% (78.6%)		(2)

TABLE II. (*Continued*)

B. Phage 186

Mutant	Size (and position) of		Phenotype[h]	Reference[i]
	Deletion[f]	Insertion[f,g]		
del1	6.1% (67.9–74.0%)	—	Att⁻, Int⁻, CI⁻	(1)
ins1	—	4.2% (73.5%)	CI⁻	(2,3,4)
ins2	—	4.2% (73.8%)	CI⁻	(2,3)
ins3	—	4.2% (70.3%)	Int⁻	(2,3,4)
Hy2	64.2% (0–64.2%)	79.0%		
Hy5	65.4% (0–65.4%)	75.0%		

C. Phage P4

Mutant[j]	Size (and position) of		Phenotype[m]	Reference[n]
	Deletion[k]	Insertion[l]		
del1	4.3% (78.8–83.1%)	—	CII	(1,2,3,8)
del2	6.9% (65.5–72.2%)	—	Int⁻	(1,2,8)
del10	8.1% (84.8–92.9%)	—	Gop	(3,4,5,8)
Hy1	29.1% (69.4–98.6%)	2.9%	Gop	(1,2,6,9)
Hy17	30.6% (69.4–100%)	26%	Gop	(7)
Hy213	33% (67–100%)	23%	nt	(7)

[a]Vir = able to multiply on a lysogen.
[b]Given in % of P2 map (see Fig.2).
[c]vir37 is a duplication of P2 DNA; *sig5* is *IS2*; the other insertions are of bacterial origin.
[d]See Fig. 2, Table 3, and Section VII.
[e](1) Chattoraj and Inman, 1972; (2) Chattoraj *et al.*, 1975; (3) Hyde and Bertani, 1975; (4) Chattoraj and Bertani, 1980; (5) Nicoletti and Bertani, 1983; (6) Ljungquist *et al.*,1984; (7) Chattoraj and Inman, 1974, (8) Haggård-Ljungquist, personal communication; (9) Lindqvist, 1981b.
[f]Given in % of 186 map; see Fig. 2.
[g]The insertion in *ins1* and *ins3* is *IS3*; in Hy2 and Hy5 it is P2 DNA.
[h]See Fig. 2 and Table 3.
[i](1) Finnegan and Egan, 1981; (2) Bradley *et al.*, 1975; (3) Younghusband *et al.*, 1975; (4) Saint, 1979.
[j]*del10* was originally isolated by G. Bertani; all Hy phages carry the P4 *vir1* mutation.
[k]Given in % of P4 map; position at 69.4% corresponds to the rightmost *Eco*RI site.
[l]The insertion in Hy1 is λ DNA; in Hy17 and Hy213 it is P2 DNA.
[m]See Fig. 2 and Table 3; nt = not tested.
[n]First reference for original description of mutant or hybrid; further references for additional information. (1) Souza *et al.*, 1978; (2) Kahn and Hopkins, 1978; (3) Raimondi *et al.*, 1985; (4) Kahn *et al.*, 1980; (5) Pierson and Kahn, 1984; (6) Thomas *et al.*, 1974; (7) Lindqvist, 1981a; (8) Calendar *et al.*, 1981; (9) Ghisotti *et al.*, 1983.

the scale, P4 phasmids containing inserts of human DNA, together totaling 37–40 kb, all packaged into a P2-size head, are found to be infectious (Kurnit *et al.*, in preparation).

2. Phage 186

A search for deletion mutants of phage 186 using the same procedure as for P2 (Bradley *et al.*, 1975) produced instead a series of heat-resistant mutants, three of which turned out to be carrying insertions (Younghus-band *et al.*, 1975) (Table II). Two of the insertions, *ins1* and *ins3*, are derivatives of *IS3* (Saint, 1979; Kalionis *et al.*, 1986a). In the other cases, heat resistance is not correlated with any obvious physical change (Younghusband *et al.*, 1975). A deletion, *del1*, covering the *int* and *CI* genes, has also been characterized (Finnegan and Egan, 1981) (Table II).

3. Phage P4

The three most widely used P4 deletions, *del1*, *del2*, and *del10*, are listed in Table II. Raimondi *et al.* (1985) have described an additional set of eight such mutants. All 11 appeared spontaneously and are located in the left 40% of the P4 map—i.e., in the "nonessential" region of the P4 genome. All show an increased heat stability as compared to wild-type P4, and all but *del1* and *del2* were selected for this property. Heat stability increases with the size of the deletion (Raimondi *et al.*, 1985). The largest deletion found, *del22*, removes about 1.7 kb of DNA, suggesting that P4 molecules smaller than about 9.8 kb cannot be packaged. The largest molecule to be packaged into a P4-size head is a kanamycin-resistant derivative of 14 kb (Goldstein, personal communication).

B. Genetic Organization

1. Phage P2

The DNA molecule of P2 can be displayed as a linear structure termi-nating with the cohesive ends. To date, about 60% has been sequenced (Haggård-Ljungquist, personal communication). The overall organization resembles that of most other temperate phages, with the genes for the virion proteins to the left and those for DNA synthesis to the right (Fig. 2). So far, a total of 27 genes have been defined by mutation (Lindahl, 1969a; Sunshine *et al.*, 1971), although there is room for more, particu-larly at the far right end of the chromosome. There are about 3 kb of DNA between the end of gene *B* at 80.3% (Haggård-Ljungquist *et al.*, 1987) and *ori* at 89% and an additional 3.5 kb between *ori* and the right end. Only two genes have been found in this 6.5-kb region: *old*, which lies within 500 base pairs of the extreme right end (Calendar, personal communica-tion), and *A*. In a preliminary sequencing of the region, Haggård-Ljung-quist (personal communication) has found four open reading frames be-fore the *A* gene and one after. Another open reading frame coding for a small basic protein has been found between genes *cox* and *B* (Haggård-Ljungquist *et al.*, 1987). Finally, both gene products *FI* and *FII* are still ascribed to the same gene (Christie and Calendar, 1985).

The known genes, together with the size and function of their gene

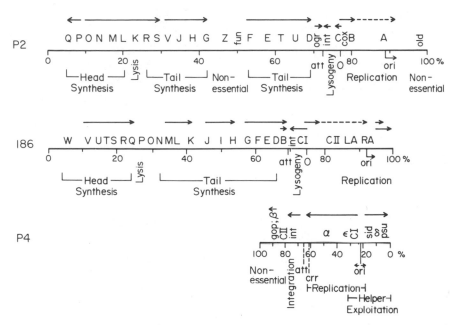

FIGURE 2. Genetic maps of phages P2, 186, and P4. The continuous lines represent double-stranded DNA molecules broken at the *cos* sites. The three maps are in scale with each other and aligned so that the left ends have a homologous single-stranded terminus (Appendix B). The genes and their directions of transcription, when known, lie above the line. Gene products are listed in Table III. Sites necessary for the initiation of replication (*ori* and *crr*), repressor binding regions (*O*), and phage attachment sites (*att*), as well as the general functions of the genes, are given below the line. In the case of P2 and 186, the genes have been oriented on the DNA molecule using specific physical sites (Appendix A) measured from the left end of the molecules. Phage P4, on the other hand, has been partially sequenced starting from the right end, so the distances are given in percent from that end instead.

products, are listed in Table III. They can be grouped into three classes: those essential for lytic multiplication (most of the genes designated by letter), those involved in lysogeny (*int*, *C*, and *cox*), and those of unknown but nonessential function (*old*, *Z*, and *fun*). The latter genes can be deleted without disturbing either the lytic multiplication of the phage or its ability to establish lysogeny (Bertani, 1975) and are not found in all members of the P2 group (see Section IV.D).

The order of the genes has been established by three-point crosses, stimulating recombination with ultraviolet light irradiation (Lindahl, 1969a). The genes have been positioned on the chromosome by heteroduplex mapping of deletions and insertions (Chattoraj and Inman, 1972, 1974b; Bertani, 1975; Chattoraj *et al.*, 1975; Hyde and Bertani, 1975; Chattoraj and Bertani, 1980), by marker rescue from cloned restriction fragments (Chattoraj, 1977; Westöö and Ljungquist, 1979, 1980; Saint and Egan, 1979a; Ljungquist and Bertani, 1983), and by sequencing (Christie

TABLE III. Genes and Gene Products

Gene	Product mol. wt. (kD)	Function	Reference
Phage P2			
old	29.5	λ exclusion	Lindahl et al., 1970; Gibbs et al., 1983
A	86	Replication	Lindahl, 1974; Haggård-Ljungquist, personal communication
B	18	Replication	Lindahl, 1974
cox	10	Excision	Lindahl and Sunshine, 1972
C	11	Repression	Ljungquist et al., 1984
int	35	Integration	Lindahl, 1969; Ljungquist and Bertani, 1983
ogr	8	Late-gene control	Sunshine and Sauer, 1975; Birkeland and Lindqvist, 1986; Christie et al., 1986
D	47	Tail	Ljungquist and Bertani, 1983
U	28	Tail	Ljungquist and Bertani, 1983
T	90	Tail fibers?	Lengyel et al., 1974; Gibbs et al., 1983
E	—	Stabilization of T protein	Lengyel et al., 1974
FI	46	Sheath	Lengyel et al., 1974
FII	20	Tube	Lengyel et al., 1974; Gibbs et al., 1983
fun	—	FUDR sensitivity	Bertani, 1964
Z	—	fun control	Bertani, 1976
G	—	Tail	Lengyel et al., 1974
H	71	Collar	Lengyel et al., 1974
J	—	Tail	Lengyel et al., 1974
V	23	Tail	Lengyel et al., 1974; Gibbs et al., 1983
S	—	Tail length	Lengyel et al., 1974
R	—	Tail length	Lengyel et al., 1974
K	—	Lysis	Lindahl, 1971
L	—	DNase-resistant heads	Lengyel et al., 1973; Pruss and Calendar, 1978
M	28	Packaging	Lengyel et al., 1973; Bowden and Modrich, 1985
N	44	Major capsid protein	Lengyel et al., 1973
O	30	Cleavage of N gene product	Lengyel et al., 1973; Gibbs et al., 1983
P	65	Packaging	Lengyel et al.,1973; Bowden and Modrich, 1985
Q	32	Packaging	Lengyel et al., 1973; Pruss and Calendar, 1978; Barrett, as quoted in Bowden and Modrich, 1981; Christie and Calendar, 1985

TABLE III. (*Continued*)

Gene	Product mol. wt. (kD)	Function	Reference
Phage 186			
RA	72	DNA synthesis	Hocking and Egan, 1982b; Sivaprasad, 1984
LA	38	DNA synthesis	Hocking and Egan, 1982b; Sivaprasad, 1984
CII	—	Lysogeny	Hocking and Egan, 1982c
CI	21	Repressor	Woods and Egan, 1974; Kalionis *et al.*, 1986a
int	37	Integration	Bradley *et al.*, 1975; Kalionis *et al.*, 1986a
B	8	Late-gene control	Hocking and Egan, 1982b; Kalionis *et al.*, 1986b
N–D	—	Tail synthesis	Hocking and Egan, 1982a
P	—	Lysis	Hocking and Egan, 1982b
W–Q	—	Head synthesis	Hocking and Egan, 1982a
Phage P4			
psu	21	Polarity suppression (protein 4)	Sauer *et al.*, 1981; Dale *et al.*, 1986
δ	19	Transactivation	Souza *et al.*, 1977; Lin, 1984
sid	27	Head size determination (protein 3)	Shore *et al.*, 1978; Lin, 1984
CI	15	P4 repression	Calendar *et al.*, 1981; Lin, 1984
ε	11	Derepression of helper	Geisselsoder *et al.*, 1981; Lin, 1984
Orf106	12	DNA replication	Flensburg and Calendar, 1987, and personal communication
α	85	DNA primase (protein 1)	Gibbs *et al.*, 1973; Barrett *et al.*, 1976, 1983; Flensburg and Calendar, 1987
int	51	Integration	Pierson and Kahn, 1984; Pierson and Kahn, in preparation
CII	31	Host survival[a]	Calendar *et al.*, 1981; Dehò, 1983; Dehò and Zangrossi, personal communication
β	—	Host survival[b]	Gibbs *et al.*, 1973; Dehò, 1983
gop	—	Blocks growth in E. coli pin mutants[b]	Ghisotti *et al.*, 1983; Dehò, 1983; Dehò and Zangrossi, personal communication

[a]Possibly a repressor of *gop*.
[b]β and *gop* may be identical.

and Calendar, 1983; Ljungquist *et al.*, 1984; Christie and Calendar, 1985; Haggård-Ljungquist *et al.*, 1987). Because of the idiosyncracies of the P2 recombination system (Lindahl, 1969b; Bertani, 1975; see Section IV.E), the *old* gene was first placed at the far left end of the linear map. Its physical location at the right end was established when a deletion affecting the *old* gene became available (Bertani, 1975).

2. Phage 186

Using the sequences of the cohesive ends as guides, the DNA molecules of phages 186 and P4 can be oriented relative to P2. Phage 186 has 26 known genes (Table III), which have been ordered by marker rescue frequency (Hocking and Egan, 1982c). The organization is much the same as in P2 (Fig. 2), although equivalents of P2 genes *cox*, *B*, and the nonessential genes *old*, *Z*, and *fun* have not been found. On the other hand, gene *CII* is not found in P2. The rightmost 20% of the chromosome contains only three known genes—*CII*, *LA*, and *RA*. Sequencing of the major control region of 186 (Kalionis *et al.*, 1986a) has revealed three open reading frames—one between genes *B* and *int*, and two, coding for potential DNA-binding proteins, immediately to the right of *CI*. Sequencing rightward to the cohesive end has been completed and shows a further 10 open reading frames (Egan, personal communication). The strands of the 186 DNA molecule have been oriented (Kalionis and Egan, 1981), and three insertions and a deletion have been localized by electron microscopy (Younghusband *et al.*, 1975; Finnegan and Egan, 1981). More detailed physical mapping of the genes on the DNA was achieved by marker rescue from cloned restriction fragments (Finnegan and Egan, 1979; Appendix A) and by the use of some of the P2–186 hybrids (Saint and Egan, 1979a; Finnegan and Egan, 1979; see below).

3. Phage P4

Since about 80% of the P4 DNA has been sequenced starting from the right end (Lin, 1984; Dale *et al.*, 1986; Flensburg and Calendar, 1987; Pierson and Kahn, 1987), base pairs are numbered beginning from this end, and all map positions are given as percentage of the distance from the same end. This represents a change in convention for P4, as the majority of papers quoted in this review use either the opposite map orientation or the opposite end as zero position.

When the identical cohesive ends of P2 and P4 are aligned (Lindqvist, 1981a), the functionally equivalent *ogr* and δ genes are also oriented in the same direction (Fig. 2). The organization of the P4 genome is strikingly different from that of P2 (Fig. 2), however. There is an essential core (at position 22% to 64%), comprising slightly less than half of the molecule, containing the genetic information for the replication of P4 DNA and for the control of early P4 functions. It also includes gene ϵ, which is responsible for derepression of the helper phage and is therefore essential for P4 growth in a helper lysogen. To the right of this core lie the genes that affect the expression of "late" helper genes. Hence two segments of the P4 genome, one responsible for DNA replication and the other for helper exploitation, overlap. Together they account for almost two-thirds of the P4 genome and carry all the information needed for the multiplication of phage P4. The remaining left third is nonessential for lytic growth. It includes the genes needed for integration and at least two others of unknown but expendable function.

The P4 genome has been mapped on the basis of recombination frequencies in phage crosses (Calendar et al., 1981; Geisselsoder et al., 1981; Dehò, 1983; Lin, 1983), by marker rescue from cloned restriction fragments (Goldstein et al., 1975; Kahn and Hopkins, 1978; Souza et al., 1978; Kahn et al., 1980; Calendar et al., 1981; Sauer et al., 1981; Raimondi et al., 1985), by heteroduplex analysis of deletion mutants (Souza et al., 1978; Lindqvist, 1981a,b), and increasingly now by DNA sequencing, as already mentioned.

The eight or nine P4 genes recognized so far are listed in Table III. All are identified by point mutations. The nonessential region is known to encode two further proteins—gene product 2 of Barrett et al. (1976) with an apparent molecular mass of 45 kd (Souza et al., 1978; Kahn et al., 1980; Calendar et al., 1981; Alano et al., 1986; Ghisotti, Tronconi, Dehò, and Sironi, personal communication), and a protein with the apparent molecular mass of 15 kd (Ghisotti, Tronconi, Dehò, and Sironi, personal communication). A hypothetical P4 gene enabling P4 to complement P2 B^- mutants (Barrett et al., 1976; Six and Lindqvist, 1978) must reside outside of the nonessential region (Six, unpublished). The position of another putative P4 gene, kil, held responsible for host cell killing by the mutant P4 cl405 (Alano et al., 1986) also remains unknown.

C. Hybrids, Plasmids, and Phasmids

The first P2 hybrid, P2 Hy dis, was produced by an exchange between P2 and a defective prophage in E. coli B (Cohen, 1959). The hybrid acquired a new immunity specificity as well as two insertions in the early region resulting in a phage with 2.2% more DNA than wild-type P2 (Chattoraj and Inman, 1973a).

A series of 12 hybrids between P2 and 186 were isolated by mixed infection of an E. coli K12 host, selecting for 186 immunity and P2 host range (Bradley et al., 1975; Hocking and Egan, 1982d). The positions of the novel joints, located genetically (Bradley et al., 1975; Hocking and

Egan, 1982d) and in some cases physically (Younghusband *et al.*, 1975), ranged between genes *J* and *B* on the 186 map. Some of the hybrids possess a combination of tail genes from both phages, suggesting the possibility of extensive interchangeability between these genes. Hybrids lacking P2 genes *E, T, U,* and *D* still had P2 host range (Hocking and Egan, 1982d). The hybrids were not characterized with respect to cohesive ends. Analysis of the hybrids suggests unequal crossing over and the possibility that they are produced by illegitimate recombination (Bradley *et al.*, 1975; Younghusband *et al.*, 1975). Similarly, P2–P3 hybrids were obtained by selecting for P3 immunity and P2 host range, but these remain to be analyzed (Six, unpublished).

A segment of P2 DNA containing the *int* gene and the *att* site has been cloned into the plasmid pBR322 (Ljungquist and Bertani, 1983). The resultant construct integrates efficiently and stably into the host chromosome, where it can be amplified *in situ*, together with the surrounding host DNA (Bertani *et al.*, 1981; Bertani and Bertani, in preparation).

A "phasmid" consisting of plasmid pBR322 cloned into an *Eco*RI site on P2 retains the replication systems of both elements and resistance to two antibiotics as well as the ability to multiply like a phage or integrate into the host chromosome (Nicoletti and Bertani, 1983).

P4-derived hybrids, with P4 heads, can be constructed *in vitro* by replacing nonessential P4 DNA with foreign DNA of similar size. Two of P4's *Eco*RI sites, about 3.4 kb apart (70–99%; Figs. 2, 3) are especially useful for this purpose. Exchange of this *Eco*RI fragment for one from phage λ generated Hy1 (Table II). Similarly, its replacement with bacterial or plasmid DNA allowed Ow and Ausubel (1980, 1983) to construct a series of P4 derivatives that are specialized transducing phages (see Section V.H).

Lindqvist (1981a) constructed six "P4-size" P2-P4 hybrids, ranging in size from 84% to 96% of the P4 genome, by *in vitro* recombination using *Eco*RI sites in the two phages. Approximately one-third of the P4 DNA was replaced by a similarly sized segment of DNA from the left end of the P2 chromosome. This was accompanied in the case of all six hybrids, including Hy17 (Fig. 3), by a spontaneous deletion of some P2 DNA, so that the P2 moiety of the hybrid retained only an intact (and functional) *Q* gene and part of gene *P*. Unexpectedly, Lindqvist found very similar hybrids *in vivo*. Hy213 (Table II) and four apparently identical hybrids may have resulted from site-specific recombination as their P4 moiety ends close to, and possibly within, the P4 *att* site. Furthermore, an octomer (tGGGGGCA) contained in the fivefold repeats found in the P4 *att* region (Pierson and Kahn, 1987) also occurs in P2 gene *P* (sequence data from G. Christie, personal communication).

Theoretically, a "P2-size," helper-independent P2–P4 hybrid could be generated by site-specific *in vivo* recombination, provided the P2 moiety carried a *sir* mutation to allow packaging (see Section V.B), but this has not been observed. Instead, Lindqvist (1981b) constructed the

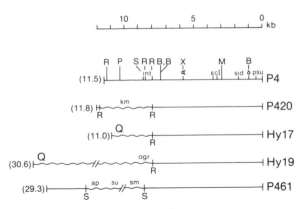

FIGURE 3. Physical maps of P4 and structures of derivatives P420, Hy17, Hy19, and P461. The straight lines represent P4 DNA, the wavy lines represent non-P4 DNA, and the numbers in parentheses give the size of the DNA in kilobases (kb). Symbols for restriction sites: For P4, all known unique sites are shown. *Pst*I and *Pvu*II, both sites at ≈10.4 kb (=P), *Sal*I at 8.595 kb (=S), *Xma*I at 5.789 kb (=X), *Mlu*I at 3.015 kb (=M9), as well as the *Eco*RI sites (=R) at 8.005, 8.480, and ≈11.4 kb and the *Bam*HI (=B) sites at 0.983, 7.376, and 7.389 kb. For the P4 derivatives, only the sites involved in constructing the hybrids are shown; they correspond to the P4 *Eco*RI sites at 8.005 and 11.4 kb and the P4 *Sal*I site. Genetic symbols: For P4, the already sequenced genes—*int*, α, ε, *CI*, *sid*, δ, and *psu*—are indicated (except for orf106 between α and ε). For the P4 derivatives, only a few genes on the non-P4 moieties are shown. These include P2 genes *Q* and *ogr* (*Q* is the only complete P2 gene of Hy17; Hy19 carries all P2 genes from *Q* to *ogr*), and the antibiotic resistance-conferring genes *km*, *ap*, *su*, and *sm* (= resistance to kanamycin, ampicillin, sulfonamide, and streptomycin, respectively).

helper-independent hybrid, Hy19 (Fig. 3), by *Eco*RI site fusion of the rightmost two-thirds of the P4 chromosome, containing the essential P4 genes, to the leftmost three-fourths of the P2 chromosome, containing all P2 late genes and gene *ogr* (Fig. 3). This *in vitro* recombination was followed by two spontaneous events—one generating *del19* in the P2 moiety, and the other blocking expression of P4 late genes, which is necessary to allow packaging (see Section V.B).

In addition, several hybrid "phasmids" that retain both the replication system of P4 and that of a plasmid have been constructed. The P4-size phasmid P420 was generated by replacing the 3.4-kb *Eco*RI fragment of P4 with the 3.6-kb *col*E1-derived, kanamycin-resistant plasmid pMK20 (Kahn and Helinski, 1978) (Fig. 3). Kahn *et al.* (1980) obtained several deletion mutants, including P422, from phasmid P420 and used them to map the right two-thirds of the P4 genome. A 29-kb (i.e., P2-size) phasmid, P461, was prepared by joining P4 and pJW7 at their unique *Sal*I sites (Six and Williams, unpublished) (Fig. 3). Plasmid pJW7 is a cointegrate of pBR313 and RSF1010 that confers resistance to four antibiotics: tetracycline, ampicillin, streptomycin, and sulfonamide. The tetracycline gene is disrupted in P461, but the *in vivo* fusion of P4 with pJW7 yielded the cointegrate P463, which expresses all four antibiotic resistances (Six and Williams, unpublished).

IV. LIFE CYCLES OF P2-LIKE PHAGES

A. Replication

1. General Features

The replication of P2 DNA is unidirectional and begins at a unique site designated *ori*, which is located 89% of the distance from the left end of the molecule (Schnös and Inman, 1971) (Fig. 2). It proceeds rightward (Fig. 2) and requires the products of two phage genes, *A* and *B* (Lindqvist, 1971; Lindahl, 1974) as well as the host functions *dnaB, dnaE, dnaG* (Bowden *et al.*, 1975), and *rep* (Calendar *et al.*, 1970) (Table IV). The product of phage gene *A* is a *cis*-acting protein (Lindahl, 1970); i.e., phages with mutations in gene *A* cannot be complemented by other phages with wild-type *A* genes.

These features of the P2 replication system—unidirectional replication and the requirements for a *cis*-acting phage protein and the host *rep* function—are also characteristic of the otherwise unrelated phage φX-174 (Baas and Jansz, 1972; Francke and Ray, 1972; Denhardt *et al.*, 1967), with which P2 shares a common host, *E. coli* C.

2. *In Vivo* DNA Forms

Although the DNA in P2 phage particles is linear, the predominant *in vivo* forms are circular. Following injection, P2 DNA is found in both covalently closed and nicked open-circular configurations (Lindqvist, 1971). The latter forms are associated with fast-sedimenting host cell components, probably membranes (Ljungquist, 1973, 1976; Geisselsoder, 1976; Chattoraj, 1978). In the electron microscope, replicating molecules appear as circles with tails (Schnös and Inman, 1971; Chattoraj, 1978).

TABLE IV. Host Genes Required
for Replication[a,b]

	Required by		
Host gene	P2	186	P4
dnaA	−	+	−
dnaB	+	+	−
dnaC	−	+	−
dnaE	+	nt	+
dnaG	+	nt	−
rep	+	+	−

[a]Key: +, required; −, not required; nt, not tested.
[b]References: Calendar *et al.*, 1970; Lane and Denhardt, 1974; Bowden *et al.*, 1975; Hooper and Egan, 1981; Egan, personal communication.

The tails are rarely of more than genome length, however, and long concatamers have never been observed. If the infecting phage is deficient in head formation, covalently closed circular DNA accumulates (Pruss and Calendar, 1978). Finally, the preferred DNA substrate for packaging into phage heads is a covalently closed monomeric circle (Pruss et al., 1975).

3. Initiation

The DNA molecules associated with cell membranes were found to have unique, single-stranded breaks in the ori region (Chattoraj, 1978). Both membrane attachment and the appearance of a single-strand break are associated with gene A activity (Ljungquist, 1976; Geisselsoder, 1976). Thus, the product of gene A, a protein of molecular mass 86 kD (Saha and Haggård-Ljungquist, personal communication), is believed to initiate replication by introducing a single-strand break at ori. It has been suggested (Schnös and Inman, 1971) that ori may actually lie within gene A, as is the case for ϕX-174 (Baas and Jansz, 1972). Recent sequencing in this region (Saha and Haggård-Ljungquist, personal communication) confirms that gene A extends from 83.4% to 90.6% on the P2 chromosome and should therefore cover the ori site. The effect of purified ϕX-174 gene A protein on P2 DNA has not been reported, but the two phage proteins do not show obvious sequence similarities (Haggård-Ljungquist, personal communication). Still, it might be possible to make viable hybrids by exchanging DNA segments that contain both ori and gene A. The gene A-dependent initiation system of P2 can substitute for the dnaA initiation system of E. coli (Lindahl et al., 1971) (see Section IV.D).

The product of gene B has been characterized both on gels (Lengyel and Calendar, 1974) and by sequencing the DNA (Haggård-Ljungquist et al., 1987). It is a weakly basic protein of 18.7 kD or 166 amino acid residues that is produced continuously and in large amounts throughout the latent period (Lengyel and Calendar, 1974). According to Funnell and Inman (1983), it is required for lagging strand synthesis. The cis-dominant rlb1 mutation (Sunshine et al., 1975) that makes P2 partially independent of the host dnaB function lies within gene B (Haggård-Ljungquist et al., 1987). Thus, following the introduction of a single-strand break at the ori site, replication may be primed by an interaction between the host dnaB and the phage gene B products.

The dependence of P2 replication on phage gene B can be eliminated by a bacterial mutation, sub (Sunshine and Six, 1986), which maps at 10 min on the E. coli C chromosome.

4. Synthesis and Termination

Following initiation, replication proceeds according to a modified rolling circle mechanism (Chattoraj, 1978), using the combined activities of DNA polymerase (dnaE), primase (dnaG), and the rep unwinding protein. There is some evidence for discontinuous DNA synthesis (Kai-numa-Kuroda and Okazaki, 1975; Kurosawa and Okazaki, 1975).

A round of replication would presumably terminate at *ori* again, and the product would be released and circularized. It has been suggested that the latter steps could also be activities of the gene *A* protein (Pruss *et al.*, 1975), which might remain attached to the nascent DNA throughout the replication cycle.

5. Phage 186

The replication of 186 DNA is puzzling. It resembles that of P2 in many respects and yet contains elements of the *E. coli* system. As in P2, the replication is unidirectional (Chattoraj and Inman, 1973b). The *ori* site of 186 has been located 92.9% from the left end of the molecule (Fig. 2), and, in the electron microscope, the replicating molecules have a similar tailed appearance. Phage 186 also depends on the host *rep* function (Lane and Denhardt, 1974) (Table IV).

Phage 186 gene *A*, concerned with DNA replication (Hocking and Egan, 1982b), is now divided into two genes—left *A* (*LA*) and right *A* (*RA*). Only gene *RA* product is absolutely required for replication from 186 *ori* (Sivaprasad, 1984), although gene *LA* product is stimulatory. Phage 186 does not seem to have an equivalent of P2 gene *B*, but instead needs two additional host functions, *dnaA* and *dnaC* (Hooper and Egan, 1981), to replicate. Unlike P2, the replication of 186 is strongly inhibited by ultraviolet irradiation of the host prior to infection (Hooper *et al.*, 1981). Finally, by considering the genetic and physical maps and transcription patterns, Finnegan and Egan (1981) argued that the 186 *ori* site was probably located to the right and outside of gene *A*. In fact, it lies within gene *RA* (Sivaprasad, 1984).

Like gene *A* of P2, 186 gene *RA* complements other mutations poorly (Hocking and Egan, 1982b). In addition, the two genes seem to have some sequence similarity (Haggård-Ljungquist, personal communication; Egan, personal communication). How the host genes *dnaA* and *dnaC*, known to be required for the initiation of DNA synthesis in *E. coli* (Hirota *et al.*, 1970; Kobori and Kornberg, 1982), are involved in phage 186 replication is not clear. The 186 *ori* region does not contain binding sites for the *dnaA* protein (Sivaprasad, 1984; Fuller *et al.*, 1984). The *dnaC* protein might make up for the lack of a P2 gene *B*-like product. It would be interesting to see if 186 can replicate in a *dnaC⁻* strain that also contains the *sub* mutation that alleviates the need for P2 gene *B* product (see section on initiation).

B. Morphogenesis, Packaging, and Lysis

Nearly two-thirds of the genes of P2 are involved in the synthesis of the head and tail structures, which are made independently. Upon infection of a suitable host, phages defective in head synthesis produce morphologically recognizable tails, and tail-defective mutants produce mature, DNA-filled heads (Lengyel et al., 1973, 1974). When these structures are mixed together in an in vitro reconstitution system, fully infectious particles are obtained (Lindahl, 1974).

1. Synthesis of Proheads

Mutations in head genes O or N result in a decrease in the number of head structures seen (Lengyel et al., 1973). Both the N and O gene products are cleaved during morphogenesis (Lengyel et al., 1973; Pruss et al., 1974a), but only derivatives of the N protein (and possibly very small pieces of O protein; Calendar, personal communication) appear in the capsid (see Section II.B). The cleavage reaction is DNase-resistant and does not require ATP (Pruss et al., 1974a). If the other minor components are present, the combined action of the N and O proteins produces an empty prohead structure, which contains all the proteins of the capsid but has a slightly rounded, rather than an icosahedral shape (Bowden and Modrich, 1985).

2. Packaging of DNA

Phages with mutations in genes M, P, or Q produce rounded, empty proheads (Lengyel et al., 1973). When proheads are mixed together with purified M protein and covalently closed DNA, a complex is formed (Bowden and Modrich, 1981). The addition of purified P protein and ATP to the complex leads to the appearance of DNA-filled, icosahedral heads (Bowden and Calendar, 1979; Bowden and Modrich, 1981). The role of the Q gene product has yet to be established.

The terminase reaction, which converts the covalently closed DNA to the linear form found in the capsid, has been studied in an in vitro system (Bowden and Calendar, 1979; Bowden and Modrich, 1985). It requires proheads and the M and P proteins. The M gene presumably codes for the ter nuclease that generates single-stranded cohesive ends from the cos site, since the M protein is not needed for packaging when linear DNA is used. P2 M protein is also active on circularized 186 or P4 DNA (Bowden and Modrich, 1985). The P and Q proteins are still required for in vitro packaging even when linear DNA is used (Bowden and Calendar, 1979). The P protein is associated with a DNA-dependent ATPase activity (Bowden and Modrich, 1985). Models for the action of ter enzymes have been proposed (Wang and Brezinski, 1973; Murray et al., 1977; Bowden and Modrich, 1981).

The packaging of P2 DNA is unusual in that the preferred DNA substrate is a covalently closed monomer, and only one cos site is needed (Pruss et al., 1975). Linear concatemers or circular dimers of P2 DNA are used much less efficiently. Using trimeric P4 DNA, Bowden and Modrich

(1985) showed that neither superhelicity of the substrate nor a hypo-thetical movement of the terminase from a binding site to the site of nicking could account for the requirement for a covalently closed mono-mer.

The logistics of inserting a linearized version of the DNA into a preformed protein shell is shared with other double-stranded DNA phages (Earnshaw and Casjens, 1980), as is the problem of how a specific cohesive end becomes associated with the tail (see Section II.D).

3. Synthesis of Tails

The tails of the P2-like phages are very complex and require the activities of 11 genes to be synthesized. Among the visible structures are a collar, tube, sheath, and baseplate to which is attached a single spike and six tail fibers (Fig. 1). Two of the major tail structures, the tube and the sheath, are affected by mutations in gene F (see Table I), but the coding sequences for the 46-kD sheath protein, FI, and the smaller FII protein have not yet been localized. Only mutations in genes R and S produce aberrant structures—giant tails and giant sheaths, respectively. Gene L mutants produce tails as well as DNA-filled heads which look normal. The heads are sensitive to DNase, however, and the mutants serve as tail rather than head donors in *in vitro* reconstitution experi-ments (Pruss and Calendar, 1978). Mutations in any of the other genes produce few recognizable structures (Lengyel *et al.*, 1974).

4. Particle Assembly and Lysis

In a complete medium at 37°C, P2-infected bacteria begin to lyse about 25 min after infection and release approximately 100 active phage particles. Lysis requires the product of gene K (Lindahl, 1971). Under standard conditions, lysates of P2 contain a significant fraction of defec-tive particles which appear to be tailless (Bertani *et al.*, 1978). A muta-tion, lg (large plaques), thought to be in gene F, simultaneously reduces the proportion of such particles and increases the burst size (Bertani *et al.*, 1978). When infecting a ρ^- host, P2 will produce a considerable propor-tion of small P4-size heads (Geisselsoder *et al.*, 1978).

5. Phage 186

The seven head genes and 11 tail genes of phage 186 have been characterized in an *in vitro* reconstitution system and by electron micros-copy (Hocking and Egan, 1982a). Phages with mutations in genes Q, R, S, T, U, V, and W produce mature tails; those with mutations in genes D, E, F, G, H, J, K, L, M, and N produce DNA-filled heads. Nothing is known about capsid composition. Phages with mutations in genes T and U pro-duce only tails, no visible head structures. These genes could be the equivalent of P2 genes N and O, and thus one could code for the precursor of the major capsid protein. Gene N mutants produce giant tails and might correspond to P2 gene R mutants. The gene that codes for 186 terminase has not been identified as yet; covalently closed circular 186 DNA can be cleaved in vitro by P2 terminase (Bowden and Modrich, 1985).

Phage 186-infected bacteria begin to lyse 37 min after infection in a complete medium at 37°C (Hooper et al., 1981). Lysis requires an active gene P product (Hocking and Egan, 1982b).

C. Regulation

1. Repressor

The repressor gene of P2, gene C, was originally defined by temperature-sensitive mutants (Bertani, 1968). It has recently been cloned (Westöö and Ljungquist, 1980) and sequenced (Ljungquist et al., 1984). The binding of the protein to DNA has been studied in an in vitro system (Lundqvist and Bertani, 1984). The monomer is a nonbasic protein of 11 kD or 99 amino acid residues. Most mutations affecting the repressor are located within the coding sequence and give clear-plaque phenotypes. One, c1, affects instead the level of repressor and appears to interfere with ribosomal binding. An unusual C gene mutation that does not have a clear-plaque phenotype was isolated in a screening for excisionless mutants and was originally designated as cox1 (Lindahl and Sunshine, 1972). It has been rechristened sly1 (for spontaneous lysis; Ljungquist et al., 1984) to distinguish it from mutations that directly affect excision (Six and Lindqvist, 1978).

P2 is often characterized as a noninducible phage. Ultraviolet light or other treatments sufficient to induce phage λ do not affect P2 repressor (Bertani, 1968); i.e., P2 lysogens remain immune. As expected, the C gene does not contain the ala-gly sequence that is cleaved by the recA protease of the host (Little and Mount, 1982). As the sly1 mutation does not make P2 lysogens more immune than usual (G. Bertani, personal communication), it might be interpreted as a change that makes the repressor resistant to inactivation by the still unknown event that triggers spontaneous lysis in this system. P2 lysogens can also be derepressed by infection with phage P4, an interaction that is not affected by the sly1 mutation (Six and Lindqvist, 1978) (see Section V.D).

The active form of the P2 repressor is a dimer (Lundqvist and Bertani, 1984). It binds to an operator region located a few nucleotides to the right of gene C (Fig. 2) and controls the only known early operon in P2, which includes genes cox and B. The operator region is defined by virulent mutations that make the phage insensitive to repressor. This region contains two 8-bp repeats that are presumably included in the binding sites.

These span the promoter (pE) for the early cox-B operon (Haggård-Ljung-quist et al., 1987), supporting the idea that competition with the host RNA polymerase for DNA-binding sites is the most likely mechanism for the P2 repressor. Recent DNase I protection studies using partially purified P2 repressor and E. coli RNA polymerase confirm this arrangement (Saha et al., 1987a). There is some sequence similarity between the P2 operator region and the operators for the biotin genes of E. coli (Ljung-quist et al., 1984).

2. Transcription of Genes Involved in the Lytic Cycle

Transcription in P2 is rifampicin-sensitive (Barrett et al., 1972; Lind-qvist, 1974), suggesting that it depends on the host RNA polymerase. The genes essential for lytic multiplication are controlled directly or indirectly by repressor. Following infection of a suitable host, transcription begins in the right half of the chromosome, presumably in the cox-B region (Funnell and Inman, 1982), and then spreads to the left half, where the late genes are located (Lindqvist and Bøvre, 1972; Geisselsoder et al., 1973). There is some evidence that genes B and cox are directly controlled by repressor (Bertani, 1968, 1980). Recently, Saha et al. (1987b) have proposed additional control through autoregulation by the cox gene product. Whether gene A is part of that operon or is regulated independently is still an open question, although there appears to be a termination signal between genes B and A (Haggård-Ljungquist et al., 1987).

The late genes have been divided into four groups on the basis of strongly polar mutations (Lindahl, 1971; Sunshine et al., 1971) that are thought to define blocks of cotranscribed genes. The genetic observations suggested that genes P and Q were transcribed in a different direction from the others. This was confirmed when the transcripts were hybridized to separated phage DNA strands (Lindqvist and Bøvre, 1972; Geisselsoder et al., 1973) and excludes the possibility that the late genes are expressed by an extension of the transcription from the early promoter. Lengyel and Calendar (1974) found that all four of the late transcripts appeared almost simultaneously, suggesting that transcription was initiated independently for each block of genes rather than in a sequential manner. More recently, Christie and Calendar (1985) have observed that polar amber mutations in gene O stimulate transcription in the other late gene clusters, as if they were repressed by one of the products of the O operon. The lack of a ribosome-binding site for the V gene cluster results in a lower level of translation for this operon (Christie and Calendar, 1985).

3. Late-Gene Control

The late genes of P2 are activated after replication has begun. Mutations in either of the phage genes needed for replication, A or B, reduce transcription of the late genes (Geisselsoder *et al.*, 1973; Lengyel and Calendar, 1974; Funnell and Inman, 1982). Originally, this was thought to indicate a direct involvement of the *A* and *B* gene products in late-gene regulation, although most evidence now suggests that it is more likely due to the configuration of the replicating DNA or a dosage effect of the *ogr* or late genes. If replication is blocked by using a *rep⁻* host instead, there is also some reduction even though the *A* gene product is present (Christie and Calendar, 1983). In addition, it has been observed the a "phasmid" consisting of phage P2 fused to the multicopy plasmid pBR322 (Nicoletti and Bertani, 1983) is able to multiply and produce phage even when the phage moiety carries a mutation in gene *A*. Thus, phage late-gene products can also be synthesized in the absence of the *A* gene product. Finally, phage P4 can activate the synthesis of P2 late-gene products from nonreplicating P2 DNA (see Section V.D). These observations suggested that P2 late genes were under some other type of control.

When the promoter regions for the late-gene transcription units were sequenced (Christie and Calendar, 1983, 1985), they were found to differ considerably from the *E. coli* consensus sequence (Appendix B). They resemble each other, however, and the surrounding regions exhibit further similarities: an inverted repeat at the −57 positions (Dale *et al.*, 1986) and one or more copies of a 10-bp sequence with the consensus − TATTCA(GT)GAC− lying within the leader sequences or N-terminal coding regions of three out of the four units (Appendix B). Additional experiments implicated an interaction between bacterial RNA polymerase and a phage gene product, *ogr*.

Although P2 can replicate in a *rpoA109* host, the transcription of its late genes is blocked (Sunshine and Sauer, 1975). The *rpoA109* strain has a single amino acid substitution in the α subunit of its DNA-dependent RNA polymerase (Fujiki *et al.*, 1976). Thus, P2 might provide a model system for the study of interactions between regulatory proteins and the α subunit. Not all *rpoA* mutations affect P2, however. It is able to multiply normally in the recently described *phs* mutants of *E. coli* (Rowland *et al.*, 1985).

A dominant mutation, located between the late gene *D* and the *att* site, restores the ability of P2 to multiply in the *rpoA109* strain (Sunshine and Sauer, 1975). A number of such mutations have been isolated and define the *ogr* gene of P2. The lack of conditional lethal *ogr* mutations threw some doubt on whether the gene was essential, but a recently described deletion of the *ogr* region has proved to be lethal (Birkeland and Lindqvist, personal communication). The *ogr* gene product may modify RNA polymerase so that it can interact with the promoters of the late-gene transcription units.

The *ogr⁺* gene has been cloned and sequenced (Birkeland and Lindqvist, 1986; Christie *et al.*, 1986). Its product is a basic polypeptide of molecular mass 8.3 kD or 72 amino acid residues. It is unlike *E. coli* σ factor or any of a number of regulatory proteins that modify the activity of host RNA polymerase (Christie *et al.*, 1986), but it is structurally similar to (Kalionis *et al.*, 1986b; Appendix B), and functionally interchangeable with, the *B* gene product of phage 186 (Hocking and Egan, 1982d; Sauer *et al.*, 1982) and the δ gene product of P4 (Sauer *et al.*, 1982). The P2 *ogr* gene has a consensus *E. coli* promoter upstream and a ρ-independent termination sequence downstream to it (Pritchard and Egan, 1985; Christie *et al.*, 1986). The former is consistent with the recent demonstration that the *ogr* gene is transcribed *in vitro* (Pritchard and Egan, 1985) using *E. coli* DNA-dependent RNA polymerase. In addition, in contrast to experiments reported earlier, Birkeland and Christie (personal communication) have observed that *ogr*-deficient P2 can be complemented *in vivo* by *A⁻* mutants of P2. Their success is most likely explained by the use of a deletion which avoids the problem of interference between an active *ogr⁺* protein and a defective gene product. There does not seem to be a transcription stop signal between genes *D* and *ogr*; hence, it may also be transcribed together with gene *D*, and it opens the possibility that it may stimulate its own transcription when it activates the late genes.

4. Transcription of Other Genes

As already mentioned, the *cox* gene, which is involved in prophage excision (see Section IV.D), is transcribed as part of the early operon and is most likely repressor-controlled. Although excision is never very efficient in P2 (see Section IV.D), the early expression of *cox* ensures that at least some copies of P2 DNA are synthesized free of the host chromosome.

Transcription of gene *C* begins at a promoter, pC (see Appendix B; an alternative −35 region has been suggested by Kalionis *et al.*, 1986a), located between the operator region and the *cox* gene and proceeds right to left (Ljungquist *et al.*, 1984) (Fig. 2). Thus, it converges with the transcription of the early *cox-B* operon from pE and overlaps it for about 30 nucleotides. An early attempt to detect regulation of *C* gene transcription was negative (Nilsson and Bertani, 1977). Recently, however, Saha *et al.* (1987a) have found that low levels of repressor both enhance the binding of RNA polymerase to pC and stimulate transcription from this promoter. When the level of repressor is increased, some reduction in transcription from the pC region has been detected (Saha *et al.*, 1987a). Saha *et al.* (1987b) have suggested further that transcription from pC might also be controlled by the product of the *cox* gene, which was implicated previously in the induction of P4 by P2 (Six and Lindqvist, 1978) (see Section V.E).

The transcription of the *int* gene is taken up in Section IV.D.

Genes *old*, *Z*, and *fun* are expressed in immune lysogens and are presumed to have repressor-independent, *E. coli* consensus promoters.

5. Phage 186

Temperature-sensitive clear mutants have long been known for phage 186. These define the *CI* gene which presumably codes for a repressor protein. Recent DNA sequencing data (Kalionis *et al.*, 1986a) suggest that the *CI* gene product is a protein of 21 kD, i.e., about twice the size of the P2 repressor. Its 192 amino acid residues show no significant similarity to either the P2 *C*, λ *CI*, or λ *cro*-like group of DNA-binding proteins (Dodd and Egan, 1987).

Virulent mutants have been isolated (Hocking and Egan, 1982a) and mapped to the right end of the chromosome (Hocking and Egan, 1982d). The operator region is thought to lie to the right of gene *CI* at about 76% (Finnegan and Egan, 1981) (Fig. 2). Sequencing in this region reveals several repeats that may be repressor-binding sites (Pritchard and Egan, 1985; Kalionis *et al.*, 1986a).

Phage 186 was originally classified as a noninducible phage, because it did not exhibit zygotic induction. Since then, it has been found to be induced by ultraviolet irradiation, nalidixic acid, and mitomycin C (Woods and Egan, 1974). The lack of zygotic induction was traced to a transient inability of the recipient bacteria to support phage multiplication (Woods and Egan, 1981). The refractory period is long enough to allow establishment of stable lysogeny. Both induction and spontaneous phage production are dependent on the host *recA* system. Noninducible (*tum*⁻) 186 mutants have been isolated (Woods and Egan, 1974). Kalionis *et al.* (1986a) reported that the sequence of *CI* does not display the similarity seen in the carboxy-terminal domain of known *recA* protease substrates, although it does have an *ala-gly* linkage near the carboxy-terminal end. Phage 186 lysogens cannot be induced by phage P4 (Sauer *et al.*, 1982; see Section V.D), another indication that 186 repressor is very different from that of P2.

Mutations in a second gene designated *CII* also result in a clear-plaque phenotype (Hocking and Egan, 1982d). The role of this gene in lysogenization has not been studied.

The first transcripts found following derepression of a 186 lysogen hybridize with the right half of the chromosome (Finnegan and Egan, 1981). After about 20 min, transcription of the late genes begins with a concomitant decrease in early-gene transcription. Most of the late genes have been assigned to four transcription units based on polarity groups (Hocking and Egan, 1982a) (Fig. 2). The direction of transcription of gene *D* is rightward (Kalionis *et al.*, 1986b).

Four transcripts were obtained in an *in vitro* system using host DNA-dependent RNA polymerase (Pritchard and Egan, 1985). All are synthesized in the rightward direction and are derived from (1) the gene *B* region, (2) the early repressor-controlled region, and (3) a region at the far right that has no known genetic markers. This region produces two overlapping transcripts and is controlled by a DNA sequence similar to a binding site (SOS box) for the *lexA* protein (Little and Mount, 1982). The promoters for these transcripts are compared with those of P2 in Appendix B.

The role of gene *A* (*RA*) in activating the late genes of phage 186 is similar to the situation described above for P2. Late gene transcription is depressed in *A⁻* mutants (Finnegan and Egan, 1981), but transcription can be activated in such mutants if the phage is replicating under the control of another replicon—e.g., a plasmid (Kalionis *et al.*, 1986b).

The main control of late-gene transcription, however, is via gene *B*, whose product is functionally interchangeable with the *ogr* and δ gene products of P2 and P4, respectively (Hocking and Egan, 1982d; Sauer *et al.*, 1982; Appendix B). The complete sequence of the gene is known (Kalionis *et al.*, 1986b). Its product is a protein of the same size as the *ogr* protein of P2—i.e., 8.3 kD. Its 72 amino acid residues show 64% identity with P2 *ogr* and 45% with the first 40 amino acid residues of the P4 δ protein. Unlike P2, wild-type 186 can multiply on the *rpoA109* strain (Sauer, 1979) and *amber* mutants in gene *B* were isolated together with those in other essential genes (Hocking and Egan, 1982a).

In addition to the *in vitro* transcription mentioned above, a low level of *B* gene transcription has been detected *in vivo* by Kalionis and Egan (1986b). Because the transcription is enhanced in a *B⁻* mutant, they have suggested that gene *B* may be repressed by its own product and have further proposed that two inverted repeats found overlapping the promoters for gene *B* might be binding sites for the repressor. Interestingly enough, these repeats contain the same 10-bp sequence found associated with the P2 late genes (see Appendix B), although they are found upstream rather than downstream to the transcription start. This sequence is not found preceding P2 gene *ogr*.

Late in infection the transcription of gene *B* may also originate from the late region (Kalionis *et al.*, 1986b).

D. The Prophage

1. Bacterial Attachment Sites

Prophage P2 may occupy any of at least 10 different sites on the bacterial chromosome (Table V), although there are site preferences and differences between hosts. The preferred site in *E. coli* strain C, site I, is located at 48 min, between the bacterial genes *metG* and *his* (Fig. 4). Other sites in *E. coli* C have been detected only in double lysogens where site I has also been occupied. Site II, located at 85 min near the *metE* gene, is the next most preferred. The P2 prophage sites in *E. coli* C have been used to study DNA replication in that organism (Jonasson, 1973).

E. coli K12 lacks site I but has instead site H, which lies on the other side of the *his* gene, at 44 min. There is no strongly preferred site in strain

TABLE V. Bacterial Attachment Sites

Site	Map location (min)	Cotransducible with	Remarks
P2I	48	metG	Preferred in *E. coli* C. Bertani and Six, 1958; Calendar and Lindahl, 1969
P2H	44	his	Only in *E. coli* K. Kelly, 1963
P2II	85	metE	Kelly, 1963; Calendar and Lindahl, 1969
P2III	32		Bertani and Six, 1958; Six, 1966
P2E	62		Six and Kahn, unpublished
P2gal	16.5	gal	Kuempel and Duerr, 1978
P2serB	100	serB	Kuempel et al., 1978
P2IV-IX			Six, 1960, 1966, 1968, and unpublished
186	51	pheA	Woods and Egan, 1974
P4	97	supP	Calendar et al., 1981

K12, although site II, which is equivalent to the site II found in *E. coli* C, is occupied more frequently than than the others.

A P2 attachment site linked to the *his* gene of *K. pneumoniae* has also been reported (Streicher *et al.*, 1972).

2. Integration

P2 integrates via the so-called Campbell model by site-specific recombination between a bacterial *att* site and the *att* site of the cir-

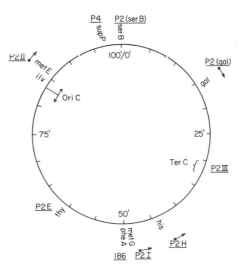

FIGURE 4. Prophage attachment sites. A generalized map of the *E. coli* chromosome including both strains C and K12. The locations of the various prophage attachment sites together with some genes known to be closely linked, and the origin (*oriC*) and termination (*terC*) of bacterial replication, are marked. The arrows indicate the direction of replication if initiated from the prophage (compare with Fig. 2).

cularized phage DNA (Calendar and Lindahl, 1969). The *recA* host system is not required. The orientation of the prophage at sites I, II, and H has been determined (Calendar and Lindahl, 1969) (Fig. 4), and the phage *att* site has been found to lie between genes *D* and *int* (Fig. 2). A number of P2 deletions have overlapping left ends beginning at 72.2% from the left end of the linear map (Hyde and Bertani, 1975). Assuming that the deletions have arisen when the phage was in the prophage state, 72.2% would mark the position of the phage *att* site. This region has been sequenced (Haggård-Ljungquist, personal communication), but the extent of the *att* site is still unknown. The hybrid phage-host *att* sites at the ends of the prophage have been cloned (Bertani, unpublished) but not yet sequenced. Phages with altered site specificity (*saf*) have been isolated from lysogens with a prophage at site II (Six, 1966). The *saf* mutation has been localized to the presumed phage *att* region (Haggård-Ljungquist, personal communication).

The integration of phage P2 into site I in *E. coli* C is very efficient (Bertani, 1980). The only phage product known to be required is that of the *int* gene (Lindahl, 1969b; Choe, 1969). The gene has been cloned (Ljungquist and Bertani, 1983) and found to produce a protein of 35 kD in minicells. Its direction of transcription has been determined (Ljungquist and Bertani, 1983) (Fig. 2). The gene is expressed regardless of its orientation in the plasmid and thus is presumed to have its own promoter, although this has not yet been identified. It is also expressed when P2 superinfects immune lysogens (Bertani, 1970), suggesting that it is constitutive.

The *int* gene has been sequenced recently (Haggård-Ljungquist, personal communication). When the amino acid sequences of a number of site-specific recombinases were compared (Argos *et al.*, 1986), the P2 *int* protein was found to be related to the *int* gene products of phages 186 and P22 but not to that of P4.

The *int* gene product is also involved in prophage excision and site-specific recombination between lytically multiplying phages.

3. Excision

In addition to the *int* gene product, prophage excision requires the product of a second gene, *cox* (Lindahl and Sunshine, 1972). Phage mutated in the *cox* gene lysogenize as well as or better than wild-type phage (Bertani, 1980) and also recombine with higher frequency in the *att* region (see Section III.A.5). The *cox* gene product may interact with that of the *int* gene to improve the specificity of the *int* protein for the phage-host hybrid *att* sites at the ends of the prophage, at the same time reducing its ability to act on pure phage *att* sites. The *cox* gene has recently been sequenced (Haggård-Ljungquist *et al.*, 1987) and found to code for a slightly basic protein of 91 amino acid residues. The gene appears to be repressor-controlled (Bertani, 1980) and is cotranscribed with gene B (Haggård-Ljungquist et al., 1987). Its product has also been implicated in the control of C gene transcription and in autoregulation of the early operon (Saha et al., 1987b) as well as in the induction of P4 by P2 (Six and Lindqvist, 1978) (see Section V.E).

In spite of the combined activities of the int and cox genes, prophage excision in P2 is inefficient. Following inactivation of the repressor by exposure to high temperature, only about 1% of the derepressed bacteria produce phage (Bertani, 1968). This appears to be due to insufficient int gene product, as induction approaches 100% if the heat-treated bacteria also carry a multicopy plasmid containing an active int^+ gene (Ljungquist and Bertani, 1983). Increased excision also results when double lysogens with two prophages in tandem at the same bacterial attachment site are formed. These strains segregate single lysogens at high frequency unless the int gene in the center of the structure is inactivated by a mutation (Choe, 1969; Bertani, 1971). In contrast, P2 double lysogens with prophages at distinct sites are very stable. These results might mean that the level of expression of the P2 int gene depends on whether the gene has phage DNA or host DNA downstream to it.

The proportion of P2 lysogens producing phage can also be raised to almost 100% by the cis-dominant phage mutation, nip1 (Calendar et al., 1972; Bertani, 1980), with the cox gene product still being required as well. The nip1 mutation appears to lie within the coding region of the int gene (Haggård-Ljungquist, personal communication; I. Dodd, personal communication). Its presence does not increase the amount of int protein produced in a minicell system (Ljungquist and Bertani, 1983). The nip1 mutation may make the int protein better suited to carry out recombination between the prophage ends. The int and cox gene products also interact in site-specific recombination between lytically multiplying phages (Section IV.E).

The induction of phage 299 has been reported to be abortive like that of P2 (Golub and Zwenigorodsky, 1969), suggesting its int gene may be similarly controlled.

4. Eduction

When prophage P2 occupies site H in E. coli K12, it generates deletions that include his and at least eight other adjacent genes (Kelly and Sunshine, 1967; Sunshine and Kelly, 1971; Templin et al., 1972; Neuhard and Thomassen, 1976). This phenomenon has been called eduction. One end of the deletion is always determined by the prophage site, whereas the other is variable. Although the "educed" genes are not essential to the host, alterations in the pools of deoxyribonucleotides have been observed when the *dcd* gene was deleted (Neuhard and Thomassen, 1976). Eduction depends on the *int* gene product and is increased by the presence of the *nip1* mutation (Sunshine, 1972). It is independent of the *cox* gene product or the RecA system of the host. Eduction, involving the *his* gene as well as some of the genes for nitrogen fixation, has also been observed in *K. pneumoniae* (Streicher *et al.*, 1972).

5. Integrative Suppression

The integration of an independent replicon into the chromosome of *E. coli* may confer on the bacteria the ability to replicate (integrative suppression; Nishimura *et al.*, 1971) even under conditions where the bacterial replication system is inactive. The replication is found to initiate at, and have the properties of, the integrated element. This was first demonstrated for P2 by Lindahl *et al.* (1971), using a temperature-sensitive *dnaA* strain of *E. coli* K12. The suppressed bacteria were found to be carrying a prophage close to the *metE* gene (site II), and the replication was found to be dependent on the gene *A* product of the phage.

Suppression has also been reported to occur when the prophage is located near the *serB* gene and to be dependent on bacterial *rep* function (Lindahl, in Kuempel *et al.*, 1978). These two sites are not far from the origin of replication of the host (Bird *et al.*, 1972). Integration at other sites, such as H (Kuempel *et al.*, 1977) and gal (Kuempel and Duerr, 1978), which are closer to the terminus region (Louarn *et al.*, 1977), does not result in suppression, although replication is initiated within the prophage. In both suppressed and nonsuppressed strains, the replication may begin unidirectionally like that of the phage, but it eventually becomes bidirectional like that of the host and terminates when the replication fork reaches the terminus at 30–35 min. The phages recovered from integratively suppressed strains carry insertions (Lindahl *et al.*, 1971). In one of these, P2 *sig5*, the new sequence is identical to the *IS2* insertion element (Saha and Haggård-Ljungquist, personal communication).

Suppression of a replication defect can also be demonstrated for a "phasmid" prepared by fusing phage P2 with a multicopy plasmid pBR322 through an *Eco*RI restriction site (Nicoletti and Bertani, 1983). This construct retains both the phage and the plasmid replication specificities. It can produce phage in a *polA*⁻ host in which the replication of pBR322 is restricted, and to a limited extent in *rep*⁻ strains in which P2 by itself cannot multiply. It can also replicate when the P2 moiety carries a mutation in gene *A*, one of the genes necessary for phage replication.

6. Exclusion of λ (Gene *old*)

Phage λ cannot replicate in the presence of P2 prophage owing to a complicated interplay between the gene products of both phages and those of the host. Sironi (1969), Lindahl *et al.* (1970), and Sironi *et al.* (1971) noted that P2 makes tiny, clear plaques on and is unable to lysogenize *recB⁻ recC⁻* bacterial hosts. Phages with mutations in the *old* gene are able to grow on such strains (Sironi, 1969; Lindahl *et al.*, 1970), producing large turbid sectors in the wild-type plaques and forming stable lysogens. It was found that the *recB⁻ recC⁻* mutants were killed by the activity of the *old⁺* gene product. The *old⁺* gene has recently been cloned (Finkel *et al.*, 1986) and has been found to be lethal when transferred into *recB⁻ recC⁻* strains, but the details of the interaction are not yet understood. Lindahl *et al.* (1970) suggested that modification of the host DNA by the P2 *old⁺* gene product might interfere with replication unless removed by the action of the *recB recC* genes. Shinomija and Sakaki (1979) observed, however, that a temperature-sensitive *recB⁻* lysogen was not killed by a P2 *old⁺* prophage when incubated at the nonpermissive temperature.

The *old⁺* gene also interferes with the multiplication of phage λ which is inhibited at an early stage following infection of a P2 lysogen (Lindahl *et al.*, 1970; Sironi *et al.*, 1971; Cohen and Chang, 1971; Brégégère, 1974). Bacterial protein synthesis is disrupted, and several species of transfer RNA are inactivated (Brégégère, 1974). Aside from an *old⁺* P2 prophage, inactivation requires the λ gene products *O* and *P* (Brégégère, 1976), the λ replication origin, and the host *dnaB* gene product (Brégégère, 1976, 1978). Derivatives of λ (*spi⁻*) that lack the nonessential genes *red* and *gam* (Sironi *et al.*, 1971) and have a *chi* recombinational hot spot (Malone and Chattoraj, 1975) are able to multiply in *rec⁺* P2 *old⁺* lysogens. Strains carrying the cloned *old⁺* gene in low copy number also inhibit λ and can be used to select for the Spi-phenotype (Finkel *et al.*, 1986). The λ *gam* gene product has been shown to inhibit the product of the *recB* and *recC* genes, DNA exonuclease V (Sironi *et al.*, 1971; Unger and Clark, 1972; Sakaki *et al.*, 1973), and it has been suggested (Sironi *et al.*, 1971) that in the course of its multiplication λ converts the host cell to a RecBC phenotype which then makes it susceptible to the P2 *old⁺* gene product.

Based on these observations, a cloning system using a λ vector has been developed (see Maniatis *et al.*, 1982). The replacement of λ genes *gam* and *red* by the cloned DNA allows the resultant phage to be selected on a P2 lysogen. This technique has found wide application.

The *old* gene has also been implicated in the increased sensitivity to X-rays shown by P2 lysogens (Ghisotti *et al.*, 1979). Both λ exclusion and X-ray sensitivity are suppressed by mutations in a bacterial gene, *pin*, mapping at 12 min on the *E. coli* chromosome (Ghisotti *et al.*, 1983). This gene is distinct from the *sbc* mutations that suppress *recBC* (Templin *et al.*, 1972).

The P2-related phage, HK-239 (Dhillon and Dhillon, 1973), that is serologically identical to P2, also excludes λ.

7. Genes Z and fun

Two nonessential genes, Z and fun, are located among the genes for tail synthesis (Fig. 2). This region of the P2 chromosome can be deleted ($del2$: Chattoraj et al., 1975) without disturbing either the multiplication of the phage or its ability to form lysogens. The fun^+ gene makes P2 unusually sensitive to 5-fluorodeoxyuridine (FUDR) (Bertani, 1964). P2 is the only member of the family known to have a Fun$^+$ phenotype (Bertani, unpublished).

Mutations in gene Z give a clear-plaque phenotype and constitute some 10–15% of all the clear mutations isolated in P2 (Bertani, 1976). Z mutants are able to lysogenize $E.$ $coli$ C but render the host cells susceptible to a low-molecular-weight substance that is produced by the cells themselves and accumulates in the medium (Bertani, 1978). The clear-plaque phenotype is thus due to killing of the host rather than to a defect in lysogenization. Z mutations can be suppressed by closely linked secondary mutations (Bertani, 1976). Suppressed Z mutants form stable lysogens that have an FUDR-resistant (Fun$^-$) phenotype (Bertani, unpublished), suggesting that the suppressor mutations are in the fun gene. The function of the Z^+ gene product may be to control the expression of gene fun.

8. Phage 186

Prophage 186 has been located at 51 min on the $E.$ $coli$ map, between genes $nalB$ and $pheA$ (Woods and Egan, 1974). This is presumably a preferred location as several independently isolated lysogens all gave the same result. The ability of phage 186 to integrate is destroyed by the $ins3$ insertion at 70.3% (Bradley et al., 1975), thus localizing the int gene. Sequencing in this region reveals a potential int protein of molecular mass 37 kD or 336 amino acid residues (Kalionis et al., 1986a) that appears to be related to the int proteins of P2 and P22 (Argos et al., 1986).

That 186 is inducible (Woods and Egan, 1974) suggests that, unlike the case of P2, the int gene of 186 is expressed efficiently following derepression of the prophage. Hocking and Egan (1982c) found that the 186 int gene was repressed by CI gene product, and recent sequencing (Kalionis et al., 1986a) shows that there are no transcription stop signals between CI and int; in fact, the genes overlap by a couple of nucleotides (Appendix B). Thus, the int gene is presumed to be transcribed from pC, the promoter for gene CI, although how it is regulated is still not clear.

Phage 186 appears to have an Old$^-$ phenotype. The phage gives turbid plaques on $recB^-$ strains and, when present as a prophage, does not inhibit λ (Woods and Egan, 1974).

Under conditions of limited glucose, prophage 186 has been found to confer a growth advantage on the host (Edlin et al., 1977).

E. Recombination

1. Phage P2

The unusually low frequencies of recombination observed with P2 (Bertani and Bertani, 1971) are obtained for lytically multiplying phages in mixed infection. The majority of recombinants in such crosses are produced by site-specific recombination, mediated by the *int* gene product, and confined to the phage *att* sites (Lindahl, 1969b). Recombination between mutations in genes *D* and *C*, which are separated by about 2 kb of DNA, approaches 0.2% and appears to be limited by the amount of *int* gene product available: the frequency of recombination obtained for *int*[+] and *int*[−] parental phages is intermediate between that obtained for *int*[+] only or *int*[−] only (Lindahl, 1969b). In addition, when recombination is carried out in the presence of an *int*[+] gene cloned into the multicopy plasmid pBR322, the frequency is 10 times higher (Bertani *et al.*, 1981; Ljungquist and Bertani, 1983). It can also be increased 5–20 times by using parental phages that are *cox*[−] (Lindahl and Sunshine, 1972), suggesting that the *cox* gene product interferes in some way with *int*-mediated recombination (Bertani, 1980). This effect of *cox* is no longer seen when excess *int* gene product is supplied by the multicopy *int*[+] plasmid (Ljungquist and Bertani, 1983).

Recombination between markers in genes *L* and *D*, which are separated by about 15 kb DNA, occurs with a frequency of about 0.01%, regardless of whether the host is *recA*[+] or *recA*[−] (Hudnik-Plevnik and Bertani, 1980). This low frequency seems to be associated with P2 replication, as recombination within an integrated prophage (Wiman *et al.*, 1970) or nonintegrated, but nonreplicating P2 DNA (G. Bertani, personal communication) is higher. Furthermore, when crosses are made between derivatives of the P2–P4 hybrid Hy19 (Section III.C), in which the left two-thirds of the P2 chromosome is joined to the P4 replication system, the frequency of recombination between markers in genes *L* and *D* increases to 1–2% (G. Bertani and Lindqvist, personal communication). This result is dependent on the host bacteria being *recA*[+]. These observations have led to the hypothesis that the P2 mode of replication makes DNA inaccessible to the recombination systems of the host (Hudnik-Plevnik and Bertani, 1980). Recombination in P2 can also be stimulated by irradiation with ultraviolet light. This effect is seen only in *recA*[+] hosts (Hudnik-Plevnik and Bertani, 1980) and might be a result of the temporary inhibition of replication produced by irradiation as well as activation of repair systems.

In the lytic cycle, recombination probably takes place between circular monomers, as these are the main *in vivo* forms of P2 DNA that are observed (Section IV.A). In addition, the genetic map has been found to be circular (Bertani, 1975). In any case, a single reciprocal recombination event would lead to a circular dimer which is packaged with very low efficiency by the P2 *ter* system (Pruss *et al.*, 1975; see Section IV.B). Thus, any dimers formed would have to be resolved by a second recombinational event. Bertani (1975) obtained evidence that, at least in the case where the first recombinational event is *int*-mediated, a second event occurs at or near to the *ori* site, and Bertani *et al.* (1981) suggested that it might be related to the initiation of replication. Hudnik-Plevnik and Bertani (1980) observed that artificially prepared dimers gave rise to somewhat higher frequencies of recombination than monomers, as if dimer formation might also be limiting.

The short sequences called *chi* sites that give rise to recombinational "hot spots" in phage λ through the activity of the host RecBC system (Smith and Stahl, 1985) have not been found in the approximately 20 kb of P2 DNA sequenced so far (Haggård-Ljungquist, personal communication).

2. Phage 186

Phage 186 exhibits the same low frequency of recombination as P2, with *int*-mediated site-specific recombination at about 0.2% and non-*int* recombination at 0.01% (Hocking and Egan, 1982c). However, covalently closed circular 186 DNA is cut by the *uvrA* and *recA* host functions when psoralen-damaged 186 phages superinfect a 186 lysogen (Ross and Howard-Flanders, 1977), a situation in which 186 is nonreplicating. Thus, as in the case of P2, replicating 186 DNA may be inaccessible to bacterial recombination enzymes, even though the two phages exhibit differences in replication requirements (see Section IV.A). The observation by Mandel and Kornreich (1972) that recombination between a pair of 186 mutants was increased 10-fold in mixed infection with λ *red*[+] phages has not been followed up.

V. THE LIFE CYCLE OF PHAGE P4

A. Replication

1. Replication Requirements

Although P4 depends on a helper to produce phage particles, its DNA replication is autonomous (Lindqvist and Six, 1971) and differs from that of the P2-like phages in a number of ways. First of all, it is bidirectional, beginning at a unique origin (*ori*) located about 22% from the right end of the 11.5-kb molecule (Krevolin *et al.*, 1985) (Fig. 2). The DNA in this region is rich in A–T base pairs and contains several repeats of 12 or 13 nucleotides (Lin, 1984). Deletion analysis has revealed a second region, *crr* (Fig. 2), located 4.7 kb to the left of *ori*, that is also required in *cis* (Krevolin *et al.*, 1985). DNA sequencing shows *crr* to be located just beyond the transcriptional terminator for gene α and to consist of two direct 120-bp repeats that are separated by 60 bp. Each repeat contains three copies of an octamer found also six times in *ori*. Either of the repeat sequences suffices for replication to occur, and *crr* can also function when inverted or when its distance from *ori* is changed (Flensburg and Calendar, 1987).

Replication of P4 requires the function of its gene α (Gibbs *et al.*, 1973) and possibly also that of another P4 coding sequence, *orf106*, which is located between genes α and ε and can encode a 12-kD polypeptide (Flensberg and Calendar, personal communication). Only one host gene, *dnaE*, appears to be required. The host's *rep* gene and the functions used for the priming of host DNA replication are not needed (Lindqvist and Six, 1971; Barrett *et al.*, 1972; Bowden *et al.*, 1975; Krevolin and Calendar, 1985) (see Table IV).

Phage P4 can complement P2 mutants that are defective in gene *B*, which is necessary for P2 DNA replication (Six and Lindqvist, 1978), suggesting the possibility that P4 possesses an as yet unidentified gene, the equivalent of P2 gene *B*, that may also be involved in P4 DNA replication.

Gene α extends from base pair 4674 to base pair 7007. This sequence corresponds to a polypeptide of 777 amino acid residues with a molecular mass of 84.8 kD. The product of gene α has been partially purified. It is a rifamycin-resistant RNA polymerase (Barrett *et al.*, 1972, 1983) that appears early in infection and, *in vitro*, will synthesize poly G in the presence of an appropriate, artificially prepared template. No other transcribing activities have been detected. This P4-encoded protein, thought to be a DNA primase, has been shown to play an essential role in an *in vitro* system designed to study P4 DNA replication (Krevolin *et al.*, 1985). Besides P4 DNA and the partially purified α protein, the system contains also *E. coli* DNA polymerase III holoenzyme and *E. coli* single-strand binding protein. Only supercoiled P4 DNA was found to act as template.

2. Synthesis and Termination

Replicating P4 DNA molecules are seen in the electron microscope as structures with long (2 kb) single-stranded regions adjacent to the replication fork, apparently the result of discontinuous replication (Krevolin *et al.*, 1985). The size distribution of Okazaki fragments obtained from P4-infected, DNA polymerase I-deficient bacteria shows no discrete classes, suggesting that such replicative intermediates begin and end at random locations on the DNA molecule (Kahn and Hanawalt, 1979). The finished product of the replication is a covalently closed P4 DNA monomer (Lindqvist and Six, 1971) that, in the presence of a helper, can be packaged into a phage head. In the absence of a helper, P4 DNA replication will continue past the end of the P4 latent period (Lindqvist and Six, 1971; Six and Lindqvist, 1978), possibly indefinitely, and may lead to the establishment of P4 genomes as high-copy-number plasmids (see Section V.F).

B. Morphogenesis, Packaging, and Lysis

1. Helper Dependence

The production of P4 virions depends on all the known late gene products of the helper phage—18 in the case of P2 (Six, 1975) and 20 in the case of phage 186 (Sauer *et al.*, 1982). These genetic observations are corroborated by the findings that all P2 virion proteins are also present in the P4 virion (Table I) and that P4 always displays the host range and antigenicity of its latest helper (Six and Klug, 1973; Sauer *et al.*, 1982; Poon and Dhillon, 1986). Given the scope of P4's helper dependence, it can be assumed that the phage will follow the morphopoietic pathways of the helper but with one major exception—the determination of the size of its capsid. The DNA molecule of P4 is only about one-third the size of that of the helper. Thus, the phage requires a smaller capsid of suitable size.

2. Head Size Determination (Gene *sid*)

Head size is determined by a P4 function rather than by some characteristic of the DNA to be packaged. Shore *et al.* (1978) identified the responsible P4 gene, *sid*, by a mutation, *sid1*, that abolishes P4's ability to specify the assembly of small heads. The mutation reduces the burst size of P4 (Diana *et al.*, 1978; Geisselsoder *et al.*, 1978), but it is not lethal. Analysis of *sid* protein synthesis (Lee, 1981) and DNA sequencing (Lin, 1984) showed the *sid* gene (located from base pair 2060 to 1326) to encode a 27-kD polypeptide, hence accounting for protein 3 of Barrett *et al.* (1976), and also identified *sid1* as an *amber* mutation, which Kurnit *et al.* (in preparation) found to be suppressible by *supF*.

The mechanism by which the *sid* function controls head size is not yet understood. An early suggestion (Geisselsoder *et al.*, 1978) that *sid* would exert a transcriptional control, via antitermination, appears less attractive now. P4 does antagonize ρ-mediated termination via the function of its *psu* gene (see Section V.D), but *psu*⁻ mutants themselves remain Sid⁺ (Sauer *et al.*, 1981). The Psu deficiency noted for P4 *sid1* presumably implies that *sid1* is polar on *psu*; another Sid⁻ mutant, P4 *sid2*, remains Psu⁺ (Kurnit *et al.*, in preparation). Nevertheless, the host's ρ function does appear to influence head size determination. For even in the absence of P4, Geisselsoder *et al.* (1978) found P2 to produce a majority of small heads and proheads when infecting a ρ-deficient host. As the ρ gene is known to be pleiotropic, it seems possible that the *sid* function antagonizes a ρ function different from termination. Possibilities for the mode of *sid* action considered by Barrett *et al.* (1976) include a role of the *sid* gene product as a scaffolding protein, as a modifier of the processing of the major head protein of P2, or as a component of the P4 capsid. These authors reported P4 heads to contain some P4 protein 4 as well as a small amount of P4 protein 3, later identified as *psu* and *sid* protein, respectively (see Table I), but the significance of these findings remains to be elucidated.

Because the *sid* gene induces the formation of capsids too small to package P2 DNA, P4 will interfere with the production of P2 in mixed infection (Diana *et al.*, 1978). P2 mutants designated *sir* have been selected because they are impervious to the action of P4 *sid*; i.e., they assemble large heads even in the presence of P4 (Six *et al.*, in preparation). Three such mutations were found to be missense mutations and were mapped to the middle of the *N* gene, indicating that the gene for the major P2 head protein also carries information essential for the determination of head size. Katsura (1983) reached a similar conclusion in the case of head size determination by phage λ.

3. Packaging of DNA

The *in vivo* packaging of P4 DNA into P4-size heads, being a helper-dependent process, is assumed to proceed from circular molecules. An *in vitro* packaging system accepts mature linear DNA (Pruss *et al.*, 1975), but circular molecules remain the preferred substrate (Pruss *et al.*, 1975).

A special situation obtains when P4 DNA has to be packaged into large, P2-size heads. For *in vivo* packaging of P4 *sid*, it has been shown that such heads usually contain two or three P4 genomes; single genomes, packaged into large heads, could account for at most 1% of the viable phage progeny (Shore *et al.*, 1978). If packaging occurs *in vitro*, then two or three mature DNA monomers may be packaged together into a P2 head (Pruss *et al.*, 1974b; Goldstein *et al.*, 1974), or multimeric, mainly trimeric, circular DNA may serve as packaging substrate (Pruss *et al.*, 1975).

Presumably *in vivo* packaging into P2-size heads proceeds from covalently closed dimers or trimers, filling the heads with the corresponding mature multimeric molecules, rather than with two or three monomers. So far, however, this has been documented only by Bowden and Modrich (1985), who obtained covalently linked trimeric DNA from P4 *sid* virions. Multimeric P4 DNA circles must occasionally be generated in P4-infected cells (Diana *et al.*, unpublished, as quoted in Geisselsoder *et al.*, 1978) and will be selected for packaging into large heads. Multimers can persist through subsequent rounds of lytic multiplication, since the helper's terminase will cut even trimeric P4 DNA only once (Bowden and Modrich, 1985). *In vivo*-produced P4 *sid* virions contain mainly dimers (Shore *et al.*, 1978), although trimers are preferred for *in vitro* packaging (Pruss *et al.*, 1975).

The size of DNA known to be packageable into P4 heads ranges from about 9.7 kb (for Hy8; Lindqvist, 1981a; see Section III) to about 14 kb (for a P4 kanamycin-resistant derivative; Shore, as quoted by Kurnit et al., in preparation), a spread of 1 : 1.4, the same as reported for the λ packaging system (Feiss et al., 1977).

4. Lysis

As in the case of the other late functions of the lytic cycle, P4 depends on its helper for lysis of the host cell (Six, 1975; Sauer et al., 1982). In cells mixedly infected with P4 and helper, the latent period is normally that characteristic of the helper, and the burst produced is mixed, with the two phages contributing roughly equal numbers of particles and the total burst size being close to 100. However, if P4 has to activate the expression of its helper's late genes, either because the helper is replication-deficient or because it is present as a prophage, then the latent period is prolonged, and essentially only P4 is produced. Typical values for P4 infection of a P2 lysogen are a latent period of about 60 min and a burst size of about 100 P4. Because of the poor excision of the helper (see section IV.D) and the effect of the sid gene on head size (see Section V.B), only about one helper particle per 10^6 P4 will be produced (Six and Klug, 1973; Six, 1975).

C. Regulation

There is evidence that P4 lytic multiplication is under a trans-acting negative control. The replication of superinfecting P4 DNA is blocked in wild-type P4 lysogens, regardless of whether a helper prophage is present (Six and Klug, 1973) or not (Six and Lindqvist, 1978). The latter observation also shows that a helper is not required for P4 to express immunity. In addition, P4 is zygotically inducible (Calendar et al., 1981), but no temperature-inducible mutants have been found.

Calendar et al. (1981) demonstrated two complementing classes of clear plaque—forming mutants, corresponding to genes CI and CII. In a deletion analysis of the P4 hybrid, P420 (see Section III), Kahn et al. (1980) found that immunity to superinfection was associated with the CI region. DNA sequencing of this region (Lin, 1984) reveals an open reading frame encoding a polypeptide of 15 kD or 137 amino acid residues. The carboxy-terminal one-third of the molecule contains 22% arginine and is thus very basic. All CI mutations sequenced so far fall into this reading frame, including those that have been selected for the Ash phenotype (Lin, 1984; Lane and Six, unpublished; see Section V.D). Of the eight mutational sites identified, seven are clustered within a 16-bp interval in the first 40% of the gene, and the eighth is 21 bp further upstream. Unexpectedly, two of these mutations do not alter the amino acid sequence encoded by this gene. Nevertheless, the phenotype of a *CI amber* mutation (so identified by sequencing) responds to *amber* suppressors (Lane and Six, unpublished), giving indirect genetic evidence that the gene is translated and that the gene product is a protein. Although P4 has not been demonstrated to be inducible by ultraviolet light, the hypothetical *CI* gene product contains three of the *ala-gly* sequences that are cleaved by the *recA* protease (Little and Mount, 1982).

So far, no mutations defining the repressor-binding sites have been isolated. The mutation designated *vir1* (Lindqvist and Six, 1971) appears a likely candidate, as it greatly reduces the repressibility of genes α and ε, but it is probably a promoter rather than an operator mutation (see below; promoters). The region around the early promoter, pLe (see below; promoters), contains some repeated sequences (Lin, 1984), but whether these represent repressor-binding sites remains to be established.

1. Transcription Patterns

The transcription of P4, like that of its helper P2, is sensitive to rifamycin, presumably reflecting its dependence on the transcriptase of the host (Lindqvist, 1974). Harris and Calendar (1978) found all early transcription to be leftward (see Fig. 2) and late transcription to go in both directions, with the rightward transcription depending on the functions of genes α and δ.

The presence of a helper P2, either as prophage or as coinfecting phage, greatly stimulates P4 transcription, causing transcripts to appear earlier and in larger amounts (Lindqvist, 1974; Harris and Calendar, 1978). This "reciprocal transactivation" of P4 will be taken up again in Section V.E. In the presence of a helper, rightward transcription no longer requires the δ function but retains its dependence on the α function (Harris and Calendar, 1978). Hence, rightward transcription may depend on P4 replication.

2. Promoters

Two early promoters, pI and pLe, both resembling the *E. coli* consensus sequence (Appendix B), have been identified. pI precedes the *int* gene (Pierson and Kahn, 1987) and is most likely an *int* promoter. It is located at 66.4% (base pair 7660–7689; Flensburg and Calendar, personal communication; see Fig. 2) in the nonessential region of the P4 chromosome. Earlier, Harris and Calendar (1978) had found that leftward *in vitro* transcription originated in this region, and other *in vitro* studies by Lindqvist and Williams (1979) revealed that three strong binding sites for the bacterial RNA polymerase were located here.

The promoter pLe, located at 26% (base pair 2915–2944; Lin, 1984), appears to be the promoter for genes *CI*, as well as ε and α (Dehò, personal communication). This suggests that there ought to be a mechanism that allows expression of only the *CI* gene when the other genes are repressed. The *vir1* mutation (Lindqvist and Six, 1971), at 22% (base pair 2544; Lin, 1984), is a C to T base change that generates another promoter for early leftward transcription, pV (Appendix B), upstream to pLe (Dehò, personal communication). Transcription from pV should extend to genes α and ε, since *vir1* renders the expression of these genes immunity-insensitive (Six, unpublished). For P4 wild type, by contrast, a very similar transcript originates only at late times from a promoter, pLl (Appendix B), located very close to the *vir1* site and probably overlapping the pV sequence. Hence, for wild-type P4, the origin of the *CI*-ε-α transcript apparently shifts from pLe to pLl (Dehò, personal communication).

The promoter for the (late) rightward transcription, pR, was found at 18% (base pair 2121–2093; Lin, 1984; Dale *et al.*, 1986). It resembles the *E. coli* consensus even less than pLl (Appendix B). It is not surprising, therefore, that its efficient use apparently depends on the function of either P4 gene δ or P2 gene *ogr* (Dale *et al.*, 1986).

Pierson and Kahn (1987) found another potential promoter for the *int* gene, PIl, about 90 bp downstream from pI. The pIl sequence resembles that of P2 late promoters, including the 10-bp consensus sequence found downstream to the transcription start site (see Appendix B). For its possible significance, see Section V.F.

3. RpoA and *org*

The *rpoA109* mutation that blocks P2 late gene expression (Section IV.C) also interferes with the P2-assisted growth of P4, albeit to a lesser degree (Sunshine and Six, unpublished), and it is not clear to what extent this effect simply reflects the helper dependence of P4. But P4 mutants with *rpoA109* suppressors, called *org*, have been isolated, and two such mutants were found to carry the same missense mutation in gene δ (at 8% or base pair 951; Lane, Six, and Sunshine, unpublished).

D. P4 Effects on Helper

Given P4's profound dependence on a helper, a variety of interactions between the two phages can be expected. Indeed, the existence of these functional and regulatory interrelations between two genomes that otherwise show so little DNA sequence similarity is one of the most interesting aspects of the P2–P4 system.

The natural hosts for phage P4 are presumably bacteria lysogenic for one or another of the P2-like phages rather than bacteria that have been simultaneously infected with the helper phage as well. This means that P4 has to be able to activate the expression of the helper prophage genes.

P4 can achieve this goal by either of two pathways, one requiring helper DNA replication and the other not.

1. Derepression

The principal mechanism to activate the expression of a helper's genes is to derepress the prophage (Six and Lindqvist, 1978). Derepression will trigger *in situ* replication of the prophage, thus boosting the helper gene dosage and activating expression of the helper's late genes.

The P4 gene ε has been identified (Geisselsoder *et al.*, 1981) as being responsible for the derepression of P2. It is located in the middle of the essential region of the P4 genome (Fig. 2) and extends from base pair 3468 to 3755 with base pair 3489 being the site of a C to T transition that defines the mutation *am104* (Lin, 1984). This sequence encodes a polypeptide of 95 amino acid residues, starting with a GUG codon. It overlaps slightly the *CI* gene upstream to it but uses a different reading frame. A single base pair insertion in *CI* apparently has no effect on the function of ε and provides further evidence that ε is a separate gene. The nature of the ε function remains to be elucidated; the gene product may act as an antirepressor. The ε function can be overwhelmed—for example, when P4 infects bacteria carrying the P2 repressor gene cloned into a multicopy plasmid (Westöö and Ljungqvist, 1980).

How wide is the action spectrum of P4's hypothetical antirepressor? The P2 family of phages includes at least six immunity specificities: P2, Hy dis, P3, W-φ, φ-D145, and 186 (Bertani and Bertani, 1971). P4 can grow well in lysogens of P2 and its homoimmune derivatives PK and 299 (Bertani and Bertani, 1971; Six and Klug, 1973) as well as in lysogens of Hy dis and W-φ (Six and Lindqvist, 1978). The ability of P4 to form plaques with φ-D145 prophage as helper is temperature-sensitive (Bertani and Bertani, 1971). P4 cannot form plaques on, or derepress, P3 or 186 lysogens (Sauer *et al.*, 1981; Six, unpublished). Mutations in the *CI* gene, called *ash* for adaptation to secondary helper, enable P4 to form plaques on P3 lysogens. The *ash* mutation may allow the ε gene to be expressed more strongly or for a longer time (Lin, 1983, 1984; Lin and Six, unpublished). No comparable mutants have been found for adaptation to 186 lysogens.

Barclay and Dove (1978a) isolated a P2 mutant, P2 *sos*, that cannot be derepressed by P4. The *sos* mutation is dominant in P2 double lysogens; in nonlysogenic hosts, it affects the ability of P2 neither to multiply nor to help P4. It is possible that the *sos* mutation alters the P2 repressor, but unfortunately no further studies on this mutant are available.

If the ε gene product is an antirepressor and interacts directly with the repressor of P2 and not with that of phage 186, then the sequences of these genes may provide some clues as to the mechanism of action. In any case, it must be different from the mechanism of spontaneous derepression of P2, since P4 can still derepress lysogens carrying P2 *sly1* (Six and Lindqvist, 1978; see Section III.C).

2. Transactivation

Derepression alone can account for P2 late-gene activation only if the P2 genome is replication-proficient. The requirement for DNA replication as a precondition for the expression of P2 late genes does not apply when P4 is present. P4 can directly transactivate the late genes of a nonreplicating helper such as P2 (Six, 1975). Using a replication-deficient P2 as helper will lengthen the latent period of P4 by about 20 min, but it will not adversely affect the P4 burst size. Similarly, P4 was found able to transactivate a derepressed, replication-deficient 186 (Sauer *et al.*, 1982). Gibbs *et al.* (1983) showed that extracts from P4-infected (nonlysogenic) bacteria could stimulate the P2 DNA-directed synthesis of late P2 proteins in an *in vitro* system. Similarly, Valla and Lindqvist (1978) obtained preliminary results suggesting that such *in vitro* transactivation could also be detected at the level of P2 transcription. A P4-promoted association of nonreplicating P2 DNA with the bacterial membrane fraction may be related to transactivation (Ljungquist, 1976).

Souza *et al.* (1978) identified the gene, δ, responsible for transactivation of both P2 and 186 (Sauer *et al.*, 1982). It extends from base pair 1329 to 829 (Lin, 1984), overlapping slightly the *sid* gene upstream. Hence a possible translational coupling of δ to *sid*, as well as ρ-dependent polarity of *amber* mutations, may explain why P4 *sid1* is transactivation deficient (Dehò, as quoted by Sauer *et al.*, 1981). Four missense mutations that abolish the δ function have been sequenced ($\delta35$ by Lin, 1984; $\delta1$, $\delta4$, and $\delta6$ by Halling, Zylbert, and Calendar, personal communication).

The δ function can substitute for that of P2's *ogr* gene and that of the *B* gene of phage 186 (Sauer *et al.*, 1982). Christie and Calendar (1984) found that P4-transactivated transcription starts from the same sites as those chosen by P2 itself, at least for the promoters of genes *O* and *P*. As already mentioned (Section V.C), δ also resembles *ogr* in that the bacterial *rpoA109* mutation interferes with its function and in that this gene can acquire suppressing mutations (called *org* rather than *ogr*).

The δ gene product also exhibits some structural similarity to the gene products of P2 *ogr* and 186 *B:* the sequence of the first 40 amino acid residues shows 47% identity with the P2 *ogr* protein (Christie *et al.*, 1986) and 45% with 186 *B* (Kalionis *et al.*, 1986b). The δ gene product is somewhat more than twice the size of the other two, however, and its amino acid sequence resembles a dimer of the *ogr* protein (Halling and Calendar, personal communication). Perhaps this dimer structure explains why δ, unlike *ogr*, can transactivate even nonreplicating P2 genomes.

Transactivation also depends on the function of P4's α gene (Lindqvist *et al.*, 1978; Gibbs *et al.*, 1983) but perhaps only indirectly, in that transcription of δ depends on the α function (Harris and Calendar, 1978), possibly because it requires P4 DNA replication.

Under most circumstances, the δ function does not seem essential for P4's lytic growth. It therefore appears to be of limited significance, and the δ gene may be a remnant of P4's evolutionary past, although it does extend the P4 host range somewhat (e.g., to Rep⁻ hosts) and may account for the P4 production in P2 hosts containing excess repressor (Westöö and Ljungquist, 1980) and perhaps also for the spontaneous P4 production by double lysogens of P4 and 186 or P4 and P3 (Six and Sunshine, unpublished).

3. Polarity Suppression

The rightmost gene on the P4 map, *psu*, endows P4 with the ability to suppress polar effects of transcriptional termination signals, in particular those associated with certain *amber* mutations in P2 late genes (Barrett *et al.*, 1976; Sunshine *et al.*, 1976). Sauer *et al.* (1981) identified the P4 gene responsible and showed the *psu* gene product to be identical with protein 4 of Barrett *et al.* (1976). According to the DNA sequence (Dale *et al.*, 1986), the gene extends from base pair 755 to 186 and hence encodes a polypeptide of 190 amino acid residues; the mutation *psu1* is a double *amber* (at base pairs 697 and 358), whereas *psu3* is a missense mutation (at base pair 250).

The mechanism of action of gene product *psu* is not known. Since missense mutations in δ cause some reduction in polarity suppression, whereas *psu* mutations do not affect transactivation, the *psu* function may be performed by a complex of the δ and *psu* gene products (Sauer *et al.*, 1981). Targets of this function are not only the ρ-dependent terminators in the P2 *amber* mutants, but they also include the terminator of the *E. coli trp* operon (Lagos *et al.*, 1986). Unlike the antitermination function of phage λ's *N* gene, the *psu* function is nonessential (except under very contrived experimental conditions), although its lack does reduce the P4 burst size somewhat (Sauer *et al.*, 1981). Lagos *et al.* (1986) discuss the possible role of a δ-*psu* antagonism for the control of P4 gene expression.

4. Head Size Determination

The role of P4's *sid* gene in head size determination was considered in Section V.B.

5. Possible Pleiotropy of Gene ε

The mutation *am104* in gene ε is pleiotropic, apparently causing a delay in the onset of the *sid* function and preventing P4 from using a gene

A defective, heat-derepressed P2 prophage as helper (Diana *et al.*, 1978; Geisselsoder *et al.*, 1981). Whether *am104* exhibits polar effects has not been investigated. It should be noted, however, that the region between genes ε and α contains two open reading frames of unknown function, with coding capacities for 151 and 106 amino acids, respectively (Lin, 1984; Flensburg and Calendar, personal communication). The situation is further complicated by the fact, discovered later on, that the *am104* mutant also carries the *ash9* mutation (Lin, 1983; Lin and Six, unpublished).

6. Additional Observations

Barclay and Dove (1978b) isolated mutants of *E. coli* C that do not allow P4 to use prophage P2 as a helper, although the mutants, when nonlysogenic, remain permissive for P2. They also isolated P4 *gog* mutants that are able to grow in the mutant hosts when lysogenic for P2. Which genes were mutated in the host and in P4, respectively, is not known.

Similarly, Six and Sunshine (unpublished) isolated an *E. coli* C strain with a mutation, *lpf1*, that interferes with P4's ability to use P2 as a helper without blocking the growth of P2 itself. They mapped *lpf1* very close to *rpoA109* and also noticed that several *ash* mutations of P4 could suppress *lpf1*.

The ability of P4 to complement gene *B*-defective mutants of P2 has already been mentioned in Section V.A.

E. Helper Effects on P4

1. Induction of P4

Not only can P4 derepress P2 lysogens, the converse also holds. The infection of P4 lysogens with P2 induces the production of P4 (Six and Lindqvist, 1978) in most bacteria. Thus, derepression as well as efficient P4 prophage excision must occur. The function of the P2 *cox* gene is necessary to obtain induction (Six and Lindqvist, 1978). This gene is known to be involved in P2 prophage excision; how it can also, directly or indirectly, affect P4 induction is not known. However, a recent suggestion (Saha *et al.*, 1987b) that *cox* gene product may antagonize the expression of P2 gene *C* should be considered. The *cox* function is not needed for P2 to act as a helper or for the spontaneous P4 production by P2–P4 double lysogens. Among P2-related phages, P2 Hy dis and P3 can induce P4, whereas phage W-φ and Hy5, which carries the early genes of 186 (Section III.C), cannot (Six and Sunshine, unpublished).

2. Transactivation of P4 by P2

A comparison of P4 transcription levels in P4-infected P2 lysogens versus nonlysogens provided the first evidence for the transactivation of

P4 by P2 (Lindqvist, 1974). Harris and Calendar (1978) could show that it is the transcription of the P4 late genes that is stimulated by P2 and that this transcription becomes independent of P4's δ function (itself late). These findings agree well with those of Barrett *et al.* (1976) that in mixedly infected bacteria, P2 stimulates and accelerates the production of specific P4 proteins, later shown to be the products of genes *sid* and *psu*, and with those of Souza *et al.* (1977) that even δ-defective P4 mutants will produce late P4 proteins in the presence of P2. Hence, the ability of P2 to transactivate P4 plays an important role in P4's lytic growth cycle.

It seems likely that the P2 *ogr* gene, which is essential for P2 late-gene expression, is also responsible for transactivating P4 late genes. Indeed, Dale *et al.* (1986) found that production of *ogr* from an expression vector activates P4 late gene transcription. Although there seems to be little resemblance between the late-gene promoters of P4 and P2 (see Appendix B), at least in the -10 and -35 regions, Dale *et al.* (1986) can recognize additional sequence similarities further upstream (a dyad symmetry centered around the -57 position) that are shared by all these promoters.

Is the P2 *ogr* (or the equivalent 186 *B*) function essential for the lytic pathway of P4 δ$^+$? The available evidence suggests that it is not, as a 186 *B*$^-$ mutant (*Bam17*) is an efficient helper for P4 (Sauer *et al.*, 1982). Similarly, with a 186 *Bam17*-P2 (Ogr$^-$) hybrid as helper, P4 phage production showed a near-normal latent period as well as phage yields (Six and Sunshine, unpublished). In the case of P2 as helper for P4, some, though weaker, evidence derives from experiments with a host carrying the *rpoA109* mutation. This mutation blocks the wild-type *ogr* function of P2 (see Section IV.C) but nevertheless allows *ogr*$^+$ genomes to help P4, at least under certain conditions (Sauer *et al.*, 1982; Sunshine and Six, unpublished). Interference by nonfunctional *ogr*$^+$ protein with the δ function may complicate matters. Clearly, experiments with the P2 *ogr* deletion mutant could settle this issue.

This leaves the question if perhaps other helper functions could be involved in allowing efficient expression of P4 late genes, possibly by triggering a positive feedback loop in which the δ function could autoactivate the further expression of P4 late genes (including δ). Indeed, studies of P2 prophage deletions suggest that the growth of P4 requires the function of an as yet unidentified P2 early gene (Barclay and Dove, 1978a).

F. The Prophage

Phage P4 can lysogenize in either the absence or presence of a helper such as prophage P2. Two types of P4 lysogens have to be distinguished: (1) lysogens that carry a single P4 prophage (or rarely 2 prophages) inserted into the bacterial chromosome, and (2) lysogens that carry multiple copies of the P4 genome as plasmids, with or without the presence of an integrated copy. Apparently the two types of lysogens correspond to different regulatory states of the P4 genome. Lysogenization by wild-type P4 normally leads to single-copy integrants that display the typical superinfection immunity of "classical" lysogens and we shall consider these first.

1. Bacterial Attachment Sites

Calendar *et al.* (1981) located the primary P4 attachment site on the *E. coli* K12 chromosome very close to *supP* (now *leuX*)—i.e., at about 97.1 min on the 100-min K12 map (Bachmann, 1983; Fig. 4)—and found this site to be indistinguishable from the one on the *E. coli* C chromosome previously recognized by Six and Klug (1973). Pierson and Kahn (1987) have since found that (in *E. coli* C) P4 integrates at the 3' end of the *supP* (*leuX*) gene. Calendar *et al.* (1981) also recognized, but did not map, secondary P4 sites on the K12 chromosome that were occupied under conditions requiring the presence of two P4 (mutant) prophages. Using other selective conditions, Ow and Ausubel (1983) could demonstrate the existence of a P4 site on the *K. pneumoniae* chromosome.

2. Integration

Like P2, P4 inserts itself into the chromosome by site-specific recombination that occurs between a bacterial *att* site and the *att* site on the circularized P4 chromosome. It does not depend on the host's *recA* system but requires the function of a *trans*-acting P4 gene, *int*. The *int* gene and the *att* site are found very close to each other at 73% and 67%, respectively, on the map (Fig. 2). Hence, P4 hybrid genomes lacking the part of the P4 DNA to the left of the *Eco*RI site at 68.6% are *int*⁻ and *att*⁺ (Calendar *et al.*, 1981; Pierson and Kahn, 1984).

Pierson and Kahn (1987) have sequenced the P4 *int* gene and its *att* region (*attP*), as well as the primary integration site (*attB*), on the *E. coli* K12 chromosome. They find that *attP* contains a 20-bp core fragment (GAGTCCGGCCTTCGGCACCA) that also occurs in *attB* and is flanked by fivefold repeats (not present in *attB*) with the whole *att* region extending over about 300 bp. An open reading frame extending from base pair 7716 to 9038 can be assigned to the *int* gene. According to the amino acid residue sequence predicted by the open reading frame, P4 integrase belongs to the family of integrases recognized by Argos *et al.* (1986) and resembles the integrase of φ80 more closely than others, including the P2 integrase. Depending on the start codon (ATG) chosen, the predicted size of the P4 integrase ranges from 48 to 51 kD. Two possible promoter sequences (pI and PII; see also Section V.C) precede the *int* gene, and Pierson and Kahn (1987) suggest roles for both of them in the control of *int* gene expression. pI, which resembles the *E. coli* consensus sequence (Appendix B), is located close to *att* and thus may allow autoregulation of the *int* gene, since binding of integrase to *att* may interfere with the binding of RNA polymerase to pI.

The other possible promoter, PII, located about 90 bp downstream from pI, resembles P2 late promoters (Appendix B) and therefore may not be recognizable by unmodified polymerase. But in P4 lysogens infected with P2, the *ogr* function of P2 could conceivably cause a strong *int* gene expression from PII. Since the *int* function appears to be required also for P4 excision (see below), such an *ogr*-mediated effect of P2 could be important for the induction of P4 lysogens by P2. Furthermore, Pierson and Kahn (1987) note that for a P4 prophage integrated at its primary site (i.e., inserted into the distal portion of *supP*), transcription from the *supP* promoter could possibly extend beyond *supP* to read the *int* gene. This might provide the P4 prophage with a means to monitor the physiological state of its host.

Surprisingly, P4 appears not to need its *int* function for inserting itself into the *K. pneumoniae* chromosome, although the *int*⁻ *att*⁺ P4 hybrid studied uses its *att* site for prophage establishment, and the latter remains *recA*-independent. Either a host function can substitute for that of *int* or the presence of a cryptic P4-related prophage supplying *int* function could account for these findings (Ow and Ausubel, 1983).

Pierson and Kahn (1987) recognized that the *E. coli* K12 sequence downstream of *supP* (determined by Yoshimura *et al.*, 1984) contains a region resembling the P4 *int* gene and speculate that this may indicate the presence of a cryptic P4-related prophage in K12, although they found no such sequence in the *attB* site of strain C.

3. Excision

P4 production by cells carrying only an integrated P4 genome—the spontaneous P4 release by cells lysogenic for P4 and a helper (Six and Klug, 1973) and the induction of P4 from P4 lysogens by infection with helper phage (Six and Lindqvist, 1978)—presumably depends on P4 excision. Lack of P4 release from cells lysogenic for P2 and an *int* deletion mutant of P4 (P4 Hy1; Calendar *et al.*, 1981) suggests that the P4 *int* function is required also for excision; no P4 gene dedicated to excision has been found. There is no evidence that P4 excision requires a helper function. Indeed, the generation of multicopy P4 plasmids from an integrated P4 genome, which occurs when cultures of a P4 *vir1* α *ts* lysogen are shifted from a nonpermissive temperature to a lower temperature allowing α function (Lagos and Goldstein, 1984), shows that P4 excision can occur in the absence of a helper. Transfer of a P4 prophage, by conjugation or transduction, into a recipient lacking P4 does not lead to noticeable P4 excision (Calendar *et al.*, 1981), suggesting that a P4 excision function, if it exists, is not under the control of P4 immunity.

4. The CII, gop, and β Genes

P4 lysogens are obtained following infection only if the CII gene, located at approximately 81% on the map, is functional. Infection with P4 CII mutants will kill the host even in the absence of a helper prophage. The CII point mutations are recessive and can be suppressed by mutations in the gop gene, which is located to the left of CII at about 90% on the map (Calendar et al., 1981; Fig. 2). By definition, gop mutations allow P4 to grow in pin3 mutant hosts (Ghisotti et al., 1983; see Section IV.D). The mechanisms involved are not known. It is possible that gop is the same gene as β, especially since most Ts+ revertants of β ts mutants become Gop (Ghisotti et al., 1983). P4 β ts mutants cannot grow at nonpermissive temperatures, but the phenotype of the original β ts mutant (then called Bts; Gibbs et al., 1973) also includes the killing of nonlysogenic bacteria at nonpermissive temperatures. Hence, the CII gene may be a negative control gene for the β-gop gene, and the latter, if not checked by the CII function, may kill the host, possibly after P4 prophage establishment.

5. P4 Cointegrates

Phage P4 can insert itself, though very rarely, into plasmid pJW7 (see Section III.C) by a crossover event occurring at or near the P4 att site and at one of at least two sites in the plasmid (Williams and Six, unpublished). P2–P4 hybrids such as Hy213 (Lindqvist, 1981a) presumably arose, as pointed out in Section III.C, from a recombinational event between P2 and P4, involving the att site of P4 and a suitable site in P2 gene P (followed by the ter function-mediated deletion of most of the P2 genome from the cointegrate). Whether these cointegrations actually depend on the att site and/or int function of P4 remains to be tested.

6. The Plasmid Lysogenic State

To maintain themselves as plasmids, P4 genomes must be capable of indefinite autonomous replication. It is therefore not surprising that in the absence of a helper (prophage)—i.e., when infecting nonlysogenic cells—P4 will establish a plasmid state, provided it carries a mutation that interferes with P4's self-repression, such as vir1 (Calendar et al., 1981; Goldstein et al., 1982) or certain CI mutations (cI405; Dehò et al., 1984) and several other ash mutations (Lin, 1983; Six, unpublished). On the other hand, Dehò et al. (1984) found that even lacking such mutations, P4 can assume the multicopy plasmid state—though it does so only rarely (in about 0.3% of cells lysogenized with wild-type P4)—whereas infections with P4 vir1 or P4 cI405 generate mostly multicopy lysogens with a copy number, for all three P4 genotypes, of about 40. Multicopy lysogens of wild-type P4, thus established, convert spontaneously, at a relatively low rate, to single-copy integrants or, more rarely yet, lose P4 entirely. Multicopy P4 *vir1* lysogens similarly convert to a low-copy-number state (with an integrated copy plus about 3 plasmid copies), whereas P4 *cI405* lysogens appear incapable of undergoing such conversions. Conversion in the opposite direction (to multicopy lysogens) requires induction, which can be achieved by various means including superinfection with P2 *cox*$^+$ or P4 *vir1*. For P4 *vir1* lysogens growing in a rich medium, the copy number can be controlled to assume high, low, or intermediate values by the choice of the growth conditions (Lagos and Goldstein, 1984), whereas P4 wild-type lysogens cannot be similarly influenced (Dehò *et al.*, 1984).

The presence of an integrated P4 genome is compatible with that of multiple plasmid copies (Calendar *et al.*, 1981; Goldstein *et al.*, 1982; Dehò *et al.*, 1984). Lagos and Goldstein (1984) found that P4 *vir1 del2*, which is *int*$^-$ and probably also *att*$^-$, is unable to lysogenize and suggested that an integrated P4 genome might be essential as a "master copy" for the maintenance of the multicopy lysogenic state.

However, Dehò *et al.* (1984) found that not all ($\leq 80\%$) multicopy lysogens of P4 *int*$^+$ *att*$^+$ carry an integrated copy. Furthermore, *att*$^-$ derivatives of P4 *vir1* exist as multicopy plasmids in *E. coli* (Ow and Ausubel, 1983) as well as in *K. pneumoniae* (Ow and Ausubel, 1980). Thus, the maintenance of P4 plasmids appears to depend on various physiological and genetic factors, some not yet identified. This may also explain why only Lin (1983) and Six (unpublished) found P4's δ function to interfere with lysogenization by P4 *vir1*.

P4 may maintain a multicopy plasmid state even if the host carries a P2 prophage, as found for P4 *vir1* (Calendar *et al.*, 1981) and several P4 *ash* mutants (Lin and Six, unpublished). This implies that gene expression for P4 plasmids is regulated, as will be considered below.

In multicopy plasmid lysogens, P4 does not appear to be as stringently repressed as it is in single-copy integrants. Superinfecting P4 will simply join the P4 plasmid pool, and superinfecting P2 can induce the lysogens (as long as they are not immune to P2), even if it is defective in its *cox* (*sin*) function (Dehò *et al.*, 1984; see Section V.E). However, there is evidence that the gene expression of P4 plasmids remains regulated and that in plasmid lysogens at least some P4 genes are not fully expressed. These include genes with the following functions: (1) the *sid* function, responsible for P4's interference with P2 growth, since only P2 *cox*$^+$ elicits severe interference when infecting P4 *CI-ash* multicopy lysogens (Six and Sunshine, unpublished); (2) the ε function (and possibly also the δ function), since P2 lysogens carrying multicopy P4 plasmids are stable (as already mentioned above); (3) the *kil* function. This function is responsible for P4 *cI405* infections killing bacteria that are not lysogenic for P4, although P4 *cI405* plasmid lysogens are viable. P4 *cI405 kil*$^-$ mutants have been isolated (Alano *et al.*, 1986).

Superinfecting P4 apparently becomes subject to the regulatory regimen exerted in plasmid lysogens; i.e., superinfecting wild-type P4 will not cause a switch to stringently repressed, single-copy integrants. In addition, plasmid lysogens are immune to killing by P4 *cI405* (Alano et al., 1986), and those carrying a helper prophage are immune as well to initiation of lytic growth by superinfecting P4 *vir*+ (Lin and Six, unpublished).

These findings, and further results of Alano et al. (1986), can be summarized in the following, very tentative general pattern of possible sequences of regulatory states that the P4 genome may experience. When P4 infects a host (not carrying P4), there will be an initial uncommitted state of P4 gene expression and replication. About 30 min later, a fraction of the infected cells will become multicopy plasmid lysogens. The P4 genomes in the remaining (majority of) infected cells may be considered to be in the "temperate phage state." About an hour later, some of these cells will have entered the single-copy-integrated (stringently repressed) state.

In the other cells, P4 will follow the lytic pathway, provided a helper is present. In its absence, the fate of these cells will depend on the expression of P4's *kil* function. If the latter is not expressed, the cells will survive and become stable lysogens. There is, of course, also the possibility that the P4 genomes will be lost; but the rate of loss appears to be quite low, since lysogenization frequencies for hosts lacking a helper appear to be quite high (Six and Klug, 1973; Calendar et al., 1981; Dehò et al., 1984; Alano et al., 1986). The presence of a helper genome will undoubtedly modify to some extent the P4 regulatory pattern by regulatory interactions and by providing the means for the lytic growth of P4.

7. Filamentation

Under certain conditions, P4 will interfere with host cell division, causing filamentous cells to appear. A necessary condition for filament induction appears to be that the level of P4 self-repression is reduced (to below that characteristic for P4 wild type in the single-copy-integrated state). The necessary conditions can be met for certain P4 lysogens. This allowed Dehò et al. (1984) to depend on filamentation to recognize multicopy plasmid lysogens. All such lysogens, regardless of the P4 genotype (wild type, *vir1*, or *cI405*) and in contrast to the corresponding single-copy integrants, formed small colonies consisting of filamentous bacteria; this presumably accounts for the typical "rosette" shape of such colonies. Goldstein et al. (1982) and Lagos and Goldstein (1984), however, did not find rosette formation for P4 *vir1* multicopy lysogens, indicating that reduction of the P4 repression level—or, at any rate, the multicopy plasmid state—is not sufficient to ensure filamentation.

Lysogens of most P4 *CI-ash* mutants can undergo filamentation whether they harbor detectable P4 plasmids or not. In this case, however, filamentation appears to be temperature-dependent: it is suppressed at high temperature (42°C) and most strongly exhibited at low temperature (30°C) (Lin, 1983).

The mechanism responsible for P4-induced filamentation appears not to be connected to the host's SOS response (Lin, 1983). According to Lagos et al. (1986), this filamentation is likely to result from P4's *psu* function antagonizing the ρ function of the host.

G. Recombination

Recombination between P4 phages resembles that between P2 phages in several respects (Dehò, 1983). The genetic map is circular, and recombination frequencies are, in general, quite low. Also, P4's *int* system apparently makes a major contribution to overall recombination; if markers are selected from opposite (*att–cos*) arms of the P4 chromosome, recombination frequencies are 10- to 100-fold higher than when the selected markers are from the same arm. On the other hand, recombination frequencies between markers on the same arm are 100-fold lower if the host is RecA$^-$, indicating that P4 DNA is more accessible than P2 to bacterial recombination systems (Dehò, personal communication). There is no evidence so far that P4 possesses its own general recombination system.

Rather wide variations notwithstanding, an efficiency for general recombination (i.e., excluding *int*-promoted recombination) of about $1/10^8$ to $1/10^7$ per base pair appears characteristic of P4 and may be compared with values of about $1/10^8$ for P2 and about $1/10^6$ for the P2–P4 hybrid Hy19 (see Section IV.E). In this regard, it may be relevant that the P4 crosses, but not the others, took place in cells lysogenic for P2. Hence, of the three recombination efficiencies mentioned above, only the Hy19 value, not the P2 or the P4 value, refers to recombination occurring in the absence of P2 early genes (and their functions).

H. P4 as a Cloning Vehicle

P4, in conjunction with its helper (in particular P2), offers some promise as a versatile cloning vector, as may be seen from the outline of P4 biology just given and as already noted by Kahn and Helinski (1978), Ow and Ausubel (1980, 1983), Calendar et al. (1981), Goldstein et al. (1982), and Lagos and Goldstein (1984). Several restriction sites are already available for cloning purposes in the nonessential region of the P4 chromosome, including unique sites for *Pst*I, *Sal*I, and *Pvu*II (Fig. 3).

Cloned DNA can be propagated either by the lytic P4 cycle or as a multicopy plasmid or as integrated, single-copy prophage. If in circular form, such DNA may be taken up directly by competent host bacteria. Otherwise, it may be introduced by infecting cells with phage particles packaged *in vitro* according to established procedures (Pruss *et al.*, 1974, 1975).

For *in vitro* packaging and for propagation by the lytic cycle, two kinds of phage heads are available—the P4 and the P2. A P4 head will allow cloning of an insert of 2 to perhaps 4 kb of foreign DNA (if nonessential P4 DNA is deleted). Ow and Ausubel (1980, 1983) used phages with P4 heads to clone the *his* and *nif* genes of *K. pneumoniae* and the *tetR* gene of pACYC 184. Use of a P2 head for *in vivo* packaging (i.e., during lytic growth) requires that P4 carry either a *sid* mutation or the helper a *sir* mutation. Under these conditions, the size of acceptable inserts should be about 20–25 kb, or possibly even somewhat larger. Kurnit *et al.* (in preparation) used a P4 *sid* derivative to clone a 25-kb human DNA fragment. Dehò and Zangrossi (personal communication) used a P2 *sir* mutant as helper in conjunction with a P4 *sid*⁺ vector.

The lytic cycle may be initiated either by (an insert-carrying) P4 infecting or transfecting cells lysogenic for a helper or by a helper infecting cells lysogenic for (an insert-carrying) P4.

To aid in the selection of such P4 lysogens, antibiotic resistance genes have been incorporated into the P4 genome (e.g., tetR, kanR; Ow and Ausubel, 1983; Lagos *et al.*, 1986). P4's own replication mechanism can be replaced with that of another replicon, such as *colE1*, without the modified vector losing its character as a "phasmid" (Kahn *et al.*, 1980; Lindqvist and Lund, personal communication).

The host range of P4 is known to include, besides its original host species *E. coli* and *Sh. dysenteriae* (Six and Klug, 1973), *K. pneumoniae* (Ow and Ausubel, 1980, 1983) and *Pseudomonas putida* (for a P4-*Pseudomonas* plasmid hybrid; Dehò and Zangrossi, personal communication). In addition, cosmid vectors have been designed for introducing cloned DNA into bacteria into which P2-like phage particles can inject their DNA. Their usefulness was demonstrated in work with *Rhizobium meliloti*, which does not permit growth of P2 itself (Kahn and Timblin, 1984; Kahn *et al.*, in preparation).

ACKNOWLEDGMENTS. The authors are indebted to Rich Calendar, Gianni Dehò, Barry Egan, Richard Goldstein, Elisabeth Haggård-Ljungquist, Conrad Halling, Mike Kahn, and Mel Sunshine for their generosity with comments and unpublished data; to Norman Horowitz for the use of his word processor and expertise; and to the Energy Conservation and Utilization Technology Division of the Department of Energy and the National Institutes of Health (grant AI-04043) for financial support.

VI. APPENDIXES

A. Physical Maps of Selected Restriction Sites and Other Features of P2 and 186

1. Phage P2 DNA[a]

Uncut by enzymes *Hind*III or *Xho*I
Cut once by *Bal*I, *Pvu*II, *Sma*I, *Xba*I, and *Sna*BI
Cut twice by *Sal*I
Cut three times by *Ava*I, *Bam*HI, *Bgl*II, *Eco*RI, *Kpn*I, and *Pst*I
Cut 6 times by *Mlu*I
Cut 10 times by *Hpa*I

Percent from left end	Enzyme	Gene or site located
0		
0.8	*Bam*HI	
5.4	*Sal*I	
6.6	*Bam*HI	Cuts gene *P*
7.4	*Pvu*II	Cuts gene *P*
10.5	*Eco*RI	Cuts gene *O*
12.8	*Kpn*I	Cuts gene *N*
13.5	*Pst*I	Cuts gene *N*
17.4	*Hpa*I	
18.8	*Mlu*I	Cuts gene *L*
29.3	*Bal*I	
33.4	*Hpa*I	
36.8	*Sal*I	
37.7	*Ava*I (*Sma*I)	
43.2	*Hpa*I	
45.3	*Bam*HI	
47.5	*Eco*RI	
48.7	*Hpa*I	
50.0	*Xba*I	
51.2	*Bgl*II	
56.0	*Hpa*I	
57.6	*Hpa*I	
62.6	*Pst*I	Cuts gene *T*
65.8	*Kpn*I	
72.2		Attachment site (*att*)
75.4	*Bgl*II	Cuts gene *int*
76.3	*Hpa*I	
76.7	*Pst*I	Cuts gene *C*
77.2	*Bgl*II	
79.3	*Hpa*I	Cuts gene *B*
79.9	*Eco*RI	Cuts gene *B*
88.7	*Hpa*I	Cuts gene *A*
89.0		Replication origin (*ori*)
95.8	*Ava*I	Cuts gene *old*
97.2	*Ava*I	Cuts gene *old*

Percent from left end	Enzyme	Gene or site located
98.4	KpnI	
98.7	HpaI	

2. Phage 186 DNA[b]
   Uncut by XhaI
   Cut once by BglII and XhoI
   Cut twice by HindIII
   Cut three times by EcoRI
   Cut seven times by BamHI
   Cut 22 times by PstI

Percent from left end	Enzyme	Gene or site located
0		} no known genes
2.3	EcoRI	} geneW
10	BamHI	} gene V
13.3	EcoRI	} genes U-R
22.3	BamHI	} gene Q
25.3	BamHI	} genes P-N
32.7	BamHI	cuts gene L
37.0	BamHI	} genes M-L
37.6	HindIII	} genes L-G
58.7	BamHI	
61.3	HindIII	
65.4		Hy5; cuts gene E
65.5	PstI	cuts gene D
		} gene B
67.6	XhoI	
67.9		left end of Del1
67.9		attachment site (att)?
69.1	KpnI	
70.2	SacI	
70.3		Ins3; cuts gene int
73.1	SalI	
73.6		Ins1; cuts gene CI
73.8		Ins2; cuts gene CI
74.9		right end of Del1
77.4	PstI	
81	BglII	
84.6	PstI	cuts gene LA
87.5	PstI	cuts gene RA
92.0	EcoRI	
92.9		replication origin (ori)
93.8	PstI	
95.8	BamHI	} no known genes
100		

[a]Data compiled from Saint and Egan, 1979; Westöö and Ljungquist, 1979; Haggård-Ljungquist, personal communication; Six, unpublished data.
[b]Data compiled from Younghusband et al., 1975; Saint and Egan, 1979a,b; Finnegan and Egan, 1979, 1981; Sivaprasad, 1984; Kalionis et al., 1986a.

B. Selected Sequences

1. Cohesive Ends[a]

a. Left

```
P2   5' - GGCGAGGCGGGGAAAGCACTGCGCGC ---
                                 ACGCGCG ---
299  5' - . . . . . . . . . . . . T . . . . . . . . . . ---
186  5' - . . . . T . . . . . . . . . T . . . . . . . ---
P4   5' - . . . . . . . . . . . . . . . . C . . . . . . ---
```

b. Right

```
P2   --- GCGGGCG
     --- CGCCCGCCCGCTCCGCCCCTTTCGTG  - 5'
299    -- . . . . . . T . . . . . . . . . . A . . . . .  - 5'
186  --- G . A . . . T . . . . A . . . . . . . . . . . A  - 5'
P4   --- TCG . . . . . . . . . . . . . . . . . . . . .  - 5'
```

2. Phage Promoters and Other Regulatory Sequences[b]

			−35	−10
E. coli consensus sequence:			TTGACA	TATAAT
Phage	Promoter	Gene(s) controlled	−35	−10
P2	pC	*C*	ATGAAT	TATAAT
P2	pE	*cox, B, (A?)*	TTGACA	TAGTAT
P2	pOgr	*ogr*	TTGTTT	TAAAAT
P2	pF	*F, E, T, U, D*	ATAGCC	GAAAAT
P2	pO	*O, N, M, L, K, R, S*	ATGGCG	GAAACT
P2	pP	*P, Q*	TTAGCG	TAGCCT
P2	pV	*V, J, H, G*	ATAGCA	CAATCT

Additional sequences found near P2 late gene promoters:
```
pP  at position:   +7  TATTCATCAC
                  +24  TATTCATGAC
pO                +28  TATTCAGGAC
pV                +23  TATTCAGGAA
```

Inverted repeat at position −57:
```
pP   TGGCTTATCACTGACACA
pO   TGTGTCAGTGATAAGCCA
pV   TGTCTGGTAGTCTACAAA
pF   TGTGCTGTCGATTAGCCA
```

186	pL	*CI, int*	TTGCGA	CATGAT
186	pR	*(CII, A?)*	TTTACT	TATATT
186	pB	*B*	TTCACA	TATCAT

Inverted repeats overlapping:
```
−10 of pB: TTTATGATTA - - - TATTCACGAA
−35 of pB: ATGATGAATA - - - TATTCACAAA
```

P4	pI	*int*	TTGAAA	CATAAT
P4	pVe	*CI, ε, α*	TTGCGT	TAAAAT
P4	pLe	*CI, ε, α*	TTGCCT	TATAGT
P4	pIl	*int*	AGACCG	AAACCT
P4	pLl	*CI, ε, α*	TTGCGT	CAAAAT
P4	pR	*sid, δ, psu*	TCGTGT	CACAAT

Inverted repeat at position −57 of pR:

TGTGTCAGGGCTGGCACA

The P2 late gene promoters and P4 pR have been identified by S1 mapping; the others are based on the DNA sequence.

3. Amino-Terminal Ends and Control Regions of P2 Genes *P*, *O*, *V*, and *F^c*

P:
```
GTA CAG CAG CGC CGC CTG ACG ACG CGG GTC GTG TAA AAG AGT GGT
Tyr Leu Leu Ala Ala Gln Arg Arg Pro Asp His Leu Leu Thr Thr

GTC TGT GGT GAT GGT CAT  GAATACCTCGCCGTGATGAATACACGGCAAGGCTA
Asp Thr Thr Ile Thr Met
                    +24                 +7              −10
                                           −57
CTGAGTCGCGCCCCGCGATCGCTAAGGTGCTGTTGTGTCAGTGATAAGCCATCCGGGAC
                    −35                       −57
          −35                      −10
TGATGGCGGAGGATGCGCATCGTCGGGAAACTGATGCCGACATGTGACTCCTCTAATCA
```

O:
```
       +28                          Met Ala Lys Lys Ala Ser Lys Phe Phe Arg
CTATTCAGGACTCCTGACA ATG GCA AAA AAA GTC TCA AAA TTC TTT CGT

Ile Gly Val Glu Gly Asp Thr Cys Asp Gly Arg Val Ile Ser Ala
ATC GGC GTT GAG GGT GAC ACC TGT GAC GGG CGT GTC ATC AGT GCG

Gln Asp Ile Gln Glu Met Ala Glu Thr Phe Asp Pro Arg Val Tyr
CAG GAT ATT CAG GAA ATG GCC GAA ACC TTT GAC CCG CGT GTC TAT

Gly Cys Arg Ile Asn Leu Glu His Leu Arg Gly Ile Leu Pro Asp
GGT TGC CGC ATT AAC CTG GAA CAT CTG CGC GGC ATC CTG CCT GAC

Gly Ile Phe Lys Arg Tyr Gly Asp Val Ala Glu Leu Lys Ala Glu
GGT ATT TTT AAG CGT TAT GGC GAT GTG GCC GAA CTG AAG GCC GAA

Lys Ile Asp Asp Asp Ser Ala Leu Lys Gly Lys Trp Ala Leu Phe
AAG ATT GAC GAT GAT TCG GCG CTG AAA GGC AAA TGG GCG CTG TTT

Ala Lys Ile Thr Pro Thr Asp Asp Leu Ile Ala Met Asn Lys Ala
GCG AAA ATC ACC CCG ACC GAT GAC CTT ATC GCG ATG AAC AAG GCC

Ala Gln Lys Val Tyr Thr Ser Met Glu Ile Gln Pro Asn Phe Ala
GCG CAG AAG GTC TAC ACC TCA ATG GAA ATT CAG CCG AAC TTT GCC

Asn Thr Gly Lys Cys Tyr Leu Val Gly Leu Ala Val Thr Asp Asp
AAC ACC GGC AAA TGT TAT CTG GTG GGT CTG GCC GTC ACC GAT GAC

Pro Ala Ser Leu Gly Thr Glu Tyr Leu Glu Phe  ----
CCG GCA AGC CTC GGC ACG GAA TAC CTG GAA TTC  ----
```

V:
```
-TTAGCCCCCACACATTAGTCACATTATAGCTGACCATTACGCTCTCCTTGAATGTTGT
  −57                    −35                     −10
CTGGTAGTTCTACAAATGAATCCAGATAGCATAACTTTTATATATTGTGCAATCTCACA
                         +23
       Met Asn Thr Leu Ala Asn Phe Gln Glu Leu Ala Arg Ala Leu
TGC ATG AAC ACT CTC GCA AAT ATT CAG GAA CTC GCG CGC GCA CTG

Arg Asn Met Ile Arg Thr Gly Ile Ile Val Glu Thr Asp Leu Asn
CGC AAC ATG ATT CGC ACT GGC ATT ATC GTC GAA ACC GAC CTT AAC

Ala Gly Arg Cys Arg Val Gln Thr Gly Gly Met Cys Thr Asp Trp
GCC GGT CGC TGC CGC GTG CAG ACC GGC GGC ATG TGC ACC GAC TGG
```

Leu Gln Trp Leu Thr His Arg Ala Gly Arg Ser Arg Thr Trp Trp
CTT CAG TGG CTG ACC CAT CGC GCA GGA CGT TCG CGC ACA TGG TGG

Ala Pro Ser Val Gly Glu Gln Val Leu Ile Leu Gly Ile   ----
GCA CCT TCC GTG GGG GAA CAG GTG CTG ATT CTG GGA ATT   ----

F: --GTACAAATCAGGGCAGGTGAGCGAATTGCCCGCCTTTTCTTTACCGGTGGTTGTGC
        −57   −35   −10
     TGTCGATTAGCCAACCGGGACAAATAGCCTGACATCTCCGGCGCAACTGAAAATACCAC
                                      Met Ser Asp Tyr His His Gly Val
     TCACCCATTAACCACGGAGTTAAACGG ATG AGT GAC TAT CAT CAC GGC GTG

Gln Val Leu Glu Ile Asn Glu Gly Thr Arg Val Ile Ser Thr Val
CAG GTG CTG GAG ATT AAC GAG GGC ACC CGC GTC ATT TCC ACC GTA

Ser Thr Ala Ile Val Gly Met Val Cys Thr Ala Ser Asp Ala Asp
TCC ACG GCC ATT GTC GGC ATG GTC TGC ACG GCC AGC GAT GCA GAT

Ala Glu Thr Phe Pro Leu Asn Lys Pro Val Leu Ile Thr Asn Val
GCG GAA ACC TTC CCC CTC AAT AAA CCT GTG CTG ATT ACC AAT GTG

Gln Ser Ala Ile Ser Lys Ala Gly Lys Lys Ala Thr Leu Ala Ala
CAG AGC GCA ATT TCA AAG GCC GGT AAA AAA GGC ACG CTG GCG GCA

Ser Leu Gln Ala Ile Ala Asp Gln Ser Lys Pro Val Thr Val Val
TCG TTG CAG GCC ATC GCT GAC CAG TCA AAA CCG GTC ACC GTT GTC

Met Arg Val Glu Asp Gly Thr Gly Asp Asp Glu Glu Thr Lys Leu
ATG CGC GTG GAA GAC GGC ACC GGT GAT GAC GAG GAA ACG AAA CTC

Ala Gln Thr Val Ser Asn Ile Ile Gly Thr Thr Asp Glu Asn Gly
GCG CAG ACC GTT TCC AAT ATC ATC GGC ACC ACC GAT GAA AAC GGT

Gln Tyr ----
CAG TAC ----

The −35 and −10 regions of the promoters are indicated. The consensus sequence
TATTCAGGAC appears at positions +7, +23, +24, and +28. An inverted repeat, found
also in the control region of P4 *sid*, centers around −57.

4. The Amino-Terminal End and Control Region of P4 Gene *sid*[d]

                        −57   −35
     ----GAGTCTCCTGTGTCAGGGCTGGCACATCTGCAATGCGTCGTGTTGTTGTCCGGTG
            −10   Met Ser Asp His
     TACGTCACAATTTTCTTAACCTGAAGTGACGAGGAGCCGGAAA ATG TCT GAC CAC

Thr Ile Pro Glu Tyr Leu Gln Pro Ala Leu Ala Gln Leu Glu Lys
ACT ATC CCT GAA TAT CTG CAA CCC GCA CTG GCA CAA CTG GAA AAG

Ala Arg Ala Ala His Leu Glu Asn Ala Arg Leu Met Asp Glu Thr
GCC AGA GCC GCC CAT CTT GAG AAC GCC CGC CTG ATG GAT GAG ACC

Val Thr Ala Ile Glu Arg Ala Glu Gln Glu Lys Asn Ala Leu Ala
GTC ACG GCC ATT GAA CGG GCA GAG CGA GAA AAA AAT GCG CTG GCG

Gln Ala Asp Gly Asn Asp Ala Asp Asp Trp Arg Thr Ala Phe Arg
CAG GCC GAC GGA AAC GAC GCT GAC GAC TGG CGC ACG GCC TTT CGT

Ala Ala Gly Gly Val Leu Ser Asp Glu Leu Lys Gln Arg His
GCA GCC GGT GGT GTC CTG AGC GAC GAG CTG AAA CAG CGC CAC ----

The −10 and −35 regions of the promoter are indicated, as well as an inverted repeat
centered around −57.

5. Carboxy-Terminal Ends of the P2 and 186 D Genes[e]

```
P2 D    Ala  Gln  Ala  Lys  Trp  Asp  Lys  Leu  Gln  Arg  Gly  Val  Ala  Glu  Phe
        GCT  CAG  GCG  AAG  TGG  GAT  AAA  CTG  CAA  CGG  GGC  GTT  GCG  GAG  TTC

186 D   ----                          Leu  Gln  Arg  Gly  Val  Ala  Glu  Phe
        ----                          ...  ..G  ..A  ...  ...  ...  ...  ..T
```

```
P2 D    Ser  Ile  Ser  Leu  Ala  Thr  Gly  Arg  Ala  Asp  Ile  Tyr  Thr  Glu  Thr
        TCT  ATC  AGC  CTA  GCT  ACC  GGT  CGG  GCA  GAT  ATT  TAC  ACG  GAA  ACA

186 D   Ser  Ile  Thr  Leu  Ala  Leu  Gly  Arg  Ala  Asp  Leu  Phe  Pro  Glu  Thr
        ..A  ..T  .CG  ..G  ..G  CTT  ...  ...  A..  ..T  ...  T.A  .T.  C.T  ..G  ...
                                                                        |
                                                                   Dam23,T
```

```
P2 D    Pro  Val  Lys  Val  Ser  Gly  Phe  Lys  Arg  Val  Ile  Asp  Glu  Gln  Asp
        CCG  GTC  AAA  GTG  TCT  GGC  TTT  AAG  CGC  GTC  ATA  GAC  GAG  CAG  GAC

186 D   Pro  Val  Arg  Val  Ser  Gly  Phe  Lys  Arg  Val  Ile  Asp  Glu  Gln  Ala
        ...  ..G  CGC  ..A  ..A  ...  ...  ...  ...  ...  ...  ..T  ...  ...  ..G
```

```
P2 D    Trp  Thr  Ile  Thr  Lys  Val  Thr  His  Phe  Leu  Asn  Asn  Ser  Gly  Phe
        TTG  ACA  ATC  ACT  AAG  GTG  ACA  CAT  TTT  CTG  AAT  AAT  AGC  GGC  TTC

186 D   Trp  Leu  Ile  Ser  Lys  Val  Thr  His  Asn  Leu  Asn  Asn  Ser  Gly  Phe
        .GG  TT.  ...  .G.  ...  ..A  ..T  ..C  AA.  ...  ...  ...  ...  ...
```

```
P2 D    Thr  Thr  Ser  Leu  Glu  Leu  Glu  Val  Arg  Leu  Ser  Asp  Val  Glu  Tyr
        ACG  ACG  TCC  TTA  GAG  CTT  GAG  GTC  AGG  CTT  TCT  GAT  GTG  GAG  TAC

186 D   Thr  Thr  Gly  Leu  Glu  Leu  Glu  Val  Lys  Leu  Ser  Asp  Val  Glu  Tyr
        ...  ...  GGC  ...  ...  ...  ...  ..T  .AA  ..C  ...  ...  ...  ...
                                               |
                                          Dam14,T
```

```
P2 D    Gln  Thr  Glu  ----  Asp  Asp  Glu       ----
        CAA  ACA  GAA  ----  GAT  GAT  GAG  TGA  ----

186 D   Gln  Ala  Glu  Ser  Asp  Asp  Glu       ----
        A.C  G.G  ...  TCG  ...  ...  ..A  .A.  ----
```

6. Control Genes P2 ogr, 186 B, and P4 δ[f]

```
P2 ogr  Met  Phe  His  Cys  Pro  Leu  Cys  Gln  His  Ala  Ala  His  Ala  Arg  Thr
        ATG  TTT  CAT  TGT  CCT  TTA  TGC  CAG  CAT  GCC  GCA  CAT  GCG  CGT  ACA

186 B   Met  Phe  His  Cys  Pro  Lys  Cys  His  His  Ala  Ala  His  Ala  Arg  Thr
        ...  ...  ...  ...  ..G  AAG  ...  ..T  ...  ...  ...  ...  ...  ..A  ...

P4 δ    Met  Ile  Tyr  Cys  Pro  Ser  Cys  Gly  His  Val  Ala  His  Thr  Arg  Arg
        ...  A..  T.C  ...  ..G  .CG  ..T  GGA  ...  .TT  ..T  ..C  A.C  ...  CGC
```

```
P2 ogr  Ser  Arg  Tyr  Ile  Thr  Asp  Thr  Thr  Lys  Glu  Arg  Tyr  His  Gln  Cys
        AGT  CGC  TAT  ATC  ACT  GAC  ACG  ACA  AAA  GAG  CGT  TAT  CAT  CAG  TGC

186 B   Ser  Arg  Tyr  Leu  Thr  Glu  Asn  Thr  Lys  Glu  Arg  Tyr  His  Gln  Cys
        ..C  ...  ...  C.A  ..C  ..A  .AC  ..T  ...  ..A  ..C  ..C  ..C  ...  ...
                                                                      |
                                                                  Bam57,T

P4 δ    Ala  His  Phe  Met  Asp  Asp  Gly  Thr  Lys  Ile  Met  Ile  Ala  Gln  Cys
        GCA  .AT  .TC  ..G  GAC  ..T  GGC  ..C  ..G  ATA  ATG  AT.  GCA  ...  ...
```

P2 ogr
| Gln | Asn | Val | Asn | Cys | Ser | Ala | Thr | Phe | Ile | Thr | Tyr | Glu | Ser | Val- |
| CAG | AAC | GTG | AAT | TGC | AGC | GCC | ACG | TTC | ATC | ACT | TAT | GAG | TCG | GTA |

ogr52,G

186 B
| Gln | Asn | Ile | Asn | Cys | Ser | Cys | Thr | Phe | Met | Thr | Met | Glu | Thr | Ile |
| ... | ... | A . C | .. C | .. T | .. T | TGT | ... | .. T | .. G | .. A | ATG | .. A | A .. | A .. |

P4 δ
| Arg | Asn | Ile | Tyr | Cys | Ser | Ala | Thr | Phe | Glu | Ala | Ser | Glu | Ser | Phe |
| . G . | .. T | A . T | T .. | ... | TCT | .. G | .. A | .. T | GAA | G . G | AG . | .. A | AGC | T . T |

P2 ogr
| Gln | Arg | Tyr | Ile | Val | Lys | Pro | Gly | Glu | Val | His | Ala | Val | Arg | Pro |
| CAG | CGA | TAC | ATC | GTG | AAG | CCG | GGA | GAA | GTC | CAC | GCC | GTA | AGG | CCG |

186 B
| Glu | Arg | Phe | Ile | Val | Thr | Pro | Gly | Ala | Ile | Asp | Pro | Ala | Pro | Pro |
| G .. | . C | . TT | .. T | .. T | . CT | ... | ... | . CC | A . T | G .. | C . G | . C . | CC . | .. T |

Bam17,T

P4 δ
| Phe | Ser | Asp | Ser | Lys | Asp | Ser | Gly | Met | Glu | Tyr | Ile | Ser | Gly | Lys |
| TTC | TCT | G .. | . GT | AAA | G . T | T : A | ... | ATG | . AA | T .. | ATT | TC . | G . C | AAA |

P2 ogr
| His | Pro | Leu | Pro | Ser | Gly | Gln | Gln | Ile | Met | Trp | Met | | ---- |
| CAC | CCG | TTG | CCA | TCA | GGG | CAG | CAA | ATT | ATG | TGG | ATG | TAA | ---- |

186 B
| His | Pro | Thr | Val | Gly | Gly | Gln | Arg | Pro | Leu | Trp | Leu | | ---- |
| ... | ... | ACT | GTC | GGT | .. T | ... | GG | CCA | T .. | ... | C . C | . G . | ---- |

P4 δ
| Gln | Arg | Tyr | Arg | Asp | Ser | Leu | Thr | Ser | Ala | Ser | Cys | Gly | Met | Lys |
| .. G | AGA | . AC | . GC | GAT | TCA | . T . | ACG | TCA | GCC | . CC | TGC | GGT | ATG | AAA |

P4 δ
| Arg | Pro | Lys | Arg | Met | Leu | Val | Thr | Gly | Tyr | Cys | Cys | Arg | Arg | Cys |
| CGC | CCG | AAA | AGA | ATG | CTT | GTT | ACC | GGA | TAT | TGT | TGT | CGG | AGA | TGT |

P4 δ
| Lys | Gly | Leu | Ala | Leu | Ser | Arg | Thr | Ser | Arg | Arg | Leu | Ser | Gln | Glu |
| AAA | GGC | CTT | GCA | CTG | TCA | AGA | ACA | TCG | CGG | CGT | CTG | TCT | CAG | GAA |

δ35,A

P4 δ
| Val | Thr | Glu | Arg | Phe | Tyr | Val | Cys | Thr | Asp | Pro | Gly | Cys | Gly | Leu |
| GTC | ACC | GAG | CGT | TTT | TAT | GTG | TGC | ACG | GAT | CCG | GGC | TGT | GGT | CTG |

P4 δ
| Val | Phe | Lys | Thr | Leu | Gln | Thr | Ile | Asn | Arg | Phe | Ile | Val | Arg | Pro |
| GTG | TTT | AAA | ACG | CTT | CAG | ACC | ATC | AAC | CGC | TTC | ATT | GTC | CGC | CCG |

P4 δ
| Val | Thr | Pro | Ala | Asn | Trp | Gln | Asn | Ala | Cys | Met | Lys | Asn | Arg | Asn |
| GTG | ACG | CCG | GCG | AAC | TGG | CAG | AAC | GCC | TGC | ATG | AAA | AAC | AGG | AAC |

P4 δ
| Cys | Arg | Gln | Tyr | Gly | | ---- |
| TGC | CGC | CAG | TAC | GGT | TAA | ---- |

[a]Data compiled from Padmanaban and Wu, 1972; Wang et al, 1973; Murray and Murray, 1973; Padmanaban et al., 1974; Murray et al., 1977; Lindqvist, 1981a.
[b]Data compiled from Christie and Calendar, 1983, 1985; Ljungquist et al., 1984; Lin, 1984; Birkeland and Lindqvist, 1986; Christie et al., 1986; Dale et al., 1986; Haggård-Ljungquist et al., 1987; Kalionis et al., 1986a,b; Dehò, personal communication; Pierson and Kahn, 1987.
[c]Data compiled from Christie and Calendar, 1983, 1985; Dale et al., 1986.
[d]Data from Dale et al., 1986.
[e]Data compiled from Christie et al., 1986; Kalionis et al., 1986b; Haggård-Ljungquist, personal communication.
[f]Data compiled from Lin, 1984; Birkeland and Lindqvist, 1986; Christie et al., 1986; Kalionis et al., 1986b.

REFERENCES

Alano, P., Dehò, G., Sironi, G., and Zangrossi, S., 1986, Regulation of the plasmid state of the genetic element P4, *Mol. Gen. Genet.* **203:**445.

Argos, P., Landy, A., Abremski, K., Egan, J. B., Haggård-Ljungquist, E., Hoess, R. H., Kahn, M. L., Kalionis, B., Narayana, S. V. L., Pierson, L. S. III, Sternberg, N., and Leong, J. M., 1986, The integrase family of site-specific recombinases: Regional similarities and global diversity, *EMBO J.* **5:**433.

Baas, P. D., and Jansz, H. S., 1972, φX-174 replicative form DNA replication: Origin and direction, *J. Mol. Biol.* **63:**569.

Bachmann, B. J., 1983, Linkage map of *Escherichia coli* K-12, edition 7, *Microbiol. Rev.* **47:**180.

Barclay, S. L., and Dove, W. F., 1978a, Mutations of bacteriophage P2 which prevent activation of P2 late genes by satellite phage P4, *Virology* **91:**321.

Barclay, S. L., and Dove, W. F., 1978b, Mutants of *E. coli* in which bacteriophage P4 cannot activate the late genes of its helper, bacteriophage P2, *Virology* **91:**336.

Barrett, K. J., Gibbs, W., and Calendar, R., 1972, A transcribing activity induced by satellite phage P4, *Proc. Natl. Acad. Sci. USA* **69:**2986.

Barrett, K. J., Marsh, M. L., and Calendar, R., 1976, Interactions between a satellite bacteriophage and its helper, *J. Mol. Biol.* **106:**683.

Barrett, K. J., Blinkova, A., and Arnold, G., 1983, The bacteriophage P4 α gene is the structural gene for bacteriophage P4-induced RNA polymerase, *J. Virol.* **48:**157.

Bertani, G., 1951, Studies on lysogenesis. I. The mode of phage liberation by lysogenic *Escherichia coli*, *J. Bacteriol.* **62:**293.

Bertani, G., 1958, Lysogeny, *Adv. Virus Res.* **5:**151.

Bertani, G., 1975, Deletions in phage P2. Circularity of the genetic map and its orientation relative to the DNA denaturation map, *Mol. Gen. Genet.* **136:**107.

Bertani, G., and Bertani, L. E., 1974, Constitutive expression of bacteriophage P2 early genes resulting from a tandem duplication, *Proc. Natl. Acad. Sci. USA* **71:**315.

Bertani, G., and Chattoraj, D. K., 1980, Tandem pentuplication of a DNA segment in a derivative of bacteriophage P2: Its use in the study of the mechanism of DNA annealing, *Nucleic Acids Res.* **8:**1339.

Bertani, G., and Six, E. W., 1958, Inheritance of prophage P2 in bacterial crosses, *Virology* **6:**357.

Bertani, G., Ljungquist, E., Jagusztyn-Krynicka, K., and Jupp, S., 1978, Defective particle assembly in wild type P2 bacteriophage and its correction by the *lg* mutation, *J. Gen. Virol.* **38:**251.

Bertani, G., and Ljungquist, E., 1984, P2, in: *Genetic Maps 1984* (S. J. O'Brien, ed.), Vol. 3, pp. 55–61, Cold Spring Harbor Laboratory, Cold Spring Harbor, NY.

Bertani, L. E., 1964, Lysogenic conversion by bacteriophage P2 resulting in an increased sensitivity of *Escherichia coli* to 5-fluorodeoxyuridine, *Biochim. Biophys. Acta* **87:**631.

Bertani, L. E., 1968, Abortive induction of bacteriophage P2, *Virology* **36:**87.

Bertani, L. E., 1970, Split-operon control of a prophage genome, *Proc. Natl. Acad. Sci. USA* **65:**331.

Bertani, L. E., 1971, Stabilization of P2 tandem double lysogens by *int* mutations in the prophage, *Virology* **46:**426.

Bertani, L. E., 1976, Characterization of clear mutants belonging to the *Z* gene of phage P2, *Virology* **71:**85.

Bertani, L. E., 1978, Cold-sensitive mutations in the *Z* gene of prophage P2 that result in increased sensitivity of lysogens to a low molecular weight product of the host bacteria, *Mol. Gen. Genet.* **166:**85.

Bertani, L. E., 1980, Genetic interaction between the *nip1* mutation and genes affecting integration and excision in phage P2, *Mol. Gen. Genet.* **178:**91.

Bertani, L. E., and Bertani, G., 1970, Preparation and characterization of temperate, noninducible bacteriophage P2 (host: *Escherichia coli*), *J. Gen. Virol.* **6:**201.

Bertani, L. E., and Bertani, G., 1971, Genetics of P2 and related phages, *Adv. Genet.* **16**:199–237.

Bertani, L. E., Ljungquist, E., and Bertani, G., 1981, Site-specific recombination in bacteriophage P2, in: *Microbiology 1981* (D. Schlessinger, ed.), pp. 61–63, American Society for Microbiology, Washington.

Bird, R., Louarn, J., Martuscelli, J., and Caro, L., 1972, Origin and sequence of chromosome replication in *Escherichia coli*, *J. Mol. Biol.* **70**:549.

Birkeland, N. K., and Lindqvist, B. H., 1986, Coliphage P2 late control gene *ogr* DNA sequence and product identification, *J. Mol. Biol.* **188**:487.

Bowden, D. W., and Calendar, R., 1979, Maturation of bacteriophage P2 DNA *in vitro:* A complex, site-specific system for DNA cleavage, *J. Mol. Biol.* **129**:1.

Bowden, D. W., and Modrich, P., 1981, *In vitro* studies on the bacteriophage P2 terminase system, *Prog. Clin. Biol. Res.* **64**:223.

Bowden, D. W., and Modrich, P., 1985, *In vitro* maturation of circular bacteriophage P2 DNA, *J. Biol. Chem.* **260**:6999.

Bowden, D. W., Twersky, R. S., and Calendar, R., 1975, *Escherichia coli* deoxyribonucleic acid synthesis mutants: Their effect upon bacteriophage P2 and satellite bacteriophage P4 deoxyribonucleic acid synthesis, *J. Bacteriol.* **124**:167.

Bradley, C., Ling, O. P., and Egan, J. B., 1975, Isolation of phage P2-186 intervarietal hybrids and 186 insertion mutants, *Mol. Gen. Genet.* **140**:123.

Brégégère, F., 1974, Phage P2-λ interference. Inhibition of protein synthesis involves transfer RNA inactivation, *J. Mol. Biol.* **90**:459.

Brégégère, F., 1976, Phage P2-lambda interference. II. Effects on the host under the control of lambda genes *O* and *P*, *J. Mol. Biol.* **104**:411.

Brégégère, F., 1978, Phage P2-lambda interference. III. Essential role of an early step in initiation of lambda replication, *J. Mol. Biol.* **122**:113.

Calendar, R., 1986, Viral transactivation, *Biotechnology* **4**:1074.

Calendar, R., and Lindahl, G., 1969, Attachment of prophage P2: Gene order at different host chromosomal sites, *Virology* **39**:867.

Calendar, R., Lindqvist, B., Sironi, G., and Clark, A. J., 1970, Characterization of *rep*⁻ mutants and their interaction with P2 phage, *Virology* **40**:72.

Calendar, R., Lindahl, G., Marsh, M., and Sunshine, M., 1972, Temperature-inducible mutants of P2 phage, *Virology* **47**:68.

Calendar, R., Six, E. W., and Kahn, F., 1977a, Temperate coliphage P2 as an insertion element, in: *DNA Insertion Elements, Plasmids, and Episomes* (A. I. Bukhari, J. A. Shapiro, and S. L. Adhya, eds.), pp. 395–402, Cold Spring Harbor Laboratory, Cold Spring Harbor, NY.

Calendar, R., Geisselsoder, J., Sunshine, M. G., Six, E., and Lindqvist, B. H., 1977b, The P2-P4 transactivation system, in: *Comprehensive Virology* (H. Fraenkel-Conrat and R. R. Wagner, eds.), Vol. 8, pp. 329–344, Plenum Press, New York.

Calendar, R., Ljungquist, E., Dehò, G., Usher, D. C., Goldstein, R., Youderian, P., Sironi, G., and Six, E. W., 1981, Lysogenization by satellite phage P4, *Virology* **113**:20.

Calendar, R., Kahn, M., Six, E., Goldstein, R., Lindqvist, B., Dehò, G., Inman, R., Jiang, R.-Z., Lin, C.-S., Lee, S.-J., Lagos, R., Christie, G., Dale, E., and Pierson, L. S., 1984, P4, in: *Genetic Maps 1984* (S. J. O'Brien, ed.), Vol. 3, pp. 62–65, Cold Spring Harbor Laboratory, Cold Spring Harbor, NY.

Calendar, R., Christie, G., Dale, E., and Halling, C., 1985, Reciprocal transactivation by P2 and P4 phages, in: *Sequence Specificity in Transcription and Translation* (R. Calendar and L. Gold, eds.), pp. 75–82, Alan R. Liss, New York.

Chattoraj, D. K., 1977, Genetic and physical map of bacteriophage P2, in: *DNA Insertion Elements, Plasmids, and Episomes* (A. I. Bukhari, J. A. Shapiro, and S. L. Adhya, eds.), pp. 733–736, Cold Spring Harbor Laboratory, Cold Spring Harbor, NY.

Chattoraj, D. K., 1978, Strand-specific break near the origin of bacteriophage P2 replication, *Proc. Natl. Acad. Sci. USA* **75**:1685.

Chattoraj, D. K., and Bertani, G., 1980, Further physical characterization of deletion and substitution mutants affecting the control of lysogeny in bacteriophage P2, *Mol. Gen. Genet.* **178:**85.

Chattoraj, D. K., and Inman, R. B., 1972, Position of two deletion mutations on the physical map of bacteriophage P2, *J. Mol. Biol.* **66:**423.

Chattoraj, D. K., and Inman, R. B., 1973a, Electron microscope heteroduplex mapping of P2 *Hy dis* bacteriophage DNA, *Virology* **55:**174.

Chattoraj, D. K., and Inman, R. B., 1973b, Origin and direction of replication of bacteriophage 186 DNA, *Proc. Natl. Acad. Sci. USA* **70:**1768.

Chattoraj, D. K., and Inman, R. B., 1974a, Location of DNA ends in P2, 186, P4 and lambda bacteriophage heads, *J. Mol. Biol.* **87:**11.

Chattoraj, D. K., and Inman, R. B., 1974b, Tandem duplication in bacteriophage P2: Electron microscopic mapping, *Proc. Natl. Acad. Sci. USA* **71:**311.

Chattoraj, D. K., Younghusband, H. B., and Inman, R. B., 1975, Physical mapping of bacteriophage P2 mutations and their relation to the genetic map, *Mol. Gen. Genet.* **136:**139.

Chattoraj, D. K., Oberoi, Y. K., and Bertani, G., 1977, Restriction of bacteriophage P2 by the *Escherichia coli* RI plasmid, and *in vitro* cleavage of its DNA by the *EcoRI* endonuclease, *Virology* **81:**460.

Choe, B. K., 1969, Integration defective mutants of bacteriophage P2, *Mol. Gen. Genet.* **105:**275.

Christie, G. E., and Calendar, R., 1983, Bacteriophage P2 late promoters: Transcription initiation sites for two late mRNAs, *J. Mol. Biol.* **167:**773.

Christie, G. E., and Calendar, R., 1984, *Trans*-activation of bacteriophage P2 late genes by satellite bacteriophage P4, in: *Microbiology 1984* (L. Leive and D. Schlessinger, eds.), pp. 108–110, American Society for Microbiology, Washington.

Christie, G. E., and Calendar, R., 1985, Bacteriophage P2 late promoters. II. Comparison of the four late promoter sequences, *J. Mol. Biol.* **181:**373.

Christie, G. E., Haggård-Ljungquist, E., Feiwell, R., and Calendar, R., 1986, Regulation of bacteriophage P2 late gene expression, *Proc. Natl. Acad. Sci. USA* **83:**3238.

Cohen, D., 1959, A variant of phage P2 originating in *E. coli* strain B, *Virology* **7:**112.

Cohen, S. N., and Chang, A. C. Y., 1971, Genetic expression in bacteriophage λ. IV. Effects of P2 prophage on λ inhibition of host synthesis and λ gene expression, *Virology* **46:**397.

Dale, E., Christie, G. E., and Calendar, R., 1986, Organization and expression of the satellite bacteriophage P4 late gene cluster and the sequence of the polarity suppression gene, *J. Mol. Biol.* **192:**793.

Dehò, G., 1983, Circular genetic map of satellite bacteriophage P4, *Virology* **126:**267.

Dehò, G., Ghisotti, D., Alano, P., Zangrossi, S., Borrello, M. G., and Sironi, G., 1984, Plasmid mode of propagation of the genetic element P4, *J. Mol. Biol.* **178:**191.

Denhardt, D. T., Dressler, D. H., and Hathaway, A., 1967, The abortive replication of φX-174 DNA in a recombination-deficient mutant of *E. coli*, *Proc. Natl. Acad. Sci. USA* **57:**813.

Dhillon, E. K. S., and Dhillon, T. S., 1973, HK239: A P2 related temperate phage which excludes mutants of T4, *Virology* **55:**136.

Dhillon, E. K. S., Dhillon, T. S., Lam, Y. Y., and Tsang, A. H. C., 1980, Temperate coliphages: Classification and correlation with habitats, *Appl. Environ. Microbiol.* **39:**1046.

Dhillon, T. S., and Dhillon, E. K. S., 1972, Studies on bacteriophage distribution. II. Isolation and host range based classification of phages active on three species of *Enterobacteriaceae*, *Jpn. J. Microbiol.* **16:**297.

Dhillon, T. S., and Dhillon, E. K. S., 1981, Incidence of lysogeny, colicinogeny, and drug resistance in *Enterobacteria* isolated from sewage and from rectum of humans and some domesticated species, *Appl. Environ. Microbiol.* **41:**894.

Dhillon, T. S., Dhillon, E. K. S., Chan, H. C., Li, W. K., and Tsang, A. H. C., 1976, Studies on bacteriophage distribution—virulent and temperate phage content of mammalian feces, *Appl. Environ. Microbiol.* **32:**68.

Diana, C., Dehò, G., Geisselsoder, J., Tinelli, L., and Goldstein, R., 1978, Viral interference at the level of capsid size determination by satellite phage P4, *J. Mol. Biol.* **126**:433.

Dodd, I. B., and Egan, J. B., 1987, Systematic method for the detection of potential λ *cro*-like DNA binding regions in proteins, *J. Mol. Biol.*, **194**:557.

Earnshaw, W. C., and Casjens, S. R., 1980, DNA packaging by the double-stranded DNA bacteriophages, *Cell* 21:319.

Earnshaw, W. C., and Harrison, S. C., 1977, DNA arrangement in isometric phage heads, *Nature* **268**:598.

Edlin, G., Lin, L., and Bitner, R., 1977, Reproductive fitness of P1, P2, and Mu lysogens of *Escherichia coli*, *J. Virol.* **21**:560.

Feiss, M., Fisher, R. A., Crayton, M. A., and Egner, C., 1977, Packaging of the bacteriophage lambda chromosome: Effect of chromosome length, *Virology* 77:281.

Finkel, S., Halling, C., and Calendar, R., 1986, Selection of lambda *Spi⁻* transducing phages using the P2 *old* gene cloned onto a plasmid, *Gene* **46**:65.

Finnegan, J., and Egan, J. B., 1979, Physical map of the coliphage 186 chromosome. I. Gene content of the *Bam*HI, *Pst*I and other restriction fragments, *Mol. Gen. Genet.* **172**:287.

Finnegan, J., and Egan, J. B., 1981, *In vivo* transcription studies of coliphage 186, *J. Virol.* **38**:987.

Flensburg, J., and Calendar, R., 1987, Bacteriophage P4 DNA replication: Nucleotide sequence of the P4 primase gene and the *cis* replication region, *J. Mol. Biol.* **195**:439.

Fraenkel-Conrat, H., 1985, Phages of prokaryotes (Bacteria and Cyanobacteria), in: *The Viruses: Catalogue, Characterization, and Classification* (H. Fraenkel-Conrat and R. R. Wagner, eds.), pp. 171–222, Plenum Press, New York.

Francke, B., and Ray, D. S., 1972, *Cis*-limited action of the gene *A* product of bacteriophage φX-174 and the essential bacterial site, *Proc. Natl. Acad. Sci. USA* **69**:475.

Fujiki, H., Palm, P., Zillig, W., Calendar, R., and Sunshine, M., 1976, Identification of a mutation within the structural gene for the α subunit of DNA-dependent RNA polymerase of *E. coli*, *Mol. Gen. Genet.* **145**:19.

Fuller, R. S., Funnell, B. E., and Kornberg, A., 1984, The *dnaA* protein complex with the replication origin (*oriC*) and other DNA sites, *Cell* 38:889.

Funnell, B. E., and Inman, R. B., 1982, Physical evidence for early transcription in intracellular phage P2 DNA, *J. Mol. Biol.* **154**:85.

Funnell, B. E., and Inman, R. B., 1983, Bacteriophage P2 DNA replication. Characterization of the requirement of the gene *B* protein *in vivo*, *J. Mol. Biol.* **167**:311.

Geisselsoder, J., 1976, Strand-specific discontinuity in replicating P2 DNA, *J. Mol. Biol.* **100**:13.

Geisselsoder, J., Mandel, M., Calendar, R., and Chattoraj, D.K., 1973, *In vivo* transcription patterns of temperate coliphage P2, *J. Mol. Biol.* **77**:405.

Geisselsoder, J., Chidambaram, M., and Goldstein, R., 1978, Transcriptional control of capsid size in the P2:P4 bacteriophage system, *J. Mol. Biol.* **126**:447.

Geisselsoder, J., Youderian, P., Dehò, G., Chidambaram, M., Goldstein, R. N., and Ljungquist, E., 1981, Mutants of satellite virus P4 that cannot derepress their P2 helper, *J. Mol. Biol.* **148**:1.

Geisselsoder, J., Sedivy, J. M., Walsh, R. B., and Goldstein, R., 1982, Capsid structure of satellite phage P4 and its P2 helper, *J. Ultrastruct. Res.* **79**:165.

Ghisotti, D., Zangrossi, S., and Sironi, G., 1979, X-ray sensitivity of *Escherichia coli* lysogenic for bacteriophage P2, *Mol. Gen. Genet.* **169**:229.

Ghisotti, D., Zangrossi, S., and Sironi, G., 1983, An *Escherichia coli* gene required for bacteriophage P2-λ interference, *J. Virol.* **48**:616.

Gibbs, W., Goldstein, R. N., Wiener, R., Lindqvist, B., and Calendar, R., 1973, Satellite bacteriophage P4: Characterization of mutants in two essential genes, *Virology* **53**:24.

Gibbs, W., Eisen, H., and Calendar, R., 1983, *In vitro* activation of bacteriophage P2 late gene expression by extracts from phage P4-infected cells, *J. Virol.* **47**:392.

Goldstein, R., Lengyel, J., Pruss, G., Barrett, K., Calendar, R., and Six, E., 1974, Head size determination and the morphogenesis of satellite phage P4, *Curr. Top. Microbiol. Immunol.* **68**:59.

Goldstein, R., Thomas, M., and Davies, R., 1975, EcoRI endonuclease cleavage map of bacteriophage P4 DNA, *Virology* **66**:420.

Goldstein, R., Sedivy, J., and Ljungquist, E., 1982, Propagation of satellite P4 as a plasmid, *Proc. Natl. Acad. Sci. USA* **79**:515.

Golub, E. I., and Zwenigorodsky, V. I., 1969, Defective thermal induction of a non-inducible bacteriophage, *Virology* **39**:919.

Haggård-Ljungquist, E., Kockum, K., and Bertani, L. E., 1987, DNA sequences of bacteriophage P2 early genes *cox* and *B* and their regulatory sites, *Mol. Gen. Genet.* **208**:52.

Harris, J. D., and Calendar, R., 1978, Transcription map of satellite coliphage P4, *Virology* **85**:343.

Hirota, Y., Mordoh, J., and Jacob, F., 1970, On the process of cellular division in *Escherichia coli*. III. Thermosensitive mutants of *Escherichia coli* altered in the process of DNA initiation. *J. Mol. Biol.* **53**:369.

Hocking, S. M., and Egan, J. B., 1982a, Genetic studies of coliphage 186. I. Genes associated with phage morphogenesis. *J. Virol.* **44**:1056.

Hocking, S. M., and Egan, J. B., 1982b, Genetic studies of coliphage 186. II. Genes associated with phage replication and host cell lysis, *J. Virol.* **44**:1068.

Hocking, S. M., and Egan, J. B., 1982c, Genetic map of coliphage 186 from a novel use of marker rescue frequencies, *Mol. Gen. Genet.* **187**:87.

Hocking, S. M., and Egan, J. B., 1982d, Genetic characterization of twelve P2–186 hybrid bacteriophages, *Mol. Gen. Genet.* **187**:174.

Hooper, I., and Egan, J. B., 1981, Coliphage 186 infection requires host initiation functions *dnaA* and *dnaC*, *J. Virol.* **40**:599.

Hooper, I., Woods, W. H., and Egan, B., 1981, Coliphage 186 replication is delayed when the host cell is UV irradiated before infection, *J. Virol.* **40**:341.

Hudnik-Plevnik, T., and Bertani, G., 1980, Recombination in bacteriophage P2: *recA*-dependent enhancement by ultraviolet irradiation and by transfection with mixed DNA dimers, *Mol. Gen. Genet.* **178**:131.

Hyde, J. M., and Bertani, G., 1975, Structure and position of a complex chromosomal aberration in bacteriophage P2, *J. Gen. Virol.* **28**:415.

Inman, R. B., Schnös, M., Simon, L. D., Six, E. W., and Walker, D. H. Jr., 1971, Some morphological properties of P4 bacteriophage and P4 DNA, *Virology* **44**:67.

Jacob, F., and Wollman, E. L., 1961, The location of some other prophages, in: *Sexuality and the Genetics of Bacteria*, pp. 85–91, Academic Press, New York.

Jonasson, J., 1973, Evidence for bidirectional chromosome replication in *Escherichia coli* C based on marker-frequency analysis by DNA/DNA hybridization with P2 and lambda prophages, *Mol. Gen. Genet.* **120**:69.

Kahn, M., and Hanawalt, P., 1979, Size distribution of DNA replicative intermediates in bacteriophage P4 and in *Escherichia coli*, *J. Mol. Biol.* **128**:501.

Kahn, M., and Helinski, D. R., 1978, Construction of a novel plasmid-phage hybrid: Use of the hybrid to demonstrate ColEI DNA replication *in vivo* in the absence of a ColEI-specified protein, *Proc. Natl. Acad. Sci. USA* **75**:2200.

Kahn, M., and Hopkins, A., 1978, Restriction endonuclease cleavage map of bacteriophage P4 DNA, *Virology* **85**:359.

Kahn, M. L., and Timblin, C. R., 1984, Gene fusion vehicles for the analysis of gene expression in *Rhizobium meliloti*, *J. Bacteriol.* **158**:1204.

Kahn, M., Ow, D., Sauer, B., Rabinowitz, A., and Calendar, R., 1980, Genetic analysis of bacteriophage P4 using P4-plasmid ColE1 hybrids, *Mol. Gen. Genet.* **177**:399.

Kainuma-Kuroda, R., and Okazaki, R., 1975, Mechanism of DNA chain growth. XII. Asymmetry of replication of P2 phage DNA, *J. Mol. Biol.* **94**:213.

Kalionis, B., and Egan, J. B., 1981, Orientation of separated DNA strands of coliphage 186 relative to its genetic map, *Gene* **15**:95.

Kalionis, B., Dodd, I. B., and Egan, J. B., 1986a, Control of gene expression in the P2-related temperate coliphages. III. DNA sequence of the major control region of phage 186, *J. Mol. Biol.* **191**:199.

Kalionis, B., Pritchard, M., and Egan, J. B., 1986b, Control of gene expression in the P2-related temperate coliphages. IV. Concerning the late control gene and control of its transcription, *J. Mol. Biol.* **191**:211.

Katsura, I., 1983, Structure and inherent properties of the bacteriophage head shell, *J. Mol. Biol.* **171**:297.

Kelly, B., 1963, Localization of P2 prophage in two strains of *Escherichia coli*, *Virology* **19**:32.

Kelly, B. L., and Sunshine, M. G., 1967, Association of temperate phage P2 with the production of *histidine*-negative segregants by *Escherichia coli*, *Biochem. Biophys. Res. Commun.* **28**:237.

King, J., and Laemmli, U., 1973, Bacteriophage T4 tail assembly: Structural proteins and their genetic identification, *J. Mol. Biol.* **75**:315.

Kobori, J. A., and Kornberg, A., 1982, The *Escherichia coli dnaC* gene product. II. Purification, physical properties and role in replication, *J. Biol. Chem.* **257**:13736.

Krevolin, M.D., and Calendar, R., 1985, The replication of bacteriophage P4 DNA *in vitro*. Partial purification of the P4 α gene product, *J. Mol. Biol.* **182**:509.

Krevolin, M. D., Roof, D., Kahn, M., Corless, C., Young, J., and Calendar, R., 1983, Satellite bacteriophage P4: Initiation of DNA replication *in vivo* and *in vitro*, in: *Microbiology 1983* (D. Schlessinger, ed.), pp. 100–103, American Society for Microbiology, Washington.

Krevolin, M. D., Inman, R. B., Roof, D., Kahn, M., and Calendar, R., 1985, Bacteriophage P4 DNA replication. Location of the P4 origin, *J. Mol. Biol.* **182**:519.

Kuempel, P. L., and Duerr, S. A., 1978, Chromosome replication in *Escherichia coli* is inhibited in the terminus region near the *rac* locus, *Cold Spring Harbor Symp. Quant. Biol.* **43**:563.

Kuempel, P. L., Duerr, S. A., and Seeley, N. R., 1977, Terminus region of the chromosome in *Escherichia coli* inhibits replication forks, *Proc. Natl. Acad. Sci. USA* **74**:3927.

Kuempel, P. L., Duerr, S. A., and Maglothin, P. D., 1978, Chromosome replication in an *Escherichia coli dnaA* mutant integratively suppressed by prophage P2, *J. Bacteriol.* **134**:902.

Kurosawa, Y., and Okazaki, R., 1975, Mechanism of DNA chain growth. XIII. Evidence for discontinuous replication of both strands of P2 phage DNA, *J. Mol. Biol.* **94**:229.

Lagos, R., and Goldstein, R., 1984, Phasmid P4: Manipulation of plasmid copy number and induction from the integrated state, *J. Bacteriol.* **158**:208.

Lagos, R., Jinag, R.-Z., Kim, S., and Goldstein, 1986, ρ-Dependent transcription termination of a bacterial operon is antagonized by an extrachromosomal gene product, *Proc. Natl. Acad. Sci. USA* **83**:9561.

Lane, H. E. D., and Denhardt, D. T., 1974, The *rep* mutation. III. Altered structure of the replicating *Escherichia coli* chromosome, *J. Bacteriol.* **120**:805.

Lee, S.-J., 1981, Altered patterns of gene expression by satellite phage P4 mutants unable to regulate their P2 helper, B.A. Thesis, Harvard University, Cambridge, MA.

Lengyel, J. A., and Calendar, R., 1974, Control of bacteriophage P2 protein and DNA synthesis, *Virology* **57**:305.

Lengyel, J. A., Goldstein, R. N., Marsh, M., Sunshine, M., and Calendar, R., 1973, Bacteriophage P2 head morphogenesis: Cleavage of the major capsid protein, *Virology* **53**:1.

Lengyel, J. A., Goldstein, R. N., Marsh, M., and Calendar, R., 1974, Structure of the bacteriophage P2 tail, *Virology* **62**:161.

Lennox, E. S., 1955, Transduction of linked genetic characters of the host by bacteriophage, P1, *Virology* **1**:190.

Lin, C. S., 1983, Genetic and molecular studies of bacteriophage P4: *ash* mutants and DNA sequence between genes *psu* and *alpha*, Ph.D. Thesis, University of Iowa, Iowa City.

140   L. ELIZABETH BERTANI and ERICH W. SIX

Lin, C-S., 1984, Nucleotide sequence of the essential region of bacteriophage P4, *Nucleic Acids Res.* **12**:8667.
Lindahl, G., 1969a, Genetic map of bacteriophage P2, *Virology* **39**:839.
Lindahl, G., 1969b, Multiple recombination mechanisms in bacteriophage P2, *Virology* **39**:861.
Lindahl, G., 1970, Bacteriophage P2: Replication of the chromosome requires a protein which acts only on the genome that coded for it, *Virology* **42**:522.
Lindahl, G., 1971, On the control of transcription in bacteriophage P2, *Virology* **46**:620.
Lindahl, G., 1974, Characterization of conditional lethal mutants of bacteriophage P2, *Mol. Gen. Genet.* **128**:249.
Lindahl, G., and Sunshine, M., 1972, Excision-deficient mutants of bacteriophage P2, *Virology* **49**:180.
Lindahl, G., Sironi, G., Bialy, H., and Calendar, R., 1970, Bacteriophage lambda: Abortive infection of bacteria lysogenic for phage P2, *Proc. Natl. Acad. Sci. USA* **66**:587.
Lindahl, G., Hirota, Y., and Jacob, F., 1971, On the process of cellular division in *Escherichia coli:* Replication of the bacterial chromosome under control of prophage P2, *Proc. Natl. Acad. Sci. USA* **68**:2407.
Lindberg, A. A., 1973, Bacteriophage receptors, *Annu. Rev. Microbiol.* **27**:205.
Lindqvist, B., 1971, Vegetative DNA of temperate coliphage P2, *Mol. Gen. Genet.* **110**:178.
Lindqvist, B. H., 1974, Expression of phage transcription in P2 lysogens infected with helper-dependent coliphage P4, *Proc. Natl. Acad. Sci. USA* **71**:2752.
Lindqvist, B. H., 1981a, Recombination between satellite phage P4 and its helper P2 I. *In vivo* and *in vitro* construction of P4::P2 hybrid satellite phage, *Gene* **14**:231.
Lindqvist, B. H., 1981b, Recombination between satellite phage P4 and its helper P2. II. *In vitro* construction of a helper-independent P4::P2 hybrid phage, *Gene* **14**:243.
Lindqvist, B. H., and Bøvre, K., 1972, Asymmetric transcription of the coliphage P2 during infection, *Virology* **49**:690.
Lindqvist, B. H., and Six, E. W., 1971, Replication of bacteriophage P4 DNA in a nonlysogenic host, *Virology* **43**:1.
Lindqvist, B. H., and Williams, R. C., 1979, Distribution of RNA polymerase binding sites on the P4 chromosome, *Virology* **96**:274.
Little, J. W., and Mount, D. W., 1982, The SOS regulatory system of *Escherichia coli, Cell* **29**:11.
Liu, L. F., Perkocha, L., Calendar, R., and Wang, J. C., 1981a, Knotted DNA from bacteriophage capsids, *Proc. Natl. Acad. Sci. USA* **78**:5498.
Liu, L. F., Davis, J. L., and Calendar, R., 1981b, Novel topologically knotted DNA from bacteriophage P4 capsids: Studies with DNA topoisomerases. *Nucleic Acids Res.* **9**:3979.
Ljungquist, E., 1973, Interaction of phage P2 DNA with some fast-sedimenting host components during infection, *Virology* **52**:120.
Ljungquist, E., 1976, Association of nonreplicating P2 DNA to fast-sedimenting cell material following infection with satellite phage P4, *Virology* **73**:402.
Ljungquist, E., and Bertani, L. E., 1983, Properties and products of the cloned *int* gene of bacteriophage P2, *Mol. Gen. Genet.* **192**:87.
Ljungquist, E., Kockum, K., and Bertani, L. E., 1984, DNA sequences of the repressor gene and operator region of bacteriophage P2, *Proc. Natl. Acad. Sci. USA* **81**:3988.
Louarn, J., Patte, J., and Louarn, J.-M., 1977, Evidence for a fixed termination site of chromosome replication in *Escherichia coli* K12, *J. Mol. Biol.* **115**:295.
Lundqvist, B., and Bertani, G., 1984, Immunity repressor of P2: Identification and DNA-binding activity, *J. Mol. Biol.* **178**:629.
Malone, R. E., and Chattoraj, D. K., 1975, The role of *Chi* mutations in the *Spi⁻* phenotype of phage lambda: Lack of evidence for a gene *delta, Mol. Gen. Genet.* **143**:35.
Mandel, M., and Kornreich, B., 1972, The effect of λ *red* genes on recombination of phage 186, *Virology* **49**:300.

Maniatis, T., Fritsch, E. F., and Sambrook, J., 1982, *Molecular Cloning*, pp. 24–25, Cold Spring Harbor Laboratory, Cold Spring Harbor, NY.

Murray, K., and Murray, N. E., 1973, Terminal nucleotide sequences of DNA from temperate coliphages, *Nature New Biol.* **243:**134.

Murray, K., Isaksson-Forsen, A. G., Challberg, M., and Englund, P. T., 1977, Symmetrical nucleotide sequences in the recognition sites for the *ter* function of bacteriophages P2, 299, and 186, *J. Mol. Biol.* **112:**471.

Neuhard, J., and Thomassen, E., 1976, Altered deoxyribonucleotide pools in P2 eductants of *Escherichia coli* K-12 due to deletion of the *dcd* gene, *J. Bacteriol.* **126:**999.

Nicoletti, M., and Bertani, G., 1983, DNA fusion product of phage P2 with plasmid pBR322: A new phasmid, *Mol. Gen. Genet.* **189:**343.

Nilsson, E., and Bertani, L. E., 1977, Restoration of immunity in lysogens carrying prophage P2, derepressed at high temperature, *Mol. Gen. Genet.* **156:**297.

Nishimura, Y., Caro, L., Berg, C., and Hirota, Y., 1971, Chromosome replication in *Escherichia coli*. IV. Control of chromosome replication and cell division by an integrated episome, *J. Mol. Biol.* **55:**441.

Ow, D. W., and Ausubel, F. M., 1980, Recombinant P4 bacteriophages propagate as viable lytic phages or as autonomous plasmids in *Klebsiella pneumoniae*, *Mol. Gen. Genet.* **180:**165.

Ow, D. W., and Ausubel, F. M., 1983, Conditionally replicating plasmid vectors that can integrate into *Klebsiella pneumoniae* chromosome via P4 site-specific recombination, *J. Bacteriol.* **155:**704.

Padmanabhan, R., 1977, Chemical synthesis of an octanucleotide complementary to a portion of the cohesive end of P2 DNA and studies on the stability of duplex formation with P2 DNA, *Biochemistry* **16:**1996.

Padmanabhan, R., and Wu, R., 1972, Nucleotide sequence analysis of DNA. IV. Complete nucleotide sequence of the left-hand cohesive end of coliphage 186 DNA, *J. Mol. Biol.* **65:**447.

Padmanabhan, R., Wu, R., and Calendar, R., 1974, Complete nucleotide sequence of the cohesive ends of bacteriophage P2 deoxyribonucleic acid, *J. Biol. Chem.* **249:**6197.

Pierson, L. S. III, and Kahn, M. L., 1984, Cloning of the integration and attachment regions of bacteriophage P4, *Mol. Gen. Genet.* **195:**44.

Pierson, L. S. III and Kahn, M. L., 1987, Integration of satellite bacteriophage P4 in *E. coli*: DNA sequences of the phage and host regions involved in site-specific recombination, *J. Mol. Biol.* **196:**487.

Poon, A. P. W., and Dhillon, T. S., 1986, Assignment of two new host range types to the P2-family of temperate coliphages, *J. Gen. Virol.* **67:**789.

Pritchard, M., and Egan, J. B., 1985, Control of gene expression in P2-related coliphages: The *in vitro* transcription pattern of coliphage 186, *EMBO J.* **4:**3599.

Pruss, G., Barrett, K., Lengyel, J., Goldstein, R., and Calendar, R., 1974a, Phage head size determination and head protein cleavage *in vitro*, *J. Supramol. Struct.* **2:**337.

Pruss, G., Goldstein, R., and Calendar, R., 1974b, *In vitro* packaging of satellite phage P4 DNA, *Proc. Natl. Acad. Sci. USA* **71:**2367.

Pruss, G. J., Wang, J. C., and Calendar, R., 1975, *In vitro* packaging of covalently-closed circular monomers of bacteriophage DNA. *J. Mol. Biol.* **98:**465.

Pruss, G. J., and Calendar, R., 1978, Maturation of bacteriophage P2 DNA, *Virology* **86:**454.

Raimondi, A., Donghi, R., Montaguti, A., Pessina, A., and Dehò, G., 1985, Analysis of spontaneous deletion mutants of satellite bacteriophage P4, *J. Virol.* **54:**233.

Richards, K. E., Williams, R. C., and Calendar, R., 1973, Mode of DNA packing within bacteriophage heads, *J. Mol. Biol.* **78:**255.

Ross, P., and Howard-Flanders, P., 1977, Initiation of recA$^+$-dependent recombination in *Escherichia coli* (λ). II. Specificity in the induction of recombination and strand cutting in undamaged covalent circular bacteriophage 186 and lambda DNA molecules in phage-infected cells. *J. Mol. Biol.* **117:**159.

Rowland, G. C., Giffard, P. M., and Booth, I. R., 1985, *phs* locus of *Escherichia coli*, a mutation causing pleiotropic lesions in metabolism is an *rpoA* allele, *J. Bacteriol.* **164**:972.

Saha, S., Lundqvist, B., and Haggård-Ljungquist, E., 1987a, Autoregulation of bacteriophage P2 repressor, *EMBO J.* **6**:809.

Saha, S., Haggård-Ljungquist, E., and Nordström, K., 1987b, The cox protein of bacteriophage P2 inhibits the formation of the repressor protein and autoregulates the early operon, *EMBO J.* **6**:3191.

Saint, R. B., 1979, Ph.D. Thesis, Adelaide University, Adelaide, Australia.

Saint, R. B., and Egan, J. B., 1979a, Restriction cleavage maps of coliphages 186 and P2, *Mol. Gen. Genet.* **171**:79.

Saint, R. B., and Egan, J. B., 1979b, A method which facilitates the ordering of DNA restriction fragments, *Mol. Gen. Genet.* **171**:103.

Sakaki, Y., Karu, A. E., Linn, S., and Echols, H., 1973, Purification and properties of the γ-protein specified by bacteriophage λ: An inhibitor of the host *recBC* recombination enzyme, *Proc. Natl. Acad. Sci. USA* **70**:2215.

Sauer, B. L., 1979, Regulation of late gene expression in temperate coliphage P2, Ph.D. Thesis, University of California, Berkeley.

Sauer, B., Ow, D., Ling, L., and Calendar, R., 1981, Mutants of satellite bacteriophage P4 that are defective in the suppression of transcription polarity, *J. Mol. Biol.* **145**:29.

Sauer, B., Calendar, R., Ljungquist, E., Six, E., and Sunshine, M. G., 1982, Interaction of satellite phage P4 with 186 phage helper, *Virology* **116**:523.

Schnös, M., and Inman, R. B., 1971, Starting point and direction of replication in P2 DNA, *J. Mol. Biol.* **55**:31.

Shinomija, S., and Sakaki, Y., 1979, Prophage P2 does not kill *recB* bacteria, *Biochem. Biophys. Res. Commun.* **86**:167.

Shore, D., Dehò, G., Tsipis, J., and Goldstein, R., 1978, Determination of capsid size by satellite bacteriophage P4, *Proc. Natl. Acad. Sci. USA* **75**:400.

Sironi, G., 1969, Mutants of *Escherichia coli* unable to be lysogenized by the temperate phage P2, *Virology* **37**:163.

Sironi, G., Bialy, H., Lozeron, H. A., and Calendar, R., 1971, Bacteriophage P2: Interaction with phage lambda and with recombination-deficient bacteria, *Virology* **46**:387.

Sivaprasad, A. V., 1984, Ph.D. Thesis, Adelaide University, Adelaide, Australia.

Six, E. W., 1960, Prophage substitution and curing in lysogenic cells superinfected with heteroimmune phage, *J. Bacteriol.* **80**:728.

Six, E. W., 1963, A defective phage depending on phage P2, *Bacteriol. Proc.* p. 138.

Six, E. W., 1966, Specificity of P2 for prophage site I on the chromosome of *Escherichia coli* strain C, *Virology* **29**:106.

Six, E. W., 1968, Prophage site specificities of P2 phages, *Bacteriol. Proc.* p. 159.

Six, E. W., 1975, The helper dependence of satellite bacteriophage P4: Which gene functions of bacteriophage P2 are needed by P4?, *Virology* **67**:249.

Six, E. W., and Klug, C. A. C., 1973, Bacteriophage P4: A satellite virus depending on a helper such as prophage P2, *Virology* **51**:327.

Six, E. W., and Lindqvist, B. H., 1978, Mutual derepression in the P2–P4 bacteriophage system, *Virology* **87**:217.

Skalka, A., and Hanson, P., 1972, Comparisons of the distribution of nucleotides and common sequences in deoxyribonucleic acid from selected bacteriophages, *J. Virol.* **9**:583.

Smith, G. R., and Stahl, F. W., 1985, Homologous recombination promoted by *chi* sites and *recBC* enzyme of *Escherichia coli*, *Bioessays* **2**:244.

Souza, L., Calendar, R., Six, E. W., and Lindqvist, B. H., 1977, A transactivation mutant of satellite phage P4, *Virology* **81**:81.

Souza, L., Geisselsoder, J., Hopkins, A., and Calendar, R., 1978, Physical mapping of the satellite phage P4 genome, *Virology* **85**:335.

Streicher, S. L., Gurney, E. G., and Valentine, R. C., 1972, The nitrogen fixation genes, *Nature* **239**:495.

Sunshine, M. G., 1972, Dependence of eduction on P2 *int* product, *Virology* **47**:61.

Sunshine, M. G., and Kelly, B., 1971, Extent of host deletions associated with bacteriophage P2-mediated eduction, *J. Bacteriol.* **108:**695.

Sunshine, M. G., and Sauer, B., 1975, A bacterial mutation blocking P2 late gene expression, *Proc. Natl. Acad. Sci. USA* **72:**2770.

Sunshine, M. G., and Six, E., 1986, *sub*, A host mutation that specifically allows growth of replication-deficient gene *B* mutants of coliphage P2, *Mol. Gen. Genet.* **204:**359.

Sunshine, M. G., Thorn, M., Gibbs, W., and Calendar, R., 1971, P2 phage *amber* mutants: Characterization by use of a polarity suppressor, *Virology* **46:**691.

Sunshine, M. G., Usher, D., and Calendar, R., 1975, Interaction of P2 bacteriophage with the *dnaB* gene of *Escherichia coli*, *J. Virol.* **16:**284.

Sunshine, M. G., Six, E. W., Barrett, K., and Calendar, R., 1976, Relief of P2 bacteriophage *amber* mutant polarity by the satellite bacteriophage P4. *J. Mol. Biol.* **106:**673.

Templin, A., Kushner, S. R., and Clark, A. J., 1972, Genetic analysis of mutations indirectly suppressing *recB* and *recC* mutations, *Genetics* **72:**205.

Thomas, M., Cameron, J. R., and Davis, R. W., 1974, Viable molecular hybrids of bacteriophage lambda and eukaryotic DNA, *Proc. Natl. Acad. Sci. USA* **71:**4579.

Unger, R. C., and Clark, A. J., 1972, Interaction of the recombination pathways of bacteriophage λ and its host *Escherichia coli* K12: Effects on exonuclease V activity, *J. Mol. Biol.* **70:**539.

Valla, S., and Lindqvist, B. H., 1978, In vitro transcription in *E. coli* crude lysates prepared on cellophan discs, *Nucleic Acids Res.* **5:**2665.

Wang, J. C., and Brezinski, D. P., 1973, Alignment of two DNA helices: A model for recognition of DNA base sequences by the termini-generating enzymes of phage λ, 186, and P2, *Proc. Natl. Acad. Sci. USA* **70:**2667.

Wang, J. C., Martin, K. V., and Calendar, R., 1973, On the sequence similarity of the cohesive ends of coliphage P4, P2 and 186 deoxyribonucleic acid. *Biochemistry* **12:**2119.

Westöö, A., and Ljungquist, E., 1979, A restriction cleavage map of bacteriophage P2, *Mol. Gen. Genet.* **171:**91.

Westöö, A., and Ljungquist, E., 1980, Cloning of the immunity repressor determinant of phage P2 in the pBR322 plasmid, *Mol. Gen. Genet.* **178:**101.

Wiman, M., Bertani, G., Kelly, B., and Sasaki, I., 1970, Genetic map of *Escherichia coli* strain C, *Mol. Gen. Genet.* **107:**1.

Wolfson, J. S., McHugh, G. L., Hooper, D. C., and Swartz, M. N., 1985, Knotting of DNA molecules isolated from deletion mutants of intact bacteriophage P4. *Nucleic Acids Res.* **13:**6695.

Woods, W. H., and Egan, J. B., 1974, Prophage induction of noninducible coliphage 186, *J. Virol.* **14:**1349.

Woods, W. H., and Egan, J. B., 1981, The transient inability of the conjugating female cell to host 186 infection explains the absence of zygotic induction for 186, *J. Virol.* **40:**335.

Yoshimura, M., Inokuchi, H., and Ozeki, H., 1984, Identification of transfer RNA suppressors in *Escherichia coli*. IV. Amber suppressor *Su6* a double mutant of a new species of leucine tRNA, *J. Mol. Biol.* **177:**627.

Younghusband, H. B., and Inman, R. B., 1974, Base sequence homologies between bacteriophage P2 and 186 DNAs, *Virology* **62:**530.

Younghusband, H. B., Egan, J. B., and Inman, R. B., 1975, Characterization of the DNA from bacteriophage P2–186 hybrids and physical mapping of the 186 chromosome, *Mol. Gen. Genet.* **140:**101.

CHAPTER 3

Strategies of Bacteriophage DNA Replication

France Keppel, Olivier Fayet, and Costa Georgopoulos

I. INTRODUCTION

There is little doubt that the bulk of our understanding of the fundamental process of DNA replication comes from studies on the replication of the various bacteriophages and *E. coli*. The bacteriophages have adapted or evolved a plethora of replication strategies. The only two common themes that one can uncover in studying these diverse replication strategies are the well-documented facts that all known DNA polymerases (1) can only polymerize deoxyribonucleotides in the 5' to 3' direction, and (2) are unable to initiate DNA replication *de novo*, instead requiring a free 3'-hydroxyl moiety of DNA or RNA to extend upon. The formation of the free 3'-hydroxyl end is the key step in DNA replication, and bacteriophages have evolved a wide variety of strategies of creating them. These include the formation of RNA primers by RNA polymerases and primases, the introduction of nicks in double-stranded DNA, the use of a terminal protein covalently linked to the first nucleotide of the DNA genome, and the formation of a hairpin structure at the two 3' ends of linear double-stranded DNA. Because of the vastness of the subject to be

FRANCE KEPPEL • Department of Molecular Biology, University of Geneva, Geneva 1211, Switzerland. OLIVIER FAYET • Centre de Recherche de Biochimie et de Genetique Cellulaires du CNRS, Toulouse, France 31062. COSTA GEORGOPOULOS • Department of Cellular, Viral, and Molecular Biology, University of Utah School of Medicine, Salt Lake City, Utah 84132.

145

covered, we will utilize examples of only a few of the bacteriophages that we consider to be both novel and interesting. Examples of DNA replication strategies of these and other bacteriophages can be found in the pioneering textbooks by Arthur Kornberg (1980, 1982); in the reviews by Wickner (1978b), Tomizawa and Selzer (1979), Mitra (1980), Nossal (1983), Marians (1984), and McMacken et al. (1987); and in the articles on individual bacteriophages found in this volume.

A. Replication Control

Bacteriophages, like all known organisms, control the rate of replication of their chromosomes primarily at the level of initiation. The replicon hypothesis, first proposed by Jacob et al. (1963), was the first to suggest that all genetic elements consist of individual units of replication, called replicons. Every replicon was thought to contain a unique origin of DNA replication, a cis-acting "activator" site, at which DNA replication is specifically initiated through the interaction with a trans-acting "initiator" protein(s) (Jacob et al., 1963). Although the positive control aspect of the replicon hypothesis has been shown to be entirely consistent with the DNA replication of all known bacteriophages, there is also negative modulation at the level of the initiation of replication that is used by bacteria and plasmids to control their intracellular copy number (Pritchard, 1985; Yarmolinsky and Sternberg, 1988; see Section III.B).

Many bacteriophages, such as λ, contain a unique origin of replication, usually designated ori. Special features of such ori regions include (1) binding sites for specific initiator protein(s), and (2) adjacent stretches of AT-rich regions, presumably to aid in unwinding of DNA. Some bacteriophages, especially the larger ones, such as T4 (see article by G. Mosig and F. Eiserling, this volume), utilize alternative replication pathways and, in addition, appear to possess accessory functions that are not absolutely necessary for growth on a given bacterial host under some laboratory conditions.

Figure 1 depicts bidirectional replication of an idealized linear DNA duplex molecule, beginning at a unique ori site and primed by RNA. The RNA primer is synthesized by either a host- or bacteriophage-coded RNA polymerase or a primase enzyme and elongated into DNA by a host- or bacteriophage-coded DNA polymerase enzyme. The leading and lagging strand syntheses may be primed by different enzymatic reactions. Eventual removal of the RNA primer by an enzyme such as E. coli DNA polymerase I allows a DNA ligase enzyme to ligate together the DNA pieces that make up lagging strand synthesis. Since all DNA replication proceeds in the 5' to 3' direction, the 3' ends of the parental molecule cannot be completely replicated, as shown in the bottom part of Fig. 1.

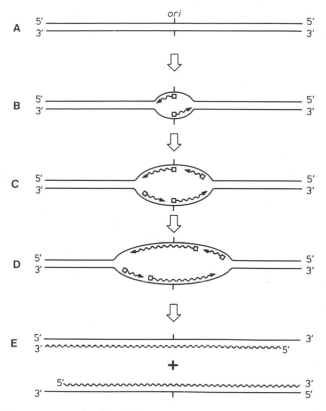

FIGURE 1. Bidirectional replication of an idealized linear DNA duplex. (A) Initiation takes place at a specific origin of replication, called *ori*. (B) Leading strand synthesis in the 5' to 3' direction is initiated. The RNA primer used to initiate DNA replication is shown as □; the newly synthesized DNA daughter strand is shown as ∿. (C) Lagging strand synthesis is initiated. (D) The RNA primer is removed, and the two contiguous DNA segments are ligated together. (E) Replication reaches the ends of the linear molecular to produce the two daughter molecules shown. Notice that the 3'-hydroxyl ends of each parental strand cannot be completely replicated in this fashion (see also Section IV.A.1).

B. Temperate versus Lytic Bacteriophages

The various strategies that bacteriophages utilize to replicate their DNA depend to a great extent on whether they are temperate or virulent. Obviously, a temperate bacteriophage cannot irreversibly damage its host early in its infection cycle, before the decision to lysogenize or lyse the host bacterium is made. This caution extends to the use of host DNA replication components, which are transiently taken over by the temperate bacteriophages (see Section III.A). In this regard, it is interesting that lysogenization by some temperate bacteriophages—such as λ, P1, P4, and Mu—endows the lysogenic host with a potential selective advantage under limiting nutrient conditions (Edlin *et al.*, 1975; Edlin and Bitner,

1977). Lysogeny is a form of passive propagation of the prophage: as the host chromosome replicates, so does the integrated prophage. In the case in which the prophage DNA is maintained extrachromosomally as a plasmid (Yarmolinsky and Sternberg, 1988; see Section III.B), the bacteriophage-coded replication machinery is distinct from that used during the lytic cycle. In addition, the plasmid prophages must code for a partitioning system in order to be stably inherited. An artificially induced plasmid prophage state of a λ derivative, λ *dv*, which lacks such a partitioning system, is readily lost under nonselective conditions (Matsubara, 1981). In the case of the temperate bacteriophages, which insert their prophages into the host chromosome, an efficient mechanism must exist to ensure that prophage replication is turned off, even in the presence of all *trans*-acting replication functions, since replication of adjacent host chromosome sequences would endanger lysogen viability. Bacteriophage λ has solved this problem in an elegant way (see Section III.A).

It is to the advantage of the virulent bacteriophages to exhibit large burst sizes and relatively short infectious cycles, so that they can readily infect a given bacterial population. This is partly accomplished by irreversibly diverting all bacterial resources to bacteriophage metabolism: the host RNA polymerase is usually modified shortly after infection to accommodate bacteriophage-coded factors (e.g., T4) or inactivated and replaced by a bacteriophage-coded enzyme (e.g., T7). Of equal importance to the virulent bacteriophages is increasing the intracellular levels of the deoxyribonucleotides to satisfy the need for fast and vigorous DNA replication. The large virulent bacteriophages, such as T4 and T7, induce deoxyribonucleases capable of degrading the host chromosome to mononucleotides that can be subsequently utilized as bacteriophage DNA precursors. Bacteriophage T7 can thereby manufacture up to 200 T7 progeny DNA molecules, even in the absence of additional nucleotide sources. Bacteriophage T4 not only induces the synthesis of additional enzymes to rapidly produce deoxynucleotide triphosphates, but has also evolved a giant replication complex consisting of both replication proteins and precursor-manufacturing enzymes. By this method, rapid accessibility of deoxynucleotide triphosphate precursors to the bacteriophage DNA polymerizing system is assured.

Most, if not all, large virulent bacteriophages have evolved efficient complex DNA replication machineries. Such machineries appear to be assembled and stabilized through diverse but very specific protein-protein and DNA-protein interactions among the constituent members (see Section IV.A.2).

C. Circular versus Linear Genomes

The genomes of most, if not all, temperate bacteriophages assume circular DNA forms after infection of sensitive bacteria. Bacteriophages, like λ and P4, achieve a circular state by pairing complementary cohesive ends, whereas others, such as P1 and P22, use generalized or site-specific recombination of their terminally redundant ends. The advantages of possessing a circular genome include (1) a single, unidirectional DNA initiation event allows complete replication of the genome. Linear genomes not only require bidirectional replication but, in addition, cannot completely replicate their ends (Fig. 1); (2) protection from degradation by host-coded exonucleases. Linear genomes, such as T4, protect their ends with a terminal pilot protein (reviewed by Goldberg, 1983). Without it, the bacteriophage genome is subject to exonucleolytic attack by the host exo V (recBCD) enzyme; (3) easy integration, through a single reciprocal recombinational event, of the temperate bacteriophage genome into the host chromosome; (4) relative ease of unwinding or overwinding of the DNA helix through the action of topoisomerases; and (5) bidirectional replication from a single *ori* site may enhance the chances of survival of a damaged parental DNA molecule. This is because such limited DNA damage (e.g., a thymine dimer) may block unidirectional but not bidirectional propagation of a replication fork.

D. DNA Modification

Many of the virulent bacteriophages, as well as some of the temperate bacteriophages, protect their genomes from host-induced restriction by modifying some of the bases of their DNA. The classic case is bacteriophage T4, which not only replaces all cytosine residues by hydroxymethylcytosine (HMC) but, in addition, modifies all HMC moieties by the covalent attachment of glucose residues (reviewed by Revel, 1983). In some instances, such a specific modification of bases appears to impart specificity to the interaction between bacteriophage-coded enzymes and their DNA (e.g., the varying specificity of the T4-coded topoisomerase enzyme for cytosine- or HMC-containing DNA) (Kreuzer and Alberts, 1984). An additional potential role for such modification could be to divert the modified bases specifically for use by the bacteriophage-coded polymerizing enzymes, as opposed to those of the host machinery.

The modification of DNA bases by temperate bacteriophages could pose a problem if such DNA modification were lethal for the host. Caution would have to be taken not to express the DNA modification function(s) before the decision to lyse or lysogenize was made. Bacteriophage Mu presents a beautiful example of how such fine tuning of expression can take place. The bacteriophage-coded mom function, in conjunction with the host-coded dam methylase enzyme, modifies approximately 20% of the adenine residues on Mu DNA (Swinton *et al.*, 1983). The expression of the *mom* gene is specifically regulated at the level of transcription, through repression by the host-coded mutH enzyme (Seiler *et al.*, 1986). However, when bacteriophage Mu enters the lytic cycle, the increased number of Mu DNA molecules titrates out the intracellular levels of mutH protein, thus allowing expression of the *mom* gene, with subsequent modification of the adenine residues.

E. Role of RNA Transcription

In the case of most bacteriophage replication systems, there seems to be a requirement for RNA transcription of the *ori* site(s) in order to initiate leading strand synthesis. The RNA can serve as a primer in DNA chain elongation, as in the case of T4 and T7 (Fuller and Richardson, 1985a; Luder and Mosig, 1982; see Sections IV.A.1 and 2). In this case, there is no need for opening up of the DNA helix, since RNA polymerases can bind and initiate transcription efficiently on double-stranded DNA. Alternatively, the role of RNA transcription can be an indirect one, somehow serving to "activate" the origin of replication. This activation could be a consequence of an opening up of the DNA helix to allow single-stranded binding protein (ssb) and other DNA replication proteins to bind to single-stranded regions. Such binding could trigger the series of events that lead to RNA primer formation by the various primase systems. A third possibility is that RNA transcription may be required to remove potential protein inhibitors bound at or near the *ori* site (McMacken *et al.*, 1986). In all instances, lagging strand synthesis does not necessarily require unwinding of the double helix, since the helix is already opened by leading strand synthesis.

In addition to a positive role in initiation of DNA replication, transcription by RNA polymerase appears to exert a negative effect in certain systems, e.g., it has been recently shown that the *ori* γ site of plasmid R6K is inactivated by transcription that initiates immediately downstream and is directed towards *ori* γ (Patel and Bastia, 1986).

F. Redundant Protein Functions

In some instances, it appears that similar protein functions can be carried out by more than one protein. An example of this in *E. coli* is offered by the *rep* and *uvrD* genes, both of which code for DNA helicases that unwind DNA duplex in the 3' to 5' direction (Scott *et al.*, 1977; Kuhn *et al.*, 1979; Matson, 1986; Yarronton and Gefter, 1979). It appears that *E. coli* can tolerate mutations in either of these two genes, but the double mutant *uvrD⁻ rep⁻* is inviable (Taucher-Scholz *et al.*, 1983). One simple interpretation of these results is that the rep protein and the uvrD (helicase II) protein perform overlapping, but essential, duties. It is therefore not surprising that Gilchrist and Denhardt (1987) have shown that the rep and uvrD proteins are 40% identical at the amino acid sequence level.

Another example of potentially overlapping functions is offered by the bacteriophage T7–*E. coli* system. Wild-type T7 bacteriophage grows well on both *optA*⁺ and *optA*⁻ *E. coli* strains. However, a T7 strain lacking *1.2* gene activity can only grow on *optA*⁺ bacteria (Saito and Richardson, 1981a). These results suggest that the 1.2 protein of T7 and the *optA* gene product of *E. coli* are required at the same step of the T7 growth cycle but that one can substitute for the other. Interestingly, certain deletions of bacteriophage T4 also require a functional *optA* gene product (Gauss *et al.*, 1983), suggesting that T4 also codes for a product whose function is analogous to that of *optA*. This product has recently been shown to be the 3' to 5' dexA exonuclease of T4 (Gauss *et al.*, 1987). A cloned and expressed *dexA* gene allows both T7 *1.2*⁻ and T4 *dexA*⁻ mutants to grow on *optA*⁻ hosts (Gauss *et al.*, 1987).

G. One Gene, Two Polypeptides

Many of the well-studied bacteriophages have been shown to possess some genes whose products are necessary for DNA replication and whose transcription and translation give rise to two different polypeptides. In the majority of the cases, as in the *A* or *II* gene of single-stranded bacteriophages, the *69* gene of T4 and the *4* gene of T7, the shorter polypeptide is contained within the carboxyl end of the larger one. The shorter polypeptide does not appear to result from processing of the larger one. Rather, it appears to be translated from independent translational initiation signals contained within the larger polypeptide coding sequence (reviewed by Normark *et al.*, 1983).

In the case of the *O* gene of bacteriophage λ, both potential polypeptides seem to be initiated at the same translational start site, and, at least *in vitro*, the larger polypeptide is probably the result of occasional translational readthrough of the UGA termination codon (Yates *et al.*, 1977). Although the function, if any, of the larger O polypeptide is not known, (assuming that it is synthesized *in vivo*), it has been observed that bacterial ribosomal mutations that drastically reduce translational readthrough simultaneously block bacteriophage λ growth (Engelberg-Kulka *et al.*, 1979).

Among the consequences of bacteriophages having evolved the synthesis of two different polypeptides that contain virtually identical sequences are the following: (1) the common domains may allow the proteins to interact with each other to build large heteromeric aggregates (Shaw and Murialdo, 1980), and (2) the regions of nonhomology of the two polypeptides may allow them to interact with different host- or bacteriophage-coded components (Mosig *et al.*, 1986). If the two polypeptides are expressed differentially, this may provide additional flexibility to such interactions, allowing the bacteriophage to adapt to changing intracellular conditions as the infection cycle proceeds.

H. *Cis*-Acting Replication Proteins

With some bacteriophages it has been shown that the DNA replication initiation-specific proteins (i.e., the proteins that specifically recognize the *ori* site) are *cis*-acting; that is, such proteins act only on the DNA molecule from which their mRNA was transcribed. This has been observed not only with double-stranded temperate bacteriophages, such as P2 (Lindahl, 1970), but also with single-stranded bacteriophages such as φX174 and fl (see Section II). In the case of bacteriophage λ, the *cis*-acting property is not absolute. Rather, it appears that the λ O protein acts *in trans* when in excess, but *in cis* when its levels are limiting (Kleckner and Signer, 1977; see Section III.A).

Interesting features of the *cis*-acting proteins and their corresponding *ori* sites include (1) the *ori* site is usually found within the structural gene that codes for the *cis*-acting protein; (2) both the DNA binding domain of the *cis*-acting protein and the *ori* site are coded for by the promoter-proximal part of the gene. Since transcription and translation are coupled in prokaryotes, it could be that the *cis*-acting protein can bind to its *ori* sequence before the whole polypeptide is synthesized. A consequence of such a DNA sequence overlap could be that some nucleotide substitutions may affect the ability of the *cis*-acting protein to bind, by simultaneously altering its target (i.e., *ori*) and its DNA binding capacity (i.e., through an amino acid substitution); and (3) many, but not all, *cis*-acting proteins nick the DNA at the corresponding *ori* site, thus providing the DNA replication apparatus with a 3'-hydroxyl end to initiate DNA synthesis. Examples of such site-specific nicking include both double-stranded (e.g., P2; Geisselsoder, 1976; Chattoraj, 1978) and single-stranded bacteriophages (e.g., φX174 and fl; see Section II).

One of the advantages of possessing a *cis*-acting DNA replication protein is obvious: it minimizes nonproductive DNA-protein interactions, resulting in faster initiation of DNA synthesis. However, it appears that such a strategy is selfish, since a fellow defective bacteriophage can be helped only at very high levels of the *cis*-acting protein. As mentioned above, such a situation is observed with the bacteriophage λ O protein (Kleckner and Signer, 1977).

I. Conservation of Replication Proteins

In a recent publication, Argos *et al.* (1986) have identified a strong homology between the DNA polymerase I enzyme of *E. coli* and T7 DNA polymerase enzyme. Similarly, the protein sequences of the corresponding ssb proteins of *E. coli* and T7 show extensive regions of conservation. Interestingly, segmental homologies were found between the DNA polymerase enzymes of adenovirus and φ29, two viruses that employ similar DNA replication strategies (see Section IV.B.2). These are but a few examples of homologies of sequence and structure among replication proteins with analogous functions.

The reasons for conservation of some amino acid sequences are clear. DNA polymerases must recognize and bind to the four deoxyribonucleotides, and ssb proteins must recognize and bind nonspecifically to single-stranded DNA. Other reasons are less obvious. For example, most lambdoid phages possess *ori* sites of different base sequence, which are recognized specifically by the λ O protein equivalent (reviewed by Furth and Wickner, 1983; see Section III.A). Hence, there is no need for conservation of O protein sequence among lambdoid phages beyond the ability to bind to double-stranded DNA. However, the λ P protein equivalent has been more extensively conserved, presumably because it must interact with both the O protein and the host dnaB protein (see Section III.A).

J. Building of "Replication Machines"

Most of the large, virulent bacteriophages code for various DNA replication components that have evolved together to produce processive, efficient, and accurate replication machines (Alberts, 1984). An obvious advantage of such an arrangement is their complete independence from the host DNA replication machinery. In most instances, the components are all bacteriophage-coded (with the exception of the host-coded thioredoxin of the T7 DNA replication machinery; see below) and can only function with each other. Examples include interactions among DNA polymerases, primases, and ssb proteins. Such strong interactions could assure that the short RNA primer synthesized by a primase is passed on to the DNA polymerase instead of dissociating from the DNA template. An excellent example of this is the recently demonstrated protein-protein interaction between the T7 DNA polymerase and primase proteins (Nakai and Richardson, 1986a,b). The case of T4 is also notable in that the DNA polymerase may associate with various analogous protein components (such as different helicases) to accommodate the various DNA replication modes of the bacteriophage (Alberts, 1984; Nossal and Alberts, 1983; see Chapter 9, this volume). In addition, it appears that the polymerizing system is part of a huge replication complex which contains both host- and T4-coded deoxyribonucleotide triphosphate-synthesizing enzymes (reviewed in Mathews and Allen, 1983).

K. Multifunctional Proteins

In biosynthetic pathways it makes good sense to incorporate as many biosynthetic steps as possible in a single polypeptide. This way, not only is each product rapidly passed directly onto the next active site, but also coordinate expression of the activities is assured. A recent publication has documented the presence of at least four enzymatic functions in a single polypeptide chain (Freund and Barry, 1987).

The prototype of a multifunctional DNA replication protein is the DNA polymerase I enzyme of *E. coli*. In a single polypeptide chain, it possesses the following three enzymatic activities: (1) a 5' to 3' nucleotide triphosphate polymerizing activity; (2) a 5' to 3' exonucleolytic ("nick-translating") activity; and (3) a 3' to 5' exonucleolytic ("proofreading") activity (Kornberg, 1980). Contrary to the polymerase I situation, the 3' to 5' proofreading activity of the *E. coli* polymerase III enzyme resides on a separate subunit from that encoding the polymerizing activity (Scheuermann and Echols, 1984). Similarly, both the helicase and RNA primase activities of bacteriophage T7 reside in a single polypeptide chain (Matson *et al.*, 1983), whereas those for the T4 (Hinton *et al.*, 1986; Selick *et al.*, 1986) and the *E. coli* (Kornberg, 1980, 1982) systems reside on two different polypeptides.

What are the advantages or disadvantages of coding for two or more activities in a single polypeptide instead of multiple, interacting polypeptides? Obvious advantages for multiple activities residing in a single polypeptide include (1) assurance of coordinate expression at the transcriptional and translational levels, and (2) since the two protein domains are already together, no lag in assembly or waste of enzymatic activity occurs. The disadvantages include built-in inflexibility, in the sense that the two domains are not free from each other to readily associate with other proteins and separately participate in the formation of different replication complexes. In some instances, the rationale behind two different activities residing on the same polypeptide chain is not obvious. A classic example is RNA ligase activity of T4, which resides on a polypeptide whose other function is to ensure the attachment of the tail fibers to the baseplate of the virion (Snopek *et al.*, 1977).

II. REPLICATION OF SINGLE-STRANDED DNA MOLECULE BACTERIOPHAGES M13, fd, fl, G4, AND φX174

A. General Considerations

The smallest known DNA bacteriophages of *E. coli* possess circular single-stranded DNA genomes of similar size. In all cases, the packaged virion strand is the plus (+) strand, which codes for the various mRNA species. Although these bacteriophages can be divided into two structural groups, isometric and filamentous, their genomes replicate by employing overall analogous strategies (see below, and Chapters 1 and 6, this volume). The isometric bacteriophages, such as φX174, S13, and G4 are about 5500 nucleotides long and grow lytically on the hosts they infect (Sanger *et al.*, 1978). In spite of the similarities in DNA structures, these viruses differ in morphology and life-style from the filamentous bacteriophages, such as fd, M13, and fl. Filamentous bacteriophages are about 6400 nucleotides long (Beck et al., 1978; Beck and Zink, 1981; Hill and Petersen, 1982; Van Wezenbeek et al., 1980), grow exclusively on E. coli male bacteria (Loeb, 1960), and are the only coliphages that do not kill their host during a productive bacteriophage infection (Marvin and Hohn, 1969). Instead, infected cells continuously release bacteriophage progeny, without a detectable effect on cell growth and viability.

It has recently been shown that in some instances a filamentous bacteriophage may integrate its DNA in the host at a specific site and exist as a typical prophage (Kuo et al., 1986). Nucleotide sequence comparisons reveal that the isometric bacteriophages have diverged more among themselves than the filamentous bacteriophages; however, the gene order is always maintained (Beck et al., 1978; Godson, 1979; Beck and Zink, 1981; Hill and Petersen, 1982; Van Wezenbeek et al., 1980). The filamentous bacteriophages may have diverged less, because they do not kill their hosts, so there may be some limitations to the types of mutations that can be tolerated in this symbiotic relationship. In addition, filamentous bacteriophages have well-conserved intergenic regions that appear to contain signals for DNA replication and gene expression (Zinder and Horiuchi, 1985; Rasched and Oberer, 1986; see below).

The replication cycle of these small bacteriophages has been extensively studied. Because of their limited coding capacity, it was originally reasoned that analysis of the replication of single-stranded bacteriophages would provide valuable information about the process of E. coli replication itself (Kornberg, 1980). Subsequent work has indeed justified this expectation and has led to many insights into the process of DNA initiation in E. coli. The mechanism of DNA replication in circular single-stranded DNA bacteriophages involves three steps that can be briefly summarized as follows: (1) The synthesis of the complementary strand (c-strand) on the viral strand (v-strand) template, which converts the single-stranded chromosome to a duplex replicative form (RF). This stage is entirely carried out by bacterial proteins. (2) The RF molecules are duplicated, by a process that requires both viral and host proteins. According to Horiuchi and Zinder (1976), the duplication of RF does not involve a distinct mechanism of duplex DNA replication (see below). (3) The final stage is the asymmetric synthesis of the v-strand on the duplex RF template, which results in the accumulation and packaging of viral single-stranded DNA molecules. A combination of bacteriophage and host proteins is also involved in this final step. Thus, there may be only two kinds of DNA synthesis for both types of bacteriophages, c-strand and v-strand synthesis (Fig. 2): the v-strands are copied to yield duplex molecules which then, in turn, serve as template for viral single-stranded DNA synthesis (Horiuchi and Zinder, 1976; Eisenberg et al., 1976), and the cycle is repeated. However, in the case of the isometric bacteriophages, such as ϕX174, there is a distinct phage of v-strand DNA synthesis late in infection, which is coupled to the act of DNA packaging (see below).

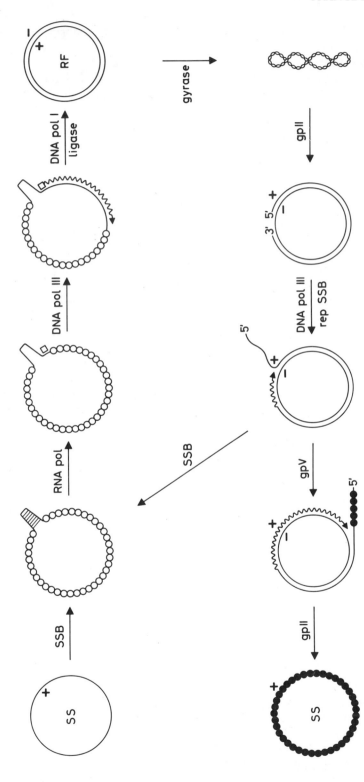

FIGURE 2. Schematic representation of the two mechanisms of replication of bacteriophage M13. The upper part shows the discontinuous synthesis of the c-strand (−), and the lower part shows the continuous synthesis of the v-strand (+). ○, SSB; □, RNA primer; ●, gpV. See text for details.

B. Complementary Strand Synthesis

1. Filamentous Bacteriophages

The synthesis of the c-strand is a model for discontinuous DNA replication, since it requires, in all cases, the synthesis of an RNA primer to initiate the synthesis of a DNA chain. This event has been looked upon as analogous to the formation of an Okazaki fragment during bacterial DNA replication, particularly since only host proteins are involved. For both filamentous and isometric bacteriophages, the DNA must first be covered with the host ssb protein (Wickner and Hurwitz, 1974; Schekman *et al.*, 1975; Zechel *et al.*, 1975). Bouché *et al.* (1975) have demonstrated that ssb is absolutely required for the synthesis of a specific RNA primer at the G4 c-strand origin. Additional studies have shown that ssb participates in the assembly or stabilization of nucleoprotein structures that form at origins of DNA replication prior to the initial priming event (Wickner, 1977; Stayton *et al.*, 1982). Two different mechanisms of transcription have been identified for priming DNA synthesis on single-stranded viral DNA in *E. coli*. The first mechanism, used by filamentous bacteriophages, depends exclusively on transcription of a short, unique RNA primer by the *E. coli* RNA polymerase holoenzyme. In M13, this transcription is specific for the c-strand origin both *in vivo* and *in vitro* (Brutlag *et al.*, 1971; Geider and Kornberg, 1974). RNA primer synthesis is initiated at the *ori* site in the intergenic region located between genes *IV* and *II* (Horiuchi and Zinder, 1976). The nucleotide sequence of this region is highly conserved among filamentous bacteriophages and possesses the potential for forming five hairpin structures (Fig. 3) (Schaller, 1978; Zinder and Horiuchi, 1985; Rasched and Oberer, 1986). Geider and Kornberg (1974) originally proposed that the double-stranded hairpin region in M13 DNA could act as a promoter for RNA polymerase. This hypothesis was not substantiated, how-

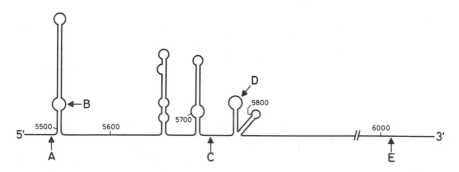

FIGURE 3. Schematic representation of the secondary structure of filamentous bacteriophage origin of replication. (A) End of gene *IV*. (B) Position of rho-dependent termination site. (C) Site of the initiation of c-strand synthesis. (D) Site of initiation of v-strand synthesis. (E) Start site of gene *II*. Adapted from Schaller (1978).

ever, since it has been shown that synthesis of filamentous bacteriophage RNA primer starts in an apparently single-stranded DNA region at nucleotide 5756 and extends into the third hairpin region, terminating at nucleotide 5728 (Fig. 3) (Geider et al., 1978; Schaller, 1978). The nucleotide sequences around this origin region have been completely conserved in bacteriophages M13, fl, and fd (Van Wezenbeek et al., 1980). The specificity of the priming event requires the σ^{70} subunit of RNA polymerase holoenzyme, as shown by reconstituting RNA polymerase from purified core enzyme and purified σ^{70} subunit (Kaguni and Kornberg, 1982; Stayton et al., 1982). However, the filamentous bacteriophage origin region lacks a typical RNA polymerase promoter sequence. RNA polymerase holoenzyme could be attracted at this specific site through both DNA and ssb protein interactions. The original suggestion that a novel form of RNA polymerase, form III, is responsible for recognition of this site (Wickner and Kornberg, 1974) has been withdrawn (Kaguni and Kornberg, 1982; Stayton et al., 1982).

2. Isometric Bacteriophages

Isometric bacteriophages use an entirely different mechanism of priming, relying instead exclusively on the E. coli dnaG primase for synthesis of RNA primers. However, initiation of c-strand replication differs considerably between G4 and φX174, both in terms of host function requirements and in unique versus multiple priming sites on the viral DNAs. The initiation of the c-strand of G4 DNA was found to be relatively simple, since only three proteins—ssb, dnaG, and DNA polymerase III— are required to perform the reaction in vitro (Zechel et al., 1975). Starting at a unique ori site on the ssb-coated bacteriophage DNA, dnaG synthesizes an oligoribonucleotide that is elongated by the DNA polymerase III holoenzyme into the full-length c-strand (Bouché et al., 1978; Meyer et al., 1978). Since the dnaG primase does not normally initiate RNA transcription on either single-stranded DNA or single-stranded DNA coated with ssb, it must recognize a unique feature of the ori DNA region complexed with ssb. Such a feature could be the special "presentation" of the ori DNA sequence when complexed with ssb protein (analogous to the presentation of single-stranded DNA when complexed with the dnaB protein; see below).

The priming of φX174 DNA is considerably more complex, and RNA primer synthesis has been shown to occur at multiple sites both in vivo and in vitro (Baas et al., 1978; McMacken and Kornberg, 1978). In addition to ssb and dnaG, six E. coli proteins are necessary for priming φX174 DNA: dnaB, dnaC, i (dnaT), n, n', and n" (Table I) (Meyer et al., 1978). The nomenclature of the various factors is confusing, primarily because two different laboratories have been involved in their purification and characterization. It has recently been demonstrated that the dnaT protein corresponds to protein 1, which in turn is identical to factor X (Table I) (Wickner

TABLE I. Comparison of Proteins Required for DNA Replication of
Single-Stranded Bacteriophages[a]

Type of replication	G4	φX174	M13, fd, fl	
Complementary strand synthesis	ssb	ssb	ssb	Only host proteins required
	dnaG	dnaG	RNA polymerase holoenzyme	
		dnaB		
		dnaC		
		dnaT (i,X)		
		n (Z or W)		
		n' (Y)		
		n" (Z or W)		
	DNA pol III	DNA pol III	DNA pol III	
Viral strand synthesis	A	A	II	Viral proteins
			V	
			X	
	rep	rep	rep	Host proteins
	ssb	ssb	ssb	
	DNA pol III	DNA pol III	DNA pol III	

[a]See text for details and various nomenclatures used.

and Hurwitz, 1974; Arai et al., 1981b; Masai et al., 1986). It is also clear that factor Y is identical to protein n' (Table I) (Kornberg, 1980).

Although the combination of factors Z and W appears to correspond to proteins n and n", the exact equivalence has not been determined yet (Arai et al., 1981a; Kornberg, 1980; Marians, 1984; Wickner and Hurwitz, 1975b; Sumida-Yasumoto et al., 1978). Studies of the interactions of these proteins among themselves and with φX174 DNA indicate that priming requires the ordered formation of various prepriming intermediates. Specifically, proteins n, n', and n" act at an early, prepriming stage of the φX174 DNA replication by facilitating the assembly of the primosome, a mobile multiprotein priming apparatus (McMacken et al., 1977; Arai and Kornberg, 1981a; Arai et al., 1981a). Protein n', which has an ATPase activity, recognizes a 55-base DNA fragment located between φX174 genes F and G. This fragment, which has the potential for forming a 44-nucleotide-long hairpin structure, is homologous to both the origin used by the dnaG primase on single-stranded G4 and the bacteriophage λ ori (Fiddes et al., 1978).

Arai et al. (1981a) suggested that prepriming proteins n and n" subsequently interact with the n' protein, already bound to DNA to form a nucleoprotein complex that can in turn bind the dnaB protein (itself activated by ATP and the dnaC protein) in a reaction that requires ATP and protein i (dnaT). Once assembled, the primosome moves rapidly in the 5' to 3' direction along the viral DNA, the opposite direction from that of DNA chain elongation (Arai and Kornberg, 1981a). At various apparently random nucleotide sites, the dnaG primase locates the dnaB-DNA complex and makes an RNA primer that can be utilized to initiate DNA chains (McMacken et al., 1977; Arai and Kornberg, 1981a). Thus, whereas the assembly of the prepriming complex takes place at a unique site on φX174 DNA, as on G4 DNA, the actual priming event itself can occur at multiple, random sites. Once the primosome has moved away from its original site of assembly, there is no evidence for the functional presence of any of the proteins except dnaB and dnaG.

It has been proposed that the ATP hydrolysis by protein n' provides the energy for primosome movement (Arai et al., 1981a). However, recent studies on both bacteriophage λ and E. coli oriC replication in vitro suggest that the dnaB protein itself may be responsible for the lagging strand translocation of a primosomelike complex in the 5' to 3' direction along single-stranded DNA (LeBowitz et al., 1985; LeBowitz and McMacken, 1986; Baker et al., 1986). Apparently, purified dnaB protein is able to translocate and unwind the DNA helix in front of it by using its nucleoside triphosphatase activity (LeBowitz and McMacken, 1986).

Elongation of the c-strand on the primed template is carried out in all cases by the host-coded DNA polymerase III holoenzyme (McHenry and Kornberg, 1977). After replication is complete, subsequent steps in RF synthesis include removal of the RNA primer, gap filling by DNA polymerase I and ligation by E. coli DNA ligase (Schekman et al., 1975; Dasgupta and Mitra, 1977). The in vitro replication of φX174 provided a functional assay to identify and purify various bacterial replication proteins. The majority of the proteins required to synthesize the φX174 c-strand were originally thought to be required for replication of the E. coli chromosome. However, recent biochemical studies have demonstrated that oriC-containing plasmids can be replicated in an in vitro system that, in addition to dnaB protein, contains the dnaC protein but none of the i (dnaT), n, n', or n" proteins (Funnell et al., 1986; Baker et al., 1986; Kornberg et al., 1986). Nevertheless, it could still be that the dnaB protein requires these proteins for binding to single-stranded DNA at sites away from oriC. For example, Minden and Marians (1985) have shown in a purified in vitro system that pBR322 lagging strand synthesis requires all of the proteins previously shown to be required for the assembly of a primosome structure on φX174.

C. DNA Structures at the Origin

Although the details about protein-protein interactions are still uncertain, the proteins implicated in single-stranded DNA bacteriophage replication have all been identified, and their mode of action has been more or less characterized. However, the roles of secondary structures formed by the viral single-stranded DNA at their respective origins are virtually unknown. For example, insertion of the transposable element Tn5 in the genome of fd demonstrated that parts of the intergenic region (e.g., the first hairpin on the 5′ end) are dispensable for replication (Schaller, 1978). However this result does not distinguish between requirements for sequences or structures. A different approach to this problem is to analyze the secondary structure of bacteriophage DNA by electron microscopy. The results obtained by Edlin and Ihler (1981) indicate that both φX174 and G4 DNA are folded into similar structures. Interestingly, the major structural difference between these two bacteriophages corresponds to the c-strand origins of replication, which are recognized by different host proteins in φX174 and G4. Since the sequences of φX174 and G4 have diverged about 35%, the overall conservation of secondary structure suggests that it may play an important function. This function may be the alignment of the various protein components, to allow for proper protein-protein and protein-DNA interactions, leading both to the stabilization of the complex and to its efficient utilization as substrate for DNA initiation. Interestingly, analogous folded structures can be seen with single-stranded RNA coliphages as well (Jacobson et al., 1985).

D. Nucleases Involved in Viral Strand Synthesis

Synthesis of the v-strand is much less complicated, since it does not involve de novo chain initiation but simply an extension from a 3′-hydroxyl end. The v-strand is synthesized continuously by a rolling-circle type of mechanism for both isometric and filamentous bacteriophages. The initial event is a site-specific cleavage of the v-strand in supercoiled replicative form DNA by a bacteriophage-coded enzyme—i.e., the gene A product for isometric bacteriophages and the gene II product for filamentous bacteriophages. The nuclease activity requires Mg^{2+} and a specific recognition sequence in negatively supercoiled or single-stranded DNA. Such a nicking event creates a 3′-hydroxyl terminus, which serves as the primer for DNA elongation by DNA polymerase III (Eisenberg and Kornberg, 1979). Bacteriophage φX174 gpA is covalently bound to the 5′ end of the nicked v-strand, whereas bacteriophage fl gpII, although not covalently bound, forms a tight complex with the complementary strand at its cleavage site (Sanhueza and Eisenberg, 1985; Meyer et al., 1981). It has been proposed that the generation of the gpA-DNA complex provides a specific entry site for the rep protein (Duguet et al., 1978). This protein is an E. coli helicase able to unwind double-stranded DNA by traveling in the 3′ to 5′ direction on single-stranded DNA, creating a replication fork (Eisenberg and Kornberg, 1979). The ssb protein also participates in the reaction by binding to and stabilizing the single-stranded DNA generated by the unwinding reaction. Surprisingly, it has been shown in vitro that excess ssb restricts gpA to cleavage at the origin of φX174. This inhibition by ssb may help gpA to discriminate between the origin region and potential additional cleavage sites (Van Mansfeld et al., 1986). After synthesis of a new copy of the v-strand, gpA or gpII is able to cut the displaced single-strand at the origin and ligate the two appropriate ends to form a circular v-strand. Thus, both gpA and gpII function as site-specific breaking and closing enzymes (Reinberg et al., 1983).

Another analogy between the A and II genes resides in the peculiar property of containing a second gene within their coding sequence. The second genes—A* for bacteriophage φX174 and X for bacteriophage fl— encode proteins that start at internal AUG codons and therefore correspond to the C-terminal portions of the gpA and gpII polypeptides (Linney and Hayashi, 1973; Yen and Webster, 1981). When gpA* is overproduced on a plasmid, host DNA synthesis is severely inhibited, and cellular division ceases (Cosalanti and Denhardt, 1985). Although the mechanism of such interference is not known, it has been shown that expression of gpA* does not interfere with either transcription or translation of the host (Cosalanti and Denhardt, 1985). The gpA* protein is an endonuclease that is only active on single-stranded DNA. It can generate 30 discrete fragments when incubated with φX174 single-stranded DNA but displays a strong preference for the origin sequence (Langeveld et al., 1979, 1981). However, gpA can cleave both single-stranded and double-stranded φX174 DNA, provided the latter is supercoiled (Franke and Ray, 1972; Langeveld et al., 1978). The specificity of the gpA* nuclease is thus much more relaxed than that of gpA, although both proteins produce 3'-hydroxyl and 5'-blocked termini. Langeveld et al. (1979, 1981) have suggested that the ratio of gpA to gpA* determines the mode of φX174 DNA replication in the infected cell. No activity has yet been found for the corresponding protein X of the filamentous bacteriophages. However, a very elegant site-directed mutagenesis experiment of the overlapping genes II and X has allowed Fulford and Model (1984) to demonstrate that protein X is required for bacteriophage DNA synthesis in vivo.

E. Viral Strand Synthesis

1. Filamentous Bacteriophages

Gene V protein plays two roles in the v-strand synthesis of filamentous bacteriophages. First, it determines whether the replication will produce single-stranded or double-stranded viral DNA by binding to the v-strand (Fig. 2). The v-strand, once associated with gpV, can no longer be primed to yield RF molecules. Gene V protein may both protect the v-strand from nucleases and serve as a prepackaging protein facilitating bacteriophage assembly at the cell membrane (Webster and Cashman, 1973; Pratt et al., 1974). It is interesting to note that, in contrast to the

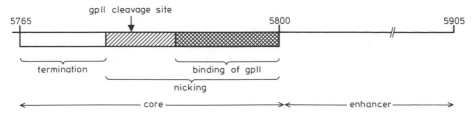

FIGURE 4. Schematic representation of the v-strand origin of bacteriophage fl. The functional v-strand origin is 140 nucleotides long and located between positions 5765 and 5905 (see Fig. 3). The core region is essential for both initiation and termination of DNA replication, whereas the enhancer region is required exclusively for initiation. Adapted from Horiuchi (1986). See text for details.

cases for T4 gp32 and *E. coli* ssb, the binding of gpV to single-stranded DNA inhibits replication. Second, gene *V* protein negatively regulates the synthesis of gpII by binding to gene *II* mRNA (Model *et al.*, 1982; Yen and Webster, 1982). Thus, gpV controls both types of DNA synthesis (c-strand and v-strand) and, ultimately, protein synthesis, since mRNAs are transcribed from double-stranded DNA. The control of DNA synthesis is especially important, since it has been proposed that the ratio of single strand to RF synthesis is what allows the filamentous bacteriophages to grow in synchrony with their hosts (Zinder and Horiuchi, 1985). For example, as an infected host divides, enough RF replicating structures must be present to assure that both daughter cells will continue to be infected and release filamentous bacteriophage.

2. Isometric Bacteriophages

The situation with the isometric bacteriophages, such as φX174, has to be different, since they undergo a lytic cycle and the progression of the infection has to be timed perfectly. Hence, RF synthesis must be completely halted late in infection, and DNA synthesis must be totally shifted to v-strand synthesis. The mechanism by which this is accomplished is very elegant (Fujisawa and Hayashi, 1977; Sims *et al.*, 1978) and is coupled to the presence of high levels of gpC (a bacteriophage-coded, single-stranded DNA-binding protein; Aoyama *et al.*, 1983b), gpJ (a highly basic structural protein of the bacteriophage; Freymeyer *et al.*, 1977), and prohead (a precursor to the mature bacteriophage head made up of gpF, gpG, gpH, and gpD proteins; Mukai *et al.*, 1979). The last steps in φX174 v-strand synthesis have been accomplished *in vitro* with purified components (Aoyama *et al.*, 1983a; Aoyama and Hayashi, 1986). The events that are thought to lead to the exclusive synthesis of encapsidated v-strands are the following. Accumulation of high amounts of gpC allows it to compete with ssb for binding to single-stranded DNA and to the *ori*-gpA-rep assembled complex. The consequences of such binding are twofold. First, the conversion of v-strands to RF is completely suppressed, because the primosome cannot be assembled. Second, the *ori*-gpA-rep-gpC complex is thought to facilitate binding of gpJ and the mature prohead. Such proper positioning of the prohead allows, in an as yet undetermined manner, the simultaneous synthesis and packaging of v-strands (Aoyama and Hayashi, 1986).

F. DNA Sequences at the Origin

1. Isometric Bacteriophages

DNA sequences involved in viral replication have been studied recently using genetic engineering techniques. The comparison of the viral origin DNA sequences of bacteriophages ϕX174, G4, St-1, and U3 revealed a conserved region of 30 nucleotides around the gpA cleavage sites, extending from nucleotide 4299 to 4328 (Baas *et al.*, 1981; Sanger *et al.*, 1978). By constructing synthetic oligonucleotides homologous to portions of the 30-nucleotide conserved region, Van Mansfeld *et al.* (1980) were able to show that the decamer 5'–CAACTTGATA–3' is cleaved upon incubation with ϕX174 gpA. This result indicates that the recognition sequence for gpA lies within residues 1 to 10 of the conserved sequence extending from nucleotides 4299 to 4308 (Sanger *et al.*, 1978). However, when cloned in a plasmid, the first 27 bp of the origin region is required not only for the cleavage of double-stranded DNA (Baas *et al.*, 1981; Fluit *et al.*, 1984, 1986) but also for termination of a round of rolling-circle DNA replication coupled to DNA packaging (Fluit *et al.*, 1986). These results have been interpreted as indicating that gpA interacts first with a binding region that is located downstream of the recognition sequence (Baas *et al.*, 1981; Van Mansfeld *et al.*, 1986). After binding, gpA may unwind the DNA helix in such a way that the recognition sequence becomes exposed in a single-stranded form so it can be cleaved. The cleavage takes place between nucleotides 4305 and 4306 (Sanger *et al.*, 1978). The A protein becomes covalently attached to the 5' end of nucleotide 4306 (Langeveld *et al.*, 1978; Van Mansfeld *et al.*, 1984; Roth *et al.*, 1984; Sanhueza and Eisenberg, 1985). The 3'-hydroxyl end of nucleotide 4305 serves as the primer for initiating DNA synthesis (Langeveld *et al.*, 1978). The unwinding reaction may be facilitated by an AT-rich sequence (bp 11 to 17), which separates the recognition site (bp 1 to 10) from the binding site (bp 18 to 30). Additionally, it seems reasonable to postulate that the 20-nucleotide sequence flanking the minimal gpA protein recognition sequences is important, since it has been conserved among the isometric bacteriophages. Indeed, analysis of mutants with preselected base changes in the origin region shows that all mutations within the recognition sequence are lethal, whereas mutations generated in the AT-rich spacer region appear to be viable (Baas *et al.*, 1981). Interpretation of these data is complicated, because the gene *A* coding sequence overlaps with its target sequence (Johnson and Sinsheimer, 1974). The results obtained with one base change could therefore be due to the interaction of an altered recognition sequence with a mutated protein (Brown *et al.*, 1982). This may explain why different approaches have given different answers to the question of which nucleotides are essential for recognition by gpA (Baas *et al.*, 1981; Heidekamp *et al.*, 1981; Brown *et al.*, 1982).

2. Filamentous Bacteriophages

The DNA sequences required for the replication of filamentous bacteriophages are easier to study, since they are all located in a noncoding DNA region (Van den Hondel *et al.*, 1976). This 508-nucleotide-long region lies between the end of gene *IV* and the beginning of gene *II* (Fig. 3) and appears to be well conserved (Zinder and Horiuchi, 1985). The first regulatory element at the 5' end is a transcription termination signal (Moses and Model, 1984; Smits *et al.*, 1984), whose function may be to prevent any mRNA transcription from entering the region (Zinder and Horiuchi, 1985). The intergenic region contains the sequences involved in both c-strand and v-strand synthesis (Suggs and Ray, 1977; Geider *et al.*, 1978). The sequence necessary to initiate c-strand synthesis lies between nucleotides 5610 and 5740 and can form two possible hairpins (Fig. 3). This 130-nucleotide-long fragment represents the DNA left after nuclease digestion of a complex formed with *E. coli* RNA polymerase, ssb, and v-strand DNA (Schaller *et al.*, 1976; Gray *et al.*, 1978). While important, this region is not absolutely essential as shown by deletion experiments (Kim *et al.*, 1981; Cleary and Ray, 1981). Mutant bacteriophages lacking one or both potential hairpin structures form small plaques and give reduced progeny yields. In accordance with this, the rate of conversion of single-stranded DNA to RF is reduced in these mutants, both *in vivo* and *in vitro* (Kim *et al.*, 1981). These results suggest that there may be an alternative initiation mechanism for c-strand synthesis.

The functional origin of v-strand synthesis has been defined by cloning different portions of the intergenic region of M13 and fl into pBR322 (Cleary and Ray, 1980; Dotto *et al.*, 1981). When gene *II* function is provided *in trans*, a functional v-strand replication origin can direct replication of the chimeric plasmid under conditions not permissive for pBR322 replication and thereby confer ampicillin resistance to its host. Deletion and insertion of DNA sequences in the vicinity of the v-strand origin have established two distinct functional domains within the 140 nucleotide minimal origin (Cleary and Ray, 1981; Dotto *et al.*, 1982). First, there is a core region of about 40 nucleotides that is absolutely required for v-strand synthesis. The second domain, named replication enhancer sequence, is implicated exclusively in v-strand initiation (Fig. 4) (Johnston and Ray, 1984). Disruption of the enhancer sequence does not completely abolish the function of the origin but reduces it to 1% of its original level (Dotto *et al.*, 1984). Accordingly, plasmids containing altered enhancer sequences can no longer interfere with bacteriophage replication by competing for available levels of gpII in infected cells. Surprisingly, the site most frequently used for cloning in the filamentous bacteriophage vectors lies within this enhancer region. Dotto and Zinder (1984a) reasoned that these cloning vectors contain mutations elsewhere in their genomes that can compensate for the disruption of this enhancer. Analysis of different vectors verified this by demonstrating the presence of suppressor mutations that lead to both qualitative and quantitative changes in gpII (Dotto and Zinder, 1984a,b; Kim and Ray, 1985).

The core region of the v-strand origin can be divided into two distinct but partially overlapping DNA signals: a region required for termination of replication, and a region required for initiation, which consists of the sequences involved in gpII recognition and cleavage (Dotto *et al.*, 1984; Horiuchi, 1986). Gene *II* protein plays a central role in both initiation and termination of v-strand synthesis. It initiates replication by nicking the v-strand at nucleotide position 5780 (Meyer *et al.*, 1979) and terminates replication by cleaving and ligating the nascent single-stranded DNA tail created by the rolling-circle type of replication. By inserting an additional origin into fl, Horiuchi (1980) found that replication starts at one origin and terminates at the other. This result demonstrates that the v-strand origin contains signals for both initiation and termination of DNA replication. Further analysis delineated more precisely the DNA sequences involved in termination and initiation of v-strand synthesis (Fig. 4) (Dotto *et al.*, 1982). Recently, Horiuchi (1986) has reported the binding of gpII to the fl origin *in vitro* (Fig. 4). The specific complex can be trapped on nitrocellulose filters and is formed equally well with either linear or superhelical DNA. This is somewhat surprising, since gpII, as mentioned above, is able to nick only superhelical DNA molecules. However, the presence of the nicking site is not necessary for the binding of gpII as judged by the ability of various deletions of the origin sequence to bind gpII *in vitro* (Horiuchi, 1986). Thus, there is a rather good correlation between the ability of gpII to bind to the various origin sequence variants *in vitro* and their observed inhibition of viral growth *in vivo* (Horiuchi, 1986).

III. REPLICATION OF CIRCULAR DOUBLE-STRANDED BACTERIOPHAGES

A. Bacteriophage λ

Bacteriophage λ, discovered by Lederberg (1951), is probably the best-studied temperate bacteriophage. Its genome, consisting of 48,502 bp, has been sequenced (Sanger *et al.*, 1982), and it has been the subject of two books (Hershey, 1981; Hendrix *et al.*, 1983) and many reviews (e.g., Skalka, 1977; Herskowitz and Hagen, 1980; Furth and Wickner, 1983; Friedman *et al.*, 1984b). Among its other characteristics, λ exemplifies the special problem that all temperate bacteriophages that integrate into the host chromosome must face: once integrated, they must cease replicating immediately, because local DNA replication would be detrimental to the host chromosome. Bacteriophage λ has solved part of this problem by manufacturing an unstable λ O initiator protein and by building in an absolute requirement for RNA transcription for initiation of DNA replication (see below). Such a transcriptional event is completely blocked by the λ cI repressor in the immune state.

1. Overall Strategy

Unlike the large virulent bacteriophages, and even unlike the temperate bacteriophage P4, λ relies almost exclusively on the host RNA priming system, mediated by the dnaG and dnaB proteins (Kornberg, 1980), for initiation of its DNA replication. To attract the host replication machinery to its unique origin of replication, *ori*λ, bacteriophage λ uses only two of its proteins—λ O and λ P (Ogawa and Towizawa, 1968). The λ O protein specifically binds to *ori*λ (Tsurimoto and Matsubara, 1981a,b) and to λ P (Tomizawa, 1971; Zylicz *et al.*, 1984). In turn, the λ P protein has been shown to interact with a variety of host-coded proteins, including dnaB (Wickner, 1978a; Klein *et al.*, 1980; Tsurimoto and Matsubara, 1982a,b; McMacken *et al.*, 1983), a key participant in the formation of RNA primer by the dnaG primase (Arai and Kornberg, 1979) and in unwinding the DNA helix (LeBowitz and McMacken, 1986).

There is a small paradox here. On the one hand, the λ P-dnaB protein interaction must be strong enough to displace dnaB from its host protein analogue dnaC (Wickner and Hurwitz, 1975a) and divert it to *ori*λ. On the other hand, once the dnaB protein has reached *ori*λ, it must somehow disengage itself from the λ P-dnaB complex. To disrupt the λ P-dnaB interaction, λ utilizes three *E. coli* heat shock proteins—dnaJ, dnaK, and grpE (see below). Through multiple protein-protein and DNA-protein interactions, and with the possible *in vivo* participation of RNA transcription from the p_R promoter, the strong λ P-dnaB interaction is weakened, and dnaB is positioned on single-stranded regions near *ori*λ. Through its helicase activity (LeBowitz and McMacken, 1986), the dnaB protein unwinds the DNA near *ori*λ (Dodson *et al.*, 1986), and the single-stranded regions are stabilized by the binding of the host-coded ssb protein. The dnaG primase locates the dnaB-DNA structure and synthesizes RNA primers that are extended into DNA by the DNA polymerase III holoenzyme (Kornberg, 1980).

Bacteriophage P2 also requires the *E. coli* dnaB function for its DNA replication (Sunshine *et al.*, 1975). Mutations in the *dnaB* gene that block P2 replication can be bypassed by mutations in the P2 *B* gene. In analogy with λ, this finding suggests an interaction between the B and *dnaB* gene products. Recently, Sunshine and Six (1986) have characterized an *E. coli* mutant, *sub*-1, which allows bacteriophage P2 to grow in the absence of functional B protein. The authors have considered two interesting possibilities to explain their finding: (1) The *sub* gene product is normally an inhibitor of P2 DNA replication. In this case the role of the B protein would be to antagonize sub's inhibitory action. (2) The *sub* gene product plays a positive role in P2 DNA replication and needs to be somehow "modified" by the B protein before it can act. The *sub*-1 mutant product would need no such modification for its action. The elucidation of the mode of action of the *sub* gene product should provide us with additional, interesting insights into the strategies of replication.

Another unique feature of bacteriophage λ's strategy is that it possesses the ability to transiently increase the rate of synthesis of a small group of host proteins following infection (Drahos and Hendrix, 1982; Kochan and Murialdo, 1982). These include the so-called heat shock proteins (reviewed by Neidhardt *et al.*, 1984). The heat shock proteins include the dnaJ, dnaK, and grpE proteins (essential for λ DNA replication; see below) and the groES and groEL proteins (essential for λ head morphogenesis; Georgopoulos *et al.*, 1973; Friedman *et al.*, 1984b). The ability of bacteriophage λ to induce the heat shock response depends on an active host-coded htpR (rpoH) protein (Tilly *et al.*, 1985). The htpR (rpoH) protein has recently been shown to be a subunit of RNA polymerase, σ^{32}, which endows the core enzyme with ability to recognize heat shock promoters (Grossman *et al.*, 1984). It has recently been shown that overproduction of the λ cIII protein alone is sufficient to induce the synthesis of the heat shock proteins (Bahl *et al.*, 1987). It appears that this induction is partly mediated through a stabilization of the σ^{32} polypeptide (Bahl *et al.*, 1987).

2. The Origin of λ DNA Replication

The position of *ori*λ was first defined with respect to the partial denaturation map of λ DNA as the site of λ DNA replication in partially replicated molecules (Schnös and Inman, 1970; Stevens *et al.*, 1971). From this position, located approximately 82% from the left end of the genome, bidirectional DNA replication was observed (Schnös and Inman, 1970; Stevens *et al.*, 1971). However, unidirectional replication with a bias toward the right has also been observed (Schnös *et al.*, 1982), especially under conditions of low thymidine concentrations (Valenzuela and Inman, 1981). More precise mapping of the *ori*λ was subsequently achieved through subcloning into other lambdoid bacteriophages (Moore *et al.*, 1977) or plasmids (Lusky and Hobom, 1979a,b).

Important features of *ori*λ include the following: (1) four adjacent, 19-bp, directly repeated sequences (Grosschedl and Hobom, 1979; Hobom *et*

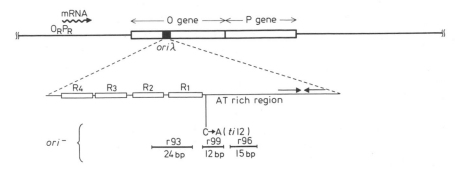

FIGURE 5. Features of the λ DNA replication system. The top line indicates the relative position of the p_R promoter, the O and P genes, and the oriλ site. The second line illustrates key features of oriλ including the R1, R2, R3, and R4 19-bp repeats, the AT-rich region, and the location of the inverted repeat to its right. The oriλ⁻ mutations shown in the lower part of the diagram block λ DNA replication. See text for details.

al., 1978; Moore et al., 1978, 1981) are found spanning positions 39,033 to 39,119 (Sanger et al., 1982) on the λ map. (These 19-bp repeats themselves appear to contain an inverted repeat sequence.) Interestingly, the ori λ sequences are contained within the λ O structural gene (Fig. 5). Purified λ O protein specifically binds to these four sequences (Tsurimoto and Matsubara, 1981a,b, 1982a,b). The lambdoid phages φ80 and 82 contain, respectively, four and five such analogous repeats of different base composition at equivalent positions in their genomes. DNA restriction fragments that contain the four repeated sequences exhibit anamolous electrophoretic mobility (Zahn and Blattner, 1985a), consistent with sequence-specific DNA bending observed in other systems (Wu and Crothers, 1984). Recently, it has been shown that the binding of λ O protein to a single 19 bp ori λ repeat induces a bend in the DNA helix (Zahn and Blattner, 1985b). In this regard it is interesting that Dodson et al. (1985) have observed by electron microscopy that λ O binding to ori leads to a shortening of the length of the DNA molecule, consistent with some type of folding of the DNA around the λ O protein. (2) Immediately adjacent and to the right of the R1 repeat, an approximately 40-bp AT-rich region is found (Fig. 5). This region displays a strikingly asymmetric distribution of purines and pyrimidines, including a run of 18 purines in a row, shown on the top strand of Fig. 5. The significance of this region in λ DNA replication is demonstrated not only by its conservation among the various lambdoid bacteriophages examined but also by the isolation of ori⁻ mutations in it (see below and Fig. 5). (3) Immediately to the right of the AT-rich region, there is an inverted repeat DNA sequence that is capable of forming a 12-bp stem and a 4-base loop hairpin structure (Fig. 5). Its importance, if any, in λ DNA replication has not been demonstrated, although a similar structure in the same relative position can be formed in other lambdoid origins of replication (Grosschedl and Hobom, 1979; Hobom *et al.*, 1978; Moore *et al.*, 1978, 1981). (4) A need for supercoiling, both *in vivo* and *in vitro*,is suggested by the fact that gyrase inhibitors block λ replication. Although the λ O protein is capable of binding to linear DNA fragments containing *ori* λ, the need for supercoiling may reflect an additional requirement for a specific spatial arrangement of all DNA sequences and interacting proteins at *ori*λ (reviewed by Echols, 1986; Gellert and Nash, 1987). Such a need for supercoiling may explain the fact that bacteriophage λ does not normally reinitiate DNA synthesis *in vivo* or *in vitro* while another round is in progress (Schnös and Inman, 1970). This could be related to the recent finding by Inman and Schnös (1987) that the replicated portion of a theta (θ) structure is less supercoiled than the unreplicated parental DNA portion.

3. Mutations in *ori*λ

Mutations in *ori*λ were isolated because they allowed *E. coli* lysogens containing a λ *c*Its*N*⁻ prophage to survive at high temperature. Upon thermal induction, such lysogens fail to excise but are able to initiate DNA replication at *ori*λ, an event that eventually leads to host killing (Eisen *et al.*, 1968). Bacteriophage mutations in *ori*λ, λ O, λ P, or host genes required for λ DNA replication (see below) allow bacterial survival (Eisen *et al.*, 1968; Dove *et al.*, 1971; Rambach, 1973; Saito and Uchida, 1977). Rambach (1973) searched specifically for *ori*λ⁻ mutations by demanding that the mutant prophage still be capable of supplying functional λ O and λ P proteins *in trans* to a superinfecting heteroimmune bacteriophage. Many of the *ori*λ⁻ mutations have been sequenced, and some of them are shown in Fig. 5 (Denniston-Thompson *et al.*, 1977; Scherer, 1978). Notice that r93, r96, and r99 are in frame deletions of the λ O gene coding sequence, which still code for functional λ O protein (Denniston-Thompson *et al.*, 1977).

4. Bacteriophage-Coded Replication Proteins

a. The λ O Protein

Studies over the subsequent years established that the λ O protein (299 amino acid residues; see Table II) and its equivalents in other lambdoid bacteriophages was the one that provided specificity to lambdoid bacteriophage DNA replication (reviewed by Skalka, 1977; Furth and Wickner, 1983). M. Furth and co-workers (Furth and Yates, 1978; Furth *et al.*, 1978) carried out elegant studies in which hybrid O genes were created between pairs of the λ, φ80, and 82 lambdoid bacteriophages. These hybrid molecules carried genetic information from one parent at the amino-terminal coding portion of the gene and from another parent at the

TABLE II. Proteins Involved in λ DNA Replication

	M_r monomer	Native form	Map position	Relevant properties
Bacteriophage-coded				
λ O	33,800	Dimer	38,686–39,583[a]	Binds specifically to oriλ; interacts with λ P
λ P	26,500	Dimer	39,582–40,281	Interacts with dnaB, dnaK, dnaJ, grpE, and λ O
Host-coded				
dnaB	52,300	Hexamer	92 min[b]	Binds to single-stranded DNA; NTPase activity; interacts with dnaC, dnaJ, and λ P
dnaG	65,600	Monomer	67 min	Makes RNA primers on single-stranded DNA
dnaJ	41,100	Dimer	0.5 min	Binds to single- and double-stranded DNA; interacts with dnaB, dnaK, and λ P
dnaK	69,100	Monomer	0.5 min	5'-nucleotidyl phosphatase activity; interacts with dnaJ, grpE, λ O, and λ P; autophosphorylates
grpE	25,000	Monomer	57 min	Interacts with dnaK and λ P
ssb	18,800	Tetramer	92 min	Binds cooperatively to and stabilizes single-stranded DNA

[a]Coordinates on λ DNA sequence (Sanger et al., 1982).
[b]Location on the E. coli genetic map (Bachmann, 1983).

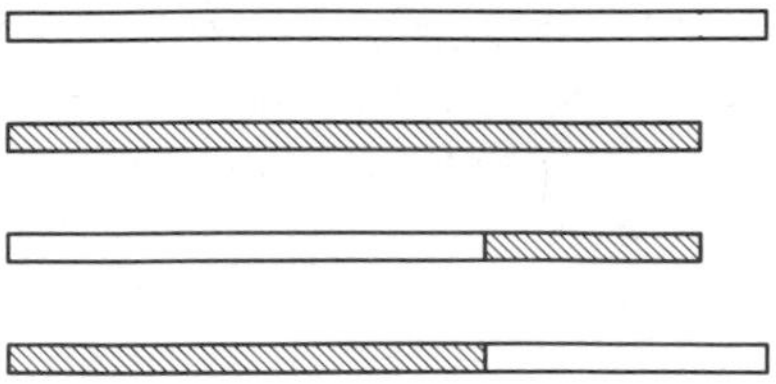

O protein type		Mr	Specificity	
			ori	P
λ		34,500	λ	λ:φ80
φ80		31,000	φ80	φ80
λ : φ80		31,000	λ	φ80
φ80 : λ		34,500	φ80	λ:φ80

FIGURE 6. Structure and function of the O protein of lambdoid bacteriophages. The ability of the λ O and φ80 O wild-type proteins and their hybrid derivatives to interact with their respective *ori* sequences and P proteins is shown. Figure taken essentially from Furth and Yates (1978).

carboxyl-terminal region (Fig. 6). It was shown that the specificity determinant in DNA replication resided in the amino-terminal portion of each hybrid protein. The carboxyl-terminal part of the λ O protein was shown to be the domain that determines interaction with the λ P protein, inasmuch as it dictated whether a P protein from λ or φ80 could be effectively utilized in the hybrid O protein studies mentioned above (Fig. 6) (Furth *et al.*, 1978).

The studies of Tsurimoto and Matsubara (1981a,b, 1982a,b) clearly demonstrated that purified λ O protein binds specifically to *ori*λ. It appears that the λ O protein binds first to the two 19-bp repeats and then to the outside ones. Such order of λ O binding may reflect either a difference in the sequence of the 19-bp repeats and/or the tertiary DNA structure of the *ori*λ region. Zahn and Blattner (1985b) have shown that λ O protein can bind to a single 19-bp repeat.

The amino-terminal portion of the λ O protein, consisting of 165 amino acid residues, has been overproduced and purified. This λ O protein fragment, corresponding to about half of the entire O protein, was shown to be sufficient for binding to *ori*λ sequences (Zahn and Blattner, 1985b), confirming the existence of two protein domains in λ O protein from the studies described above. Since the native structure of the λ O protein is a dimer (Tsurimoto *et al.*, 1982; Zylicz *et al.*, 1984), the above study suggests that the amino-terminal domain of the λ O protein is capable of not only binding to *ori*λ but probably also of dimerizing.

The λ O protein has been observed to be extremely labile, with an intracellular half-life of less than 2 min (Gottesman *et al.*, 1981; Kuypers *et al.*, 1980; Lipinska *et al.*, 1980; Wyatt and Inokuchi, 1974). As mentioned above, such a short half-life for λ O could be related to the need to quickly arrest bacteriophage DNA replication after integration, assuming enough λ cI repressor has accumulated. Both the extreme lability of the λ O protein and its binding to its own DNA-coding sequence probably contribute to the observation that the λ O protein acts *in cis* under limiting protein conditions (Kleckner and Signer, 1977).

b. The λ P Protein

From the DNA sequence of the λ P gene (Schwarz *et al.*, 1980; Sanger *et al.*, 1982), the λ P protein is predicted to consist of 233 amino acids totaling 26,500 M_r per monomer, consistent with that found for the purified protein (Tsurimoto and Matsubara, 1982a,b; see Table II). The native form of the λ P protein appears to be a dimer (Zylicz *et al.*, 1984). Unlike the λ O protein, λ P protein is fairly stable (Wyatt and Inokuchi, 1974; Lipinska *et al.*, 1980).

The key role that the λ P protein plays in λ DNA replication is to attract the host DNA replication apparatus specifically to *ori*λ. It accomplishes this through its interactions with the λ O protein as well as with a variety of host proteins. These include a direct interaction with the dnaB protein (Wickner, 1978b; Klein *et al.*, 1980; Tsurimoto and Matsubara, 1982a,b; McMacken *et al.*, 1983), the key protein, whose presence on single-stranded DNA allows the dnaG primase to initiate RNA primer synthesis (Arai and Kornberg, 1979). In this regard, it is perhaps not surprising that excess λ P protein inhibits *E. coli* DNA replication *in vivo* (Klinkert and Klein, 1979). In addition, the λ P protein has been shown to physically interact with the host dnaK protein, since it inhibits the ATPase activity of the dnaK protein (Zylicz *et al.*, 1983) and it binds specifically to a dnaK affinity column (M. Zylicz and C. Georgopoulos, unpublished results). The λ P protein has also been shown by genetic means to functionally interact with the host-coded dnaJ, dnaB, dnaK, and grpE proteins (Georgopoulos and Herskowitz, 1971; Georgopoulos, 1977; Georgopoulos *et al.*, 1980; Saito and Uchida, 1977; Sunshine *et al.*, 1977). The evidence consists of the isolation of mutations in the λ P gene, called π, which permit bacteriophage λ to bypass either the *dnaB⁻-*, *dnaJ⁻-*, *dnaK⁻-*, or *grpE⁻*-imposed block on its DNA replication. In some instances, it has been demonstrated that there are allele-specific suppression patterns (Georgopoulos *et al.*, 1980), supporting the idea of specific protein-protein interactions. Many of the π mutations, which exhibit altered interaction with certain *dnaB⁻* missense mutants, have been sequenced and shown to cluster in a limited region of the P gene (Schafer *et al.*, 1983). Such a region could code for the λ P protein domain necessary for interaction with the dnaB protein. Surprisingly, deletions of the carboxyl-terminal portion of the P gene can also lead to a π phenotype (Schafer *et al.*, 1983; Schwarz *et al.*, 1980). The mechanism by which these deletions bypass the host-imposed block on λ DNA replication is not known. Nevertheless, the existence of these deletions has shown that the last 63 amino acids of the λ P protein are not absolutely essential for its function in λ DNA replication.

5. Host-Coded Proteins

Bacteriophage λ relies exclusively on the *E. coli* RNA priming and DNA polymerizing systems for replication of its genome. Below we summarize pertinent facts about the host proteins whose functional presence is absolutely necessary for *in vivo* λ DNA replication (see Table II).

a. The dnaB Protein

The *dnaB* gene was originally discovered because mutations in it blocked *E. coli* DNA replication (Kornberg, 1980). It was subsequently shown that the *dnaB* gene product was essential for the *in vitro* conversion of φX174 single-stranded DNA to the duplex replicative form (Schekman *et al.*, 1972), a property used as a functional assay for its subsequent purification (Wickner *et al.*, 1974; Reha-Krantz and Hurwitz, 1978; Ueda *et al.*, 1978). The native form of the dnaB protein appears to be a hexamer (Arai *et al.*, 1981a,b,c; Reha-Krantz and Hurwitz, 1978) of 52,300-m$_r$ subunits, as deduced from the sequence of the *dnaB* gene (Nakayama *et al.*, 1984). The purified dnaB protein has been shown (1) to possess a single-stranded DNA-dependent nucleoside triphosphatase activity (Wickner *et al.*, 1974), (2) to bind to single-stranded DNA (Arai and Kornberg, 1981c), (3) to bind to the *E. coli* dnaC protein in an approximately 1:1 subunit ratio (Kobori and Kornberg, 1982; Lanka and Schuster, 1983; Wickner and Hurwitz, 1975a), (4) to possess a 5' to 3' direction helicase activity capable of unwinding duplex DNA in a processive fashion (LeBowitz and McMacken, 1986), and (5) to be absolutely essential for dnaG primase action on single-stranded DNA (with the exception of the ssb-coated G4 single-stranded DNA mentioned above) by apparently engineering a DNA secondary structure that can be recognized by the dnaG protein (Arai and Kornberg, 1981c).

b. The dnaK and dnaJ Proteins

The *dnaJ* and *dnaK* genes were originally discovered because mutations in them efficiently blocked bacteriophage λ DNA replication *in vivo* (Georgopoulos and Herskowitz, 1971; Georgopoulos, 1977; Saito and Uchida, 1977; Sunshine *et al.*, 1977). The following have subsequently been demonstrated. (1) Mutations in the λ *P* gene compensate for such blocks, suggesting that the P protein interacts with both the dnaJ and dnaK proteins. A direct protein-protein interaction has been demonstrated between λ P and dnaK and λ O and dnaK (Zylicz *et al.*, 1983; M. Zylicz and C. Georgopoulos, unpublished results). (2) Neither the dnaJ nor the dnaK protein is required for the reconstitution of *oriC* plasmid DNA replication in a purified system (Funnell *et al.*, 1986). (3) The two genes form an operon at 0.5 min of the *E. coli* genetic map (Bachmann, 1983; Yochem *et al.*, 1978), with the order being promoter-*dnaK-dnaJ*. (4) The two gene products appear to be dispensable for bacterial growth at low temperature, since each can be deleted or insertionally inactivated (Paek and Walker, 1987; E. Craig, P. Kang, S. Sell, and C. Georgopoulos, unpublished results). However, *E. coli* bacteria with deleted or insertionally inactivated *dnaJ* or *dnaK* genes grow more slowly than their corresponding parent strains at permissive temperatures and tend to accumulate extragenic suppressors. (5) Mutations in either gene interfere with bacterial growth at high temperature, resulting in an inhibition of both RNA and DNA syntheses (Itikawa and Ryu, 1979; Saito and Uchida, 1977, 1978; Wada *et al.*, 1982). (6) The native form of the dnaJ protein is a dimer (Zylicz *et al.*, 1985) of 40,900-M_r monomers as determined by the DNA sequence of the gene (Bardwell *et al.*, 1986; Ohki *et al.*, 1986). The native form of the dnaK protein appears to be a monomer, although oligomeric forms may exist (Zylicz and Georgopoulos, 1984). The *dnaK* gene sequence predicts a 69,000-M_r for the dnaK protein monomer (Bardwell and Craig, 1984), in agreement with its denatured molecular weight (Zylicz and Georgopoulos, 1984). (7) Both proteins belong to the so-called heat shock class of *E. coli* proteins (Bardwell *et al.*, 1986; Georgopoulos *et al.*, 1982; reviewed by Neidhardt *et al.*, 1984). Interestingly, the dnaK protein is 48% identical at the amino acid sequence level with the hsp70 heat shock protein of eukaryotes (Bardwell and Craig, 1984). (8) The dnaK protein has been shown to be a negative modulator of the heat shock response, since *dnaK⁻* mutants overproduce heat shock proteins at all temperatures (Tilly *et al.*, 1983; Paek and Walker, 1987). Moreover, the overproduction of the dnaK protein dampens the heat shock response (Tilly *et al.*, 1983). Similarly, *dnaJ⁻* mutants appear to overproduce heat shock proteins at all temperatures (S. Sell and C. Georgopoulos, unpublished results). (9) The purified dnaJ protein possesses both single-stranded and double-stranded DNA binding activities, with no apparent sequence preference (Zylicz *et al.*, 1985). The purified dnaK protein exhibits both an autophosphorylating (Zylicz *et al.*, 1983) and 5'-nucleotidyl transferase activity (Bochner *et al.*, 1986). (10) It has recently been shown that mutations in either the *dnaJ* or *dnaK* gene interfere with normal phosphorylation of the host threonyl- and glutamyl-tRNA synthetase enzymes (Wada *et al.*, 1986).

c. The grpE Protein

The *grpE* gene was also discovered through the analysis of *E. coli* mutants that failed to support λ DNA replication (Saito and Uchida, 1977). The grpE protein is thought to interact with the λ P replication protein, since mutations in the *P* gene compensate for the *grpE⁻*-imposed block on λ DNA replication (Saito and Uchida, 1977). It has been shown that (1) the *grpE* gene maps at 56 min on the *E. coli* map and codes for a 24,000-M_r protein (Saito *et al.*, 1978); (2) the *grpE* operon is monocistronic and under heat shock regulation (Ang *et al.*, 1986a,b; D. Ang, S. Sharma, and C. Georgopoulos, unpublished results); (3) in analogy with the *dnaJ* and *dnaK* genes, a mutation in *grpE* blocks both host RNA and DNA syntheses at high temperature (Ang *et al.*, 1986a,b); (4) the grpE and dnaK proteins intimately interact (see below); (5) the purified grpE protein undergoes autophophorylation when incubated with ATP (C. Johnson, personal communication); and (6) the purified grpE protein behaves as a monomer in solution (D. Ang, M. Zylicz, and C. Georgopoulos, unpublished results). The precise role that grpE protein plays in λ DNA replication is not known. It appears to be completely dispensable in the purified systems described below. However, a recent observation by C. Alfano and R. McMacken (personal communication) suggests that the grpE requirement is bypassed only when high levels of dnaK protein are present in the reaction.

6. Transcriptional Activation at *ori* λ

It has been demonstrated that, in addition to possessing an intact *ori* site and functional host- and bacteriophage-coded proteins, transcription initiated at the p_R promoter and reaching *ori*λ is essential for initiation of bacteriophage λ DNA replication (Thomas and Bertani, 1964; Dove et al., 1969, 1971). In agreement with this, insertional mutations that prevent transcription initiated at the p_R promoter from entering the *ori* λ region also block bacteriophage λ DNA replication (Eisen et al., 1982). The precise role of transcriptional activation has not been elucidated. Some of the p_R transcripts may be used *in vivo* as primers for rightward leading strand synthesis. Another possibility is that such transcription helps to open up the DNA helix at *ori*λ (Hobom et al., 1978) or to remove inhibitors at *ori*λ (McMacken et al., 1986; see below).

Many of the features of transcriptional activation at *ori*λ have been delineated through the isolation of λ mutants that bypass the requirement for p_R-promoted transcription for DNA replication. The isolation of such mutants was achieved by selecting for λ bacteriophages, which can replicate in the presence of active λ cI repressor (Dove et al., 1969, 1971). The λ O and P proteins were provided *in trans* by a heteroimmune helper phage. One of these mutants, λ *ri*c5b, has been studied in detail. It was originally shown to map near *ori*λ and to allow constitutive rightward transcription from this region (Nijkamp et al., 1971). Surprisingly, the initiation site for this transcription is located approximately 100 bases to the right of *ori*λ with transcription heading in the rightward direction (Furth et al., 1982). DNA sequencing of *ri*c5b has confirmed this conclusion by demonstrating the presence of two point mutations, creating a better promoter sequence, near the site of the new transcription initiation (Moore and Blattner, 1982). Although it is not clear how the new rightward transcription at *ri*c5b helps promote DNA replication (unless it directly affects the λ O-P-dnaB complex assembled at *ori*λ; see below), it has been shown by Furth et al. (1982) that *ri*c5b functioned even when coupled to *ori*82, provided that an intact O protein from bacteriophage 82 was provided *in trans*. This result suggests that DNA replication in the *ri*c5b mutant requires both an intact *ori*λ region and the appropriate functional corresponding O protein.

7. Early versus Late Replication Modes in λ

The form of λ DNA that can be packaged appears to be more than unit length (reviewed by Feiss and Becker, 1983). More than unit-length molecules can be formed either through a recombinational event between single molecules or by a rolling-circle type of replication (Eisen *et al.*, 1968; Gilbert and Dressler, 1968). Early in λ infection, monomer-length molecules replicating in the θ form are found, whereas late in infection, rolling-circle (σ) forms predominate (reviewed in Skalka, 1977; Furth and Wickner, 1983). About half of the σ forms were shown to originate at or near *ori*λ and, in analogy with θ form replication, to replicate in either direction (Bastia *et al.*, 1975; Better and Freifelder, 1983; Takahashi, 1975b). Very little is known about the factors that govern whether the θ or σ mode is used in λ DNA replication, except that under limiting O and P protein levels, the σ form predominates (Bastia *et al.*, 1975; Takahashi, 1975a). The following simple model explains why many, if not all, σ forms initiate at or near *ori*λ. It could be that a uni-directionally replicating DNA molecule fails to terminate when it reaches *ori*λ. Instead, the replicating complex displaces the 5' end of the newly replicated strand (which is perhaps bound to λ O protein). Such displacement and subsequent elongation would result in a rolling-circle type of DNA replication (Eisen *et al.*, 1968; Gilbert and Dressler, 1968).

8. Termination of λ DNA Replication

Obviously the rolling-circle type of replication does not require any specific termination event. In those instances in which O form replication has been carefully examined, it appears that no specific termination site, other than where two replication forks collide, can be identified (Valenzuela *et al.*, 1976). This holds true even for λ *dv* plasmid DNA replication (Matsubara, 1981). Furthermore, λ deletion derivatives that lack the nonessential DNA region located diametrically opposite *ori*λ replicate normally. The two daughter λ DNA molecules are usually catenated (Sogo *et al.*, 1976) and can be subsequently uncatenated by the host gyrase enzyme (Gellert, 1981).

9. *In Vitro* λ Replication Systems

Recently, Fuller *et al.* (1981) pioneered the use of an *in vitro E. coli* crude extract, called fraction II, capable of faithfully replicating *oriC*-containing plasmids. This fraction II system was subsequently shown by various laboratories to replicate exogenously added λ plasmid DNA molecules (Anderl and Klein, 1982; Tsurimoto and Matsubara, 1982a,b; Wold *et al.*, 1982). The requirements for such λ DNA replication mimicked the *in vivo* conditions for θ form replication including (1) the presence of functional forms of the λ O and P replication proteins, (2) supercoiled substrate DNA, (3) specificity for *oriλ* as opposed to other origins such as *ori82*, and (4) a transcriptional requirement, since rifampicin inhibited the reaction. Furthermore, DNA replication starts at or near *oriλ* and proceeds bidirectionally. The elegant studies of Tsurimoto and Matsubara (1984) further demonstrated that, in this fraction II system, bidirectional DNA replication was initiated just outside of the minimal *oriλ* region and proceeded toward it (as judged by the position of the RNA:DNA transition points). These authors observed a marked bias for leftward DNA replication, as opposed to rightward DNA replication in the *in vivo* studies of Schnos *et al.* (1982) and in the *in vitro* purified system of Dodson *et al.* (1986) (see below).

This *in vitro* λ fraction II replication system has also proved to be invaluable as an assay for purifying to homogeneity a variety of host proteins essential for λ DNA replication. This can be done by preparing a fraction II extract from mutant bacteria, such as *dnaK756*, and following the presence of the dnaK protein during the various purification steps by its ability to complement such mutant extracts for λ DNA replication. In this way the dnaB, dnaJ, dnaK, and grpE proteins have been purified to homogeneity (Zylicz *et al.*, 1983, 1985; Zylicz and Georgopoulos, 1984; Ang *et al.*, 1986a; M. Zylicz, D. Ang, S. Sell, and C. Georgopoulos, unpublished results).

10. Protein-Protein Interactions in λ DNA Replication

A number of protein-protein interactions among the λ- and host-coded replication proteins have been documented over the past few years. Many of these interactions were originally suggested by genetic studies and have been subsequently demonstrated *in vitro* with purified proteins.

a. Viral-Viral

The λ O and λ P replication proteins have been shown to interact. This interaction was originally inferred from the genetic studies of Tomizawa (1971), who demonstrated that certain mutations in the *P* gene compensate for an *Ots* mutation. This conclusion was verified biochemically by demonstrating that (1) the purified λ O and λ P proteins cosediment in metrizamide gradients, and (2) the λ P protein binds to λ DNA if, and only if, the λ O protein is already bound to it (Zylicz *et al.*, 1984).

b. Host-Viral

As mentioned above, the λ P replication protein has been implicated from genetic studies as interacting with at least four host-coded proteins—dnaB, dnaJ, dnaK, and grpE (Georgopoulos and Herskowitz, 1971; Georgopoulos, 1977; Saito and Uchida, 1977; Sunshine *et al.*, 1977). This genetic conclusion has been verified conclusively only with the dnaB and dnaK proteins. In the case of λ P and dnaB, it has been shown that the two proteins physically interact since (1) they cosediment, (2) the λ P protein inhibits the NTPase activity of the dnaB protein, and (3) the λ P protein protects dnaB from heat inactivation (Wickner, 1978b; Klein et al., 1980; Tsurimoto et al., 1982; McMacken et al., 1983). The λ P and dnaK purified proteins have been shown to interact since (1) the λ P protein inhibits the ATPase activity of dnaK protein, and (2) the λ O and λ P protein bind specifically to a dnaK affinity column (Zylicz et al., 1983; M. Zylicz and C. Georgopoulos, unpublished results).

c. Host-Host

The dnaJ and dnaK proteins are thought to interact, because mutations in the *dnaK* gene can compensate for the temperature-sensitive phenotype of the *dnaJ*259 mutation (S. Sell, personal communication). The dnaJ and dnaB proteins also interact, since purified dnaB protein binds specifically to a dnaJ affinity column (M. Zylicz, personal communication).

It has recently been shown, both genetically and biochemically, that the grpE and dnaK proteins interact. The genetic evidence consists of the demonstration that mutations in the *dnaK* gene compensate for the temperature-sensitive phenotype of the *grpE*280 mutation (C. Johnson and C. Georgopoulos, unpublished results). The biochemical evidence consists of the demonstration that (1) the dnaK and grpE proteins form a complex in glycerol gradients, (2) grpE protein binds tightly to a dnaK affinity column, and (3) antibodies to dnaK protein quantitatively coprecipitate grpE protein from *E. coli* extracts. In all instances, the physical interaction between grpE and dnaK is disrupted by ATP (Ang et al., 1986a,b; D. Ang, G. N. Chandrasekhar, C. Johnson, M. Zylicz, and C. Georgopoulos, unpublished results).

A report in the literature (D'Ari et al., 1975) can be interpreted as pointing to a functional interaction between the dnaB and dnaK proteins. The authors found that synthesis of the ban protein of bacteriophage P1 (the dnaB protein analogue) in *E. coli dnaK*756 mutant bacteria allows bacteriophages to propagate at 37°C. One explanation is that the mixed dnaB-ban oligomer (Lanka et al., 1978; Reeve et al., 1980) restores a productive interaction with the mutant dnaK756 protein.

11. DNA Replication with Purified Proteins

Two DNA replication systems have been devised in the past few years that specifically utilize the λ O and P replication proteins. The first system is concerned with initiation of DNA replication on ssb-coated M13 single-stranded DNA (LeBowitz et al., 1985). Normally, initiation on such molecules is carried out through the formation of an RNA primer by the host *E. coli* RNA polymerase (Brutlag *et al.*, 1971; Kornberg, 1980; see above). However, in a DNA sequence-independent manner, it has been shown that (1) the λ O and P proteins allow the attachment of the dnaB protein onto ssb-coated M13 DNA, and (2) the dnaJ and dnaK proteins (with the participation of a triphosphate as a source of energy) allow the subsequent dissociation of the dnaB protein from such a complex and its binding to single-stranded DNA. The dnaB protein thereby positioned is capable of movement on the ssb-coated DNA (LeBowitz *et al.*, 1985). Antibodies against the λ O, λ P, dnaJ, and dnaK proteins do not block dnaB activity after dnaB has gained access to single-stranded DNA, suggesting that only dnaB protein is present in this mobile preprimosome structure (LeBowitz and McMacken, 1984). The dnaB-DNA complex attracts the dnaG primase, at apparently random sites, thus allowing the synthesis of RNA primers (LeBowitz *et al.*, 1985). The further addition of DNA polymerase III, the eighth purified protein in the system, allows the extension of these RNA primers into DNA (LeBowitz *et al.*, 1985).

The λ O and P proteins in conjunction with the host dnaB, dnaJ, dnaK, and ssb proteins and ATP have been recently shown to allow localized unwinding of λ DNA at *oriλ* (Dodson *et al.*, 1986). The minimal *oriλ* DNA sequence required for the unwinding of DNA consists of at least two 19-bp λ O binding sites and the AT-rich region adjacent to it. The λ O protein binding to *oriλ* leads to its self-aggregation and to the formation of an O-some structure (Dodson *et al.*, 1985). At least 20 molecules of λ O protein per *oriλ* structure are required for DNA unwinding to occur (Dodson *et al.*, 1986). The addition of λ P and dnaB to the O-some generates a larger structure (Dodson *et al.*, 1985). The subsequent addition of the dnaJ, dnaK, and ssb proteins and ATP allows partial unwinding of DNA at *oriλ*. However, this partial unwinding is asymmetrical with respect to *oriλ*, since the majority of the molecules preferentially unwind toward the right. It is not clear why the unwinding reaction is unidirectional in this system. Addition of gyrase enzyme did not alter the unidirectionality (Dodson *et al.*, 1986). It is thought that, in this system, the unwinding reaction is carried out by the dnaB protein through its helicase activity (LeBowitz and McMacken, 1986) and that the role of ssb includes a stabilization of the single-stranded DNA formed by this unwinding reaction (Dodson *et al.*, 1986).

It has recently been shown by McMacken *et al.* (1986) that addition of purified dnaG primase, gyrase, and DNA polymerase III to the just described unwinding system allows the replication of λ plasmid DNA *in vitro*. This replication system is absolutely dependent, as expected, on an *oriλ* sequence and supercoiling of the DNA substrate. The most surprising aspect of this system is that no need for transcription by RNA polymerase is observed. A host factor has been purified on the basis of its inhibition of this nine-protein λ replication system and shown to be the HU DNA binding protein (McMacken *et al.*, 1986; Rouvière-Yaniv and Gros, 1975). The interpretation of these results is that in the nine-protein purified system there is no need for RNA polymerase transcription, because no HU inhibitory activity is present. The precise level at which HU protein blocks DNA replication in this system is not certain, although preliminary evidence suggests that it interferes with the assembly of the λ O–λ P–dnaB complex at oriλ (McMacken et al., 1986; see below). The HU inhibitory action could be related to its recently discovered ability to allow formation of nucleosomelike structures with altered DNA helical pitch (Broyles and Pettijohn, 1986). The role of transcription by RNA polymerase in the crude fraction II system would then be simply to displace the HU protein from its binding sites around oriλ, thus allowing the assembly of the appropriate replication complex (McMacken et al., 1986). The role of gyrase would be to relieve the positive supercoiling caused by the excessive unwinding of the double helix (reviewed by Gellert, 1981).

12. Summary of the Steps Required in λ DNA Replication

The steps in λ DNA replication, partly shown in Fig. 7, can be summarized as follows: (1) The λ O protein binds specifically to oriλ and forms an O-some structure. (2) The λ P protein in a complex with the dnaB protein locates the λ O protein at oriλ and binds to it. According to McMacken et al. (1986), the inhibitory action of HU protein prevents the formation of the λ O–λ P–dnaB complex. The role of transcription by RNA polymerase would then be to "sweep away" HU molecules bound at critical sites near oriλ (McMacken et al., 1986). (3) The dnaJ, dnaK, and grpE proteins associate with the existing protein complex at oriλ through both protein-protein and protein-DNA interactions. (4) These protein-protein and protein-DNA interactions, together with energy from triphosphate hydrolysis, "weaken" the tight λ P–dnaB interaction, thereby allowing dnaB protein to bind to a nearby single-stranded DNA region. DNA sequences closely resembling the consensus dnaB protein-binding sequence (5′–GATCTNTTNTTTT–3′; Kornberg et al., 1986) are found near oriλ (R. McMacken, personal communication). Perhaps dnaB protein enters single-stranded DNA at such sites. Since both the dnaK and dnaB proteins are capable of NTP hydrolysis, it is not clear which protein (if not both) is involved in the nucleotide triphosphate hydrolysis needed in this reaction. (5) The dnaB protein, utilizing its helicase action, unwinds DNA near oriλ (LeBowitz and McMacken, 1986). The ssb protein stabilizes such an open DNA structure. (6) The dnaG protein locates the dnaB-DNA structure and makes an RNA primer. (7) The DNA polymerase III holoenzyme extends this RNA primer into DNA.

B. Bacteriophage P1

Bacteriophage P1 is well known for its ability to mediate generalized transduction of the E. coli chromosome (Lennox, 1955; Ikeda and Tomizawa, 1965). The molecular genetics of this bacteriophage have recently

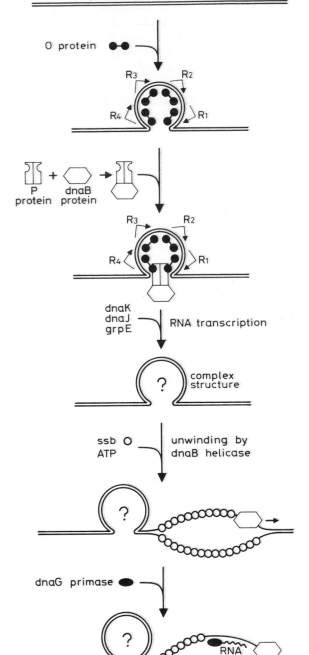

R4   R3   R2   R1   AT rich region

O protein

R3   R2
R4   R1

P protein + dnaB protein

R3   R2
R4   R1

dnaK
dnaJ   RNA transcription
grpE

?   complex
            structure

ssb O   unwinding by
ATP   dnaB helicase

?

dnaG primase

?   RNA

DNA polymerase III
dNTPs
gyrase

DNA replication

been reviewed by Sternberg and Hoess (1983), and it is also the object of a detailed contribution (Yarmolinsky and Sternberg, 1988). Therefore, we will concentrate briefly on the novel aspects of its replication. Notable among these is the peculiar property of being maintained and propagated as a stable plasmid during the prophage state.

The P1 genome, as found in mature virions, is a linear, double-stranded DNA molecule about 90 kb in size which is terminally redundant (over 7–12% of its genome) and circularly permuted (although not completely; Yarmolinsky and Sternberg, 1988). Upon infection, the viral DNA is circularized (Fig. 8) via a recA-mediated recombination between the terminal repeats or via the bacteriophage-coded cre-*lox* site-specific recombination system (Sternberg *et al.*, 1981). Two main modes of replication can then be used: the lytic or the prophage plasmid mode. To carry out these different types of replication, P1 possesses different replication mechanisms (at least 2 and more probably 4; Yarmolinsky and Sternberg, 1988). However, only one of them, the *oriR*-repA system, has been extensively studied.

1. Replication during Lytic Growth

P1 replication during lytic growth is under the control of a DNA replication initiation system, *oriL*, which is totally distinct from the *oriR* replicon used for plasmid replication (see below). The genes involved and the origin(s) used in the lytic replication mode are not yet defined. Observations by electron microscopy suggest the existence (as in replication) of two types of replication intermediates, the θ and σ structures (Fig. 8; Sternberg and Hoess, 1983). The latter form, probably resulting from a rolling-circle type of replication (Fig. 8), generates long concatemers that are suitable substrates for the P1 processive headful packaging system. One of the P1-coded gene products that should play a role in vegetative bacteriophage DNA replication is ban. The ban function was originally discovered because a *cis*-acting mutation, named *bac*, allowed its constitutive expression during the lysogenic state (D'Ari *et al.*, 1975; Ogawa, 1975). The expressed ban protein can completely substitute for a defective *E. coli* dnaB protein (D'Ari *et al.*, 1975; Ogawa, 1975). The ban protein has been shown to be similar in size to dnaB, to cross-react with antibodies directed against dnaB, and to form a mixed complex with dnaB subunits (Lanka *et al.*, 1978; Reeve *et al.*, 1980). It seems reasonable to assume that the ban protein plays a role in bacteriophage P1 DNA replication analogous to that dnaB protein—namely, to assist RNA priming by dnaG primase (or a bacteriophage-coded analogous function) by enabling it to gain success to single-stranded DNA (see above).

FIGURE 7. The series of events that lead to DNA initiation at *ori*λ. See text for a detailed description of the various steps.

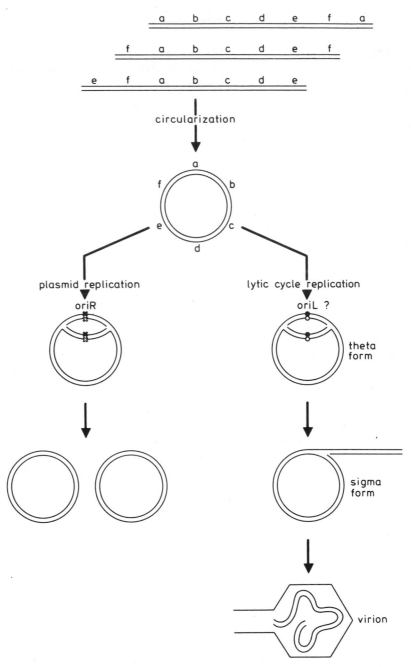

FIGURE 8. The two main pathways used by bacteriophage P1 for its DNA replication. Upon infection, the circularly permuted and terminally repeated molecules are circularized via generalized or site-specific recombination. This circular structure can be replicated by the lytic replicon (*oriL*) or maintained by the *oriR* replicon as a low-copy-number plasmid prophage. In the former case, a rolling-circle type of synthesis produces concatemers that are eventually cut to the proper headful size by the encapsidation process.

2. The *oriR* Replicon and Plasmid Prophage Replication

If, following P1 infection, enough repressor is produced, the lytic functions will be repressed, and P1 will establish a low-copy-number, stable plasmid prophage state actively controlling its own replication. Two *cis*-acting sites (*oriR* and *incA*) and the product of the *repA* gene have been shown to be essential for plasmid replication and copy number control, and the mechanism of their action has been partly uncovered. However, no *in vitro* P1 plasmid DNA replication system is available (by contrast with bacteriophages like λ, T7, or ϕX174), and hence the exact molecular mechanisms of the initiation reaction at *oriR* are not known.

The *oriR* replicon, localized within a short 1.5-kb segment of the P1 genome, is composed of three elements (Abeles *et al.*, 1984) (Fig. 9): an origin (*oriR*), a gene coding for an initiator protein (*repA*), and a control locus (*incA*). The origin is within a 245-bp segment containing several structural features probably important for its activity (Chattoraj *et al.*, 1985b). At one end (left end in Fig. 9), two potential binding sites for the *E. coli* dnaA protein, 5'-TTAT$^C/_A$CA$^C/_A$A–3' (Fuller *et al.*, 1984), are followed by an AT-rich region containing four 7-bp direct repeats (5'–AGATCC$^A/_C$–3'). Note that the latter repeat contains the *E. coli* dam methylase recognition sequence 5'–GATC–3' (Marinus, 1984). A fifth GATC dam methylation site is also present nearby (Fig. 9). It has been established that these two types of host factor recognition sequences are important for functioning of the P1 origin (Austin *et al.*, 1985; Hansen and Yarmolinsky, 1986). Further to the left, five other 19-bp direct repeats are found (*incC* incompatibility determinant). Surprisingly, nine more of these 19-bp repeats are localized within a 285-bp segment, found immediately to the left of the *repA* gene. These nine repeats constitute the *incA* incompatibility determinant (Abeles *et al.*, 1984). The *repA* gene, located between *incC* and *incA*, codes for a 32,000-Mr polypeptide. Interestingly, its promoter lies within the 19-bp repeats, specifically between repeats 10 and 12 (Fig. 9) (Abeles, 1986). Three more potential dnaA protein-binding sites exist between the promoter and the coding sequence of the gene. The repA protein is a *trans*-acting factor essential for initiation at *oriR* (initiator protein; Austin *et al.*, 1985). Its active form is a dimer, found in very low concentration in cells lysogenic for P1 (about 10 dimers per cell; Yarmolinsky and Sternberg, 1988). The presence of the repA protein in such low amounts makes it a rate-limiting factor for initiation (Pal and Chattoraj, 1986).

Besides this positive effect on plasmid DNA replication, repA also acts as a negative element in two ways. It autorepresses its own synthesis at the transcriptional level, and, more surprisingly, it inhibits initiation when present at elevated levels (Chattoraj *et al.*, 1985a,b; Pal and Chattoraj, 1986). The target of repA is the 19-bp sequence repeated 12 times in the *oriR* replicon as evidenced by the capacity of purified repA to bind *in vitro* to the *incC* and *incA* regions (Abeles, 1986). The current model for

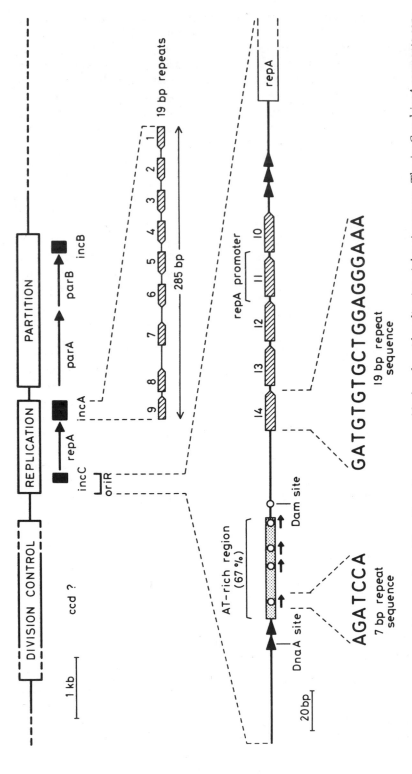

FIGURE 9. Structure of bacteriophage P1 *oriR* replicon responsible for plasmid replication and maintenance. The *incC* and *incA* segments contain sets of five and nine 19-bp repeats that are marked by numbers from 1 to 14. The five dam methylation sites of *oriR* are indicated by open circles, and the potential dnaA binding sites are represented by solid triangles. For more details see Abeles *et al.* (1985) and Yarmolinsky and Sternberg (1988).

control of P1 plasmid replication integrates the known properties of the *incA*, *incC*, and *repA* components of the *oriR* replicon (Chattoraj *et al.*, 1985a; Abeles, 1986; Yarmolinsky and Sternberg, 1988). The *incA* repeats, in view of their negative effect on replication, are presumably the first to be occupied by repA. The subsequent occupation of the *incC* sites, at the appropriate level, would allow DNA initiation to take place. When in large excess, the initiator protein could saturate the binding capacity of *incC* and thus inhibit initiation of DNA synthesis by perhaps preventing access and/or proper interaction with other necessary bacteriophage- or host-coded proteins at the origin. In agreement with these models is the finding that deletion of all or part of *incA* results in a higher copy number for P1-derived plasmids (Chattoraj *et al.*, 1984). Conversely, the introduction of extra copies of *incA* destabilizes a resident P1-derived plasmid (Chattoraj *et al.*, 1985a). An excess of *incA* sequences presumably renders unlikely the possibility that a sufficient amount of the limiting repA molecules will bind to the *incC* region of the P1 plasmid, to initiate DNA replication in the time interval between bacterial divisions. This suggests, quite unexpectedly, that the autoregulatory control of *repA* expression cannot adjust the intracellular concentration of repA to the elevated number of its binding sites. Such an apparent paradox can be explained by assuming that the repA protein has two different domains: one for DNA initiation and the other for autorepression. Binding at *incA* would inhibit the initiator function while leaving unaffected the autorepressor function.

A basic property of the intact *oriR* replicon is that it limits the number of P1 plasmids to one or two molecules per cell (Prentki *et al.*, 1977). Strikingly, the origin regions of other low-copy-number plasmids (like F and pSC101) have structural and functional features (dam methylase and dnaA-binding sites, reiterated sequences, and autoregulated initiator proteins) reminiscent of the P1 replicon (Yarmolinsky and Sternberg, 1988). Another similarity between F and P1 is the presence of genes and sites that control their accurate distribution to daughter cells. The *par* system allows the binding of P1 to a hypothetical mitotic apparatus (Abeles *et al.*, 1985), whereas the *ccd* system may ensure the coupling of cell division to plasmid replication (Ogura and Hiraga, 1983; Yarmolinsky and Sternberg, 1988).

C. Bacteriophage P4

Although bacteriophage P4 was originally isolated from an *E. coli* strain (Six and Klug, 1973), it was subsequently found to be able to infect other gram-negative bacterial species (Bertani and Bertani, 1970; Six and Klug, 1973; Ow and Ausubel, 1980). A characteristic feature of this bacteriophage is its absolute need for a helper bacteriophage, P2 or a P2 relative, to accomplish its lytic cycle (Six and Klug, 1973). The helper pro-

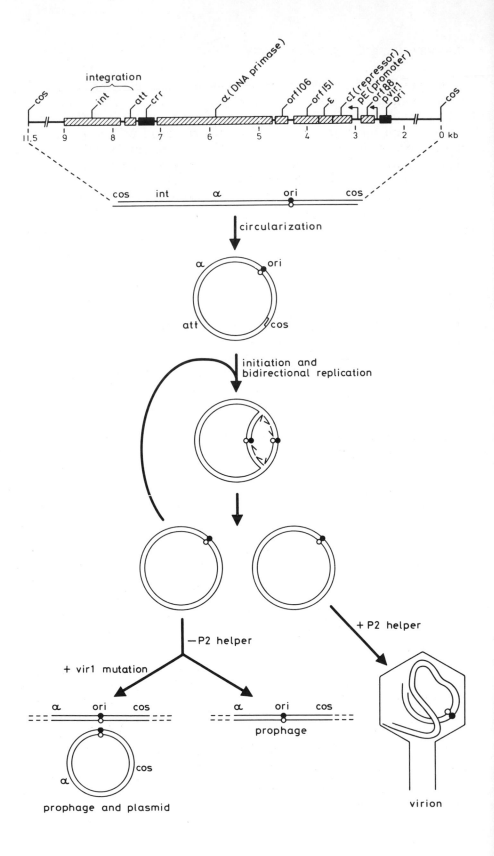

vides the proteins necessary for manufacturing the P4 capsid and tail structure and lysing the host cell (Six, 1975). Rather surprisingly, P4 and P2 do not show any homology at the DNA level except for their 19-base-long cohesive ends and a few adjacent base pairs (Wang *et al.*, 1973; Lindquist, 1974, 1981). Bacteriophage P4 has a relatively small genome, 11.5 kb long, which codes for functions necessary for its own replication, for functions altering the normal pattern of helper gene expression, and for functions enabling it to lysogenize its host (Calendar *et al.*, 1984). The novelty of P4 DNA replication is that, although it possesses a small genome, it (1) codes for its own DNA primase required for both leading and lagging DNA synthesis and (2) exhibits a strict *in cis* requirement for a site located away from its unique origin of replication.

1. *In Vivo* Replication

Replication intermediates of P4 were isolated and analyzed by electron microscopy (Krevolin *et al.*, 1985). This allowed the determination of the mode of replication of this bacteriophage and the precise mapping of the replication initiation site (Fig. 10). Upon infection, the linear genome is circularized via annealing of the 19-base complementary ends. Site-specific initiation occurs, possibly via the formation of a DNA or RNA displacement loop, in a region located 2.6 kb from the right end of the genetic map (Fig. 10). Replication then proceeds, generally in both directions, although some molecules appear to be replicated unidirectionally without any evident preferred direction. At the replication forks, both strands are synthesized: one continuously, and the other discontinuously, through formation of Okazaki fragments (Kahn and Hanawalt, 1979; Kornberg, 1980; Krevolin *et al.*, 1985). The end products of this first round of replication are two covalently closed circular molecules that are subsequently replicated in the same manner (Lindquist and Six, 1971; Kahn and Hanawalt, 1979). By contrast with other bacteriophages (e.g., λ, T4, and T7), concatemeric molecules are not formed during replication of P4. These are probably not necessary, since circular monomeric P4 DNA is a preferred substrate for packaging (at least *in vitro*) when extracts of P4-infected cells

---

FIGURE 10. Genetic organization of the minimal region of P4 genome required for autonomous replication and the replicative cycle of the intact bacteriophage. The minimal P4 replicon spans the region between the origin (*ori*) and the *cis*-required region *crr*. It contains the α gene coding for a DNA primase and other open reading frames coding for products of unknown function (*orf 88, 106, 151*). The *cI* gene directs the synthesis of a transcriptional repressor of bacteriophage-coded genes, necessary for maintenance of P4 as a stable prophage integrated in the host chromosome via the *att* site and the *int* gene product. When cI-mediated repression cannot be achieved because of the promoter created by the *vir1* mutation, P4 can be maintained in two forms: as an integrated prophage and as a plasmid. Finally, when a P2 helper is present, infection results in the production of many P4 virions per cell. See text for further details.

are used (Pruss *et al.*, 1975). The final product of packaging is a mature virion containing a P4 DNA molecule linearized by site-specific (*cos* site) staggered cuts, which regenerate the cohesive ends (Fig. 10).

In the absence of P2 helper, replication of P4 takes place, but without concomitant virion production (Lindquist and Six, 1971; Kahn and Hana-walt, 1979). P4 codes for a repressor (product of the *cI* gene) and possesses a site-specific recombination system (*int* gene and *att* site; Fig. 10). Therefore, infection can result in lysogenization by integration at a host attachment site located near the 97-min region of the chromosome (Cal-endar *et al.*, 1981). In addition, if P4 carries the *virI* mutation, which creates a promoter between the *ori* site and *orf88* (Fig. 10) (Lin, 1984), it can maintain itself as a plasmid (Goldstein *et al.*, 1982). However, in this case, a copy of the bacteriophage is also found inserted into the bacterial chromosome (Lagos and Goldstein, 1984).

2. Genes Involved in P4 Replication

P4 DNA synthesis requires the presence of a functional host *dnaE* gene product (Bowden *et al.*, 1975). This result as well as those of *in vitro* studies (see below) suggest that the host DNA polymerase III holoenzyme is the polymerase active at the P4 replication fork. The *dnaA, dnaB, dnaC,* and *dnaG* gene products are not required (Bowden *et al.*, 1975). Therefore, the bacteriophage must code for its own origin-specific initia-tion protein and enzyme(s) necessary for the priming of Okazaki frag-ments. The finding that the *rep* gene of *E. coli* is dispensable for P4 replication (in contrast to the case for its helper bacteriophage P2) sug-gests that the bacteriophage may synthesize its own helicase or that it can effectively utilize another host-coded helicase (Lindquist and Six, 1971).

So far, only one P4-coded protein, the α gene product (Fig. 10), has been shown to be essential for *in vivo* P4 replication (Gibbs *et al.*, 1973). The protein is a 88,000-M_r polypeptide possessing a rifampicin-resistant RNA polymerase activity that has been shown to utilize GTP for the synthesis of poly(rG) on (1) poly (dG) poly(dC) or (2) poly(dI) poly(dC) template (Barrett *et al.*, 1972, 1983). This property has led to the proposal that the α protein is a DNA primase involved in the initiation of P4 replication (Krevolin and Calendar, 1985). Since the dnaG/dnaB priming system of *E. coli* is not necessary for *in vivo* P4 DNA replication, the α protein most likely primes both leading and lagging strand synthesis.

3. The Origin Region: Definition of the Initiation Site (*ori*) and of a *cis*-Acting Region (*crr*)

The position of the *ori* site of P4 DNA replication was shown by electron microscopy to be located near coordinate 2.6 kb on the physical map of the bacteriophage (Fig. 10) (Krevolin *et al.*, 1985). However, when the replication ability of deleted derivatives of P4 (carried on a colE1 replicon) was assayed in a *polA*(Ts) strain, it was discovered that another region of P4 had to be present on the same molecule for the proper functioning of *ori*. This *cis*-acting region, consisting of about 300 bp, is located 4 kb away from *ori* and is called *crr* (Fig. 10) (Krevolin *et al.*, 1985). Its sequence includes two 120-bp direct repeats (G. Flensburg and R. Calendar, personal communication). Each direct repeat contains three copies of the sequence 5′–TGTTCACC–3′. Interestingly, this octameric sequence is also repeated six times in the 300-bp *ori*-containing segment where replication starts. In addition, the *ori* region carries a yeast consensus origin sequence (5′–TTTATATTT–3′), another sequence repeated three times (5′–CTTTAA$^G/_A$TG–3′), and a potential α protein priming site (CCCCCC) (R. Calendar, personal communication).

The exact roles of the *ori* and *crr* structural regions in P4 DNA replication remain to be determined. Most likely, the *ori* and *crr* regions are brought together through protein-protein interactions, probably of the protein bound to the octameric repeat sequences. Such a spatial arrangement would be important in creating the proper DNA structure at *ori*, to allow the occurrence of the series of events that lead to α protein entry on single-stranded DNA, the formation of RNA primer, and initiation of DNA replication.

4. *In Vitro* Replication of P4 DNA

An *in vitro* system replicating supercoiled P4 DNA is now available. DNA synthesis is initiated at the P4 origin, requires the *crr* region, and can take place in the presence of partially purified α protein, *E. coli* DNA polymerase III holoenzyme, *E. coli* ssb, the four dNTPs, ATP, and GTP (Krevolin and Calendar, 1985). This system should prove useful in elucidating, at the molecular level, the exact roles that these replication proteins play in the priming event as well as the exact roles of the *ori* and *crr cis*-acting sites.

IV. REPLICATION OF DOUBLE-STRANDED LINEAR BACTERIOPHAGES

A. Replication of DNA Molecules with Terminal Repeats and Internal Origins

1. Bacteriophage T7

Bacteriophages T7 and T4 are model systems for the study of the replication of linear genomes with terminal repeats. A detailed analysis of T7 replication, which is the simpler system, is presented in this chapter, whereas only the distinctive features of T4 are described. The replica-

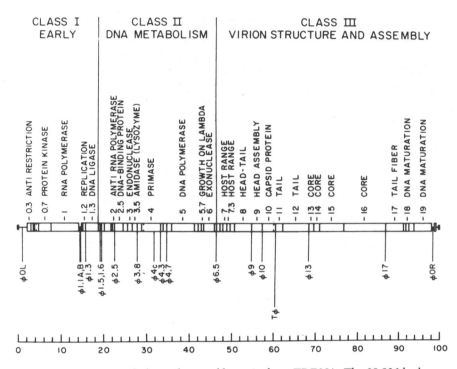

FIGURE 11. Genetic and physical map of bacteriophage T7 DNA. The 39,936-bp-long genome is divided into 100 units. The position of each gene is shown, as are the functions of
some of them. The 17 T7 RNA polymerase-specific promoters (symbolized by φ) are also
shown. The primary origin of replication coincides with the position of the φ1.1A and φ1.1B
promoters. Reproduced from Studier and Dunn (1982), with permission from the publisher
and the authors.

tion of bacteriophage T4 is reviewed ably and in detail by G. Mosig and F.
Eiserling (this volume).

T7 is a virulent bacteriophage of *E. coli*, originally isolated by Demerec and Fano (1945), that has been extensively characterized at the
genetic and biochemical levels (for a review see the article by R. Hausmann, this volume). Its genome, as found in the virion, is a linear molecule of double-stranded DNA whose complete nucleotide sequence
(39,936 bp) has been determined (Dunn and Studier, 1981, 1983). A simplified genetic and physical map of T7 DNA is presented in Fig. 11: the
identification numbers and the functions of 27 genes (out of approximately 50) are indicated, as are the positions of the 17 T7 RNA polymerase-specific promoters. At both ends of the genome, a 160-bp segment
forms a perfect direct repeat (TR). The novelties of T7 DNA replication
include (1) RNA priming by its own RNA polymerase as well as its own
primase, (2) extensive replication through recombination, and (3) a well-
engineered, highly efficient DNA replication complex consisting of few
interacting proteins.

a. In Vivo Replication

T7 has evolved a very efficient way to reproduce itself (Studier, 1972; McCorquodale, 1975; Hausmann, 1976). Twelve to fifteen minutes after infection at 37°C, the host cell is lysed, liberating on the average 200 bacteriophage progeny. Replication is initiated 4–6 min after infection (following expression of class II genes; see Fig. 11) and proceeds at a high rate nearly until lysis occurs. At this time about 300–400 bacteriophage genome equivalents have been synthesized (Kelly and Thomas, 1969; Langman and Paetkau, 1978). Most of the necessary nucleotides are de-rived from degradation of the host chromosome.

The main features of T7 DNA replication are summarized in Fig. 12. In contrast with other bacteriophages such as λ, P1, and P4, no obligatory formation of a circular intermediate is found. Three major stages can be distinguished: (1) site-specific initiation, (2) movement of the replication forks in both directions along a linear template, and (3) formation and processing of concatemers (Fuller et al., 1982).

Initiation occurs at the primary origin located at a position approx-imately 15% on the genetic map (Fig. 11). This step, as will be detailed below, involves the synthesis of an RNA primer by the T7 DNA-depen-dent RNA polymerase enzyme. Bidirectional replication from this site generates eye-form DNA molecules that can be visualized by electron microscopy (Dressler et al., 1972). Termination, occurring first on the left side of the origin, gives rise to Y-form molecules (Wolfson et al., 1972). Reinitiation of DNA synthesis can take place, before completion of the first round of replication, either within an eye-form or within a Y-form template molecule. However, such reinitiation at the two potential sites existing in an eye or Y form seems to be asynchronous (Dressler et al., 1972). The products of the first round of replication are unit-length linear molecules (possessing an eye form if reinitiation has occurred). As a con-sequence of the linearity of the genome and the primer requirement for DNA polymerase activity (Kornberg, 1980), the progeny molecules must differ at their ends from the parental templates. The left end of one should have a 3' single-stranded tail, as should the right end of the other (Figs. 1, 12) (Watson, 1972). The sizes of the single-stranded tails will depend on the position of the leftmost and rightmost sequences used by the T7 RNA primase (gene 4 product; Fig. 11 and Table III) to prime DNA Okazaki fragment synthesis (see below). Two complementary ends will be generated if the single-stranded region, on each daughter molecule, extends over all or most of one of the 160-bp terminally repeated seg-ment.

The pairing of these ends will generate a hydrogen-bond-linked di-mer, which could be converted to a covalently linked dimer by the action of DNA repair enzymes. A similar mechanism will generate a tetramer after replication of the dimer molecules (Watson, 1972). The existence of linear concatemers of T7 DNA has indeed been demonstrated (Kelly and

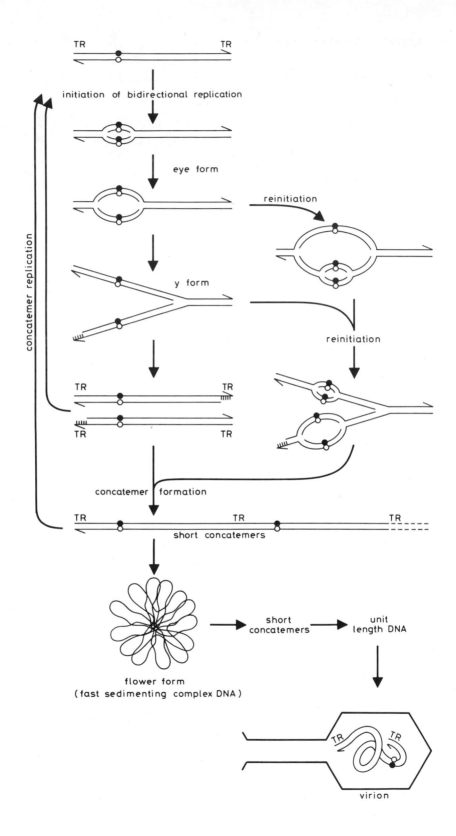

TR   TR

initiation of bidirectional replication

eye form

reinitiation

y form

reinitiation

TR   TR

TR   TR

concatemer replication

concatemer formation

TR   TR   TR

short concatemers

short concatemers → unit length DNA

flower form
(fast sedimenting complex DNA)

virion

TR   TR

TABLE III. Proteins Involved in Bacteriophage T7 DNA Replication *in Vivo*

Type of protein	T7 Gene	E. coli Gene	M_r $(\times 10^{-3})$	Relevant properties
Genes essential for initiation and elongation of DNA replication				
RNA polymerase	*1*		98.1	RNA synthesis at T7 promoters,
helicase-primase	*4A*		62.6	5′ to 3′ migration on single-
	4B		55.7	stranded DNA, unwinding of double-stranded DNA, and synthesis of short RNA primers
DNA polymerase	*5*		79.7	Limited DNA synthesis and 3′ to 5′ exonuclease activity on single- and double-stranded DNA
DNA polymerase accessory subunit		*trxA*	12	Thioredoxin confers high processivity to the DNA-synthesizing activity of gene 5 product and stimulates its 3′ to 5′ exonuclease activity on double-stranded DNA
Genes essential for concatemer stability and processing				
Host RNA polymerase inhibitor	*2*		7	Inhibition of *E. coli* RNA polymerase activity
Endonuclease	*3*		17	Endonucleolytic cleavage of single-stranded DNA
Exonuclease	*6*		40	5′ to 3′ exonucleolytic cleavage of double-stranded DNA
Genes replaceable by E. coli functions				
Unknown	*1.2*		10	Unknown activity replaceable by the *optA*+ gene of *E. coli*
DNA ligase	*1.3*		41.1	Ligation of DNA at nicks; replaceable by the *lig*+ gene of *E. coli*
DNA binding	*2.5*		25.6	Single-stranded DNA-binding activity replaceable by the *ssb*+ gene of *E. coli*

FIGURE 12. The T7 DNA replication cycle. The primary origin of replication is indicated (8), as is the 160-bp terminally repeated sequence (TR). After infection of the host cell, bidirectional replication of the linear T7 DNA is initiated repeatedly at the primary origin. The progeny molecules associate in a head-to-tail fashion, probably through the generated cohesive ends, to give rise to short concatemers that are again replicated by the same process. A higher-order concatemeric structure (flower form) then appears. It is processed first to short concatemers and finally to unit-length genomes.

Thomas, 1969; Schlegel and Thomas; 1972, Serwer, 1974a; Frohlich *et al.*, 1975). As expected, they are composed of unit-length genomes linked in a head-to-tail fashion (Serwer *et al.*, 1982; DeWyngaert and Hinkle, 1980). Other mechanisms, in addition to the one proposed above, could *a priori* explain the occurrence of such structures: for example, a rolling-circle type of replication (Eisen *et al.*, 1968; Gilbert and Dressler, 1968) or homologous recombination between the terminal repeats. However, no evidence exists either for circular intermediates in T7 replication or for the involvement of the two T7 gene products essential for recombination in concatemer formation (genes 3 and 6) (Lee and Miller, 1974; Miller *et al.*, 1976; Lee *et al.*, 1976; Paetkau *et al.*, 1977). Soon after infection, short concatemers are formed, and subsequently most of T7 DNA is found within a fast sedimenting DNA complex. This stable DNA complex (i.e., resistant to ionic detergent, pronase, and phenol), when observed by electron microscopy, has a flower form (Fig. 12) in which double-stranded DNA loops emanate from a dense central core (Paetkau *et al.*, 1977; Langman and Paetkau, 1978). The loops have an average length of 0.71 bacteriophage equivalents of DNA, and each complex is made up of about 200 such loops. Thus, these structures must contain approximately 140 bacteriophage genomes at a time where the average cellular content is approximately 200 bacteriophage equivalents (Paetkau *et al.*, 1977).

Apparently replication, as well as recombination, occurs within such a flower form complex, both processes probably being favored by its compactness and the close proximity of the many genomes (Paetkau *et al.*, 1977; Langman and Paetkau, 1978). Its exact structure and the way it forms are still unknown, but it must be composed, at least in part, of concatemers, since head-to-tail dimers and tetramers are released from it by treatment with S1 nuclease (Serwer *et al.*, 1982). This fast-sedimenting complex, as a true replication intermediate, has a transient existence during the infective cycle. It disappears progressively, being converted to short concatemers and then to unit-length T7 DNA molecules that are eventually packaged into bacteriophage heads (Fig. 12) (Paetkau *et al.*, 1977; Serwer, 1974b).

The processing of concatemers gives rise to DNA molecules identical to the initial infecting molecule; i.e., the 160-bp terminal repeat must be present at both ends of the packaged molecule. Watson (1972) proposed a model in which two staggered nicks, created by a site-specific endonuclease, are produced on each side of the terminally repeated sequence at a dimer junction. Strand displacement synthesis by T7 DNA polymerase from the two 3'-hydroxyl ends (provided they are recessed relative to the 5' ends on the opposite strands) should finally yield two unit-length genomes, each containing two copies of the terminal 160-bp sequence. The products of genes 18 and 19 are probably directly involved in this process (Fig. 11) (Richardson *et al.*, 1986). The DNA sequence at a concatemer junction has some peculiar features that could be functionally important, in a yet undetermined manner, for the processing (Studier and Dunn, 1982). On the left side of the junction, the ϕOR promoter is followed by gene 19.5 and a 159-bp segment (SRR) containing 12 regularly spaced copies of the sequence 5'–CCTAAAG–3' (or slight variants of it.) On the other side of the 160-bp terminal repetition (TR) separating the two bacteriophage genomes, there is a 164-bp region (SRL) analogous to SRR, since it also harbors 12 copies of the 5'–CCTAAAG–3' sequence. The ϕOL promoter and three E. coli RNA polymerase promoters (A1, A2, A3) directing rightward transcription of T7 class I early genes are adjacent to SRL (Fig. 11). Another minor host RNA polymerase promoter (AO) is present, but it directs transcription in the opposite orientation, into SRL. As described in the next paragraph, two of the secondary T7 origins of replication appear to be associated with the ϕOR and ϕOL promoters.

b. Secondary Origins of Replication

Bacteriophage T7 DNA has several origins of replication, whose functioning can be demonstrated under certain conditions. The contribution, if any, of these secondary origins to in vivo wild-type bacteriophage replication is not known, but, as in the case of the primary origin, their positions seem to coincide with some of the T7 RNA polymerase promoters. One, located near the left end of the molecule (around the ϕOL promoter), is utilized when the primary origin is deleted (Fig. 11) (Tamanoi et al., 1980; Dunn and Studier, 1981). Other T7-specific origins of replication were found among hybrid plasmids containing various fragments of T7 DNA. The only plasmids that can replicate in bacteriophage-infected cells are those containing the $\phi 1.1A$ and $\phi 1.1B$ promoters (primary origin) or the ϕOR, $\phi 6.5$, or $\phi 13$ promoter regions (Fig. 11) (Richardson et al., 1986).

c. Genes Involved in T7 Replication

Genetic analysis revealed that the products of seven genes are strictly required for in vivo T7 DNA synthesis (see Table III, Fig. 11). Six are bacteriophage-coded (genes 1, 2, 3, 4, 5, and 6), and one is an E. coli gene (trxA). However, only four gene products are needed for in vitro site-specific DNA initiation (products of genes 1, 5, and trxA) and the basic reactions (i.e., leading and lagging strand synthesis) at the replication fork (products of genes 4, 5, and trxA). This is in clear contrast to other bacteriophages, for which the same reactions require either more bacteriophage-coded proteins (e.g., T4) or multisubunit host complexes (e.g., bacteriophage λ or primosome formation on single-stranded $\phi X174$ DNA) as well as the pol III holoenzyme of E. coli (Kornberg, 1980, 1982; Nossal, 1983).

d. T7 RNA Polymerase and Initiation of DNA Replication

T7 RNA polymerase is the product of gene *1*. Its primary function is the transcription of most of the bacteriophage genes (the class II and class III genes shown in Fig. 11). It recognizes specific promoter sequences consisting of 23 highly conserved base pairs located from nucleotides -17 to $+6$, relative to the RNA start site (for a review see Studier and Dunn, 1982). Seventeen such promoters are found in T7 DNA (Fig. 11), and all of them are transcribed to the right. T7 RNA polymerase has also been shown to be essential for initiation of DNA replication (Hinkle, 1980). This role is well documented biochemically in the case of the primary origin, whose sequence is shown in Fig. 13. The essential features of this region are the two promoters $\phi 1.1A$ and $\phi 1.1B$ (at least one must be

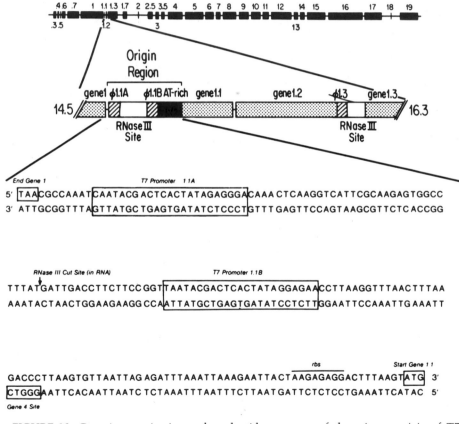

FIGURE 13. Genetic organization and nucleotide sequence of the primary origin of T7 DNA replication. The elements essential for origin activity are the two T7 RNA polymerase-specific $\phi 1.1A$ and $\phi 1.1B$ promoters and the 61-bp AT-rich sequence immediately to the right of $\phi 1.1B$. Reproduced from Fuller *et al.* (1982), with permission from the publisher and the authors.

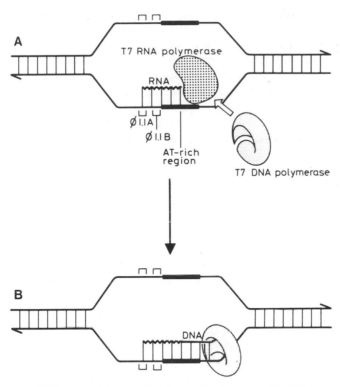

FIGURE 14. Model for the initiation of rightward leading strand T7 DNA replication. (A) The T7 RNA polymerase initiates the synthesis of an RNA chain at the φ1.1A or φ1.1.B promoter. (B) The T7 DNA polymerase displaces the RNA polymerase and uses as a primer, for limited DNA synthesis, the 3' end of the short transcript.

intact; Matson *et al.*, 1983) and the nearby 61-bp AT-rich region (Saito *et al.*, 1980). Site-specific initiation can be obtained *in vitro* with T7 DNA (or with plasmids carrying the primary origin), two purified proteins (T7 RNA polymerase and T7 DNA polymerase), and nucleotides (rNTPs and dNTPs) (Romano *et al.*, 1981; Fuller and Richardson, 1985a). The first step in the reaction is the synthesis by T7 RNA polymerase of a short transcript originating either from φ1.1A or φ1.1B (Fig. 14). The T7 DNA polymerase then displaces the RNA polymerase and uses the 3'-hydroxyl end of the transcript as a primer for limited DNA synthesis. The resulting nascent DNA chains have 10–60 ribonucleotides covalently linked to their 5' ends. The position of the transition point between RNA and DNA is variable, albeit not random. *In vitro* (Fuller and Richardson, 1985a) and also *in vivo* (T. Okazaki, personal communication), it occurs in three regions: between the φ1.1A and φ1.1B promoters, within or next to φ1.1B, and within the AT-rich region. As detailed later on, bidirectional propagation of DNA replication requires two additional proteins: the gene *4* helicase product, and a single-stranded DNA binding protein.

e. T7 Gene 4 Product; A Helicase-Primase

The gene 4 product is found in two forms of different molecular weights (58,000 and 66,000 M_r) that copurify (Hinkle and Richardson, 1975; Scherzinger *et al.*, 1977b; Lechner and Richardson, 1983; Fischer and Hinkle, 1980; Matson and Richardson, 1983). These species may arise from two potential translation initiation events, occurring 189 bases apart in the same reading frame (Dunn and Studier, 1981, 1983). For the moment, no functional differences are known for the two polypeptides. For example, it is not known if both polypeptides are needed *in vivo* for T7 DNA replication. By itself, the gene 4 protein is a multifunctional enzyme that (1) hydrolyzes 5' nucleotide triphosphates (Kolodner and Richardson, 1977; Matson and Richardson, 1983), (2) unwinds double-stranded DNA (helicase activity; Hinkle and Richardson, 1975; Kolodner and Richardson, 1978; Kolodner *et al.*, 1978; Matson *et al.*, 1983), and (3) synthesizes RNA primers at specific recognition sequences on single-stranded DNA templates (primase activity; Scherzinger *et al.*, 1977a,b; Romano and Richardson, 1979a,b; Tabor and Richardson, 1981). The gene 4 protein binds to single-stranded DNA, nonspecifically (Fig. 15) in the presence of a nucleotide triphosphate, preferably dTTP (Matson and Richardson, 1985). The continuous hydrolysis of dTTP to dTDP allows the protein to translocate in the 5' to 3' direction along the DNA. While moving, the protein can catalyze the unwinding of duplex DNA, provided the strand to be displaced has a single-stranded tail of seven nucleotides or more at its 3' end (Fig. 15) (Matson *et al.*, 1983). The gene 4 protein also synthesizes, in the presence of rNTPs, tetraribonucleotide primers (pp-pACCC/A) at specific sites (3'–CTGGG/T–5') on the strand to which it is bound. T7 DNA polymerase uses the 3'-hydroxyl of the tetraribonucleotide as a primer for polymerizing deoxyribonucleotides (Richardson *et al.*, 1986). It has recently been shown that the gene 4 primase and the T7 DNA polymerase physically interact, since they form a protein-protein complex *in vitro* (Nakai and Richardson, 1986a). Such an intimate interaction may help the T7 DNA polymerase locate the RNA primers synthesized by the gene 4 primase (Nakai and Richardson, 1986a,b).

f. T7 DNA Polymerase

The T7 DNA polymerase is composed of two polypeptides, strongly associated in a stoichiometry of one to one, which are the gene 5 product of T7 and, surprisingly, the *E. coli* thioredoxin, product of the *trxA* gene (Tables III, IV) (Modrich and Richardson, 1975; Mark and Richardson, 1976; Holmgren, 1985). As is the case with other DNA polymerases, the T7 enzyme is able to add deoxyribonucleotides to only a preexisting 3'-hydroxyl end, which can be provided by either an RNA or a DNA molecule. It also possesses single- and double-stranded 3' to 5' exonuclease activities (Adler and Modrich, 1979; Hori *et al.*, 1979). The two polypep-

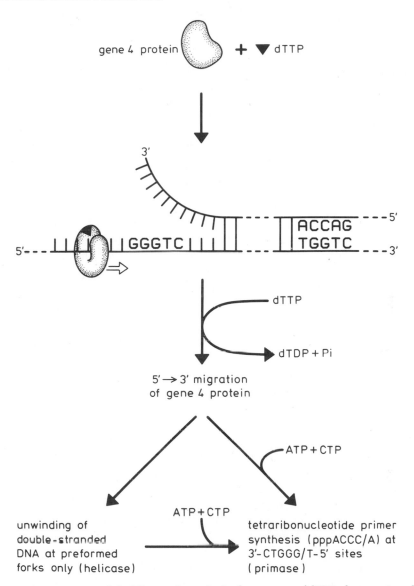

FIGURE 15. Activities of the T7 gene 4 protein. In the presence of dTTP, the gene 4 product binds to single-stranded DNA, then moves along in a 5' to 3' direction by hydrolyzing dTTP to dTDP. This results in an unwinding of the double-stranded DNA structure. In addition, the gene 4 protein synthesizes short RNA primers (pppACCC/A) at specific sites (3'–CTGGG/T–5').

tides can be purified separately. The isolated *E. coli* thioredoxin does not possess any DNA polymerase, DNA binding, or exonuclease activities. The isolated gene 5 product shows a normal level of 3' to 5' single-stranded DNA exonuclease activity but low levels of the double-stranded exonuclease and DNA polymerase activities (Adler and Modrich, 1979;

TABLE IV. Properties of the Two Forms of T7 DNA Polymerase

3' to 5' exonuclease activity	T7 DNA polymerase (T7 gene 5 protein + E. coli thioredoxin)	
	Form I (− EDTA) (low)	Form II (+ EDTA) (high, ×30)
Polymerase activity on nicked, double-stranded circular DNA	Limited DNA synthesis (strand displacement and template switching), stimulated by gene 4 protein	No DNA synthesis even when gene 4 product is present
Polymerase activity on nicked, double-stranded circular DNA with a protruding 5'-ended, single-stranded tail	Limited DNA synthesis (strand displacement and template switching), stimulated by gene 4 protein	Rapid and extensive rolling-circle type of synthesis only when gene 4 protein is present
Putative function in vivo	Recombination and processing of concatemers	DNA synthesis at the replication fork

Hori et al., 1979). This DNA synthesis is distributive, leading to the addition of very few nucleotides to each primer. Addition of purified thioredoxin to purified gene 5 protein restores a fully functional DNA polymerase with its characteristic very high processivity, probably by stabilizing the complex that the DNA polymerase forms with the primer-template DNA substrate (Richardson et al., 1986, Tabor et al., 1986) In this regard, thioredoxin plays a role analogous to that of the T4 DNA polymerase accessory proteins 44/62 and 45 (Nossal and Alberts, 1983; see below).

Thioredoxin was originally isolated as a cofactor necessary for ribonucleotide reductase activity (Laurent et al., 1964). The finding that thioredoxin participates in T7 DNA replication (Modrich and Richardson, 1975; Mark and Richardson, 1976) was made possible because of the isolation of E. coli tsnC mutants, which blocked T7 DNA replication (Chamberlin, 1974). The tsnC and trxA loci were subsequently shown to be identical. Thioredoxin has also been shown to be essential for the correct assembly of the filamentous E. coli bacteriophages fl, fd, and M13 (Russel and Model, 1984, 1985). An elegant site-directed mutagenesis study demonstrated that the reducing potential of thioredoxin is not necessary for bacteriophage assembly (Russel and Model, 1986). This same conclusion has been extended to the role of thioredoxin in T7 DNA polymerase function (Huber et al., 1986). Instead, it appears that the defect of these mutant thioredoxin proteins is a reduced affinity for the gene 5 DNA polymerase (Huber et al., 1986). Interestingly, the thioredoxin mutations that affect both fl assembly and interaction with the gene 5 DNA polymerase map on the same hydrophobic surface of the protein, previously implicated as being important in protein-protein interactions (Eklund et al., 1984). The tight association of the host-coded thioredoxin protein with that of the T7 gene 5-coded DNA polymerase, although rare, is not without precedent. A similar tight association between the Qβ-coded RNA polymerase and the host-coded elongation factor Tu has been previously documented (for a review see Blumenthal and Carmichael, 1979).

The T7 DNA polymerase can be purified in alternative forms, called form I and form II, that are functionally different in spite of their apparent physical and chemical identity (Fischer and Hinkle, 1980; Engler and Richardson, 1983; Engler et al., 1983; Lechner and Richardson, 1983; Lechner et al., 1983). Form II is obtained when 0.1 mM EDTA is included in the buffers used during purification. Omission of this chelating agent yields form I or a mixture of the two forms. In addition, form I can be prepared directly by prolonged dialysis of form II in the absence of EDTA. The properties of the two forms are summarized in Table IV. The essential differences are their template specificity and their mode of DNA synthesis. Form I, whose activity is stimulated by gene 4 protein, is able to carry out limited strand displacement synthesis at nicks and thus could be involved in recombination and processing of concatemers. Form II by itself has a gap-filling activity but is unable to perform strand displacement synthesis, perhaps because of its enhanced exonucleolytic activity. When form II is associated with gene 4 protein, it can accomplish an extensive and rapid rolling-circle type of synthesis on a nicked double-stranded template, provided there is a single-stranded 5'-ended tail at the nick for binding the helicase-primase enzyme. Thus, form II is a good candidate for carrying out efficient DNA synthesis at the T7 replication fork, as discussed below.

g. The Replication Fork

The current model for the establishment of T7 replication fork is outlined in Fig. 16. Form II of T7 DNA polymerase, once it has displaced the T7 RNA polymerase, is able to extend the RNA primer to the right end of the T7 DNA molecule without dissociating from its template (Fuller et al., 1982; Lechner et al., 1983; Richardson et al., 1986). However, this leading-strand synthesis relies absolutely on the functional cooperation, probably via a direct protein-protein interaction (Nakai and Richardson, 1986a,b; Richardson et al., 1986), of the polymerase with the gene 4 product, whose helicase activity is necessary to efficiently separate the parental strands. Lagging-strand synthesis is initiated at regular intervals from RNA primers synthesized by the gene 4 protein. The pppACCC/A tetraribonucleotides are used as primers for Okazaki fragment synthesis by the form II DNA polymerase, using its gap-filling activity. To complete lagging-strand synthesis, the Okazaki fragments have to be processed (RNA primer removal) and joined together. These reactions can be

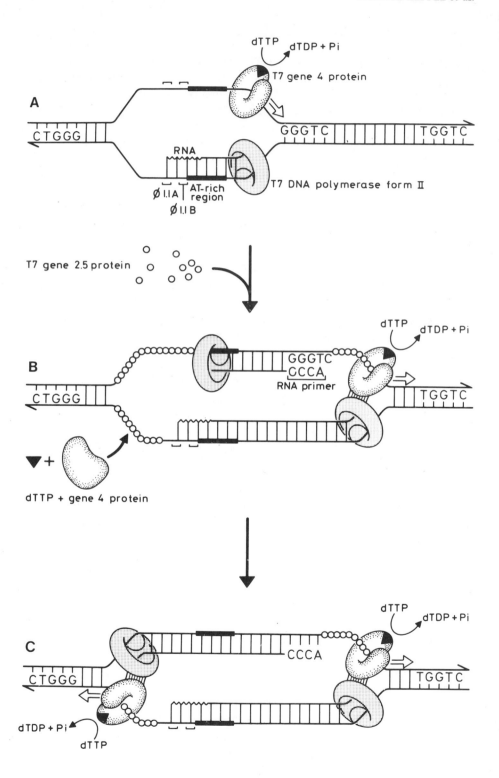

achieved *in vitro* by the sequential action of three enzymes (Engler and Richardson, 1983). The gene 6 product is a 5' to 3' double-stranded exonuclease (Fig. 11, Table III) whose RNase H activity can hydrolyze RNA in RNA/DNA hybrids (Shinozaki and Okazaki, 1977, 1978). The created gap is repaired by the form II DNA polymerase, and the remaining nick is sealed by the host DNA ligase or by the T7 DNA ligase, the gene *1.3* product (Fig. 11, Table III) (Masamune *et al.*, 1971; Studier, 1973). Another T7-specified protein, the gene *2.5* product (Fig. 11, Table III) probably participates *in vivo* for proper functioning of the replication fork, although it can be replaced by the *E. coli ssb* gene product. The gene *2.5* protein is a single-stranded DNA-binding protein that stimulates T7 DNA polymerase-synthesizing activity (Scherzinger *et al.*, 1973; Reuben and Gefter, 1974; Romano and Richardson, 1979a). In addition, the gene *2.5* protein (or the *E. coli* ssb protein, but not the T4 gene *32* single-stranded binding product) is required *in vitro* for establishment of a leftward moving replication fork (Fuller and Richardson, 1985b). Its role in that event is probably to locally unwind the DNA duplex to the left of the φ*1.1A* promoter, to allow binding of the gene *4* product. The helicase and primase activities of this protein will in turn permit the polymerase to extend DNA synthesis to the left of the primary origin.

h. Other T7 Gene Products Participating in in Vivo DNA Replication

Gene *1.2* codes for a function nonessential for bacteriophage T7 growth, since it is replaceable by the host *optA* gene product (Fig. 11, Table III) (Saito and Richardson, 1981a,b). When both genes are inactivated, *in vivo* T7 DNA replication is prematurely arrested, and the newly synthesized DNA is degraded. *In vitro*, the gene *1.2* product or the *optA* product is required for proper T7 DNA packaging. However, so far no specific role has been assigned to the gene *1.2* protein, in spite of the fact that it has been purified to near homogeneity (Richardson *et al.*, 1986).

Gene *2* amber mutants do not produce viable bacteriophage progeny upon infection of a nonpermissive host, even though a substantial amount of DNA synthesis takes place. The replicated DNA is found in molecules slightly shorter than unit-length T7 DNA (Center, 1975) as a consequence of concatemer degradation (DeWyngaert and Hinkle, 1980;

FIGURE 16. Model for the establishment of rightward and leftward T7 DNA replication forks at the primary origin. (A) The gene *4* product binds to the single-stranded region created by the priming reaction (see Fig. 14) and forms a complex with the DNA polymerase form II. (B) The gene *4* protein in this complex unwinds duplex DNA, allowing extension of leading strand synthesis by the T7 DNA polymerase moiety. It also synthesizes short RNA primers which can be used by other DNA polymerase molecules for lagging-strand synthesis. (C) Binding of single-stranded DNA binding protein molecules (T7 gene *2.5* product or *E. coli* ssb protein) results in limited unwinding, sufficient to allow the binding of a molecule of gene *4* protein and the subsequent assembly of a second replication complex.

Mooney et al., 1980). Gene 2 protein forms a tight complex with E. coli RNA polymerase. This results in the inhibition of host gene transcription. More unexpectedly, the gene 2 product–RNA polymerase complex protects the left end of the T7 genome (i.e., the region where E. coli RNA polymeraselike promoters are found) within concatemers from nucleases and in particular from gene 3 endonuclease.

Nucleases coded by genes 3 and 6 of T7 (Fig. 11, Table III) are essential for bacteriophage propagation. One of their functions is to degrade the host DNA in order to provide most of the nucleotides necessary for efficient replication of bacteriophage DNA (Sadowski and Kerr, 1970; Langman and Paetkau, 1978). They also play a more direct role in replication (see below) and in recombination (Miller, 1975; Lee et al., 1976; Tsujimoto and Ogawa, 1977, 1978; Lee and Sadowski, 1981).

The gene 3 product is an endonuclease that has a strong specificity for single-stranded DNA (Center and Richardson, 1970; Sadowski, 1971). In its absence, bacteriophage DNA synthesis does take place, and concatemers are formed. However, the newly synthesized DNA is found exclusively within a fast-sedimenting complex that is not further processed (Paetkau et al., 1977; Langman and Paetkau, 1978). In addition, the gene 3 endonuclease is not required, at least in vitro, for the conversion of short concatemers to unit-length genomes. Thus, the gene 3 endonuclease is likely to be involved in an early stage of DNA maturation: the conversion of the complex DNA to short concatemers. It has recently been shown that purified gene 3 endonuclease has a strong preference for cleaving either Y- or X-shaped DNA molecules resembling Holliday structures (De Massy et al., 1987). This activity is analogous to the T4 endo-VII enzyme (Mizuuchi et al., 1982; Lilley and Kemper, 1984; Jensch and Kemper, 1986; see below). Gene 3 endonuclease is involved, then, in the resolution of the highly branched DNA structures seen at late stages of the T7 DNA replication cycle. The enzyme cleaves two opposing strands near or at the branch point to give rise to linear molecules. Some of these products are substrates for T4 DNA ligase, demonstrating that they are precisely cleaved at the base of the stem structure (De Massey et al., 1987). Site specificity could be conferred to the gene 3 protein by interaction with the host RNA polymerase bound to a promoter in the left end region of a bacteriophage genome within a concatemeric structure. Such an interaction would have to be precisely timed to avoid premature degradation of the replicating T7 DNA. The gene 2 protein possibly contributes to such a control (DeWyngaert and Hinkle, 1979; Mooney et al., 1980).

The exonuclease encoded by gene 6 removes nucleotides from the 5' terminus of double-stranded DNA (Kerr and Sadowski, 1972a,b). During the DNA replication cycle, T7 exonuclease appears to be required for the stabilization of the long concatemeric structures. When gene 6 is defective, T7 DNA replication proceeds until short concatemers are formed. They are then rapidly fragmented to pieces shorter than unit length (Miller *et al.*, 1976). One explanation is that the gene 6 exonuclease is needed for the repair of structures (e.g., possibly the junctions between Okazaki fragments) that can be degraded by the gene 3 endonuclease.

2. Bacteriophage T4

T4 is the prototype of a large, virulent bacteriophage. Originally discovered by Demerec and Fano (1945), it was one of the first bacteriophages chosen by the Max Delbruck school to study various aspects of molecular genetics and biochemistry. An excellent book with reviews on various aspects of T4 biology has recently been published (Mathews *et al.*, 1983), and a detailed article by G. Mosig and F. Eiserling on T4 can be found in this volume. Specific reviews on DNA replication include articles by Alberts *et al.* (1982), Nossal and Alberts (1983), and Alberts (1984). The interesting features of bacteriophage T4 DNA replication include the use of modified DNA bases, complete independence from the host DNA replication machinery, multiple DNA replication mechanisms, and the construction of specific DNA replication machineries that function properly only in the presence of specific bacteriophage-coded components (i.e., they will not accept components from either the bacteriophage T7 or *E. coli* DNA replication systems; see below).

a. Background

Bacteriophage T4 possesses an approximately 166-kb linear genome (Kutter and Rüger, 1983), which is terminally redundant (about 3% of its genome). It packages its DNA by a "headful" mechanism (Streisinger *et al.*, 1967), without apparent preference for a specific *pac* site to initiate its encapsidation process (Kalinski and Black, 1986). As a consequence, the T4 genome is circularly permuted (Streisinger *et al.*, 1964).

The bacteriophage T4 chromosome encodes for two types of unusual modifications which render it resistant to digestion by most deoxyribonucleases. The first is the replacement of all cytosine residues with 5-hydroxymethylcytosine (HMC) (Wyatt and Cohen, 1953). To accomplish the complete replacement of cytosine by HMC on its DNA, T4 induces the synthesis of a dCTPase enzyme (the product of gene *59*) and a dCMP hydroxymethylase enzyme (the product of gene *42*) (reviewed by Mathews and Allen, 1983). The replacement of C by HMC has led to the evolution of T4-coded proteins which recognize different sequences on HMC- as opposed to C-containing DNA, as exemplified by the T4 topoisomerase enzyme (Kreuzer and Alberts, 1984). The second is the α or β glucosylation of all of the HMC residues in T4 DNA. Both glucosylation and methylation of T4 DNA are carried out by bacteriophage-coded enzymes on completed polynucleotide chains (reviewed by Revel, 1983; Hattman, 1983).

Since T4 is a lytic bacteriophage, it is to its advantage to utilize all

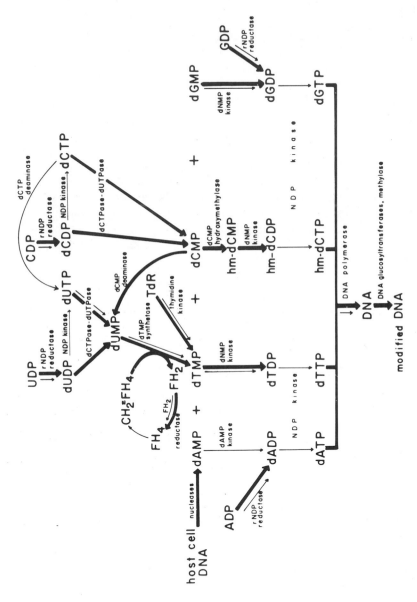

FIGURE 17. The synthesis of DNA nucleotides in T4-infected *E. coli*. The enzymatic reactions catalyzed by bacteriophage-coded enzymes are shown with thick arrows, those by the host-coded enzymes with light arrows. Reproduced from Mathews and Allen (1983), with permission from the publisher and the authors.

available sources of deoxyribonucleotides for its DNA replication. Accordingly, T4 induces two cytosine-specific deoxyribonucleases (the *denA* and *denB* gene products; reviewed by Snustad *et al.*, 1983), which initiate the degradation of the host chromosome. Of these two enzymes, the *denA*-coded protein appears to play the major role in host DNA breakdown (Carlson and Overvatn, 1986). Next, the gene *46*- and *47*-coded exonuclease degrades the host DNA fragments into acid-soluble components (reviewed by Snustad *et al.*, 1983). In addition to utilizing the nucleotides derived from host DNA breakdown, bacteriophage T4 also synthesizes a number of other DNA precursor biosynthetic enzymes, which contribute to the production of deoxyribonucleotides (reviewed by Mathews and Allen, 1983). Often these bacteriophage-coded enzymes overlap in activity with the corresponding host-coded ones (e.g., dTMP synthetase and dNMP kinase). Figure 17 summarizes the flow of DNA precursors from both host DNA breakdown and *de novo* synthesis.

There are two interesting sets of observations about DNA precursor biosynthesis. The first is the demonstration in two laboratories of the presence of a dNTP-synthesizing multienzyme complex, sedimenting as an aggregate in sucrose gradients (Chiu and Greenberg, 1968; Reddy *et al.*, 1977; reviewed by Mathews and Allen, 1983). It has been possible to identify the presence of most T4-coded as well as several of the host-coded enzymes involved in DNA precursor biosynthesis in this fast-sedimenting aggregate (reviewed in Mathews and Allen, 1983). The role of the multienzyme complex may be to facilitate rapid synthesis of deoxyribonucleotides by limiting the distance that the various intermediate molecules have to travel to reach the catalytic site of the next enzyme. In addition, the multienzyme complex appears to synthesize the dNTPs in the same ratio as is found in T4 DNA (Flanegan and Greenberg, 1977). The second interesting aspect of the multienzyme complex is that various polypeptides in this complex appear to functionally interact with components of the replicating machinery. This conclusion is based on (1) the altered fidelity of DNA replication exhibited by temperature-sensitive mutations in gene *42* (Chiu and Greenberg, 1973; Drake, 1973), (2) the fact that mutations in gene *42* can be compensated by mutations in gene *43*, which codes for the T4 DNA polymerase (Chao *et al.*, 1977; Karam *et al.*, 1983), and (3) allele-specific suppression between mutations in genes *41/61* (which code for the helicase/primase system of T4; see below) and mutations in *frd* (which codes for dihydrofolate reductase; MacDonald and Hall, 1984).

b. The in Vitro Building of T4 DNA Replication Machineries

The combined efforts of the B. Alberts and N. Nossal laboratories have allowed over the past years the delineation of minimal *in vitro* DNA replication systems made up of purified components (reviewed in Alberts *et al.*, 1982; Alberts, 1984; Nossal and Alberts, 1983). Table V summa-

TABLE V. Properties of Bacteriophage T4 DNA
Replication Proteins

Protein function	T4 gene		M_r monomer
DNA polymerase	43		110,000
Single-stranded DNA binding; helix-destabilizing protein	32		34,500
Polymerase accessory proteins	44 ⎱ 62 ⎰ 45	complex	34,000 20,000 24,500
Helicase	41		58,000
RNA primase	61		40,000
Topoisomerase II proteins	39 ⎫ 52 ⎬ 60 ⎭	complex	56,000 46,000 17,000
Helicase	dda		47,000
Recombination, repair	uvsX uvsY		39,000 16,000
DNA replication	69 69* 61.1		46,000 25,000 6,000

rizes the properties of some T4-coded proteins that play a major role in bacteriophage T4 DNA replication and recombination.

i. Five-Protein System. The T4 DNA polymerase (gp43) is responsible for all bacteriophage DNA replication, including repair (reviewed by Nossal and Alberts, 1983; Bernstein and Wallace, 1983). The purified gp43 enzyme is a 110,000-M_r monomer capable of 5' to 3' nucleotide polymerizing (Goulian et al., 1968) and 3' to 5' "proofreading" exonuclease activities (Brutlag and Kornberg, 1972). The enzyme is capable of copying primed single-stranded DNA and of repairing single-stranded gaps, albeit with limited processivity. However, it is not capable of catalyzing strand displacement on duplex DNA, unlike other enzymes such as DNA polymerase I (Nossal, 1974). Both the processivity of gp43 and its exonuclease activity are stimulated specifically by either the gp32 protein or the gp44/gp62 and gp45 proteins (Huberman et al., 1971; Piperno and Alberts, 1978; Bedinger and Alberts, 1983; Venkatesan and Nossal, 1982; Mace and Alberts, 1984b).

The gp32 protein binds to single-stranded DNA in a cooperative fashion and is capable of destabilizing but not melting double-stranded DNA (Alberts and Frey, 1970). It specifically stimulates the polymerization activity of gp43 but not that of other polymerases by direct protein-protein interactions with gp43 (as judged by its cosedimentation with gp43 and the specific retention of gp43 on a gp32 affinity column; see

Table VI) and by its ability to eliminate potentially inhibitory secondary structures in DNA (Huberman *et al.*, 1971; Piperno and Alberts, 1978; Huang *et al.*, 1981; Roth *et al.*, 1982; Formosa *et al.*, 1983). Genetic studies, mostly consisting of isolating extragenic suppressors, have demonstrated that gp32 functionally interacts with many T4-coded proteins (summarized in Mosig, 1983; Karam *et al.*, 1983; see article by G. Mosig and F. Eiserling, this volume). Many of these interactions have now been demonstrated biochemically by affinity chromatography (Table VI).

The gp44/gp62 protein complex has an ATPase activity that is greatly stimulated by the binding of gp45 (Piperno and Alberts, 1978; Piperno *et al.*, 1978; Mace and Alberts, 1984a). The gp44/gp62 and gp45 protein complex stimulates both the polymerizing and exonuclease activities of gp43 (but not those of other polymerases) by "clumping" it down on DNA (Mace and Alberts, 1984b; Bedinger and Alberts, 1983; Nossal and Alberts, 1983; Selick *et al.*, 1986).

Through its interactions with gp32, gp44/gp62, and gp45, the T4 DNA polymerase is capable of both high processivity and strand displacement on double-stranded DNA templates (Nossal and Peterlin, 1979; Liu *et al.*, 1978). This constitutes the five-protein "core" DNA replication system (Nossal and Alberts, 1983).

ii. Six-Protein System. The addition of gp41 to the five-protein "core" DNA replication system allows it to proceed on double-stranded DNA at almost physiological rates (Morris *et al.*, 1979a,b) because of gp41's helicase activity (Venkatesan *et al.*, 1982; Liu and Alberts, 1981a). The gp41 helicase utilizes the energy derived from GTP or ATP hydrolysis to unwind the DNA by advancing along the lagging strand. Thus, the gp43, gp44/gp62, gp45, gp32, and gp41 six-protein system is a good example of leading strand synthesis at a replication fork (Alberts *et al.*, 1982; Nossal and Alberts, 1983).

TABLE VI. Proteins That Bind to a gp32 Affinity Column[a]

Protein	Function
gp32	Single-stranded DNA binding; helix-destabilizing
gp43	T4 DNA polymerase
gp45	T4 DNA polymerase accessory protein
gpuvsX	T4 recombination
gpuvsY	T4 recombination
gpdda	Helicase
gp46/gp47	Exonuclease; T4 recombination
RNase H	Removes RNA from RNA:DNA hybrids
BP-1	Unknown; T4-coded; 30,000 M_r
BP-2	Unknown; host-coded; 32,000 M_r

[a]Reproduced from Alberts (1984), with permission from the publisher and the author.

iii. Seven-Protein System. The six-protein replication system is still not capable of lagging strand synthesis on the displaced DNA strand, because it has no capacity for RNA primer formation. This activity is supplied by the addition of gp61, a protein capable of forming RNA primers at specific DNA sequences on single-stranded DNA (Silver and Nossal, 1982; Hinton and Nossal, 1985; Hinton *et al.*, 1986; Cha and Alberts, 1986; Selick *et al.*, 1986). The gp41 and gp61 proteins function together to augment each others' respective helicase and primase activities. Together they constitute a "primosome" capable of movement and synthesis of the pentanucleotide primers used in initiating discontinuous DNA synthesis *in vivo* (Nossal, 1980; Liu and Alberts, 1980; reviewed in Hinton *et al.*, 1986; Selick *et al.*, 1986). It appears that the gp41/gp61 complex requires the presence of the 5'–GTT–3' and 5'–GCT–3' trinucleotide sequences for efficient synthesis of RNA primers (Cha and Alberts, 1986; Selick *et al.*, 1986). However, since hydroxymethylation of cytosine residues prevents the *in vitro* recognition of the 5'–GCT–3' sites by the primosome (Liu and Alberts, 1981b), it could be that *in vivo* only the 5'–GTT–3' sites are effectively utilized (Selick *et al.*, 1986). The seven-protein system is therefore capable of both leading and lagging strand synthesis on naked double-stranded DNA at physiological *in vivo* rates. However, it is still not capable of *de novo* initiation of DNA synthesis.

It is thought that two interacting DNA polymerizing complexes are found *in vivo* at each replication fork—one performing leading-strand synthesis and the other performing lagging-strand synthesis (Alberts *et al.*, 1982; Selick *et al.*, 1986; Hinton *et al.*, 1986). Such a mechanism would clearly allow for maximal rates of DNA synthesis at each fork.

iv. Eight-Protein System. Double-stranded T4 DNA is not naked *in vivo* as it is in the *in vitro* studies with purified components. Proteins such as RNA polymerase and other DNA-binding proteins (both host- and T4-coded) are bound to it. It has been shown that the seven-protein system described above is not capable of moving past an RNA polymerase molecule bound onto DNA. However, the addition of another T4-coded helicase, gpdda (Table V), endows the replication complex with the ability to move swiftly past such RNA polymerase-imposed blocks (Bedinger *et al.*, 1983; Jongeneel *et al.*, 1984). However, since the *dda* gene is dispensable for T4 growth on wild-type *E. coli* (Gauss *et al.*, 1983), it is obvious that *in vivo* other bacteriophage- or host-coded helicases can substitute in this particular reaction. For gpdda helicase action, the presence of all proteins from the five-protein "core" system is required, suggesting some direct protein-protein interactions. In accordance with this, Tables VI and VII show that the gpdda helicase binds specifically onto both a gp32 affinity column and a gpuvsX affinity column (Formosa *et al.*, 1983; Formosa and Alberts, 1984).

v. Seven-Protein Recombination-Dependent DNA Replication System. Recently, an elegant *in vitro* recombination-dependent DNA rep-

TABLE VII. Proteins That Bind to a gpuvsX Protein Affinity Column[a]

Protein	Function	Major elution position (M NaCl)
gpuvsX	Genetic recombination; properties similar to recA protein	0.45–2.0
gpuvsY	Genetic recombination	0.45
gp32	Binds single-stranded DNA; helix-destabilizing	0.05–0.15
gpdda	DNA helicase	0.05
gp42	dCMP hydroxymethylase	0.15
Host protein	Unknown; 32,000 M_r	0.45

[a]Reproduced from Formosa and Alberts (1984), with permission from the publisher and the authors.

lication system, made up of the five-protein "core" system, supplemented with the gpdda helicase and the T4-coded gpuvsX protein, has been developed (Fig. 18) (Formosa and Alberts, 1986b). The gpuvsX protein binds cooperatively to single-stranded DNA, possesses a DNA-dependent ATPase activity, and catalyzes pairing and strand exchange between a DNA single strand and its double-stranded homologue (Yonesaki and Minagawa, 1985; Yonesaki et al., 1985; Hinton and Nossal, 1986; Formosa and Alberts, 1986a,b). The E. coli ssb and recA proteins (the gp32 and gpuvsX analogues, respectively) cannot substitute in this seven-protein replication system, indicating that there is a need for specific protein-protein interactions (Formosa and Alberts, 1986b). In accordance with this, both gp32 and gpdda bind specifically to a gpuvsX affinity column (Table VII) (Formosa et al., 1983; Formosa and Alberts, 1984). It is interesting to note that, although the recA and uvsX genes do not show significant homology at the DNA level, their products are 38% homologous at the protein sequence level (Fujisawa et al., 1985).

Figure 18 summarizes some of the steps thought to take place in this replication system. The gpuvsX protein allows synapsis, formation of a D loop, and branch migration of the free single-stranded molecule on its double-stranded homologue. DNA synthesis is initiated at the 3'-hydroxyl invasive end by the minimal replication complex and proceeds with the aid of the gpdda helicase and gp32 proteins. The novel feature of this reaction is that, under the conditions employed, the DNA product synthesized is almost exclusively single-stranded, leaving the parental molecule intact. The authors suggest that this conservative mode of DNA synthesis may be used in vivo in various T4 DNA processes, including strand-switching during replication of damaged DNA as well as repair of double-stranded breaks (Formosa and Alberts, 1986b). Any interpretation of the in vivo significance of this reaction, however, is clearly premature, not only because of the absence of other protein components implicated from in vivo work (such as gpuvsY; Bernstein and Wallace, 1983), but also

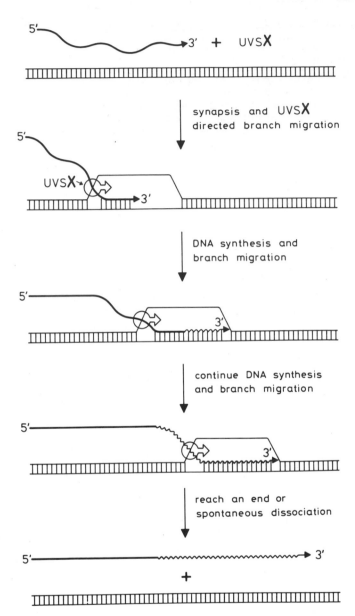

FIGURE 18. Hypothetical series of events during T4 DNA replication promoted by genetic recombination. The synapsis event between the free single-stranded molecule and its double-stranded homologue is initiated by the gpuvsX protein. Notice that the action of gpuvsX is such that the newly synthesized DNA strand remains unpaired. The released single-stranded DNA molecules can reanneal with their complementary counterparts in the cell to form double-stranded DNA. Alternatively, the T4 primosomal system may initiate RNA primer formation, leading to double-strand formation. The functioning of such a T4 recombination-dependent replication system is specific for the gpuvsX and other T4-coded proteins; the recA protein of the host cannot substitute in their process (Formosa and Alberts, 1986b).

because of the additional arguments raised in the article by G. Mosig and F. Eiserling (this volume).

c. Origins and Modes of T4 DNA Replication in Vivo

Up to now, it has been extremely difficult to analyze the various modes of T4 DNA replication in vivo, primarily because they are so interdependent (reviewed by Mosig, 1983; Nossal and Alberts, 1983; Alberts, 1984; see article by G. Mosig and F. Eiserling, this volume). The only unifying theme is their absolute dependence on gp43, the T4 DNA polymerase enzyme. Here we will briefly highlight a few of the known facts about T4 DNA replication in vivo. The reader is referred for more details to the article by G. Mosig and F. Eiserling (this volume).

i. Primary Origins of DNA Replication. Several laboratories, starting with Mosig's (1970), have attempted, with a combination of physical and genetic studies, to define the first events of T4 DNA replication in vivo. The results from the various laboratories have identified at least six "origins," some of which appear to coincide with recombinational hot spots (progress up to 1983 has been critically summarized by Kozinski, 1983; Yee and Marsh, 1985; see article by G. Mosig and F. Eiserling, this volume). One of the few generally accepted facts is that DNA replication at primary origins requires transcription by the unmodified host RNA polymerase (Luder and Mosig, 1982).

The best-characterized primary origin at the molecular level is oriA discovered and studied in G. Mosig's laboratory (Fig. 19) (Mosig et al., 1981; MacDonald et al., 1983; MacDonald and Mosig, 1984). These authors have been able to show that oriA maps in the 69 structural gene. This is intriguing, because it has been shown that 69^- mutations result in a DNA negative phenotype (MacDonald and Mosig, 1984) and because the location of oriA in 69 is reminiscent of the situation in other DNA replication systems mentioned before, such as λ and φX174, where the corresponding ori region is located in the coding sequence for the protein that binds to it and initiates the series of events leading to initiation of DNA replication. Gene 69 codes, in the same reading frame, for two proteins, gp69 and gp69*, a situation often encountered with other initiator proteins (see Introduction). The two mRNA species coding for the two proteins are transcribed from different promoters—the gp69-coding one from a gpmot-middle promoter (see Brody et al., 1983), and the gp69*-coding one from an immediate early promoter (MacDonald and Mosig, 1984). Another interesting observation is that gp69, a membrane protein, has patches of homology with the E. coli initiator protein dnaA (Mosig and MacDonald, 1986). Finally, an RNA:DNA copolymer that is coded from this region can be isolated early after T4 infection. All these facts have been taken into account in a model for T4 primary DNA replication proposed by Mosig et al. (1986).

Recently, a plasmid recombination system has been developed [based

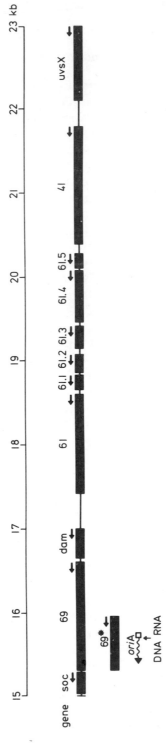

FIGURE 19. A genomic region of bacteriophage T4 important for DNA replication. The numbers on the top indicate position on the T4 physical map (Mathews *et al.*, 1983). The arrows indicate the direction of transcription. The *oriA* site, contained within the gene *69* coding sequence, is shown on the left. The RNA primer used to initiate DNA replication is made by the unmodified host RNA polymerase (for details see text and article by G. Mosig and F. Eiserling, this volume). The existence of the *61.1, 61.2, 61.3, 61.4,* and *61.5* genes has been determined through DNA sequencing. Disruption of these genes does not interfere with bacteriophage growth except in the case of *61.1,* which leads to a minute plaque phenotype and a slow rate of DNA synthesis (Selick *et al.*, 1986). The *41/61* gene products constitute the helicase/primase system (see text for details).

on original observations on T4:plasmid DNA recombination made by Mattson *et al.* (1983)] that allows for site-directed inactivation of T4 genes (Selick *et al.*, 1986). Using this system, Selick *et al.* (1986) have shown that the carboxyl-terminal end of gp69 (which includes the gp69* coding sequence) is dispensable for bacteriophage T4 growth. In contrast, the amino-terminal end of gp69 is essential for T4 growth, a result in agreement with previous genetic studies on gene *69*. The *69* gene is embedded in a region of the T4 genome that codes for other DNA replication proteins such as gp41 and gp61 (see Fig. 19). By DNA sequencing, Selick *et al.* (1986) defined the open reading frames designated *61.1*, *61.2*, *61.3*, *61.4*, and *61.5* (Fig. 19). By employing the site-directed inactivation scheme mentioned above, Selick *et al.* (1986) have shown that inactivation of only the *61.1* reading frame interferes with T4 growth, specifically at the level of DNA replication. Interestingly, *61.1* codes for a 54-amino acid protein with good homology to conserved sequences of other DNA binding proteins. Why was not gene *61.1* identified in early genetic studies, such as those by Epstein *et al.* (1963)? Probably because, on the one hand, its small coding sequence makes it an infrequent target for mutagenesis, and, on the other hand, inactivation of the gene leads to a leaky, minute plaque phenotype (Selick *et al.*, 1986). Most likely, there are other T4 genes, not yet identified, whose products may be essential for T4 DNA replication *in vivo*.

ii. DNA Replication by Recombination: A Secondary Initiation Mode. Since T4 DNA molecules are terminally redundant and circularly permuted, the 3'-hydroxyl ends created by the first round of replication (Fig. 1) can invade their double-stranded homologues (Fig. 18). The resulting D-loop structure can serve as origins of DNA replication (Fig. 18) (Dannenberg and Mosig, 1983). Host RNA polymerase is modified soon after infection (reviewed by Rabussay, 1983), at which time RNA transcription from early T4 promoters ceases so that DNA replication relies on recombination, since recombination-deficient mutants arrest DNA replication at this point (Hosoda *et al.*, 1971).

As a consequence of extensive recombination, the final T4 DNA progeny is highly branched (Broker and Lehman, 1971). Before packaging can be completed, the Holliday structures are probably processed by the gene *49*-coded nuclease capable of resolving X- of Y-shaped branched structures like the T7 gene *3* endonuclease (Mizuuchi *et al.*, 1982; Lilley and Kemper, 1984; Jensch and Kemper, 1986; De Massy *et al.*, 1987). In the absence of extensive recombination, the gp49 activity may no longer be required, since mutations in *uvsX* suppress *49*$^-$ mutations (Shah and DeLorenzo, 1977). For more detailed information on the relationship between recombination and DNA replication in T4, the reader is referred to the article by G. Mosig and F. Eiserling (this volume).

iii. Tertiary Origins of DNA Replication. A new mode of DNA initiation, called "tertiary," has been observed by Kreuzer and Alberts (1985, 1986). This mode is distinguished by the two previously described modes because (1) it is independent of the T4 recombination system, since it operates in 46^-47^- infections (Kreuzer and Alberts, 1985), and (2) unlike "primary" origins, it is insensitive to rifampicin (Kreuzer and Alberts, 1985).

This mode was discovered through the isolation of T4 DNA recombinant plasmid clones that can replicate effectively after T4 infection (Kreuzer and Alberts, 1985, 1986). Again, as is the case with most T4 studies, there are many possible interpretations and pitfalls in these experiments. For example, T4 origins that require HMC for functioning will not be selected with this scheme. Also, very strong origins cloned on such multicopy plasmids should drastically interfere with helper T4 DNA replication. Such interference will lead to the underproduction of bacteriophage structural components, coded by the helper bacteriophage, with the concomitant underrepresentation of such plasmids in subsequent selections.

Some of these putative "tertiary" origins have been analyzed in molecular detail (Kreuzer and Menkens, 1986). A few resemble gpmot-dependent middle promoters (reviewed by Brody *et al.*, 1983). Surprisingly, these promoters can function in the absence of any DNA homology with the superinfecting helper bacteriophage (Kreuzer and Menkens, 1986). The last observation proves that initiation of DNA replication at such "tertiary" origins is not the consequence of a recombinational event.

In summary, the exact nature and significance of all the replication events in T4 have not been worked out. The difficulties encountered stem not only from the presence of the HMC modification of its DNA, which has hampered molecular studies until very recently (Mathews *et al.*, 1983), but also on the ability of T4 to carry out multiple, occasionally overlapping strategies for its DNA replication. This complexity is undoubtedly due to its large genome, independence from the host DNA replication machinery, and selection for better growth on its various bacterial hosts.

B. Replication through Initiation at the Ends

1. Bacteriophage N4

N4 is a lytic bacteriophage that propagates on *E. coli* K12 strains (for a detailed review on this bacteriophage, see Chapter 7, this volume). The virion DNA consists of a 72-kb, double-stranded, linear DNA molecule with terminal repeats and 3′ single-stranded ends. A 400- to 450-bp segment is directly repeated at the ends. Whereas the left end is unique and has a seven-base overhang (3′–CCATAAA–5′), the right end shows some variability. Five different species of ends (1 major and 4 minor) are found; they differ by increments of 10 bp over a 50-bp region. In addition, a 3′-hydroxyl overhang, two or three bases long, is found at the right extremity. Another unique feature of N4 is that it packages a DNA-dependent RNA polymerase molecule(s) in its capsid. Upon infection, this bacteriophage-coded polymerase is injected along with the bacteriophage DNA, initiates transcription of the early genes, and participates in the initiation of DNA replication.

The novelty of bacteriophage N4 resides in its use of three different transcription mechanisms and in its replication mode based on 3'-hydroxyl single-stranded ends for priming of DNA synthesis.

a. In Vivo Replication

A characteristic of N4 infection is the delayed lysis of the bacteria, especially in liquid medium (Schito, 1973). This allows the production of up to 3000 bacteriophages per infected cell. Upon infection, host DNA synthesis is rapidly arrested (after 8 min at 37°C), but, in contrast to the cases for bacteriophages T4 and T7, the host chromosome is not degraded (Schito et al., 1969), although some selective shutoff of its gene expression does occur (Rothman-Denes et al., 1972). The early steps of in vivo N4 replication are not known precisely. Most of the information about initiation of DNA synthesis has been derived from in vitro studies (see below), and it is not clear how applicable these studies are to the in vivo situation. Newly synthesized DNA is found, in part, in short fragments subsequently chased into unit-length DNA (Guinta et al., 1986b). This indicates that N4 uses a discontinuous mode of DNA synthesis, possibly lagging-strand type of synthesis. Physical analysis of the structure of replicating N4 DNA (utilizing restriction endonucleases) suggests that it is, at least in part, in the form of head-to-tail concatemers, each bacteriophage genome being separated from the others by one copy of the terminal repeat (L. B. Rothman-Denes, personal communication). However, there may still be circular intermediates with one copy of the terminal repeat at some stage in the replication cycle. The direct repeats at the ends of the molecules allow the formation of head-to-tail concatemers as outlined above for bacteriophage T7. Sequence-specific nicking at the ends, probably carried out by the packaging machinery, can give rise to the mature DNA structures found in the virions.

b. Host Genes Involved in N4 Replication

Various E. coli genes implicated in chromosomal DNA synthesis were examined for their importance in in vivo N4 replication (Guinta et al., 1986b). Most of them (dnaA, dnaB, dnaC, dnaE, dnaG, rep) are dispensable for efficient bacteriophage production. This suggests that the bacteriophage codes for its own DNA polymerase, primase, and, possibly, helicase activities. However, N4 replication requires the host-coded lig gene product (DNA ligase) and the 5' to 3' exonuclease activity of the polA gene product. Therefore, processing of N4 Okazaki fragments probably relies mostly on the host-coded machinery. Finally, DNA gyrase (*gyrA* and *gyrB* gene products) and ribonucleotide reductase (*dnaF* gene product) are also required (Guinta *et al.*, 1986b).

c. The N4 Replication Genes

The products of at least five bacteriophage-coded genes are essential for *in vivo* DNA replication (Guinta *et al.*, 1986b). The *dnp* cistron codes for a 90,000-M_r DNA polymerase, and the *dbp* gene product is a 30,000-M_r, single-stranded, DNA-binding protein. Mutations in the *dns* gene, coding for a 78,000-M_r polypeptide of unknown function, also lead to a DNA negative phenotype, as do mutations inactivating the 5' to 3' exonuclease activity of the 45,000-M_r product of the *exo* gene (Guinta *et al.*, 1986a). As already mentioned, N4 possesses a virion-encapsidated RNA polymerase. This large protein (320,000 M_r), encoded by the *vrp* gene, is directly involved in DNA synthesis, in addition to being essential for early gene transcription. The exact role of the N4 RNA polymerase in replication is not known, except that both the *E. coli* DNA gyrase and ssb proteins are required for *in vivo* transcription by vrp (L. B. Rothman-Denes, personal communication). No other single-stranded DNA-binding protein can substitute for ssb, strongly suggesting that there could be protein-protein interactions with the N4 RNA polymerase. The gyrase and ssb proteins may help prepare the proper single-stranded DNA template required for initiation of RNA transcription by the N4 RNA polymerase (Falco *et al.*, 1978; Haynes and Rothman-Denes, 1985).

d. In Vitro Replication

N4-specific DNA synthesis can be obtained with a cell-free extract of infected bacteria (Rist *et al.*, 1983, 1986). Synthesis depends on the addition of N4 DNA, $MgCl_2$ and the four dNTPs. It requires at least the functional products of the *dnp*, *dbp*, and *exo* genes, which cannot be replaced by functionally equivalent proteins from other DNA replication systems. A simpler replication assay, requiring only the dnp, dbp, and exo proteins, has recently been developed (L. B. Rothman-Denes, personal communication). The two systems behave identically in terms of DNA template and origin specificity. The physical analysis of the replication products leads to a possible model for the early steps in N4 DNA replication (Fig. 20). The 5' to 3' exonuclease removes nucleotides from the two recessed 5' ends. The longer, 3' single-stranded ends then form two hairpin structures, thus providing 3'-hydroxyl primers that are elongated by the N4 DNA polymerase. The further steps in N4 replication, such as the priming of lagging-strand synthesis and the formation of concatemers, remain to be determined, as is the exact role of the virion-encapsidated DNA-dependent RNA polymerase.

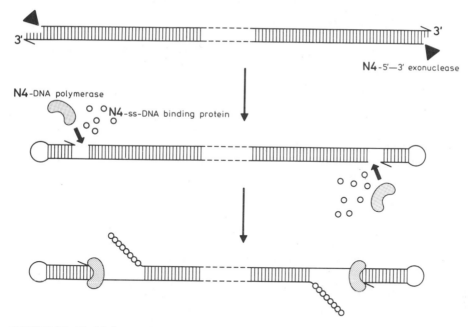

FIGURE 20. Model for *in vitro* initiation of N4 DNA replication. The preexisting 3′ protruding ends are increased in length by the action of the N4-coded 5′ to 3′ exonuclease. Terminal hairpins are formed, providing two 3′-hydroxyl primers for the N4 DNA polymerase. This results in the synthesis of one strand from both ends, with the help of the N4 single-stranded DNA binding protein.

2. Bacteriophage φ29

The *Bacillus subtilis* bacteriophage φ29 possesses a linear double-stranded DNA of about 18 kb with a viral protein, gp3 (the product of gene 3), covalently linked to its two 5′ ends (Anderson and Mosharrafa, 1968; Ito, 1978; Salas *et al.*, 1978). φ29 is a perfect example of how to solve the problem of replicating the ends of linear DNA molecules. All known DNA polymerases add new nucleotides to the 3′-hydroxyl end of preexisting polynucleotide chains and cannot initiate *de novo* synthesis of a new chain. Hence, the end of the DNA strand that serves as the template for lagging-strand synthesis cannot be replicated (see Fig. 1). A novel mechanism of priming, first proposed for adenovirus (Rekosh *et al.*, 1977), has been shown to occur in bacteriophage φ29 (Harding *et al.*, 1978; Inciarte *et al.*, 1980). The original model described by Rekosh *et al.* (1977) predicted the use of the terminal protein as the actual primer for DNA replication. Specifically, it was proposed that the terminal protein reacts with a dNTP molecule to form a protein-dNMP complex. Such a complex would provide the 3′-hydroxyl end needed for elongation by the DNA polymerase (Rekosh *et al.*, 1977).

a. In Vitro Replication

All features of the above model have been verified in the case of φ29 DNA replication, since a complex between protein gp3 and 5'-dAMP has been shown to be formed *in vitro* after incubation of φ29-infected cells with dATP (Penalva and Salas, 1982; Blanco *et al.*, 1983). In addition, synthesis of full-length φ29 DNA can be achieved *in vitro* by incubating purified φ29 DNA polymerase (gp2) and terminal protein (gp3) with φ29 DNA-gp3 complex as template (Blanco and Salas, 1985). Restriction analysis of the *in vitro*–synthesized φ29 DNA showed that initiation can take place at either DNA end, since the terminal fragments were labeled preferentially to the internal ones (Blanco and Salas, 1985). Pulse-chase experiments, followed by analysis of the labeled DNA on alkaline sucrose gradients, confirmed that full-length φ29 DNA was replicated by elongation from each end (Blanco and Salas, 1985). However, it was not demonstrated in these experiments whether replication could start at both ends of the same DNA molecule. The rate of elongation in this *in vitro* minimal system is about a 100-fold lower (by analogy with the rate of DNA replication in *B. subtilis*) than *in vivo*, suggesting that other factors are needed to replicate φ29 efficiently *in vivo*. The addition of host factors to this *in vitro* minimal system appears to stimulate the initiation step rather than the elongation one (Blanco and Salas, 1985).

b. φ29 Gene Products Involved in DNA Replication

Although not much is known about the stimulatory host factors, it has been found, by using conditional mutants of φ29, that the products of five bacteriophage-coded genes (2, 3, 5, 6, and 17) are required for *in vivo* DNA synthesis of φ29 (Carrascosa *et al.*, 1976). Data from *in vitro* experiments indicate that gp2 and gp6 are involved not only at the initiation step but probably throughout elongation (Matsumo *et al.*, 1984; Blanco and Salas, 1985). Moreover, these two proteins interact, since they form a complex in glycerol gradients and copurify during several purification steps (Matsumo *et al.*, 1984). Gp6, although not essential *in vitro*, stimulates the formation of the replication complex by decreasing the K_m value for dATP binding by gp3 (Blanco *et al.*, 1986). It has recently been shown that gp6 is a DNA-binding protein. However, it does not seem to bind preferentially to specific DNA sequences. Instead, it appears to recognize specific features of the DNA at the ends of φ29 DNA, since the protection patterns of restriction fragments containing either the ends of φ29 DNA or internal fragments are different (Salas *et al.*, 1986).

c. DNA Template Requirements for Replication

Apart from proteins, template requirements were analyzed for the formation of the initiation complex. It was found that an intact DNA template is not needed, since gp3-containing fragments including as little as 73 bp from the left end and 269 bp from the right end can be used as templates *in vitro* (Garcia *et al.*, 1984). Another piece of evidence comes from the cloning of the terminal fragments from the left and right φ29 DNA ends on the same plasmid. The plasmid was constructed so that terminal sequences can be recreated after the appropriate restriction enzyme digestion. Fragments containing the recreated ends, but not the circular parental molecule or plasmids linearized at different sites, are active templates for the *in vitro* initiation reaction (Gutierrez *et al.*, 1986a). The activity of the φ29 end-containing fragments is about 15% of that of φ29 gp3-DNA, demonstrating that the parental terminal protein is not absolutely required for the *in vitro* initiation reaction. Hence, this result does indicate that gp2 protein interacts with φ29 DNA ends less efficiently than with the gp3-DNA complex.

In apparent contradiction with this result, previous experiments showed that proteinase K-treated φ29 DNA is completely inactive as a template in an *in vitro* reaction complemented with cell extracts (Penalva and Salas, 1982; Garcia *et al.*, 1984). It could either be that the presence of the terminal protein protected the bacteriophage DNA from degradation in the crude extracts used in the latter experiments or that the end product of proteinase K treatment specifically interferes with gp2 binding at the ends (Gutierrez *et al.*, 1986b). It would be of interest to find out if *in vitro*–packaged φ29 DNA molecules that do not contain the terminal protein (having been treated with proteinase K) are infectious.

Terminal φ29 DNA fragments are active templates for the formation of the initiation complex, so the ends of φ29 DNA may contain sequences that allow the initiation of replication to occur. Double-stranded DNA is essential for the recognition of these sequences, since terminal fragment-separated strands are poor templates (Gutierrez *et al.*, 1986b). Preliminary evidence suggests that the 6-bp inverted terminal repeats at the ends of φ29 DNA may be important for the initiation of replication (Gutierrez *et al.*, 1986a,b). These sequences may play a role in recognition by either gp2 or gp3. It is interesting to note that similar sequences are present at the ends of DNA molecules from φ29-related bacteriophages and of some *Streptococcus pneumoniae* bacteriophages (Yoshikawa *et al.* 1985; Salas, 1988).

d. Model of φ29 DNA Replication

The current model of φ29 initiation of DNA replication is represented in Fig. 21. The terminal protein, gp3, and the DNA polymerase protein, gp2, interact with φ29 DNA containing gp3 covalently attached to both 5' ends. The gp2-gp3 complex could be stabilized at the ends of the φ29 DNA-gp3 template through both protein-protein and protein-DNA interactions. In the presence of dATP, the DNA polymerase cata-

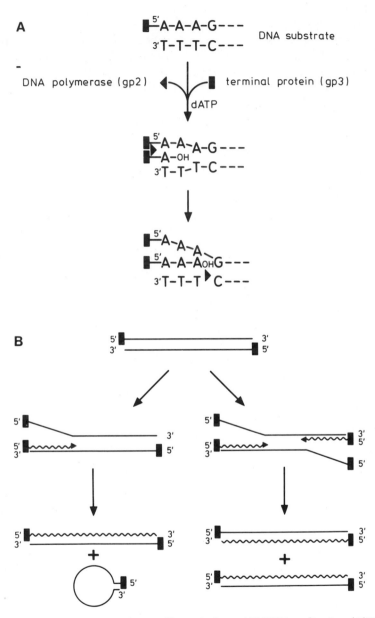

FIGURE 21. Schematic representation of bacteriophage φ29 DNA replication. (A) The current model of protein-primed initiation, in which the DNA polymerase gp2 protein catalyzes the formation of a covalent bond between dAMP and the terminal protein gp3. (B) The two possible modes of replication. Replication starting at one end is drawn on the left part of the diagram, and replication starting at both ends of the genome is shown on the right.

lyzes the formation of a covalent bond between protein gp3 (the serine residue at position 232) and 5'-dAMP. This reaction is stimulated *in vitro* by the φ29 protein gp6. As a result of these protein-protein and protein-DNA interactions, the 3'-hydroxyl of the dAMP moiety is positioned in such a way that it can serve as the primer for subsequent chain elongation. Replication is then thought to proceed by strand displacement (Inciarte *et al.*, 1980; Watabe *et al.*, 1982), although its exact mechanism is not known. For example, it has so far not been possible to distinguish between two alternate modes of replication (Fig. 21). In one mode, displacement synthesis would proceed to completion, resulting in the formation of a daughter duplex and the release of the parental strand. Formation of a panhandle structure through the inverted terminal repeats could provide a replication origin for the unreplicated parental strand. In the other mode, replication would start at both ends of the genome before the parental strand was completely displaced. In such doubly initiated molecules, both parental strands would serve as templates for daughter-strand synthesis.

Both pathways of replication are compatible with electron microscopic pictures of φ29 DNA-replicating molecules (Inciarte *et al.*, 1980; Sogo *et al.*, 1982). In addition, the same mechanisms could apply on circular DNA molecules held together by the terminal proteins at the ends of bacteriophage DNA (Salas, 1988). In principle, there is no requirement for a discontinuous mode of DNA synthesis in φ29 DNA replication. All nascent daughter strands grow from their 5' termini toward the 3' termini and thus can be elongated without the need for the synthesis and joining of Okazaki fragments. Discontinuous DNA synthesis cannot entirely be ruled out, although there is no evidence for internal initiation, as judged by electron microscopy (Inciarte *et al.*, 1980; Sogo *et al.*, 1982). The use of an *E. coli* bacteriophage PRD1 (analogous in all studied respects to φ29; Bamford and Mindich, 1984) may help elucidate the potential involvement of host proteins in the DNA synthesis of these bacteriophages because of our better understanding of both the genetics and the biochemistry of *E. coli* DNA replication compared to *Bacillus subtilis*.

This type of protein-primed initiation of replication is not uncommon, since it occurs in a variety of bacteriophages, viruses, and plasmids (Salas, 1988). The best-studied example is adenovirus, whose DNA replication mechanism is analogous to that of φ29, with minor exceptions. For example, the 5' ends of adenovirus DNA are covalently linked to a terminal protein through a serine residue (Robinson *et al.*, 1973; Rekosh *et al.*, 1977). Although the nucleotide involved in initiation is dCTP rather than dATP (Challberg *et al.*, 1980), the replication of the viral genome occurs by a similar strand displacement mechanism (Lechner and Kelly, 1977). In addition, a cellular protein, named nuclear factor 1, may play an analogous role to that of gp6 (Nagata *et al.*, 1982).

C. Replication via Transposition in the Host Chromosome: Bacteriophage Mu

1. General Considerations

Bacteriophage Mu was first discovered by Taylor (1963), who noticed its ability to cause mutations by integrating at various sites in the *E. coli* genome. Since its discovery, the temperate bacteriophage Mu has been shown to be remarkably efficient at transposing into seemingly random sites in many bacterial genomes and to mediate a variety of DNA rearrangements, including inversions, deletions, duplications, and replicon fusions (for reviews see Toussaint and Resibois, 1983; Bukhari, 1976; Kleckner, 1981; Grindley and Reed, 1985; Mizuuchi and Craigie, 1986; Harshey, 1988). The interest in Mu biology intensified when it first became apparent that it is a member of the transposonlike family of DNA elements. The transposable elements include those like Tn5 and Tn10 that apparently transpose by a conservative mechanism (Berg, 1983; Kleckner *et al.*, 1984; Bender and Kleckner, 1986; for reviews see Grindley and Reed, 1985; Derbyshire and Grindley, 1986; Mizuuchi and Craigie, 1986). However, recent data suggest that Tn5 transposition may indeed proceed through a recA-dependent replicative intermediate (Ahmed, 1986). On the other hand, the Tn3-like elements transpose exclusively by a replicative mechanism (Grindley, 1983), which involves a duplication of the element and rearrangement of the host DNA flanking the element (reviewed in Kleckner, 1981; Toussaint and Resibois, 1983; Grindley and Reed, 1985). Bacteriophage Mu utilizes both mechanisms of transposition. Following infection, it integrates randomly by conservative transposition (Liebart *et al.*, 1982; Akroyd and Symonds, 1983; Harshey, 1984a,b). The lytic infection that follows proceeds exclusively by replicative transposition (Ljungquist and Bukhari, 1977; Chaconas *et al.*, 1981; Pato and Reich, 1985).

The Mu bacteriophage is an excellent system for studying both conservative and replicative transposition because of the ready availability of bacteriophage DNA and mini-Mu derivatives (Faelen *et al.*, 1978b), the ease of bacteriophage genetic analysis, and above all, its extremely high frequency of transposition compared to the other transposons. This has allowed the detection of replicative intermediates *in vivo* (Resibois *et al.*, 1982a,b; Harshey *et al.*, 1982) as well as *in vitro* (Mizuuchi, 1983, 1984; Craigie and Mizuuchi, 1985a; Craigie *et al.*, 1985). Below, we will discuss only those features of bacteriophage Mu DNA structure and protein function that are essential for understanding the transposition phenomenon. In a nutshell, it appears that the symmetric transposition model originally proposed by Shapiro (1979) accounts perfectly for replicative transposition of Mu, and the modification proposed by Ohtsubo *et al.* (1980) accounts for its conservative transposition. The accumulated data do not favor the various asymmetric models of transposition previously proposed (Grindley and Sherratt, 1978; Harshey and Bukhari, 1981; Galas and Chandler, 1981; reviewed by Grindley and Reed, 1985, Mizuuchi and Craigie, 1986; Derbyshire and Grindley, 1986).

2. Mu Bacteriophage DNA

The mature Mu virion contains a linear DNA molecule of approximately 39 kb. Unlike bacteriophage λ, it does not possess cohesive ends, and unlike bacteriophage P22, it does not contain terminally repeated sequences. Instead, it possess approximately 37 kb of unique, Mu-specific DNA embedded in approximately 1.7 kb of host DNA, with 50–150 bp on the left end and 1.5 kb or so on the right end. These host DNA sequences differ from molecule to molecule (reviewed by Bukhari, 1976; Toussaint and Resibois, 1983) and reflect the life-style of the bacteriophage: replicative transposition during lytic growth, followed by a "headful" mechanism of packaging, starting at the left end and proceeding to the right. Because of this heterogeneity, Mu has no obvious way of circularization following infection. However, circular intracellular forms of Mu DNA can be seen in the electron microscope, even in the absence of protein synthesis (Harshey and Bukhari, 1983; Puspurs et al., 1983). Apparently, the two ends of Mu are held together by a 64,000-M_r protein that is injected into the host along with the bacteriophage DNA. This interaction may allow the linear Mu DNA to undergo the supercoiling detected under the electron microscope. It is interesting that Craigie et al. (1985) have shown in an in vitro transposition assay that the donor Mu DNA must be supercoiled for transposition to take place (see below). The structural gene that codes for this 64,000-M_r protein has not been conclusively identified. Since it binds to the ends, it could be a truncated form of the A protein (see below). However, recently Gloor and Chaconas (1986) have presented evidence suggesting the N gene codes for the 64,000-M_r protein. Surprisingly, the N protein has been previously shown to be a component of the tail (Giphart-Gassler et al., 1981).

Unlike the 9- to 40-bp inverted repeats normally found at the ends of transposons (Calos and Miller, 1980; Kleckner, 1981; Grindley and Reed, 1985), bacteriophage Mu DNA possesses only the same 2-bp repeat (TG . . . CA) found at the ends of most transposons (Fig. 22) (Kahmann and Kamp, 1979; Calos and Miller, 1980; Kleckner, 1981). The rest of the sequences at the ends of Mu DNA appear dissimilar except for a perfect 8-bp inverted repeat found further in from the two ends (Fig. 22). In spite of this apparent lack of homology, footprinting experiments with purified A transposase protein (see below) revealed the presence of six binding sites—L1, L2, L3, R1, R2, and R3 (Fig. 22)—near the two ends of Mu DNA and allowed the identification of a consensus sequence (Craigie et al., 1984). The importance of these sites in the transposition process has been demonstrated by sequence deletion experiments. Deletion of either the attL or attR ends completely blocks the replicative capacity of Mu pro-

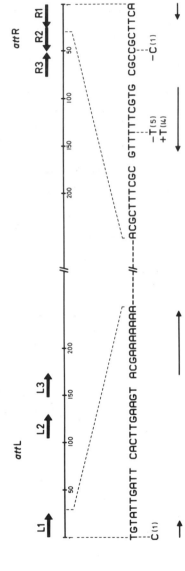

FIGURE 22. Sequences at the ends of Mu DNA. The regions designated L1, L2, L3, R1, R2, and R3 refer to the postulated A protein binding sites (Craigie *et al.*, 1984). Arrows indicate the relative orientation of the sites. Numbers indicate distance, in nucleotides, from the respective ends of Mu. The lower part of the figure shows the DNA sequence of the last 30 residues at the ends of Mu. Arrows indicate the positions of the perfect inverted repeats. Nucleotide changes that eliminate capacity to transpose (Burlingame *et al.*, 1986) are also shown. Numbers in parentheses indicate numbers of mutant isolates.

phage (Van de Putte *et al.*, 1978; Waggoner *et al.*, 1981). Furthermore, analysis of Bal31-generated deletions established the need for the L1, L2, L3, R1, and R2 repeats for efficient transposition (Groenen *et al.*, 1985).

The genetic mutational analysis performed by Burlingame *et al.* (1986) has proved the importance of the TG . . . CA terminal repeat, as well as the 8-bp inverted repeat in Mu transposition (Fig. 22). Note that the majority of the mutational events occur in the R1 repeat, which binds A transposase weakly compared to L1 (Craigie *et al.*, 1984). Presumably, any further weakening in A transposase action may have a more pronounced effect on R1 than L1 binding. Recently, the transposition of mini-Mu containing only one intact end has been studied in detail (Groenen *et al.*, 1986). It has been shown that the low frequency of transposition observed in this system proceeds essentially through the normal Mu transposition mechanism, except that an alternative DNA sequence, partly homologous to the A protein–binding site, is employed as a second end. In agreement with previous mutagenic studies (Burlingame *et al.*, 1986) the final base pair of the utilized sequence was always found to be T/A (Groenen *et al.*, 1986).

Efficient transposition requires that both Mu termini be on the same molecule and in inverted orientation both *in vivo* (Schumm and Howe, 1981) and *in vitro* (Mizuuchi, 1983; Craigie *et al.*, 1985). In an elegant experiment, however, Craigie and Mizuuchi (1986) demonstrated that the Mu ends can be on separate molecules or in direct repeat orientation on the same molecule and still function efficiently as substrates for transposition. What appears to be important is that the topology of the DNA molecules has to favor the proper alignment of the two ends.

3. The A Transposase Protein

Genetic and biochemical evidence has demonstrated that the A gene product is absolutely essential *in vivo* and *in vitro* for Mu DNA integration, transposition, or other DNA rearrangements (Wijffelman and Lotterman, 1977; Faelen *et al.*, 1978a; O'Day *et al.*, 1978; reviewed by Toussaint and Resibois, 1983; Craigie and Mizuuchi, 1985a). The A gene has been sequenced (Harshey *et al.*, 1985), and its 75,000-M_r gene product has been purified to homogeneity (Craigie and Mizuuchi, 1985b). The purified A protein has been shown to bind *in vitro* to six sites on Mu DNA— three at each end, as indicated in Fig. 22 (Craigie *et al.*, 1984). Surprisingly, the purified Mu c repressor protein also binds to these six sites, albeit with reduced affinity (Craigie *et al.*, 1984). Such binding may play an important biological role during bacteriophage infection by preventing A transposase action when the intracellular c repressor levels are high (Craigie *et al.*, 1984). The A protein has been shown to possess an unstable activity *in vivo* (Pato and Reich, 1982), to be required in stoichiometric amounts, and to act primarily *in cis* (Pato and Reich, 1984). This stoichiometric requirement may be due to the inability of the A protein to recycle after a round of transposition, perhaps because of proteolytic cleavage of a 10,000-M_r fragment from its carboxyl terminus, which has so far been observed only in minicells (M. Betermier, M. Chandler, and A. Toussaint, personal communication).

Although transposition is generally abolished in A^- mutants, certain deletions in the carboxyl terminus appear to allow conservative integration during infection but to completely abolish replicative transposition (Harshey, 1984a, 1985; A. Toussaint, personal communication). This last observation is interesting, because it suggests the possibility of a carboxyl domain in the A protein that may allow it to interact with other bacteriophage- or host-coded proteins necessary for the replicative integration process (see below). Equally tantalizing is the observation that a 33,000-M_r polypeptide, coded in phase by the carboxyterminal part of the gene, is synthesized early after Mu infection (M. Betermier and M. Chandler, personal communication). It could be that this short polypeptide sequesters the host-coded DNA replication components early in infection, thereby preventing replicative integration, and instead allowing conservative integration. From all the gathered data, there is little doubt that the A transposase plays the key role in Mu transposition by being a multifunctional protein able to bring the ends of Mu together, align them with the target sequences, and initiate cleavage and transfer reactions with the help of the host HU and other proteins (see below).

4. The B Protein

Mutations in the B gene have been shown to block Mu DNA replication in vivo (Wijffelman and Lotterman, 1977) and to lower the transposition frequency approximately 100-fold compared to wild type (O'Day et al., 1978; Faelen et al., 1978a). The B gene has been sequenced (Miller et al., 1984), and its 35,000-M_r product has been purified to homogeneity (Chaconas et al., 1985b).

Previous reports suggested that the B protein is not essential for the lysogenization process (O'Day et al., 1978), which may be equivalent to the conservative mode of Mu integration. However, Chaconas et al. (1985a), using the incorporation of ^{32}P-labeled Mu bacteriophage DNA into the host chromosome as a measure of integration, have presented data suggesting that the B protein may be necessary for conservative integration. Briefly, it appears that long B amber fragments, lacking 18 amino acids from the carboxyl end, are capable of supporting Mu DNA integration into the host chromosome. However, shorter B amber fragments, lacking 66 amino acids, do not exhibit any Mu DNA integration activity. In addition, all B amber fragments are incapable of supporting Mu replicative transposition. (A complication with this experiment is that incorporation of the ^{32}P-labeled Mu DNA into the host chromosome is not seen for a long time, until a least 30 min following bacteriophage infection.)

These results suggest the possibility that the carboxyl-terminal domain of the B protein is necessary for replicative transposition, perhaps through its ability to interact with and recruit the host DNA replication machinery at the site of Mu DNA (see below). Alternatively, this domain may be necessary for interaction with a different domain on either the B or A polypeptides to catalyze replicative transposition. This domain of the B protein may be sequestered during the first conservative integration event, perhaps through a protein-protein interaction with the 64,000-M_r protein that is injected along with Mu DNA and capable of binding to its two ends, as discussed above. Following Mu DNA integration, the 64,000-M_r protein cannot interfere, since there are no free Mu ends to bind to, thus allowing B protein to resume its function in replicative integration.

5. Host Requirements for Mu Growth

By screening the effects of known mutations in the genes whose products are required for host DNA synthesis, it has been established that the *E. coli* dnaB, dnaC, dnaE, and *dnaG* gene products are absolutely necessary for Mu DNA replication (Toussaint and Faelen, 1974; Wijffelman and Van de Putte, 1977; Toussaint and Resibois, 1983; Resibois *et al.*, 1984). These results indicate that bacteriophage Mu relies on the lagging-strand primer synthesizing system of *E. coli*, as well as the host DNA polymerase III activity, for replicating its DNA. In addition, it has been shown that the *E. coli* himA, hipD, gyrA, and *gyrB* gene products are necessary for Mu growth (Friedman *et al.*, 1984a; Goosen *et al.*, 1984; Miller and Friedman, 1980; Ross *et al.*, 1986). However, because of their pleiotropic effects on gene expression, it is not clear whether these *E. coli* gene products affect bacteriophage Mu DNA replication directly or indirectly. For example, it has been shown that the *E. coli* integration host factor (made up of the *himA* and *hipD*-gene products) positively controls the expression of early Mu gene expression (Goosen *et al.*, 1984; Krause and Higgins, 1986) and therefore does not seem to participate directly in Mu DNA replication.

It has recently been shown that the dnaK function of *E. coli* is essential for bacteriophage Mu growth, although not necessarily for Mu DNA replication *per se*; rather it appears to be essential for late mRNA transcription (M. Pato and A. Toussaint, personal communication). Interestingly, the *E. coli* dnaJ function is also essential for bacteriophage Mu growth, provided the bacteriophage is deficient in expression of a region located between genes *B* and *C*. This last observation suggests the possibility that bacteriophage Mu codes for a dnaJ protein analogue (M. Pato and A. Toussaint, personal communication). Recent *in vitro* work has established a requirement for the *E. coli* HU DNA-binding protein in Mu DNA replication (Craigie *et al.*, 1985; see below). However, since *E. coli* mutants in HU do not exist yet, it has not been possible to directly investigate its role in *in vivo* Mu DNA replication.

6. *In Vivo* DNA Replication

Following infection of wild-type *E. coli* by wild-type Mu, a few percent of the bacteriophage establish the lysogenic state. It has been demonstrated that the first event in this process is the conservative transposition of Mu DNA into the host chromosome (Liebart *et al.*, 1982; Akroyd and Symonds, 1983; Harshey, 1984a). In this regard, the Mu conservative transposition process is exactly analogous to that of transposon Tn*10* (Morisato and Kleckner, 1984; Bender and Kleckner, 1986).

It was originally reported that when the A protein was provided *in trans* by a cloned *A* gene, simple insertions were predominantly observed (Harshey, 1983). However, it was subsequently shown that the original *A* clone used in these studies carried a deletion near the end of the *A* gene coding sequence (Harshey, 1985). Hence, it appears that a truncated A protein, missing part of its carboxyl domain, can efficiently participate in simple insertions but not in replicative transpositions (Harshey, 1985; M. Betermier, M. Chandler, and A. Toussaint, personal communication). This carboxyl domain of the A protein may therefore be important in interactions with other bacteriophage (e.g., B protein) or host components (e.g., DNA polymerase III enzyme), essential for replicative transposition (see below).

It was originally shown by Ljungquist and Bukhari (1977) that the original Mu-host DNA junction fragments are conserved after prophage induction. The original suggestion that Mu replicated by repetitive transposition into the host DNA has been verified (Chaconas *et al.*, 1980, 1981; Harshey and Bukhari, 1981; Resibois *et al.*, 1982a,b). For Mu transposition to occur, both the left and right ends have to be intact (Van de Putte *et al.*, 1978; Waggoner *et al.*, 1981) and in the proper orientation (Schumm and Howe, 1981). The ends of Mu must also play a role in termination of Mu DNA replication, since the host DNA does not seem to be replicated (Van de Putte *et al.*, 1978; Waggoner and Pato, 1978).

The electron microscopic observations of Harshey *et al.* (1982) and Resibois *et al.* (1982a,b) are consistent with Shapiro's (1979) model of Mu transposition, although there does appear to be a bias in the direction of DNA replication in favor of the left end over the right end in wild-type Mu. This bias has been verified by hybridization with Okazaki DNA fragments to the separated Mu strands (Wijffelman and Van de Putte, 1977; Goosen, 1978; Resibois *et al.*, 1984). It could be that since the A protein acts preferentially *in cis*, it acts first at the left end, where its structural gene is located (Pato and Reich, 1984). Alternatively, it could be that DNA initiations are simultaneous from both DNA ends but that the movement of the DNA replication fork from the right end is slower. For example, there may be fewer primosome assembly sites for lagging-strand synthesis on the right end than on the left end. The observation that a mini-Mu derivative replicates equally well from both ends (Resibois *et al.*, 1984) is consistent with both explanations.

7. *In Vitro* DNA Replication

Two *in vitro* Mu DNA transposition systems that seem to mimic the *in vivo* situation faithfully have been developed. One employs the cellophane disk system originally developed by Schaller *et al.* (1972). Mu DNA replication in this system appears to be (1) extensions of replication forks that had already initiated *in vivo*, (2) semiconservative, (3) continuous synthesis in the 5' to 3' direction and discontinuous synthesis in the 3' to 5' direction, and (4), in agreement with the *in vivo* situation, bias toward replication from the left end (Higgins *et al.*, 1983a,b). The second system employs a modified fraction II extract (Fuller *et al.*, 1981) in the presence of purified A and B proteins, to detect the actual transposition process of a plasmid-borne mini-Mu element into well-defined donor molecules, such as bacteriophage λ DNA or φX174 RF (Mizuuchi, 1983, 1984). In an elegant study, Mizuuchi (1984) and Craigie and Mizuuchi (1985a) carefully analyzed the distribution of newly synthesized Mu DNA strands in the *in vitro* transposition products. They concluded that all Mu transposition is initiated through a pair of strand transfer reactions, which result in the covalent attachment of the 3' ends of Mu DNA to the 5' staggered ends of the target DNA, exactly as predicted by Shapiro's model (Fig. 23). Replication of this intermediate resulted in cointegrate formation, whereas failure to replicate resulted in a simple insertion into the target DNA (Fig. 23) (Mizuuchi, 1984; Craigie and Mizuuchi, 1985a; Mizuuchi and Craigie, 1986). Remarkably, once the Mu transposition intermediate was formed, only *E. coli* proteins were subsequently required for its conversion to a cointegrate form or simple insertion (Craigie and Mizuuchi, 1985a).

In subsequent experiments, Craigie *et al.* (1985) were able to prepare a Mu transposition intermediate structure by simply incubating the donor and acceptor DNAs with purified Mu A and B proteins, *E. coli* HU protein, ATP, and Mg^{2+}. In this simple system, both Mu ends must be present on the same molecule, the ends must be in the same orientation as that found in bacteriophage Mu DNA, the donor DNA must be supercoiled, and the acceptor DNA can be in any duplex form (Craigie *et al.*, 1985). From this work it can be concluded that once the pair of 3'-hydroxyl acceptor ends are created at the host-Mu DNA junctions, they can be elongated by the host replication machinery to give rise to a cointegrate structure (Fig. 23). The A protein, with the help of the B protein, brings the ends of Mu together with the target sequence, makes the necessary staggered cuts on Mu DNA and target DNA, performs the two strand transfer reactions, and positions the remaining 3'-hydroxyl ends of the target DNA so that they become accessible to the host DNA replication machinery (Fig. 23).

Once the host DNA polymerase III enzyme has extended these 3'-hydroxyl ends into Mu DNA, the exposed single-stranded regions are coated with ssb protein. The *E. coli* lagging-strand priming system (con-

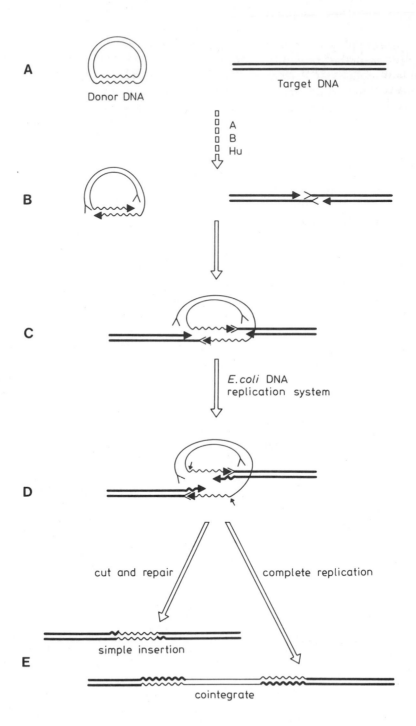

sisting of at least the dnaB and dnaG proteins) can be used to synthesize RNA primers on these ssb-coated DNA strands. The exact role that the HU protein plays in this minimal transposition system is not understood. Its role could be limited to a nonspecific condensation of the DNA molecules (Broyles and Pettijohn, 1986). It is unlikely that specific protein-protein interactions between the HU protein and the other components are involved, since the HU protein analogue from blue-green algae can substitute efficiently in both the Mu (Craigie et al., 1985) and E. coli oriC system (Dixon and Kornberg, 1984). An additional role that the A and B proteins may play would be to physically block propagation of the replication forks into the adjacent target sequences, thus permitting the duplication of Mu-specific DNA sequences only. Although the details of the nature of the replication complex assembled at the ends of Mu remain to be worked out, the general outline of the Mu transposition process has been magnificently documented.

What determines the decision between a simple and a replicative insertion? As mentioned above, either the intracellular levels of the putative cleaved form of the A protein or its putative in phase $33,000\text{-}M_r$ polypeptide made in minicells (M. Betermier and M. Chandler, personal communication) may play a role in such a decision. For example, either of the two A protein forms may be able to perform (1) the recognition and bringing together of the Mu ends and target DNA, (2) the nicking, and (3) the strand transfer reactions required. However, these two A protein forms may be unable to interact with either the B protein or the host DNA replication machinery to allow initiation of Mu DNA replication. Appropriate DNA processing, involving additional cleavage, repair, and ligation of such "stalled" replication intermediates would result in simple, conservative Mu insertions.

A transposase-mediated excision activity has been observed under conditions that overproduce Tn10 transposase (Morisato and Kleckner, 1984). Interestingly, Harshey (1984b) has also reported that induction of a plasmid-borne truncated A gene leads to double-strand breaks at the ends of Mu. As mentioned above, Tn10 transposes exclusively through a con-

---

FIGURE 23. Steps in bacteriophage Mu DNA transposition. The depicted steps are essentially those predicted by Shapiro's (1979) transposition model. The Mu-coded A and B proteins together with the host-coded HU protein assemble the Mu ends and the chosen target DNA sequence. The broken arrow at top indicates that the cleavage events may be transient and that the two DNA molecules are not separated but held into close proximity by the transposition protein complex. The free 3'-hydroxyl ends, belonging to target DNA (see text for details), are used to prime DNA replication directed toward the Mu DNA sequences. When the replication complex reaches the Mu ends, it terminates, and a cointegrate structure is eventually formed, as shown on the bottom left. However, anywhere along the DNA replication cycle, a simple Mu insertion can be formed, provided the appropriate cuts (indicated by arrows), repair, and ligation take place (see text for more details). >, 5'PO₄; ▶, 3'OH; ⋀⋀, Mu parental DNA; ⋀⋀⋀, newly replicated DNA; ▬, target DNA; —, Mu adjacent DNA.

servative mechanism, and this truncated A polypeptide leads exclusively to conservative Mu insertions. Whether these double-stranded cleavages represent inherent activities of these polypeptides or reflect the further processing of *bona fide* Shapiro-type replicative transposition intermediates (Fig. 23) remains to be determined.

ACKNOWLEDGMENTS. We thank all of our colleagues who supplied us with published and unpublished information about their work; K. Tilly for a critical reading of the manuscript; R. Bullock, J. Adamson, and M. Visini for cheerful help with the preparation of the manuscript; and O. Jenni and Y. Delotto for the beautiful art work. Research in the authors' laboratories is supported by grants from the National Institutes of Health (to C.G.) and the Swiss National Foundation (to Lucien Caro).

REFERENCES

Abeles, A. L., 1986, P1 plasmid replication: Purification and DNA-binding activity of the replication protein repA, *J. Biol. Chem.* **261:**3548.

Abeles, A. L., Snyder, K. M., and Chattoraj, D. K., 1984, P1 plasmid replication: Replicon structure, *J. Mol. Biol.* **173:**307.

Abeles, A. L., Friedman, S. A., and Austin, S. J., 1985, Partition of unit-copy miniplasmids to daughter cells. III. The DNA sequence and functional organization of the P1 partition region, *J. Mol. Biol.* **185:**261.

Adler, S., and Modrich, P., 1979, T7-induced DNA polymerase: Characterization of associated exonuclease activities and resolution into biologically active subunits, *J. Biol. Chem.* **254:**11605.

Ahmed, A., 1986, Evidence for replicative transposition of Tn5 and Tn9, *J. Mol. Biol.* **191:**75.

Akroyd, J. E., and Symonds, N., 1983, Conservative transposition of bacteriophage Mu?, *Nature* **303:**84.

Alberts, B. M., 1984, The DNA enzymology of protein machines, *Cold Spring Harbor Symp. Quant. Biol.* **49:**1.

Alberts, B. M., and Frey, L., 1970, T4 bacteriophage gene 32: A structural protein in the replication and recombination of DNA, *Nature* **227:**1313.

Alberts, B. M., Barry, J., Bedinger, P., Formosa, T., Jongeneel, C. V., and Kreuzer, K. N., 1982, Studies on DNA replication in the T4 bacteriophage *in vitro* system, *Cold Spring Harbor Symp. Quant. Biol.* **47:**655.

Anderl, A., and Klein, A., 1982, Replication of λdv DNA *in vitro*, *Nucleic Acids Res.* **10:**1733.

Anderson, D. L., and Mosharrafa, E. T., 1968, Physical and biological properties of phage φ29 deoxyribonucleic acid, *J. Virol.* **2:**1185.

Ang, D., Chandrasekhar, G. N., Johnson, C., Zylicz, M., and Georgopoulos, C., 1986a, Genetic and biochemical analysis of the *Escherichia coli grpE* gene and its product, in: *Mechanisms of DNA Replication and Recombination*, UCLA Symposia on Molecular and Cellular Biology, New Series, Vol. 47 (T. Kelly and R. McMacken, eds.), pp. 521–532, Alan R. Liss, New York.

Ang, D., Chandrasekhar, G. N., Zylicz, M., and Georgopoulos, C., 1986b, The *grpE* gene of *Escherichia coli* codes for heat shock protein B25.3, essential for DNA replication at all temperatures and host viability at high temperature, *J. Bacteriol.* **167:**25.

Aoyama, A., and Hayashi, M., 1986, Synthesis of bacteriophage φX174 *in vitro*: Mechanism of switch from DNA replication to DNA packaging, *Cell* **47:**99.

Aoyama, A., Hamatake, R. K., and Hayashi, M., 1983a, *In vitro* synthesis of bacteriophage φX174 by purified components, *Proc. Natl. Acad. Sci. USA* **80:**4195.

Aoyama, A., Hamatake, R. K., Mukai, R., and Hayashi, M., 1983b, Purification of φX174 gene *C* protein, *J. Biol. Chem.* **258:**5798.

Arai, K., and Kornberg, A., 1979, A general priming system employing only dnaB protein and primase for DNA replication, *Proc. Natl. Acad. Sci. USA* **76:**4308.

Arai, K., and Kornberg, A., 1981a, Unique primed start of phage φX174 replication and mobility of the primosome in a direction opposite chain synthesis, *Proc. Natl. Acad. Sci. USA* **78:**69.

Arai, K., and Kornberg, A., 1981b, Mechanism of dnaB protein. II. ATP hydrolysis by dnaB protein dependent on single- or double-stranded DNA, *J. Biol. Chem.* **256:**5253.

Arai, K., and Kornberg, A., 1981c, Mechanism of dnaB protein action. III. Allosteric role of ATP in the alteration of structure by dnaB protein in priming replication, *J. Biol. Chem.* **256:**5260.

Arai, K., Low, R., Kobori, J., Shlomai, J., and Kornberg, A., 1981a, Mechanism of dnaB protein action. V. Association of dnaB protein, n' and other prepriming proteins in the primosome of DNA replication, *J. Biol. Chem.* **256:**5273.

Arai, K., McMacken, R., Yasuda, S., and Kornberg, A., 1981b, Purification and properties of *Escherichia coli* protein i, a prepriming protein in φX174 DNA replication, *J. Biol. Chem.* **256:**5281.

Arai, K., Yasuda, S., and Kornberg, A., 1981c, Mechanism of dnaB protein action. I. Crystallization and properties of dnaB protein, an essential replication protein in *Escherichia coli, J. Biol. Chem.* **256:**5247.

Argos, P., Tucker, A. D., and Philipson, L., 1986, Primary structural relationships may reflect similar DNA replication strategies, *Virology* **149:**208.

Austin, S. J., Mural, R. J., Chattoraj, D. K., and Abeles, A. L., 1985, *Trans-* and *cis-*acting elements for the replication of P1 miniplasmids, *J. Mol. Biol.* **183:**145.

Baas, P. D., Teertstra, W. R., and Jansz, H. S., 1978, Bacteriophage φX174 RF DNA replication *in vivo:* A biochemical study, *J. Mol. Biol.* **125:**167.

Baas, P. D., Heidekamp, F., Van Mansfeld, A. D. M., Jansz, M. S., Van der Marel, G. A., Veneman, G. H., and Van Boom, J. H., 1981, Essential features of the origin of bacteriophage φX174 RF DNA replication: A recognition and a key sequence for φX gene *A* protein, in: *The Initiation of DNA Replication*, UCLA Symposia on Molecular and Cellular Biology, Vol. 22 (D. S. Ray, ed.), pp. 195–209, Academic Press, New York.

Bachmann, B., 1983, Linkage map of *Escherichia coli* K-12, edition 7, *Microbiol. Rev.* **47:**180.

Bahl, H., Echols, H., Strauss, D. B., Court, D., Crowl, R., and Georgopoulos, C. P., 1987, Induction of the heat shock response of *E. coli* through stabilization of σ32 by the phage λ cIII protein, *Genes Dev.* **1:**57.

Baker, T. A., Sekimizu, K., Funnell, B. E., and Kornberg, A., 1986, Extensive unwinding of the plasmid template during staged enzymatic initiation of DNA replication from the origin of the *Escherichia coli* chromosome, *Cell* **45:**53.

Bamford, D. H., and Mindich, L., 1984, Characterization of the DNA-protein complex at the termini of the bacteriophage PRD1 genome, *J. Virol.* **50:**309.

Bardwell, J. C. A., and Craig, E. A., 1984, Major heat shock gene of *Drosophila* and the *Escherichia coli* heat inducible *dnaK* gene are homologous, *Proc. Natl. Acad. Sci. USA* **81:**848.

Bardwell, J. C. A., Tilly, K., Craig, E. A., King, J., Zylicz, M., and Georgopoulos, C., 1986, The nucleotide sequence of the *Escherichia coli* K12 *dnaJ* gene: A gene that encodes a heat shock protein, *J. Biol. Chem.* **261:**1782.

Barrett, K., Gibbs, W., and Calendar, R., 1972, A transcribing activity induced by satellite phage P4, *Proc. Natl. Acad. Sci. USA* **69:**2986.

Barrett, K., Blinkova, A., and Arnold, G., 1983, The P4 α gene is the structural gene for the P4-induced RNA polymerase, *J. Virol.* **48:**157.

Bastia, D., Sueoka, N., and Cox, E., 1975, Studies on the late replication of phage lambda:

Rolling-circle replication of the wild type and a partially suppressed strain, Oam29 Pam80, *J. Mol. Biol.* **98**:305.

Beck, E., and Zink, B., 1981, Nucleotide sequence and genome organization of bacteriophages fl and fd, *Gene* **16**:35.

Beck, E., Sommer, R., Auerswald, E. A., Kurz, C., Zink, B., Osterburg, H., Schaller, H., Sugino, K., Sugisaki, H., Okamoto, T., and Takanami, M., 1978, Nucleotide sequence of bacteriophage fd DNA, *Nucleic Acids Res.* **5**:4495.

Bedinger, P., and Alberts, B. M., 1983, The 3' to 5' proofreading exonuclease of bacteriophage T4 DNA polymerase is stimulated by other T4 DNA replication proteins, *J. Biol. Chem.* **258**:9649.

Bedinger, P., Hochstrasser, M., Jongeneel, C. V., and Alberts, B. M., 1983, Properties of the T4 bacteriophage DNA replication apparatus: The T4 dda helicase is required to pass a bound RNA polymerase molecule, *Cell* **34**:115.

Bender, J., and Kleckner, N., 1986, Genetic evidence that Tn*10* transposes by a non-replicative intermediate, *Cell* **45**:801.

Berg, D. E., 1983, Structural requirements for IS*50*-mediated gene transposition, *Proc. Natl. Acad. Sci. USA* **80**:792.

Bernstein, C., and Wallace, S. S., 1983, DNA repair, in: *Bacteriophage T4* (C. Mathews, E. Kutter, G. Mosig, and P. Berger, eds.), pp. 138–151, American Society for Microbiology, Washington.

Bertani, E., and Bertani, G., 1970, Preparation and characterization of temperate, non inducible bacteriophage P2, *J. Gen. Virol.* **6**:201.

Better, M., and Freifelder, D., 1983, Studies on the replication of *Escherichia coli* phage λ DNA. I. The kinetics of DNA replication and requirements for the generation of rolling circles, *Virology* **126**:168.

Blanco, L., and Salas, M., 1985, Replication of phage φ29 DNA with purified terminal protein and DNA polymerase: Synthesis of full length φ29 DNA, *Proc. Natl. Acad. Sci. USA* **82**:6404.

Blanco, L., Garcia, J. A., Penalva, M. A., and Salas, M., 1983, Factors involved in the initiation of phage φ29 DNA replication *in vitro:* Requirement of the gene 2 product for the formation of the protein p3-dAMP complex, *Nucleic Acids Res.* **11**:1309.

Blanco, L., Gutierrez, J., Lazaro, J. M., Bernad, A., and Salas, M., 1986, Replication of phage φ29 DNA *in vitro:* Role of the viral protein p6 in initiation and elongation, *Nucleic Acids Res.* **14**:4923.

Blumenthal, T., and Carmichael, G. G., 1979, RNA replication: Function and structure of Qβ-replicase, *Annu. Rev. Biochem.* **48**:525.

Bochner, B. R., Zylicz, M., and Georgopoulos, C., 1986, *Escherichia coli* dnaK protein possesses a 5'-nucleotidase activity that is inhibited by AppppA, *J. Bacteriol.* **168**:931.

Bouché, J.-P., Zechel, K., and Kornberg, A., 1975, dnaG gene product, a rifampicin-resistant RNA polymerase, initiates the conversion of a single-stranded coliphage DNA to its duplex replicative form, *J. Biol. Chem.* **250**:5995.

Bouché, J.-P., Rowen, L., and Kornberg, A., 1978, The RNA primer synthesized by primase initiates phage G4 DNA replication, *J. Biol. Chem.* **253**:765.

Bowden, D. W., Twersky, R. S., and Calendar, R., 1975, *Escherichia coli* DNA synthesis mutants: Their effect upon bacteriophage P2 and satellite bacteriophage P4 DNA synthesis, *J. Bacteriol.* **124**:167.

Brody, E., Rabussay, D., and Hall, D. H., 1983, Regulation of transcription of prereplicative genes, in: *Bacteriophage T4* (C. Mathews, E. Kutter, G. Mosig, and P. Berger, eds.), pp. 32–39, American Society for Microbiology, Washington.

Broker, T. R., and Lehman, I. R., 1971, Branched DNA molecules intermediates in T4 recombination, *J. Mol. Biol.* **60**:131.

Brown, D. R., Reinberg, D., Schmidt-Glenewinkel, T., Roth, M., Zipursky, S. L., and Hurwitz, J., 1982, DNA structures required for φX174 A protein-directed initiation and termination of DNA replication, *Cold Spring Harbor Symp. Quant. Biol.* **47**:701.

Broyles, S. S., and Pettijohn, D. E., 1986, Interactions of the *Escherichia coli* HU protein with DNA. Evidence for formation of nucleosome-like structures with altered DNA helical pitch, *J. Mol. Biol.* **187**:47.

Brutlag, D., and Kornberg, A., 1972, Enzymatic synthesis of deoxyribonucleic acid, *J. Biol. Chem.* **247**:241.

Brutlag, D., Schekman, R., and Kornberg, A., 1971, A possible role for RNA polymerase in the initiation of M13 DNA synthesis, *Proc. Natl. Acad. Sci. USA* **68**:2826.

Bukhari, A. I., 1976, Bacteriophage Mu as a transposition element, *Annu. Rev. Genet.* **10**:389.

Burlingame, R. P., Obukowicz, M. G., Lynn, D. L., and Howe, M. M., 1986, Isolation of point mutations in bacteriophage Mu attachment regions cloned in a λ::mini-Mu phage, *Proc. Natl. Acad. Sci. USA* **83**:6012.

Calendar, R., Ljungquist, E., Deho, G., Goldstein, R., Youderian, P., Sironi, G., and Six, E. W., 1981, Lysogenization by satellite phage P4, *Virology* **113**:20.

Calendar, R., Kahn, M., Six, E., Goldstein, R., Lindqvist, B., Deho, G., Inman, R., Jiang, R.-Z., Lin, C.-S., Lee, S.-J., Lagos, R., Christie, G., Dale, E., and Pierson, L. S., 1984, Bacteriophage P4, in: *Genetic Maps,* (S. J. O'Brien, ed.), pp. 62–65, Cold Spring Harbor Laboratory, Cold Spring Harbor, NY.

Calos, M. P., and Miller, J. H., 1980, Transposable elements, *Cell* **20**:579.

Carlson, K., and Overvatn, A., 1986, Bacteriophage T4 endonucleases II and IV, oppositely affected by dCMP hydroxymethylase activity, have different roles in the degradation and in the RNA polymerase-dependent replication of T4 cytosine-containing DNA, *Genetics* **114**:669.

Carrascosa, J. L., Camacho, A., Moreno, F., Jimenez, F., Mellado, R. P., Vinuela, E., and Salas, M., 1976, *Bacillus subtilis* phage φ29: Characterization of gene products and functions, *Eur. J. Biochem.* **66**:229.

Center, M. S., 1975, Role of gene 2 in bacteriophage T7 DNA synthesis, *J. Virol.* **16**:94.

Center, M. S., and Richardson, C. C., 1970, An endonuclease induced after infection of *Escherichia coli* with bacteriophage T7, *J. Biol. Chem.* **245**:6285.

Cha, T.-A., and Alberts, B. M., 1986, Studies of the DNA helicase-RNA primase unit from bacteriophage T4: A trinucleotide sequence on the DNA template starts RNA primer synthesis, *J. Biol. Chem.* **261**:7001.

Chaconas, G., Harshey, R. M., and Bukhari, A. I., 1980, Association of Mu containing plasmids with the *E. coli* chromosome upon prophage induction, *Proc. Natl. Acad. Sci. USA* **77**:1778.

Chaconas, G., Harshey, R. M., Sarvetnick, N., and Bukhari, A. I., 1981, The predominant end products of prophage Mu transposition during the lytic cycle are replicon fusions, *J. Mol. Biol.* **150**:341.

Chaconas, G., Giddens, E. B., Miller, J. I., and Gloor, G., 1985a, A truncated form of the bacteriophage Mu B protein promotes conservative integration, but not replicative transposition, of Mu DNA, *Cell* **41**:857.

Chaconas, G., Gloor, G., and Miller, J. L., 1985b, Amplification and purification of the bacteriophage Mu encoded B transposition protein, *J. Biol. Chem.* **260**:2662.

Challberg, M. D., Desiderio, S. V., and Kelly, T. J. Jr., 1980, Adenovirus DNA replication *in vitro:* Characterization of a protein covalently linked to nascent DNA strands, *Proc. Natl. Acad. Sci. USA* **77**:5105.

Chamberlin, M., 1974, Isolation and characterization of prototrophic mutants of *Escherichia coli* unable to support the intracellular growth of T7, *J. Virol.* **14**:509.

Chao, J., Leach, M., and Karam, J., 1977, *In vivo* functional interaction between DNA polymerase and dCMP-hydroxymethylase of bacteriophage T4, *J. Virol.* **24**:557.

Chattoraj, D. K., 1978, Strand-specific break near the origin of bacteriophage P2 DNA replication, *Proc. Natl. Acad. Sci. USA* **75**:1685.

Chattoraj, D. K., Cordes, K., and Abeles, A. L., 1984, Plasmid P1 replication: Negative control by repeated DNA sequences, *Proc. Natl. Acad. Sci. USA* **81**:6456.

Chattoraj, D. K., Abeles, A. L., and Yarmolinsky, M. B., 1985a, P1 plasmid maintenance a paradigm of precise control, in: *Plasmids in Bacteria* (D. R. Helinski, S. N. Cohen, B. D. Elewell, D. A. Jackson, and A. Hollaender, eds.), pp. 355–381, Plenum Press, New York.

Chattoraj, D. K., Snyder, K. M., and Abeles, A. L., 1985b, P1 plasmid replication: Multiple functions of repA protein at the origin, *Proc. Natl. Acad. Sci. USA* **82**:2588.

Chin, C.-S., 1984, Nucleotide sequence of the essential region of bacteriophage P4, *Nucleic Acids Res.* **12**:8667.

Chiu, C. S., and Greenberg, G. R., 1968, Evidence for a possible direct role of dCMP hydroxymethylase in T4 phage DNA synthesis, *Cold Spring Harbor Symp. Quant. Biol.* **33**:351.

Chiu, C. S., and Greenberg, G. R., 1973, Mutagenic effects of temperature-sensitive mutants of gene *42* of bacteriophage T4. *J. Virol.* **12**:199.

Cleary, J. M., and Ray, D. S., 1980, Replication of the plasmid pBR322 under the control of a cloned replication origin from the single-stranded DNA phage M13, *Proc. Natl. Acad. Sci. USA* **77**:4638.

Cleary, J. M., and Ray, D. S., 1981, Deletion analysis of the cloned replication origin region from bacteriophage M13, *J. Virol.* **40**:197.

Cosalanti, J., and Denhardt, D. T., 1985, Expression of the cloned bacteriophage φX174 *A** gene in *Escherichia coli* inhibits DNA replication and cell division, *J. Virol.* **53**:807.

Craigie, R., and Mizuuchi, K., 1985a, Mechanism of transposition of bacteriophage Mu: Structure of a transposition intermediate, *Cell* **41**:867.

Craigie, R., and Mizuuchi, K., 1985b, Cloning of the *A* gene of bacteriophage Mu and purification of its product, the Mu transposase, *J. Biol. Chem.* **260**:1832.

Craigie, R., and Mizuuchi, K., 1986, Role of DNA topology in Mu transposition: Mechanism of sensing the relative orientation of two DNA segments, *Cell* **45**:793.

Craigie, R., Mizuuchi, M., and Mizuuchi, K., 1984, Site-specific recognition of the bacteriophage Mu ends by the Mu A protein, *Cell* **39**:387.

Craigie, R., Arndt-Jovin, D. J., and Mizuuchi, K., 1985, A defined system for the DNA strand-transfer reaction at the initiation of bacteriophage Mu transposition: Protein and DNA substrate requirements, *Proc. Natl. Acad. Sci. USA* **82**:7570.

Dannenberg, R., and Mosig, G., 1983, Early intermediates in bacteriophage T4 DNA replication and recombination, *J. Virol.* **45**:813.

D'Ari, R. A., Jaffé-Brochet, A., Touati-Schwartz, D., and Yarmolinsky, M., 1975, A dnaB analogue specified by bacteriophage P1, *J. Mol. Biol.* **94**:341.

Dasgupta, S., and Mitra, S., 1977, The role of DNA polymerase I–associated 5' exonuclease in replication of coliphage M13 replicative-form DNA, *Biochem. Biophys. Res. Commun.* **78**:1108.

De Massy, B., Weisberg, R. A., and Studier, F. W., 1987, Gene 3 endonuclease of bacteriophage T7 resolves conformationally branched structures in double-stranded DNA, *J. Mol. Biol.* **193**:359.

Demerec, M., and Fano, U., 1945, Bacteriophage-resistant mutants in *Escherichia coli*, *Genetics* **30**:119.

Denniston-Thompson, K., Moore, D. D., Kruger, K., Furth, M., and Blattner, F. R., 1977, Physical structure of the replication origin of bacteriophage lambda, *Science* **198**:1051.

Derbyshire, K. M., and Grindley, N. D. F., 1986, Replicative and conservative transposition in bacteria, *Cell* **47**:325.

DeWyngaert, M. A., and Hinkle, D. A., 1979, Bacterial mutants affecting phage T7 DNA replication produce RNA polymerase resistant to inhibition by the T7 gene 2 protein, *J. Biol. Chem.* **254**:11247.

DeWyngaert, M. A., and Hinkle, D. A., 1980, Characterization of the defects in bacteriophage T7 DNA synthesis during growth in *Escherichia coli* mutant tsnB, *J. Virol.* **33**:780.

Dixon, N. E., and Kornberg, A., 1984, Protein HU in the enzymatic replication of the chromosomal origin of *Escherichia coli*, *Proc. Natl. Acad. Sci. USA* **81**:424.

Dodson, M., Roberts, J., McMacken, R., and Echols, H., 1985, Specialized nucleoprotein structures at the origin of replication of bacteriophage λ: Complexes with λ O protein and with λ O, λ P, and *Escherichia coli* dnaB proteins, *Proc. Natl. Acad. Sci. USA* **82**:4678.

Dodson, M., Echols, H., Wickner, S., Alfano, C., Mensa-Wilmot, K., Gomes, B., LeBowitz, J. H., Roberts, J. D., and McMacken, R., 1986, Specialized nucleoprotein structures at the origin of replication of bacteriophage λ: Localized unwinding of duplex DNA by six-protein reaction, *Proc. Natl. Acad. Sci. USA* **83**:7638.

Dotto, G. P., and Zinder, N. D., 1984a, Increased intracellular concentration of an initiator protein markedly reduces the minimal sequence required for initiation of DNA synthesis, *Proc. Natl. Acad. Sci. USA* **81**:1336.

Dotto, G. P., and Zinder, N. D., 1984b, Reduction of the minimal sequence for initiation of DNA synthesis by qualitative or quantitative changes of an initiator protein, *Nature* **311**:5983.

Dotto, G. P., Enea, V., and Zinder, N. D., 1981, Functional analysis of bacteriophage fl intergenic region, *Virology* **114**:463.

Dotto, G. P., Horiuchi, K., and Zinder, N. D., 1982, Initiation and termination of phage fl plus-strand synthesis, *Proc. Natl. Acad. Sci. USA* **79**:7122.

Dotto, G. P., Horiuchi, K., and Zinder, N. D., 1984, The functional origin of bacteriophage fl DNA replication. Its signals and domains, *J. Mol. Biol.* **172**:507.

Dove, W., Hargrave, E., Ohashi, M., Haugli, F., and Guha, A., 1969, Replicator activation in lambda, *Jpn. J. Genet.* (Suppl.) **44**:11.

Dove, W., Inokuchi, H., and Stevens, W., 1971, Replication control in phage lambda, in: *The Bacteriophage Lambda* (A. D. Hershey, ed.), pp. 747–771, Cold Spring Harbor Laboratory, Cold Spring Harbor, NY.

Drahos, D. J., and Hendrix, R. W., 1982, Effect of bacteriophage lambda infection on synthesis of groE protein and other *Escherichia coli* proteins, *J. Bacteriol.* **149**:1050.

Drake, J. W., 1973, The genetic control of spontaneous and induced mutation rates in bacteriophage T4, *Genetics* (Suppl.) **73**:45.

Dressler, D., Wolfson, J., and Magazin, M., 1972, Initiation and reinitiation of DNA synthesis during replication of bacteriophage T7, *Proc. Natl. Acad. Sci. USA* **69**:998.

Duguet, M., Yarranton, G., and Gefter, M., 1978, The rep protein of *Escherichia coli:* Interaction with DNA and other proteins, *Cold Spring Harbor Symp. Quant. Biol.* **43**:335.

Dunn, J. J., and Studier, F. W., 1981, Nucleotide sequence from the genetic left end of bacteriophage T7 DNA to the beginning of gene 4, *J. Mol. Biol.* **148**:303.

Dunn, J. J., and Studier, F. W., 1983, The complete nucleotide sequence of bacteriophage T7 DNA and the location of T7 genetics elements, *J. Mol. Biol.* **166**:477.

Echols, H., 1986, Multiple DNA-protein interactions governing high-precision DNA transactions, *Science* **233**:1050.

Edlin, G., and Bitner, R., 1977, Reproductive fitness of P1, P2 and Mu lysogens of *Escherichia coli, J. Virol.* **21**:560.

Edlin, G., Lin, L., and Kudrna, R., 1975, Lambda lysogens of *E. coli* reproduce more rapidly than non-lysogens, *Nature* **255**:735.

Edlin, T. D., and Ihler, G. M., 1981, Conservation and divergence in single-stranded phage DNA secondary structure: Relations to origins of DNA replication, in: *The Initiation of DNA Replication,* UCLA Symposia on Molecular and Cellular Biology, Vol. 22, (D. S. Ray, ed.), pp. 223–243, Academic Press, New York.

Eisen, H., Pereira da Silva, L., and Jacob, F., 1968, The regulation and mechanism of DNA synthesis in bacteriophage lambda, *Cold Spring Harbor Symp. Quant. Biol.* **33**:755.

Eisen, H., Barrand, P., Spiegelman, W., Reichardt, L. F., Heinemann, S., and Georgopoulos, C., 1982, Mutants in the *y* region of bacteriophage λ constitutive for repressor synthesis: Their isolation and the characterization of the Hyp phenotype, *Gene* **20**:71.

Eisenberg, S., 1980, Cleavage of φX174 single-stranded DNA by gene *A* protein and formation of a tight protein-DNA complex, *J. Virol.* **35**:409.

Eisenberg, S., and Kornberg, A., 1979, Purification and characterization of φX174 gene *A* protein. A multifunctional enzyme of duplex DNA replication, *J. Biol. Chem.* **254**:5328.

Eisenberg, S., Scott, J. F., and Kornberg, A., 1976, Enzymatic replication of viral and complementary strands of duplex DNA of phage φX174 proceeds by separate mechanisms, *Proc. Natl. Acad. Sci. USA* **73**:3151.

Eklund, H., Cambillau, C., Sjöberg, B.-M., Holmgren, A., Jörnvall, H., Höög, J.-O., and Bränden, C.-I., 1984, Conformational and functional similarities between glutaredoxin and thioredoxins, *EMBO J.* **3**:1443.

Engelberg-Kulka, H., Dekel, L., Israeli-Reches, M., and Belfort, M., 1979, The requirement of nonsense suppression for the development of several phages, *Mol. Gen. Genet.* **170**:155.

Engler, M. J., and Richardson, C. C., 1983, Bacteriophage T7 DNA replication; synthesis of lagging strands in a reconstituted system using purified proteins, *J. Biol. Chem.* **258**:11197.

Engler, M. J., Lechner, R. L., and Richardson, C. C., 1983, Two forms of the DNA polymerase of bacteriophage T7, *J. Biol. Chem.* **258**:11165.

Epstein, R. H., Bolle, A., Steinberger, C., Kellenberger, E., Boy de la Tour, E., Chevalley, R., Edgar, R., Susman, M., Denhardt, C., and Lielausis, I., 1963, Physiological studies of conditional lethal mutants of bacteriophage T4D, *Cold Spring Harbor Symp. Quant. Biol.* **28**:375.

Faelen, M., Huisman, O., and Toussaint, A., 1978a, Involvement of phage Mu-1 early functions in Mu mediated chromosomal rearrangements, *Nature* **271**:580.

Faelen, M., Resibois, A., and Toussaint, A., 1978b, Mini-Mu: An insertion element derived from temperate phage Mu-1, *Cold Spring Harbor Symp. Quant. Biol.* **43**:1169.

Falco, S. C., Zivin, R., and Rothman-Denes, L. B., 1978, Novel template requirements of N4 virion RNA polymerase, *Proc. Natl. Acad. Sci. USA* **75**:3220.

Feiss, M., and Becker, A., 1983, DNA packaging and cutting, in: *Lambda II* (R. W. Hendrix, J. W. Roberts, F. W. Stahl, and R. A. Weisberg, eds.), pp. 305–330, Cold Spring Harbor Laboratory, Cold Spring Harbor, NY.

Fiddes, J. C., Barrel, B. G., and Godson, G. N., 1978, Nucleotide sequences of the separate origins of synthesis of bacteriophage G4 viral and complementary DNA strands, *Proc. Natl. Acad. Sci. USA* **75**:1081.

Fischer, H., and Hinkle, D. C., 1980, Bacteriophage T7 DNA replication *in vitro:* Stimulation of DNA synthesis by T7 RNA polymerase, *J. Biol. Chem.* **255**:7956.

Flanegan, J. B., and Greenberg, G. R., 1977, Regulation of deoxyribonucleotide biosynthesis during *in vivo* bacteriophage T4 replication, *J. Biol. Chem.* **252**:3019.

Fluit, A. C., Baas, P. D., Van Boom, J. H., Veneeman, G. H., and Jansz, H. S., 1984, Gene *A* protein cleavage of recombinant plasmids containing the φX174 replication origin, *Nucleic Acids Res.* **12**:6443.

Fluit, A. C., Baas, P. D., and Jansz, H. S., 1986, Termination and reinitiation signals of bacteriophage φX174 rolling circle DNA replication, *Virology* **154**:357.

Formosa, T., and Alberts, B. M., 1984, The use of affinity chromatography to study proteins involved in bacteriophage T4 genetic recombination, *Cold Spring Harbor Symp. Quant. Biol.* **49**:363.

Formosa, T., and Alberts, B. M., 1986a, Purification and characterization of the T4 bacteriophage uvsX protein, *J. Biol. Chem.* **261**:6107.

Formosa, T., and Alberts, B. M., 1986b, DNA synthesis dependent on genetic recombination: Characterization of a reaction catalyzed by purified bacteriophage T4 proteins, *Cell* **47**:793.

Formosa, T., Burke, R. L., and Alberts, B. M., 1983, Affinity purification of T4 bacteriophage proteins essential for DNA replication and genetic recombination, *Proc. Natl. Acad. Sci. USA* **80**:2442.

Franke, B., and Ray, D. S., 1972, *Cis*-limited action of the gene *A* product of bacteriophage φX174 and the essential bacterial site, *Proc. Natl. Acad. Sci. USA* **69**:475.

Freund, J. N., and Barry, B. P., 1987, The *rudimentary* gene of *Drosophila melanogaster* encodes four enzymic functions, *J. Mol. Biol.* **193**:1.

Freymeyer, D. K. II, Shank, P. R., Edgell, M. H., Hutchison, C. A. III, and Vanaman, T. C., 1977, Amino acid sequence of small core protein from bacteriophage φX174, *Bio-chemistry* **16:**4550.

Friedman, D. I., Plantefaber, L. C., Olson, E. J., Carver, D., O'Dea, M. H., and Gellert, M., 1984a, Mutations in the DNA *gyrB* gene that are temperature sensitive for labmda site-specific recombination, Mu growth, and plasmid maintenance, *J. Bacteriol.* **157:**490.

Friedman, D. I., Olson, E. J., Tilly, K., Georgopoulos, C., Herskowitz, I., and Banuett, F., 1984b, Interactions of bacteriophage and host macromolecules in the growth of bacte-riophage λ, *Microbiol. Rev.* **48:**299.

Fröhlich, B., Powling, A., and Knippers, R., 1975, Formation of concatemeric DNA in bacte-riophage T7 infected bacteria, *Virology* **65:**455.

Fujisawa, H., and Hayashi, M., 1977, Assembly of bacteriophage φX174: Identification of a virion capsid precursor and of a model for the functions of bacteriophage gene products during morphogenesis, *J. Virol.* **24:**303.

Fujisawa, H., Yonesaki, T., and Minagawa, T., 1985, Sequence of the T4 recombination gene, *uvsX*, and its comparison with that of the *recA* gene of *Escherichia coli*, *Nucleic Acids Res.* **13:**7473.

Fulford, W., and Model, P., 1984, Gene *X* of bacteriophage f1 is required for phage DNA synthesis. Mutagenesis of in-frame overlapping genes, *J. Mol. Biol.* **178:**137.

Fuller, C. W., and Richardson, C. C., 1985a, Initiation of DNA replication at the primary origin of bacteriophage T7 by purified proteins: Site and direction of initial DNA syn-thesis, *J. Biol. Chem.* **260:**3185.

Fuller, C. W., and Richardson, C. C., 1985b, Initiation of DNA replication at the primary origin of bacteriophage T7 by purified proteins: Initiation of bidirectional synthesis, *J. Biol. Chem.* **260:**3197.

Fuller, C. W., Beauchamp, B. B., Engler, M. J., Lechner, R. L., Matson, S. W., Tabor, S., White, J. H., and Richardson, C. C., 1982, Mechanisms for the initiation of bacteriophage T7 DNA replication, *Cold Spring Harbor Symp. Quant. Biol.* **47:**999.

Fuller, R. S., Kaguni, J. M., and Kornberg, A., 1981, Enzymatic replication of the origin of the *Escherichia coli* chromosome, *Proc. Natl. Acad. Sci. USA* **78:**7370.

Fuller, R. S., Funnell, B. E., and Kornberg, A., 1984, The dnaA protein complex with the *E. coli* chromosomal replication origin (oriC) and other DNA sites, *Cell* **38:**889.

Funnell, B. E., Baker, T. A., and Kornberg, A., 1986, Complete enzymatic replication of plasmids containing the origin of the *Escherichia coli* chromosome, *J. Biol. Chem.* **261:**5616.

Furth, M. E., and Wickner, S. H., 1983, Lambda DNA replication, in: *Lambda II* (R. W. Hendrix, J. W. Roberts, F. W. Stahl, and R. A. Weisberg, eds.), pp. 145–174, Cold Spring Harbor Laboratory, Cold Spring Harbor, NY.

Furth, M., and Yates, J., 1978, Specificity determinants for bacteriophage lambda DNA replication. II. Structure of O proteins of λ-φ80 and λ-82 hybrid phages and of a λ mutant defective in the origin of replication. *J. Mol. Biol.* **126:**227.

Furth, M., McLeester, C., and Dove, W., 1978, Specificity determinants for bacteriophage lambda DNA replication. I. A chain of interactions that controls the initiation of replication, *J. Mol. Biol.* **126:**195.

Furth, M., Dove, W., and Meyer, B., 1982, Specificity determinants for bacteriophage λ DNA replication. III. Activation of replication in ori^c mutants by transcription outside of ori, *J. Mol. Biol.* **154:**65.

Galas, D. J., and Chandler, M., 1981, On the molecular mechanisms of transposition, *Proc. Natl. Acad. Sci. USA* **78:**4858.

Garcia, J. A., Penalva, M. A., Blanco, L., and Salas, M., 1984, Template requirements for initiation of phage φ29 DNa replication *in vitro*, *Proc. Natl. Acad. Sci. USA* **81:**80.

Gauss, P., Doherty, D. H., and Gold, L., 1983, Bacterial and phage mutations that reveal helix-unwinding activities required for bacteriophage T4 DNA replication, *Proc. Natl. Acad. Sci. USA* **80:**1669.

Gauss, P., Gayle, M., Winter, R. B., and Gold, L., 1987, The bacteriophage T4 *dexA* gene:

Sequence and analysis of a gene conditionally required for DNA replication, *Mol. Gen. Genet.* **206**:24.

Geider, K., and Kornberg, A., 1974, Conversion of the M13 viral single-strand to the double-stranded replicative forms by purified proteins, *J. Biol. Chem.* **249**:3999.

Geider, K., Beck, E., and Schaller, H., 1978, An RNA transcribed from DNA at the origin of phage fd single-strand to replicative form conversion, *Proc. Natl. Acad. Sci. USA* **75**:645.

Geisselsoder, J., 1976, Strand-specific discontinuity in replicating P2 DNA, *J. Mol. Biol.* **100**:13.

Gellert, M., 1981, DNA topoisomerases, *Annu. Rev. Biochem.* **50**:879.

Gellert, M., and Nash, H., 1987, Communication between segments of DNA during site-specific recombination, *Nature* **325**:401.

Georgopoulos, C. P., 1977, A new bacterial gene (*groPC*) which affects λ DNA replication, *Mol. Gen. Genet.* **151**:35.

Georgopoulos, C. P., and Herskowitz, I., 1971, *Escherichia coli* mutants blocked in lambda DNA synthesis, in: *The Bacteriophage Lambda* (A. D. Hershey, ed.), pp. 553–564, Cold Spring Harbor Laboratory, Cold Spring Harbor, NY.

Georgopoulos, C. P., Hendrix, R. W., Casjens, S. R., and Kaiser, A. D., 1973, Host participation in bacteriophage lambda head assembly, *J. Mol. Biol.* **76**:45.

Georgopoulos, C., Tilly, K., Yochem, J., and Feiss, M., 1980, Studies with the *Escherichia coli dnaJ* and *dnaK* genes, in: *Mechanistic Studies of DNA Replication and Genetic Recombination* (B. Alberts, ed.), pp. 609–617, Academic Press, New York.

Georgopoulos, C., Tilly, K., Drahos, D., and Hendrix, R., 1982, The B66.0 protein of *Escherichia coli* is the product of the *dnaK* gene, *J. Bacteriol.* **149**:1175.

Ghisotti, D., Zangrossi, S., Sironi, G., 1983, An *Escherichia coli* gene required for bacteriophage P2-λ interference, *J. Virol.* **48**:616.

Gibbs, W., Goldstein, R. N., Wiener, R., Lindqvist, B., and Calendar, R., 1973, Satellite bacteriophage P4: Characterization of mutant in two essential genes, *Virology* **53**:24.

Gilbert, W., and Dressler, D., 1968, DNA replication: The rolling circle model, *Cold Spring Harbor Symp. Quant. Biol.* **33**:473.

Gilchrist, C. A., and Denhardt, D. T., 1987, *Escherichia coli rep* gene: Sequence of the gene, the encoded helicase, and its homology with uvrD, *Nucleic Acids Res.* **15**:465.

Giphart-Gassler, M., Wijffelman, C., and Reeve, N., 1981, Structural polypeptides and products of late genes of bacteriophage Mu: Characterization and structural aspects, *J. Mol. Biol.* **145**:139.

Gloor, G., and Chaconas, G., 1986, The bacteriophage Mu *N* gene encodes the 64 kd virion protein which is injected with and circularizes infecting Mu DNA, *J. Biol. Chem.* **261**:16682.

Godson, G. N., 1979, Comparative DNA-sequence analysis of the G4 and φX174 genomes, in: *The Single-Stranded DNA Phages* (D. Denhardt, D. Dressler, and D. Ray, eds.), pp. 671–695, Cold Spring Harbor Laboratory, Cold Spring Harbor, NY.

Goldberg, E., 1983, Recognition, attachment, and injection, in: *Bacteriophage T4* (C. Mathews, E. Kutter, G. Mosig, and P. Berger, eds.), pp. 32–39, American Society for Microbiology, Washington.

Goldstein, R., Sedivy, J., and Ljungquist, E., 1982, Propagation of satellite phage P4 as a plasmid, *Proc. Natl. Acad. Sci. USA* **79**:515.

Goosen, T., 1978, Replication of bacteriophage Mu: Direction and possible location of the origin, in: *DNA Synthesis, Present and Future* (I. Molineux and M. Kohiyama, eds.), pp. 121–126, Plenum Press, New York.

Goosen, N., Van Heuvel, M., Moolenaar, G. F., and Van de Putte, P., 1984, Regulation of Mu transposition. II. The *Escherichia coli* himD protein positively controls two repressor promoters and the early promoter of bacteriophage Mu, *Gene* **32**:419.

Gottesman, S., Gottesman, M., Shaw, J., and Pearson, M., 1981, Protein degradation in *E. coli*. The *lon* mutation and bacteriophage lambda N and cII protein stability, *Cell* **24**:225.

Goulian, M., Lucas, Z. J., and Kornberg, A., 1968, Enzymatic synthesis of deoxyribonucleic acid. XXV. Purification and properties of deoxyribonucleic acid polymerase induced by infection with phage T4, *J. Biol. Chem.* **243**:627.

Gray, C. P., Sommer, R., Polke, C., Beck, E., and Schaller, H., 1978, Structure of the origin of DNA replication of bacteriophage fd, *Proc. Natl. Acad. Sci. USA* **75**:50.

Grindley, N. D. F., 1983, Transposition of Tn3 and related transposons, *Cell* **32**:3.

Grindley, N. D. F., and Reed, R. R., 1985, Transpositional recombination in prokaryotes, *Annu. Rev. Biochem.* **54**:863.

Grindley, N. D. F., and Sherratt, D. J., 1978, Sequence analysis at IS1 insertion sites: Models for transposition, *Cold Spring Harbor Symp. Quant. Biol.* **43**:1257.

Groenen, M. A. M., Timmer, E., and Van de Putte, P., 1985, DNA sequences at the ends of the genome of bacteriophage Mu essential for transposition, *Proc. Natl. Acad. Sci. USA* **82**:2087.

Groenen, M. A. M., Kokke, M., and Van de Putte, P., 1986, Transposition of mini-Mu containing only one of the ends of bacteriophage Mu, *EMBO J.* **13**:3687.

Grosschedl, R., and Hobom, G., 1979, DNA sequences and structural homologies of the replication origins of lambdoid bacteriophages, *Nature* **277**:621.

Grossman, A. D., Erickson, J. W., and Gross, C. A., 1984, The *htpR* gene product of *E. coli* is a sigma factor for heat shock promoters, *Cell* **38**:383.

Guinta, D., Lindberg, G., and Rothman-Denes, L. B., 1986a, Bacteriophage N4-coded 5' to 3' exonuclease: Purification and characterization, *J. Biol. Chem.* **261**:10736.

Guinta, D., Stambouly, J., Falco, S. C., Rist, J. K., and Rothman-Denes, L. B., 1986b, Host- and phage-coded functions required for coliphage N4 DNA replication, *Virology* **150**:33.

Gutierrez, J., Garcia, J. A., Blanco, L., and Salas, M., 1986a, Cloning and template activity of the origins of replication of phage φ29 DNA, *Gene* **43**:1.

Gutierrez, J., Vinos, J., Prieto, I., Méendez, E., Hermoso, J. M., and Salas, M., 1986b, Signals in the φ29 DNA-terminal protein template for the initiation of phage φ29 DNA replication, *Virology* **155**:474.

Hansen, E. B., and Yarmolinsky, M. B., 1986, Host participation in plasmid maintenance: Dependence upon *dnaA* of replicons derived from P1 and F, *Proc. Natl. Acad. Sci. USA* **83**:4423.

Harding, N. E., Ito, J., and David, G. S., 1978, Identification of the protein firmly bound to the ends of bacteriophage φ29 DNA, *Virology* **84**:279.

Harshey, R. M., 1983, A switch in the transposition products of Mu DNA mediated by proteins: Cointegrates versus simple insertions, *Proc. Natl. Acad. Sci. USA* **80**:2012.

Harshey, R. M., 1984a, Transposition without duplication of infecting bacteriophage Mu DNA, *Nature* **311**:580.

Harshey, R. M., 1984b, Non-replicative DNA transposition: Integration of infecting bacteriophage Mu, *Cold Spring Harbor Symp. Quant. Biol.* **49**:273.

Harshey, R. M., 1985, Two mechanisms of Mu DNA transposition, in: *Microbiology 1985* (L. Leive, ed.), pp. 292–294, American Society for Microbiology, Washington.

Harshey, R. M., 1988, Phage Mu, in: *The Bacteriophages*, Vol. 1 (R. Calendar, ed.), pp. 193–234, Plenum Press, New York.

Harshey, R. M., and Bukhari, A. I., 1981, A mechanism of DNA transposition, *Proc. Natl. Acad. Sci. USA* **78**:1090.

Harshey, R. M., and Bukhari, A. I., 1983, Infecting bacteriophage Mu DNA forms a circular DNA-protein complex, *J. Mol. Biol.* **167**:427.

Harshey, R. M., McKay, R., and Bukhari, A. I., 1982, DNA intermediates in transposition of phage Mu, *Cell* **29**:561.

Harshey, R. M., Baldwin, D. L., Getzoff, E. D., Miller, J. L., and Chaconas, G., 1985, Primary structure of phage Mu transposase: Homology to Mu repressor, *Proc. Natl. Acad. Sci. USA* **82**:7676.

Hattman, S., 1983, DNA modification: Methylation, in: *Bacteriophage T4* (C. Mathews, E. Kutter, G. Mosig, and P. Berger, eds.), pp. 152–155, American Society for Microbiology, Washington.

Hausmann, R., 1976, Bacteriophage T7 genetics, *Curr. Top. Microbiol. Immunol.* **75**:77.

Haynes, L. L., and Rothman-Denes, L. B., 1985, N4 virion RNA polymerase sites of transcription initiation, *Cell* **41**:597.

Heidekamp, F., Baas, P. D., Van Boom, J. H., Veeneman, G. H., Zipursky, S. L., and Jansz, H. S., 1981, Construction and characterization of recombinant plasmid DNAs containing sequence of the origin of bacteriophage φX174 DNA replication, *Nucleic Acids Res.* **9**:3335.

Hendrix, R. W., Roberts, J. W., Stahl, F. W., and Weisberg, R. A. (eds.), 1983, *Lambda II*, Cold Spring Harbor Laboratory, Cold Spring Harbor, NY.

Hershey, A. D. (ed.), 1981, *The Bacteriophage Lambda*, Cold Spring Harbor Laboratory, Cold Spring Harbor, NY.

Herskowitz, I., and Hagen, D., 1980, The lysis-lysogeny decision of phage λ: Explicit programming and responsiveness, *Annu. Rev. Genet.* **14**:399.

Higgins, N. P., Manlapaz-Ramos, P., Gandhi, R. T., and Olivera, B. M., 1983a, Bacteriophage Mu: A transposing replicon, *Cell* **33**:623.

Higgins, N. P., Moncecchi, D., Manlapaz-Ramos, P., and Olivera, B. M., 1983b, Bacteriophage Mu DNA replication *in vitro*, *J. Biol. Chem.* **258**:4293.

Hill, D. F., and Petersen, G. P., 1982, Nucleotide sequence of bacteriophage fl DNA, *J. Virol.* **44**:32.

Hinkle, D. C., 1980, Evidence for direct involvement of T7 RNA polymerase in bacteriophage DNA replication, *J. Virol.* **34**:136.

Hinkle, D. C., and Richardson, C. C., 1975, Bacteriophage T7 deoxyribonucleic acid replication *in vitro*: Purification and properties of the gene 4 protein of bacteriophage T7, *J. Biol. Chem.* **250**:5523.

Hinton, D. M., and Nossal, N. C., 1985, Bacteriophage T4 DNA replication protein 61: Cloning of the gene and purification of the expressed protein, *J. Biol. Chem.* **260**:11696.

Hinton, D. M., and Nossal, N. G., 1986, Cloning of the bacteriophage T4 *uvsX* gene and purification and characterization of the T4 uvsX recombination protein, *J. Biol. Chem.* **261**:5663.

Hinton, D. M., Richardson, R. W., and Nossal, N. G., 1986, Bacteriophage T4 DNA replication: Role of the T4 41 and 61 protein primase-helicase and the T4 uvsX recombination protein, in: *Mechanisms of DNA Replication and Recombination*, UCLA Symposia on Molecular and Cellular Biology, New Series, Vol. 47 (T. Kelly and R. McMacken, eds.), pp. 173–182, Alan R. Liss, New York.

Hobom, G., Grosschedl, R., Lusky, M., Scherer, G., Schwartz, E., and Kössel, H., 1978, Functional analysis of the replicator structure of lambdoid bacteriophage DNAs, *Cold Spring Harbor Symp. Quant. Biol.* **43**:165.

Holmgren, A., 1985, Thioredoxin, *Annu. Rev. Biochem.* **54**:237.

Hori, K., Mark, D. F., and Richardson, C. C., 1979, Deoxyribonucleic acid polymerase of bacteriophage T7. XV. Characterization of the exonuclease activities of the gene 5 protein and the reconstituted polymerase, *J. Biol. Chem.* **254**:11598.

Horiuchi, K., 1980, Origin of DNA replication of bacteriophage fl as the signal for termination, *Proc. Natl. Acad. Sci. USA* **77**:5226.

Horiuchi, K., 1986, Interaction between gene *II* protein and the DNA replication origin of bacteriophage fl, *J. Mol. Biol.* **188**:215.

Horiuchi, K., and Zinder, N. D., 1976, Origin and direction of synthesis of bacteriophage fl DNA, *Proc. Natl. Acad. Sci. USA* **73**:2341.

Hosoda, J., Mathews, E., and Jansen, B., 1971, Role of genes 46 and 47 in bacteriophage T4 replication. I. *In vivo* deoxyribonucleic acid replication, *J. Virol.* **8**:372.

Huang, C. C., Hearst, J. E., and Alberts, B. M., 1981, Two types of replication proteins increase the rate at which T4 DNA polymerase traverses the helical regions in a single-stranded DNA template, *J. Biol. Chem.* **256**:4087.

Huber, H. E., Russel, M., Model, P., and Richardson, C. C., 1986, Interaction of mutant thioredoxins of *Escherichia coli* with the gene 5 protein of phage T7. The redox capacity of thioredoxin is not required for stimulation of DNA polymerase activity, *J. Biol. Chem.* **261**:15006.

Huberman, J., Kornberg, A., and Alberts, B. M., 1971, Stimulation of T4 bacteriophage DNA polymerase by the protein product of T4 gene *32*, *J. Mol. Biol.* **62**:39.

Ikeda, H., and Tomizawa, J.-I., 1965, Transducing fragments in generalized transduction by P1. I. Molecular origin of the fragments, *J. Mol. Biol.* **14**:85.

Inciarte, M. R., Salas, M., and Sogo, J. M., 1980, Structure of replicating DNA molecules of *Bacillus subtilis* bacteriophage ϕ29, *J. Virol.* **34**:187.

Inman, R. B., and Schnös, M., 1987, Electron microscopic identification of supercoiled regions in complex DNA structures, *J. Mol. Biol.* **193**:377.

Itikawa, H., and Ryu, J.-I., 1979, Isolation and characterization of a temperature-sensitive *dnaK* mutant of *Escherichia coli* B, *J. Bacteriol.* **138**:339.

Ito, J., 1978, Bacteriophage ϕ29 terminal protein: Its association with the 5' termini of the ϕ29 genome, *J. Virol.* **28**:895.

Jacob, F., Brenner, S., and Cuzin, F., 1963, On the regulation of DNA replication in bacteria, *Cold Spring Harbor Symp. Quant. Biol.* **28**:329.

Jacobson, A. B., Kumar, H., and Zuker, M., 1985, Effect of spermidine on the conformation of bacteriophage MS2 DNA: Electron microscopy and computer modeling, *J. Mol. Biol.* **181**:517.

Jensch, F., and Kemper, B., 1986, Exonuclease VII resolves Y-junctions in branched DNA *in vitro*, *EMBO J.* **5**:181.

Johnson, P. H., and Sinsheimer, R. L., 1974, Structure of an intermediate in the replication of bacteriophage ϕX174 deoxyribonucleic acid: The initiation site for DNA replication, *J. Mol. Biol.* **83**:47.

Johnston, S., and Ray, D. S., 1984, Interference between M13 and *ori*M13 plasmids is mediated by a replication enhancer sequence near the viral strand origin, *J. Mol. Biol.* **177**:685.

Jongeneel, C. V., Bedinger, P., and Alberts, B. M., 1984, Effects of the bacteriophage T4 dda protein on DNA synthesis catalyzed by purified T4 replication proteins, *J. Biol. Chem.* **259**:12933.

Kaguni, J., and Kornberg, A., 1982, The σ subunit of RNA polymerase holoenzyme confers specificity in priming M13 viral DNA replication, *J. Biol. Chem.* **257**:5437.

Kahmann, R., and Kamp, D., 1979, Nucleotide sequences of the attachment sites of bacteriophage Mu DNA, *Nature* **280**:247.

Kahn, M., and Hanawalt, P., 1979, Size distribution of DNA replicative intermediates in bacteriophage P4 and in *Escherichia coli*, *J. Mol. Biol.* **128**:501.

Kalinski, A., and Black, L. W., 1986, End structure and mechanism of packaging of bacteriophage T4 DNA, *J. Virol.* **58**:951.

Karam, J. D., Trajanowska, M., and Baucom, M., 1983, Interactions of T4-induced enzymes *in vivo*: Inferences from intergenic suppression, in: *Bacteriophage T4* (C. Mathews, F. Kutter, G. Mosig, and P. Berger, eds.), pp. 334–341, American Society for Microbiology, Washington.

Kelly, T. J. Jr., and Thomas, C. A. Jr., 1969, An intermediate in the replication of bacteriophage T7 DNA molecules, *J. Mol. Biol.* **44**:459.

Kerr, C., and Sadowski, P. D., 1972a, Gene 6 exonuclease of bacteriophage T7. I. Purification and properties of the enzyme, *J. Biol. Chem.* **247**:305.

Kerr, C., and Sadowski, P. D., 1972b, Gene 6 exonuclease of bacteriophage T7. II. Mechanism of the reaction, *J. Biol. Chem.* **247**:311.

Kim, M. H., and Ray, D. S., 1985, Mutational mechanisms by which an inactive replication origin of bacteriophage M13 is turned on are similar to mechanisms of activation of ras proto-oncogenes, *J. Virol.* **53**:871.

Kim, M. H., Hines, J. C., and Ray, D. S., 1981, Viable deletions of the M13 complementary stand origin, *Proc. Natl. Acad. Sci. USA* **78**:6784.

Kleckner, N., 1981, Transposable elements in prokaryotes, *Annu. Rev. Genet.* **15**:341.

Kleckner, N., and Signer, E., 1977, Genetic characterization of plasmid formation of N⁻ mutants of bacteriophage λ, *Virology* **79**:160.

Kleckner, N., Morisato, D., Roberts, D., and Bender, J., 1984, Mechanism and regulation of Tn*10* transposition, *Cold Spring Harbor Symp. Quant. Biol.* **49**:235.

Klein, A., Lanka, E., and Schuster, E., 1980, Isolation of a complex between the P protein of phage λ and the dnaB protein of *Escherichia coli, Eur. J. Biochem.* **105**:1.

Klinkert, J., and Klein, A., 1979, Cloning of the replication gene P of bacteriophage lambda: Effects of increase P-protein synthesis on cellular and phage DNA replication, *Mol. Gen. Genet.* **171**:219.

Kobori, J. A., and Kornberg, A., 1982, The *Escherichia coli dnaC* gene product. III. Properties of the dnaB-dnaC protein complex, *J. Biol. Chem.* **257**:13770.

Kochan, J., and Murialdo, H., 1982, Stimulation of groE synthesis in *Escherichia coli* by bacteriophage lambda infection, *J. Bacteriol.* **149**:1166.

Kolodner, R., and Richardson, C. C., 1977, Replication of duplex DNA by bacteriophage T7 DNA polymerase and gene *4* protein is accompanied by hydrolysis of nucleoside 5′-triphosphates, *Proc. Natl. Acad. Sci. USA* **74**:1525.

Kolodner, R., and Richardson, C. C., 1978, Gene *4* protein of bacteriophage T7, characterization of the product synthesized by the T7 DNA polymerase and gene *4* protein in the absence of ribonucleoside 5′-triphosphates, *J. Biol. Chem.* **253**:574.

Kolodner, R., Masamune, Y., Leclerc, J. E., and Richardson, C. C., 1978, Gene *4* protein of bacteriophage T7. Purification, physical properties and stimulation of T7 DNA polymerase during the elongation of polynucleotide chains, *J. Biol. Chem.* **253**:566.

Kornberg, A., 1980, *DNA Replication,* W. H. Freeman & Co., San Francisco.

Kornberg, A., 1982, *1982 Supplement to DNA Replication,* W. H. Freeman & Co., San Francisco.

Kornberg, A., Baker, T. A., Bertsch, L. L., Brambill, D., Funnell, B. E., Lasken, R. S., Maki, H., Maki, S., Sekimizu, K., and Wahle, E., 1986, Enzymatic studies of replication of oriC plasmids, in: *Mechanisms of DNA Replication and Recombination,* UCLA Symposia on Molecular and Cellular Biology, New Series, Vol. 47 (T. Kelly and R. McMacken, eds.), pp. 137–149, Alan R. Liss, New York.

Kozinski, A. W., 1983, DNA metabolism *in vivo:* Origins of T4 DNA replication, in: *Bacteriophage T4* (C. Mathews, E. Kutter, G. Mosig, and P. Berget, eds.), pp. 111–119, American Society for Microbiology, Washington.

Krause, H. M., and Higgins, N. P., 1986, Positive and negative regulation of the Mu operator by Mu repressor and *E. coli* integration host factor, *J. Mol. Biol.* **261**:3744.

Kreuzer, K. N., and Alberts, B. M., 1984, Site-specific recognition of bacteriophage T4 DNA by T4 type II DNA topoisomerase and *Escherichia coli* DNA gyrase, *J. Biol. Chem.* **259**:5339.

Kreuzer, K. N., and Alberts, B. M., 1985, A defective phage system reveals bacteriophage T4 replication origins that coincide with recombination hotspots, *Proc. Natl. Acad. Sci. USA* **82**:3345.

Kreuzer, K. N., and Alberts, B. M., 1986, Characterization of a defective phage system for the analysis of bacteriophage T4 DNA replication origins, *J. Mol. Biol.* **188**:185.

Kreuzer, K. N., and Menkens, A. E., 1986, Plasmid model systems for the initiation of bacteriophage T4 DNA replication, in: *Mechanisms of DNA Replication and Recombination,* UCLA Symposia on Molecular and Cellular Biology, New Series, Vol. 47 (T. Kelly and R. McMacken, eds.), pp. 451–471, Alan R. Liss, New York.

Krevolin, M., and Calendar, R., 1985, The replication of bacteriophage P4 DNA *in vitro:* Partial purification of the P4 α gene product, *J. Mol. Biol.* **182**:509.

Krevolin, M., Inman, R., Roof, D., Kahn, M., and Calendar, R., 1985, Phage P4 DNA replication: Locations of the P4 origin and an additional essential region, *J. Mol. Biol.* **182**:519.

Kuhn, B., Abdel-Monem, M., Krell, H., and Hoffmann-Berling, H., 1979, Evidence for two mechanisms for DNA unwinding catalyzed by DNA helicases, *J. Biol. Chem.* **254**:11343.

Kuo, T.-T., Chao, Y.-S., Lin, Y.-H., Lin, B.-Y., Liu, L.-F., and Feng, T.-Y., 1986, Integration of the DNA of filamentous bacteriophage Cflt into the chromosomal DNA of its host, *J. Virol.* **61**:60.

Kutter, E. M., and Rüger, W., 1983, Map of the T4 genome and its transcription control sites, in: *Bacteriophage T4* (C. Mathews, E., Kutter, G. Mosig, and P. Berget, eds.), pp. 277–290, American Society for Microbiology, Washington.

Kuypers, B., Reiser, W., and Klein, A., 1980, Cloning of the replication gene *O* of *E. coli* bacteriophage lambda and its expression under the control of the *lac* promoter, *Gene* **10**:195.

Lagos, R., and Goldstein, R., 1984, Plasmid P4: Manipulation of plasmid copy number and induction from the integrated state, *J. Bacteriol.* **158**:208.

Langeveld, S. A., Van Mansfeld, A. D. M., Baas, P. D., Janz, H. S., Van Arkel, G. A., and Weisbeek, P. J., 1978, Nucleotide sequence of the origin of replication in bacteriophage ϕX174 RF DNA, *Nature* **271**:417.

Langeveld, S. A., Van Mansfeld, A. D. M., De Winter, J. M., and Weisbeek, P. J., 1979, Cleavage of single-stranded DNA by the A and A* proteins of bacteriophage ϕX174, *Nucleic Acids Res.* **7**:2177.

Langeveld, S. A., Van Mansfeld, A. D. M., Van der Erde, A., Van de Pol, J. M., Van Arkel, G. A., and Weisbeek, P. J., 1981, The nuclease specificity of the bacteriophage ϕX174 A* protein, *Nucleic Acids Res.* **9**:545.

Langman, L., and Paetkau, V., 1978, Purification and structure of recombining and replicating bacteriophage T7 DNA, *J. Virol.* **25**:562.

Lanka, E., and Schuster, H., 1983, The dnaC protein of *Escherichia coli*. Purification, physical properties and interaction with dnaB protein, *Nucleic Acids Res.* **11**:987.

Lanka, E., Mikolajczyk, M., Schlicht, M., and Schuster, H., 1978, Association of the prophage P1 ban protein with the dnaB protein of *Escherichia coli*, *J. Biol. Chem.* **253**:4746.

Laurent, T. C., Moore, E. C., and Reichard, P., 1964, Enzymatic synthesis of deoxyribonucleotides. IV. Isolation and characterization of thioredoxin, the hydrogen donor from *Escherichia coli* B, *J. Biol. Chem.* **239**:3436.

LeBowitz, J. H., and McMacken, R., 1984, The bacteriophage λ O and P protein initiators promote the replication of single-stranded DNA, *Nucleic Acids Res.* **12**:3069.

LeBowitz, J. H., and McMacken, R., 1986, The *Escherichia coli* dnaB replication protein is a DNA helicase, *J. Biol. Chem.* **261**:4738.

LeBowitz, J. H., Zylicz, M., Georgopoulos, C., and McMacken, R., 1985, Initiation of DNA replication on single-stranded DNA templates catalyzed by purified replication proteins of bacteriophage λ and *Escherichia coli*, *Proc. Natl. Acad. Sci. USA* **82**:3988.

Lechner, R. L., and Kelly, T. J., 1977, The structure of replicating adenovirus 2 DNA molecules, *Cell* **12**:1007.

Lechner, R. L., and Richardson, C. C., 1983, A preformed topologically stable replication fork: Characterization of leading strand synthesis catalyzed by T7 DNA polymerase and T7 gene 4 protein, *J. Biol. Chem.* **258**:11185.

Lechner, R. L., Engler, M. J., and Richardson, C. C., 1983, Characterization of strand displacement synthesis catalyzed by bacteriophage T7 DNA polymerase, *J. Biol. Chem.* **258**:11174.

Lederberg, E. M., 1951, Lysogenicity in *E. coli* K12, *Genetics* **36**:560.

Lee, D., and Sadowski, P. D., 1981, Genetic recombination of bacteriophage T7 *in vivo* studied by use of a simple physical assay, *J. Virol.* **40**:839.

Lee, M., and Miller, R. C. Jr., 1974, T7 exonuclease (gene 6) is necessary for molecular recombination of bacteriophage T7, *J. Virol.* **14**:1040.

Lee, M. C., Miller, R. C. Jr., Scraba, D., and Paetkau, V., 1976, The essential role of bacteriophage T7 endonuclease (gene 3) in molecular recombination, *J. Mol. Biol.* **104**:883.

Lennox, E. S., 1955, Transduction of linked genetic characters of the host by bacteriophage P1, *Virology* **1**:190.

Liebart, J. C., Ghelardini, P., and Paolozzi, L., 1982, Conservative integration and bacteriophage Mu DNA into pBR322 plasmid, *Proc. Natl. Acad. Sci. USA* **79**:4362.

Lilley, D. M. J., and Kemper, B., 1984, Cruciform-resolvase interactions in supercoiled DNA, *Cell* **36**:413.

Lindahl, G., 1970, Bacteriophage P2: Replication of the chromosome requires a protein which acts only on the genome that coded for it, *Virology* **42**:522.

Lindquist, B. H., 1974, Expression of phage transcription in P2 lysogens infected with helper-dependent coliphage P4, *Proc. Natl. Acad. Sci. USA* **71**:2752.

Lindquist, B. H., 1981, Recombination between satellite phage P4 and its helper P2. I. *In vivo* and *in vitro* construction of P4::P2 hybrids, *Gene* **14**:231.

Lindquist, B. H., and Six, E. W., 1971, Replication of bacteriophage P4 DNA in a nonlysogenic host, *Virology* **43**:1.

Linney, E., and Hayashi, M., 1973, Two proteins of gene *A* of φX174, *Nature New Biol.* **245**:6.

Lipinska, B., Podhajska, A., and Taylor, K., 1980, Synthesis and decay of λ DNA replication proteins in minicells, *Biochem. Biophys. Res. Commun.* **92**:120.

Liu, C.-C., and Alberts, B. M., 1980, Pentaribonucleotides of mixed sequence are synthesized and efficiently prime *de novo* DNA chain starts in the T4 bacteriophage DNA replication system, *Proc. Natl. Acad. Sci. USA* **77**:5698.

Liu, C.-C., and Alberts, B. M., 1981a, Characterization of the DNA-dependent GTPase activity of T4 gene *41* protein, an essential component of the T4 bacteriophage DNA replication apparatus, *J. Biol. Chem.* **256**:2813.

Liu, C.-C., and Alberts, B. M., 1981b, Characterization of RNA primer synthesis in the T4 bacteriophage *in vitro* DNA replication system, *J. Biol. Chem.* **256**:2821.

Liu, C.-C., Burke, R. L., Hibner, U., Barry, J., and Alberts, B. M., 1978, Probing DNA replication mechanisms with the T4 bacteriophage *in vitro* system, *Cold Spring Harbor Symp. Quant. Biol.* **43**:469.

Ljungquist, E., and Bukhari, A. I., 1977, State of prophage Mu DNA upon induction, *Proc. Natl. Acad. Sci. USA* **74**:3143.

Loeb, T., 1960, Isolation of a bacteriophage specific for the F$^+$ and Hfr for mating types of *Escherichia coli* K-12, *Science* **131**:932.

Luder, A., and Mosig, G., 1982, Two alternative mechanisms for initiation of DNA replication forks in bacteriophage T4: Priming by RNA polymerase and by recombination, *Proc. Natl. Acad. Sci. USA* **79**:1101.

Lusky, M., and Hobom, G., 1979a, Inceptor and origin of DNA replication in lambdoid coliphages. I. The λ DNA minimal replication system, *Gene* **6**:137.

Lusky, M., and Hobom, G., 1979b, Inceptor and origin of DNA replication in lambdoid coliphages. II. The λ DNA maximal replication system, *Gene* **6**:173.

MacDonald, P. M., and Hall, D. H., 1984, Genetic evidence for physical interactions between enzymes of nucleotide synthesis and proteins involved in DNA replication in bacteriophage T4, *Genetics* **107**:343.

MacDonald, P. M., and Mosig, G., 1984, Regulation of a new bacteriophage T4 gene, *69*, that spans one origin of DNA replication, *EMBO J.* **3**:2863.

MacDonald, P. M., Seaby, R. M., Brown, W., and Mosig, G., 1983, Initiator DNA from a primary origin and induction of a secondary origin of bacteriophage T4 DNA replication, in: *Microbiology 1983* (D. Schlessinger, ed.), pp. 111–116, American Society for Microbiology, Washington.

Mace, D. C., and Alberts, B. M., 1984a, The complex of T4 bacteriophage gene *44* and *62* replication proteins forms an ATPase that is stimulated by DNA and by T4 gene *45* protein, *J. Mol. Biol.* **177**:279.

Mace, D. C., and Albert, B. M., 1984b, Characterization of the stimulatory effect of T4 gene *45* protein and the gene *44/62* protein complex on DNA synthesis by T4 DNA polymerase, *J. Mol. Biol.* **177**:313.

Marians, K., 1984, Enzymology of DNA replication in prokaryotes, *Crit. Rev. Biochem.* **17**:153.

Marinus, M. G., 1984, Methylation of prokaryotic DNA, in: *DNA Methylation* (A. Razin, H. Cedar, and A. D. Riggs, eds.), pp. 81–109, Springer-Verlag, New York.

Mark, D. F., and Richardson, C. C., 1976, *Escherichia coli* thioredoxin: A subunit of bacteriophage T7 DNA polymerase, *Proc. Natl. Acad. Sci. USA* **73**:780.

Marvin, D. A., and Hohn, B., 1969, Filamentous bacterial viruses, *Bacteriol. Rev.* **33**:172.

Masai, H., Bond, M. W., and Arai, K.-I., 1986, Cloning of the *Escherichia coli* gene for primosomal protein i: The relationship to dnaT, essential for chromosomal DNA replication, *Proc. Natl. Acad. Sci. USA* **83**:1256.

Masamune, Y., Frenkel, G. D., and Richardson, C. C., 1971, A mutant of bacteriophage T7 deficient in polynucleotide ligase, *J. Biol. Chem.* **246**:6874.

Mathews, C. K., and Allen, J. R., 1983, Enzymes and proteins of DNA metabolism, in: *Bacteriophage T4* (C. Mathews, E. Kutter, G. Mosig, and P. Berget, eds.), pp. 59–70, American Society for Microbiology, Washington.

Mathews, C. K., Kutter, E., Mosig, G., and Berget, P. (eds.), 1983, *Bacteriophage T4*, American Society for Microbiology, Washington.

Matson, S. W., 1986, *Escherichia coli* helicase II (*uvrD* gene product) translocates unidirectionally in a 3' to 5' direction, *J. Biol. Chem.* **261**:10169.

Matson, S. W., and Richardson, C. C., 1983, DNA-dependent nucleoside 5' triphosphatase activity of the gene 4 protein of bacteriophage T7, *J. Biol. Chem.* **258**:14009.

Matson, S. W., and Richardson, C. C., 1985, Nucleotide dependent binding of the gene 4 protein of bacteriophage T7 to single-stranded DNA, *J. Biol. Chem.* **260**:2281.

Matson, S. W., Tabor, S., and Richardson, C. C., 1983, The gene 4 protein of bacteriophage T7, characterization of the helicase activity, *J. Biol. Chem.* **258**:14017.

Matsubara, K., 1981, Replication control system in lambda dv, *Plasmid* **5**:32.

Matsumo, K., Saito, T., Kim, C. I., Ando, T., and Hirokawa, H., 1984, Bacteriophage φ29 DNA replication *in vitro*: Participation of the terminal protein and the gene 2 product in elongation, *Mol. Gen. Genet.* **196**:381.

Mattson, T., Van Houwe, G., Bolle, A., and Epstein, R., 1983, Fate of cloned bacteriophage T4 DNA after phage T4 infection of clone-bearing cells, *J. Mol. Biol.* **170**:343.

McCorquodale, D. J., 1975, The T-odd bacteriophages, *Crit. Rev. Microbiol.* **5**:101.

McHenry, C. S., and Kornberg, A., 1977, DNA polymerase III holoenzyme of *Escherichia coli*: Purification and resolution into subunits, *J. Biol. Chem.* **252**:6478.

McMacken, R., and Kornberg, A., 1978, A multienzyme system for priming the replication of φX174 viral DNA, *J. Biol. Chem.* **253**:3313.

McMacken, R., Ueda, K., and Kornberg, A., 1977, Migration of *Escherichia coli* dnaB protein on the template DNA strand as a mechanism in initiating DNA replication, *Proc. Natl. Acad. Sci. USA* **74**:4190.

McMacken, R., Wold, M. S., LeBowitz, J. H., Roberts, J. D., Mallory, J. B., Wilkinson, J. A. K., and Loehrlein, C., 1983, Initiation of DNA replication *in vitro* promoted by the bacteriophage λ O and P replication proteins, in: *Mechanisms of DNA Replication and Recombination*, UCLA Symposia on Molecular and Cellular Biology, New Series, Vol. 10 (N. Cozzarelli, ed.), pp. 819–848, Alan R. Liss, New York.

McMacken, R., Alfano, C., Gomes, B., LeBowitz, J. H., Mensa-Wilmot, K., Roberts, J. D., and Wold, M., 1986, Biochemical mechanisms in the initiation of bacteriophage λ DNA replication, in: *Mechanisms of DNA Replication and Recombination*, UCLA Symposia on Molecular and Cellular Biology, New Series, Vol. 47 (T. Kelly and R. McMacken, eds.), pp. 227–246, Alan R. Liss, New York.

McMacken, R., Silver, L., and Georgopoulos, C., 1987, DNA replication in: *Escherichia coli and Salmonella typhimurium: Cellular and Molecular Biology* (J. Ingraham, K. Low, B. Magasanik, F. Neidhardt, M. Schaechter, and M. Umbarger, eds.), pp. 564–612, American Society for Microbiology, Washington.

Meyer, R. R., Shlomai, J., Kobori, J., Bates, D. L., Rowen, L., McMacken, R., Ueda, K., and Kornberg, A., 1978, Enzymatic conversion of single-stranded φX174 and G4 circles to duplex forms: Discontinuous replication, *Cold Spring Harbor Symp. Quant. Biol.* **43**:289.

Meyer, T. F., Geider, K., Kurz, C., and Schaller, H. M., 1979, Cleavage site of bacteriophage fd gene *II* protein in the origin of viral strand replication, *Nature* **278**:365.

Meyer, T. F., Baumel, I., Geider, K., and Bedinger, P., 1981, Replication of phage fd RF with fd gene 2 protein and phage T4 enzymes, *J. Biol. Chem.* **256**:5810.

Miller, H. I., and Friedman, D. I., 1980, An *E. coli* gene product required for lambda site-specific recombination, *Cell* **20**:711.

Miller, J. L., Anderson, S. K., Fujita, D. J., Chaconas, G., Baldwin, D. L., and Harshey, R. M., 1984, The nucleotide sequence of the *B* gene of bacteriophage Mu, *Nucleic Acids Res.* **12**:8627.

Miller, R. C. Jr., 1975, Replication and molecular recombination of T-phages, *Annu. Rev. Microbiol.* **29**:355.

Miller, R. C. Jr., Lee, M., Scraba, D. G., and Paetkau, V., 1976. The role of bacteriophage T7 exonuclease (gene 6) in genetic recombination and production of concatemers, *J. Mol. Biol.* **101**:223.

Minden, J. S., and Marians, K. J., 1985, Replication of pBR322 DNA *in vitro* with purified proteins. Requirement for topoisomerase I in the maintenance of template specificity, *J. Biol. Chem.* **260**:9316.

Mitra, S., 1980, DNA replication in viruses, *Annu. Rev. Genet.* **14**:347.

Mizuuchi, K., 1983, *In vitro* transposition of bacteriophage Mu: A biochemical approach to a novel replication reaction, *Cell* **35**:785.

Mizuuchi, K., 1984, Mechanism of transposition of bacteriophage Mu: Polarity of the strand transfer reaction at the initiation of transposition, *Cell* **39**:395.

Mizuuchi, K., and Craigie, R., 1986, Mechanism of bacteriophage Mu transposition, *Annu. Rev. Genet.* **20**:385.

Mizuuchi, K., Kemper, B., Hays, J., and Weisberg, R. A., 1982, T4 endonuclease VII cleaves Holliday structures, *Cell* **29**:357.

Model, P., McGill, C., Mazur, B., and Fulford, W. D., 1982, The replication of bacteriophage f1: Gene *V* protein regulates the synthesis of gene *II* protein, *Cell* **29**:329.

Modrich, P., and Richardson, C. C., 1975, Bacteriophage T7 deoxyribonucleic acid replication *in vitro:* Bacteriophage T7 DNA polymerase: An enzyme composed of phage- and host-specified subunits, *J. Biol. Chem.* **250**:5515.

Mooney, P. Q., North, R., and Molineux, I. J., 1980, The role of T7 gene 2 protein in DNA replication, *Nucleic Acids Res.* **8**:3043.

Moore, D., and Blattner, F., 1982, Sequence of λric5b, *J. Mol. Biol.* **154**:82.

Moore, D., Denniston-Thompson, K., Furth, M., Williams, B., and Blattner, F., 1977, Construction of chimeric phages and plasmids containing the origin of replication of bacteriophage lambda, *Science* **198**:1041.

Moore, D. D., Denniston-Thompson, K., Kruger, K., Furth, M., Williams, B., Daniels, D., and Blattner, F. R., 1978, Dissection and comparative anatomy of the origins of replication of lambdoid phages, *Cold Spring Harbor Symp. Quant. Biol.* **43**:155.

Moore, D. D., Denniston-Thompson, K., and Blattner, F. R., 1981, Sequence organization of the origins of DNA replication in lambdoid coliphages, *Gene* **14**:91.

Morisato, D., and Kleckner, N., 1984, Transposase promotes double-strand breaks and single-strand joints at Tn10 termini *in vivo, Cell* **39**:181.

Morris, C. F., Hama-Inaba, H., Mace, D., Sinha, N. K., and Alberts, B. M., 1979a, Purification of the gene 43, 44, 45 and 62 proteins of the bacteriophage T4 DNA replication apparatus, *J. Biol. Chem.* **254**:6787.

Morris, C. F., Moran, L. A., and Alberts, B. M. 1979b, Purification of gene 41 protein of bacteriophage T4, *J. Biol. Chem.* **254**:6797.

Moses, P. B., and Model, P., 1984, A *rho*-dependent transcription termination signal in bacteriophage f1, *J. Mol. Biol.* **172**:1.

Mosig, G., 1970, A preferred origin and direction of bacteriophage T4 DNA replication, *J. Mol. Biol.* **53**:503.

Mosig, G., 1983, Relationship of T4 DNA replication and recombination, in: *Bacteriophage T4* (C. Mathews, E. Kutter, G. Mosig, and P. Berget, eds.), pp. 120–130, American Society for Microbiology, Washington.

Mosig, G., and MacDonald, P., 1986, A new membrane-associated DNA replication protein, the gene 69 product of bacteriophage T4, shares a patch of homology with the *Escherichia coli* dnaA protein, *J. Mol. Biol.* **189**:243.

Mosig, G., Luder, A., Rowen, L., MacDonald, P., and Bock, S., 1981, On the role of recombination and topoisomerase in primary and secondary initiation of T4 DNA replication, in: *The Initiation of Replication* (D. Ray, ed.), pp. 277–295, Academic Press, New York.

Mosig, G., MacDonald, P. M., Powell, D., Trupin, M., and Gary, T., 1986, A membrane protein involved in initiation of DNA replication from the *OriA* region of phage T4 in: *Mechanisms of DNA Replication and Recombination*, UCLA Symposia on Molecular and Cellular Biology, New Series, Vol. 47 (T. Kelly and R. McMacken, eds.), pp. 403–414, Alan R. Liss, New York.

Mukai, R., Hamatake, R. K., and Hayashi, M., 1979, Isolation and identification of bacteriophage ϕX174 prohead, *Proc. Natl. Acad. Sci. USA* **76**:4877.

Nagata, K., Guggenheimer, R. A., Enomoto, T., Lichy, J. H., and Hurwitz, J., 1982, Adenovirus DNA replication *in vitro:* Identification of a host factor that stimulates synthesis of the preterminal protein-dCMP complex, *Proc. Natl. Acad. Sci. USA* **79**:6438.

Nakai, H., and Richardson, C. C., 1986a, Interactions of the DNA polymerase and gene 4 protein of bacteriophage T7. Protein-protein and protein-DNA interactions involved in RNA-primed DNA synthesis, *J. Biol. Chem.* **261**:15208.

Nakai, H., and Richardson, C. C., 1986b, Dissection of RNA-primed DNA synthesis catalyzed by gene 4 protein and DNA polymerase of bacteriophage T7. Coupling of RNA primer and DNA synthesis, *J. Biol. Chem.* **261**:15217.

Nakayama, N., Arai, N., Bond, M. W., Kaziro, Y., and Arai, K., 1984, Nucleotide sequence of *dnaB* and the primary structure of the dnaB protein from *Escherichia coli, J. Biol. Chem.* **259**:97.

Neidhardt, F. C., VanBogelen, R. A., and Vaughn, V., 1984, The genetics and regulation of heat shock proteins, *Annu. Rev. Genet.* **18**:295.

Nijkamp, H., Szybalski, W., Ohashi, M., and Dove, W., 1971, Gene expression by constitutive mutants of coliphage lambda, *Mol. Gen. Genet.* **114**:80.

Normark, S., Bergstrom, S., Edlund, T., Grundstram, T., Jaurin, B., Lindberg, F. P., and Olslon, O., 1983, Overlapping genes, *Annu. Rev. Genet.* **17**:499.

Nossal, N. G., 1974, DNA synthesis on a double-stranded DNA template by the T4 bacteriophage DNA polymerase and the T4 gene 32 DNA unwinding protein, *J. Biol. Chem.* **249**:5668.

Nossal, N. G., 1980, RNA priming of DNA replication by bacteriophage T4 proteins, *J. Biol. Chem.* **255**:2176.

Nossal, N. G., 1983, Prokaryotic DNA replication systems, *Annu. Rev. Biochem.* **53**:581.

Nossal, N. G., and Alberts, B. M., 1983, The mechanism of DNA replication catalyzed by purified bacteriophage T4 DNA replication proteins, in: *Bacteriophage T4* (C. Mathews, E. Kutter, G. Mosig, and P. Berget, eds.), pp. 71–81, American Society for Microbiology, Washington.

Nossal, N. G., and Peterlin, B. M., 1979, DNA replication by bacteriophage T4 proteins: The T4, 43, 32, 44-62, and 45 proteins are required for strand displacement synthesis at nicks in duplex DNA, *J. Biol. Chem.* **254**:6032.

O'Day, K. J., Schultz, D., and Howe, M. M., 1978, A search for integration deficient mutants of bacteriophage Mu-1, in: *Microbiology 1978* (D. Schlessinger, ed.), pp. 48–51, American Society for Microbiology, Washington.

Ogawa, T., 1975, Analysis of the *dnaB* function of *Escherichia coli* K12 and the *danB*-like function of P1 prophage, *J. Mol. Biol.* **94**:327.

Ogawa, T., and Tomizawa, J.-I., 1968, Replication of bacteriophage DNA. I. Replication of DNA of lambdoid phage defective in early functions, *J. Mol. Biol.* **38**:217.

Ogura, T., and Hiraga, S., 1983, Mini-F plasmid genes that couple host cell division to plasmid proliferation, *Proc. Natl. Acad. Sci. USA* **80**:4784.

Ohki, M., Tamura, F., Nishimura, S., and Uchida, H., 1986, Nucleotide sequence of the *Escherichia coli dnaJ* gene and purification of its gene product, *J. Biol. Chem.* **261**:1778.

Ohtsubo, E., Zenilman, M., Ohtsubo, H., McCormick, M., Machida, C., and Machida, Y.,

1980, Mechanism of insertion and cointegration mediated by IS1 and Tn3, *Cold Spring Harbor Symp. Quant. Biol.* **45**:283.

Ow, D., and Ausubel, F., 1980, Recombinant P4 bacteriophages propagate as viable lytic phages or as autonomous plasmids in *Klebsiella pneunomiae, Mol. Gen. Genet.* **180**:165.

Paek, K.-H., and Walker, G. C., 1987, *Escherichia coli dnaK* null mutants are inviable at high temperature, *J. Bacteriol.* **169**:283.

Paetkau, V., Langman, L., Bradley, R., Scraba, D., and Miller, R. C. Jr., 1977, Folded, concatenated genomes as replication intermediates of bacteriophage T7 DNA, *J. Virol.* **22**:130.

Pal, S. K., and Chattoraj, D. K., 1986, repA protein is rate limiting for P1 plasmid replication, in: *Mechanisms of DNA Replication and Recombination,* UCLA Symposia on Molecular and Cellular Biology, New Series, Vol. 47 (T. Kelly, and R. McMacken, eds.), pp. 441–450, Alan R. Liss, New York.

Patel, I., and Bastia, D., 1986, A replication origin is turned off by an origin-"silencer" sequence, *Cell* **47**:785.

Pato, M. L., and Reich, C., 1982, Instability of transposase activity: Evidence from bacteriophage Mu DNA replication, *Cell* **29**:219.

Pato, M. L., and Reich, C., 1984, Stoichiometric use of the transposase of bacteriophage Mu, *Cell* **36**:197.

Pato, M. L., and Reich, C., 1985, Synchronization of bacteriophage Mu replicative transposition: Products of the first round after induction, in: *Genome Rearrangement* (M. Simon and I. Herskowitz, eds.), pp. 27–35, Alan R. Liss, New York.

Penalva, M. A., and Salas, M., 1982, Initiation of phage φ29 DNA replication *in vitro:* Formation of a covalent complex between the terminal protein p3 and 5'-dAMP, *Proc. Natl. Acad. Sci. USA* **79**:5522.

Piperno, J. R., and Alberts, B. M. 1978, An ATP stimulation of T4 DNA polymerase mediated via T4 gene *44/62* and *45* proteins: The requirement for ATP hydrolysis, *J. Biol. Chem.* **253**:5174.

Piperno, J. R., Kallen, R. G., and Alberts, B. M., 1978, Analysis of a T4 DNA replication protein complex: Studies of the DNA recognition site for T4 gene *44/62* and *45* protein-catalyzed ATP hydrolysis, *J. Biol. Chem.* **253**:5180.

Pratt, D., Laws, P., and Griffith, J., 1974, Complex of bacteriophage M13 single-stranded DNA and gene 5 protein, *J. Mol. Biol.* **82**:425.

Prentki, P., Chandler, M., and Caro, L., 1977, Replication of the prophage P1 during the cell cycle of *E. coli, Mol. Gen. Genet.* **152**:71.

Pritchard, R. H., 1985, Control of chromosome replication in bacteria, in: *Plasmids in Bacteria* (D. R. Helinski, S. N. Cohen, D. B. Clewell, D. A. Jackson, and A. Hollaender, eds.), pp. 277–282, Plenum, New York.

Pruss, G. J., Wang, J. C., and Calendar, R., 1975, *In vitro* packaging of covalently closed circular monomers of bacteriophage DNA, *J. Mol. Biol.* **98**:465.

Puspurs, A. H., Trun, N. J., and Reeve, J. N., 1983, Bacteriophage Mu DNA circularizes following infection, *EMBO J.* **2**:345.

Rabussay, D., 1983, Phage-evoked changes in RNA polymerase, in: *Bacteriophage T4* (C. Mathews, E. Kutter, G. Mosig, and P. Berger, eds.), pp. 167–173, American Society for Microbiology, Washington.

Rambach, A, 1973, Replicator mutants of bacteriophage λ: Characterization of two subclasses, *Virology* **54**:270.

Rasched, I., and Oberer, E., 1986, FF coliphages: Structural and functional relationships, *Microbiol. Rev.* **50**:401.

Reddy, G. P. V., Singh, A., Stafford, M. E., and Mathews, C. K., 1977, Enzyme association in T4 phage DNA precursor synthesis, *Proc. Natl. Acad. Sci. USA* **74**:3152.

Reeve, J. N., Lanka, E., and Schuster, H., 1980, Synthesis of P1 ban protein in minicells infected by P1 mutants, *Mol. Gen. Genet.* **177**:193.

Reha-Krantz, L. J., and Hurwitz, J., 1978, The *danB* gene product of *Escherichia coli.* I. Purification, homogeneity, and physical properties, *J. Biol. Chem.* **253**:4043.

Reinberg, D., Zipursky, S. L., Weisbeek, P., Brown, D., and Hurwitz, J., 1983, Studies on the φX A protein-mediated termination of leading strand DNA synthesis, *J. Biol. Chem.* **258**:529.

Rekosh, D. M. K., Russel, W. C., Bellet, A. J. D., and Robinson, A. J., 1977, Identification of a protein linked to the ends of adenovirus DNA, *Cell* **11**:283.

Resibois, A., Toussaint, A., and Colet, M., 1982a, DNA structures induced by mini-Mu replication, *Virology* **117**:329.

Resibois, A., Colet, M., and Toussaint, A., 1982b, Localisation of mini-Mu in its replication intermediates, *EMBO J.* **1**:965.

Resibois, A., Pato, M., Higgins, P., and Toussaint, A., 1984, Replication of bacteriophage Mu and its mini-Mu derivatives, in: *Proteins Involved in DNA Replication* (U. Hübscher and S. Spaderi, eds.), pp. 69–76, Plenum, New York.

Reuben, R. C., and Gefter, M. L., 1974, A DNA-binding protein induced by bacteriophage T7: Purification and properties of the protein, *J. Biol. Chem.* **249**:3843.

Revel, H. R., 1983, DNA modification: Glucosylation, in: *Bacteriophage T4* (C. Mathews, E. Kutter, G. Mosig, and P. Berger, eds.), pp. 156–165, American Society for Microbiology, Washington.

Richardson, C. C., Beauchamps, B. B., Huber, H. E., Ikeda, R. A., Myers, J. A., Nakai, H., Rabkin, S. D., Tabor, S., and White, J., 1986, Bacteriophage T7 DNA replication, in: *Mechanisms of DNA Replication and Recombination*, UCLA Symposia on Molecular and Cellular Biology, New Series, Vol. 47 (T. Kelly, and R. McMacken, eds.), pp. 151–172, Alan R. Liss, New York.

Rist, J. K., Guinta, D. R., Sugino, A., Stambouly, J., Falco, S. C., and Rothman-Denes, L. B., 1983, Bacteriophage N4 replication, in: *Mechanisms of DNA Replication and Recombination*, UCLA Symposia on Molecular and Cellular Biology, New Series, Vol. 10 (N. R. Cozarelli, ed.), pp. 245–254, Alan R. Liss, New York.

Rist, J. K., Pearle, M., Sugino, A., and Rothman-Denes, L. B., 1986, Development of an *in vitro* bacteriophage N4 DNA replication system, *J. Biol. Chem.* **261**:10506.

Robinson, A. J., Younghusband, H. B., and Bellet, A. J. D., 1973, A circular DNA-protein complex from adenovirus, *Virology* **56**:54.

Romano, L. J., and Richardson, C. C., 1979a, Requirements for synthesis of ribonucleic acid primers during lagging-strand synthesis by the DNA polymerase and gene 4 protein of bacteriophage T4, *J. Biol. Chem.* **254**:10476.

Romano, L. J., and Richardson, C. C., 1979b, Characterization of the ribonucleic acid primers and the deoxyribonucleic acid product synthesized by the DNA polymerase and gene 4 protein of bacteriophage T7, *J. Biol. Chem.* **254**:10483.

Romano, L. J., Tamanoi, F., and Richardson, C. C., 1981, Initiation of DNA replication at the primary origin of bacteriophage T7 by purified proteins: Requirements for T7 RNA polymerase, *Proc. Natl. Acad. Sci. USA* **78**:4107.

Ross, W., Shore, S. H., and Howe, M. M., 1986, Mutants of *Escherichia coli* defective for replicative transposition of bacteriophage Mu, *J. Bacteriol.* **167**:905.

Roth, A. C., Nossal, N. G., and Englund, P. T., 1982, Rapid hydrolysis of deoxynucleoside triphosphates accompanies DNA synthesis by T4 DNA polymerase and T4 accessory proteins 44/62 and 45, *J. Biol. Chem.* **257**:1267.

Roth, M. J., Brown, D. R., and Hurwitz, J., 1984, Analysis of bacteriophage φX174 gene A protein-mediated termination and reinitiation of φX DNA synthesis. II. Structural characterization of the covalent φX A protein-DNA complex, *J. Biol. Chem.* **259**:10556.

Rothman-Denes, L. B., Haselkorn, R., and Schito, G. C., 1972, Selective shutoff of catabolite-sensitive host synthesis by bacteriophage N4, *Virology* **50**:95.

Rouvière-Yaniv, J., and Gros, F., 1975, Characterization of a novel, low-molecular-weight DNA-binding protein from *Escherichia coli*, *Proc. Natl. Acad. Sci. USA* **72**:3428.

Russel, M., and Model, P., 1984, Replacement of the *fip* gene of *Escherichia coli* by an inactive gene cloned on a plasmid, *J. Bacteriol.* **159**:1034.

Russel, M., and Model, P., 1985, Thioredoxin is required for filamentous phage assembly, *Proc. Natl. Acad. Sci. USA* **82**:29.

Russel, M., and Model, P., 1986, The role of thioredoxin in filamentous phage assembly. Construction, isolation and characterization of mutant thioredoxins, *J. Biol. Chem.* **261**:14997.

Sadowski, P. D., 1971, Bacteriophage T7 endonuclease. I. Properties of the enzyme purified from T7 phage-infected *Escherichia coli* B, *J. Biol. Chem.* **246**:209.

Sadowski, P. D., and Kerr, C., 1970, Degradation of *Escherichia coli* B deoxyribonucleic acid after infection with DNA-defective amber mutants of bacteriophage T7, *J. Virol.* **6**:149.

Saito, H., and Richardson, C. C., 1981a, Genetic analysis of gene *1.2* of bacteriophage T7: Isolation of a mutant of *Escherichia coli* unable to support the growth of T7 gene *1.2* mutants, *J. Virol.* **37**:343.

Saito, H., and Richardson, C. C., 1981b, Processing of mRNA by ribonuclease III regulates expression of gene *1.2* of bacteriophage T7, *Cell* **27**:533.

Saito, H., and Uchida, H., 1977, Initiation of the DNA replication of bacteriophage lambda in *Escherichia coli* K12, *J. Mol. Biol.* **113**:1.

Saito, H., and Uchida, H., 1978, Organization and expression of the *dnaJ* and *dnaK* genes of *Escherichia coli* K12, *Mol. Gen. Genet.* **164**:1.

Saito, H., Nakamura, Y., and Uchida, H., 1978, A transducing lambda phage carrying *grpE*, a bacterial gene necessary for labmda DNA replication, and two ribosomal protein genes, *rpsP*(S16) and *rp18*(L19), *Mol. Gen. Genet.* **165**:247.

Saito, H., Tabor, S., Tamanoi, F., and Richardson, C. C., 1980, Nucleotide sequence of the primary origin of bacteriophage T7 DNA replication: Relationship to adjacent genes and regulatory elements, *Proc. Natl. Acad. Sci. USA* **77**:3917.

Salas, M., 1988, Phages with protein attached to the DNA ends, in: *The Bacteriophages*, Vol. 1 (R. Calendar, ed.), pp. 169–192, Plenum Press, New York.

Salas, M., Mellado, R. P., and Vinuela, E., 1978, Characterization of a protein covalently linked to the 5′ termini of the DNA of *Bacillus subtilis* phage ϕ29, *J. Mol. Biol.* **119**:269.

Salas, M., Prieto, I., Gutierrez, J., Blanco, L., Zaballos, A., Lazaro, J. M., Martin, G., Bernad, A., Garmendia, C., Mellado, R. P., Escarmis, C., and Hermoso, J. M., 1986, Replication of phage ϕ29 DNA primed by the terminal protein, in: *Mechanisms of DNA Replication and Recombination*, UCLA Symposia on Molecular and Cellular Biology, New Series, Vol. 47 (T. Kelly and R. McMacken, eds.), pp. 215–225, Alan R., Liss, New York.

Sanger, F., Coulson, A. R., Friedman, T., Air, G. M., Barrell, B. G., Brown, N. L., Fiddes, J. C., Hutchinson, C. A. III, Slocombe, P. M., and Smith, M., 1978, The nucleotide sequence of bacteriophage ϕX174, *J. Mol. Biol.* **125**:225.

Sanger, F., Coulson, A. R., Hong, G. F., Hill, D. F., and Petersen, G. B., 1982, Nucleotide sequence of bacteriophage λ DNA, *J. Mol. Biol.* **162**:729.

Sanhueza, S., and Eisenberg, S., 1985, Bacteriophage ϕX174 A protein cleaves single-stranded DNA and binds to it covalently through a tyrosyl-dAMP phosphodiester bond, *J. Virol.* **53**:695.

Schafer, A., Anderl, K., Reiser, W., and Klein, A., 1983, Initiation of bacteriophage λ DNA replication, in: *Microbiology 1983* (D. Schlessinger, ed.), pp. 96–99, American Society for Microbiology, Washington.

Schaller, H., 1978, The intergenic region and the origins for filamentous phage DNA replication, *Cold Spring Harbor Symp. Quant. Biol.* **43**:401.

Schaller, H., Otto, B., Nusslein, V., Huf, J., Herrmann, R., and Bonfoeffer, F. R., 1972, Deoxyribonucleic acid replication *in vitro*, *J. Mol. Biol.* **63**:183.

Schaller, H., Uhlmann, A., and Geider, K., 1976, A DNA fragment from the origin of single-strand to double-strand DNA replication of bacteriophage fd, *Proc. Natl. Acad. Sci. USA* **73**:49.

Schekman, R., Wickner, W., Westergaard, O., Brutlag, K., Geider, L., Bertsch, L., and Kornberg, A., 1972, Initiation of DNA synthesis: Synthesis of ϕX174 replicative form requires RNA synthesis resistant to rifampicin, *Proc. Natl. Acad. Sci. USA* **69**:2691.

Schekman, R., Weiner, J. H., Weiner, A., and Kornberg, A., 1975, Ten proteins required for conversion of ϕX174 single-stranded DNA to duplex form *in vitro*, *J. Biol. Chem.* **250**:5859.

Scherer, G., 1978, Nucleotide sequence of the O gene and of the origin of replication in bacteriophage lambda DNA, *Nucleic Acids Res.* **5**:3141.

Scherzinger, E., Liftin, F., and Jost, E., 1973, Stimulation of T7 DNA polymerase by a new phage coded protein, *Mol. Gen. Genet.* **123**:247.

Scherzinger, E., Lanka, E., and Hillenbrand, G., 1977a, Role of bacteriophage T7 DNA primase in the initiation of DNA strand synthesis, *Nucleic Acids Res.* **4**:4151.

Scherzinger, E., Lanka, E., Morelli, G., Seiffert, D., and Yuki, A., 1977b, Bacteriophage T7 induced DNA-priming protein, a novel enzyme involved in DNA replication, *Eur. J. Biochem.* **72**:543.

Scheuermann, R. H., and Echols, H., 1984, A separate editing exonuclease for DNA replication: The ϵ subunit of *Escherichia coli* DNA polymerase III holoenzyme, *Proc. Natl. Acad. Sci. USA* **81**:7747.

Schito, G. C., 1973, The genetics and physiology of coliphage N4, *Virology* **55**:254.

Schito, G. C., Pesce, A., and Satto, G., 1969, Filament formation in *E. coli* cells infected with UV-inactivated N4 bacteriophage, *Gen. Microbiol.* **17**:141.

Schlegel, R. A., and Thomas, C. A. Jr., 1972, Some special structural features of intracellular bacteriophage T7 concatemers, *J. Mol. Biol.* **68**:319.

Schnös, M., and Inman, R., 1970, Position of branch points in replicating lambda DNA, *J. Mol. Biol.* **51**:61.

Schnös, M., Denniston, K., Blattner, F., and Inman, R., 1982, Replication of bacteriophage λ DNA: Examination of variants containing double origins and observation of a bias in directionality, *J. Mol. Biol.* **159**:441.

Schumm, J. W., and Howe, M. M., 1981, Mu-specific properties of λ phages containing both ends of Mu depend on the relative orientation of Mu end DNA fragments, *Virology* **114**:429.

Schwarz, E., Scherer, G., Hobom, G., and Kossel, H., 1980, The primary structure of phage λ P gene completes the nucleotide sequence of the plasmid λdvh93, *Biochem. Int.* **1**:386.

Scott, J. F., Eisenberg, S., Bertsch, L. L., and Kornberg, A., 1977, A mechanism of duplex DNA replication revealed by enzymatic studies of ϕX174: Catalytic strand separation in advance of replication, *Proc. Natl. Acad. Sci. USA* **74**:193.

Seiler, A., Blocker, H., Frank, R., and Kahnmann, R., 1986, The *mom* gene of bacteriophage Mu: The mechanism of methylation-dependent expression, *EMBO J.* **5**:2719.

Selick, H. E., Barry, J., Cha, T. A., Munn, M., Nakanishi, M., Wong, M. L., and Alberts, B. M., 1986, Studies of the T4 bacteriophage DNA replication system, in: *Mechanisms of DNA Replication and Recombination*, UCLA Symposia on Molecular and Cellular Biology, New Series, Vol. 47 (T. Kelly and R. McMacken, eds.), pp. 183–214, Alan R. Liss, New York.

Serwer, P., 1974a, Fast sedimenting bacteriophage T7 DNA from T7 infected *Escherichia coli*, *Virology* **59**:70.

Serwer, P., 1974b, Complexes between bacteriophage T7 capsids and T7 DNA, *Virology* **59**:89.

Serwer, P., Greenshaw, G. A., and Allen, J. L., 1982, Concatemers in a rapidly sedimenting, replicating bacteriophage T7 DNA, *Virology* **123**:474.

Shah, D. B., and DeLorenzo, L., 1977, Suppression of gene 49 mutations of bacteriophage T4 by a second mutation in gene X: Structure of pseudo revertant DNA, *J. Virol.* **24**:794.

Shapiro, J. A., 1979, Molecular model for the transposition and replication of bacteriophage Mu and other transposable elements, *Proc. Natl. Acad. Sci. USA* **76**:1933.

Shaw, J. E., and Murialdo, H., 1980, Morphogenetic genes C and Nu3 overlap in bacteriophage λ, *Nature* **283**:30.

Shinozaki, K., and Okazaki, T., 1977, RNA linked nascent DNA pieces in T7 phage-infected *E. coli* cells. I. Role of gene 6 exonuclease in removal of the linked RNA, *Mol. Gen. Genet.* **154**:263.

Shinozaki, K., and Okazaki, T., 1978, T7 gene 6 exonuclease has an RNase H activity, *Nucleic Acids Res.* **5**:4245.

Silver, L. L., and Nossal, N. G., 1982, Purification of bacteriophage T4 gene 61 protein: A protein essential for synthesis of RNA primers in the T4 *in vitro* DNA replication system, *J. Biol. Chem.* **257**:11696.

Sims, J., Koths, K., and Dressler, D., 1978, Single-stranded phage replication: Positive- and negative-strand DNA synthesis, *Cold Spring Harbor Symp. Quant. Biol.* **43**:349.

Six, E. W., 1975, The helper dependence of satellite bacteriophage P4: Which gene functions of bacteriophage P2 are needed by P4?, *Virology*, **67**:249.

Six, E. W., and Klug, C., 1973, Bacteriophage P4: A satellite virus depending on a helper such as prophage P2, *Virology* **51**:327.

Skalka, A., 1977, DNA replication—Bacteriophage lambda, *Curr. Top. Microbiol. Immunol.* **78**:201.

Smits, M. A., Jansen, J., Konings, R. N. H., and Schoenmakers, J. G. G., 1984, Initiation and termination signals for transcription in bacteriophage M13, *Nucleic Acids Res.* **12**:4071.

Snopek, T. J., Wood, W. B., Conley, M. P., Chen, P., and Cozzarelli, N. R., 1977, Bacterio- phage T4 RNA ligase is gene 63 product, the protein that promotes tail fiber attachment to the baseplate, *Proc. Natl. Acad. Sci. USA* **74**:3355.

Snustad, D. P., Snyder, L., and Kutter, E., 1983, Effects on host genome structure and expression, in: *Bacteriophage T4* (C. Mathews, E. Kutter, G. Mosig, and P. Berger, eds.), pp. 40–55, American Society for Microbiology, Washington.

Sogo, J., Greenstein, M., and Skalka, A., 1976, The circle mode of replication of bacterio- phage lambda: The role of covalently closed templates and the formation of mixed catenated dimers, *J. Mol. Biol.* **103**:537.

Sogo, J. M., Garcia, J. A., Penalva, M. A., and Salas, M., 1982, Structure of protein-containing replicative intermediates of *Bacillus subtilis* phage φ29 DNA, *Virology* **116**:1.

Stayton, M. M., Bertsch, L., Biswas, S., Burgers, P., Dixon, N., Flynn, J. E. Jr., Fuller, R., Kaguni, J., Kobori, J., Kodaira, M., Low, R., and Kornberg, A., 1982, Enzymatic recogni- tion of DNA replication origins, *Cold Spring Harbor Symp. Quant. Biol.* **47**:693.

Sternberg, N., and Hoess, R., 1983, The molecular genetics of bacteriophage P1, *Annu. Rev. Genet.* **17**:123.

Sternberg, N., Hamilton, D., Austin, S., Yarmolinsky, M., and Hoess, R., 1981, Site-specific recombination and its role in the life cycle of bacteriophage P1, *Cold Spring Harbor Symp. Quant. Biol.* **45**:297.

Stevens, W., Adhya, S., and Szybalski, W., 1971, Origin and bidirectional replication in coliphage lambda, in: *The Bacteriophage Lambda* (A. D. Hershey, ed.), pp. 515–533, Cold Spring Harbor Laboratory, Cold Spring Harbor, NY.

Streisinger, G., Edgar, R. S., and Denhardt, G. H., 1964, Chromosome structure in phage T4. I. Circularity of the linkage map, *Proc. Natl. Acad. Sci. USA* **51**:775.

Streisinger, G., Emrich, J., and Stahl, M. M., 1967, Chromosome structure in phage T4. III. Terminal redundancy and length determination, *Proc. Natl. Acad. Sci. USA* **57**:292.

Studier, F. W., 1972, Bacteriophage T7, *Science* **176**:367.

Studier, F. W., 1973, Genetic analysis of non essential bacteriophage T7 genes, *J. Mol. Biol.* **79**:227.

Studier, F. W., and Dunn, J. J., 1982, Organization and expression of bacteriophage T7 DNA, *Cold Spring Harbor Symp. Quant. Biol.* **47**:669.

Suggs, S. V., and Ray, D. S., 1977, Replication of bacteriophage M13. XI. Localization of the origin for M13 single-strand synthesis, *J. Mol. Biol.* **110**:147.

Sumida-Yasumoto, G., Ikeda, J.-E., Benz, E., Marians, K. J., Vicuna, R., Sugrue, S., Zipursky, S. L., and Hurwitz, J., 1978, Replication of φX174 DNA: *In vitro* synthesis of φX RFI DNA and circular single-stranded DNA, *Cold Spring Harbor Symp. Quant. Biol.* **43**:311.

Sunshine, M., and Six, E., 1986, *sub*, a host mutation that specifically allows growth of replication-deficient gene *B* mutants of coliphage P2, *Mol. Gen. Genet.* **204**:359.

Sunshine, M., Usher, D., and Calendar, R., 1975, Interaction of P2 bacteriophage with the *dnaB* gene of *Escherichia coli*, *J. Virol.* **16**:204.

Sunshine, M., Feiss, M., Stuart, J., and Yochem, J., 1977, A new host gene (*groPC*) necessary for lambda DNA replication, *Mol. Gen. Genet.* **151**:27.

Swinton, D., Hattman, S., Crain, P. F., Cheng, C.-S., Smith, D. L., and McCloskey, J. A., 1983, Purification and characterization of the unusual dexoynucleoside, α-N-(9-β-D-2′-deoxyribofuranosylpurin-6-yl) glycinamide, specified by the phage Mu modification function, Proc. Natl. Acad. Sci. USA 80:7400.

Tabor, S., and Richardson, C. C., 1981, Template recognition sequence for RNA primer synthesis by the gene 4 protein of bacteriophage T7, Proc. Natl. Acad. Sci. USA 78:205.

Tabor, S., Huber, H. E., and Richardson, C. C., 1986, Escherichia coli thioredoxin: An accessory protein for bacteriophage T7 DNA polymerase, in: Thioredoxin and Glutaredoxin: Structure and Function (A. Holmgren, C. I. Branden, H. Jornvall, and B. M. Sjoberg, eds.), pp. 285–300, Raven Press, New York.

Takahashi, S., 1975a, Physiological transition of a coliphage λ DNA replication, Biochim. Biophys. Acta 395:306.

Takahashi, S., 1975b, The starting point and direction of rolling-circle replication intermediates of coliphage λ DNA, Mol. Gen. Genet. 142:137.

Tamanoi, F., Saito, H., and Richardson, C. C., 1980, Physical mapping of primary and secondary origins of bacteriophage T7 DNA replication, Proc. Natl. Acad. Sci. USA 77:2656.

Taucher-Scholz, G., Abdel-Monem, M., and Hoffmann-Berling, H., 1983, Functions of DNA helicases in Escherichia coli, in: Mechanisms of DNA Replication and Recombination, UCLA Symposium on Molecular Biology, Vol. 10 (N. Cozzarelli, ed.), pp. 65–76, Academic Press, New York.

Taylor, A. L., 1963, Bacteriophage-induced mutation in Escherichia coli, Proc. Natl. Acad. Sci. USA 50:1043.

Thomas, R., and Bertani, L., 1964, On the control of the replication of temperate bacteriophages superinfecting immune hosts, Virology 24:241.

Tilly, K., McKittrick, N., Zylicz, M., and Georgopoulos, C., 1983, The dnaK protein modulates the heat shock response of Escherichia coli, Cell 34:641.

Tilly, K., Chandrasekhar, G. N., Zylicz, M., and Georgopoulos, C., 1985, Relationship between the bacterial heat shock response and bacteriophage lambda growth, in: Microbiology 1985 (L. Leive, cd.), pp. 322–326, American Society for Microbiology, Washington.

Tomizawa, J.-I., 1971, Functional cooperation of genes O and P, in: The Bacteriophage Lambda (A. D. Hershey, ed.), pp. 549–552, Cold Spring Harbor Laboratory, Cold Spring Harbor, NY.

Tomizawa, J.-I., and Selzer, G., 1979, Initiation of DNA synthesis in Escherichia coli, Annu. Rev. Biochem. 48:554.

Toussaint, A., and Faelen, M., 1974, The dependence of phage Mu-1 upon the replication functions of E. coli K12, Mol. Gen. Genet. 131:209.

Toussaint, A., and Resibois, A., 1983, Phage Mu: Transposition as a life style, in: Mobile Genetic Elements (J. A. Shapiro, ed.), pp. 105–158, Academic Press, New York.

Tsujimoto, Y., and Ogawa, H., 1977, Intermediates in genetic recombination of bacteriophage T7 DNA, J. Mol. Biol. 109:423.

Tsujimoto, Y., and Ogawa, H., 1978, Intermediates in genetic recombination of bacteriophage T7 DNA: Biological activity and the roles of gene 3 and gene 5, J. Mol. Biol. 125:255.

Tsurimoto, T., and Matsubara, K., 1981a, Purification of bacteriophage λO protein that specifically binds to the origin of replication, Mol. Gen. Genet. 181:325.

Tsurimoto, T., and Matsubara, K., 1981b, Purified bacteriophage λO protein binds to four repeating sequences at the λ replication origin, Nucleic Acids Res. 9:1789.

Tsurimoto, T., and Matsubara, K., 1982a, Replication of λdv plasmid in vitro promoted by purified λO and P proteins, Proc. Natl. Acad. Sci. USA 79:7639.

Tsurimoto, T., and Matsubara, K., 1982b, Replication of bacteriophage λ DNA, Cold Spring Harbor Symp. Quant. Biol. 47:681.

Tsurimoto, T., and Matsubara, K., 1984, Multiple initiation sites of DNA replication flanking the origin region of λdv genome, Proc. Natl. Acad. Sci. USA 81:7402.

Tsurimoto, T., Hase, T., Matsubara, H., and Matsubara, K., 1982, Bacteriophage lambda initiators: Preparation from a strain that overproduces the O and P proteins, *Mol. Gen. Genet.* **187**:79.

Ueda, K., McMacken, R., and Kornberg, A., 1978, dnaB protein of *Escherichia coli:* Purification and role in the replication of φX174 DNA, *J. Biol. Chem.* **253**:261.

Valenzuela, M., and Inman, R., 1981, Direction of bacteriophage λ DNA replication in a thymine requiring *Escherichia coli* K-12 strain. Effect of thymidine concentration, *Nucleic Acids Res.* **9**:6975.

Valenzuela, M., Freifelder, D., and Inman, R., 1976, Lack of a unique termination site for the first round of bacteriophage lambda DNA replication, *J. Mol. Biol.* **102**:569.

Van den Hondel, C. A., Pennings, L., and Schoenmakers, J. G. G., 1976, Restriction-enzyme-cleavage maps of bacteriophage M13. Existence of an intergenic region on the M13 genome, *Eur. J. Biochem.* **68**:55.

Van de Putte, P., Giphart-Gassler, M., Goosen, T., Van Meeteren, A., and Wijffelman, C., 1978, Is integration essential for Mu development?, in: *Integration and Excision of DNA Molecules* (P. Hofschneider and P. Starlinger, eds.), pp. 33–40, Springer-Verlag, Berlin.

Van Mansfeld, A. D. M., Langeveld, S. A., Baas, P. D., Jansz, H. S., Van der Marel, G. A., Veeneman, G. H., and Van Boom, J. H., 1980, Recognition sequence of bacteriophage φX174 gene A protein—an initiator of DNA replication, *Nature* **288**:561.

Van Mansfeld, A. D. M., Van Teefelen, H. A. A. M., Baas, P. D., Veeneman, G. H., Van Boom, J. H., and Jansz, H. S., 1984, The bond in bacteriophage φX174 gene A protein–DNA complex is a tyrosyl-5'-phosphate ester, *FEBS Lett.* **173**:351.

Van Mansfeld, A. D. M., Van Teeffelen, H. A., Fluit, A. C., Baas, P. D., and Jansz, H. S., 1986, Effect of ssb protein on cleavage of single-stranded DNA by φX gene A protein and A* protein, *Nucleic Acids Res.* **14**:1845.

Van Wezenbeek, P. M. G. F., Hulsebos, J. J. M., and Schoenmakers, J. G. G., 1980, Nucleotide sequence of the filamentous bacteriophage M13 DNA genome: Comparison with phage fd, *Gene* **11**:129.

Venkatesan, M., and Nossal, N. C., 1982, Bacteriophage T4 gene 44/62 and gene 45 polymerase accessory proteins stimulate hydrolysis of duplex DNA by T4 DNA polymerase, *J. Biol. Chem.* **257**:12435.

Venkatesan, M., Silver, L. L., and Nossal, N. G., 1982, Bacteriophage T4 gene 41 protein, required for the synthesis of RNA primers, is also a DNA helicase, *J. Biol. Chem.* **257**:12426.

Wada, M., Kadokami, Y., and Itikawa, H., 1982, Thermosensitive synthesis of DNA and RNA in *dnaJ* mutants of *Escherichia coli* K12, *Jpn. J. Genet.* **57**:407.

Wada, M., Sekine, K., and Itikawa, H., 1986, Participation of the *dnaK* and *dnaJ* gene products in phosphorylation of glutaminyl-tRNA synthetase and threonyl-tRNA synthetase of *Escherichia coli* K-12, *J. Bacteriol.* **168**:213.

Waggoner, B. T., and Pato, M. L., 1978, Early events in the replication of Mu prophage DNA, *J. Virol.* **27**:587.

Waggoner, B. T., Pato, M. L., Toussaint, A., and Faelen, M., 1981, Replication of mini-Mu prophage DNA, *Virology* **113**:379.

Wang, J. C., Martin, K. V., and Calendar, R. H., 1973, On the sequence similarity of the cohesive ends of coliphage P4, P2 and 186 DNA, *Biochemistry* **12**:2119.

Watabe, K., Shih, M. F., Sugino, A., and Ito, J., 1982, *In vitro* replication of bacteriophage φ29 DNA, *Proc. Natl. Acad. Sci. USA* **70**:5245.

Watson, J. D., 1972, Origin of concatameric T7 DNA, *Nature New Biol.* **239**:197.

Webster, R. E., and Cashman, J. S., 1973, Abortive infection of *Escherichia coli* with the bacteriophage fl: Cytoplasmic membrane proteins and the fl DNA–gene 5 protein complex, *Virology* **55**:20.

Wickner, S., 1977, DNA or RNA priming of bacteriophage G4 DNA synthesis by *Escherichia coli* dnaG protein, *Proc. Natl. Acad. Sci. USA* **74**:2815.

Wickner, S., 1978a, DNA replication proteins of *Escherichia coli* and phage λ, *Cold Spring Harbor Symp. Quant. Biol.* **43**:303.

Wickner, S., 1978b, DNA replication proteins of E. coli, Annu. Rev. Biochem. **47:**1163.

Wickner, S., and Hurwitz, J., 1974, Conversion of φX174 viral DNA to double-stranded forms by E. coli proteins, Proc. Natl. Acad. Sci. USA **71:**4120.

Wickner, S., and Hurwitz, J., 1975a, Interaction of Escherichia coli dnaB and dnaC(D) gene products in vitro, Proc. Natl. Acad. Sci. USA **72:**921.

Wichner, S., and Hurwitz, J., 1975b, Association of φX174 DNA-dependent ATPase activity with an E. coli protein, replication factor Y, required for in vitro synthesis of φX174 DNA, Proc. Natl. Acad. Sci. USA **72:**3342.

Wickner, W., and Kornberg, A., 1974, A novel form of RNA polymerase from Escherichia coli, Proc. Natl. Acad. Sci. USA **71:**4425.

Wickner, S., Wright, M., and Hurwitz, J., 1974, Association of DNA-dependent and independent ribonucleoside triphosphatase activities with the dnaB gene product of Escherichia coli, Proc. Natl. Acad. Sci. USA **71:**783.

Wijffelman, C., and Lotterman, B., 1977, Kinetics of Mu DNA synthesis, Mol. Gen. Genet. **151:**169.

Wijffelman, C., and Van de Putte, P., 1977, Asymmetric hybridization of Mu strands with short fragments synthesized during Mu DNA replication, in: DNA Insertion Elements, Plasmids and Episomes (A. I. Bukhari, J. A. Shapiro, and S. L. Adhya, eds.), pp. 329–33, Cold Spring Harbor Laboratory, Cold Spring Harbor, NY.

Wold, M., Mallory, J., Roberts, J., LeBowitz, J., and McMacken, R., 1982, Initiation of bacteriophage λ DNA replication in vitro with purified λ replication proteins, Proc. Natl. Acad. Sci. USA **79:**6176.

Wolfson, J., Dressler, D., and Magazin, M., 1972, Bacteriophage T7 DNA replication: A linear replicating intermediate, Proc. Natl. Acad. Sci. USA **69:**499.

Wu, H. M., and Crothers, D. M., 1984, The locus of sequence-directed and protein-induced DNA bending, Nature **308:**509.

Wyatt, G. R., and Cohen, S. S., 1953, The bases of the nucleic acids of some bacterial and animal viruses: The occurrence of 5-hydroxymethylcytosine, Biochem. J. **55:**774.

Wyatt, W., and Inokuchi, H., 1974, Stability of lambda O and P replication functions, Virology **58:**313.

Yarmolinsky, M. B., and Sternberg, N., 1988, Bacteriophage P1, in: The Bacteriophages, Vol. 1 (R. Calendar, ed.), pp. 291–438, Plenum Press, New York.

Yarronton, G. T., and Gefter, M. L., 1979, Enzyme-catalyzed DNA unwinding studies on Escherichia coli rep protein, Proc. Natl. Acad. Sci. USA **76:**1658.

Yates, J., Gette, W., Furth, M., and Nomura, M., 1977, Effects of ribosomal mutations on the readthrough of a chain termination signal: Studies on the synthesis of bacteriophage λ O gene protein in vitro, Proc. Natl. Acad. Sci. USA **74:**689.

Yee, J.-K., and Marsh, R. C., 1985, Locations of bacteriophage T4 origins of replication, J. Virol. **54:**271.

Yen, T. S. B., and Webster, R. E., 1981, Bacteriophage f1 gene II and X proteins. Isolation and characterization of the products of two overlapping genes, J. Biol. Chem. **256:**11259.

Yen, T. S. B., and Webster, R. E., 1982, Translational control of bacteriophage f1 gene II and gene X proteins by gene V protein, Cell **29:**337.

Yochem, J., Uchida, H., Sunshine, M., Saito, H., Georgopoulos, C., and Feiss, M., 1978, Genetic analysis of two genes, dnaJ and dnaK, necessary for Escherichia coli and bacteriophage lambda DNA replication, Mol. Gen. Genet. **164:**9.

Yonesaki, T., and Minagawa, T., 1985, T4 phage gene uvsX product catalyzes homologous DNA pairing, EMBO J. **4:**3321.

Yonesaki, T., Ryo, Y., Minagawa, T., and Takahashi, H., 1985, Purification and some of the functions of the products of the bacteriophage T4 recombination genes, uvsX and uvsY, Eur. J. Biochem. **148:**127.

Yoshikawa, H., Garvey, K. J., and Ito, J., 1985, Nucleotide sequence analysis of DNA replication origins of the small Bacillus bacteriophages: Evolutionary relationships, Gene **37:**125.

Zahn, K., and Blattner, F. R., 1985a, Sequence-induced DNA curvature at the bacteriophage λ origin of replication, *Nature* **317:**451.

Zahn, K., and Blattner, F. R., 1985b, Binding and bending of the λ replication origin by the phage O protein, *EMBO J.* **4:**3605.

Zechel, K., Bouché, J.-P., and Kornberg, A., 1975, Replication of phage G4: A novel and simple system for the initiation of deoxyribonucleic acid synthesis, *J. Biol. Chem.* **250:**4684.

Zinder, N. D., and Horiuchi, K., 1985, Multiregulatory element of filamentous bacteriophages, *Microbiol. Rev.* **49:**101.

Zylicz, M., and Georgopoulos, C., 1984, Purification and properties of the *Escherichia coli* dnaK replication protein, *J. Biol. Chem.* **259:**8820.

Zylicz, M., LeBowitz, J. H., McMacken, R., and Georgopoulos, C., 1983, The dnaK protein of *Escherichia coli* possesses an ATPase and autophosphorylating activity and is essential in an *in vitro* DNA replication system, *Proc. Natl. Acad. Sci. USA* **80:**6431.

Zylicz, M., Gorska, I., Taylor, K., and Georgopoulos, C., 1984, Bacteriophage λ replication proteins: Formation of a mixed oligomer and binding to the origin of λ DNA, *Mol. Gen. Genet.* **196:**401.

Zylicz, M., Yamamoto, T., McKittrick, N., Sell, S., and Georgopoulos, C., 1985, Purification and properties of the dnaJ replication protein of *Escherichia coli*, *J. Biol. Chem.* **260:**7591.

CHAPTER 4

Regulation of Phage Gene Expression by Termination and Antitermination of Transcription

DAVID I. FRIEDMAN

I. INTRODUCTION

Successful viral infection generally requires the sequential expression of sets of genes. Studies of a number of viruses have identified a variety of strategies for obtaining temporal regulation (e.g., see Rabussay and Geiduschek, 1977; McKnight and Tjian, 1986). Most of these strategies involve transcriptional control. The classically described strategies operate at initiation of transcription (Jacob and Monod, 1961; Ptashne, 1986).

In another strategy, first described for phage λ, the same promoters used for transcription of genes expressed early in the infection are used to transcribe genes expressed later through a process of termination and subsequent antitermination of transcription (Roberts, 1969). Operons exhibiting this type of control are arranged so that genes located promoter-proximal to the termination signal can be expressed maximally while genes promoter-distal to the termination signal are unexpressed or poorly expressed. These latter sets of genes are expressed when some physiological or developmental change eliminates the activity of the termination signal. The nature of the termination signals and the nature of the ef-

DAVID I. FRIEDMAN • Department of Microbiology and Immunology, University of Michigan Medical School, Ann Arbor, Michigan 48109-0620.

fector factors vary greatly (Platt, 1986; Von Hippel *et al.*, 1984; Kolter and Yanofsky, 1982). It is the purpose of this article to review the subject of transcription antitermination in the regulation of gene expression in phage. It will primarily focus on the studies of the regulation of gene expression in coliphage λ.

Although this review addresses the question of gene expression in phage, it should be emphasized that transcription termination as a mechanism of gene regulation is not limited to phages. In bacteria many operons involved in biosynthetic processes are regulated by a system of transcription termination and readthrough called attenuation which was originally described for the *his* operon by Kasai (1979) and subsequently described for many other biosynthetic operons (reviewed by Yanofsky, 1981). And there is evidence that this type of regulatory mechanism is operative in eukaryotic cells (Bentley and Groudine, 1986; Nepveu and Marcu, 1986).

Phages of *B. subtilis* have also been studied in some detail. Although termination signals have been identified in phage φ29 (Barthelemy *et al.*, 1987), there is no evidence that *B. subtilis* phages employ termination-antitermination to achieve gene regulation (Doi and Wang, 1986; R. Losick, personal communication). In assessing these observations, it should be noted that polarity, a phenomenon reflecting transcription termination, is not observed in *B. subtilis* (Shimotsu and Henner, 1986). Details of polarity will be discussed below.

The emphasis of this chapter will be on the antitermination component of the regulation in two coliphage families, λ and P2. Although there is some evidence that this mode of regulation is operative in coliphage T4 (Brody *et al.*, 1983), there have not been any recent advances in the study of these systems that require a detailed review (L. Gold, personal communication). The termination component has been reviewed in a number of recent articles (Platt, 1986; Von Hippel *et al.*, 1984). On the other hand, there have been substantial advances in the study of antitermination in coliphage λ, and I therefore begin with a discussion of that topic.

II. COLIPHAGE LAMBDA

A. A General Primer

Gene expression from λ is temporally regulated by transcription termination and antitermination. A schematic representation of the patterns of λ transcription is presented in Fig. 1. In brief, two phage-encoded proteins are involved in this regulation, the products of the *N* gene, gpN (gene product), and the *Q* gene, gpQ. In addition to these phage functions, host-encoded proteins, Nus, also appear to be necessary. The λ antitermination systems have been the subject of a number of reviews (Roberts, 1988; Imamoto and Nakamura, 1986; Friedman *et al.*, 1984; Friedman

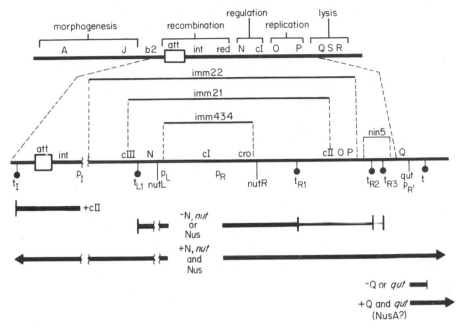

FIGURE 1. Genetic map of phage λ showing placement of relevant genes. This map is not drawn to scale. Top: Relative locations of representative genes. Clusters of genes encoding functionally related products are identified. Middle: An expansion of the portion of the map encoding the major regulatory functions (the "immunity region"). The extents of substituted DNAs in the hybrid phages of λ and P22, 21, and 434 discussed in this review are indicated above the expanded map of the control region. The locations of important sites (promoters, terminators, a deletion, and antiterminators) and genes are indicated. Bottom: The transcription patterns of the early promoters in the presence and absence of gpN, as well as the *int* promoter in the presence of cII, are shown. The transcription patterns of the late promoter in the presence and absence of gpQ is also shown.

and Gottesman, 1983; Ward and Gottesman, 1982; Greenblatt, 1981), and the reader is referred to these articles for more substantive coverage of the subject.

1. Transcripts

During lytic growth, numerous transcripts are produced (Friedman and Gottesman, 1983; Szybalski *et al.*, 1983, 1970; Szybalski, 1977). This discussion will focus only on those transcripts relevant to the subject of antitermination. Transcription of early operons initiates at two promoters, p_L and p_R. Two short transcripts are synthesized—a 12S from p_L (Roberts, 1969; Lozeron *et al.*, 1976) and a 7S from p_R. Each encodes an important regulatory protein; the 12S, gpN (Franklin and Bennet, 1979), and the 7S, Cro (Heinemann and Spiegelman, 1970; Kourilsky *et al.*, 1970; Kumar *et al.*, 1970). The sizes of these transcripts result from the action of the *E. coli*–encoded Rho termination protein at terminators t_{L1}

and t_{R1} (Court et al., 1980; Richardson et al., 1977; Brunel and Davison, 1975; Roberts, 1969). For discussions of the nature and action of the Rho protein, see the reviews by Platt (1986) and Von Hippel et al. (1984).

Transcription of late genes, which initiates at the p_R' promoter, terminates at the t_R' terminator in the absence of gpQ (Sklar et al., 1975; Blattner and Dahlberg, 1972), which explains earlier observations that gpQ is required for late gene expression (Dove, 1966; Joyner et al., 1966). In the presence of the Q gene product, this transcription extends past the t_R' terminator through the late genes (Roberts, 1975; Blattner and Dahlberg, 1972).

2. Terminators

The precise location of termination for the early p_L message is of some controversy both because there are multiple termination sites and because there is extensive processing of this message (Hyman and Honigman, 1986; Szybalski et al., 1983; Das et al., 1983b; Lozeron et al., 1977, 1976; Kourilsky et al., 1971). Recent studies demonstrate that efficient Rho-dependent termination results from a combination of two adjacent signals, t_{L1B} and t_{L1C} (Hyman and Honigman, 1986; Das et al., 1983b; Drahos and Szybalski, 1981).

Rho-dependent termination at t_{R1} is inefficient, with 40% of the transcripts proceeding through t_{R1} (Court et al., 1980; Dambly-Chaudiere et al., 1983; Luk and Szybalski, 1982; Szybalski et al., 1969) and the O and P genes eventually terminating in a region called nin (Greenblatt et al., 1981; Court and Sato, 1969). In vitro studies demonstrated that transcription from p_R terminates in five clusters in the region of t_{R1} (Bear et al., 1985; Lau et al., 1982). These findings stand in contradiction to the results of in vivo studies that demonstrated a unique termination site at t_{R1}. This discrepancy is not explainable on the basis of RNA processing, since there appears to be no processing of this transcript (Court et al., 1980; Lozeron, cited by Friedman and Gottesman, 1983). However, it is entirely possible that additional factors influence the in vivo reaction, limiting it to a unique site.

Attempts to identify specific sequences required for Rho-mediated termination in this region have proved to be somewhat elusive (Bear et al., 1985). Sequences in the cro gene were implicated in Rho action by binding studies (Bektesh and Richardson, 1980) as well as functional studies (Lau and Roberts, 1985). More recently, studies employing complementary oligodeoxynucleotides have identified two specific regions near the 3' end of the p_R message terminating at t_{R1} that may be important in Rho action (Chen et al., 1986). Interestingly, these sequences are near the boxA, B, and C sequences that have been implicated in transcription antitermination (see Section II.E).

The N protein modifies RNA polymerase so that transcription initiating at p_L and p_R overrides t_{L1} and t_{R1} as well as downstream termination signals (Lozeron et al., 1976; Kumar et al., 1971; Kourilsky et al.,

1971; Nijkamp *et al.*, 1970; Luzzati, 1970; Roberts, 1969; Thomas, 1966). N-resistant termination signals are located in the *b2* region (Gottesman *et al.*, 1980). Variants of λ that can grow in the absence of N function, *nin* (*N-in*dependent), have been isolated (Court and Sato, 1969). These phages have deletions between *P* and *Q* (see Fig. 1) [e.g., *nin5*, a 2800-bp deletion (Daniels *et al.*, 1983; Fiandt *et al.*, 1971)] so that gpN is no longer required for *Q* expression.

3. The *nin* Region

a. t_{R2}

Recent studies confirm the presence of at least two termination signals in the *nin* region (Leason, 1986; M. Gottesman, personal communication). One signal, called t_{R2}, has the hyphenated dyad symmetry (stem loop structure) typical of a terminator (Kröger and Hobom, 1982). Two mutations in the region eliminate t_{R2} termination activity. One is a deletion of the entire region of dyad symmetry (Kroeger and Hobom, 1982; unpublished studies in this laboratory); the other is a point mutation in one of the arms of the stem-loop structure (Leason, 1986). *In vitro* studies show that termination at t_{R2} is partially NusA-dependent (Schmidt and Chamberlin, 1987).

b. *roc*

A second region of termination was identified in the study of a 2-kb deletion, *roc*, that maps to the right of the t_{R2} structure (Leason, 1986). Although this region could contain more than one terminator, for purposes of this discussion it will be assumed that there is one terminator, which will be called t_{R3}. Elimination of both the t_{R2} and t_{R3} signals is necessary but not sufficient for λ N-independent growth. Elimination of the termination signals in this region should be sufficient for N-independent growth for three reasons: (1) All of the functions required for lytic growth that require gpN for their expression ultimately require antiterminated transcription from pR. (2) t_{R1} is a weak terminator and by itself poses no physiologically significant barrier to effective downstream gene expression. (3) The *Q* gene, located downstream of $t_{R2}-t_{R3}$, encodes an antitermination function that modifies additional transcription initiating at the p_R' promoter located downstream of the *Q* gene. The *nin* deletion removes this region of termination and thus allows N-independent expression of *Q* and, therefore, expression of all late genes.

B. The Lambdoid Phages

Lambda is one member of a family of related phages (Campbell and Botstein, 1983). The other lambdoid phages have served as useful tools in both the genetic and biochemical analysis of λ, because they share with λ a common genome organization as well as limited amounts of DNA homology. However, in many cases, genes having analogous activities differ substantially in sequence, and their products will only function with phages of the same species. For example, lambdoid phages 21 and λ have N genes that encode antitermination functions and have been mapped to the same relative position on their respective genomes (Franklin, 1985a; Hilliker and Botstein, 1976; Friedman et al., 1973). However, as will be discussed in the section on N, the N product of one will not efficiently complement an N defect of the other.

Hybrid lambdoid phages can be constructed, because the lambdoid phages share regions of homology scattered throughout their genomes (Botstein and Herskowitz, 1974; Gemski et al., 1972; Szpirer et al., 1969; Liedke-Kulke and Kaiser, 1967; Kaiser and Jacob, 1957). Hybrid phages can be used to mix and match genes and sites of action; these hybrid phages have proved invaluable in the study of transcription antitermination (see Fig. 1).

C. The N Antitermination Protein

The previous discussion makes it apparent that the N gene product, gp$N$, is a central factor in the regulation of expression of early λ genes by transcription antitermination. N, the first gene in the p_L operon, encodes a 12,200-dalton highly basic protein (Greenblatt and Li, 1981a; Franklin and Bennett, 1979). Early studies identified gp$N$ as an important regulatory factor stimulating expression of phage gene products. In the absence of gp$N$, transcription of the λ genome is reduced by 98%, with transcription primarily limited to the genes, cro and N, immediately downstream of the early promoters (Lozeron et al., 1976; Kumar et al., 1970; Kourilsky et al., 1970; Heinemann and Spiegelman, 1970; Nijkamp et al., 1970; Luzzati, 1970; Roberts, 1969).

1. Action of gp$N$

Roberts (1969) first postulated a role for gp$N$ in transcription antitermination (see also Szybalski et al., 1969). Surprisingly, the in vitro studies that led Roberts to this highly novel concept did not involve gp$N$! In these elegant studies, the E. coli transcription termination protein Rho and the Rho-dependent termination signals on the λ genome (t_{R1} and t_{L1}) were identified. Roberts, studying in vitro transcription initiating at p_R and p_L, inferred that Rho-terminated transcripts are the same as those formed in vivo in the absence of gp$N$. Thus, based on this intuitive argument, Roberts developed the concept of regulation of gene expression by the process of transcription termination and antitermination, a mechanism subsequently shown to operate in the regulation of some bacterial operons (see reviews by Morgan, 1986; Yanofsky, 1981). Luzatti (1970) provided direct evidence that gpN regulates gene expression from p_L by transcription antitermination.

This action of gpN explains why polarity is not observed in λ gene expression. Polarity results when a mutation in one gene reduces the expression of other genes in that operon that are located promoter-distal to the mutated gene (Ames and Hartman, 1963; Franklin and Luria, 1961; Jacob and Monod, 1961). Experiments from a number of laboratories demonstrated that N-modified transcription overcomes the effects of polar mutations in bacterial operons fused to the early λ promoters (Segawa and Imamoto, 1976; Adhya et al., 1974; Franklin, 1974).

2. A Model of Polarity

A role for gpN in overcoming polarity is consistent with one model of polarity (Adhya and Gottesman, 1978). According to this model, polar mutations activate normally silent Rho-dependent termination signals. Because polar mutations terminate translation prior to the transcription termination signal, the RNA downstream of the site of translation termination will be free of ribosomes. This "naked" RNA is postulated to serve as an efficient substrate for binding Rho. The bound Rho, in turn, winds its way toward the 3' end of the RNA and terminates transcription at a site where the RNA polymerase has paused (provided there is no translation initiation signal between the translation stop and transcription termination signals). Genes in the same operon located distal to the polar mutation and activated terminator will thus be poorly transcribed and, in turn, inefficiently expressed. The N-modified transcription overcomes the transcription termination signals, allowing transcription to proceed into downstream genes. Genes distal to the polar mutation are thus expressed normally when transcription is N-modified.

3. Mutations

Two types of mutation have been important in the study of gpN action—null and altered action. The null type of mutation results in a loss of function and includes nonsense, missense, and deletion mutations (Franklin, 1985b). Studies with λ derivatives carrying null mutations in N demonstrated a major role for gpN in phage gene expression. As discussed, transcription of λ in the absence of effective gpN is severely reduced, being primarily limited to the early genes located proximal to Rho-dependent termination signals (see Fig. 1).

Null mutations, nonsense and missense, that impose phenotypes similar to those seen with the null N mutations of λ have been identified in phages P22 (Hilliker and Botstein, 1976) and 21 (H. Inokuchi and W. F. Dove, cited by Franklin, 1985b; Friedman et al., 1973b). That these mutations have been mapped to the same relative position as λ N suggests that they define the N gene equivalents of phages P22 and 21. Mutations conferring properties similar but not identical to mutations in the λ N gene have been identified in φ80 (Gilbert and Lozeron, 1983). These mutations are not, however, in the gene that sequence analysis identified as a likely candidate for the N gene of that phage (Kanemoto et al., 1987; Tanaka and Matsushiro, 1985).

Altered action mutations, pun, are missense mutations that change gpN so that it functions with mutant host factors that fail to function with wild-type gpN (see Section II.D for discussions of host Nus proteins and a special class of N mutations, mar). For example, the punA1 mutation has been mapped to the N gene, between two amber mutations. The resulting protein is active in hosts carrying either the nusA1 or nusE71 mutation (Schauer, 1985; Friedman and Ponce-Campos, 1975). Other mutations in N exhibiting similar phenotypes have been isolated and sequenced (Schauer et al., 1987; Franklin, 1985b; Friedman and Olson, 1983; Hilliker et al., 1978). The isolation of pun mutations suggests an interaction between gpN and host factors. Such an interaction was demonstrated in vitro between gpN and the E. coli NusA protein by Greenblatt and Li (1981a).

4. Structure of N Genes

Our knowledge of the structure of the N gene is primarily the result of work from the laboratory of N. Franklin. Franklin and Bennett (1979) determined the nucleotide sequence of the N gene and found that it encoded an 11.8-kD protein. Probably because of its highly basic nature, when the N protein is subjected to SDS-PAGE, it runs with an apparent size of 14 kD (Shaw et al., 1978; Greenblatt et al., 1980). The N protein has been purified and characterized as basic and asymmetric (Ishii et al., 1980a; Greenblatt et al., 1981). To relate the structure and function of gpN, Franklin compared gpN of λ with the N analogues of related lambdoid phages 21 and P22 on the basis of DNA sequence. The genes encoding N_{21} and N_{P22} map at sites analogous to the map position of the λ N gene (Hilliker and Botstein, 1976; Friedman et al., 1973b). The sequence analysis revealed open reading frames that translated into small basic proteins equidistant from p_L in all three phages. In the case of the P22 N (called gene 24), a known 24 amber mutation (Hilliker and Botstein, 1976), resulted in a CAG to TAG change in the open reading frame identified as the 24 gene (Franklin, 1985b).

Comparison of the sequences of the three N genes (λ, 21, and P22) revealed very little homology except in the case of λ and 21, where there is a match of 22 of 34 amino acids at the carboxy termini (Franklin, 1985a). On the basis of charge, sequence homologies, and potential structure, Franklin aligned the amino acid sequences of the three proteins (derived from their nucleotide sequences) and identified five areas of similarity. Lettered from A to E, these areas are located consecutively from the amino termini of the N proteins. Three areas are of particular interest. Area B is an 18–amino acid region rich in arginine and lysine residues. Because four of 18 amino acids in the B region are common to the three proteins, this region served as a primary focus for aligning the three N proteins. The region has potential to form an α helical structure and is demonstrably important for gpN action, since four missense and two poorly suppressible nonsense mutations are found in the B region of the λ N gene. Analysis of the amino acid sequences of the D region also suggests possible α helical structure. All of the *pun* mutations are located in the C region of the λ N gene, suggesting that this region is important for gpN interaction with Nus proteins.

A sequence identified as the N gene of phage ϕ80 has also been determined (Tanaka and Matsushiro, 1985). Like the other N genes, the protein encoded by the putative N gene of ϕ80 is small and basic and contains many arginine residues. A 12-kD protein corresponding to the sequence of the putative ϕ80 N has recently been isolated (Kanemoto *et al.*, 1987). This protein has antitermination activity in an *in vitro* transcription system using ϕ80 DNA as the template.

Recent studies suggest that the *nun* gene of phage HKO22, because of its location on the HKO22 genetic map and peculiar activity, may be related to the N family structure (R. Weisberg and M. Gottesman, personal communication). Because of its unique action on λ transcription, Nun will be discussed in a separate section.

5. Coda

Although the model that gpN acts by antitermination was postulated based on information gained from *in vitro* transcription studies done in the absence of gpN, elucidation of this novel role also relied heavily on genetic studies. In a similar way, the studies to be discussed in the following sections defining the host contributions to as well as the role of sites on the phage genome on transcription antitermination have relied on genetic as well as biochemical methods.

D. Host Factors

In addition to gpN, a number of host proteins are required for the N antitermination reaction. Initially, these host factors were identified by mutations in *E. coli* genes, *nus*, that cause a failure of λ growth due to a failure of the N antitermination system. The name given to the genes identified by such mutations, *nus*, reflects this phenotype—*N-utilization substance*. The products of the previously uncharacterized *nus* genes were subsequently identified by *in vitro* experiments. Table I summarizes information on the *nus* genes and their products. Since this subject has been extensively reviewed (Imamoto and Nakamura, 1986; Friedman *et al.*, 1984; Friedman and Gottesman, 1983), this discussion will only

TABLE I. *nus* Genes[a]

nus Allele	Gene	Map position	Product	Role in host	Other relevant phenotypes of mutations in this gene
nusA	*nusA*	min 69	55,000 M_r	Transcription termination and antitermination	Conditional lethal
nusB	*nusB*	min 11	15,000 M_r	Transcription termination and antitermination	Conditional lethal Suppression of *nusA* and *nusE* mutations
nusC	*rpoB*	min 82	β subunit RNA polymerase	Transcription	Suppression of N mutants (*lycA*) Enhancer of Nus phenotype (*snu*)
nusD	*rho*	min 85	Rho	Transcription termination	Hyperdegradation of proteins
nusE	*rpsJ*	min 72	Ribosomal protein S10	Translation	—

[a]Genes in which mutations have been isolated that result in a failure in the action of the λ *N* gene product.

summarize older material while focusing on the results of more recent studies.

The phenotype used to identify *E. coli* with *nus* mutations (Friedman, 1971) is a failure to support the growth of λ derivatives that require gpN (N-dependent phages) while allowing growth of λ derivatives that do not require gpN (N-independent phages such as λ*nin5*) (Court and Sato, 1969). The *nus* genes have been mapped to different locations on the *E. coli* chromosome, and all play roles in bacterial transcription or translation (see Table I). *In vitro* experiments rule out one possible explanation for the isolation of *nus* mutations at multiple loci. According to this explanation, there is only one true *nus* gene, and the phenotype of the other *nus* mutations results from a failure of their products to support expression of the true *nus* gene. If this were the case, however, there would be no *in vitro* complementation following the mixing of extracts from the various mutants, because all of the extracts would be missing the same Nus function. Supernatant extracts prepared from various strains (Nus$^+$ and Nus$^-$) were tested for their ability to support GalK synthesis in a coupled transcription-translation system (Das and Wolska, 1984). The plasmid used as a template had a termination signal placed between the promoter and *galK* gene. It was found that extracts from *nusA1*, *nusB5*, and *nusE71* mutants do show pairwise complementation, demonstrating that each mutant synthesizes the other Nus proteins.

1. nusA

a. Genetics

Mapping studies located the *nusA* gene at min 69 on the *E. coli* chromosome (Friedman and Baron, 1974). The *nusA1* mutation, employed in this mapping, was the first *nus* mutation isolated (Friedman, 1971) and exhibits a strong Nus⁻ phenotype (failure to support gpN action) at higher temperatures (above 42°C) and a weaker Nus⁻ phenotype at lower temperatures (Friedman, 1971). The defect in the *nusA1* mutant is not due to a lowered level of NusA expression, but, as was previously discussed, is due to the expression of an altered protein (Greenblatt and Li, 1981a). Isolation of conditional lethal mutations in the *nusA* gene demonstrates that NusA is an essential function (Schauer *et al.*, 1987; Nakamura *et al.*, 1986; Nakamura and Uchida, 1983). Moreover, it is essential at both low and high temperatures, since both *cs-* and *ts*-lethal mutations in the *nusA* gene have been isolated.

A natural variant of *nusA* was identified in studies with a hybrid *E. coli* in which the wild-type *nusA* allele had been replaced with the *nusA* gene from the closely related enteric bacterium *Salmonella typhimurium* (this allele will be referred to as *nusA*ˢᵃˡ) (Friedman and Baron, 1974; Baron *et al.*, 1970). This hybrid exhibits a Nus⁻ phenotype. However, it appears to be more defective, since unlike *nusA1* mutants, the *nusA*ˢᵃˡ hybrid fails to support the action of gpN at all temperatures.

Comparison of the nucleotide sequences of the two natural *nusA* genes reveals much homology. Most of the significant differences occur between the 5′ two-thirds of the genes (Schauer, 1985; Ishii *et al.*, 1984a; Saito *et al.*, 1986). Strikingly, the change resulting in the *nusA1* mutation is located in one of the runs of bases in which significant differences between the two natural alleles are observed (Saito *et al.*, 1986). It is likely that these changes define a functional domain of NusA involved in recognition of gpN (see Fig. 2).

There are two reasons for inferring an important functional role for the 5′ two-thirds of the *nusA* gene: (1) A. Granston (unpublished studies, this laboratory) has used the cloned *nusA* genes from *E. coli* and *S. typhimurium* to construct hybrid genes on plasmids (see Fig. 2). He finds that a hybrid with the 5′ two-thirds from *E. coli* (*hy1*) complements *nusA* mutants for both gpN action and bacterial viability. However, when only the 5′ one-tenth of *nusA* is from *E. coli* (*hy3*) or the 5′ two-thirds is from *S. typhimurium* (*hy2*), the cloned hybrid only reverses the effects on bacterial viability. (2) A cloned fragment from *E. coli* that expresses only the 5′ three-fourths of the *nusA* gene of *E. coli* (to a Pst1 site) complements the *nusAcs10* mutant for growth at low temperature (Schauer *et al.*, 1987) and both the *NusA1* and *nusA*ˢᵃˡ for gpN action.

The *nusA* gene is in an operon that includes at least four other genes—an F-met tRNA, two as yet unidentified proteins, and *infB*

S.t.
E.C.

M - N - K - E - I - L - A - V - V - E - A - V - S - N - E - K - A - L - P - R
                                                     R
                                                     E
                                                     I
                                                     K

Q - E - Y - K - K - K - T - A - T - A - L - A - S - E - L - A - E - F - I - K
|E|
|Q|

I - D - V - R - R - V - [E/Q] - I - D - R - K - S - G - D - F - D - T - F - R - R - [S/W]

◁ *hy3* (PvuI)

E - [F/Y] - R - A - A - E - L - T - I - E - K - T - P - [M/Q] - T - V - E - [E/D] - V - [L/I/V]

E - S - L - N - [V/L] - G - D - Y - V - E - D - Q - I - E - S - V - T - F - D - R

[W/M/V/V] - A - R - [A/E] - A - E - R - V - [E/K] - [A/Q] - [A/V] - I - [I/V] - [G/Q] - K - A - T - Q - T - T

V - D - Q - F - R - E - H - E - G - E - I - I - T - G - V - V - K - V - [N/R/I/D]

S - D - E - R - L - I - V - A - E - A - N - N - G - L - D - L - S - I - N - [S/C/I/R]

R - V - K - T - F - A - L - A - T - [V/A] - F - [A/V] - A - C - [C/S] - [M/I] - [L/P] - F - [D/N] - [G/K/R/R]

                          nusA11 ↓T   ↓A *nusA1*

R - F - L - E - I - L - M - E - P - K - S - R - T - V - F - L - Q - A - [V/G]

E - V - P - E - I - G - E - E - V - I - E - I - N - A - A - A - R - D - P - [G/I/S/R]

V - C - A - G - V - P - D - I - R - K - D - N - T - K - V - A - T - K - A - R

M - R - [R/G] - A - R - V - Q - A - V - S - [Y/T] - [Q/E] - L - G - G - E - R - [F/I] - D - [I/L/V/L]

A - V - D - A - P - A - M - [R/A] - N - I - V - F - Q - A - P - N - D - D - W - L

I - V - V - D - E - D - K - H - T - M - D - I - A - V - E - A - G - N - L - [A/I/Q/I/A]

                         ◁ *hy1, hy2* (NcoI)

L - E - W - G - S - L - Q - S - A - L - R - V - N - Q - G - N - R - G - I - A

V - M - T - V - D - D - L - Q - A - K - H - Q - A - E - A - H - A - A - I - [E/D/I/T/I/F]

   ◁ Δ*pKR324* (PstI)

F - G - E - E - V - L - V - T - A - F - [E/D] - E - D - I - D - L - Y - K - T - [F/S/I/T]

T - L - E - E - L - A - T - V - P - M - K - E - L - L - E - I - [D/E] - G - L - [D/I/E/I/P]

[D/A/Q/I/E] - Q - A - [L/L/I] - T - A - L - A - N - K - A - R - E - R - L - A - E - V - T - P

E - [A/E] - S - L - G - D - N - K - P - A - D - D - L - L - N - L - E - G - V - [D/J/R/I/D]

Q - [Q/E] - A - L - D - E - L - T - C - V - G - R - A - A - L - K - F - A - [M/L] - D
|I|
|G|
|I|

I - D - [H/D] - L - A - D - I - E - G - L - T - D - E - K - A - G - A - L - I - [I/M/A/I/A]

A - E - D - G - F - W - C - I - N - R - A

(Nakamura and Mizusawa, 1985; Ishii *et al.*, 1984a,b). A sequence conforming to the consensus *E. coli* promoter sequence is found 5' of the F-met tRNA gene (Ishii *et al.*, 1984b). *In vitro* and *in vivo* transcription studies are consistent with this being the promoter of the operon (Nakamura and Mizusawa, 1985; Ishii *et al.*, 1984b). Expression of this operon is, in part, regulated by NusA; higher levels of NusA result in a reduction in expression (Friedman *et al.*, 1985; Plumbridge *et al.*, 1985).

b. General Physiological Role

The NusA protein is capable of playing a number of different and what appear to be contradictory roles in transcription. Studies by Kung *et al.* (1975) identified a protein, called L and later shown to be NusA (Greenblatt *et al.*, 1980), that stimulates β-galactosidase synthesis in a coupled *in vitro* transcription-translation system. Although the precise role of NusA in this reaction was not determined, it was suggested that NusA might reduce Rho-dependent transcription termination within the *lacZ* gene (Kung *et al.*, 1975). Subsequently, it has been shown that NusA can also play an antagonistic role, facilitating pausing or termination of transcription (reviewed by Platt, 1986; Von Hippel *et al.*, 1984).

c. Role in Antitermination

The discussion in this section will be limited to the relatively well understood NusA-gpN interactions, although *in vitro* studies have also implicated a role for NusA protein in the action of the gpQ antitermination function; this subject will be discussed in a subsequent section on gpQ action. Although there is substantial evidence that NusA can act at some terminators to stimulate transcription termination (Schmidt and Chamberlin, 1987; Nakamura *et al.*, 1986; Lau *et al.*, 1984; Greenblatt *et al.*, 1981; Ward and Gottesman, 1981), there is now overwhelming evidence that NusA functions as an essential component of the N-antitermination complex. This rules out an alternative model in which NusA's only role in this antitermination reaction is as a termination factor whose action is opposed by gpN. I will next summarize the evidence for this statement.

FIGURE 2. Comparison of the amino acid sequences of the *nusA* genes of *E. coli* and *S. typhimurium* as translated from the DNA sequences. The single-letter code is used to identify amino acids. The differences in the two sequences are boxed for easy identification. The upper letter represents the amino acid found in the *S. typhimurium* gene, and the lower letter the amino acid found at the corresponding position in the *E. coli* gene. Arrows identify the changes caused by the *nusAll* and *nusAl* mutations (Y. Nakamura, personal communication). Junction points for hybrid *nusA* proteins are shown (A. Granston, unpublished studies this laboratory): hy3, 5' *E. coli*—3' *S. typhimurium*; hyl, 5' *E. coli*—3' *S. typhimurium*; hy2, 5' *S. typhimurium*—3' *E. coli*. Also shown is a Pst1 site used to create a *nusA* gene truncated at the 3' end. Diagram kindly supplied by A. Granston.

Experiments with *E. coli* carrying either a mutant or natural variant *nusA* gene provided *in vivo* evidence that NusA is required for N-mediated antitermination (Friedman, 1971; Friedman and Baron, 1974; Schauer *et al.*, 1987). Studies of λ growth in diploid *nusA*[+]/*nusA1* or *nusA*[+]/*nusA*[Sal] hosts demonstrated that the wild-type *E. coli* allele is dominant; λ grows normally in the diploid bacteria. It is argued that the fact that both the *nusA1* and the *nusA*[Sal] alleles are recessive to the wild type means that the failure of gpN action in the mutants results from the inability of the variant NusA products to support the antitermination reaction.

The hybrid bacterium has been employed in another type of experiment that supports a positive role for NusA in antitermination. A variant of λ that carries two mutations in N (*punA1,133*) was isolated that can grow poorly in the hybrid (*nusA*[Sal]) bacterium (Friedman and Olson, 1983). However, λ*punA1,133* grows well if the hybrid bacterium contains a plasmid from which *nusA*[Sal] is overproduced (Schauer *et al.*, 1987). Obviously, if NusA is part of the termination reaction that is antagonized by the N antitermination complex, overproduction of such an inhibitory function should, if anything, result in a greater inhibitory effect. The fact that overproduction of a NusA product, under conditions where it is normally not effective with a λ gpN, supports gene expression past terminators argues that NusA is required for the antitermination reaction; i.e., NusA[Sal] can only weakly interact in the antitermination complex even with the mutant gpN, but increasing the amount of NusA[Sal] results, through mass action, in the formation of an active antitermination complex.

In vitro studies are consistent with the *in vivo* genetic studies. First, NusA and gpN have been shown to physically associate (Greenblatt and Li, 1981a). Second, using extracts from a *nusA1* mutant, it has been shown that N-facilitated readthrough of a transcription termination signal requires the addition of wild-type NusA protein (Goda and Greenblatt, 1985; Das and Wolska, 1984). The latter experiments are open to the same criticism as the *in vivo* genetic studies, in that they rely on a *nusA1* mutant to provide extracts free of NusA activity. However, recent studies from the Das and Greenblatt laboratories support a positive role for NusA in N-mediated antitermination. W. Whalen and A. Das (personal communication) find that NusA and gpN are the only auxillary proteins required for antitermination at *nut* sites. J. Li and J. Greenblatt (personal communication) have removed NusA quantitatively from an S100 extract by passing the extract through a column loaded with anti-NusA antibody. The treated extract fails to support gpN action.

Results from experiments with *E. coli* carrying conditional lethal (*ts*) *nusA* mutations have been advanced to argue that NusA is not a required factor for the gpN antitermination reaction (Nakamura *et al.*, 1986; Nakamura and Uchida, 1983). The following summarizes the important results of these experiments. First, at the high, nonpermissive temperature, λ is able to grow in hosts with the *nusAts11* mutation as measured by single-step growth experiments. Second, λ fails to form plaques on a bacterial lawn of a strain that is a *nusAts11/nusA1* diploid at 42°C. It was argued that the *nusAts11* gene product could not be functioning at high temperature since the *nusA1* allele is dominant. In trying to explain how these interesting observations can be rationalized in view of the overwhelming evidence arguing that NusA is required for gpN action, I offer the following commentary. First, the haploid and diploid strains were tested under different conditions, single-step growth versus lawn plating, making it difficult to compare the experiments. Second, there is no evidence that gpN is required for λ growth in the *nusAts11* mutant at high temperature; i.e., it has not been reported that a λ N⁻ phage does not grow in the mutant host at the nonpermissive temperature. Obviously, if gpN is not required, then the presence of the *nusA1* allele would have no effect on growth even if NusA is a required factor for gpN action. Because of these questions relating to the results of experiments with the *nusAts11* mutant, it is not possible to definitively assess whether the reported studies argue against a positive role for NusA in the N-mediated antitermination reaction.

A dialectic approach permits a conciliatory resolution to the problem. It is conceivable that NusA acts in both transcription termination *and* antitermination, depending on the nature of the interacting factors. Thus, in the cases of N-imposed antitermination, NusA is directed toward antitermination, whereas in the case of λ termination at t_{R1} (Nakamura *et al.*, 1986; Lau *et al.*, 1984) and t_{R2} (Schmidt and Chamberlin, 1987; Greenblatt *et al.*, 1980), NusA is directed toward termination. NusA protein *per se*, according to this model, would not determine which pathway of activity is chosen; other factors ultimately throw the switch toward termination or antitermination. What throws the switch, of course, is the critical question.

2. *nusB*

The *nusB* gene, also known as *groNB*, has been mapped to min 11 (Friedman *et al.*, 1976; Keppel *et al.*, 1974) and encodes a protein with a molecular weight of 15 kD (Strauch and Friedman, 1981; Swindle *et al.*, 1981). First identified because of its role in gpN action, the *nusB* gene product, NusB, was subsequently shown to be involved in both termination (Kuroki *et al.*, 1982; Ward and Gottesman, 1981) and antitermination of bacterial transcription (Sharrock *et al.*, 1985a; M. Cashel and M. Gottesman, personal communication). Some *nusB* mutations confer both a Nus⁻ (failure to support action of λ gpN) and a cold-sensitive phenotype (Georgopoulos *et al.*, 1980). The fact that cold-resistant revertants of these mutations also have a Nus⁺ phenotype demonstrates that NusB is a protein essential for *E. coli* viability. The *nusB* gene has been cloned and sequenced (Swindle *et al.*, 1984; Ishii *et al.*, 1984c). It contains an open reading frame encoding a 15,689-M_r protein. The resulting amino acid sequence matches the N-terminal amino acid sequence derived from the purified NusB protein (Maekawa *et al.*, 1985).

In vitro studies prove that the NusB protein is required for N-mediated antitermination. Gosh and Das (1984), employing an S30-coupled transcription-translation system, demonstrated that purified NusB protein specifically complemented a *nusB⁻* extract for gpN-mediated antitermination. Horwitz *et al.* (1987) have used a TSK60 gel permeation column to isolate transcription complexes in order to study the requirements for the formation and the components of the N antitermination complex. These studies suggest that NusB may be necessary for the participation of one signal in the RNA, *boxA*, required for N-mediated antitermination (see Section II.E).

3. *rpoB-nusC*

A number of mutations that influence gpN action have been mapped to min 82 in the *rpoB* gene (encoding the β subunit of RNA polymerase). One of the originally identified mutations that conferred a Nus phenotype, *groN785*, was initially mapped to *rpoB* (Georgopoulos, 1971a,b). However, the change in *rpoB* was later shown to be only one of three mutations that collectively cause the GroN phenotype (Greenblatt and Li, 1981a; C. Georgopoulos, personal communication). *E. coli* carrying another class of *rpoB* mutations, *ron*, fails to support the growth of λ derivatives that have a *mar* mutation in their N gene even though they support the growth of wild-type λ (Ghysen and Pironio, 1972). It has been suggested by N. Franklin (personal communication) that this indicates a direct interaction between polymerase and gpN—i.e., the Ron polymerase requires higher levels of gpN than the wild-type enzyme, and N genes containing *mar* mutations might express lower levels of active gpN.

As in the case of the polymerase component of the *groN* mutant, other *rpoB* mutations by themselves have little effect on gpN action, although they can enhance the effects of *nus* mutations. The *snu* class of *rpoB* mutations was selected for their ability to enhance the effect of the *NusA1* mutation on gpN action; λ will not plate on the *snu9-nusA1* double mutants even at low temperature (Baumann and Friedman, 1976). Although the *snu* mutations confer a similar enhancement when combined with other *nus* mutations, by themselves they have no influence on λ lytic growth.

Another class of *rpoB* mutants has been identified because it causes a delay in λ lytic growth (Sternberg, 1976). Again, combining one of these mutations with *nus* mutations results in a more stringent Nus phenotype.

The *nusC60* mutant exhibits a more restrictive Nus⁻ phenotype, and, in contrast to the previously discussed mutants, the responsible mutations have all been mapped to the *rpoB* gene (unpublished experiments, this laboratory). Fine-structure mapping has revealed that *nusC60* is composed of three mutations, all of which map in *rpoB* (D. Jin and C. Gross, personal communication). *In vitro* studies show that the NusC60 polymerase is extremely inactive (unpublished results, this laboratory; J. Greenblatt, personal communication).

A class of *rpoB* mutants has been described that exhibits a phenotype opposite to the phenotype discussed above. A mutation of this class, *lycA*, permits the host to support the growth of λ derivatives that express little or no gpN activity (Lecocq and Dambly, 1976). Greenblatt (1984) ascribes this phenotype of the *lycA* mutant to the inability of the mutant polymerase to recognize pause signals.

4. *rho-nusD*

One mutation yielding a Nus phenotype has been mapped to the *rho* locus, min 85. This mutation was found in the HDF026 mutant originally isolated because it failed to support growth of T4 (Simon *et al.*, 1979). The *rho* mutation in the HDF026 mutant causes the bacterium to be hyperdegradative for proteins.

The HDF026 mutant exhibits only a marginal Nus⁻ phenotype; λ wild type grows normally in this mutant, whereas λr32, a λ derivative with an IS2 element adjacent to *cII* (Brachet *et al.*, 1970), fails to grow. Because the IS2 contains a strong Rho-dependent terminator (De Crombrugghe *et al.*, 1973), it is thought that λr32 requires higher than normal levels of gpN activity for antitermination (Tomich and Friedman, 1977). Hyperdegradation of gpN is not the cause of the Nus phenotype of HDF026, since the half-life of gpN is the same in an HDF026 mutant as in a wild-type isogenic control (Gottesman *et al.*, 1981). The defect in HDF026 specifically affects Rho-dependent terminators (Das *et al.*, 1983a).

5. *rpsJ-nusE*

Perhaps the *nus* mutation that presents the most interesting and perplexing problems of interpretation is *nusE71*, an allele of *rpsJ* that has been mapped to min 72 and encodes ribosomal protein S10 (Friedman *et al.*, 1981). *In vitro* studies show that either purified S10 or the 30S ribosomal subunit protein will complement extracts made from a *nusE71* mutant for N-antitermination activity (Das *et al.*, 1985; Horwitz *et al.*, 1987). The isolation of a mutation that confers a Nus⁻ phenotype in a ribosomal protein gene suggests that the ribosome or some of its component parts are involved in N-mediated antitermination. Although not conclusive, the bulk of the experimental evidence argues against a role for the complete ribosome. A ribosomal involvement would not be surprising; it has been shown that the translating ribosome plays a central role in attenuation, another termination-antitermination regulatory mechanism that controls expression of many bacterial biosynthetic operons (Yanofsky, 1981). Moreover, the isolation of a second-site suppressor in another gene encoding a ribosomal protein that partially reverses the Nus⁻ phenotype of the *nusE71* mutation is consistent with ribosomal involvement (see below). Two results from *in vitro* experiments testing N-modified antitermination also suggest the possibility of a role for ribosomes (Das and Wolska, 1984; A. Das, personal communication). First, it was shown that gp*N* binds tightly to ribosomes and that some *nus* mutations influence this binding. In both *nus*⁺ and *nusB5* extracts, gp*N* is found associated with both the large and small ribosomal subunits, whereas in *nusA1* and *nusE71* extracts, gp*N* is only found associated with the large subunit. Second, it was found that washed ribosomes from Nus⁻ bacteria could complement both S30 and S100 extracts from Nus mutants.

Nevertheless, results of a number of experiments have argued against a direct role for the translating ribosome in gp*N* action. Translation initiation can be prevented or prematurely terminated upstream of the usual termination site (which is immediately 5' to the *nutR* region) without significantly affecting the N reaction at *nutR* (Olson *et al.*, 1984; Warren and Das, 1984). This suggests that translation adjacent to *nut* is not required for gp*N* action; however, it does not definitively rule out a role for ribosomes. For instance, it is conceivable that ribosomes could be directed to the *nut* site by a special signal not requiring translation.

Results from *in vitro* studies on N-mediated antitermination in partially purified coupled transcription-translation systems have been advanced as arguments that ribosomes are not likely to be involved in gp*N* action (Goda and Greenblatt, 1985; Das and Wolska, 1984; Ishii *et al.*, 1980b). The basis of these arguments is that the S100 extracts used in these studies should be ribosome-free. However, such extracts are likely to contain at least low levels of ribosomal contamination; up to 40% of the cellular ribosomes could be found in S100 preparations (F. Imamoto, personal communication). In the case of complementation of NusE⁻ extracts, the added S10 need not act as a free protein but could become part of the ribosome by exchanging with bound protein. However, more recent studies using stringent methods for purification show that extracts measurably free from contaminating ribosomes do function efficiently in the cell-free antitermination system (A. Das, personal communication; J. Greenblatt and V. Chen, personal communication). Although these studies obviously raise a strong argument against possible ribosomal involvement, it is important to keep in mind that the *in vitro* process may differ in a qualitative manner from the *in vivo* reaction; i.e., the strength as well as distances between and numbers of terminators that must be overcome in the test vectors is different from those in the phage. However, *in vitro* studies show that in the absence of ribosomes, N-modified transcription can override as many as four consecutive termination signals (A. Das, personal communication).

6. Combinations of *nus* Mutations

When *nus* mutations are combined in the same host, a more restrictive Nus$^-$ phenotype is observed (Friedman *et al.*, 1983). The *nusB5* (as well as other *nusB* mutations isolated in this laboratory) and *nusE71* mutations, like the *nusA1* mutation, impose a stronger Nus$^-$ phenotype at higher temperatures (42°C) than at lower temperatures (32°C); λ derivatives with wild-type gpN activity form plaques on lawns of *E. coli* carrying one of these mutations at 32°C but not at 42°C. When these mutations are combined in pairs, wild-type λ fails to form plaques on lawns of the double mutants even at 32°C. Lambda derivatives with the *punA1* mutation in *N* can grow in either *nusA1* or *nusE71* single mutants at 42°C but fail to grow in the *nusA1-nusE71* double mutant (Schauer *et al.*, 1987). As will be discussed in the section on the Q gene, the *nusA1-nusC60* double mutant fails to support the action of the λ Q antitermination function (unpublished results from this and the J. Roberts laboratories).

7. Suppressors of *nus* Mutations

Selecting second-site suppressors of mutations has proved to be a powerful tool for analyzing the physiological role of the gene identified by the original mutation. As discussed by Jarvik and Botstein (1975), the isolation of such suppressors suggests protein-protein interactions. Thus, identification of a second-site suppressor with a known physiological function can provide a useful clue to the role of the gene product being studied. The interactions suggested by the genetic studies can eventually be confirmed by appropriate biochemical studies.

a. Host Suppressors of nusA

Suppressors of two classes of *nusA* mutations have been isolated: (1) those that reverse the effect of a mutation that causes a failure in gpN action, and (2) those that overcome the lethality of conditional-lethal (*ts* and *cs*) mutations.

Suppressors that reverse the block in gpN action imposed by the *nusA1* mutation (the Nus$^-$ phenotype) will be examined first. Based on the Nus$^-$ phenotype of *nusA1*, Ward *et al.* (1983) isolated second-site suppressors employing a selection in which *gal* operon expression depends on gpN action and therefore also on the bacterium being phenotypically Nus$^+$ (Fig. 3). Localized mutagenesis with a specialized transducing phage was employed by these workers in the isolation of mutations in *nusB* that suppress the effect of the *nusA1* mutation on gpN action. Two types of suppressors in *nusB* were isolated. One, *nusB101*, suppresses the *nusA1* block of gpN$_\lambda$ action, and the other, *nusB201*, suppresses the block of gpN$_{21}$ action. Remarkably, these suppressors are specific; e.g., *nusB101* does not suppress the effect of *nusA1* on the action

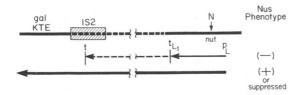

FIGURE 3. Selection for revertants of the Nus$^-$ phenotype using a fusion of the *gal* operon to the p_L promoter with an intervening IS2 element (Ward *et al.*, 1983). A functional Nus-gpN complex is required for expression of the *gal* genes because of a strong Rho-dependent terminator in the IS2. Nus$^-$ derivatives are therefore Gal$^-$, and revertants that are phenotypically Nus$^+$ can be selected as Gal$^+$ mutants.

of gpN$_{21}$. These results suggest interactions between (1) NusA and NusB and (2) NusB and gpN (Ward *et al.*, 1983).

Employing this selection procedure without localized mutagenesis, Gottesman and Ward (M. Gottesman, personal communication) identified another gene that could be mutated to yield a second-site suppressor of *nusA1*. This gene, *U*, maps at min 90 on the *E. coli* chromosome. The precise nature of the mutated gene has not been determined. Both the *nusB* and *U* suppressors also suppress the Nus$^-$ phenotype of *E. coli* carrying the *nusE71* mutation (Ward *et al.*, 1983; M. Gottesman, personal communication). Thus, these suppressors are not allele-specific and therefore cannot be cited as evidence for protein-protein interactions.

A second class of suppressors overcomes the effects of conditional lethal *nusA* mutations. These mutations, called *sna* (suppressor of *nusA*), have been isolated both for *nusAts* (Nakamura *et al.*, 1986) and *nusAcs* mutations (Schauer, 1985; unpublished experiments, this laboratory). Although the mapping of the suppressor mutations has not been definitively finished, preliminary mapping results place suppressors of the *nusAts11*, *sna* mutations, near the *rplKAJL-rpoBC* (min 90) and *rpsS-pnp* (min 69) loci (Nakamura *et al.*, 1986). Mutations suppressing *nusAcs10* have been mapped on both sides of the *argG* gene near *nusA* (unpublished experiments, this laboratory). One of these two mutations, which is necessary but not sufficient for suppression, maps within or immediately upstream of the *metY* gene, which is located promoter-proximal to the *nusA* gene in the *nusA-infB* operon (A. Granston, D. Carver, and L. Eades, unpublished experiments, this laboratory). The *metY* gene encodes a minor F-met tRNA (Ishii *et al.*, 1984b).

Another suppressor of the *nusAcs10* mutation was identified in an unusual manner (M. Craven, D. Alessi, A. Schauer, D. Friedman and D. Henner, unpublished results). A cloned fragment of *B. subtilis* DNA was found to complement the *cs* defect. Analysis of the nucleotide sequence of the gene responsible for complementation revealed that it is >50% homologous, at the amino acid level, with an *E. coli* gene previously identified as an open reading frame, *orfE*, located promoter-proximal to the *pyrE* gene at min 81 (Poulsen *et al.*, 1984). The cloned *E. coli orfE* gene can complement the *nusAcs10* mutation, but only when it is expressed from a promoter other than its natural promoter. This suggests that NusA may control the expression of the *orfE* gene product. Neither the *E. coli* nor the *B. subtilis orfE* genes complement the *nusAts11* defect for growth at high temperature. Current studies are directed toward understanding whether the *orfE* gene product is an essential function for the cell or indirectly influences the expression or action of other gene products. The observation that the *orfE* gene product suppresses the effect of a *cs*, but not a *ts*, mutation may reflect the fact that *nusA* is a cold-shock protein (Jones *et al.*, 1987).

Three particularly interesting findings about these suppressors emerge from these studies: (1) Many of the suppressors map in regions encoding factors involved in translation; (2) those that suppress the Nus⁻ phenotype of *nusA1* also show the same suppression for the *nusE71* mutation; and (3) they have little or no effect on the phenotype of *nusB* or *nusC* mutants.

b. Host Suppressors of nusE71

A number of second-site suppressors of the *nusE71* mutation have been isolated (Schauer, 1985). These mutations reverse the block in gpN action imposed by *nusE71*. The method of selection (see Fig. 3) for suppressors of *nus* mutations employed by Ward *et al.* (1983) was adapted to uncover second-site suppressors of the *nusE71* mutation. The selection was directed toward isolating mutations in genes encoding ribosomal proteins by employing the method of localized mutagenesis described by Hong and Ames (1971). Other mutations were isolated using nondirected mutagenesis techniques.

The best-described suppressor mutation, *sne16*, was isolated following localized mutagenesis directed toward the ribosomal gene cluster at min 72. This mutation has been mapped to the *rplP* gene, which encodes ribosomal protein L16 (Nomura *et al.*, 1977). Other suppressor mutations, mapping in this and other regions of the *E. coli* chromosome, have been isolated but have not been as well characterized (Schauer, 1985).

c. Joint Suppression of nusA1 and nusE71

Although the *nusA1* and *nusE71* mutations result in the alteration of proteins that appear to be functionally unrelated in terms of bacterial physiology, most second-site mutations that suppress the Nus⁻ phenotype of one of these mutations will suppress the Nus⁻ phenotype of the other. The *nusB101* mutation, selected as a suppressor of *nusA1*, also suppresses *nusE71* mutants; the double *nusB101-nusE71* host supports gpN action (Ward *et al.*, 1983; M. Gottesman, personal communication). A similar suppression of *nusE71* was observed when the *U* suppressor mapping at min 90 was examined (M. Gottesman, personal communication). The *sne16* second-site suppressor of the *nusE71* mutation also suppresses the Nus$^-$ phenotype of the *nusA1* mutation (unpublished experiments, this laboratory). This cross-suppression appears to occur only between the *nusA1* and *nusE71* mutations, since these suppressors do not affect the Nus$^-$ phenotype of mutations in other *nus* genes. However, it is not possible to determine if there is any allele specificity for suppression of either the *nusA* or *nusE* mutations, since *nusA1* and *nusE71* are the only characterized mutations in the respective genes that exhibit Nus$^-$ phenotypes.

Cosuppression of *nusA1* and *nusE71* is observed not only for second-site host mutations but also for phage mutations that were selected to overcome the inhibition imposed by either mutation. As discussed in the sections on *N* and *nut*, two types of phage mutations (other than those that eliminate the major $t_{R2}-t_{R3}$ termination region) have been identified that suppress, at least partially, the Nus$^-$ phenotype of both the *nusA1* and *nusE71* mutations. The first, *pun*, is a group of mutations in *N* (Franklin, 1985a; Schauer *et al.*, 1987; Friedman and Ponce-Campos, 1975), and the second, *boxA1* (Friedman and Olson, 1983; Schauer *et al.*, 1987), is in the *nut* region. These suppressors also do not significantly influence the Nus$^-$ phenotype of other *nus* mutations. An explanation for the diverse nature of the mutations that cosuppress the *nusA1* and *nusE71* mutations has been suggested by D. Court (personal communication). According to his hypothesis, NusA and NusE interact with a third protein, and all of the suppressors improve the action of this protein in N-mediated antitermination such that the resulting complex is functional even when one component is mutationally altered to a less active form.

d. Suppressors of nusC60

Suppressors of *nusC60* that relieve the Nus$^-$ phenotype have been isolated (D. Jin and C. Gross, personal communication). These mutations have been mapped at either of two loci—min 61 or min 82. Although the min 61 mutations have not been assigned to any identified locus, the min 82 mutations have been mapped to the *rpoB-C* genes.

e. Significance of Second-Site Suppressors

Two unexpected sets of observations on suppressors of the *nus* mutations seem significant and warrant further discussion. The first is the cosuppression by second-site suppressors of the Nus$^-$ phenotype of the *nusA1* and *nusE71* mutations. The second is the suppression of either the Nus$^-$ or conditional lethal phenotypes by mutations that map in genes whose products are involved in translation.

Although there is no definitive explanation for the wide range of suppressors that influence the phenotype of either a *nusA1* or *nusE71* host, I can offer some reasoned speculation. It seems likely that the modification of polymerase at *nut* is a concerted event with multiple proteins interacting (see Section II.E). Therefore, improvement of one interaction could nonspecifically compensate for a weakness in a second interaction. A stronger interaction at *nut* by a gpN with a *punA* alteration might compensate for either a weakened NusA or S10–NusE interaction. Consistent with this explanation is the observation that a λ *punA* phage fails to grow in a double *nusA1-nusE71* mutant (Schauer *et al.*, 1987).

A corollary to this idea is that the role of NusB in the reaction must differ in some substantive way from that of NusA or NusE. In this regard, the *in vitro* studies of Horwitz *et al.* (1987) suggest an important role for NusB in N-mediated antitermination; both the *nusA1* and *nusE71* mutations inhibit binding of NusB to the transcription complex. It is possible that all of the suppressors might improve NusB activity, obviating the effect of poor activity of other components; NusB might be the hypothetical factor whose interaction in the N reaction is improved by the suppressors of the *nusA1* and *nusE71* mutations. Arguing against a central role for NusB, however, are *in vitro* studies by W. Whalen and A. Das (personal communication) demonstrating that NusA and gpN, in the absence of other Nus factors, are sufficient to activate *nut*-facilitated antitermination. The latter studies suggest that NusA, rather than NusB, is the primary function required for antitermination.

The identification of suppressors in genes encoding translation factors, considered with the fact that one *nus* mutation has been mapped to a gene encoding a small ribosomal subunit protein, suggests that Nus action, at a minimum, could rely on some cooperative relationship with macromolecules involved in translation.

E. The Nut Site

1. Early Experiments

Roberts's antitermination model explained many of the observations on gpN action (Roberts, 1969). However, one critical set of observations remained unexplained. This resulting problem was dubbed by the cognoscenti "the paradox of *imm21*" (Herskowitz and Signer, 1970). Although phages λ and 21 express different N products, hybrid phages can be constructed that contain the N gene from one phage and terminators from the other phage. What appeared paradoxical was that although an N gene product can function to overcome an apparent heterologous termination signal in *cis*, it cannot overcome the same termination signal in *trans* (Couturier and Dambly, 1970; Herskowitz and Signer, 1970). Thus, although 21 fails to complement a λN⁻ phage, a viable hybrid phage can be constructed that has the N gene from 21 but the t_{R2}–t_{R3} region from λ.

This apparent paradox was solved by a model postulating that the sites for *recognition* of gpN on the phage genome differ from the sites of *action* of gpN (Friedman *et al.*, 1973b). Accordingly, the specificity for gpN is near the early promoters p_L and p_R in the immunity region (see Fig.

1), whereas the sites of action are at downstream terminators. Studies employing contructions in which the early λ promoters were fused to *E. coli* operons demonstrated that N-modified transcription could overcome the effects of polar mutations and other terminators on downstream gene expression (Segawa and Imamoto, 1976; Adhya *et al.*, 1974; Franklin, 1974). Since this antipolar effect of gpN requires the λ promoter to be in *cis* with the bacterial genes, these experiments were also interpreted as showing that the recognition sites for gpN were near the λ promoters.

2. The *nut* Region

The region of recognition for gpN and associated factors was identified by Salstrom and Szybalski (1978) who isolated *cis*-acting mutations that eliminate N modification of transcription from p_L without affecting initiation of transcription at p_L. These mutations, *nut*, map together downstream of p_L and upstream of N. Sequence analysis has revealed that *nut* mutations are in a region of 17 bp of hyphenated dyad symmetry (Somasekhar *et al.*, 1982) and that a similar sequence (16/17 bp) can be found in the p_R operon downstream of *cro* (Rosenberg *et al.*, 1978). In the ensuing discussion, I will refer to the sequences where various factors interact, presumably to modify polymerase into an antitermination complex, as the *nut* region.

Two types of experiments confirmed that the sequence identified in the p_R operon represents part of a functional *nut* site. First, when a region that includes the dyad symmetry is placed downstream of a non-λ promoter, *Pgal*, transcription from that promoter becomes termination-resistant in the presence of gpN (de Crombrugghe *et al.*, 1979). Second, mutations mapping in the vicinity of this dyad symmetry eliminate N modification of p_R transcription (Olson *et al.*, 1982).

Surprisingly, these latter mutations are not located in the *nut* region *per se* (Olson *et al.*, 1982). Sequence analysis shows that they are located in the 3′ region of the upstream *cro* gene (see Fig. 1). Four independently selected mutations all consist of a deletion of a single base pair in a run of AT bp in *cro* and are therefore called Δ*cro*. Moreover, this single-base pair deletion results in a shift in the reading frame of *cro*, causing translation to extend one additional amino acid beyond the normal site of termination. Since complementation studies revealed no alteration in the biological activity of the Cro protein encoded by the mutant allele, it was inferred that it is translation of four additional nucleotides into the *nut* region that interferes with the N modification reaction. Subsequent experiments, employing clones constructed in a terminator tester vector in which the reading frame can be altered so that the location of translation termination can be precisely controlled, demonstrated that the inhibition of gpN action by the Δ*cro* mutations requires translation to reach the translation termination signal at the extended 3′ end of the mutant *cro* gene (Olson *et al.*, 1984). If translation of *cro* is terminated at an upstream site, then there is no interference with the modification reaction, even though the mutation is present.

How can translation four nucleotides into the *nut* region interfere with the N modification reaction? It has been suggested that progression of ribosomes into this region hinders a protein-RNA interaction necessary for N modification (Olson *et al.*, 1982). Since the distance of the new termination site to the *nutR* hairpin loop is greater than the size of the ribosome, it was concluded that a more proximal sequence than the stem loop must be occluded. This led to the identification of the *boxA* sequence located promoter-proximal to the *nut* stem-loop structure.

Thus, the extent of the sequences involved in N-mediated alteration of polymerase appears to be greater than the hyphenated-dyad symmetry identified by the Salstrom and Szybalski (1978) work. At a minimum, two sequences are involved, the promoter-proximal *boxA* and the stem-loop structure, now referred to as *boxB*. A third region of homologies downstream of *boxB*, called *boxC*, has been identified (Friedman and Gottesman, 1983), but there is no evidence that the *boxC* sequence plays any functional roles in gp*N* action (Brown and Szybalski, 1985). The aggregate of these sequences and the surrounding sequences comprises the *nut* region.

3. *boxB*

For historical reasons, we will first discuss the *boxB* section of the *nut* region. Examination of the sequences in the positions analogous to the λ *nut* sequences of phages 21, P22, φ80, and HKO22 (Franklin, 1985; Tanaka and Matsushiro, 1985; Schwarz, 1980; J. Oberto and R. Weisberg, personal communication) all reveal regions of hyphenated dyad symmetry like *boxB* (see Fig. 4). Analysis of the sequences of these *boxB* stem loops reveals three important points: First, the *boxB* structures exhibit variations from phage to phage. Second, within these variations there are common motifs. Third, where the data are available, it can be seen that the two *boxB* structures within the same phage (in the *nutR* and *nutL* regions) have very similar sequences (see Fig. 4).

The intraphage specificity of the *boxB* sequences could reflect a functional role for *boxB* sequences recognizing their cognate N products. The interphage similarities found in the loop portion of the structure are subtle, but recognizable. All have runs of A's, and most have single translation termination codons. These limited homologies might explain how the *boxB* structures can be the gp*N* recognition elements even though, under certain conditions, heterologous N gene products are exchangeable (Schauer *et al.*, 1987; Hilliker and Botstein, 1976; N. Franklin, personal communication), and the *nun* gene product of HKO22 can act at λ *nut* sites (Gottesman and Weisberg, personal communication).

A functional role for the loop portion of *boxB* is suggested by the fact that the two Salstrom and Szybalski (1978) *nutL* mutations change a single base pair in the loop (Somasekhar *et al.*, 1982). Mutations in the

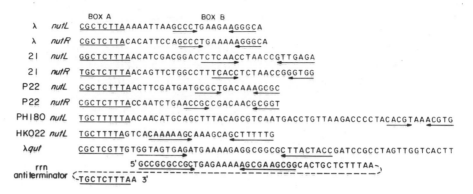

FIGURE 4. A comparison of the *nut* regions of various lambdoid phages (including related sequences adjacent (3') to the λ *qut* region). The *nut* region from the leader region of the *rrn* operons is also shown. The region of hyphenated dyad symmetry analogous to the λ *boxB* is located differently, 5' to the *boxA* sequence. The *rrn* sequence is drawn such that the *box* sequences of *rrn* are aligned with those of λ. The *boxA* sequences are underlined, and the putative *boxB* regions of hyphenated dyad symmetry are indicated by arrows. See text for the source of the sequences. Robert Weisberg's help in preparing this figure is gratefully acknowledged.

stem also cause a Nut⁻ phenotype but can be compensated by mutation in the other stem, which restores base pairing (Szybalski *et al.*, 1987).

4. *boxA*

Examination of the *nut* regions of various lambdoid phages also reveals that they contained sequences very similar to λ *boxA* in the same promoter-proximal position relative to *boxB*. Moreover, a consensus *boxA* sequence could be discerned: 5'CGCTCTT(T)A (see Fig. 4).

Studies of a λ mutant that can utilize the NusA of *S. typhimurium* (NusA^{Sal}), a NusA normally not compatible with λ growth, contribute supporting evidence that *boxA* is important for gpN action and could be involved, as discussed below, in NusA recognition (Friedman and Olson, 1983). Two mutations are required for λ to utilize NusA^{Sal}, one in *N* and the other in the *nutR*-associated boxA sequence (Friedman and Olson, 1983). The latter mutation, *boxA1*, results from a transversion, a T substituted for an A, with the resulting *boxA* sequence ending in three T's. This *boxA* sequence is close to that of phage P22 (Franklin, 1985a,b). Moreover, the *boxA* sequence of the *nutR* region of phage 21 also has the three T's. Even though both P22 and 21 can grow in the *E. coli* hybrid with NusA^{Sal}, it was striking to find that a λ derivative that could use NusA^{Sal} has a *boxA* sequence with three terminal T's.

These phages express functionally different *N* products (Hilliker and Botstein, 1976; Friedman *et al.*, 1973; Couturier and Dambly, 1970); i.e., they recognize different *nut* regions. Therefore, a sequence held in common among *nut* sites of different lambdoid phages (*boxA*) most likely defines regions of recognition for a shared host factor(s). The observation that an altered *boxA* permits λ to function with NusA^{Sal} suggested that this host factor might be NusA (Friedman and Olson, 1983). Consistent with this idea was the finding that sequences resembling the consensus *boxA* sequence are located near sites where NusA is known to act either in transcription termination or antitermination (Friedman and Gottesman, 1983). As mentioned previously, Horwitz *et al.* (1987) have studied the components of the N-mediated antitermination reaction. These studies suggest that *boxA* influences NusB activity, because in the absence of *boxA* and closely associated pairs, there is residual N-mediated antitermination, but this activity is not stimulated by the addition of NusB. However, as pointed out by Horwitz and co-workers, this does not necessarily mean that NusB acts directly with *boxA*. Its activity could be modulated by another factor; e.g., NusA.

Although many *boxA* sequences have C at their 5' ends, there are a number of significant exceptions (see Fig. 4); e.g., phage 21 has T at this position in its *nutR*. However, a recent study suggests that the consensus *boxA* sequence can be assigned a C at this position; when the 5' T in $nutR_{21}$ is changed to a C, a 21 derivative containing this altered sequence functions more effectively with NusA^{Sal} (at 43°C) and NusA1 (at 40°C) than do 21 phages with the wild-type *boxA* sequence (E. Olson, M. Craven, and D. Friedman, unpublished results). Moreover, it can be concluded from the previous discussion that the TTT arrangement at the 3' end of *boxA* is functionally more effective than the TT arrangement found in the wild-type λ *boxA*. Therefore, the optimal consensus *boxA* sequence for lambdoid phages is most likely 5'CGCTCTTTA.

Experiments using vectors designed to assess transcription termination yielded ambiguous information as to the role of *boxA* in N-mediated antitermination. Olson *et al.* (1984) found that when one bp in *boxA* was altered, antitermination activity was destroyed. The change, called *boxA5*, results in a *boxA* sequence reading 5'C*T*CTCTTA (changes here and below are italicized). Peltz *et al* (1985) altered another base pair in *boxA*, yielding the sequence 5'CG*G*TCTTA. They also found a loss of N-promoted antitermination activity with a single base pair change in *boxA* as well as other changes. The latter group reported that an intact *boxA* sequence is required only at higher temperatures (above 39°C); constructions with a *nut* region lacking a *boxA* sequence mediated N-antitermination at 30°C (see also Drahos *et al.*, 1982). They concluded that, in terms of gp*N* action, *boxA* is dispensable at low temperature. This finding is consistent with the earlier studies on *nus* mutants showing that λ growth (and thus N action) is more restricted in these mutants at higher temperatures (Friedman *et al.*, 1973a). However, another report contradicts the finding of temperature dependence for *boxA*. Brown and Szybalski (1985) reported that effective N antitermination requires both a *boxA* and *boxB* sequence when antitermination is measured at 30°C. The reason for this contradiction is not apparent, since there are no obvious differences among the plasmids, promoters, and terminators employed in these studies that could be responsible for the discrepancy. In a later study employing a series of artificially constructed *nut* regions, Hasan and Szybalski (1986b) concluded that the nature of the promoter influences the requirement for *boxA*. In this regard, it has been reported that gp*N* can, in the absence of a *nut* site, stimulate transcription from certain promoters by "about two-fold" (Drahos and Szybalski, 1981).

The experiments dscussed above employing different constructions showed that, at least at higher temperatures and perhaps at all temperatures, *boxA* is required for efficient N-mediated antitermination. However, work from another laboratory indicates that *boxA* is not necessary even at high temperature (Zuber *et al.*, 1987). These workers used constructions in expression vectors designed to test for antitermination and found that *nut* regions containing *boxB*, but deleted for the *boxA* sequence, functioned normally to facilitate N-mediated antitermination. However, recent studies employing the same vector system (D. Court, personal communication) show that the *boxA5* mutation eliminates N-mediated antitermination. Although this study demonstrates that there is no contradiction with the results of Olson *et al.* (1984), it raises a paradox relating to the functional role of *boxA*: namely, how can a single base change in *boxA* produce such a profound alteration in activity when a deletion of the sequence has no effect? M. Gottesman and co-workers (personal communication) find that a λ derivative with the *boxA5* mutation grows poorly and requires higher than normal levels of gp*N* activity to form an observable plaque. This result adds to the evidence that the *boxA5* mutation interferes with the operation of a sequence required for gp*N* action. Relevant to the paradoxical findings with *boxA* point and deletion mutations, these workers also find that the *boxA5* mutation causes the downstream t_{R1} terminator to be more active. This result suggests a complex interplay between signals and factors at *nut* influencing not only antitermination, but also termination in the absence of antitermination. In this regard, it is conceivable that *boxA5* imposes more termination at t_{R1}, rather than less antitermination activity, through its action at *nut*.

In assessing the results of the different experiments, it is important to consider the differences among the plasmid constructions employed. First, each laboratory used a different terminator signal. Olson *et al.* (1982) used a combination of λ t_{R1} and the Rho-dependent terminator found in IS2. Peltz *et al.* (1985) and Brown and Szybalski (1985) used the t_{L1} terminator. Zuber *et al.* (1987) used the t_I terminator. Second, the constructions of the first two groups had the potential for translation prior to the termination signal, but those of the last group did not. Although Zuber *et al.* (1987) suggest that translation either upstream or downstream of the *nut* region prior to the termination signal might impose a requirement for *boxA*, their recent findings with *boxA5* suggest that translation may not be an important factor in gp$N$ action. Consistent with the latter conclusion are *in vitro* studies (Greenblatt *et al.*, 1987) in which translation presumably did not occur, that demonstrated a requirement for *boxA* in the *nut* region (see below, Section II.E.5.b). Finally, in the studies of both Peltz *et al.* (1985) and Brown and Szybalski (1985), synthetic *boxA* and *boxB* cassettes were employed. The sequences between and surrounding the two boxes are not the same as those found in the phage. These additional sequences are also thought to influence N modification (Zuber *et al.*, 1987; Hasan and Szybalski, 1986a,b).

In addition to questioning the role of *boxA* in gp$N$ action, the Zuber experiments also challenge the idea that the sequence plays a role in NusA action. Those workers find that constructions lacking a *boxA* sequence fail to exhibit N-promoted antitermination in a *nusA1* host. Thus, in these experiments, the *nusA* mutation affects antitermination in the absence of the *boxA* sequence, implying that there can be NusA action in the absence of *boxA*. *In vitro* studies show that although there is a significant reduction in N-stimulated transcription in the absence of *boxA* and immediately adjacent bases, there is a residual (10%) level of stimulation without those sequences (Horwitz *et al.*, 1987).

One problem common to all of these experiments is the low levels of galactokinase expressed from the plasmids. For instance, in the experiments of Olson *et al.* (1984), maximal antitermination represents only one-fourth of the level of expression observed when the *galK* gene is directly fused to the same promoter. In assessing the results of experiments employing various plasmid constructions to test gp$N$ antitermination, it is obviously important to keep in mind that results of these experiments may not be a true reflection of what is occurring at the *nut* sites on the phage.

Arguing in favor of a role for *boxA* in NusA action as a factor in termination are the studies of Stewart and Yanofsky (1985, 1986) on attenuation in the tryptophanase operon of *E. coli*. These studies implicate a *boxA*-like sequence in NusA action as a termination factor in the attenuation process. Changes away from consensus reduce termination. In other studies, Lau and Roberts (1985) demonstrated, in an *in vitro* system, that NusA relieves Rho-imposed termination at some of the multiple termination sites in the λ t_{R1} region. A deletion of the adjacent *boxA* sequence substantially reduced this activity of NusA.

Other studies argue against this role for NusA. Studies of Chen and Richardson (1987) indicate that deletions of the *boxA* sequence have no effect on NusA interference with the *in vitro* activity of Rho at the t_{R1} terminators. Schmidt and Chamberlin (1987) have found that NusA enhances the efficiency of termination at both the t_{R2} terminator of λ and the T1 terminator of the *E. coli rrnB* operon. The latter workers pointed out that no *boxA* sequence can be identified in the regions of these terminators. However, a sequence with reasonable correspondence to what appears to be the essential bases of *boxA* is present in each of the identified structures of these terminators. This common sequence is 5'GGC-CUUU. The underlined bases represent differences from the consensus *boxA* sequence. However, it should be noted that in examining possible *boxA* sequences, the fourth and fifth nucleotides appear to vary somewhat but do maintain pyrimidines in these positions (Friedman and Gottesman, 1983), as do the sequences found in these two terminators. Whether these putative *boxA* sequences are functionally significant awaits experiments in which the effects of appropriate alterations on termination are tested.

5. Structure of the *nut* Region

a. Location and Function

The distance of the *nut* region from the upstream promoter is not critical for effective conversion to an antiterminating polymerase. This is readily apparent in the placement of the *nut* regions in the phages; nut_L sequences are located directly downstream of their respective p_L promoters, whereas the nut_R sequences have genes between themselves and their respective p_R promoters (Franklin, 1985a; Rosenberg *et al.*, 1978). However, the locations of the putative *nut* regions of the lambdoid phages are well conserved. This arrangement is very different from that of the recognition site, *qut*, for λ's other antitermination protein, gpQ. The *qut* site appears to be part of the promoter, p_R', whose transcription is altered by gpQ (see Section II.G).

b. Relative Positions of Component Elements

The *nut* regions of all lambdoid phages share a common structure. It should be emphasized that only in the case of λ are studies available that prove a functional role for the *nut* site. The sequence common to all *nut* regions (Fig. 4) is *boxA* located 5' to the *boxB* stem loop. The distances between these components vary among the different *nut* regions. Without functional studies, it can only be surmised that a stem-loop structure represents a functional *boxB*. The distance from the 3' A of *boxA* to the beginning of the loops of the *boxB* sequences varies from 13 to 19 nucleotides, suggesting that the positions of *boxA* and *boxB* sequences on the helix play no functional role, a conclusion consistent with the idea that RNA, and not DNA, is the nucleic acid sequence signaling the reaction (Olson *et al.*, 1984; Warren and Das, 1984). Constructs containing synthetic *boxA* and *boxB* modules showed that changing the distances between *boxA* and *boxB* had only a small effect on N-mediated antitermination (Brown and Szybalski, 1985).

A third region of homologies has been identified downstream of *boxB*, called *boxC*. These sequences, which contain the translation initiation codons AUG or GUG, have been shown to play no functional role in N-modified antitermination in an *in vivo* plasmid vector system (Peltz *et al.*, 1985; Brown and Szybalski, 1985) or an *in vitro* reaction (J. Greenblatt, personal communication). It is possible, however, that a more complicated signal is required to fully modify polymerase into a long-acting antitermination mode that is capable of functioning over long distances, as would be necessary for the expression of the delayed early genes of the phage.

6. Interactions at *nut*

The findings that translation into (Olson *et al.*, 1984; Warren and Das, 1984) or through (Zuber *et al.*, 1987) the *nut* region interferes with N-mediated antitermination and that the antitermination complex is sensitive to T1 ribonuclease (Horwitz *et al.*, 1987) suggest that at least part of the *nut* signal is RNA-determined. *In vitro* studies offer the most direct means for determining the nature of the interactions at the *nut* region. In essence, such studies would look at RNA polymerase and associated factors after initiation and compare the structure of a transcription complex prior to the time it traverses a *nut* region with its structure after traversing a *nut* sequence. Two schemes for examining such altered polymerase complexes will be discussed. As both are just being developed, the data discussed are very preliminary but certainly are consistent with the results of the genetic experiments that form the basis for our thinking about the role of the *nut* region.

a. Immunoprint Assay

Barik *et al.* (1987) have developed an ingenious method for determining the point beyond the promoter at which a transcription protein is associated with the transcribing RNA polymerase. In these experiments, gpN was employed as the associating protein. Using an antiserum specific for gpN, transcription complexes were precipitated from an *in vitro* antitermination reaction, and the isolated RNA was analyzed by gel electrophoresis. Significantly, only transcripts equal to or larger than the nucleotide distance extending from the transcription start site at p_R to the *nut* region were isolated from the immunoprecipitate. One likely scenario explaining these observations is that gpN accesses the transcription machinery at *nut* and proceeds along with the polymerase. Interestingly, extracts from *nus* mutants showed similar N binding. In other experiments, these workers found that when a T7 promoter was joined to a *nut* region, transcription by the T7 polymerase through *nut* did not, as in the case of the *E. coli* enzyme, result in binding of gpN to the polymerase. Thus, the N-*nut* system has specificity for the *E. coli* polymerase.

This "immunoprint" method offers a powerful technique for analyzing the antitermination complex in particular, but also interactions between RNA polymerases and proteins in general. For instance, anti-NusA antibody could be employed to determine if and where NusA binds to polymerase.

b. Chromatographic Analysis

Greenblatt and co-workers have employed HPLC on a TSK60 column to isolate modified RNA polymerase transcription complexes from S100 extracts (Greenblatt *et al.*, 1987; Horwitz *et al.*, 1987). These studies suggest not only that is a *nut* region necessary for binding gp*N* to the complex but that there is an apparent order to the addition of the modification factors.

Previous studies from the Greenblatt laboratory demonstrated that NusA associated with core polymerase but not with holoenzyme (Greenblatt and Li, 1981a). It was proposed that one molecule of NusA associates with polymerase after initiation of transcription. The recent studies have led Greenblatt to suggest that after passing through a *nut* site, polymerase with its bound NusA molecule acquires, in this order, one molecule of S10 (NusE), 0.2–0.5 molecules of NusB, then another molecule of NusA, and finally gp*N*. Thus, the N modification reaction appears to be a stoichiometric process. Although Greenblatt has shown that free NusA is found in dimers, only a monomer is bound in the initial association with polymerase. In the presence of gp*N* and a *nut* region, the ratio of NusA to polymerase is greatly increased, suggesting that NusA-gp*N* might join polymerase-NusA under the influence of *nut*. Significantly, the *nut* region required in these experiments included the *boxA* sequence. As discussed, it may be that NusB is essential for full gp*N* action by virtue of NusB's ability to interact with NusA and NusE (Horwitz *et al.*, 1987).

c. Additional Nus Factors

The *in vitro* studies have shown that the identified Nus factors are necessary, but not sufficient for optimal N modification (A. Das, personal communication). At least two additional host proteins are required. An *E. coli* mutant has been isolated that carries a mutation identifying a candidate for an additional Nus gene; this mutation does not map at any known *nus* locus (A. Das, personal communication).

7. Bacterial *nut* Region

Transcription antitermination has also been described for ribosomal RNA operons—e.g., *rrnB* of *E. coli* (reviewed by Morgan, 1986). Like λ *nut*, a region downstream of the *rrn* promoters confers termination resistance on the transcribing polymerases (see Fig. 4). This downstream region, *mirabile dictu*, contains sequences corresponding to the *boxA*, *boxB*, and *boxC* sequences found in the λ *nut* regions. However, the hyphenated dyad symmetry representing a potential *boxB* lies 5′ to the *boxA* sequence. Functional studies demonstrate a role for this *nut*-like region in antitermination (Li *et al.*, 1984; M. Cashel, personal communication; C. Squires, personal communication). Moreover, there is evidence implicating NusA and NusB in the *rrn* antitermination reaction (Sharrock *et al.*, 1985a; M. Cashel and M. Gottesman, personal communication). The component obviously missing from this catalog of factors is a bacterial analogue of gpN. Although there is no evidence for such a factor, this does not mean that such a component is not required. However, it is conceivable that the *rrn* antitermination operates in the absence of such a factor. That the λ and *rrn* antitermination systems share at least one common factor is indicated by the observation that transcription of the *nutL* region on a high-copy-number plasmid causes a reduction in the transcription of rRNA as well as growth rate (Sharrock *et al.*, 1985b). Hence, the two regions compete for at least one common factor.

F. A Model of N Action

A model of gpN action must explain not only how RNA polymerase is modified to an antitermination mode of operation but also the role of the various nucleic acid sequences and proteins implicated in the reaction. Aiding the consideration of the mechanism of gpN action is the ability to compare the activity of the closely related N systems of other lambdoid phages.

The evidence discussed above clearly shows that the *nut* region of λ is necessary and sufficient, in the presence of the appropriate factors, to impose antitermination upon RNA polymerase molecules that have initiated transcription at an upstream promoter. What is not obvious is the precise extent of the *nut* region and the roles of the various protein factors. Originally, *nut* was delineated by the hyphenated dyad symmetry identified by the Salstrom and Szybalski mutations (1978). Subsequently, additional sequences were identified as being necessary for gpN modification (Olson *et al.*, 1982). The demonstration that translation into the *nut* region interferes with the N modification reaction suggests that at least part of the nucleic acid signal is mediated by the mRNA transcript. It is conceivable that the entire signal is operating at the level of RNA. This would explain why the placement of the signals along the DNA helix can show variation among *nut* sites without apparently influencing the reaction; the helical surface of the DNA would obviously play no role in the recognition of the reacting proteins.

The apparently contradictory findings about the size of the *nut* site and the nature of the proteins involved could reflect the structure of the antitermination complex under different physiological conditions. The structure of the complex required may depend on the nature (quality) and/or the number (quantity) of the terminators that the polymerase subsequently encounters. A transcription complex partially modified owing to an incomplete nucleic acid signal or the lack of a protein factor might be active in overcoming some transcription terminators but not others. Consistent with the latter part of this argument is the observation that *in vivo* the N-modified polymerase loses potency over distance (Gottesman *et al.*, 1980), although Franklin (1974) showed that sequential terminators could be traversed with high efficiency.

The recent *in vitro* evidence elegantly confirms and extends working models derived from the extensive genetic studies. We can summarize the essential features of these models in the following steps:

1. RNA polymerase holoenzyme initiates transcription. In the phage, this would be at the early p_R and p_L promoters.
2. Transcription proceeds out, and one molecule of NusA associates with the polymerase shortly after the σ subunit of polymerase is lost (Greenblatt *et al.*, 1987).
3. The polymerase passes through the *nut* site and perhaps pauses after synthesizing the *nut* RNA (W. Whalen and A. Das, personal communication).
4. At this point the various Nus factors and gpN are mobilized. At a minimum, a component of the *nut* signal is RNA-determined. Whether the addition of Nus factors is a stoichiometric process is a matter of debate. In contradiction to the contention of the Greenblatt laboratory (Horwitz *et al.*, 1987), the Das group (A. Das, personal communication) finds that Nus factors are not added in stoichiometric amounts. It is likely that the component proteins act in a concerted manner, because changes in one factor suppress inhibitory changes in more than one other factor. For instance, a change in NusB can compensate for either a less active NusA or NusE protein. Similarly, changes in gpN can also compensate for the changes in NusA or NusE. This argues against independent allele specificity.
5. The immunoprint studies of the Das group (Barik *et al.*, 1987) suggest that, at a minimum, gpN continues to be associated with polymerase as it exits from the *nut* region. The studies of the Greenblatt group suggest that Nus factors also stay associated with polymerase. In addition, Greenblatt *et al.* (1987) have proposed that the Nus-gpN-polymerase complex remains stably bound to the *nut* RNA as the polymerase moves out from *nut*.

The mechanisms of the various interactions involved in the modification and subsequent action of the antitermination complex wait to be unraveled. In particular, three points of current contention must be resolved: (1) Is *boxA* required? (2) Is the host component central to the antitermination reaction NusA or NusB? (3) Do the factors act stoichiometrically? It is perhaps at the time of modification that the ribosomal components play a crucial role. How the modified transcription complex traverses terminators is also unknown. One simple idea is that the added factors trail (in either a real or symbolic way) the polymerase and block access to a signal required by termination factors or to the formation of a secondary structure in the RNA that might impose termination. Added to the list of unknowns is the question why some terminators are resistant to the N antitermination mechanism (Gottesman *et al.*, 1980).

It is hoped that this summary of the N antitermination system has provided the reader a useful primer into the workings of this complex system. Although there is much to be learned about the nature of the varied interactions at *nut*, it is obvious that genetic and biochemical experiments have uncovered significant information permitting, at a minimum, the definition of the next level of questions. This list includes *definitive* answers to such questions as these: Is the *nut* region signal read at the level of DNA or RNA, or are both nucleic acids involved? What are the protein-protein and protein–nucleic acid interactions? What is the precise change that renders an RNA polymerase molecule termination-resistant? Specifically, is there some type of allosteric change in one or more of the subunits of polymerase, or is the antitermination activity caused by one or more of the additional factors being bound to the polymerase?

G. The Q Transcription Antitermination Function

1. Action of gpQ

Expression of λ late genes, like that of delayed early genes, is primarily regulated by gpQ (Dove, 1966; Joyner *et al.*, 1966) through a transcription termination and antitermination mechanism (Roberts, 1975). Interestingly, even though late genes exhibit differential levels of expression, all 23 kb of late-gene DNA are transcribed from one promoter, p_R' (Daniels and Blattner, 1982). Transcription initiating at this promoter is constitutive but in the absence of the appropriate effector does not result in gene expression, because there is a strong terminator, t_R', located 194 bp downstream (Sklar *et al.*, 1975; Blattner and Dahlberg, 1972). In the presence of the activator, the λ-encoded Q gene product (gpQ) transcription initiating at p_R' becomes termination-resistant and overrides the subsequent terminators including t_R' (Roberts, 1975; Herskowitz and Signer, 1970). Thus, like N-imposed antitermination, gpQ-activation results in long-distance antitermination activity and is antipolar (Forbes and Herskowitz, 1982). Although gpQ appears to act in a manner similar to gpN, there are substantial differences between the two reactions in the requirement for host factors and the nature of the nucleic acid signal.

All of the lambdoid phages studied have Q-like antitermination functions. The Q product of λ and P22 are exchangeable (Roberts *et al.*,

1976), as are those of ϕ80 and 82 (Schleif, 1972). However, there is no exchange between members of the two pairs. Each of these phages synthesizes a leader RNA analogous to the constitutive short p_R' message of λ. However, each of the RNAs differs both in sequence and size from each other (Roberts, 1975; Roberts et al., 1976; Schechtman et al., 1980).

Although late genes are not normally expressed by a λ prophage, they can be turned on by an infecting lambdoid phage with a different immunity, provided the infecting phage expresses a compatible Q function; a process called "transinduction" (Dambly et al., 1970).

A number of studies indicated that gpQ acts preferentially in cis (Echols et al., 1976) at a site called qut (Salstrom and Szybalski, 1978) located in the region of p_R' (Grayhack et al., 1985; Somasekhar and Szybalski, 1983; Roberts, 1975; Herskowitz and Signer, 1970). In vitro studies have provided significant additional insights into the nature of the gpQ modification of polymerase (Grayhack and Roberts, 1982). This stands in contrast to in vitro studies of the gpN reaction, which have proved to be difficult to interpret because it has not been possible until recently to study the reaction with a totally purified system.

2. In Vitro Experiments

J. Roberts and co-workers have exploited the in vitro system to provide a rather complete picture of gpQ action (Yang et al., 1987; Grayhack et al., 1985; Grayhack and Roberts, 1982; Goliger and Roberts, 1987). The in vitro reaction requires gpQ, the host NusA protein, λ DNA containing the p_R' region (including the -35 and -10 sequences as well as a run of about 20 nucleotides downstream of p_R') and RNA polymerase. The specificity of the reaction was demonstrated conclusively by showing that transcription from other promoters does not antiterminate in the presence of gpQ. Moreover, fusion of a functional heterologous promoter, p_O, with all of the sequences 3' to the -6 position of p_R' failed to yield Q-mediated termination-resistant transcription (Yang et al., 1987). Thus, unlike nut, the Q recognition site, qut, cannot be separated from its promoter.

Employing a purified system with small DNA templates (e.g., 729 or 837 bp) that contain p_R', the Roberts group (J. Roberts, personal communication; Yang et al., 1987; Grayhack et al., 1985) has discovered the following additional important points about the Q reaction: (1) The Q protein does not have to be present at initiation of transcription to impose antitermination. (2) In the absence of gpQ, there is a prolonged pause (measured in minutes) at bp 16, resulting in the production of a so-called 16-mer RNA. The cause of this pause is not readily apparent from the sequence of the pause site. The pause occurs upstream of the boxA sequence identified in the qut region (see Fig. 4). (3) Extension of the paused RNA is facilitated in the presence of gpQ; extension of the 16-mer after the beginning of the pause occurs on the average within 6 min in the absence of gpQ and within 1.5 min in the presence of gpQ. (4) Interestingly, this extension is facilitated by NusA protein. (5) NusA also facilitates subsequent gpQ-mediated antitermination. (6) The gpQ-modified RNA polymerase is not terminator-specific and remains effectively modified after passing through the first of two tandem terminators.

3. The *qut* Region

The finding that the pause site is upstream from the *boxA* sequence raises a provocative, and to some disturbing, question as to the significance of the *boxA* sequence. Obviously, if *boxA* serves as a signal in the gpQ-NusA-mediated extension of the 16-mer, it would have to do so at the DNA level. This would mean that *boxA* may function differently in the *qut* region from how it does in the *nut* region (where, as we have seen, it has been postulated that the signal is read from the RNA). The role of *boxA* in the *qut* region is addressed by the finding that a deletion (+18) that deletes upstream toward the *qut* region (removing 5 bp from the 3' end of the *boxA* sequence) reduces the *in vitro* gpQ-NusA-mediated antitermination reaction by 50% (Grayhack et al., 1985) and *in vivo* by 80% (Somasekhar and Szybalski, 1987). Complicating this observation, however, is the fact that the junction created by the deletion forms a sequence maintaining what may be the essential features of *boxA*. The reconstructed *boxA* is 5'*CGC*GG*AATT* (the italicized bases are those that maintain a resemblance to the paradigm *boxA* sequence, CGCTCTTT).

Results from *in vivo* experiments are consistent with these *in vitro* findings. Employing plasmid constructions designed to study gpQ antitermination, it was shown that the same sequences are required for gpQ action *in vivo* as were shown to be necessary *in vitro* (Yang et al., 1987; Somasekhar and Szybalski, 1987). Although NusA is required for maximal Q-mediated readthrough of t_R', there are as yet no *nusA* mutations that significantly influence gpQ action. This is not surprising, since procedures for isolating *nusA* mutations have usually required that gpQ action not be hampered (Friedman, 1971). However, gpQ action is significantly curtailed in two *E. coli* multiple mutants: one carrying the *nusA1* and *nusC60* mutations (unreported experiments from this and the J. Roberts laboratories) and another a host with the *nusAts11* mutation and an outside suppressor of the *ts* phenotype (Nakamura et al., 1987).

Although the elements of the gpQ-*qut* interaction resulting in an antiterminating RNA polymerase appear to be the same both *in vivo* and *in vitro*, a higher concentration of gpQ is required for the *in vivo* reaction (Yang et al., 1987). One explanation for this difference is that the pause at the +16 position is a prerequisite for gpQ action, and this pause may be longer *in vitro*, giving more time for gpQ to act.

The boundaries of the *qut* region (i.e., the site of recognition for gpQ) were determined primarily in two ways (Yang et al., 1987; Somasekhar and Szybalski, 1983, 1987; S. Yang and J. Roberts, personal communication). The first employed deletions or additions that removed, replaced or altered the relative positions of segments of the genome in the p_R' region. The second used fusion of segments of p_R' with other promoters to yield functional hybrid promoters that could be tested for antitermination in the presence of gpQ. These studies identified the *qut* region as excluding the -35 of p_R' and extending from -17 to include sequences through $+18$ of the 6S coding region. Somasekhar and Szybalski (1987) find that transcription cannot be Q-modified if the *qut* site is separated from the p_R' promoter. Since, as previously discussed, gpQ can be added to the paused polymerase following initiation of transcription at p_R', this result suggests that the *qut* sequence may alter the initiating polymerase so that it can subsequently be modified by gpQ or that a subpopulation of modifiable RNA polymerase molecules is selected.

One of the most intriguing observations derived from the study of the 82 gpQ and its *qut* site (*modified* at the $+24$ position by a linker) is that transcription initiating at a p_R' with a modified *qut* is partially termination-resistant in the absence of gpQ (J. Goliger and J. Roberts, personal communication)! This, of course, implies that, at least for 82, there is antitermination activity associated with a modified *qut* signal independent of gpQ.

H. Retroregulation

The N-mediated antitermination process is incorporated in another mechanism of gene regulation—retroregulation. The details of this type of regulation have been extensively reviewed (Echols and Guaneros, 1983), and therefore this review will not deal in any substantive manner with the subject. The following is a brief summary of retroregulation, with emphasis on the role of transcription termination and antitermination in the process.

The λ *int* gene can be expressed from either of two promoters, p_L or p_I (see Fig. 1). Transcription from p_L is N-modified and therefore can override many termination signals, including t_I, which is downstream of the *int* gene. Transcription initiating at p_I requires stimulation by the cII protein. However, this transcription does not traverse a *nut* site and therefore cannot be N-modified. Thus, transcripts initiating at p_I terminate at t_I. The truncated p_I message obviously has a different 3' end from the readthrough p_L message. The latter RNA forms a structure at p_I that is processed by RNase III; the processing results in an increased lability of the *int* message. Thus, p_L transcription does not produce Int because of readthrough of a termination signal. This regulation is called "retro," because it depends on the formation and ultimate destruction of a message from a site beyond the regulated gene (Guarneros *et al.*, 1982; Schmeissner *et al.*, 1982; Luk *et al.*, 1982; Schindler and Echols, 1981; Belfort, 1980; Guarneros and Galindo, 1979).

Retroregulation of *int* expression provides a mechanism for controlling the site-specific recombination reactions that integrate and excise λ DNA from the bacterial chromosome. The high levels of Int required for integration are not expressed from p_L. Retroregulation allows the phage to separate the Int expression required for integration and subsequent lysogeny from the expression of p_L required for lytic growth (Echols and Guarneros, 1983). Retroregulation of *int* expression represents an example of how transcription termination and antitermination can be used to regulate expression of the same gene in different ways from different promoters.

I. Contraantitermination

Nature in her confounding manner has found another and apparently contradictory use for the *nut* region. This role for *nut* was discovered by M. Gottesman and R. Weisberg and co-workers (Robert *et al.*, 1987), who found that the prophage from lambdoid phage HKO22 (Dhillon *et al.*, 1980) inhibits the growth of λ, although λ is not repressed. In addition, functional studies show that this HKO22-imposed inhibition results from a termination of transcription.

1. The *nun* Gene

A series of studies exploring the nature of the HKO22-induced inhibition has permitted Robert *et al.* (1987) to understand the basis of this phenomenon, and the following discussion is based exclusively on their work. Mutational analysis of HKO22 demonstrates that the inhibition is imposed by a function encoded by the *nun* gene located to the left of the putative HKO22 *cI* repressor gene (inactivated by point and insertion mutations). Like other lambdoid phages, the HKO22 *cI* gene is flanked by sequences that resemble lambdoid operators. By position and size, the *nun* gene resembles the *N* genes of lambdoid phages. Surprisingly, unlike the other *N* gene products, Nun action is dispensable to HKO22 for both lytic growth and lysogeny. HKO22 phages with mutations in the *nun* gene do not inhibit λ growth, nor do they exhibit any reduction in antitermination if a polar insertion is placed downstream from *nun*.

In the presence of Nun, transcription initiating at the early λ promoters terminates at or near the *nut* sites. Moreover, this inhibition requires Nus functions. HKO22 fails to inhibit growth of λ in *nus* mutants. In these experiments λ*nin5*, a derivative able to grow in *nus⁻* hosts under normally restrictive conditions, was used. For example, λ*nin5* fails to grow in a *nusA⁺* host carrying an HKO22 prophage but does grow in an isogenic *nusA1* lysogen at the nonpermissive high temperature. The inhibition observed in the *nusA⁺* host does not require the presence of the λ *N* gene product, since a λ*bio30–7nin5* phage fails to grow in the *nus⁺*

HKO22 lysogen. Similar experiments with isogenic strains show that the *nusE71* and *nusB5* mutations have an even greater inhibitory effect on Nun action than the *nusA1* mutation.

These remarkable findings lead to the proposal that Nun acts essentially as the functional equivalent of a contra-gp*N*. This is not to say that Nun directly opposes gp*N* action, but rather that it terminates transcription at *nut* sites, apparently using much of the same molecular machinery, sites, and proteins that gp*N* employs to achieve antitermination.

2. *nun* and *nut*

Confounding the interpretation of the Nun phenomenon is the finding that Nun appears to terminate transcription only at λ *nut* sites. Phage 434 shares the same *N* gene and *nut* regions with λ, whereas phage 21 has a different *N* gene and *nut* region (Friedman *et al.*, 1973b; Eisen *et al.*, 1966). HKO22 inhibits growth of phages with the λ *nut* regions whether they carry the repressor region (called the immunity region) of 434 or λ, but it has no effect on the growth of phages with the immunity of phage 21. This specificity makes it unlikely that Nun acts as a general exclusion function such as the P22 Sie functions (Susskind and Botstein, 1978) or even λ Rex (Court and Oppenheim, 1983; Howard, 1967), which inhibits growth of a variety of competing phages.

Why HKO22 evolved such a specific inhibitory system is perplexing. I offer two hypotheses at this point and will return to the subject in the final discussion: (1) λ and HKO22 populated the same natural environment and therefore competed directly. Lambdoid phages with different *nut* regions were not present to a significant degree. HKO22 evolved the *nun* system in order to master this competition. (2) The *nun* product evolved as an antitermination function like gp*N*. gp*nun* initially acted at its own *nut* site to render transcription from the HKO22 early promoters termination-resistant. Because of putative similarities between the signals for gp*nun* and gp*N*, the former protein can recognize the λ *nut* region. However, gp*nun* interaction at *nut*λ is not functional; only a portion of the proteins and/or sites necessary for antitermination are called into play. This abortive attempt at antitermination results in premature termination of transcription at *nut*.

Four observations suggest that gp*nun* action requires, at least in part, the same factors and signals as gp*N*. First, *nut* mutations isolated as defective in gp*N* action have been shown to be defective for gp*nun* action. Second, analysis of the λ RNA synthesized in the presence of gp*nun* indicates that termination occurs at or near the *nut* site. Third, there is competition between the two proteins; the inhibitory action of gp*nun* on λ growth is overcome by overproduction of gp*N*. Fourth, as previously discussed, Nun action at *nut*λ appears to require Nus function.

A recent finding by the Gottesman group (M. Gottesman, personal communication) provides further evidence that the *nut* region signal is a factor in determining the functional activity of the transcription complex. These workers discovered that when the *nut* region contains the *boxA5* mutation, a mutation that results in a *nut* region dead to gpN action (see Section II.E.4), Nun promotes antitermination in the λ p_R operon. The reason for this role reversal is not known, but the fact that the same mutation reverses the roles of Nun and gpN suggests that a third protein (e.g., one of the Nus proteins) may actually recognize the *boxA* sequence.

Although the details of gp*nun* action are just being worked out, the Nun phenotype offers a unique tool to aid in the analysis of the N modification system. Identifying the shared components of the gp*nun* and gpN reactions versus those specific to one system should contribute further information to the ongoing effort to elucidate the functional roles of the components of the system. For instance, the fact that NusA is necessary for both gpN-mediated antitermination and gp*nun*-mediated termination is strong evidence for the model proposed above that NusA protein is neither a termination or antitermination protein, but rather must formally be an intermediary acting with other factors (proteins or sequences) to generate transcription complexes that recognize either termination or antitermination signals.

III. P2 PHAGES AND SATELLITE PHAGE P4

The P2 family of temperate phages, which are unrelated to lambdoid phages, are also able to grow in and lysogenize *E. coli* (see Bertani and Six, this volume, for details about P2 phages). The best-characterized representative of this group is phage P2. Two other phages of the P2 family have been studied to some extent—phages 186 and P4. There is evidence that these latter phages express transcription antitermination factors. Phage P4 is a satellite phage requiring a P2 or a P2-like helper for growth.

A. P2

Studies using nonsense mutations suggest that P2 does not encode an antitermination system (Sunshine *et al.*, 1971; Lindahl, 1971). This conclusion assumes that polarity would not be observed if an antitermination system were active. The late genes of P2 are expressed from four transcriptional units. Amber mutations in these operons exhibit polarity on the expression of promoter-distal genes. Late-gene expression is activated by the product of the *ogr* gene. The P2 *ogr* gene was identified by mutations (e.g., *ogr1*) that enable P2 to overcome a block in its growth imposed by a mutation (*rpoA109*) in the α subunit of the host RNA polymerase (Birkeland and Lindqvist, 1986; Christie and Calendar, 1985; Fujiki *et al.*, 1976; Sunshine and Sauer, 1975; Christie *et al.*, 1985). The *ogr* gene product acts in *trans* to stimulate transcription, but because polarity can be observed in P2 late operons, it is unlikely that it functionally resembles the λ *N* and *Q* products by having antitermination activity.

B. Phage 186

Analysis of phage 186 transcription suggests that gene expression from the P_R and P_{95} operons is regulated, at least in part, by termination and antitermination (Pritchard and Egan, 1985; J. B. Egan, personal communication). Even though protein synthesis is required for the observed antitermination, no candidate antitermination function has been identified. Analysis of the regions of apparent termination reveal terminatorlike sequences of hyphenated dyad symmetries. A thorough assessment of the significance of this antitermination will require the isolation of mutations that reduce or eliminate antitermination.

Phages P2 and 186 share similar genetic arrangements (Hocking and Egan, 1982). Thus, it is curious that even though P2 is the best-characterized phage of this family of phages, as discussed above there is no evidence that P2 has an antitermination system.

C. Satellite Phage P4

1. Helper Phage Function

Phage P4 differs from most viruses by virtue of the fact that its genome does not encode information for many of the functions it requires for lytic growth; i.e., the functions necessary for head and tail production, as well as lysis, must be supplied by a helper phage such as P2 (Six, 1975). In the presence of P4, these helper functions can be expressed even by a repressed P2 prophage. The helper genes can be activated in either of two ways by the satellite phage: (1) induction of the helper prophage and subsequent transcription controlled by helper factors (Six and Lindqvist, 1975; Geisselsoder *et al.*, 1981), or (2) transcription of helper genes controlled by a satellite phage-encoded protein, δ (a process called transactivation) (Souza *et al.*, 1977). Although P4 uses the capsid proteins expressed from the helper phage genome, studies on the P2 contribution to P4 production show that the capsid used by P4 has one-third the volume of the P2 capsid (Goldstein *et al.*, 1974).

Studies using P2 helper phages with amber mutations revealed that P4 encodes information that not only stimulates expression of helper phage genes, but suppresses polarity (Sauer *et al.*, 1981; Sunshine *et al.*, 1976). Two P4 gene products have been implicated as antitermination functions. These functions are encoded by genes *sid* and *psu* that map in the late transcription unit regulated by the δ transactivation gene product (Dale *et al.*, 1986). The δ gene is also located in this operon, which is located on the extreme right side of the standard P4 genetic map and has the order p_{sid}, *sid*, δ, *psu* (Dale *et al.*, 1986).

2. The *sid* Gene

The *sid* gene was identified by studies with the *sid1* mutation. P4*sid1* fails to direct the synthesis of small-size capsids from information encoded in the P2 genome; thus, the gene name: capsid size determination (Shore *et al.*, 1978; Geisselsoder *et al.*, 1978). Two observations led to the proposal that gp*sid* is an antitermination function: first, P4*sid1* phages fail to exhibit relief of polarity when transactivating gene expression from P2, and second, the failure of P4*sid1* to direct synthesis of small proheads can be suppressed in a host carrying the *rho102* allele. These observations led Geisselsoder *et al.* (1978) to propose that the *sid* gene product directs synthesis of small, P4-size proheads by antiterminating at a Rho-dependent termination signal(s) in a helper operon(s). According to this argument, antitermination results in increased concentrations of products of genes downstream of the termination signal, causing an alteration in the relative concentrations of proteins involved in prohead synthesis. The size of the prohead would then be determined by the relative concentrations of helper gene products. Studies with P4*psu* mutants argue against this model.

3. The *psu* Gene

The *psu* gene is located in the *sid* operon and was identified by mutations that render P4 ineffective in suppressing transcriptional polarity; this phenotype explains the derivation of its name, polarity suppression (Sauer *et al.*, 1981). Although the P4*psu*⁻ mutant is defective in polarity suppression and gives a somewhat reduced burst in the presence of a P2 helper, P4 proheads are synthesized. Thus, polarity suppression does not seem to be required for the production of P4 proheads. This makes it even more curious that a *rho* mutation suppresses the *sid1* mutation. Studies identifying *sid1* as a nonsense mutation (Lin, 1984; Lee, 1981; D. Kurnit, personal communication) offer an explanation for the failure of P4*sid1* to exhibit antipolarity. The *sid* gene is upstream of *psu* in the *sid* operon, and thus the nonsense *sid1* mutation could be polar on the expression of the downstream *psu* gene.

The ability of gp*psu* to act as an antitermination factor on bacterial operons was assessed by employing P4 derivatives that can propagate as plasmids (Lagos *et al.*, 1986). In these studies, an *E. coli* containing a *trp-lac* fusion in which *lac* expression depends on transcription from the *trp* promoter was employed. For transcription to extend into the *lac* operon, it must overcome the *trp* terminator. P4 plasmids expressing gp*psu* allow

transcription to overcome this termination. Since the plasmid constructions employed in these studies are incapable of integrating into the
bacterial chromosome, it is argued that the P4 function is acting in *trans*.
This means that either Psu action does not require a recognition signal
such as the *nut* or *qut* regions used by the λ antitermination proteins or
there is a Psu recognition sequence (*sut* or *put*?) at an appropriate position
in the *trp* operon. Lagos *et al.* (1986) have suggested that, unlike the λ
antitermination functions, the *psu* protein acts directly as an anti-Rho
function.

Tests of polarity suppression have identified only Psu as a P4 antitermination protein (Sauer *et al.*, 1981). Since *psu*⁻ derivatives grow in a
relatively normal manner, it is difficult to see how antitermination could
influence capsid formation. However, one observation is consistent with
transcription termination's having an influence on P2 capsid size: P2
infection leads to the formation of small proheads in the *rho102* host. It is
not known whether the formation of small proheads in the *rho102* host is
due directly to the overriding of a termination signal on the P2 genome or
only a change in the physiological state of the host imposed by the *rho*
mutation. The latter explanation is consistent with observations that *rho*
mutations can cause many physiological abnormalities in *E. coli*, including a failure to support growth of phage P2 (Gulletta *et al.*, 1983; Das *et
al.*, 1978).

Finally, it should be noted that even though early studies implicated
the P4 δ gene product in Psu antipolarity (Sauer *et al.*, 1981), more recent
studies argue against such an interaction (Dale *et al.*, 1986; Lagos *et al.*,
1986; N. Linderoth, personal communication).

IV. CONCLUSIONS

Before beginning a discussion of the specifics of regulation of phage
gene expression by transcription antitermination, I would like to stress
the importance of considering the rationale for the choice of one mechanism of regulation over another. For instance, it might seem curious that
expression from the λ genome is both negatively controlled by the *c*I
repressor and positively regulated by transcription antitermination functions. A deterministic explanation for these regulatory mechanisms is
offered by the "demand theory" (Savageau, 1983a). In brief, this theory
proposes that if regulation of a biological system is favored, then it will
evolve in such a way that loss of that regulation will be selected against.
Thus, temperate phages have evolved negative controls (repressors) for
the lysogenic state, because loss of control means loss of lysogeny. On the
other hand, temperate phages have evolved positive control for lytic
growth, because loss of control means loss of viability. In each case, then,
selection will be against the loss of regulation.

First identified as an important mechanism regulating expression of genes in phage λ, transcription termination-antitermination has been described as a mechanism for regulation of operons in E. coli as well as other phages. If past studies of other regulatory mechanisms can serve as a model, this type of regulation will likely be found to occur in higher organisms. Indeed, it has been postulated that gene expression from SV40 and HIV-1 may in part be governed by termination-antitermination of transcription (Hay et al., 1982; Kao et al., 1987), and this form of regulation may be operative in some eukaryotic genes (Bentley and Groudine, 1986; Nepveu and Marcu, 1986).

what advantage regulation of gene expression by termination and antitermination offers to the phage. Max Gottesman and I have addressed this point in a previous article, and those arguments still hold (Friedman and Gottesman, 1983). I will summarize them and present additional arguments.

1. One means for a phage to acquire new genes is by recombination with other genetic elements (Campbell and Botstein, 1983). In this way, phages might have incorporated relatively large changes in single steps. However, there is one obvious problem in such a strategy. If new genes are recombined within existing phage operons that contain termination signals, there could be an interruption of downstream gene expression. Thus, essential phage functions might not be expressed. By having an antitermination mechanism that modifies RNA polymerase at the beginning of an operon, the phage ensures that transcription overcomes such termination signals.

2. Retroregulation of gene expression requires a process of termination and antitermination. As discussed above, such regulation of the int gene would not be possible without N-modified transcription.

3. The nature of the phage-encoded components of the termination-antitermination system permits their clustering in a small region of the genome. Thus, in the case of the gpN, both its gene and sites of recognition, nut, are located in the central control (immunity) region. This centralization of control elements would appear to be essential for temperate phages, because they must stringently control gene expression so that the repressed prophage does not express lytic functions that could be lethal to its host. The N antitermination system permits the phage to regulate expression of genes removed from the central control region at sites near these distal genes, terminators, without having the control elements, nut, substantially removed from the control (immunity) region. Thus, all of the major control elements of λ can be centrally located in the small cassette of genes and elements called the immunity region. Obviously, this rationale does not explain the reason for gpQ regulation, since the Q gene lies distal to the

immunity region. I can offer one explanation for this regulatory scheme. Q expression ultimately depends on N expression, and, because of the vagaries of λ regulation, gp$Q$ might be an auxiliary antitermination function whose role is to replace gp$N$ after lytic growth has commenced.

4. The final argument is based on the assumption that temporal regulation of genes in an ordered and timely manner is important for maximal viral production. For instance, expression and replication of the viral genome must obviously precede packaging. Thus, packaging functions are usually expressed late in viral development. The antitermination mode of regulation does not influence initiation of transcription, since the entire regulatory machinery is placed downstream of the promoter. Therefore, the system is primed to proceed into the unexpressed genes immediately upon receipt of the appropriate signal. In essence, the RNA polymerase can be thought of as being in an "idling" mode primed to continue transcription into the forbidden regions when given the appropriate signal. Thus, antitermination offers a means to regulate genes whose products are required immediately upon demand. In the case of phage, such regulation could ensure that replication, genome processing, and packaging proceed in an orderly and timely manner.

A possible pathway for the evolution of the lambdoid antitermination mechanism is suggested by two studies in which factors involved in termination and antitermination operate in contradictory manners. First is the finding that *E. coli* proteins (NusA, NusB, and NusD) required for N-mediated antitermination are also involved in transcription termination. Second is the studies on the exceptional lambdoid phage HKO22. The Nun protein of HKO22 resembles gp$N$ of λ but functions as a termination factor at λ *nut* sites and requires at least some of the Nus factors. Moreover, the structure of the *nut* regions resembles the structure of some terminators; both have regions of hyphenated dyad symmetry and impose pausing on RNA polymerase.

Perhaps the λ*nut* sites and the HKO22 *nun* gene represent components of an early termination system. Such a system, relying on host termination factors (e.g., NusA and NusB) in addition to Nun, could conceivably have been present in the progenitor of the lambdoid phages. The need for some type of positive regulatory system with the characteristics of an antitermination system as outlined above might have resulted in the coevolution of antitermination functions and sites for their action. Speculating further, it is possible that λ evolved so that the *nut* site remained relatively unchanged, whereas the N gene diverged to a greater extent. In the case of HKO22, the opposite may have been true: the *nut* sites diverged to a greater extent than the *nun* gene. Thus, the more conserved elements of each phage can still recognize each other and, when placed together, reconstitute the original functional unit to perform its original activity—termination.

This model for the evolution of the N antitermination mechanism explains the apparent peculiarity of the Nun-*nut* interaction and explains why an antitermination system employs factors involved in termination. In this regard, based on the logic of the demand theory discussed above (Savageau, 1983b), a negative control system with the characteristics of contraantitermination (protermination), such as seen with HKO22 Nun at *nut*λ, should be found.

On this speculative note, we leave the subject looking forward to future results that will define the nature of the protein-protein and protein–nucleic acid interactions that alter the polymerase so that it recognizes termination signals or disregards such signals. Understanding these reactions may well change our concept of RNA polymerase; this molecule may be extremely fluid in structure, varying considerably depending on the nature of the signals that it encounters at initiation and during elongation of transcription.

ACKNOWLEDGMENTS. The author thanks all of the people who have worked in his laboratory on this subject. Special thanks are in order for Andrew Granston for help with the figures, and Diane Alessi and Eileen Lynch for their helpful criticism. Rich Calendar, Naomi Franklin, Mike Imperiale, Don Court, Asis Das, Max Gottesman, Jeff Roberts, Al Schauer, Jack Greenblatt, Wes Dunnick, Robert Weisberg, and Waclaw Szybalski are thanked for their helpful comments. In addition, I thank many of my other colleagues in the field for making results available and for their cooperation over the years: S. Adhya, L. Baron, M. Baumann, B. Bigelow, D. Carver, M. Chamberlin, M. Craven, D. Court, A. Das, L. Eades, J. Eagan, H. Echols, E. Flamm, C. Georgopoulos, L. Gold, L. Goldstein, J. Greenblatt, C. Gross, G. Gussin, D. Henner, I. Herkowitz, M. Howe, F. Imamoto, C. Jolly, D. Kurnit, K. Leason, B. Lindqvist, R. Losick, A. Matsushiro, D. McGrath, R. Mural, Y. Nakamura, N. Nossal, A. Oppenheim, E. Olson, S. Penner, J. Richardson, M. Rosenberg, A. Schauer, M. Strauch, T. Platt, J. Wilgus, and L. Zelig.

Ruth Douglas and Jana Gilbert are gratefully acknowledged for their careful help in preparing the manuscript. Work in the author's laboratory was supported by grants 2 R01 AI 11459-14 and 5RO1 AI 14363-10 from the National Institutes of Health.

REFERENCES

Adhya, S., and Gottesman, M., 1978, Control of transcription termination, *Annu. Rev. Biochem.* **47**:967.

Adhya, S., Gottesman, M., and de Crombrugghe, B., 1974, Release of polarity in *Escherichia coli* by gene N of phage λ: Termination and antitermination of transcription, *Proc. Natl. Acad. Sci. USA* **71**:2534.

Ames, B. N., and Hartman, P. E., 1963, The histidine operon, *Cold Spring Harbor Symp. Quant. Biol.* **28**:357.

Barik, S., Ghosh, B., Whalen, W., Lazinski, D., and Das, A., 1987, An antitermination protein engages the elongating transcription apparatus at a promoter-proximal recognition site, *Cell* **50**:885.

Baron, L. S., Penido, E., Ryman, I. R., and Falkow, S., 1970, Behavior of coliphage lambda in hybrids between *Escherichia coli* and *Salmonella*, *J. Bacteriol.* **102**:221.

Barthelemy, I., Salas, M., and Mellado, R. P., 1987, *In vivo* transcription of bacteriophage φ29 DNA: Transcription termination, *J. Virol.* **61**:1751.

Baumann, M. F., and Friedman, D. I., 1976, Cooperative effects of bacterial mutations affecting λ *N* gene expression, *Virology* **73**:128.

Bear, D. G., McSwiggen, J. A., Morgan, W. D., and Von Hippel, P. H., 1985, Mechanisms of Rho-dependent transcription termination site selection, in: *Sequence Specificity in Transcription and Translation* (R. Calendar and L. Gold, eds.), pp. 137–150, Alan R. Liss, New York.

Bektesh, S. L., and Richardson, J. P., 1980, A ρ-recognition site on phage λ *cro*-gene mRNA, *Nature* **283**:102.

Belfort, M., 1980, The cII-independent expression of phage λ *int* gene in RNase III-defective *E. coli*, *Gene* **11**:149.

Bentley, D. L., and Groudine, M., 1986, A block to elongation is largely responsible for decreased transcription of c-*myc* in differentiated HL60 cells, *Nature* **321**:702.

Birkeland, N. K., and Lindqvist, B. H., 1986, Coliphage P2 late control gene *ogr*: DNA sequence and product identification, *J. Mol. Biol.* **188**:487.

Blattner, F., and Dahlberg, J., 1972, RNA synthesis start points in bacteriophage lambda: Are the promoters and operators transcribed?, *Nature New Biol.* **237**:232.

Botstein, D., and Herskowitz, I., 1974, Properties of hybrids between *Salmonella* phage P22 and coliphage λ, *Nature* **251**:584.

Brachet, P., Eisen, H., and Rambach, A., 1970, Mutations of coliphage λ affecting the expression of replicative functions O and P, *Mol. Gen. Genet.* **108**:266.

Brody, E., Rabussay, D., and Hall, D. H., 1983, Regulation of transcription of prereplicative genes, in: *Bacteriophage T4* (C. K. Mathews, E. M. Kutter, G. Mosig, and P. B. Berget, eds.), pp. 174–183, American Society for Microbiology, Washington.

Brown, A. L., and Szybalski, W., 1985, Transcriptional antitermination activity of the synthetic *nut* elements of coliphage lambda. I. Assembly of the *nut*R recognition site from *boxA* and *nut* core elements, *Gene* **39**:121.

Brunel, F., and Davison, J., 1975, Bacterial mutants able to partly suppress the effect of *N* mutations in bacteriophage λ, *Mol. Gen. Genet.* **136**:167.

Campbell, A., and Botstein, D., 1983, Evolution of the lambdoid phages, in: *Lambda II* (R. W. Hendrix, F. W. Stahl, and R. A. Weisberg, eds.), pp. 365–380, Cold Spring Harbor Laboratory, Cold Spring Harbor, NY.

Chen, C. A., Galluppi, G. R., and Richardson, J. P., 1986, Transcription termination at λ tR1 is mediated by interaction of Rho with specific single-stranded domains near the 3′ end of *cro* mRNA, *Cell* **46**:1023.

Chen, C.-Y., and Richardson, 1987, Sequence elements essential for ρ-dependent transcription termination at λt_{R1}, *J. Biol. Chem.* **262**:11292.

Christie, G., and Calendar, R., 1985, Bacteriophage P2 late promoters. II. Comparison of the four late promoter sequences, *J. Mol. Biol.* **181**:373.

Christie, G. E., Haggard-Ljungquist, E., Feiwell, R., and Calendar, R., 1986, Regulation of bacteriophage P2 late gene expression: The *ogr* gene, *Proc. Natl. Acad. Sci. USA* **83**:3238.

Court, D., and Oppenheim, A. B., 1983, Phage lambda's accessory genes, in: *Lambda II* (R. W. Hendrix, F. W. Stahl, and R. A. Weisberg, eds.), pp. 251–277, Cold Spring Harbor Laboratory, Cold Spring Harbor, NY.

Court, D., and Sato, K., 1969, Studies of novel transducing variants of lambda: Dispensibility of genes *N* and *Q*, *Virology* **39**:348.

Court, D., Brady, C., and Rosenberg, M., 1980, Control of transcription termination: A Rho-dependent termination site in bacteriophage lambda, *J. Mol. Biol.* **138**:231.

Couturier, M., and Dambly, C., 1970, Activation sequentielle des fonctions tardives chez les bacteriophage temperes, *C. R. Acad. Sci. Paris* **270**:428.

Dale, E. C., Christie, G. E., and Calendar, R., 1986, Organization and expression of the satellite bacteriophage P4 late gene cluster, *J. Mol. Biol.* **192**:793.

Dambly, C., Couturier, M., and Thomas, R., 1968, Control of development of temperate bacteriophages. II. Control of lysosyme synthesis, *J. Mol. Biol.* **32**:67.

Dambly-Chaudiere, C., Gottesman, M., Debouck, C., and Adhya, S., 1983, Regulation of the pR operon of bacteriophage lambda, *J. Mol. Appl. Genet.* **2**:45.

Daniels, D. L., and Blattner, F. R., 1982, The nucleotide sequence of the Q gene and the Q to S intergenic region of bacteriophage lambda, *Virology* **117**:81.

Daniels, D. L., Schroeder, J. L., Szybalski, W., Sanger, F., and Blattner, F. R., 1983, A molecular map of coliphage lambda, in: *Lambda II* (R. W. Hendrix, J. W. Roberts, F. W. Stahl, and R. A. Weisberg, eds.), pp. 469–676, Cold Spring Harbor Laboratory, Cold Spring Harbor, NY.

Das, A., and Wolska, K., 1984, Transcription antitermination *in vitro* by lambda N gene product: Requirement for a phage *nut* site and the products of host *nusA, nusB,* and *nusE* genes, *Cell* **38**:165.

Das, A., Court, D., and Adhya, A., 1978, Isolation and characterization of conditional lethal mutants of *Escherichia coli* defective in transcription termination factor *rho, Proc. Natl. Acad. Sci. USA* **73**:1959.

Das, A., Gottesman, M. E., Wardwell, J., Trisler, P., and Gottesman, S., 1983a, A mutation in the *Escherichia coli rho* gene that inhibits the N protein activity of phage λ, *Proc. Natl. Acad. Sci. USA* **80**:5530.

Das, A., Shoemaker, K., Wardwell, J., and Wolska, K., 1983b, Role of *Escherichia coli nusAB* genes in lambda N protein-mediated transcription antitermination in plasmid pBR322 leading to galactokinase synthesis, in: *Microbiology 1983* (D. Schlessinger, ed.), pp. 43–48, American Society for Microbiology, Washington.

Das, A., Ghosh, B., Barik, S., and Wolska, K., 1985, Evidence that ribosomal protein S10 itself is a cellular component necessary for transcription antitermination by phage λ N protein, *Proc. Natl. Acad. Sci. USA* **82**:4070.

de Crombrugghe, B., Adhya, S., Gottesman, M., and Pastan, I., 1973, Effect of *rho* on transcription of bacterial operons, *Nature* **241**:260.

de Crombrugghe, B., Mudryj, M., DiLaura, R., and Gottesman, M., 1979, Specificity of the bacteriophage lambda *N* gene product (pN): *nut* sequences are necessary and sufficient for the antitermination by pN, *Cell* **18**:1145.

Dhillon, T. S., Dhillon, E. K. S., and Lair, A. N. C., 1980, Genetic recombination between phage HKO22, λ and φ80, *Virology* **109**:198.

Doi, R. H., and Wang, L.-F., 1986, Multiple procaryotic ribonucleic acid polymerase sigma factors, *Microbiol. Rev.* **50**:227.

Dove, W. F., 1966, Action of the λ chromosome. I. Control of functions late in bacteriophage development, *J. Mol. Biol.* **19**:187.

Drahos, D., and Szybalski, W., 1981, Antitermination and termination functions of the cloned *nutL, N* and *tL1* modules of coliphage lambda, *Gene* **16**:261.

Drahos, P., Galluppi, G. R., Caruthers, M., and Szybalski, W., 1982, Synthesis of the *nutL* DNA segments and analysis of antitermination and termination functions of coliphage λ, *Gene* **18**:343.

Echols, H., and Guarneros, G., 1983, Control of integration and excision, in: *Lambda II* (R. W. Hendrix, J. W. Roberts, F. W. Stahl, and R. A. Weisberg, eds.), pp. 75–92, Cold Spring Harbor Laboratory, Cold Spring Harbor, NY.

Echols, H., Court, D., and Green, L., 1976, On the nature of *cis*-acting regulatory proteins and genetic organization in bacteriophage: The example of Q of bacteriophage lambda, *Genetics* **83**:5.

Eisen, H. A., Fuerst, C. R., Siminovitch, L., Thomas, R., Lambert, L., Pereira da Silva, L., and Jacob, F., 1966, Genetics and physiology of defective lysogeny in K12(λ): Studies of early mutants, *Virology* **30**:224.

Fiandt, M., Hradecna, Z., Lozeron, H. A., and Szybalski, W., 1971, Electron micrographic mapping of deletions, insertions, inversion, and homologies in the DNA's of coliphages λ and ϕ80, in: *The Bacteriophage Lambda* (A. D. Hershey, ed.), pp. 329–354, Cold Spring Harbor Laboratory, Cold Spring Harbor, NY.

Forbes, D., and Herskowitz, I., 1982, Polarity suppression by the Q gene product in phage lambda, *J. Mol. Biol.* **160**:549.

Franklin, N. C., 1974, Altered reading of genetic signals fused to the N operon of bacteriophage λ: Genetic evidence for the modification of polymerase by the protein product of the *N* gene, *J. Mol. Biol.* **89**:33.

Franklin, N. C., 1985a, Conservation of genome form but not sequence in the transcription antitermination determinants of bacteriophage λ, ϕ21 and P22, *J. Mol. Biol.* **181**:75.

Franklin, N. C., 1985b, "*N*" transcription antitermination proteins of bacteriophages λ, ϕ21, and P22, *J. Mol. Biol.* **181**:85.

Franklin, N. C., and Bennett, G. N., 1979, The N protein of bacteriophage lambda, defined by its DNA sequence, is highly basic, *Gene* **8**:107.

Franklin, N. C., and Luria, S. E., 1961, Transduction by bacteriophage P1 and the properties of the lac genetic region in *E. coli* and *S. dysenteriae*, *Virology* **15**:299.

Friedman, D., 1971, A bacterial mutant affecting λ development, in: *The Bacteriophage Lambda* (A. D. Hershey, ed.), pp. 733–738, Cold Spring Harbor Laboratory, Cold Spring Harbor, NY.

Friedman, D. I., and Baron, L. S., 1974, Genetic characterization of a bacterial locus involved in the activity of the N function of phage λ, *Virology* **58**:141.

Friedman, D., and Gottesman, M., 1983, Lytic mode of lambda development, in: *Lambda II* (R. W. Hendrix, J. W. Roberts, F. W. Stahl, and R. A. Weisberg, eds.), pp. 21–51, Cold Spring Harbor Laboratory, Cold Spring Harbor, NY.

Friedman, D. I., and Olson, E. R., 1983, Evidence that a nucleotide sequence, "boxA," is involved in the action of the NusA protein, *Cell* **34**:143.

Friedman, D. I., and Ponce-Campos, R., 1975, Differential effect of phage regulator functions on transcription from various promoters: Evidence that the P22 gene *24* and the λ *N* gene products distinguish three classes of promoters, *J. Mol. Biol.* **98**:537.

Friedman, D. I., Jolly, C. T., and Mural, R. J., 1973a, Interference with the expression of the N gene product of phage λ in a mutant of *Escherichia coli*, *Virology* **51**:216.

Friedman, D. I., Wilgus, G. S., and Mural, R. J., 1973b, Gene N regulator function of phage λimm21: Evidence that a site of N action differs from a site of N recognition, *J. Mol. Biol.* **81**:505.

Friedman, D. I., Baumann, M., and Baron, L. S., 1976, Cooperative effects of bacterial mutations affecting λ N gene expression. I. Isolation and characterization of a *nus*B mutant, *Virology* **73**:119.

Friedman, D. I., Schauer, A. T., Baumann, M. R., Baron, L. S., and Adhya, S. L., 1981, Evidence that ribosomal protein S10 participates in the control of transcription termination, *Proc. Natl. Acad. Sci. USA* **78**:1115.

Friedman, D. I., Schauer, A. T., Mashni, E. J., Olson, E. R., and Baumann, M. F., 1983, *Escherichia coli* factors involved in the action of the λ gene *N* antitermination function, in: *Microbiology 1983* (D. Schlessinger, ed.), pp. 39–42, American Society for Microbiology, Washington.

Friedman, D. I., Olson, E. R., Georgopoulos, C., Tilly, K., Herskowitz, I., and Banuett, F., 1984, Interactions of bacteriophage and host macromolecules in the growth of bacteriophage λ, *Microbiol. Rev.* **48**:299.

Friedman, D. I., Schauer, A. T., Olson, E. R., Carver, D. L., Eades, L. J., and Bigelow, B., 1985, Proteins and nucleic acid sequences involved in regulation of gene expression by the bacteriophage λ N transcription antitermination function, *Microbiology* **1985**:271.

Fujiki, H., Palm, P., Zillig, W., Calendar, R., and Sunshine, M., 1976, Identification of a mutation within the structural gene for the alpha subunit of DNA-dependent RNA polymerase of *E. coli*, *Mol. Gen. Genet.* **145**:19.

Geisselsoder, J., Chidambaram, M., and Goldstein, R., 1978, Transcription control of capsid size in the P2:P4 bacteriophage system, *J. Mol. Biol.* **126**:447.

Geisselsoder, J., Youderian, P., Deho, G., Chidambaram, M., Goldstein, R., Ljungquist, E.,

1981, Mutants of satellite virus P4 that cannot derepress their bacteriophage P2 helper, *J. Mol. Biol.* **148**:1.

Gemski, P. Jr., Baron, L. S., and Yamamoto, N., 1972, Formation of hybrids between coliphage λ and *Salmonella* phage P22 with a *Salmonella typhimurium* hybrid sensitive to these phages, *Proc. Natl. Acad. Sci. USA* **69**:3110.

Georgopoulos, C. P., 1971a, A bacterial mutation affecting N function, in: *The Bacteriophage Lambda* (A. Hershey, ed.), pp. 639–645, Cold Spring Harbor Laboratory, Cold Spring Harbor, NY.

Georgopoulos, C. P., 1971b, Bacterial mutants in which the gene N function of bacteriophage lambda is blocked have an altered RNA polymerase, *Proc. Natl. Acad. Sci. USA* **68**:2977.

Georgopoulos, C. P., Swindle, J., Keppel, F., Ballivet, M., Bisig, R., and Eisen, H., 1980, Studies on the *E. coli groNB (nusB)* gene which affects bacteriophage λ N gene function, *Mol. Gen. Genet.* **179**:55.

Ghosh, B., and Das, A., 1984, nusB: A protein factor necessary for transcription antitermination *in vitro* by phage λ N gene product, *Proc. Natl. Acad. Sci. USA* **81**:6305.

Ghysen, A., and Pironio, M., 1972, Relationship between the N function of bacteriophage λ and host RNA polymerase, *J. Mol. Biol.* **65**:259.

Gilbert, W. R., and Lozeron, H. A., 1983, Regulation of transcription and DNA replication of bacteriophage φ80, *Virology* **126**:635.

Goda, Y., and Greenblatt, J., 1985, Efficient modification of *E. coli* RNA polymerase *in vitro* by the N gene transcription antitermination protein of bacteriophage lambda, *Nucleic Acids Res.* **13**:2569.

Goldstein, R., Lengyel, J., Pruss, G., Barrett, K., Calendar, R., and Six, E., 1974, Head size determination and the morphogenesis of satellite phage P4, *Curr. Top. Microbiol. Immunol.* **68**:59.

Goliger, J. A., and Roberts, J. W., 1987, Bacteriophage gene Q and Q protein, *J. Biol. Chem.* **262**:11721.

Gottesman, M. E., Adhya, S., and Das, A., 1980, Transcription antitermination by bacteriophage lambda N gene product, *J. Mol. Biol.* **140**:57.

Gottesman, S., Gottesman, M., Shaw, J. E., and Pearson, M. L., 1981, Protein degradation in *E. coli*: The *lon* mutation and bacteriophage lambda N and cII protein stability, *Cell* **24**:225.

Grayhack, E. J., and Roberts, J. W., 1982, The phage λ gene Q product: Activity of a transcription antiterminator *in vitro*, *Cell* **30**:637.

Grayhack, E. J., Yang, X., Lau, L. F., and Roberts, J. W., 1985, Phage lambda gene Q antiterminator recognizes RNA polymerase near the promoter and accelerates it through a pause, *Cell* **42**:259.

Greenblatt, J., 1981, Regulation of transcription termination by the N gene protein of bacteriophage lambda, *Cell* **24**:8.

Greenblatt, J., 1984, Regulation of transcription in *Escherichia coli*, *Can. J. Biochem. Cell Biol.* **62**:79.

Greenblatt, J., and Li, J., 1981a, The *nusA* gene protein of *Escherichia coli*: Its identification and a demonstration that it interacts with the gene N transcription anti-termination protein of bacteriophage lambda, *J. Mol. Biol.* **147**:11.

Greenblatt, J., and Li, J., 1981b, Interaction of the sigma factor and the *nusA* gene protein of *E. coli* with RNA polymerase in the initiation-termination cycle of transcription, *Cell* **24**:421.

Greenblatt, J., Malnoe, P., and Li, J., 1980a, Purification of the gene N transcription antitermination protein of bacteriophage λ, *J. Biol. Chem.* **255**:1465.

Greenblatt, J., Li, J., Adhya, S., Friedman, D. I., Baron, L. S., Redfield, B., Kung, H., and Weissbach, H., 1980b, L factor that is required for β-galactosidase synthesis is the *nusA* gene product involved in transcription termination, *Proc. Natl. Acad. Sci. USA* **77**:1991.

Greenblatt, J., McLimont, M., and Hanly, S., 1981, Termination of transcription by *nusA* gene protein of *Escherichia coli*, *Nature* **292**:215.

Greenblatt, J., Horwitz, R. J., and Li, J., 1987, Genetic and structural analysis of an elongation control particle containing the N protein of bacteriophage lambda, in: *RNA Polymerase and the Regulation of Transcription* (W. S. Renznikoff, R. R. Burgess, J. E.
Dahlberg, C. A. Gross, M. T. Record, and M. P. Wickens, eds.), pp. 357–366, Elsevier,
New York.

Guarneros, G., and Galindo, J. M., 1979, The regulation of integrative recombination by the
b2 region and the *cII* gene of bacteriophage λ, *Virology* **95**:119.

Guarneros, G., Montanez, C., Hernandez, T., and Court, D., 1982, Posttranscriptional control of bacteriophage λ *int* gene expression from a site distal to the gene, *Proc. Natl.
Acad. Sci. USA* **79**:238.

Gulletta, E., Das, A., and Adhya, S., 1983, The pleiotropic *ts15* mutation of *E. coli* is an IS1
insertion in the *rho* structural gene, *Genetics* **105**:265.

Hasan, N., and Szybalski, W., 1986a, Boundaries of the *nutL* antiterminator of coliphage
lambda and effects of mutations in the spacer region between *boxA* and *boxB*, *Gene*
50:87.

Hasan, N., and Szybalski, W., 1986b, Effect of the promoter structure on the transcription
antitermination function, *Gene* **50**:97.

Hay, N., Skolnick-David, H., and Aloni, Y., 1982, Attenuation in the control of SV40 gene
expression, *Cell* **29**:183.

Heinemann, S., and Spiegelman, W., 1970, Role of the gene *N* product in phage lambda,
Cold Spring Harbor Symp. Quant. Biol. **35**:315.

Herskowitz, I., and Signer, E. R., 1970, Control of transcription from the *r* strand of bacteriophage lambda, *Cold Spring Harbor Symp. Quant. Biol.* **35**:355.

Hilliker, S., and Botstein, D., 1976, Specificity of genetic elements controlling regulation of
early functions in temperate bacteriophages, *J. Mol. Biol.* **106**:537.

Hilliker, S., Gottesman, M., and Adhya, S., 1978, The activity of *Salmonella* phage P22 gene
24 product in *Escherichia coli*, *Virology* **86**:37.

Hocking, S. M., and Egan, J. B., 1982, Genetic map of coliphage 186 from a novel use of
marker rescue frequencies, *Mol. Gen. Genet.* **187**:87.

Hong, J. S., and Ames, B. N., 1971, Localized mutagenesis of any specific small region of the
bacterial chromosome, *Proc. Natl. Acad. Sci. USA* **68**:3158.

Horwitz, R. J., Li, J., and Greenblatt, J., 1987, An elongation control particle containing the
N gene transcriptional antitermination protein of bacteriophage lambda, *Cell* **51**:631.

Howard, B. D., 1967, Phage lambda mutants deficient in rII exclusion, *Science* **158**:1588.

Hyman, H., and Honigman, A., 1986, Transcription termination and processing sites in the
bacteriophage λ p_L operon, *J. Mol. Biol.* **189**:131.

Imamoto, F., and Nakamura, Y., 1986, *Escherichia coli* proteins involved in regulation of
transcription termination: Function, structure, and expression of the *nusA* and *nusB*
genes, *Adv. Biophys.* **21**:175.

Ishii, S., Kuroki, K., Sugino, Y., and Imamoto, F., 1980a, Purification and characterization of
the *N* gene product of bacteriophage lambda, *Gene* **10**:291.

Ishii, S., Salstrom, J., Sugino, Y., Szybalski, W., and Imamoto, F., 1980b, A biochemical assay
for the transcription-antitermination function of the coliphage λ *N* gene, *Gene* **10**:17.

Ishii, S., Ihara, M., Maekawa, T., Nakamura, Y., Uchida, H., and Imamoto, F., 1984a, The
nucleotide sequence of *nusA* and its flanking region of *Escherichia coli*, *Nucleic Acids
Res.* **12**:3333.

Ishii, S., Kuroki, K., and Imamoto, F., 1984b, tRNA^{met} gene in the leader region of the nusA
operon in *Escherichia coli*, *Proc. Natl. Acad. Sci. USA* **81**:409.

Ishii, S., Hatada, E., Maekawa, T., and Imamoto, F., 1984c, Molecular cloning and nucleotide sequence of the *nusB* gene of *E. coli*, *Nucleic Acids Res.* **12**:4987.

Jacob, F., and Monod, J., 1961, Genetic regulatory mechanisms in the synthesis of proteins,
J. Mol. Biol. **3**:318.

Jarvik, J., and Botstein, D., 1975, Conditional-lethal mutations that suppress genetic defects
in morphogenesis by altering structural proteins, *Proc. Natl. Acad. Sci. USA* **72**:2738.

Jones, P. G., VanBogelen, R. A., and Neidhardt, F. C., 1987, Induction of proteins in response
to low temperature in *Escherichia coli*, *J. Bacteriol.* **169**:2092.

Joyner, A. L., Isaacs, N., Echols, H., and Sly, W. S., 1966, DNA replication and messenger RNA production after induction of wild-type bacteriophage and mutants, *J. Mol. Biol.* **19:**174.

Kaiser, A. D., and Jacob, F., 1957, Recombination between related temperate bacteriophages and the genetic control of immunity and prophage localization, *Virology* **4:**509.

Kamen, R. I., 1975, Structure and function of the Qβ replicase, in: *RNA Phage* (N. Zinder, ed.), pp. 203–234, Cold Spring Harbor Laboratory, Cold Spring Harbor, NY.

Kanemoto, K., Tanaka, S., Miyashita, T., and Matsushiro, A., 1986, Identification and purification of the *N* gene product of bacteriophage φ80, *Mol. Gen. Genet.* **205:**523.

Kao, S.-Y., Colman, A. F., Luciw, P. A., and Peterlin, B. M., 1987, Anti-termination of transcription within the long terminal repeat of HIV-1 by *tat* gene product, *Nature* **330:**484.

Kasai, T., 1974, Regulation of the expression of the *histidine* operon in *Salmonella typhimurium*, *Nature* **249:**523.

Keppel, F., Georgopoulos, C. P., and Eisen, H., 1974, Host interference with expression of the lambda *N* gene product, *Biochimie* **56:**1503.

Kolter, R., and Yanofsky, C., 1982, Attenuation in amino acid biosynthetic operons, *Annu. Rev. Genet.* **16:**113.

Kourilsky, P., Bourguignon, M., Bouquet, M., and Gros, F., 1970, Early transcription control after induction of prophage λ, *Cold Spring Harbor Symp. Quant. Biol.* **35:**305.

Kourilsky, P., Bourguignon, M. F., and Gros, F., 1971, Kinetics of viral transcription after induction of prophage, in: *The Bacteriophage Lambda* (A. D. Hershey, ed.), pp. 647–666, Cold Spring Harbor Laboratory, Cold Spring Harbor, NY.

Kroeger, M., and Hobom, G., 1982, The *nin* region of bacteriophage lambda: A chain of interlinked genes, *Gene* **20:**25.

Kumar, S., Calef, E., and Szybalski, W., 1970, Regulation of the transcription of *Escherichia coli* phage λ by its early genes *N* and *tof*, *Cold Spring Harbor Symp. Quant. Biol.* **35:**331.

Kung, H., Spears, C., and Weissbach, H., 1975, Purification and properties of a soluble factor required for the deoxyribonucleic acid-directed *in vitro* synthesis of β-galactosidase, *J. Biol. Chem.* **250:**1556.

Kuroki, K., Ishii, S., Kano, Y., Miyashita, T., Nishi, K., and Imamoto, F., 1982, Full transcription of the tryptophan operon *in vitro* is improved by the *nusA* and *nusB* gene products, *Mol. Gen. Genet.* **185:**369.

Lagos, R., Jiang, R.-Z., Kim, S., and Goldstein, R., 1986, An extrachromosomal gene product which antagonizes Rho-dependent termination of a bacterial operon, *Proc. Natl. Acad. Sci. USA* **83:**9561.

Lau, L., Roberts, J. W., and Wu, R., 1982, Transcription terminates at the λt$_{R1}$ in three clusters, *Proc. Natl. Acad. Sci. USA* **79:**6171.

Lau, L. F., and Roberts, J. W., 1985, ρ-Dependent transcription termination at λ t$_{R1}$ requires upstream sequences, *J. Biol. Chem.* **260:**574.

Leason, K. R., 1986, Terminators involved in phage lambda lytic regulation, Ph.D. dissertation, University of Michigan, Ann Arbor.

Lecocq, J. P., and Dambly, C., 1976, A bacterial RNA polymerase mutant that renders growth independent of *N* and *cro* function at 42°, *Mol. Gen. Genet.* **145:**53.

Lee, S.-J., 1981, Altered patterns of gene expression by satellite phage P4 mutants unable to regulate their P2 helper, M.A. Thesis, Harvard University, Cambridge, MA.

Li, S. C., Squires, C. L., and Squires, C., 1984, Antitermination of *E. coli* rRNA transcription is caused by control region segment containing lambda *nut*-like sequences, *Cell* **38:**851.

Liedke-Kulke, M., and Kaiser, A. D., 1967, Genetic control of prophage insertion specificity in bacteriophage λ and 21, *Virology* **20:**465.

Lin, C.-S., 1984, Nucleotide sequence of the essential region of bacteriophage P4, *Nucleic Acids Res.* **12:**8667.

Lindahl, G., 1971, On the control of transcription in bacteriophage P2, *Virology* **46:**426.

Lozeron, H. A., Dahlberg, J. E., and Szybalski, W., 1976, Processing of the major leftward mRNA of coliphage lambda, *Virology* **71:**262.

Lozeron, H. A., Subbarao, M. N., Daniels, D. L., and Blattner, F. R., 1977, Transcriptional antitermination and RNase III-mediated processing of the major RNA transcripts of bacteriophage lambda, in: *Microbiology 1983* (D. Schlessinger, ed.) pp. 74–77, American Society for Microbiology, Washington.

Luk, K.-C., and Szybalski, W., 1982, Characterization of the cloned terminators t_{R1}, t_{L3} and t_1, and of the *nut*R antitermination site of coliphage lambda, *Gene* **20**:127.

Luk, K.-C., Dobnenski, P., and Szybalski, W., 1982, Cloning and characterization of the termination site t_I for the gene *int* transcript in phage lambda, *Gene* **17**:259.

Luzati, D., 1970, Regulation of λ exonuclease synthesis: Role of the N gene product and λ repressor, *J. Mol. Biol.* **49**:515.

Maekawa, T., Nagase, T., Imamoto, F., and Ishii, S., 1985, Purification of the NusB gene product of *Escherichia coli* K12, *Mol. Gen. Genet.* **200**:14.

McKnight, S., and Tjian, R., 1986, Transcriptional selectivity of viral genes in mammalian cells, *Cell* **46**:795.

Morgan, E. A., 1986, Antitermination mechanism in rRNA operons of *Escherichia coli*, *J. Bacteriol.* **168**:1.

Nakamura, Y., and Mizusawa, S., 1985, *In vivo* evidence that the *nusA* and *infB* genes of *E. coli* are part of the same multi-gene operon which encodes at least four proteins, *EMBO J.* **4**:527.

Nakamura, Y., and Uchida, H., 1983, Isolation of conditionally lethal amber mutations affecting synthesis of *nusA* protein of *Escherichia coli*, *Mol. Gen. Genet.* **190**:196.

Nakamura, Y., Mizusawa, S., Court, D. L., and Tsugawa, A., 1986, Regulatory defects of conditionally lethal *nusA*ts mutants of *Escherichia coli*, *J. Mol. Biol.* **189**:103.

Nakamura, Y., Tsugawa, A., Saito, M., and Egawa, K., 1987, Genetic dissection of the *nusA* protein of *Escherichia coli*, in: *RNA Polymerase and the Regulation of Transcription* (W. S. Reznikoff, R. R. Burgess, J. E. Dahlberg, C. A. Gross, M. T. Record, and M. P. Wickens, eds.), pp. 367–380, Elsevier, New York.

Nepveu, A., and Marcu, K. B., 1986, Intragenic pausing and anti-sense transcription within the murine c-*myc* locus, *EMBO J.* **5**: 2859.

Nijkamp, H. J. J., Bovre, K., and Szybalski, W., 1970, Control of rightward transcription in coliphage λ, *J. Mol. Biol.* **54**:599.

Nomura, M., Morgan, E. A., and Jaskunas, S. R., 1977, Genetics of bacterial ribosomes, *Annu. Rev. Genet.* **11**:297.

Olson, E. R., Flamm, E. L., and Friedman, D. I., 1982, Analysis of *nut*R: A region of phage lambda required for antitermination of transcription, *Cell* **31**:61.

Olson, E. R., Tomich, C. C., and Friedman, D. I., 1984, The *nusA* recognition site: Alteration in its sequence or position relative to upstream translation interferes with the action of the N antitermination function of phage λ, *J. Mol. Biol.* **180**:1053.

Peltz, S. W., Brown, A. L., Hasan, N., Podhajska, A. J., and Szybalski, W., 1985, Thermosensitivity of a DNA recognition site: Activity of a truncated *nut*L antiterminator of coliphage lambda, *Science* **228**:91.

Platt, T., 1986, Transcription termination and the regulation of gene expression, *Annu. Rev. Biochem.* **55**:339.

Plumbridge, J. A., Dondon, J., Nakamura, Y., and Grunberg-Manago, M., 1985, Effect of NusA protein on expression of the *nusA*, *infB* operon in *E. coli*, *Nucleic Acids Res.* **13**:3371.

Poulsen, P., Bonekamp, F., and Jensen, K. F., 1984, Structure of the *Escherichia coli pyrE* operon and control of *pyrE* expression by a UTP modulated intercistronic attenuation, *EMBO J.* **3**:1783.

Pritchard, M., and Egan, J. B., 1985, Control of gene expression in P2-related coliphages: The *in vitro* transcription pattern of coliphage 186, *EMBO J.* **4**:3599.

Ptashne, M., 1986, *A Genetic Switch: Gene Control and Phage* λ, Cell Press and Blackwell Scientific Publications, Palo Alto, CA.

Rabussay, D., and Geiduschek, E. P., 1977, Regulation of gene action in the development of lytic bacteriophages, in: *Comprehensive Virology 8* (F.-C. Wagner, ed.), pp. 1–150, Plenum Press, New York.

Richardson, J. P., Fink, P., Blanchard, K., and Macy, M., 1977, Bacteria with defective Rho factors suppress the effects of N mutations in bacteriophage λ, *Mol. Gen. Genet.* **153**:81.

Robert, J., Sloan, S. B., Weisberg, R. A., Gottesman, M. E., Robledo, R., and Harbrecht, D., 1987, The remarkable specificity of a new transcription termination factor suggests that the mechanisms of termination and antitermination are similar, *Cell* **51**:483.

Roberts, J. W., 1969, Termination factor for RNA synthesis, *Nature* **224**:1168.

Roberts, J. W., 1970, The ρ factor: Termination and anti-termination in lambda, *Cold Spring Harbor Symp. Quant. Biol.* **35**:121.

Roberts, J. W., 1975, Transcription termination and late control in phage lambda, *Proc. Natl. Acad. Sci. USA* **72**:3300.

Roberts, J. W., 1988, Phage lambda and the regulation of transcription termination, *Cell* **52**:5.

Roberts, J. W., Roberts, C. W., Hilliker, S., and Botstein, D., 1976, Transcription termination and regulation in bacteriophages P22 and lambda, in: *RNA Polymerase* (R. Losick, and M. Chamberlain, eds.), pp. 707–718, Cold Spring Harbor Laboratory, Cold Spring Harbor, NY.

Rosenberg, M., Court, D., Shimatake, H., Brady, C., and Wulff, D. L., 1978, The relationship between function and DNA sequence in an intercistronic regulatory region of phage λ, *Nature* **272**:414.

Saito, M., Tsugawa, A., Egawa, K., and Nakamura, Y., 1986, Revised sequence of the *nusA* gene of *Escherichia coli* and identification of *nusA(ts)* and NusA1 mutations which cause changes in a hydrophobic cluster, *Mol. Gen. Genet.* **205**:380.

Salstrom, J. S., and Szybalski, W., 1978, Coliphage λnutL⁻: A unique class of mutants defective in the site of gene N product utilization for antitermination of leftward transcription, *J. Mol. Biol.* **124**:195.

Sauer, B., Ow, D., Ling, L., and Calendar, R., 1981, Mutants of satellite bacteriophage P4 that are defective in the suppression of transcriptional polarity, *J. Mol. Biol.* **145**:29.

Savageau, M., 1983a, Regulation of differentiated cell-specific functions, *Proc. Natl. Acad. Sci. USA* **80**:1411.

Savageau, M., 1983b, Models of gene function: General methods of kinetic analysis and specific ecological correlates, in: *Foundations of Biochemical Engineering: Kinetics and Thermodynamics in Biological Systems*, ACS Symposium series 207 (H. W. Blanch, E. T. Papoutskais, and G. Stephanopoulos, eds.), pp. 3–25, American Chemical Society, Washington.

Schauer, A. T., 1985, Proteins involved in phage λ transcription antitermination, Ph.D. Dissertation, University of Michigan, Ann Arbor.

Schauer, A. T., Carver, D. L., Bigelow, B., Friedman, D. I., and Baron, L. S., 1987, The λ N antitermination system: Functional analysis of phage interactions with host NusA protein, *J. Mol. Biol.* **194**:679.

Schechtman, M. G., Snedeker, J. D., and Roberts, J. W., 1980, Genetics and structure of the late regulatory region of phage 82, *Virology* **105**:393.

Schindler, D., and Echols, H., 1981, Retroregulation of the *int* gene of bacteriophage λ: Control of translation completion, *Proc. Natl. Acad. Sci. USA* **78**:4475.

Schleif, R., 1972, The specificity of lambdoid phage late gene induction (lambdoid phage late gene specificity), *Virology* **50**:610.

Schmeissner, U., Court, D., McKenney, K., and Rosenberg, M., 1981, Positively activated transcription of λ integrase gene initiates with UTP *in vivo*, *Nature* **292**:173.

Schmidt, M., and Chamberlin, M., 1987, The *nusA* protein of *Escherichia coli* is an efficient transcription termination factor for certain terminator sites, *J. Mol. Biol.* **195**:809.

Schwarz, E., 1980, Sequenz analyse des DNA lambdoide bacteriophages, Ph.D. Thesis, University of Freiburg, Freiburg, F.R.G.

Segawa, T., and Imamoto, F., 1976, Diversity of regulation of genetic transcription. II. Specific relaxation of polarity in *in vitro* transcription of the translocated *trp* operon in bacteriophage lambda *trp*, *J. Mol. Biol.* **87**:741.

Sharrock, R. A., Gourse, R. L., and Nomura, M., 1985a, Defective antitermination of rRNA transcription and derepression of rRNA and tRNA synthesis in the *nusB5* mutant of *Escherichia coli, Proc. Natl. Acad. Sci. USA* **82**:5275.

Sharrock, R. A., Gourse, R. L., and Nomura, M., 1985b, Inhibitory effect of high-level transcription of the bacteriophage *nutL* region on transcription of rRNA in *Escherichia coli, J. Bacteriol.* **163**:704.

Shaw, J. E., Jones, B. B., and Pearson, M. L., 1978, Identification of the *N* gene protein of bacteriophage λ, *Proc. Natl. Acad. Sci. USA* **75**:2225.

Shimotsu, H., and Henner, D. J., 1986, Contruction of a single-copy integration vector and its use in analysis of regulation of the *trp* operon of *Bacillus subtilis, Gene* **43**:85.

Shore, D., Deho, G., and Goldstein, R., 1978, Determination of capsid size by satellite bacteriophage P4, *Proc. Natl. Acad. Sci. USA* **75**:400.

Simon, L. D., Gottesman, M., Tomczak, K., and Gottesman, S., 1979, Hyperdegradation of proteins in *Escherichia coli rho* mutants, *Proc. Natl. Acad. Sci. USA* **76**:1623.

Six, E., 1975, The helper dependence of satellite bacteriophage p4: Which gene functions of bacteriophage P2 are needed by P4, *Virology* **67**:249.

Six, E., and Lindqvist, B., 1978, Mutual derepression in the P2-P4 bacteriophage system, *Virology* **87**:217.

Sklar, J. L., Yot, P., and Weissman, S. M., 1975, Determination of genes, restriction sites and DNA sequences surrounding the 6s RNA template of bacteriophage lambda, *Proc. Natl. Acad. Sci. USA* **72**:1817.

Somasekhar, G., and Szybalski, W., 1983, Mapping of the Q-utilization site (*qut*) required for antitermination of late transcription in bacteriophage lambda, *Gene* **26**:291.

Somasekhar, G., and Szybalski, W., 1987, The functional boundaries of Q-utilization (*qut*) site required for antitermination of late transcription in bacteriophage lambda, *Virology* **158**:414.

Somasekhar, G., Drahos, D., Salstrom, J., and Szybalski, W., 1982, Sequence changes in coliphage lambda mutants affecting the t_{L1} and t_{L2} termination and *nutL* antitermination sites, *Gene* **20**:473.

Souza, L., Calendar, R., Six, E., and Lindqvist, B., 1977, A transactivation mutant of satellite phage P4, *Virology* **81**:81.

Sternberg, N., 1976, A class of *rif*R polymerase mutations that interfere with the activity of coliphage *N* gene product, *Virology* **73**:139.

Stewart, V., and Yanofsky, C., 1986, Role of leader peptide synthesis in tryptophanase operon expression in *Escherichia coli* K-12, *J. Bacteriol.* **167**:383.

Stewart, V., and Yanofsky, C., 1985, Evidence for transcription antitermination control of tryptophanase operon expression in *Escherichia coli* K-12, *J. Bacteriol.* **164**:731.

Strauch, M., and Friedman, D. I., 1981, Identification of the *nusB* gene product of *Escherichia coli, Mol. Gen. Genet.* **182**:498.

Sunshine, M., and Sauer, B., 1975, A bacterial mutation blocking P2 phage late gene expression, *Proc. Natl. Acad. Sci. USA* **72**:2770.

Sunshine, M., Thorn, M., Gibbs, W., Calendar, R., and Kelly, B., 1971, P2 phage amber mutants: Characterization by use of a polarity suppressor, *Virology* **46**:691.

Sunshine, M., Six, E., Barrett, K., and Calendar, R., 1976, Relief of P2 bacteriophage amber mutant polarity by the satellite bacteriophage P4, *J. Mol. Biol.* **106**:673.

Suskind, M., and Botstein, D., 1978, Molecular genetics of bacteriophage P22, *Microbiol. Rev.* **42**:385.

Swindle, J., Ajioka, J., and Georgopoulos, C., 1981, Identification of the *E. coli groNB* (*nusB*) gene product, *Mol. Gen. Genet.* **182**:409.

Swindle, J., Ajioka, J., Dawson, D., Meyers, R., Carroll, D., and Georgopoulos, C., 1984, The nucleotide sequence of the *Escherichia coli* K12 *nusB* (*groNB*) gene, *Nucleic Acids Res.* **12**:4977.

Szpirer, J., Thomas, R., and Radding, C., 1969, Hybrids of bacteriophage λ and φ 80: A study of nonvegetative functions, *Virology* **37**:585.

Szybalski, W., 1977, Initiation and regulation of transcription and DNA replication in coliphage lambda, in: *Regulatory Biology* (J. C. Copland and G. A. Marzluff, eds.), pp. 3–45, Ohio State University Press, Columbus.

Szybalski, W., Bovre, K., Fiandt, M., Guha, A., Hradecna, Z., Kumar, S., Lozeron, H. A., Maher, V. M., Nijkamp, H. J. J., Summers, W. C., and Taylor, K., 1969, Transcriptional controls in developing bacteriophage, *J. Cell. Physiol.*, **74** (Suppl. 1):33.

Szybalski, W., Bovre, K., Fiandt, M., Hayes, S., Hradecna, Z., Kumar, S., Lozeron, H. A., Nijkamp, H. J. J., and Stevens, W. F., 1970, Transcriptional units and their control in *Escherichia coli* phage λ: Operons and scriptons, *Cold Spring Harbor Symp. Quant. Biol.* **35**:341.

Szybalski, W., Drahos, D., Luk, K.-C., and Somasekhar, 1983, Modules for termination in coliphage lambda, in: *Microbiology 1983* (D. Schlessinger, ed.), pp. 35–38, American Society for Microbiology, Washington.

Szybalski, W., Brown, A. L., Hasan, N., Podhajska, A. J., and Somasekhar, G., 1987, Modular structure of the *nut* and *qut* antiterminators of transcription. Interactions between control elements of phage lambda and construction of novel regulatory circuits, in: *RNA Polymerase and the Regulation of Transcription* (W. S. Reznikoff, R. R. Burgess, J. E. Dahlberg, C. A. Gross, M. T. Record, and M. P. Wickens, eds.), pp. 381–390, Elsevier, New York.

Tanaka, S., and Matsushiro, A., 1985, Characterization and sequencing of the region containing gene *N*, the *nutL* site and t_{L1} terminator of bacteriophage φ80, *Gene* **38**:119.

Thomas, R., 1966, Control of development in temperate bacteriophages. I. Induction of prophage genes following hetero-immune super-infection, *J. Mol. Biol.* **22**:79.

Tomich, P. K., and Friedman, D. I., 1977, Isolation of mutations in insertion sequences that relieve IS-induced polarity, in: *DNA Insertion Elements, Plasmids, and Episomes* (A. I. Bukhari, J. A. Shapiro, and S. L. Adhya, eds.), pp. 99–107, Cold Spring Harbor Laboratory, Cold Spring Harbor, NY.

Von Hippel, P. H., Bear, D. G., Morgan, W. D., and McSwiggen, J. A., 1984, Protein–nucleic acid interactions in transcription: A molecular analysis, *Annu. Rev. Biochem.* **53**:389.

Ward, D. F., and Gottesman, M. E., 1981, The *nus* mutations affect transcription termination in *Escherichia coli*, *Nature* **292**:212.

Ward, D. F., and Gottesman, M. E., 1982, Suppression of transcription termination by phage lambda, *Science* **216**:946.

Ward, D. F., DeLong, A., and Gottesman, M. E., 1983, *Escherichia coli nusB* mutations that suppress *nusA1* exhibit λ N specificity, *J. Mol. Biol.* **168**:73.

Warren, F., and Das, A., 1984, Formulation of termination-resistant transcription complex at phage λ *nut* locus: Effects of altered translation and a ribosomal mutation, *Proc. Natl. Acad. Sci. USA* **81**:3612.

Yang, X., Hart, C. M., Grayhack, E., and Roberts, J. W., 1987, Transcription antitermination by phage λ gene Q protein requires a DNA segment spanning the RNA start site, *Genes Dev.* **1**:217.

Yanofsky, C., 1981, Attenuation in the control of expression of bacterial operons, *Nature* **289**:751.

Zuber, M., Patterson, T. A., and Court, D. L., 1987, Analysis of *nutR:* A site required for transcription antitermination in phage lambda, *Proc. Natl. Acad. Sci. USA* **84**:4514.

CHAPTER 5

DNA Packaging in dsDNA Bacteriophages

Lindsay W. Black

I. INTRODUCTION

Packaging of duplex DNA within the icosahedral phage head has long been of interest as the prokaryotic equivalent of chromosome condensation and, more recently, because of its usefulness *in vitro* in recombinant DNA work. Viewed in the electron microscope, the overall DNA packaging process is a striking morphological development within infected bacteria (Fig. 1). This DNA condensation results from a complex and highly evolved biological process whose mechanisms depart in numerous ways from simple self-assembly. Its molecular mechanisms have proved to be accessible to combined genetic, biochemical, and structural analyses.

Advances in understanding phage DNA packaging have allowed more recent work to emphasize five related but somewhat distinct questions: (1) the mechanism and energetics of DNA translocation into the prohead* precursor; (2) the higher-order structure(s) of the condensed DNA within the capsid; (3) the mechanism of DNA end formation by concatemer cutting at *cos* or *pac* sites and by headful cutting, and control *in vivo* of concatemer cutting and packaging; (4) the relationship of DNA packaging to global DNA metabolism and structure in infected bacteria; and (5) use of *in vitro* packaging systems in recombinant DNA constructions and cloning work. Accordingly, these interests will be treated separately in the following review.

---

*For abbreviations and terminology, see legend to Fig. 2.

LINDSAY W. BLACK • Department of Biological Chemistry, University of Maryland Medical School, Baltimore, Maryland 21201.

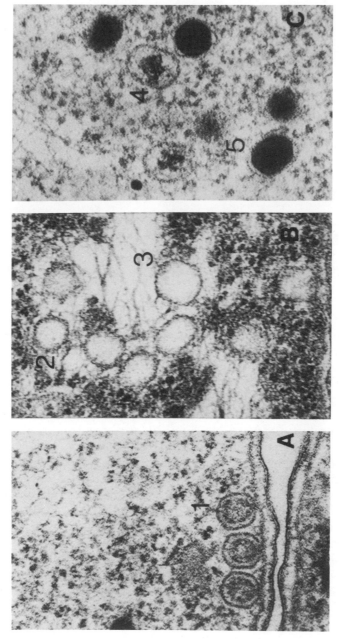

FIGURE 1. Prohead-DNA packaging; morphological development within phage T4-infected bacteria. Thin sections of phage T4-infected *E. coli* at various stages of head development reveal the principal packaging intermediates: (A) 1, Scaffold-containing immature prohead. (B) 2, Empty unexpanded mature prohead; 3, empty expanded mature prohead. (C) 4, Partially DNA-filled head; 5, DNA full head. Panels at same magnification. Courtesy A. Zachary.

Work emphasizing topic 5 (in *E. coli*) has been the subject of excellent recent reviews as well as practical guides (Murray, 1983; Hohn, 1983; Enquist and Sternberg, 1983), so the use of *in vitro* packaging systems in cloning work will be discussed here only in relationship to mechanism. There are numerous bacteriophages and DNA packaging systems, yet it is still possible to speak of a single packaging mechanism and DNA structure (topics 1 and 2) among the duplex DNA-containing icosahedral bacteriophages; whether this is the result of insufficient knowledge remains to be seen. Phages containing dsDNA displaying these broadly similar overall packaging properties include λ, T4, P22, T7 and T3, φ29, P2, T1, μ, their close relatives, and others which have been less intensively studied. On the other hand, although there are many striking similarities, topic 3 clearly includes a number of divergent mechanisms among these bacteriophages in *cos*, *pac*, and other terminase-related and headful cutting mechanisms. This area is also the best-understood aspect of the DNA packaging process in terms of molecular DNA-protein interaction mechanisms.

This review is not intended to be comprehensive or historical; a number of earlier reviews of phage head assembly convey the development of this research area. Of more recent reviews, the first listed specifically addressed the topic of phage DNA packaging; the second is a general overview of packaging in viral systems and includes the packaging of RNA and single-stranded DNA into icosahedral and helical viruses (Earnshaw and Casjens, 1980; Casjens, 1985; Feiss and Becker, 1983; Black and Showe, 1983; Kellenberger, 1980; Wood and King, 1979; Black, 1981b; Murialdo and Becker, 1978; Casjens and King, 1975; Kellenberger, 1961). Packaging into dsDNA lipid-containing bacteriophages (reviewed by Mindich, this series) is not considered in this review.

II. ENERGETICS AND MECHANISM OF DNA TRANSLOCATION

A number of early studies established that duplex concatemeric DNA is translocated into a DNA-free prohead rather than being first condensed and then coated or co-condensed with a capsid (Luftig et al., 1971; Kaiser and Masuda, 1973; Hohn and Hohn, 1974; Hohn et al., 1974; Kaiser et al., 1975). Although the latter mechanisms are thought to apply to the packaging of nucleic acid into certain icosahedral viruses (see Casjens, 1985), work thus far with the icosahedral DNA duplex containing bacteriophages supports the generalization that translocation of DNA into a preformed prohead is the universal packaging mechanism. Among these dsDNA bacteriophages, a procapsid is assembled around a protein scaffold, and this DNA-free prohead is subsequently matured, in some cases by elaborate processes, such as proteolysis and protein fusion, to a mature DNA packaging competent prohead (Figs. 1, 2). For a review of prohead assembly and processing, see Casjens and Hendrix (1988).

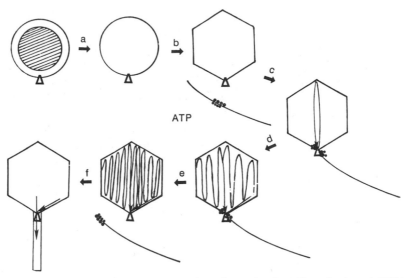

ATP

FIGURE 2. A general scheme and terminology for prohead DNA packaging. A DNA-free prohead (prehead*) consisting of a procapsid assembled around a scaffold (assembly or morphopoietic core) is generally assembled starting at a unique vertex containing the portal protein dodecamer (DNA translocating vertex protein, DNA entrance vertex protein, proximal vertex protein, connector); DNA passes through the portal protein during packaging and ejection, and the tail is connected at this vertex. The other procapsid protein essential for packaging is the major capsid protein. Following scaffold removal, protein processing, and prohead expansion (a, b), packaging can be initiated into the packaging-competent mature prohead. Although packaging initiation in some phages precedes these prohead maturation steps, these features of prohead maturation are apparently not an essential part of the packaging mechanism because the former sequence is possible. Terminases (packaging proteins, packaging-linkage proteins) are nonstructural proteins that cut the concatemeric DNA, link it to the portal protein, and package it within the prohead (c, d). When the mature head contains a headful of DNA in the packaged DNA condensate structure, headful cutting produces the second end in the mature DNA, the tail is attached, and one end descends into the tail for ejection from the capsid (e, f). [*Numerous synonymous terms are found in the literature; in this review the preferred usage (with synonomous terms in parentheses) will be followed. Terminase is an unfortunate term for all the multifunctional phage proteins in this category, since not all cleave concatemeric DNA; nevertheless it will be used because of common usage and because packaging protein is too broad. Other abbreviations: gp, gene product, gpX, gene product of gene X; dsDNA, double-stranded DNA.]

A. Early Models of DNA Translocation

The translocation and concentration of DNA within a capsid [estimated to be on the order of a 100-fold (Hohn, 1976) or a 30- to 60-fold (Kellenberger *et al.*, 1986) decrease in DNA volume within the head from the cytoplasm] has long been recognized to be energetically unfavorable. Early mechanisms proposed to account for the energetics emphasized a number of striking features of head structure and assembly. These features include DNA-binding internal proteins, peptides, polyamines, and other small molecules found packaged with the DNA in phage heads; internal prohead core or scaffolding proteins that exit or are proteolytically degraded during or prior to packaging; and procapsid expansion.

Perhaps the earliest proposal was that DNA-binding internal proteins served as condensing agents for DNA (Kellenberger et al., 1959; Kellenberger, 1961). It was also hypothesized that hydrolysis of core proteins to acid-soluble peptides could collapse the DNA into the prohead, much as ψ-DNA condensates can be formed from counterions and certain polymers (Lerman, 1971; Laemmli and Favre, 1973; Laemmli, 1975). It was supposed that in phages without proteolytic processing, scaffolding protein exit might analogously be coupled energetically to DNA entrance (King and Casjens, 1974). The presence of polyamines in the completed head and an apparent requirement for them in in vitro packaging suggested that these could be central to DNA condensation, which might, because of such counterions, occur essentially spontaneously (Eickbush and Moudrianakis, 1978; Glinert and Luftig, 1977). The expansion of the capsid shell was proposed to be energetically coupled to packaging to suck in the DNA (Hohn et al., 1974; Serwer, 1975). Yet it now appears probable that these properties per se of prohead structure or construction are peripheral to the energetics of packaging.

If a single mechanism applies among the phages, a reasonable assumption in view of numerous overall similarities in packaging and packaged DNA structure, then a number of early proposals fail because they can be eliminated in specific cases. DNA-binding internal proteins are not generally found in bacteriophage heads and, where investigated, have proved to be nonessential. In fact, mutants eliminating them are without significant effect on the kinetics of DNA packaging (Black, 1974). In some phages (e.g., P22, T7), scaffold protein exit is not a separable stage of development from packaging (King and Casjens, 1974; Roeder and Sadowski, 1977). In others, proteolysis of core proteins and exit of scaffold proteins can be uncoupled from packaging and have been shown to precede packaging (T4, λ, ϕ29). Therefore, the scaffold is implicated in the early stages of prohead assembly rather than in the mechanism of DNA packaging (Hsiao and Black, 1977; Kaiser et al., 1975; Hendrix and Casjens, 1975; D. Anderson, personal communication). The hypothesis that DNA replication is coupled to the energetics of packaging (Luftig and Lundh, 1973) appears to be ruled out both by an observed independence of replication in most if not all in vitro packaging systems and where independence of packaging upon replication has been measured in vivo (Hsiao and Black, 1977).

There is an extensive literature on the thermodynamics and structure of polyamine- and other counterion-induced collapse of phage (and nonphage) DNAs into toroidal or rodlike structures that have an overall dimensional resemblance to the capsids from which they originated (Chattoraj et al., 1978; Laemmli, 1975; Widom and Baldwin, 1980; Marx and Reynolds, 1982; Lerman, 1971; Eickbush and Moudrianakis, 1978).

Biological models based on such studies have proposed that polyamines (Eickbush and Moudrianakis, 1978; Glinert and Luftig, 1977) or packaging coupled to protein cleavage into acid-soluble peptides within the prohead could analogously collapse the DNA into the head (Laemmli and Favre, 1973). However, contrary to the latter proposed mechanism, cleavage of the T4 acid-soluble peptides has been demonstrated to be uncoupled from and to precede packaging (Hsiao and Black, 1977; Rao and Black, 1985b). Moreover, it has now been convincingly demonstrated that *E. coli* mutants entirely lacking polyamines can allow efficient T4 and T7 phage formation in their absence (Hafner *et al.*, 1979). In keeping with this observation, in well-defined phage packaging systems with highly purified reactants, polyamines to a limited extent stimulate, but are not essential for packaging, although they may stabilize the head (Hamada *et al.*, 1986a; Syvanen and Yin, 1978). Therefore, it may be that polyelectrolyte repulsion is the major energetic barrier to packaging, suggesting a requirement for counterions (Riemer and Bloomfield, 1978), although Rau *et al.* (1984) find that hydration forces predominate at the packaging densities of phage heads, accounting for DNA pressure within the head, and that varying ions, including polyamines, or concentrations of these show little effect on DNA packing forces. Nevertheless, in either case, although polyamines stimulate *in vitro* packaging, especially in crude systems, as they stimulate numerous other DNA processes *in vitro*, [e.g., recombination (Nash, 1981)], it can be concluded that polyamines are peripheral to the energetics of packaging DNA as a biological mechanism.

B. Prohead Expansion in Packaging

Among the general features of prohead structure and assembly, probably the procapsid expansion that accompanies DNA packaging among the numerous phages is the most striking. Expansion results from a change in the bonding properties of the major capsid protein in the surface lattice of the prohead and can lead to a volume increase of over 50% (summarized by Earnshaw and Casjens, 1980). Moreover, the expansion leads to major functional as well as structural changes in the prohead: increased angularity of the procapsid (Bjornsti *et al.*, 1983; Yamagishi and Okamoto, 1978; Steven *et al.*, 1976), permeability changes (Serwer, 1980), increased capsid protein-bonding stability (Steven *et al.*, 1976; Ross *et al.*, 1985), exposure of binding sites for outer capsid accessory proteins (Ishii and Yanagida, 1975, 1977; Sternberg and Weisberg, 1975), and changes in ATP- and possibly DNA-binding properties of the assembled capsid protein (Rao and Black, 1985a).

It was initially proposed that prohead expansion might be energetically coupled to packaging so that the DNA could be sucked into the head in this step by energy stored in the unexpanded shell. It was suggested that the prohead expansion is triggered by binding a packaging protein-DNA complex to the unexpanded shell, as a result of which a negative pressure differential is created owing to prohead impermeability to solvent, which would then suck the DNA into the head (Hohn et al., 1974; Serwer, 1975). In a direct test of the coupled expansion-packaging hypothesis, Rao and Black (1985b) found that T4 DNA could be packaged into fully expanded T4 proheads in vitro, the latter in fact being preferred over unexpanded proheads for packaging. These results are consistent with earlier studies in vivo which suggested that a significant portion of the T4 DNA could resume packaging into a head structure which proved to be fully expanded (Luftig et al., 1971; Wunderli et al., 1977), or could apparently be initiated into an expanded prohead (Hsiao and Black, 1977).

Subsequently, Serwer (1980) demonstrated changes in permeability in the T7 procapsid accompany maturation for packaging. Serwer (1980) on the basis of these data proposed that an osmotic pressure differential resulting from the expansion of a relatively impermeable head shell could drive packaging; consequently, there would be no direct coupling of expansion and DNA packaging. While this proposal is not eliminated by the above data, it is difficult to reconcile with the observation that expanded proheads remain active for days in aqueous solution (Rao and Black, 1985b) and that molecules considerably larger than water can enter the expanded prohead (Gope and Serwer, 1983; Serwer et al., 1983). Such observations weigh against the storage of an osmotic pressure in the expanded prohead as a major source of energy for packaging. Moreover, it has been observed that a morphological change in ϕ29 proheads (probably equivalent to if not in fact demonstrated to be an expansion) apparently results from packaging of restriction fragments corresponding to the first one-third or less of the packaged DNA (Bjornsti et al., 1983), whereas in lambda, expansion occurs between packaging those corresponding to 11% and 45% of the DNA (Hohn, 1983). These observations strongly weigh against the direct cause-and-effect relationship between expansion and packaging which is a feature of either expansion model. In addition, as summarized by Earnshaw and Casjens (1980), the volume increase of several proheads appears to be insufficient to account for packaging of more than a portion of the DNA by such a mechanism; i.e., the packaged DNA occupies considerably more space than the increase in volume.

Why is there prohead expansion if it does not serve an energetic function in DNA packaging? It can be argued that in addition to serving the demonstrated function of stabilizing the capsid (Steven et al., 1976; Carrascosa and Kellenberger, 1978; Ross et al., 1985), prohead expansion might function to (1) remove weak scaffold-procapsid interactions involved in shape specification, (2) drive polymerization along the assembly pathway, (3) expel the scaffold and create a free space for packaging, and (4) restructure the capsid protein for a DNA interacting rather than a core-interacting functional role. Clearly, more must be learned about the structure of the capsid protein and its functional role in a DNA packaging active conformation to answer this question.

C. ATP-Driven DNA Translocation Models

Because of evidence against the proposals discussed above in one or more phages, ATP-driven DNA translocation mechanisms are now favored by default. A number of quite specific models have been proposed: a symmetry-mismatch ATP-driven pump by the connector or portal vertex protein (Hendrix, 1978), an ATP topoisomerase-supercoiling pump mechanism by the terminase proteins (Black and Silverman, 1978), and an ATP-EcoK DNA-walking protein pump by the terminase proteins (Yuan et al., 1980; Earnshaw and Casjens, 1980).

The first model proposed that the mismatch between five- and six-fold symmetry at the head-tail junction allowed ATP-driven rotation of a gear (the connector) which would screw in the DNA. The second proposed that topoisomeraselike nicking and underwinding energized by ATP hydrolysis would provide a torque through relaxation of the super-helical turn, leading to translocation of DNA into the head. This model was proposed in part to explain the dependence of T4 packaging in vivo on DNA ligase and a mechanism for nick removal (Hsiao and Black, 1977). Both of these models allow translocation without leading to a high degree of supercoiling in the packaged DNA, whereas an objection to the third is that if the translocating enzyme and the prohead are fixed to each other, a highly supercoiled DNA would result from a protein tracking along the DNA as does the EcoK restriction enzyme (Yuan et al., 1980). Although topoisomerases (which might relax excessive supercoils) have been reported within animal viruses, none have so far been described within the phage head (Bauer et al., 1977). Topoisomerase inhibitors were reported to inhibit in vitro packaging in Phi29 (Guo et al., 1987a), but not P22 (Poteete et al., 1979) or T4 (Black, 1981; V. B. Rao, personal communication).

There is little evidence in direct support of any of these specific models. Nevertheless, this class of models coupling ATP hydrolysis to DNA translocation is supported by the demonstration of an ATP requirement in all in vitro DNA packaging systems (λ (Kaiser et al., 1975), T3 (Hamada et al., 1986a), P22 (Poteete et al., 1979; Strobel et al., 1984), P2 (Bowden and Calendar, 1979), T4 (Black, 1981a; Rao and Black, 1985b), Phi29 (Bjornsti et al., 1983; Guo et al., 1986). In the Phi29 in vitro packaging system, it has been determined that one ATP is hydrolyzed per 2 bp packaged (Guo et al., 1987b). The packaging time for P22 DNA was estimated to be less than 1.5 min, and probably as fast as 0.25 min, equivalent to a translocation rate of about 3 kb/sec, and packaging intermediates were not detected (Gope and Serwer, 1983). On the other hand, packaging into the ϕ29 system was apparently discontinuous, with pauses between incorporation of variable-length segments of DNA into the prohead (Bjornsti et al., 1983). However, packaging in the defined φ29 system is much faster, and intermediates could be detected only at low temperature (Guo et al., 1987a; D. Anderson, personal communication).

Packaging of mature DNA can be carried out in vitro in purified systems containing only proheads, purified terminase proteins, and small molecules (Hamada et al., 1986a; Guo et al., 1986, 1987a). It therefore appears that at least the components required for packaging of mature DNA are quite limited in number: the mature prohead, the terminase proteins (generally a large multimeric complex of 2 proteins), ATP, and various counterions. And although the prohead is a strikingly complex structure, its active components for packaging appear to be limited to two essential structural proteins—the portal protein and the major capsid protein. Mature proheads of some phages contain many more proteins, although others that employ very similar overall packaging processes need contain only these two (e.g., P22, φ29). Moreover, it is striking that in the complex proheads most, if not all, of these additional proteins can frequently be removed by mutation without loss of packaging function, as for example, the T4 internal proteins (Black, 1974). In addition, the major lambda surface capsid protein, gpD (Sternberg and Weissberg, 1977), or the T4 gpsoc, gphoc, and gp24 vertex proteins can be lost (Ishii and Yanagida, 1975; McNicol et al., 1977) yet permit production of less stable heads that are equally able to package DNA.

D. Functions of the Packaging Components

If a generalized DNA packaging scheme is abstracted from the duplex DNA-containing phages, there appear to be a number of irreducible features related to an underlying mechanism (Fig. 2). A prohead consisting of a procapsid surrounding a scaffold is first constructed. This internal structure may serve to specify the icosahedral symmetry of the procapsid, and it may exclude cellular components from the prohead or serve other assembly functions (see Casjens and Hendrix, 1988). Although for some phages, removal of the scaffold has not been clearly separated from or shown to precede the packaging event (P22), because, as discussed above, it has been demonstrated to do so in others (λ, T4, and probably φ29), scaffolding protein removal is unlikely to act directly and functionally in packaging, but more likely serves to prepare a mature prohead which is ready to accept the DNA (Fig. 2). Moreover, in no phage system have mutations been reported in genes for scaffold and internal components that have a specific effect on packaging other than gross morphological defects in head formation. In contrast, specific packaging mutations of this sort have been reported in structural genes for the portal protein of T4 (Hsiao and Black, 1977) and P22 (Casjens, personal communication), and probably the major capsid protein of λ (Katsura, 1980, 1986).

Packaging *in vivo* may be initiated into a scaffold-containing prohead (P22, T7) or into an unexpanded prohead (λ). In phage T4, although packaging *in vitro* has been demonstrated to occur into the expanded prohead (Rao and Black, 1985b), packaging *in vivo* may well be initiated into the unexpanded prohead (Schaerli and Kellenberger, 1980). The data strongly suggest, however, that there is no necessary mechanistic coupling of packaging to these maturation events. Therefore the receptacle for the DNA to be packaged *can* in some cases be a scaffoldless mature prohead whose capsid has been stabilized by expansion. The maturation of the procapsid for DNA packaging in some phages is accompanied by proteolysis and protein fusion. The proteins having a significant role in the DNA translocation stage of head assembly therefore appear to be confined to the terminase proteins, the assembled prohead DNA portal protein, and the major capsid protein of the mature procapsid, which may have undergone protein processing. There is evidence in support of a direct and active role of each of these proteins in packaging (see Fig. 2).

1. The Terminases

The terminases are ATP-binding and hydrolyzing proteins that assemble to form multimeric packaging protein complexes (see Section IV and Table I) (Guo *et al.*, 1986; Becker and Gold, 1978; Gold and Becker, 1983; Hamada *et al.*, 1984, 1986a; Bowden and Calendar, 1979; Rao and Black, 1987; Poteete and Botstein, 1979). In addition to cutting DNA at *pac* or *cos* sites, continued action of these proteins is apparently required during DNA translocation, at least in some phages. For example, some temperature-sensitive mutations in the T4 terminase components can lead to interruption of DNA packaging and accumulation of partially filled heads, arguing for continued active participation in packaging following cutting (Wunderli *et al.*, 1977). Continued action of the λ terminase is required for packaging after cutting (Becker *et al.*, 1977). Acridines interrupt packaging and lead to the accumulation of partially filled T4 proheads, and mutants that can in part overcome such arrest map in the terminase genes (Piechowski and Susman, 1967; Schaerli and Kellenberger, 1980). These observations suggest an active role of terminases in packaging as well as in cutting DNA. The terminase proteins appear to interact with the portal protein and prohead during packaging (Hsiao and Black, 1977; Guo *et al.*, 1987a; Frackman *et al.*, 1984), consistent with proposals that the terminase proteins pump DNA into the prohead through ATP hydrolysis (Black and Silverman, 1978; Earnshaw and Casjens, 1980). The observation that mature T7 and T4 DNA can be packaged without the small terminase subunit and the terminase-prohead interaction studies suggests that the large subunit in some cases carries out the essential binding and translocating functions (Hamada *et al.*, 1986a; Rao and Black, 1987; Frackman *et al.*, 1984; see Section IV).

TABLE I. Properties of Purified Bacteriophage Terminases[a,b]

Bacteriophage	λ	P2	T3 (T7)	P22	T4	φ29
Gene product names and molecular weights of terminase subunits	gpA 74,000 gpNul 21,000	gpP 65,000 gpM 28,000	gp19 67,000 gp18 10,000	gp2 63,000 gp3 17,000	gp17 67,000 gp16 18,000	gp16 39,000 (gp3 30,000)
State of purified terminase	Multimeric	Multimeric	Multimeric	Multimeric	Multimeric	Multimeric
In vitro packaging activity DNA requirements						
Specific sequence	+	+	+ (less for monomer)	Probably not	No	+ (and 5'-gp3 covalent protein)
Concatemeric DNA	+	+ (c.c. circular preferred)	+	+	+	
Mature DNA	Probably not	+ (gpM not required)	+ (gp18 not required)	+	+ (gp16 not required)	+
Endonuclease activity	+	+	n.r.	n.r.	+	+
Sequence-specific	+	+	n.r.	n.r.	n.r.	–
End formed by terminase *in vivo*	5' 12-b extension	5' 19-b extension	n.r.	Blunt end	n.r.	–
Other activities	DNA dep ATPase	DNA dep ATPase	DNA dep ATPase	ATP stabilizes	ATP stabilizes binds gp17	DNA dep ATPase
Other cutting requirements	IHF or THF	Prohead, closed circular DNA	n.r.	n.r.	n.r.	–
References	a	b	c	d	e	f

[a] Key: +, Activity found, or property required for activity; –, activity not found, or property not required for activity; n.r., not reported.

[b] References: a: λ, Gold and Becker, 1983; Murialdo and Fife, 1984; Feiss, 1986; Feiss and Becker, 1983. b: P2, Bowden and Calendar, 1979; Bowden and Modrich, 1985; Pruss and Calendar, 1978; Pruss et al., 1975. c: T3 and T7, Hamada et al., 1986a,b; Fujisawa et al., 1980 (values are for T3). d: P22, Poteete and Botstein, 1979; Strobel et al., 1984; Backhaus, 1985; Casjens et al., 1987. e: T4, Rao and Black, 1987, 1985b; Black, 1987, 1985b; G. Mosig, personal communication. f: φ29, Guo et al., 1986, 1987a,b; Bjornsti et al., 1983. P1 ends are inferred to be 3' two-base extensions (Sternberg and Coulby, 1987b). For other properties of terminases, see Figs. 4 and 5.

2. The Portal Protein

Evidence suggests that, while head expansion may not be coupled directly to packaging, the prohead is not a passive DNA receptacle. Structural proteins of the procapsid undergo complex structural transformations following assembly; the most obvious is the expansion-transformation of the capsid surface lattice. It is probable that such changes allow expression by structural proteins of activities involved in DNA translocation. In T4, the portal vertex protein can undergo a structural change which initiates DNA packaging. Mutations in its structural gene can lead to a prohead containing a defective vertex structure that does not initiate DNA packaging. This defect can be overcome by temperature shift activation of the defective portal vertex protein or by specific terminase mutations, suggesting structural association between the portal vertex structure and the terminase complex (Hsiao and Black, 1977). Similarly, the λ terminase also displays specific structural interactions with the prohead (Frackman *et al.*, 1984).

In P22, it has been found that mutational change in the portal protein can lead to apparently overfilled heads (Casjens, personal communication). These observations suggest that the portal vertex protein is intimately involved with the terminase proteins in initiating DNA packaging, in translocation, and in headful cutting. Indirect evidence thus favors a DNA-translocating or "packasome" complex located at the portal vertex, as in the symmetry-mismatch ATP pump, or the terminase-supercoiling pump (Hendrix, 1978; Black and Silverman, 1978; Bazinet and King, 1985).

Multiple functional roles of the portal vertex protein in prohead assembly and packaging argue for regulatory structural transformation. A necessary feature of head assembly is a requirement that DNA packaging initiation not occur before prohead maturation, since otherwise introduction of DNA into an unfinished head would presumably result in abortive packaging. Since in many phages an assembled portal vertex structure appears to initiate prohead assembly, this structure may first be assembled in a packaging inactive conformation which is subsequently activated in the mature prohead. Such a packaging transformation may relate to the mutant T4 portal vertex structure, which can be activated by temperature shift, following its assembly with the T4 prohead on the cytoplasmic membrane through attachment of the portal vertex (Hsiao and Black, 1977). This may also account in part for the proteolytic processing of the lambda portal vertex protein (gpB) just prior to packaging (Murialdo and Becker, 1978; Hendrix and Casjens, 1975). The portal protein displays a markedly similar overall structure among the phages studied (Bazinet and King, 1985; Jiminez *et al.*, 1985). It is possible that comparable transformation activations for packaging also occur in other phages to separate and regulate the assembly and packaging roles of the portal protein dodecamer.

3. The Major Capsid Protein

The major capsid protein also appears to play an active role in the DNA translocation mechanism. An early report suggested that a soluble conformer of gpE, the λ major capsid protein, might bind to DNA (Brody, 1973). In addition, mutations in gene E apparently block packaging of morphologically normal proheads (Katsura, 1980, 1986).

A minor proteolytically processed derivative of the T4 major capsid protein has also been shown to display both DNA binding and enzymatic activities. In certain conformational states, the protein has both DNA-dependent ATPase activity and endonuclease activities (Manne et al., 1982). Moreover, the assembled major capsid protein appears to have an identical ATP-binding site in certain of its precursor conformations. These findings suggest that the assembled major capsid protein not only is structural but, like the minor processed form released from the prohead, is enzymatic and may act both in DNA translocation in conjunction with ATP hydrolysis and in headful cutting (Rao and Black, 1985a). Recent genetic findings are consistent with this proposed role for the major capsid protein.

T7 missense mutations in the major capsid protein gene cause DNA breakdown or altered transcriptional activity of T7 DNA in certain hosts. Expression of this phenotype does not require assembly of the mutationally altered capsid protein into a head structure, and it involves a functional interrelationship with phage DNA ligase (Beck et al., 1986). A class of T4 mutations is at least formally analogous: mutations in the major capsid protein display in certain hosts altered transcriptional properties from the T4 DNA. Similar T7 phenotypes have also been observed among other host-interacting capsid missense mutations (I. J. Molineaux, personal communication). These properties are displayed by cloned mutational forms of a portion of the major T4 capsid gene which requires in-frame translation of this part of the gene to express the phenotype (Champness and Snyder, 1984; Snyder, personal communication). These complex mutant phenotypes, while not permitting an unambiguous interpretation, at least suggest that the major capsid protein is a multifunctional protein with DNA-directed enzymatic activities that are under host- and assembly-dependent regulation.

E. Relationship of Packaging to DNA Ejection

A necessary feature of packaging is the reversibility that permits DNA ejection. This requires that the DNA be packaged into a metastable conformation. It is clear that the proteins that are added to the outer capsid during maturation are not fundamentally involved in destabilizing the packaged DNA; e.g., the T4 hoc and soc proteins and the λ D proteins are not required for packaging or ejection (although λgpD is reported to be a "histonelike" protein (Witkiewicz and Schweiger, 1982). Since all of the T4 DNA and probably much of the DNA of φ29 and λ can be packaged into an expanded procapsid, head expansion probably does not serve the function of destabilizing the packaged DNA for ejection by disrupting DNA-binding sites in the capsid. In addition, underpackaged DNA, at least up to 75%, can be ejected (Feiss et al., 1977; Shore et al., 1978; Sternberg and Weissberg, 1977). The portal vertex protein-terminase translocating apparatus may simply introduce sufficient DNA under pressure (e.g., Rau et al., 1984) to allow spontaneous ejection when this translocating force is removed at the completion of packaging, when a "plug" is removed for ejection. DNA ejection could also involve more subtle changes in the major capsid protein than the expansion-transformation; e.g., it could involve hydrolysis and release of ATP from the DNA binding site in the major capsid protein during packaging and postexpansion conformational change which is not readily detectable morphologically. DNA ejection could also involve structural changes in DNA [e.g., straightening kinks (Black et al., 1985) or removal of supercoiling].

In summary, there is substantial but indirect evidence that ATP hydrolysis drives, at least in large part, DNA translocation. Terminase as well as assembled structural proteins of the prohead may express DNA-directed enzymatic activities during packaging, although their precise role in the mechanistic coupling of ATP hydrolysis to DNA motion is not known. In conjunction with ATP hydrolysis, the terminase and/or DNA portal vertex proteins could constitute a "packasome" complex which pushes the DNA into the prohead, the assembled major capsid protein could pull the DNA into the head, or the DNA could be both pushed into the head at the portal vertex and pulled in as a consequence of undergoing active structural organization by the DNA- (and ATP-) binding site of the assembled capsid protein. Bacteriophage DNA packaging continues to be an attractive model system for understanding energetic translocation of nucleic acids.

III. STRUCTURE OF PACKAGED PHAGE DNA

The most precise techniques for structural analysis of DNA (e.g., X-ray crystallography, sequencing) have not been successfully applied to determine packaged phage DNA structure. Indeed, successful analysis of three-dimensional nucleic acid structure by such techniques is lacking for the much simpler single-stranded DNA- and RNA-containing icosahedral viruses, possibly because of variability in the structure (Olson et al., 1983). Consequently, although many properties of packaged DNA organization appear to be established in a general sense, exact knowledge of this structure is conspicuously lacking, and quite divergent models have been proposed. Since this topic was last thoroughly reviewed (Earnshaw and Casjens, 1980), studies that use a number of different techniques have raised serious doubts about the validity of the then favored toroidal, spool, solenoidal, or concentric shell model for the structure of packaged phage DNA (Earnshaw and Harrison, 1977; Richards et al., 1973) and have led to a number of other models (see Fig. 5) (Black et al., 1985; Serwer, 1986; Lepault et al., 1987).

Many common features of DNA packaging mechanism and structure among the bacteriophages support the hypothesis of an essentially unitary packaged phage DNA structure. Such features include most obviously major similarities in packaging mechanism as discussed in the preceding section (ATP-dependent filling of icosahedral procapsids assembled by broadly similar mechanisms). The packaged DNA structure also allows among all these phages DNA packaging and ejection at the portal vertex through a 20-to-30-Å hole in a protein dodecamer which appears to be very similar in structure among them (Bazinet and King, 1985; Jiminez et al., 1986). The packaged structure is metastable in the sense that it allows for rapid DNA ejection through a variety of tails followed by host uptake. Probably of greater support for the hypothesis of a single structure, however, is that nearly the same degree of compaction of DNA is found among almost all of the phages (Earnshaw and Casjens, 1980). DNA is found to be packed in predominantly the B form to essentially a uniform density of 0.5 g/ml (neglecting water).

Although DNA measurements in general support such a single DNA density structure, an interesting departure has been discovered in a phage containing diputrescinyl-thymidylate that packs DNA to a density of about 0.63 g/ml (Scraba et al., 1983). This higher packaging density has been clearly shown to result from the unusual base, since mutants that lack it underpackage to the common value. Condensation studies with the isolated DNA suggest that the condensed DNA has an unusual structure (Benbasat, 1984). In a sense, these findings are the exception that proves the rule that the packaged phage DNA structure is primarily due to the properties of DNA and its interaction with the icosahedral capsid. Two other general sorts of observations are also consistent with this hypothesis. One is that phages with significant amounts (1200 molecules per head) of internal proteins (T4) and those without such components (e.g., lambda) appear to have very similar packaged DNA structures. In accordance with this, loss of these components by T4 does not significantly change the packaged structure (Black and Showe, 1983). In addition, counterion-collapsed DNA condensates have on the order of 16% less density than phage DNA (see Benbasat, 1984), and major variation in viral nucleic acid packaging density is certainly observed. Some animal icosahedral viruses display both very different DNA density and structural organization. For example, adenovirus, with an icosahedral structure not unlike that of many phages, has about one-fourth the DNA density (Ginsberg, 1979). Here DNA appears to be organized in a structure to which internal proteins make a major contribution (Newcomb et *al.*, 1984). In reovirus, on the other hand, dsRNA is packaged to a density comparable to that of the dsDNA bacteriophages (Harvey *et al.*, 1981).

A variety of physical techniques for higher-order DNA structural characterization support the hypothesis of a basicaliy unitary DNA structure among the phages. On the basis of low-angle X-ray scattering data, there appears to be a high degree of local order in packaged DNA, with overall 25-Å parallel spacing of duplex DNA segments as well as long-range order, suggesting an essentially symmetrical arrangement of DNA in shells across the head. Similar packing density is observed among the phages (Earnshaw and Harrison, 1977; Stroud *et al.*, 1981). Ordered parallel packing of DNA duplexes consistent with such results has also been observed by flow dichroism and electric linear dichroism and is similar among a number of phages (Hall and Schellman, 1982; Kosturko *et al.*, 1979). In the latter study, it was observed that packing of parallel helices according to overall icosahedral symmetry would be expected to tilt the DNA relative to the tail axis, so that an ordered arrangement would yield values consistent with the experimental values among the measured phages. Consequently, DNA packed in a highly ordered structure (e.g., toroidally, or in folded rods organized from vertex to vertex (Fig. 5a,b)) would be consistent with these measurements, although a number of other models are probably also consistent (Hall and Schellman, 1982).

These physical measurements of packaged DNA show generally similar arrangement and packaging density among phages with or without unique termination sequences (λ, T4, P22). An important difference, however, is that deletions in phages with unique mature DNA ends, such as lambda, result in packing of less DNA, and this underpackaged DNA is found to undergo general reorganization to uniform overall looser packaging (Earnshaw and Harrison, 1977). Analysis of lambda deletion and addition mutants suggests, moreover, that the head is constrained from accepting over 9% more [viability is reduced above about 5% more (Weil *et al.*, 1972, 1974; Sternberg and Weisberg, 1975)] and, less certainly, probably about 25% less DNA than the value characteristic of wild-type packaged phage (Feiss *et al.*, 1977). It is probably the cutting mechanism and/or the DNA ejection process, however, that places a lower limit on the DNA, since short restriction fragments of λ DNA can be packaged (Hohn, 1983). Physical studies of DNA structure in a number of phages thus favor similar highly ordered DNA condensate structures (e.g., Fig. 5) and are inconsistent with nonparallel or unordered structures (e.g., DNA duplexes wound randomly as in a ball of twine, or DNA organized radially outward from the center of the capsoid).

Electron microscopic observations have also been consistent with a common packaged structure among the phages. Although there is early electron microscopic evidence for a hole or reduction in DNA packaging density toward the center of the head (Cummings *et al.*, 1965), more recent and probably less artifact-prone cryoelectron microscopy does not appear to support a reduced packaging density toward the center, and suggests uniform density of packaging throughout the head (Lepault *et al.*, 1987; Adrian *et al.*, 1984). Size variants of the phage T4 head also establish that the packaged DNA structure possesses great flexibility. DNA contained within petite phage heads (Eiserling *et al.*, 1970; Mosig *et al.*, 1972) as well as giant elongated heads (Doermann *et al.*, 1973; Cummings *et al.*, 1973; Bijlenga *et al.*, 1976; Uhlenhopp *et al.*, 1974) ranges from two-thirds to over 10× normal length. Single duplex DNA molecules can therefore be packaged by the same headful mechanism into functional heads of corresponding volumes to basically same final packaging density.

In low-angle X-ray scattering and electron microscopy observations of T4 giant head phages, it was observed that the DNA appeared to be packaged parallel to the long axis of the phage head (Fig. 3B) (Earnshaw *et al.*, 1978). This work confirms early findings by X-ray crystallography and birefringence that DNA is substantially aligned parallel to the head-tail axis (Bendet *et al.*, 1960; North and Rich, 1961) (or, in the solenoidal organization, as is shown in Fig. 5A, relative to 5B). DNA has been visualized within heads, or after rapid emptying from them, as a ball or spool (Fig. 3A) (Richards *et al.*, 1973; Fujiyoshi *et al.*, 1982). The DNA appears to be released from the phage head as a bundle with relatively little supercoiling (Fig. 3C) (Earnshaw *et al.*, 1978). Rosettes and other radial-looped structures are most generally released from disrupted phage heads (Fig. 4A). Supercoiling within loops in such rosette structures released from the condensate can be demonstrated. From this and other evidence of supercoiling, it was suggested that DNA within the phage head might assume a nucleosomelike organization (Virrankoski-Costrodeza and Parish, 1980; Virrankoski-Costrodeza *et al.*, 1982).

Generally, DNA is packaged from the end opposite the end first ejected [lambda: Emmons (1974), Syvanen (1975), Feiss and Bublitz (1975), Sternberg and Weisberg (1975); T1: Gill and MacHattie (1975, 1976), MacHattie and Gill (1977); T7: Roberts *et al.* (1978), Hartman *et al.* (1979); mu: George and Bukhari (1981); and φ29: Bjornsti *et al.* (1983)]. There is also good evidence that the last end of the λ DNA to be packaged is positioned near the portal vertex and descends into the tail (Thomas, 1974; Chattoraj and Inman, 1974; Saigo and Uchida, 1974; Bode and Gillin, 1971).

However, T4 DNA appeared to be packaged and ejected from the same end; labeling of the DNA at one end *in vivo* also showed that only one end of the DNA moved into the head (Black and Silverman, 1978). The correctness of these observations has an important bearing on whether DNA is packaged by moving a mature end (by sliding) or by moving folds of DNA. The T4 result would require that DNA be packaged by moving folds or kinks of DNA into the head, since the first end is fixed. Morever, because of headful cutting, the T4 result would require

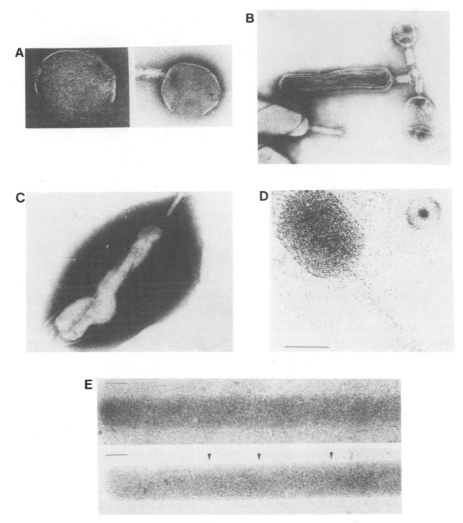

FIGURE 3. Visualization of packaged phage DNA structure by electron microscopy. (A) DNA condensate released by sudden rupture of the phage T4 capsid (Richards *et al.*, 1973). (B, C) DNA visualized running lengthwise in the T4 giant phage head and in a gently supercoiled bundle suddenly released from the ruptured capsid (Earnshaw *et al.*, 1978). (D, E) DNA visualized within phage T4 and giant phage T4 heads in unstained vitreous samples examined by cryo-electron microscopy. The bars correspond to 500 Å. From Lepault *et al.* (1987).

that both T4 ends lie near the portal vertex of the head (Black and Silverman, 1978).

That both ends of the packaged DNA are probably situated near the portal vertex is also one implication of the finding that the DNA ends of P2 or P4 heads can be ligated together to form complex knotted DNAs (Fig. 4B) (Liu *et al.*, 1981a,b). To a lesser degree, this is also true of tailed

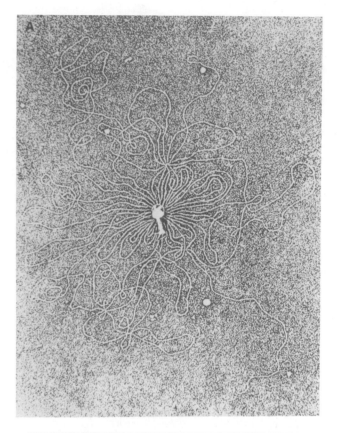

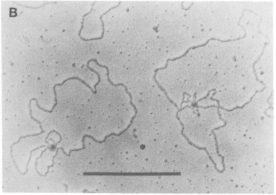

FIGURE 4. DNA structures obtained from packaged phage DNA condensates. (A) A rosette structure obtained from an osmotically shocked T2 phage particle (Kleinschmidt *et al.,* 1962). (B) P2 protein-free knotted DNA obtained by extraction and ligation of packaged phage heads (Liu *et al.,* 1981a). Scale bar: 1 μm.

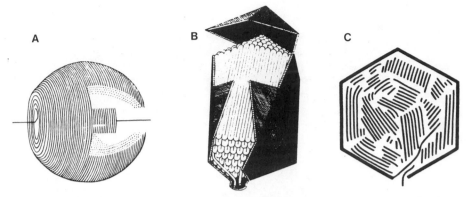

FIGURE 5. Models of the ordered arrangement of DNA inside the bacteriophage head. (A) Concentric shell, solenoid, or toroidal winding DNA model (Earnshaw and Harrison, 1977); the duplex DNA orientation should be parallel to the head-tail axis (or as shown relative to the phage head in B) (Earnshaw *et al.*, 1978). (B) The spiral fold model for packaged phage DNA, consisting of 180° folded DNA rods organized in shells (Black *et al.*, 1985). (C) A nemetic crystal model, showing local parallel packaging of duplex DNA (Lepault *et al.*, 1987).

phage P4 DNA, and the fraction isolated in knotted form increases with increasing size of DNA deletions (Wolfson *et al.*, 1985). The simplest interpretation of these findings is that the two DNA ends are in proximity and readily cohere in the packaged structure, but that one end is normally prevented from doing so by descending into the tail. The formation of knotted DNA by the extraction and ligation procedure probably does not require that DNA be packaged in knotted form within the capsid, although this possibility has not been excluded. Knotting could result from the simple passage of one duplex relative to another before ligation, if the ends are free to move, and such an explanation may be favored by the observed increased frequency with deletions (Liu *et al.*, 1981a; Haas *et al.*, 1982). Considering all of these observations as they relate to packaged DNA structure, it appears to be established that the end of the DNA to be ejected is situated near the portal vertex, and it is most likely that the other end is also located in this vicinity (see Figs. 2 and 5B).

The features of packaged DNA structure discussed above were generally consistent with the model that DNA is packaged toroidally into concentric shells with overall 25-Å spacing and with both DNA ends located near the portal vertex of the head (Fig. 5A). Such a solenoidal shell DNA structure was argued to be capable of reorganization during packaging by tightening up the loops, so that DNA might be maintained in an equilibrium conformation throughout packaging (Harrison, 1983). In the event of deletions that lead to underpackaging, generally looser packaging could follow the same organizational principle (Earnshaw and Harrison, 1977; Harrison, 1983). However, since DNA was observed to be packaged parallel to the long axis of T4 giant heads, this arrangement requires that the DNA be pulled through the shells of DNA, given the first-end-in, last-end-out packaging, and assuming that this orientation is also true in isometric phage heads (Earnshaw et al., 1978).

If DNA is toroidally wound in such concentric shells, the expectation is that the DNA should be condensed from the outside toward the inside of the head, since the most energetially unfavorable position for the DNA would be at its position of maximum curvature toward the center of the head, although there was no direct evidence in support of this predicted condensation direction (Earnshaw and Casjens, 1980). On the contrary, electron microscopic observations of packaging intermediates in thin sections tended to reveal inside-to-outside packaging in thin-sectioned materials (e.g., Fig. 1), although such images may well result from artifactual reorganization of the unfixed DNA. In fact, electron microscopic studies emphasizing fixation of the DNA most probably support the idea that DNA in packaging intermediates is uniformly distributed throughout the head (Lenk et al., 1975; Zachary and Black, 1981; Lickfeld et al., 1977; Yamagishi and Okamoto, 1978; Wunderli et al., 1977; E. Kellenberger, personal communication). Electron microscopy-autoradiography of the pattern of terminally labeled DNA released from shocked mature phage heads, however, was interpreted to suggest inside-to-outside DNA packaging (Black and Silverman, 1978).

A number of more recent studies have been in serious conflict with expectations from the concentric shell model. Restriction fragments arising throughout the entire lambda DNA molecule could be cross-linked with a bis-psoralen cross-linking agent (Haas et al., 1982; Welsh and Cantor, 1986). Their studies were not consistent with a simple toroidal, or indeed any invariant, highly organized structure, although some evidence for regular structure in cross-linking patterns between fragments was found. At the same time, it is difficult to account for the absence of cross-linking within large restriction fragments in this study. And although the DNA condensate is probably relatively immobile according to measurements of fluorescence anisotropy decay, it might have sufficient flexibility for cross-linking with a bifunctional intercalating agent to induce substantial rearrangement (Ashikawa et al., 1984). Other investigations, however, also demonstrate convincingly that, at least on a kilobase scale, every lambda DNA sequence can be cross-linked to and therefore is in contact with the capsid, a finding in clear contradiction to a simple toroidal organization of packaged phage DNA (Widom and Baldwin, 1983).

In response to these findings, Harrison (1983) suggested that DNA could be toroidally organized without a fixed condensation direction, so that shells of DNA loops could be laid down in a variable pathway from outside to inside, or from inside to outside, with no overall condensation pathway and variability from particle to particle. However, ion-etching studies with T4 and, more recently, phage lambda allow direct measurement of the condensation direction by gradual erosion of DNA from outside to inside the structure (Black *et al.*, 1985; Brown and Newcomb, 1986). By this technique, T4 and lambda DNAs are condensed from inside to outside the capsid. This technique also suggests a relatively invariant organization among individual particles (Black *et al.*, 1985; Brown and Newcomb, 1986), in contrast to the findings of Haas *et al.* (1982) and the proposal of Harrison (1983). In view of these findings, moreover, a solenoidal organization, at least of phage λ DNA, is unattractive because of the determined order of entry and exit of the λ DNA ends. Since the lambda DNA is packaged starting from the left end and exiting from the right end, a toroidal organization is difficult to reconcile with DNA ejection, given that the DNA condenses from inside to outside. This requires that DNA be pulled through the densely packaged DNA condensate shells, if λDNA is packaged parallel to the long axis, as is T4 giant DNA (see Fig. 5A). But in fact, the opposite direction of condensation had been a strong prediction of the original concentric shell organization (Earnshaw and Casjens, 1980).

Black *et al.* (1985) suggested that T4 DNA can be condensed from inside to outside because it is organized in 180° folded rods in a so-called spiral fold organization, in which DNA arrives finally in spiral shells. These 180° folds of DNA are arranged insofar as is compatible with icosahedral symmetry of the capsid parallel to the phage tail, or along the long axis of the T4 phage head, an organization also compatible with ion-etching studies of phage lambda (Fig. 5B) (Brown and Newcomb, 1986). This model was argued to be compatible with all current observations on condensed phage DNA structure, and it strongly suggests that DNA is packaged in folds rather than from an end and that kinks in DNA should be mobile and capable of reorganization in the event of deletions or during packaging; thus, intermediates in packaging may not resemble the final spiral fold structure. This structure is clearly not in good agreement with the interpretation of ball-like structures visualized in released packaged DNA (Fig. 3A) (Richards *et al.*, 1973). However, by electron microscopic techniques, kinked, single-strand nuclease-sensitive DNA condensates may be visualized as indistinguishable ball-like DNA condensates (Laemmli, 1975). In addition, DNA may rapidly reorganize after release, and the kinked DNA may not be detectable with electron microscopy.

A related folded DNA structure was also suggested by Serwer (1986). This structure was proposed to account for the observation of two types of intercalator binding sites in the DNA, the high-affinity, low-concentration sites being equated with infrequent folds in the DNA (Griess *et al.*, 1985, 1986). In this model, condensation is shown as proceeding from outside to inside the capsid, since the DNA is both gently bent and folded, and the ends of the 180° folded rods apparently coalesce so as to make a circular structure, as in the folded rod structure of Eickbush and Moudrianakis (1978). This has been reported to be inconsistent with the formation of artificial spermidine DNA condensates (Marx and Reynolds, 1982).

A recent cryoelectron microscopy study of phages λ and T4 and T4 giant phages has produced striking images of the packaged DNA condensate in vitrified unstained specimens. Electron diffraction patterns of these phages also reveal a 25-Å spacing of the packed B-form DNA, and a largely longitudinal and parallel arrangement of DNA in the giant, as well as to a lesser degree the normal T4 heads (Fig. 3D,E). Packaging density appears to be uniform within the phage head, but the 25-Å spacings appear to be differently oriented locally within the isometric λ phage heads, suggesting a liquid or nematic crystalline structure (Fig. 5C). In this model, the DNA would presumably be kinked more or less sharply to connect the microcrystalline arrays. Although this structure might allow a less sharp bend in B-form DNA, it is uncertain whether it is sufficiently symmetrical to account for the long-range order in packaged DNA across the head (e.g., Earnshaw and Harrison, 1977). It cannot be excluded that the cryomicroscopy images could result from slight deformation of a more ordered (spiral-fold or solenoidal) structure (Fig. 5A or B).

Thus, there is compelling evidence against simple solenoidal organization of the DNA, whereas many observations of overall structure are more consistent with folded DNA models of the sort proposed by Black et al. (1985). However, there is no unequivocal demonstration of non-B-form DNA within phage heads—certainly not 180° folds. A number of studies of packaged DNA have been interpreted to suggest various portions of non-B-form DNA within this structure, some of them surprisingly large fractions. These studies have measured packaged DNA reactivity with formaldehyde or bisulfite (Sklyadneva et al., 1980), with angelicin (a psoralen derivative that is supposed to be capable of binding only to bent DNA) (Kittler et al., 1980) or acridines (McCall and Bloomfield, 1976; Griess et al., 1985, 1986). Related earlier studies (reviewed by Tikchonenko, 1975) have presented evidence that packaged phage DNA has binding or reactivity that differs from extended B-form DNA; however, their support for kinks or any particular minor non-B-form DNA structure or particular model of condensed DNA is speculative. Although there is considerable evidence that less sharply bent DNA is found in other contexts (Frederick et al., 1984; Marini et al., 1982), 180° bends still appear to remain a theoretical structure in natural higher-order DNA structures (Crick and Klug, 1975). It should be noted that in contrast to the above characterized kinked structures in certain natural DNAs, DNA within the head, if bent, should not be bent at specific sequences to any significant extent. This is because of the observed packaging within capsids of DNAs with deletions and the capacity of most heads to take up duplex DNA of any sequence in transducing particles. Ends of folds may be immobilized by major capsid protein interaction, but reorganization during packaging is probably necessary to account for general reorganization in underpackaged phage heads. However, DNA organization in folds would tend to suggest a significant participation by the major capsid protein in the packaging process. If DNA is packaged as folded rods, it is uncertain to what degree the structure is invariant (as in the spiral-fold model; Fig. 5B), or variable and possibly less sharply bent, as in the nemetic crystalline structure (Fig. 5C). New techniques may be necessary to establish a definitive structure for packaged phage DNA.

IV. TERMINASE AND HEADFUL CUTTING OF CONCATEMERIC DNA IN PACKAGING

There is more exact knowledge of the mechanism of concatemer cutting in DNA packaging than of the processes involved in translocating and arranging DNA within the prohead. In general, phage replication mechanisms lead to the accumulation of DNA concatemers: tandem, covalently joined, head-to-tail arrays of mature phage DNA sequences (Fig. 6). Concatemeric DNA in the infected bacterium is found to be the substrate for DNA packaging *in vivo* and must be cut to yield mature packaged DNA [exceptions are the packaging of replicated circular DNA for phage P2, protein-terminated mature length DNA for φ29, and chromosomally integrated DNA for phage mu (Fig. 7)]. Formation of ends in mature phage DNA by packaging also in part determines replication mechanisms—e.g., for circular DNA molecules that result from reannealing the single-stranded cohesive ends, or for concatemer formation by recombination between terminally redundant sequences in replicated linear monomeric DNA. Although the mechanisms of formation of the intracellular substrates for DNA packaging by replication and recombination mechanisms will not be discussed, in this context it should be noted that in actuality intracellular concatemers of many phages are nonlinear structures containing DNA branches generated by recombinational and replicative processes (e.g., Dannenberg and Mosig, 1983); moreover, they are complexed with other macromolecules. Problems associated with packaging real *in vivo* concatemers as opposed to *in vitro* linear concatemers are discussed in the following section.

Packaging of headfuls of concatemeric DNA, where measured, has invariably been found to be directional and processive along the concatemer. Thus a variable number of proheads are packaged in series in a unidirectional sense along the concatemer following an initiating packaging cut which displays special features; e.g., more than seven, but on average 3–5 headfuls per concatemer are packaged in P22 (Adams *et al.*, 1983; Jackson *et al.*, 1978), 2–3 in lambda (Emmons, 1974; Feiss and Bublitz, 1975; Feiss *et al.*, 1985a), and about 3–4 for T1 and P1 (Gill and MacHattie, 1976; Bachi and Arber, 1977).

Concatemeric DNA is cut *in vivo* in conjunction with headful DNA packaging events by a group of phage proteins called terminases. These yield the mature phage DNA found within the capsid. Such cuts can be strictly sequence-specific, as in λ or T7; they can be initiated in a processive series from a specific packaging sequence called *pac* and there-

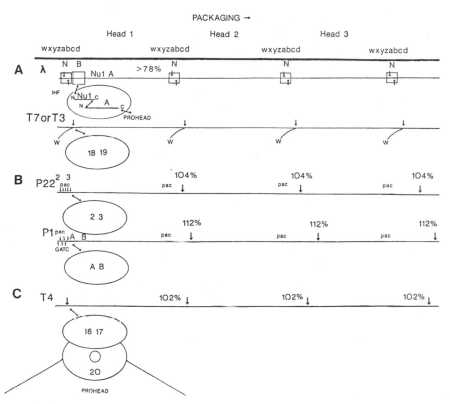

FIGURE 6. Mechanisms of processive terminase and headful cutting and packaging of dsDNA bacteriophage packaging concatemeric DNA. (Top) DNA concatemer. (A) bateriophages with identical end sequences, λ with cohesive ends, and T7 or T3, with identical direct blunt-end repeats at the ends, require repair or displacement DNA synthesis as shown. (B) Phages utilizing *pac* site mechanisms P22 and P1. Imprecise cutting at a unique *pac* sequence is followed by processive head filling of a series of heads with more than one genome length of DNA to create permuted, terminally redundant mature DNA. (C) T4, a phage using a pure head-filling mechanism, initiates packaging at random and adds 102% of the genome to the head to create randomly permuted, terminally redundant mature DNA.

after at whatever sequence results from headful measuring and cutting of DNA from the previous head (P22, P1, T1) (Tye *et al.*, 1974), or heads can be filled without any apparent sequence specificity by a pure headful mechanism (T4) (Streisinger *et al.*, 1967). The cutting mechanisms can yield blunt ends or 5′ or 3′ protruding ends in the mature DNA (Fig. 6, Table I).

The terminal cut in packaging a head that creates the second end in mature DNA is termed headful cutting. The second cut may occur at the same sequence as the initiating cut (e.g., λ) or, in a second headfilling class of bacteriophage, by a sequence-independent headful measuring cut (e.g., P22, P1, T1, T4). However, even among phages of the first type,

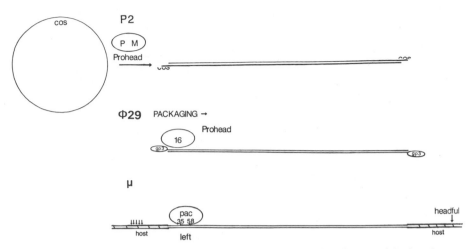

FIGURE 7. Mechanisms of terminase and headful cutting and packaging of dsDNA bacte-riophage packaging nonconcatemeric DNA. P2 terminase packages covalently closed, cir-cular DNA and produces cohesive ends. φ29 packages a 5' protein terminated linear mature DNA from the left end. μ packages host-integrated DNA from a *pac* site by a headful mechanism.

where the second cut is at the same sequence as the first, the second cutting event may show headful DNA-length dependence and display different sequence recognition requirements; e.g., in λ, the cutting of the terminal site depends on DNA length between sites (Feiss and Siegele, 1979) and displays less stringency for DNA sequence recognition of the entire terminase interaction site (Feiss, 1986). Phages of this category with fixed end sequences have cohesive ends (λ, P2) or nonpermuted terminal redundancy (T7, T3, T5).

In the second category, phages such as T4, P22, P1, T1, and mu carry out headful cutting, which is apparently entirely sequence-nonspecific but which can measure DNA length fitting a head volume to within about 1% variation in length (Kim and Davidson, 1974; Chow and Bukhari, 1977). Such phages, unlike phages of the first type, necessarily do not display underpackaged DNA-containing particles or density vari-ants. Their DNA is terminally redundant and circularly permuted, al-though not freely permuted in phages with a *pac* site. The structural signal allowing the precise and sequence-independent headful cutting mechanism is not understood, and terminase is not known to carry out the second headful, as well as the first cutting reaction, at least in all of the head-filling phages (Rao and Black, 1985a).

As will be summarized at the end of Section IV, there are many overall similarities in the terminases and the cutting mechanisms ob-served among the phages (Figs. 6, 7; Table I). Nevertheless, each phage displays characteristic features.

A. Phages with Unique Ends

1. Phage λ

DNA end formation in phage λ is perhaps the best understood (Feiss and Becker, 1983; Feiss, 1986). Phage λ mature DNA has 12 base single-strand 5' protruding complementary cohesive end sequences. These result from staggered nicks or *"ter"* cuts in concatemeric DNA which are produced by λ terminase at *"cos"* sites (cohesive end sites). Lambda terminase recognizes and nicks in a strictly sequence-specific mechanism at extended sites of about 200 bp in concatemeric λ DNA. Dissection of the terminase site reveals that there are separate nicking (N) and binding (B) sequences in the DNA at the *cos* site whose major structural features have been characterized (Miwa and Matsubara, 1983; Feiss *et al.*, 1983; Hohn, 1983) (Fig. 6).

Lambda terminase is a multimer of the λ gpNu1 and gpA proteins. The N and B sequences of the λ *cos* site are immediately adjacent and upstream (relative to packaging) to the Nu1 and A genes. The N-terminal portion of gpNu1 binds to *cos*B, its C terminus interacts with the N terminus of gpA, and the C terminus of gpA interacts with the prohead (Fig. 6). Since gpA also contains an ATP-binding site, there are at least four functional domains in the terminase. Numerous lambdoid phages display nearly identical ends and terminases. However, the dissection of functional domains in the proteins has been revealed by studying the specificity properties of λ-21 hybrids, which, except for a common nicking specificity, recognize only the homologous terminase and prohead gene products (Frackman *et al.*, 1984, 1985; Feiss *et al.*, 1985a,b; Feiss, 1986).

Packaging from λ *cos* sites in concatemeric DNA is directional (from Nu1 to R) and processive, presumably because of the asymmetric *cos* site (Feiss *et al.*, 1985a). Although cutting at all N sites is strictly sequence-specific, deletions between *cos* sites may lead to a reduction in cutting. Thus, terminase cleavage at the second and third *cos* sites requires N but does not require *cos*B, and it shows some headful cleavage dependence (Feiss and Siegele, 1979) in the sense that if the DNA length between *cos* sites 1 and 2 is reduced below about 78%, then cleavage and packaging are greatly reduced (Feiss and Bublitz, 1975; Feiss *et al.*, 1977). There are on average 2–3 head-filling events per initiating cut, with different binding cutting properties at both second and subsequent *cos* sites where *cos*B recognition is not required (Feiss *et al.*, 1985a). These properties suggest that terminase remains associated with the concatemer between cutting events, consistent with tracking along the DNA during DNA translocation and in support of an active role of terminase throughout packaging (Feiss, 1986).

A requirement for host factors in initiating terminase cuts is observed for phage λ (or phage 21). The terminase requires either IHF (in-

tergrative host factor, produced by genes *him*A and *hip*) or THF (terminase host factor—gene unknown) for activity at the first *cos* site *in vivo*
and *in vitro* (Bear *et al.*, 1984; Feiss *et al.*, 1985b; Gold and Becker, 1983;
G. Shinder, W. Parris, and M. Gold, personal communication). Consensus
sequences around the *cos* site resemble those found for IHF binding sites
around the λ*att* site, as the staggered cutting resembles the λInt cutting at
the λ*att* site. Host factors probably participate in the initial interaction of
terminase with the B recognition site, as they do for entry of Int at the *att*
site, but entry to the distal cutting sites may be provided by DNA translocation (Feiss, 1986).

   In vitro packaging of λ DNA and λ *cos* cutting by terminase are
generally consistent with these observations (Becker *et al.*, 1977; Murialdo and Fife, 1984; Becker and Gold, 1978; Gold and Becker, 1983).
Formation of a complex of terminase and *cos*-containing DNA (complex
I) is followed by binding to the prohead (complex II), and terminase must
remain associated until the completion of packaging. Cutting at *cos* depends on ATP, and terminase exhibits DNA-dependent ATPase activity.
The dependence of lambda cutting and packaging on the lambda gp*ben*
endonuclease and gp*FI* proteins is obscure. gp*FI* is apparently required *in
vivo*, and it interacts at the genetic level with the terminase genes, but it
is not required *in vitro* for packaging in the absence of single-stranded
DNA; the gp*ben* endonuclease interacts with gp*FI* and is activated by
single-stranded DNA (Benchimol *et al.*, 1982; Feiss and Becker, 1983).

   It has recently been found employing a *cos*-deficient λ packaging
system that concatemers are probably the obligatory substrate for λ *in
vitro* packaging. Although *in vivo* observations established that the substrate for packaging was concatemeric DNA, conflicting results from λ *in
vitro* packaging systems appeared to suggest that mature linear monomers and circular monomers either could or could not be packaged by
various *in vitro* packaging systems (Gold *et al.*, 1982; Hohn, 1975; Syvanen, 1975). The positive results with monomers and monomer circles
are now thought to be due to utilization of endogenous *cos*-like sequences in residual defective prophages in most *E. coli* to form concatemers. And the packaging of linear monomers shows concentration
dependence, suggesting a requirement for cohesive end annealing (Rosenberg *et al.*, 1985a,b).

   A reasonable explanation of these results is that *cos* cutting in the
absence of packaging can lead to the formation of concatemers through
annealing of cohesive ends (making use of the endogenous *cos* sites)
which can then be packaged. Consistent with the suggested model, terminase may cleave *cos* sites in the absence of packaging and prohead
structures, as demonstrated by the interaction of *chi* sites and *cos* sites
(see Section V) (Kobayashi *et al.*, 1983). In keeping with the suggested
mechanism, a number of *in vitro* systems allow *cos* cutting in extracts
producing the λ terminase components in the absence of proheads, although cutting is apparently inhibited by other phage products and has

not always been detected biochemically *in vivo* (Laski and Jackson, 1982; Gold *et al.*, 1982; Murialdo and Fife, 1984, 1987). These findings suggest an absolute requirement for λ concatemeric DNA as the substrate for *in vitro* packaging, a requirement not seen for several other phages (Table I). A packaging active λ terminase may be formed only by entry at a B site, although it may cut at distal *cos* sites without *cos*B, because translocation along the DNA provides an alternative access to *cos*N (Feiss, 1986).

2. Phages T7 and T3

Replication of the closely related phage T7 and T3 DNAs proceeds through concatemer formation by recombination within identical end sequences of synthesized linear monomers and forms very long concatemers. Both phages have identical blunt-end [160bp(T7)or 230bp(T3)] direct repeats at both termini of the mature DNA (Dunn and Studier, 1983; Fujisawa and Sugimoto, 1983). These ends are apparently created by extension synthesis at the 3′ ends of widely separated staggered nicks. If there were not such repair synthesis, half the replicated DNA would necessarily be lost (Fig. 6). Therefore, although T7 (or T3) DNA is blunt-ended and has terminal direct repeats, it is unlikely that T7 concatemeric DNA is simply cut to yield blunt ends in packaging, but terminase probably creates staggered nicks of 160 (or 230) bp. The mechanism of DNA repair synthesis and separation of the single-stranded 160 or 230 base sequence overlaps resulting from the staggered cutting is not understood. Staggered nicks of this length (Tm on the order of 85°) must apparently be separated by enzymes, and this might be accomplished by displacement DNA synthesis. In contrast, phages λ and P1, in which concerted nicking produces short, overlapped, single-stranded ends (12 and 2 bp, respectively), are thought not to require a special mechanism to separate the two cut duplexes.

Most recent work with these phages on terminase and on end formation in packaging has used a defined T3 *in vitro* packaging system. Mature T3 DNA can be packaged in a highly purified and defined packaging system consisting of proheads and the overexpressed purified terminase proteins gp18 and gp19, which lacks other T3 components (Hamada *et al.*, 1986a,b). Packaging of mature DNA does not absolutely depend on the presence of gp18 (the small subunit of terminase), and the terminase displays a prohead-stimulated ATPase activity. The terminases of T7 and T3 are homologous but differ in packaging specificity (Fujisawa *et al.*, 1980; Yamagishi *et al.*, 1985; Yamado *et al.*, 1986). Packaging of concatemers showed that the T3 system is able to discriminate against T7 sequences, and hybrid studies analogous to those of λ-21 hybrids show that the specificity determinants for this process probably reside in the 5% end sequences of T3–T7, close to the structural genes for terminase. It was concluded that the COOH terminus of the large subunit gp19 was at least in part responsible for the specific DNA sequence recognition at the T3 end sequence (Yamagishi *et al.*, 1985). However, mature DNA can be packaged efficiently in the refined system in the apparent absence of concatemer formation, and under these conditions the discrimination against T7 DNA is lost (Hamada *et al.*, 1986). It therefore appears that the T3 *in vitro* packaging systems can use mature as well as concatemeric DNA (Fujisawa *et al.*, 1980) and that, as in the case of λ, concatemer cutting imposes more stringent sequence recognition requirements for terminase (Table I). However, no nuclease activity has been found to be associated with either terminase protein.

It has recently been observed that gp18 contains the DNA-binding site, whereas gp19 contains the prohead and ATP-binding amino acid consensus sequences and interacts in the presence of ATP with the portal protein. And in the presence of ATP, the gp18 DNA and gp19 prohead interact to form a "50S" packaging complex which can package the mature T3 DNA (H. Fujisawa, personal communication).

B. Phages with *pac* Site Cutting

1. Phage P22

Phage P22 is the prototype for specific *pac* site cutting followed by processive headful cutting. This was originally revealed by the observation that its permuted DNA ends fell within a limited portion of the genome (Tye *et al.*, 1974). Following the initiating *pac* cut, cutting is processive and operates by a headful mechanism, so that 104% of a genome is packaged, with second and subsequent headfuls initiating from the other end of the headful cut (Fig. 6). Processivity of packaging is affected by the time of phage development and the levels of synthesis of the terminase proteins that are required more for first than for subsequent headfuls (Adams *et al.*, 1983).

The initiating packaging cut in a P22 concatemer is at a specific *pac* recognition site. *Pac* site cutting *in vitro* depends on the gp2 and gp3 proteins but not proheads or packaging (Jackson *et al.*, 1978; Laski and Jackson, 1982). Cutting is not precise at the *pac* site, and occurs at about 20-bp separated *end* sites within 120 bp around this site; cutting apparently creates blunt-end sites (Casjens and Huang, 1982; Backhaus, 1985). The *pac* site is within gene 3, and gene 3 mutants can also lose specificity for *pac* site cutting, suggesting that, as in the other phages (Table I), the small subunit gp3 is important for the site recognition or DNA binding (Raj *et al.*, 1974; Jackson *et al.*, 1982). A consensus sequence for the *pac* recognition site has been identified (Casjens *et al.*, 1987). As in phage λ, recognition and cutting sites are apparently distinct.

The P22 gp2 and gp3 proteins form the multimeric terminase and can probably package concatemeric DNA (Poteete *et al.*, 1979; Poteete and

Botstein, 1979). However, packaging of mature P22 DNA *in vitro* is more efficient than that of concatemeric DNA and does not requie *pac* site cutting, *pac* site recognition, or concatemer formation; both gp2 and gp3 are required. Therefore any DNA end in P22 and related phage DNA appears to be active for packaging *in vitro* by the P22 terminase (Strobel *et al.*, 1984).

2. Phage P1

Phage P1 displays overall similarity to P22 in its end formation mechanism, because it has been known for some time to employ a *pac* site and processive headful packaging mechanism. P1 fills 3–4 heads from a *pac* site within concatemeric DNA to yield permuted and 12% terminally redundant mature DNA (Fig. 6) (Bachi and Arber, 1977; Sternberg and Hoess, 1983). Two adjacent P1 genes, *A* and *B*, are essential for *pac* cleavage, and *pac* is located in the upstream gene (N. Sternberg and J. Coulby, personal communication). *Pac* site cleavage does not depend on synthesis of phage head gene products, and it appears to be due to an early gene product.

Understanding of the *pac* site mechanism has been advanced by a demonstration that cleavage (rather than for example initiation of DNA replication) occurs at the P1 *pac* site. When *pac* site cleavage (dependent upon the P1 gene 9 product) occurs within *E. coli* DNA, the end to be packaged survives, whereas the yield of the other end is reduced, even in the absence of packaging. When the *pac* site is located in a small plasmid DNA, both ends are lost, except in a *recBCD* host. Then the end recovery is comparable to that in chromosomally located *pac* site cutting. This suggests that following *pac* site cleavage, the end destined to be packaged is protected from the *recBCD* nuclease and other nucleases, probably by terminase. If the two ends are close (plasmid), then *recBCD* can traverse the DNA to degrade the *pac* site from the opposite end. If they are not (chromosome), then *recBCD* cannot traverse the DNA to reach the protected end while another nuclease degrades the unprotected end (Sternberg and Coulby, 1987a). The P1 *pac* site is contained within 161 bp, and cleavage is imprecise within about a 10-bp segment at the center of this site, apparently leaving protruding 2-bp 3' termini (Sternberg and Coulby, 1987b).

As a general mechanism, *pac* site cleavage might have evolved to produce efficient use of DNA in packaging by avoiding competitive filling by two proheads of the same mature-length DNA segment. However, the *pac* site mechanism requires precise control over frequency of *pac* site cutting (or the ability to rejoin the ends), since 100% *pac* site cutting would destroy the ability of the phage DNA to replicate by eliminating its terminal redundancy and would therefore be expected to be less efficient than random initiation and competitive packaging. DNA methylation has been proposed to be an essential regulatory mechanism for controlling *pac* site cleavage in P1 (Sternberg, 1985). It is observed that in P1 DNA there are 7 *Dam* methylation sites (GATC) in the *pac* site segment and that *pac* cleavage appears to depend on and be controlled by the methylation of these sequences (Sternberg and Coulby, 1987b). *In vitro* *pac* cleavage occurs only in fully methylated, not unmethylated or hemimethylated, *pac* site-containing DNA. *In vitro*, an unmethylated *pac* site can be cleaved if methylated by the *E. coli Dam* enzyme, and evidence suggests that *in vivo*, both *E. coli* and P1 *Dam* methylases may act at the *pac* site (N. Sternberg, personal communication). These observations therefore suggest a mechanism for control *in vivo* of P1 *pac* site cleavage: following replication, such sites are shielded until later in development, when DNA has undergone a maturation step controlled by full methylation around the *pac* site.

3. Phage T1

Phage T1 also utilizes a *pac* site, with processive and headful packaging of about three headfuls following utilization of a *pac* site. T1 terminal redundancy is about 6% (MacHattie and Gill, 1977; Gill and MacHattie, 1975, 1976; Ramsay and Ritchie, 1983). An additional mutation, *pip*, led to increased initiation at other sites and reduced the processivity of packaging (Drexler and Christensen, 1986). A prohead mutation (13.3) affected termination cutting but not the initiation of *pac* site cutting and may be in a gene similar to λ*D*; a pathway for T1 head assembly and packaging was proposed (Ramsay and Ritchie, 1984).

An *in vitro* packaging system for phage T1 has been characterized (Liebeschuetz *et al.*, 1985; Hug *et al.*, 1986). It was concluded that packaging of concatemers was most efficient and that *pac*-like sequences in T1 and related phage DNA concatemers were required for packaging. Less efficient packaging can apparently result from non-sequence-specific utilization of any DNA end in monomer-size DNA that does not require *pac*-like sequences (Liebeschuetz *et al.*, 1985; Hug *et al.*, 1986). Therefore, like phages T7, P22, and T4, T1 can package from any end in the DNA as well as from the T1 *pac* site *in vitro* (Table I). Selective formation of T1 transducing particles and of T1 particles containing λ DNA apparently results from recognition of *pac*-like sequences in the DNAs (Drexler, 1984).

4. Other *pac* Site Phages

A number of other phages, indeed perhaps most without specific end sequences, also utilize *pac* site mechanisms. Among these are phage SPP1 (Deichelbohrer *et al.*, 1982) and *Proteus mirabilis* phage 5006M (Hascoet *et al.*, 1982). In addition, a *pac* site in phage Mu has been identified (see below).

C. Phages with Non-Sequence-Specific Cutting of Concatemeric DNA

Phages T4, φ42 (Moynet and DeFillippes, 1982), and φ11 (Lofdahl *et al.*, 1981) and coliphage 15 (Lee *et al.*, 1970) apparently have randomly permuted DNAs. The techniques that have revealed specific *pac* site sequences in other phages have not revealed them in these phages. These phages have therefore been concluded to package their DNA according to a pure headful mechanism (Fig. 6). Of these, only T4 has been extensively characterized. A number of biochemical, electron microscopic, and genetic experiments argue against the existence of a T4 *pac* site (MacHattie *et al.*, 1967; Wilson *et al.*, 1979; Mosig *et al.*, 1971; Kalinski and Black, 1986), although some departure from random end sequences in T4 mature DNA has been reported (Grossi *et al.*, 1983). Nevertheless, if T4 (and other phages of this type) had multiple *pac* sites, as it does replication origins, or if it separated cutting from sequence recognition at *pac* by an extended migration of terminase along the concatemer for cutting (e.g., as does the *EcoK* restriction enzyme—Yuan *et al.*, 1980), these sequence-specific sites might not have been detected.

In many respects, T4 terminase is similar to that of the other phages (Table I). It appears that the initiating cut in T4 DNA is at least in part structurally regulated by interaction of the terminase proteins with the prohead portal protein, because cold-sensitive mutations in the structural gene for this prohead protein control formation of mature DNA ends (Hsiao and Black, 1977). Although selection of T4 sequences to be cut is unknown, there is apparently an endonuclease activity associated with the overexpressed and purified terminase proteins (Rao and Black, 1987). The small subunit gp16 is stringently required for concatemer packaging but not for packaging mature DNA, which is consistent with earlier *in vivo* observations (Wunderli *et al.*, 1977).

Phage T4 will package non-T4 DNAs *in vitro* and prefers mature to concatemeric DNA (Rao and Black, 1985b; Black, 1981, 1986). The large subunit gp17 contains the ATP-binding site, and terminase does not bind nonspecifically to DNA (T4 or DNA cellulose) (Rao and Black, 1987). Because site mutations have been discovered in the terminase g17 that are suppressed by g32 mutations, it has been proposed that recombinational intermediates serve as specific sites for packaging initiation (Mosig *et al.*, 1981). In addition, it has been observed that g32 and g17 display amino acid sequence homology (G. Mosig, personal communication).

D. Phages Packaging Nonconcatemeric dsDNA

1. Phage P2

The overall packaging properties of phage P2 (and its smaller satellite, P4) most resemble those of phage λ, except that P2 packages covalently closed circular DNA *in vivo* (λ monomer circles are not packaged *in vivo* by λ) (Fig. 7). Circular DNA is the replication product *in vivo* that accumulates in the absence of head maturation (Pruss and Calendar, 1978) and is the preferred substrate for packaging *in vitro*, although linear monomeric and concatemeric DNA can also be packaged *in vitro* (Pruss *et al.*, 1975). Phage P2 has 19 base 5' single-strand cohesive ends. These are the products of the P2 terminase, composed of proteins gpP and gpM. The headful cutting properties of P2 terminase at *cos* also resemble those of λ, since roughly a headful of DNA is required to carry out headful cutting of P4 DNA in P2 heads (Pruss *et al.*, 1975; Shore *et al.*, 1978).

The terminase gene products have been highly purified and have been shown to carry out cohesive end cutting *in vitro*: gpM, gpP, and proheads, as well as ATP are required. gpM (28K) is implicated in cutting, since in the absence of gpM *in vitro*, mature but not circular DNA can be packaged, but gpP appears to be the cutting enzyme (Bowden and Calendar, 1979). Cutting at the *cos* site depends on its location in covalently closed circular DNA-multimer circles, but linear multimers are not active. This property does not appear to reflect a requirement for superhelicity, since nicked circles are cut. The P2 terminase ATPase activity is activated by any DNA and hydrolyzes ATP to AMP (Bowden and Modrich, 1981, 1985). In certain respects these P2 terminase properties resemble those of phages using concatemeric DNA in packaging (Table I).

2. Phage φ29

Phi 29 DNA replication proceeds from either end of the linear molecule by strand displacement to generate mature molecules with a viral protein, gp3, covalently linked to the 5' termini. Because φ29 DNA is always linear and unit length, there is no need for a DNA cleavage reaction, and protein-terminated DNA is the packaging substrate *in vitro* and *in vivo*; DNA must have attached gp3 for packaging (Bjornsti *et al.*, 1982). In a sense, however, φ29 could also utilize a bipartite terminase, where one of the subunits is permanently attached to the end of the DNA (Table I).

Phi 29 *in vitro* packaging occurs with essentially *in vivo* efficiency and demonstrates that packaging proceeds from left to right along the DNA. Therefore, either the proteins at the two termini must differ or there must be recognition by the packaging protein (gp16) of a sequence downstream from the left short inverted 6-bp-long terminal repetitions found at the flush ends of φ29 (Fig. 7).

Packaging *in vitro* of φ29 DNA in a defined system has been demonstrated to depend on the single packaging protein gp16, which (except for the terminal gp3) is necessary and sufficient for DNA packaging into purified proheads (Guo *et al.*, 1986). Packaging is initiated by prohead-gp16 binding, and this complex then binds DNA-gp3. ATP hydrolysis leads to head filling as well as formation of aggregates in the gp3-φ29 DNA, although these structures have not been demonstrated to function as intermediates (Guo *et al.*, 1987a). The gp16 terminase protein has ATP and Mg^{2+} binding sites; as discussed previously, one ATP was calculated to be hydrolyzed per 2 bp packaged (Guo *et al.*, 1987b). Protein gp16 was found probably to interact with the portal protein (Guo *et al.*, 1987a), and the φ29 portal protein has also been reported to interact specifically with gp3 DNA (Herranz *et al.*, 1986).

A small RNA of φ29 has been shown to be essential for packaging *in vitro*. This RNA of about 120 nucleotides copurified with the prohead and was shown to originate from near the left, first-packaged end of the DNA. There therefore appears to be novel involvement of a specific RNA molecule to initiate the packaging process in φ29 (Guo *et al.*, 1987c).

3. Phage Mu

Bacteriophage Mu DNA is always associated with host DNA *in vivo*. Phage Mu particles contain about 37 kb of linear DNA which is heterogeneous at both left and right ends owing to attached host DNA of both varying length and sequence. The right end sequences vary between 500 and 3200 bp, whereas the left end sequences vary between 50 and 150 bp. Mu DNA insertions reduce and deletions add to the host sequence length on the right end. Phage deletions or insertions have no effect on the amount of left-end host sequences. From these and other observations, it was concluded that integrated Mu DNA *in vivo* is packaged by a headful mechanism directionally from a site toward the left end and proceeding past the right end of the phage DNA (Fig. 7) (Chow and Bukhari, 1977).

It was found that cutting at the left end varied in increments of about 11 bp, with a minimum of 56 and a maximum of about 144 bp of host DNA, the smaller segments being favored. It was proposed that the proteins at the left end measured its length in units of helical turns and cut the first left-end DNA to be packaged following completion of packaging (George and Bukhari, 1981). The *pac* site has been located between nucleotides 35 and 58 from the left-hand end of the phage DNA sequences, so that the terminase proteins of Mu would have to cut DNA about 100–250 bp upstream of their recognition stie in the host DNA. It can therefore be concluded that phage Mu terminase also has separate recognition and cutting sites and the same orientation of these sites relative to the direction of packaging as other phages (Figs. 6, 7) (Groenen and Van de Putte, 1985).

E. Common Features of DNA Maturation Processes

1. Headful Cutting

The terminal headful-measuring cutting mechanism in phages such as P22, P1, T1, T4, and Mu is not understood. Evidently this must involve structural interaction between the prohead, the DNA, and the cutting enzyme to achieve precision to within 1%. This communication is unlikely to be due simply to pausing in DNA translocation. For example, in phage T4 packaging *in vivo,* pauses in head-filling resulting from g49 endonuclease or DNA ligase mutations, or from mutations in the terminase structural genes, do not result in cutting of the concatemer (see Section V). Of course, it cannot be excluded in these cases that failure to cut the concatemer is because of abnormal DNA structure at the cutting site, deficient terminase nuclease activity, or simple rejoining of the cut ends if the head is not full. Nevertheless, various defects in DNA replication can lead to partially filled heads, either because DNA has "run out" during packaging or because of a premature headful cutting event (Black and Showe, 1983).

In phages with unique ends such as λ, it is established that terminase carries out terminal (headful) cutting, its properties probably changed by prohead interaction as discussed above (see Feiss, 1986; Feiss and Becker, 1983). Presumably this is also the case for phages T7 and T3, although the terminase cuts would appear sufficiently separated (T3, 230 bp) to be carried out by different terminase molecules. There is an imperfectly symmetrical sequence that might provide two such terminase-binding sites around the widely separated cutting sites (Dunn and Studier, 1983).

In phages P1 and P22, headful cutting is generally thought to be carried out by the terminase that receives information from the packaged prohead to signal the non-*pac*-site (headful) cutting, although there is no information about the nature of this signal or direct evidence, in fact, that headful cutting in these phages is actually carried out by the terminase. However, evidence that the portal protein of the prohead is involved in both the initiating terminase cut (phage T4) and the specificity of headful cutting (phage P22) has been discussed (Section III).

It has been proposed that in T4 the terminal headful cutting is carried out by a different enzyme from the initiating terminase (gp16 + gp17) cut. From the observation that a sequence-non-specific endonuclease present in the prohead but not the mature head was derived by protein processing from the major capsid protein, it was proposed that this enzyme was released from the head structure onto the DNA to carry out headful cutting upon completion of head filling. A speculative mechanism was that inability to relax a supertwisted molecule by a coupled translocation-supercoiling mechanism might provide a single-stranded structure in the DNA which, together with the structural change in the procapsid which releases the enzyme when the head is full, could provide a headful cut (Rao and Black, 1985; Manne *et al.,* 1982; Black *et al.,* 1981). A possibly analogous mechanism is the proposed autoproteolysis of assembled picornavirus capsid protein, which is controlled by interaction with the RNA chain during assembly (Rossman *et al.,* 1985).

2. Mechanisms of DNA End Formation

Differences in DNA end formation mechanisms among the phages have been emphasized above. These differences include formation of

unique or nonspecific end sequences in concatemeric or nonconcatemeric replicative dsDNA. Phages with nonspecific end sequences
may apparently use *pac* sequences or pure head-filling mechanisms. Also,
as summarized in Table I, mature DNA resulting from terminase action
may have 5' or 3' extensions or be blunt-ended and result from cuts
staggered by as few as zero (P22), 2 (P1), 12 (λ), 19 (P2), or as many as 230
(T3) bp. DNA may therefore be cut on opposite strands some distance
apart and without symmetrical sequences at the cutting sites (P2, T3).

Nevertheless, the formation of the mature DNA ends and the phage
terminases also show many common features. Thus far, all of the terminases appear to have separated binding and cutting sites in the DNA.
With respect to the direction of packaging along the concatemer, these
DNA interaction sites are so far either in or close to, and upstream of, the
structural genes for the terminase proteins. Packaging is directional and
processive along the DNA, and postinitiation cutting shows headful dependence which can be limited in phages with unique ends or strict in
phages that employ a head-filling mechanism (Figs. 6, 7).

These common end formation mechanisms are apparently due to
comparable terminase proteins of many phages (Table I). These proteins
all appear to hydrolyze or bind ATP, bind to the prohead portal protein
and to DNA (although some do not bind to DNA celluloses), and travel
along DNA in a unidirectional sense from a *pac, cos,* or other DNA-
binding and cutting site. Additional common features include a one-
large-one-small subunit composition motif in the apparently highly multimeric terminase found to be active in packaging, although the ratio of
these proteins in a holoenzyme is not well established (or possibly fixed)
(Hamada *et al.,* 1986b; Rao and Black, 1987; Guo *et al.,* 1986). These
terminase subunits display separation of functions in packaging; e.g., the
small λ and P22 subunits are implicated in specific DNA recognition site
binding in the concatemer. A similar property is that the small subunit is
nonessential (although efficiency may be greatly reduced) for packaging
mature DNA *in vitro* in a number of phages (T3, P2, and T4) as well as *in
vivo* (T4). In P22, distinct gp2 and gp3 roles in *pac* and headful cutting are
also suggested (Adams *et al.,* 1983). The predominant role of the small
subunit in initiating cutting of a DNA concatemer might be consistent
with the exception to the bipartite terminase structure found in the case
of φ29, which does not cut DNA. Here the second subunit can be viewed
as attached to the DNA, although it also functions in replication (Table I).
Moreover, there is evidence of further separation of functional domains
within the λ terminase polypeptides (reviewed by Feiss, 1986).

Terminases show significant differences in requirements for specific
sequences and DNA structure for activity in *in vitro* packaging systems
(Table I). Thus some terminases apparently require concatemeric DNA as
well as specific end sequences for packaging activity (λ) or end sequence
alone (P2). Other terminases can use mature as well as concatemeric
DNA for packaging (T1) and show sequence requirements only in concatemeric DNA, which is used more efficiently. Still others can appar-

ently use either concatemeric or monomeric DNA of any sequence and prefer nonspecific ends in monomeric DNA to *pac*-containing concatemers (P22, T4). Differences are also seen between λ, where a terminase-DNA complex is first formed and subsequently interacts with a prohead (Becker *et al.*, 1977), and T3, φ29, and probably T4. In phages φ29 and T3, the major terminase subunit first interacts with the prohead portal protein. This apparently activates the terminase to then associate with the DNA–small subunit complex to initiate packaging (Guo *et al.*, 1987a; H. Fujisawa, personal communication). These *in vitro* differences may relate to the poorly understood and replicated (*in vitro*) factors that control DNA binding and cutting *in vivo* by terminases in the various phages.

Many DNA sequences are now available for comparison of the terminase proteins and their binding and cutting sites (λ, P22, T3, T7, T4, φ29, P1). However, investigations of sequence homology have not been reported, or homology appears not to be great, at least between λ and P22 terminase proteins and binding sites (Backhhaus, 1985; Casjens *et al.*, 1987). As expected, the terminase protein genes display ATP and metal binding consensus sequences (Guo *et al.*, 1987b; H. Fujisawa, personal communication; G. Mosig, personal communication). A proposal has been made that the influence of flanking methylation sites on a distantly (~90 bp) located cutting site, as well as the imprecision of cutting at this site, might involve bending of the DNA by terminase molecules into a loop similar to that seen in binding of regulatory proteins (Sternberg and Coulby, 1987b). Significant features of the λ *cos* binding site recognized by terminase and IHF show some features common to operon regulatory sites for DNA binding proteins (Feiss and Becker, 1983; Feiss, 1986).

It has often been observed that the general terminase properties of translocating along DNA and making staggered or flush double-stranded cuts are analogous to those of the type I restriction enzymes. Phage DNA packaging also reveals a number of overall features seen in the transformation system for *Haemophilus* (DNA sequence-dependent, ATP energy requiring packaging of DNA into a receptacle that can bind a cell surface) (Smith *et al.*, 1981). Do such similarities reflect either a common mechanism or common origins?

V. INTERACTIONS OF DNA PACKAGING WITH OTHER DNA PROCESSES *IN VIVO*, AND DNA STRUCTURAL REQUIREMENTS FOR PACKAGING

Packaging *in vivo* must interact with numerous other DNA processes, suggesting that regulatory mechanisms governing these interactions are likely. Such interactions are described generally rather than understood at a mechanistic level. Nevertheless, these interactions suggest properties of the DNA structure required for packaging and characteristics of the packaging apparatus. A striking example of a packaging interaction with an unknown mechanism is found in the removal of cytoplasmic DNA-binding replication-recombination proteins from the packaged DNA. Proteins found with the DNA in the head enter before the DNA as part of the scaffold. Proteins found in high concentration on active intracellular DNA are presumably removed in a way that does not lead to defects (e.g., nicks, single-stranded regions) in duplex DNA entering the head. Although proteins might be stripped from the entering DNA by its passage through the 20- to 30-Å hole in the portal vertex structure, proteins of up to 67 kD are ejected from the T4 head through this structure (Black and Showe, 1983). Is it properties of the portal protein, of the duplex DNA structure required to enter the head, or of the terminases that allow these proteins to be removed?

A. Interactions *in Vivo*

In phage λ, the interaction of packaging with recombinational processes has been analyzed in depth genetically. The *chi* sequence in phage lambda DNA stimulates *recA–recBCD*–mediated recombination when correctly oriented with respect to *cos* sites (Kobayashi *et al.*, 1983). As this relates to packaging, *cos* activation of *chi* sites is separable from DNA packaging and prohead formation but requires both nicking and binding sites for terminase (Kobayashi *et al.*, 1984). *Cos* sites (or *EcoRI* sites—Stahl *et al.*, 1983) probably activate *chi* sites by providing entry points for recombination enzymes, including the *recBCD* endonuclease, at transient double-strand breaks. The directional properties of *chi* activation by *cos* can be explained by the binding of terminase to the right of the cut *cos* site. These genetic analyses therefore provide strong evidence for transient *cos* cutting in the absence of proheads, and for intimate connections between λ packaging and recombination *in vivo*. Because mature λ DNA does not accumulate *in vivo* in the absence of proheads and packaging, and recombination is not observed by rejoining between *cos* sites (Emmons, 1974), there should be rapid reannealing of the same cut ends in the absence of filling. Control over this terminase cutting and rejoining at *cos* is poorly understood (see Murialdo and Fife, 1984, 1987). The existence of terminase–single-strand DNA binding protein (gene 32) interaction mutations may also suggest participation in T4 of recombination processes in packaging-related cleavage of concatemers (Mosig *et al.*, 1981). The importance of host factors in initiating terminase cutting at *cos* and the similarity of this to recombinational cutting by λ*int* protein have been noted above (Section V).

In phage T7, RNA polymerase interaction with packaging is suggested by the observation that gp2, a protein that inactivates *E. coli* RNA polymerase, is required for *in vitro* packaging of mature T7 DNA in crude extracts; consistent with this, rifampicin can substitute for gp2 to stimulate the packaging (LeClerc and Richardson, 1979). F^+ and *Shigella* mutations interacting with T7 capsid protein mutations are possibly analogous to T4 capsid gene *gol* host interacting mutations (Section II). Because expression of these mutations does not require assembly of the capsid protein, these capsid mutations, although of unknown mechanism and connection to packaging, are apparently unconnected to this RNA polymerase interaction (Beck *et al.*, 1986; Champness and Snyder, 1984).

B. DNA Structural Requirements for Packaging

Apparently, small icosahedral virus RNAs first condense and then assemble the capsid around the condensate or cocondense the RNA and capsid. It has been hypothesized that an energetic or physical basis for the prohead mechanism may exist, as the condensation of nucleic acid is much greater in the dsDNA icosahedral bacteriophages (e.g., Hohn, 1976). There could, however, be an additional biological rationale for preferring the prohead packaging-condensation mechanism, especially for long dsDNAs. This allows the possibility of coupled DNA repair processes during packaging, whereas a prior DNA condensation mechanism does not. A significant amount of DNA is not packaged in each burst. Is this a random sample, or can damaged DNA be excluded by the packaging machinery? At the present time there is little evidence, except in extreme cases, that the packaging apparatus is able to discriminate actively against introduction of damaged DNA into the prohead.

Probably the best-understood example of DNA structure representing a roadblock to packaging arises in the case of T4 gene 49 (endonuclease VII) mutations. T4 g49 mutations lead to the accumulation of partially filled heads, apparently because of the accumulation of branches (recombinational intermediates) which can be visualized outside the partially filled head (Luftig *et al.*, 1971; Kemper and Brown, 1976). The gene 49 endonuclease is able to resolve Holliday structures in DNA as well as display other activities consistent with a role in removing such branches in the concatemeric DNA (Mizuuchi *et al.*, 1982). The phenotype of temperature-sensitive gene 49 mutations therefore demonstrates that DNA damage can arrest DNA packaging, and DNA repair processes can rescue arrested intermediates.

The precise structural requirements of DNA for its packaging are not understood; however, it is known that a number of DNA directed functions, if defective, can arrest DNA translocation into the prohead, suggesting the existence of such requirements. DNA ligase is required to complete DNA filling of T4 proheads *in vivo*. When both T4 and host DNA ligase temperature-sensitive mutant enzymes are inactivated, following the accumulation of a large DNA concatemer pool in the presence of ligase, full heads accumulate to only about 3% of the total. Restoration of ligase activity by temperature shift allows the major product, partially filled heads, to be filled to active heads. These experiments demonstrate that either the T4 or the *E. coli* ligase can satisfy the packaging requirement. Whether the lesion in DNA is a nick or more extensive damage to duplex DNA is unknown (Hsiao and Black, 1977; Zachary and Black, 1981). In phage T4 a number of "early" DNA replication-recombination functions, when altered by mutation, lead to defects in packaging as revealed by the accumulation of partially filled heads as the predominant product, suggesting that defects in the concatemer block continuation of DNA translocation (Zachary and Black, 1986).

The requirement for DNA ligase activity in T4 packaging might suggest that nicked DNA is not translocated into the head. And in phage λ, it has been observed that when DNA is nicked and packaged *in vitro*, fewer nicks are found in the DNA that is encapsidated (E. Lee and J. Hays, personal communication). However, in the defined T3 *in vitro* packaging system, nicked DNA is packaged without a reduction (H. Fujisawa, personal communication). Mature phage T5 DNA is observed to have nicks at specific sequences in one of the two strands. Mutations eliminating or increasing the frequency of these nicks have been isolated and demonstrate these to be nonessential. These mutations map in the late region, consistent with the possibility that they might be introduced into the DNA during packaging (Rogers *et al.*, 1979; Rhoades, 1984). Could certain terminases themselves be capable of introducing or even removing nicks in the DNA they package? The less well characterized phages RP1 (Donohue *et al.*, 1985), the Erwinia phage Erh1 (Kozloff *et al.*, 1981), and 13 (Reddy and Gopinathan, 1986) have nicks and single-strand gaps as well as very heterogeneous lengths of packaged DNA, suggesting that considerable departure from the duplex structure requirement is allowed in these phages.

It has long been known that heteroduplex loops are discriminated against, and it has been speculated that these could be excised during packaging (Nomura and Benzer, 1961; Benz and Berger, 1973). At the same time, it is known that heteroduplex loops of more limited extent, although discriminated against, can apparently be packaged (Drake, 1966). More recently, it has been reported that in the absence of the T4gp49 endonuclease VII, very much longer heteroduplex loops (up to 150 bp) can be packaged, suggesting that the T4 packaging machinery is able to tolerate very substantial departures from duplex DNA structure (Mosig and Powell, 1985). Packaging of such heterozygote loops is somewhat surprising, since it suggests that at some point three, or more likely, four single strands of DNA (assuming the single strand is held in a fixed folded configuration) can pass together through the 20- to 30-Å hole in the portal protein. At the same time, T7 and T4 UV-damaged DNA can be packaged, although UV dimers in T4 DNA caused slower DNA packaging *in vivo* (Kummerle and Masker, 1977; Zachary and Black, 1984). These overall observations do not lead to an obvious unitary model but might suggest that considerable departures from duplex structure are tolerated by the packaging machinery, at least in some phages, and that *in vivo* binding of repair proteins at sites of damage may arrest packaging and allow repair. With defined and simple host-component free packaging systems, it should be possible to test more directly the structural requirements for translocation into the prohead and the hypothesis of coupled DNA repair processes.

VI. CONCLUSIONS

Great progress has been made in describing the overall DNA packaging process and identifying the essential components and types of mechanisms. Nevertheless, in each area of current interest, significant general problems remain. (1) How is ATP hydrolysis energy coupled to a phage (or indeed any other) DNA translocation mechanism? How do structural proteins of the prohead participate together with terminase in a megamolecular machine to package and organize DNA? A host of questions is raised about the assembly and functions of such sophisticated multipurpose enzymatic and structural proteins. (2) The basic structure of packaged phage DNA now appears less well established than that of the nucleosome structure in chromosomes. Is DNA gently or sharply bent in the head, how invariant is this structure, and does this relate to the conformation and motion of DNA in other environments and biological processes? (3) Work in progress with purified terminases and defined and efficient packaging systems should establish further mechanistic properties of this interesting class of multifunctional enzymes including their still problematic translocation functions. (4) Recent findings that methylation of DNA, phage RNA molecules, and phage and host recombination factors and mechanisms may act in control of terminase activity and/or packaging point to a wealth of interesting molecular regulatory mechanisms connecting packaging to other DNA processes *in vivo*. The long-standing hope, mentioned at the outset, that knowledge of phage DNA packaging will bear on packaging in higher chromosomes and lead to new protein-DNA interaction mechanisms is encouraged by increased knowledge of the sophistication of the highly evolved phage DNA packaging mechanisms.

ACKNOWLEDGMENTS. Thanks are due D. Anderson, L. M. Black, R. Calendar, S. Casjens, H. Drexler, W. Earnshaw, M. Feiss, H. Fujisawa, E. Kellenberger, G. Mosig, H. Murialdo, V. B. Rao, M. Rhoades, N. Sternberg, A. Steven, D. B. Wilson, and A. Zachary for helpful comments and suggestions on this manuscript and for communication of unpublished work.

REFERENCES

Adams, M. B., Hayden, M., and Casjens, S., 1983, On the sequential packaging of bacteriophage P22 DNA, *J. Virol.* **46:**673–677.

Adrian, M., Dubochet, J., Lepault, J., and McDowall, A. W., 1984, Cryo-electron microscopy of viruses, *Nature* **308:**32–36.

Ashikawa, I., Furuno, T., Kinosita, K., Ikegami, A., Takahashi, H., and Akutsu, H., 1984, Internal motion of DNA in bacteriophages, *J. Biol. Chem.* **259:**8338–8344.

Bachi, B., and Arber, W., 1977, Physical mapping of *bg1*II, *Bam*H1, *Eco*RI, *Hind*III, and *Pst*I restriction fragments of bacteriophage P1 DNA, *Mol. Gen. Genet.* **153:**311–324.

Backhaus, H., 1985, DNA packaging initiation of *Salmonella* bacteriophage P22: Determination of cut sites within the DNA sequence coding for gene 3, *J. Virol.* **55:**458–465.

Bauer, W. R., Ressner, E. C., Kates, J., and Patzke, J. V., 1977, A DNA nicking-closing enzyme encapsidated in vaccinia virus: Partial purification and properties, *Proc. Natl. Acad. Sci. USA* **74:** 1841–1845.

Bazinet, C., and King, J., 1985, The DNA translocating vertex of DS DNA bacteriophage, *Annu. Rev. Microbiol.* **39:**109–129.

Bear, S. E., Court, D. L., and Friedman, D. I., 1984, A new accessory role for *E. coli* integration host factor (IHF): Characterization of a lambda mutant dependent upon IHF for DNA packaging, *J. Virol.* **52:**966–972.

Beck, P. J., Condreay, J. P., and Molineux, I. J., 1986, Expression of the unassembled capsid protein during infection of *Shigella sonnei* by bacteriophage T7 results in DNA damage that is repairable by bacteriophage T3, but not T7, DNA ligase, *J. Bacteriol.* **167:**251–256.

Becker, A., and Gold, M., 1978, Enzymatic breakage of the cohesive end site of phage λ DNA: Terminase (ter) reaction, *Proc. Natl. Acad. Sci. USA* **75:**4199–4209.

Becker, A., Marko, M., and Gold, M., 1977, Early events in the *in vitro* packaging of bacteriophage λ DNA, *Virology* **78:**291–305.

Benbasat, J. A., 1984, Condensation of bacteriophage phiW14 DNA of varying charge densities by trivalent counterions, *Biochemistry* **23:**3609–3619.

Benchimol, S., Lucko, H., and Becker, A., 1982, Bacteriophage λ DNA packaging *in vitro:* The involvement of the λFI gene product, single-strand DNA, and a novel λ-directed protein in the packaging reaction, *J. Biol. Chem.* **257:**5201–5210.

Bendet, I. J., Goldstein, D. A., and Lauffer, M. A., 1960, Evidence for internal organization of nucleic acid in T2 bacteriophage, *Nature* **187:**781–782.

Benz, W. C., and Berger, H., 1973, Selective allele loss in mixed infections with T4 bacteriophage, *Genetics* **73:**1–11.

Bijlenga, R. K. L., Aebi, U., and Kellenberger, E., 1976, Properties and structure of a gene 24-controlled T4 giant phage, *J. Mol. Biol.* **103:**469–498.

Bjornsti, M.-A., Reilly, B. E., and Anderson, D. L., 1982, Morphogenesis of bacteriophage Phi29 of *Bacillus subtilis:* DNA-gp3 intermediate in *in vivo* and *in vitro* assembly, *J. Virol.* **41:**508–517.

Bjornsti, M.-A., Reilly, B. E., and Anderson, D. L., 1983, Morphogenesis of bacteriophage φ29 of *Bacillus subtilis:* Oriented and quantized *in vitro* packaging of DNA protein gp3, *J. Virol.* **45:**383–396.

Black, L. W., 1974, Bacteriophage T4 internal protein mutants: Isolation and properties, *Virology* **60:**166–179.

Black, L. W., 1981a, *In vitro* packaging of bacteriophage T4 DNA, *Virology* **113:**336–344.

Black, L. W., 1981b, The mechanism of bacteriophage DNA encapsidation, in: *Bacteriophage Assembly* (M. S. DuBow, ed.), pp. 97–110, Alan R. Liss, New York.

Black, L. W., 1986, *In vitro* packaging into phage T4 particles and specific recircularization of phage lambda DNAs, *Gene* **46:**97–101.

Black, L. W., and Showe, M. K., 1983, Morphogenesis of the T4 head, in: *Bacteriophage T4*

(C. K. Mathews, E. M. Kutter, G. Mosig, and P. B. Berget, eds.), American Society for Microbiology, Washington.

Black, L. W., and Silverman, D., 1978, Model for DNA packaging into bacteriophage T4 heads, *J. Virol.* **28**:643–655.

Black, L. W., Zachary, A. L., and Manne, V., 1981, Studies of the mechanism of bacteriophage T4 DNA encapsidation, in: *Bacteriophage Assembly* (M. DuBow, ed), pp. 111–126, Alan R. Liss, New York.

Black, L. W., Newcomb, W. W., Boring, J. W., and Brown, J. C., 1985, Ion etching of bacteriophage T4: Support for a spiral-fold model of packaged DNA, *Proc. Natl. Acad. Sci. USA* **82**:7960–7964.

Bode, V. C., and Gillin, F. D., 1971, The arrangement of DNA in lambda phage heads. I. Biological consequences of micrococcal nuclease attack on a portion of the chromosome exposed in tailless heads, *J. Mol. Biol.* **62**:493–502.

Bowden, D. W., and Calendar, R., 1979, Maturation of bacteriophage P2 DNA *in vitro:* A complex, site-specific system for DNA cleavage, *J. Mol. Biol.* **129**:1–18.

Bowden, D. W., and Modrich, P., 1981, *In vitro* studies on the bacteriophage P2 terminase system, in: *Bacteriophage Assembly* (M. DuBow, ed.), pp. 223–230, Alan R. Liss, New York.

Bowden, D. W., and Modrich, P., 1985, *In vitro* maturation of circular bacteriophage P2 DNA: Purification of *ter* components and characterization of the reaction, *J. Biol. Chem.* **260**:6999–7007.

Brody, T., 1973, A DNA-binding form of the main structural protein of lambda heads, *Virology,* **54**:441–451.

Brown, J. C., and Newcomb, W. W., 1986, Ion etching of bacteriophage λ: Evidence that the right end of the DNA is located at the outside of the phage DNA mass, *J. Virol.* **60**:564–568.

Carrascosa, J. L., and Kellenberger, E., 1978, Head maturation pathway of bacteriophage T4 and T2. III. Isolation and characterization of particles produced by mutants in gene 17, *J. Virol.* **25**:831–844.

Casjens, S., 1985, Nucleic acid packaging by viruses, in: *Virus Structure and Assembly* (S. Casjens, ed.), pp. 76–147, Jones and Bartlett, Boston.

Casjens, S., and Hendrix, R., 1988, Control mechanisms in dsDNA bacteriophage assembly, in: *The Bacteriophages,* Vol. 1 (R. Calendar, ed.), pp. 15–92, Plenum Press, New York.

Casjens, S., and Huang, W. M., 1982, Initiation of sequential packaging of bacteriophage P22 DNA, *J. Mol. Biol.* **157**:287–298.

Casjens, S., and King, J., 1975, Virus assembly, *Annu. Rev. Biochem.* **44**:555–611.

Casjens, S., Huang, W. M., Hayden, M., and Parr, R., 1987, Initiation of bacteriophage P22 DNA packaging series: Analysis of a mutant which alters the DNA target specificity of the packaging apparatus, *J. Mol. Biol.* **194**:411–422.

Champness, W. C., and Snyder, L., 1984, Bacteriophage T4 *gol* site: Sequence analysis and effects of the site on plasmid transformation, *J. Virol.* **50**:555–562.

Chattoraj, D. K., and Inman, R. B., 1974, Location of DNA ends in P2, 186, P4, and lambda bacteriophage heads, *J. Mol. Biol.* **87**:11–22.

Chattoraj, D. K., Gosule, L. C., and Schellman, J. A., 1978, DNA condensation with polyamines. II. Electron microscopic studies, *J. Mol. Biol.* **121**:327–337.

Chow, L. T., and Bukhari, A. I., 1977, Bacteriophage Mu genome: Structural studies on Mu DNA and Mu mutants carrying insertions, in: *Insertion Elements, Plasmids, and Episomes* (A. I. Bukhari, J. A. Shapiro, and S. L. Adhya, eds.), pp. 295–306, Cold Spring Harbor Laboratory, Cold Spring Harbor, NY.

Crick, F. H. C., and Klug, A., 1975, Kinky helix, *Nature* **255**:530–533.

Cummings, D. J., Chapman, V. A., and Delong, S. S., 1965, An electron microsopic study of λ and λdg bacteriophage in thin sections, *J. Mol. Biol.* **14**:418–422.

Cummings, D. J., Chapman, V. A., Delong, S. S., and Couse, M. L., 1973, Structural aberrations in T-even bacteriophage. III. Induction of "lollipops" and their partial characterizations, *Virology* **54**:245–261.

Dannenburg, R., and Mosig, G., 1983, Early intermediates in bacteriophage T4 DNA replication and recombination, *J. Virol.* **45**:813–831.

Deichelbohrer, I., Messer, W., and Trautner, T. A., 1982, Genome of *Bacillus subtilis* bacteriophage SPP1: Structure and nucleotide sequence of *pac*, the origin of DNA packaging, *J. Virol.* **42**:83–90.

Doermann, A. H., Eiserling, F. A., and Boehner, L., 1973, Genetic control of capsid length in bacteriophage T4. I. Isolation and preliminary description of four new mutants, *J. Virol.* **12**:374–385.

Donohue, T. J., Chory, J., Goldsand, T. E., Lynn, S. P., and Kaplan, S., 1985, Structure and physical map of *Rhodospeudomonas sphaeroides* bacteriophage RS1 DNA, *J. Virol.* **55**:147–157.

Drake, J., 1966, Heteroduplex heterozygotes in bacteriphage T4 involving mutations of various dimensions, *Proc. Natl. Acad. Sci. USA* **55**:506–512.

Drexler, H., and Christensen, J. R., 1986, T1*pip:* A mutant which affects packaging initiation and processive packaging of T1 DNA, *Virology* **150**:373–380.

Drexler, H., 1984, Initiation by bacteriophage T1 of DNA packaging at a site between the P and Q genes of bacteriophage λ, *J. Virol.* **49**:754–759.

Dunn, J. J., and Studier, F. W., 1983, Complete nucleotide sequence of bacteriophage T7 DNA and the locations of T7 genetic clements, *J. Mol. Biol.* **166**:477–535.

Earnshaw, W. C., and Casjens, S. R., 1980, DNA packaging bv the double-stranded DNA bacteriophages, *Cell* **21**:319–331.

Earnshaw, W. C., and Harrison, S. C., 1977, DNA arrangement in isometric phage heads, *Nature* **268**:598–602.

Earnshaw, W. C., King, J., Harrison, S C., and Eiserling, F. A., 1978, The structural organization of DNA packaged within the heads of T4 wild-type, isometric and giant bacteriophages, *Cell* **14**:559–568.

Eickbush, T. H., and Moudrianakis, E. N., 1978, The compaction of DNA helices into either continuous supercoils or folded-fiber rods and toroids, *Cell* **13**:295–306.

Eiserling, F. A., Geiduschek, E. P., Epstein, R. H., and Metter, E. J., 1970, Capsid size and deoxyribonucleic acid length: The petite variant of bacteriophage T4, *J. Virol.* **6**:865–876.

Emmons, S., 1974, Bacteriophage lambda derivatives carrying two copies of the cohesive end site, *J. Mol. Biol.* **83**:511–525.

Enquist, L. W., and Sternberg, N., 1983, *In vitro* packaging of λ Dam vectors and their use in cloning DNA fragments, *Methods Enzymol.* **68**:281–298.

Feiss, M., 1986, Terminase and the recognition, cutting and packaging of chromosomes, *Trends Genet.* (April) **2**:100–104.

Feiss, M., and Becker, A., 1983, DNA packaging and cutting, in: *Lambda II* (R. W. Hendrix, J. W. Roberts, F. W. Stahl, and R. A. Weisberg, eds.), pp. 305–330, Cold Spring Harbor Laboratory, Cold Spring Harbor, NY.

Feiss, M., and Bublitz, A., 1975, Polarized packaging of bacteriophage lambda chromosomes, *J. Mol. Biol.* **94**:583–594.

Feiss, M., and Siegele, D. A., 1979, Packaging of the bacteriophage lambda chromosome: Dependence of *cos* cleavage on chromosome length, *Virology* **92**:190–200.

Feiss, M., Fisher, R. A., Crayton, M. A., and Egner, C., 1977, Packaging of the bacteriophage lambda chromosome: Effect of chromosome length, *Virology*, **77**:281–293.

Feiss, M., Widner, W., Miller, G., Johnson, G., and Christiansen, S., 1983, Structure of the bacteriophage lambda cohesive end site: Location of the sites of terminase binding (*cos*B) and nicking (*cos*N), *Gene* **24**:207–218.

Feiss, M., Sippy, J., and Miller, G., 1985a, Processive action of terminase during sequential packaging of bacteriophage λ chromosomes, *J. Mol. Biol.* **186**:759–771.

Feiss, M., Frackman, S., and Sippy, J., 1985b, Essential interaction between lambdoid phage 21 terminase and the *Escherichia coli* integrative host factor, *J. Mol. Biol.* **183**:239–249.

Frackman, S., Siegele, D. A., and Feiss, M., 1984, A functional domain of bacteriophage λ terminase for prohead binding, *J. Mol. Biol.* **180**:283–300.

Frackman, S., Siegele, D. A., and Feiss, M., 1985, The terminase of bacteriophage λ: Functional domains for cosB binding and multimer assembly, *J. Mol. Biol.* **180**:283–300.

Frederick, C. A., Grable, J., Melia. M., Samudzi, C., Jen-Jacobson, L., Wang, B.-C., Greene, P., Boyer, H. W., and Rosenberg, J. M., 1984, Kinked DNA in crystalline complex with EcoRI endonuclease, *Nature* **309**:327–331.

Fujisawa, H., and Sugimoto, K., 1983, On the terminally redundant sequences of bacteriphage T3 DNA, *Virology* **124**:251–258.

Fujisawa, H., Yamagishi, M., and Minagawa, T., 1980, *In vitro* formation of the concatemeric DNA bacteriophage T3 and its biological activity in the *in vitro* packaging reaction, *Virology* **101**:327–334.

Fujiyoshi, Y., Yamagishi, H., Kunisada, T., Sugisaki, H., Kobayashi, T., and Uyeda, N., 1982, Visualization of the DNA thread packing within bacteriophage T4 heads, *J. Ultrastruct. Res.* **79**:235–240.

George, M., and Bukhari, A. I., 1981, Heterogeneous host DNA attached to the left end of mature bacteriophage Mu DNA, *Nature* **292**:175–176.

Gill, G. S., and MacHattie, L. A., 1975, Oriented extrusion of DNA from coliphage T1 particles, *Virology* **65**:297–303.

Gill, G. S., and MacHattie, L. A., 1976, Limited permutations of the nucleotide sequence in bacteriophage T1 DNA, *J. Mol. Biol.* **104**:505–515.

Ginsberg, H. S., 1979, Adenovirus structural proteins, in: *Comprehensive Virology* (H. Fraenkel-Conrat and R. R. Wagner, eds.), pp. 409–457, Plenum Press, New York.

Glinert, S. J., and Luftig, R. B., 1977, Bacteriophage T4D head morphogenesis. VIII. DNA-protein associations in intermediate head structures that accumulate in gene 49-mutant-infected cells. *J. Virol.* **22**:758–777.

Gold, M., and Becker, A., 1983, The bacteriophage λ terminase: Partial purification and preliminary characterization of properties, *J. Biol. Chem.* **258**:14619–14625.

Gold, M., Hawkins, D., Murialdo, H., Fife, W. L., and Bradley, B., 1982, Circular monomers of bacteriophage λ DNA as substrates for *in vitro* packaging, *Virology* **119**:35–41.

Gope, R., and Serwer, P., 1983, Bacteriophage P22 *in vitro* DNA packaging monitored by agarose gel electrophoresis: Rate of DNA entry into capsids. *J. Virol.* **47**:96–105.

Griess, G. A., Serwer, P., and Horowitz, P. M., 1985, Binding of ethidium to bacteriophage T7 and T7 deletion mutants, *Biopolymers* **24**:1635–1646.

Griess, G. A., Serwer, P., Kaushal, V., and Horowitz, P. M., 1986, Kinetics of ethidium's intercalation in packaged bacteriophage T7 DNA: Effects of DNA packing density, *Biopolymers* **25**:1345–1357.

Groenen, M. A. M., and Van de Putte, P., 1985, Mapping of a site for packaging of bacteriophage mu DNA, *Virology* **144**:520–522.

Grossi, G. F., Macchiato, M. F., and Gialanella, G., 1983, Circular permutation analysis of phage T4 DNA by electron microscopy, *Z. Naturforsch.* **38c**:294–296.

Guo, P., Grimes, S., and Anderson, D., 1986, A defined system for *in vitro* packaging of DNA-gp3 of the *Bacillus subtilis* bacteriophage φ29, *Proc. Natl. Acad. Sci. USA* **83**:3505–3509.

Guo, P., Peterson, C., and Anderson, D., 1987a, Initiation events in *in vitro* packaging of bacteriophage phi29 DNA-gp3, *J. Mol. Biol.* **197**:219–228.

Guo, P., Peterson, C., and Anderson, D., 1987b, The DNA packaging protein gp16 of bacteriophage Phi29 is a prohead- and DNA-gp3-dependent ATPase, *J. Mol. Biol.* **197**:229–236.

Guo, P.. Erickson, S.. and Anderson, D., 1987c, A small viral RNA is required for *in vitro* packaging of bacteriophage phi29 DNA, *Science* **236**:690–694.

Haas, R., Murphy, R. F., and Cantor, C. R., 1982, Testing models of the arrangement of DNA inside bacteriophage λ by crosslinking the packaged DNA, *J. Mol. Biol.* **159**:71–92.

Hafner, E., Tabor, C., and Tabor, H., 1979, Mutants of *Escherichia coli* that do not contain 1,4-diaminobutane (Putrescine) or spermidine, *J. Biol. Chem.* **254**:12419–12426.

Hall, S. B., and Schellman, J. A., 1982, Flow dichroism of capsid DNA phages. I. Fast and slow T4B, *Biopolymers* **21**:1991–2010.

Hamada, K., Fujisawa, H., and Minagawa, T., 1984, Purification and properties of gene 18 product of bacteriophage T3, *Virology* **139**:251–259.

Hamada, K., Fujisawa, H., and Minagawa, T., 1986a, A defined *in vitro* system for packaging of bacteriophage T3 DNA, *Virology* **151**:119–123.

Hamada, K., Fujisawa, H., and Minagawa, T., 1986b, Overproduction and purification of the products of bacteriophage T3 genes 18 and 19, two genes involved in DNA packaging, *Virology* **151**:110–118.

Harrison, S. C., 1983, Packaging of DNA into bacteriophage heads: A model, *J. Mol. Biol.* **171**:577–580.

Hartman, P. S., Eisenstark, A., and Pauw, P. G., 1979, Inactivation of phage T7 by near-ultraviolet radiation plus hydrogen peroxide: DNA-protein crosslinks prevent DNA injection, *Proc. Natl. Acad. Sci. USA* **76**:3228–3232.

Harvey, J. D., Bellamy, A. R., Earnshaw, W. C., and Schutt, C., 1981, Biophysical studies of reovirus type 3. IV. Low-angle X-ray diffraction studies, *Virology* **112**:240–249.

Hascoet, E. C., Pretorius, G. H. J., and Coetzee, W. F., 1982, *Proteus mirabilis* phage 5006M: Restriction maps of genome in relation to headful packaging, *Virology* **123**:1–7.

Hendrix, R. W., 1978, Symmetry mismatch and DNA packaging in large bacteriophages, *Proc. Natl. Acad. Sci. USA* **75**:4779–4783.

Hendrix, R., and Casjens, S., 1975, Assembly of bacteriophage lambda heads: Protein processing and its genetic control in petit λ assembly, *J. Mol. Biol.* **91**:187–199.

Herranz, L., Salas, M., and Carrascosa, J. L., 1986, Interaction of the bacteriophage φ29 connector protein with the viral DNA, *Virology* **155**:289–292.

Hohn, B., 1975, DNA as substrate for packaging into bacteriophage lambda, *in vitro, J. Mol. Biol.* **98**:93–106.

Hohn, B., 1979, *In vitro* packaging of λ and cosmid DNA, *Methods Enzymol.* **68**:299–309.

Hohn, B., 1983, DNA sequences necessary for packaging of bacteriophage λ DNA, *Proc. Natl. Acad. Sci. USA* **80**:7456–7460.

Hohn, B., and Hohn, T., 1974, Activity of empty, headlike particles for packaging of DNA of bacteriophage λ *in vitro, Proc. Natl. Acad. Sci. USA* **71**:2372–2376.

Hohn, B., Wurtz, B., Klein, B., Lustig, A., and Hohn, T., 1974, Phage lambda DNA packaging *in vitro, J. Supramol. Struct.* **2**:302–317.

Hohn, T., 1976, Packaging of genomes in bacteriophages: A comparison of ssRNA bacteriophages and dsDNA bacteriophages, *Phil. Trans. R. Soc. Lond. B* **276**:143–150.

Hsiao, C. L., and Black, L. W., 1977, DNA packaging and the pathway of bacteriophage T4 head assembly, *Proc. Natl. Acad. Sci. USA* **74**:3652–3656.

Hug, H., Hausmann, R., Liebeschuetz, J., and Ritchie, D. A., 1986, *In vitro* packaging of foreign DNA into heads of T1, *J. Gen. Virol.* **67**:333–343.

Ishii, T., and Yanagida, M., 1975, Molecular organization of the shell of the T-even bacteriophage head, *J. Mol. Biol.* **97**:655–660.

Ishii, T., and Yanagida, M., 1977, The two dispensable structural proteins (soc and hoc) of the T4 phage capsid: Their properties, isolation and characterization of defective mutants, and their binding with the defective heads *in vitro, J. Mol. Biol.* **109**:487–514.

Jackson, E. N., Jackson, D. A., and Deans, R. J., 1978, *Eco*RI analysis of bacteriophage P22 DNA packaging, *J. Mol. Biol.* **118**:365–388.

Jackson, E. N., Laski, F., and Andres, C., 1982, Bacteriophage P22 mutants that alter the specificity of DNA packaging, *J. Mol. Biol.* **154**:551–563.

Jimenez, J., Santisteban, A., Carazo, J. M., and Carrascosa, J. L., 1986, Computer graphic display method for visualizing three-dimensional biological structures, *Science* **232**:1113–1115.

Kaiser, A.D., and Masuda, T., 1973, *In vitro* assembly of bacteriophage lambda heads, *Proc. Natl. Acad. Sci. USA* **70**:260–264.

Kaiser, A. D., Syvanen, M., and Masuda, T., 1975, DNA packaging steps in bacteriophage lambda head assembly, *J. Mol. Biol.* **91**:175–186.

Kalinski, A., and Black, L. W., 1986, End structure and mechanism of packaging of bacteriophage T4 DNA, *J. Virol.* **58**:951–954.

Katsura, I., 1980, Structure and inherent properties of the bacteriophage lambda head shell. II. Isolation and initial characterization of prophage mutants defective in gene E, *J. Mol. Biol.* **142:**387–398.

Katsura, I., 1986, Structure and inherent properties of the bacteriophage lambda head shell. V. Amber mutants in gene E, *J. Mol. Biol.* **190:**577–586.

Kellenberger, E., 1961, Vegetative bacteriophage and the maturation of the virus particles, *Adv. Virus Res.* **8:**1–61.

Kellenberger, E., 1980, Control mechanisms in the morphogenesis of bacteriophage heads, *Biosystems* **12:**201–223.

Kellenberger, E., Sechaud, J., and Ryter, A., 1959, Electron microscopical studies of phage multiplication. IV. The establishment of the DNA pool of vegetative phage and the maturation of phage particles, *Virology* **8:**478–498.

Kellenberger, E., Carlemalm, E., Sechaud, J., Ryter, A., and DeHaller, G., 1986, Considerations on the condensation and the degree of compactness in non-eukaryotic DNA-containing plasmas, in: *Bacterial Chromatin* (C. O. Gualerzi and C. L. Pon, eds.), pp. 11–25, Springer-Verlag, Berlin.

Kemper, B., and Brown, D. T., 1976, Function of gene 49 of bacteriophage T4. II. Analysis of intracellular development and the structure of very fast-sedimenting DNA, *J. Virol.* **18:**1000–1015.

Kim, J.-S., and Davidson, N., 1974, Electron microscope heteroduplex studies of sequence relations of T2, T4, and T6 bacteriophage DNAs, *Virology* **57:**93–111.

King, J., and Casjens, S., 1974, Catalytic head assembling protein in virus morphogenesis, *Nature* **251:**112–119.

Kittler, L., Hradecna, Z., and Suhnel, J., 1980, Cross-link formation of phage lambda DNA *in situ* photochemically induced by the furocoumarin derivative angelicin, *Biochim Biophys. Acta* **607:**215–220.

Kleinschmidt, A. K., Lang, D., Jacherts, D., and Zahn, R. K., 1962, Darstellung und Langenmessungen des gesamten desoxyribonucceinsaure-Inhaltes von T2-bakteriophagen, *Biochim. Biophys. Acta* **61:**857–864.

Kobayashi, I., Stahl, M. M., Leach, D. R. F., and Stahl, F. W., 1983, The interaction of *cos* with *chi* is separable from DNA packaging in recA-recBC mediated recombination of bactaeriophage lambda, *Genetics* **104:**549–570.

Kobayashi, I., Stahl, M. M., Fairfield, F. R., and Stahl, F. W., 1984, Coupling with packaging explains apparent nonreciprocality of *chi*-stimulated recombination of bacteriophage lambda by *recA* and *RecBC* functions, *Genetics* **108:**773–794.

Kosturko, L., Hogan, M., and Dattagupta, N., 1979, Structure of DNA packing of an unusual DNA in a virulent Erwinia phage, Erh I, in: *Bacteriophage Assembly* (M. S. DuBow, ed.), pp. 253–269, Alan R. Liss, New York.

Kuemmerle, N. B., and Masker, W. E., 1977, *In vitro* packaging of UV radiation-damaged DNA from bacteriophage T7, *J. Virol.* **23:**509–516.

Laemmli, U. K., 1975, Characterization of DNA condensates induced by poly(ethylene oxide) and polylysine, *Proc. Natl. Acad. Sci. USA* **72:**4288–4292.

Laemmli, U. K., and Favre, M., 1973, Maturation of the head of bacteriophage T4. I. DNA packaging events, *J. Mol. Biol.* **80:**575–599.

Laski, F., and Jackson, E. N., 1982, Maturation cleavage of bacteriophage P22 DNA in the absence of DNA packaging, *J. Mol. Biol.* **154:**565–579.

LeClerc, J. E., and Richardson, C. C., 1979, Gene 2 protein of bacteriophage T7: Purification and requirement for packaging of T7 DNA *in vitro*, *Proc. Natl. Acad. Sci. USA* **76:**4852–4856.

Lee, C. S., Davis, R. W., and Davidson, N., 1970, A physical study by electron miroscopy of the terminally repetitious, circularly permuted DNA from the coliphage particles of *Escherichia coli* 15, *J. Mol. Biol.* **48:**1–22.

Lenk, E., Casjens, S., Weeks, J., and King, J., 1975, Intracellular visualization of precursor capsids in phage P22 mutant infected cells, *Virology* **68:**182–199.

Lepault, J., Dubochet, J., Baschong, W., and Kellenberger, E., 1987, Organization of double-stranded DNA in bacteriophages: A study by cryo-electron microscopy of vitrified samples, *EMBO J.* **6**:1507–1512.

Lerman, L. S., 1971, A transition to a compact form of DNA in polymer solutions, *Proc. Natl. Acad. Sci. USA* **68**:1886–1890.

Lickfeld, K. G., Menge, B., Wunderli, H., vandenBroek, J., and Kellenberger, E., 1977, The interpretation and quantitation of sliced intracellular bacteriophages and phage-related particles, *J. Ultrastruct. Res.* **60**:148–168.

Liebeschuetz, J., Davison, P. J., and Ritchie, D. A., 1985, A coupled *in vitro* system for the formation and packaging of concatemeric T1 DNA, *Mol. Gen. Genet.* **200**:451–457.

Liu, L. F., Perkocha, L., Calendar, R., and Wang, J. C., 1981a, Knotted DNA from bacteriophage capsids, *Proc. Natl. Acad. Sci. USA* **78**:5498–5502.

Liu, L. F., Davis, J. L., and Calendar, R., 1981b, Novel topologically knotted DNA from bacteriophage P4 capsids: Studies with DNA topoisomerases, *Nucleic Acids Res.* **9**:3979–3989.

Lofdahl, S., Zabielski, J., and Philipson, L., 1981, Structure and restriction enzyme maps of the circularly permuted DNA of staphylococcal bacteriophage φ11, *J. Virol.* **37**:784–794.

Luftig, R. B., and Lundh, N. P., 1973, Bacteriophage T4 head morphogenesis. V. The role of DNA synthesis in maturation of an intermediate in head assembly, *Virology* **51**:432–442.

Luftig, R. B., Wood, W. B., and Okinaka, R., 1971, Bacteriophage T4 head morphogenesis. On the nature of gene 49 defective heads and their role as intermediates, *J. Mol. Biol.* **57**:555–573.

MacHattie, L., and Gill, G., 1977, DNA maturation by the "headful" mode in bacteriophage T1, *J. Mol. Biol.* **110**:441–465.

MacHattie, L. A., Ritchie, D. A., Thomas, C. A. Jr., and Richardson, C. C., 1967, Terminal repetition in permuted T2 bacteriophage DNA molecules, *J. Mol. Biol.* **23**:355–363.

Manne, V. S., Rao, V. B., and Black, L. W., 1982, A bacteriophage T4 DNA packaging related DNA-dependent ATPase-endonuclease, *J. Biol. Chem.* **257**:13223–13232.

Marini, J. C., Levene, S. D., Crothers, D. M., and Englund, P. T., 1982, Bent helical structure in kinetoplast DNA, *Proc. Natl. Acad. Sci. USA* **79**:7664–7668.

Marx, K. A., and Reynolds, T. C., 1982, Spermidine-condensed PhiX174 DNA cleavage by micrococcal nuclease: Torus cleavage model and evidence for unidirectional circumferential DNA wrapping, *Proc. Natl. Acad. Sci. USA* **79**:6484–6488.

McCall, P. J., and Bloomfield, V. A., 1976, Kinetics of proflavin binding to bacteriophages T2L and T4D, *Biopolymers* **15**:2323–2336.

McNicol, L. A., Simon, L. D., and Black, L. W., 1977, A mutation which bypasses the requirement for p24 in bacteriophage T4 capsid morphogenesis, *J. Mol. Biol.* **116**:261–283.

Miwa, T., and Matsubara, K., 1983, Lambda phage DNA sequences affecting the packaging process, *Gene* **24**:199–206.

Mizuuchi, K., Kemper, B., Hays, J., and Weisberg, R. A., 1982, T4 endonuclease VII cleaves Holliday structures, *Cell* **29**:357–365.

Mosig, G., and Powell, D., 1985, Heteroduplex loops are packaged in gene 49 (endonuclease VII) mutants of bacteriophage T4, *ASM Proc. Abst.* p. 209.

Mosig, G. R., Ehring, R., Schliewen, W., and Bock, S., 1971, The patterns of recombination and segregation in terminal regions of T4 DNA, *Mol. Gen. Genet.* **113**:51–91.

Mosig, G., Carnighan, J. R., Bibring, J. B., Cole, R., Bock, H.-G. O., and Bock, S., 1972, Coordinate variation in lengths of deoxyribonucleic acid molecules and head lengths in morphological variants of bacteriophage T4, *J. Virol.* **9**:857–871.

Mosig, G., Ghosal, D., and Bock, S., 1981, Interactions between the maturation protein gp17 and the single stranded DNA binding protein gp32 initiate DNA packaging and compete with initiation of secondary replication forks in phage T4, in: *Bacteriophage Assembly* (M. S. DuBow, ed.), pp. 139–151, Alan R. Liss, New York.

Moynet, D. J., and DeFilippes, F. M., 1982, Characterization of bacteriophage φ42 DNA, *Virology* **117**:475–484.

Murialdo, H., and Becker, A., 1978, Head morphogenesis of complex double-stranded deoxyribonucleic acid bacteriophages, *Microbiol. Rev.* **42**:529–576.

Murialdo, H., and Fife, W. L., 1984, The maturation of coliphage lambda DNA in the absence of its packaging, *Gene* **30**:183–194.

Murialdo, H., and Fife, W. L., 1987, Synthesis of a *trans*-acting inhibitor of DNA maturation by prohead mutants of phage λ, *Genetics***115**:3–10.

Murray, N. E., 1983, Phage lambda and molecular cloning, in: *Lambda II* (R. W. Hendrix, J. W. Roberts, F. W. Stahl, and R. A. Weisberg, eds.), pp. 395–432, Cold Spring Harbor Laboratory, Cold Spring Harbor, NY.

Nash, H. A., 1981, Integration and excision of bacteriophage λ: The mechanism of conservative site specific recombination, *Annu. Rev. Genet.* **15**:143–167.

Newcomb, W. W., Boring, J. W., and Brown, J. C., 1984, Ion etching of human adenovirus. 2. Structure of the core, *J. Virol.* **51**:52–56.

Nomura, M., and Benzer, S., 1961, The nature of the "deletion" mutants in the rII region of phage T4, *J. Mol. Biol.* **3**:684–692.

North, A. C. T., and Rich, A., 1961, X-ray diffraction studies of bacterial viruses, *Nature* **191**:1242–1245.

Olson, A. J., Bricogne, G., and Harrison, S. C., 1983, Structure of tomato bushy stunt virus. IV. The virus particle at 2.9Å resolution, *J. Mol. Biol.* **171**:61–93.

Piechowski, M. M., and Susman, M., 1967, Acridine resistance in phage T4, *Genetics* **56**:133–148.

Poteete, A. R., and Botstein, D., 1979, Purification and properties of proteins essential to DNA encapsulation by phage 22, *Virology* **95**:565–573.

Poteete, A. R., Jarvik, V., and Botstein, D., 1979, Encapsidation of phage P22 *in vitro*, *Virology* **95**:550–564.

Pruss, G., and Calendar, R., 1978, Maturation of bacteriophage P2 DNA, *Virology* **86**:454–467.

Pruss, G. J., Wang, J. C., and Calendar, R., 1975, *In vitro* packaging of covalently closed circular monomers of bacteriophage DNA, *J. Mol. Biol.* **98**:465–478.

Raj, A. S., Raj, A. Y., and Schmieger, H., 1974, Phage genes involved in the formation of generalized transducing particles in *Salmonella*-phage P22, *Mol. Gen. Genet.* **135**:175–184.

Ramsay, N., and Ritchie, D. A., 1983, Uncoupling of initiation site cleavage from subsequent headful cleavages in bacteriophage T1 DNA packaging, *Nature* **301**:264–266.

Ramsay, N., and Ritchie, D. A., 1984, Phage head assembly in bacteriophage T1, *Virology* **132**:239–249.

Rao, V. B., and Black, L. W., 1985a, Evidence that a phage T4 DNA packaging enzyme is a processed form of the major capsid gene product, *Cell* **42**:967–977.

Rao, V. B., and Black, L. W., 1985b, DNA packaging of bacteriophage T4 proheads *in vitro*: Evidence that prohead expansion is not coupled to DNA packaging, *J. Mol. Biol.* **185**:565–578.

Rao, V. B., and Black, L. W., 1988, Cloning, overexpression and purification of the terminase proteins gp16 and gp17 of bacteriophage T4: Construction of a defined *in vitro* DNA packaging system using purified terminase proteins, **200**:(in press). *J. Mol. Biol.*.

Rau, D. C., Lee, B., and Parsegian, V. A., 1984, Measurement of the repulsive force between polyelectrolyte molecules in ionic solution: Hydration forces between parallel DNA double helices, *Proc. Natl. Acad. Sci. USA* **81**:2621–2625.

Reddy, A. B., and Gopinathan, K. P., 1986, Presence of random single-strand gaps in mycobacteriophage I3 DNA, *Gene* **44**:227–234.

Rhoades, M., 1984, A bacteriophage T5 mutant with an increased frequency of single-chain interruptions, *J. Virol.* **51**:553–555.

Richards, K., Williams, R., and Calendar, R., 1973, Mode of DNA packing within bacteriophage heads, *J. Mol. Biol.* **78**:255–259.

Riemer, J., and Bloomfield, V., 1978, Packaging of DNA in bacteriophage heads: Some considerations on energetics, *Biopolymers* **17**:784–785.

Roberts, L., Sheldon, R., and Sadowski. P., 1978, Genetic recombination of bacteriophage T7 DNA *in vitro*. IV. Asymmetry of recombination frequencies caused by polarity of DNA packaging *in vitro*, *Virology* **89**:252–261.

Roeder, G. S., and Sadowski, P. D., 1977, Bacteriophage T7 morphogenesis: Phage-related particles in cells infected with wild-type and mutant T7 phage, *Virology* **76**:263–285.

Rogers, S. G., Godwin, E. A., Shinosky, E. S., and Rhoades, M., 1979, Interruption-deficient mutants of bacteriophage T5. I. Isolation and general properties, *J. Virol.* **29**:716–725.

Rosenberg, S. M., Stahl, M. M., Kobayashi, I., and Stahl, F. W., 1985a, Improved *in vitro* packaging of coliphage lambda DNA: A one-strain system free from endogenous phage, *Gene* **38**:165–175.

Rosenberg, S. M., Stahl, M. M., Kobayashi, I., and Stahl, F. W., 1985b, Clean and simple one strain *in vitro* packaging of bacteriophage λ DNA, *ASM News* **51**:386–391.

Ross, P. D., Black, L. W., Bisher, M. E., and Steven, A. C., 1985, Assembly-dependent conformational changes in a viral capsid protein: Calorimetric comparison of successive conformational states of the gp23 surface lattice of bacteriophage T4, *J. Mol. Biol.* **183**:353–364.

Rossman, M. G., Arnold, E., Erickson, J. W., Frankenberger, E. A., Griffith, J. P., Hecht, H.-J., Johnson, J. E., Kamer, G., Luo, M., Mosser, A. G., Rueckert, R. R., Sherry, B., and Vriend, G., 1985, Structure of a human common cold virus and functional relationship to other picornaviruses, *Nature* **317**:145–153.

Saigo, K., and Uchida, H., 1974, Connection of the right-hand terminus of DNA to the proximal end of the tail in bacteriophage lambda, *Virology* **61**:524–536.

Schaerli, C., and Kellenberger, E., 1980, Head maturation pathway of bacteriophages T4 and T2, V. Maturable ε-particle accumulating in acridine-treated bacteriophage T4-infected cells, *J. Virol.* **33**:830–844.

Scraba, D. G., Bradley, R. D., Leyritz-Wills, M., and Warren, R. A. J., 1983, Bacteriophage PhiW-14: The contribution of covalently bound putrescine to DNA packing in the phage head, *Virology* **124**:152–160.

Serwer, P., 1975, Buoyant density sedimentation of macromolecules in sodium iothalamate density gradients, *J. Mol. Biol.* **92**:433–448.

Serwer, P., 1980, A metrizamide-impermeable capsid in the DNA packaging pathway of bacteriophage T7, *J. Mol. Biol.* **A138**:65–91.

Serwer, P., 1986, Arrangement of double-stranded DNA packaged in bacteriophage capsids, *J. Mol. Biol.* **190**:509–512.

Serwer, P., Masker, W. E., and Allen, J. L., 1983, Stability and *in vitro* DNA packaging of bacteriophages: Effects of dextrans, sugars, and polyols, *J. Virol.* **45**:665–671.

Shore, D., Deho, G., Tsipis, J., and Goldstein, R., 1978, Determination of capsid size by satellite bacteriophage P4, *Proc. Natl. Acad. Sci. USA* **75**:400–404.

Sklyadneva, L. A., Chekanovskaya, L. A., Grigor'ev, V. B., and Tikhonenko, T. I., 1980, Investigation of bacteriophage P22 DNA structure *in situ*, *Molekulyarnaya Biol.* **15**:208–219.

Smith, H. O., Danner, D. B., and Deich, R. A., 1981. Genetic transformation, *Annu. Rev. Biochem.* **50**:41–68.

Stahl, M. M., Kobayashi, I., Stahl, F. W., and Huntington, S. K., 1983, Activation of *chi*, a recombinator, by the action of an endonuclease at a distant site, *Proc. Natl. Acad. Sci. USA* **80**:2310–2313.

Sternberg, N., 1985, Evidence that adenine methylation influences DNA-protein interactions in *Escherichia coli*, *J. Bacteriol.* **164**:490–493.

Sternberg, N., and Coulby, J., 1987a, Recognition and cleavage of the bacteriophage P1 packaging site (*pac*). I. Differential processing of the cleaved ends *in vivo*, *J. Mol. Biol.* **194**:453–468.

Sternberg, N., and Coulby, J., 1987b, Recognition and cleavage of the bacteriophage P1 packaging site (*pac*). II. Functional limits of *pac* and location of *pac* cleavage termini, *J. Mol. Biol.* **194**:469–480.

Sternberg, N., and Hoess, R., 1983, The molecular genetics of bacteriophage P1, *Annu. Rev. Genet.* **17**:123–154.

Sternberg, N., and Weissberg, R., 1975, Packaging of prophage and host DNA by coliphage λ, *Nature* **256**:97–103.

Sternberg, N., and Weissberg, R., 1977, Packaging of coliphage lambda DNA. II. The role of the gene D protein, *J. Mol. Biol.* **117**:733–759.

Steven, A. C., Couture, E., Aebi, U., and Showe, M. K., 1976, Structure of T4 polyheads. II. A pathway of polyhead transformations as a model for T4 capsid maturation, *J. Mol. Biol.* **106**:187–221.

Streisinger, G., Emrich, J., and Stahl, M. M., 1967, Chromosome structure in phage T4. III. Terminal redundancy and length determination, *Proc. Natl. Acad. Sci. USA* **57**:292–295.

Strobel, E., Behnisch, W., and Schmieger, H., 1984, *In vitro* packaging of mature phage DNA by *Salmonella* phage P22, *Virology* **133**:158–165.

Stroud, R. M., Serwer, P., and Ross, M. J., 1981, Assembly of bacteriophage T7 dimensions of the bacteriophage and its capsids, *Biophys. J.* **36**:743–757.

Syvanen, M., 1975, Processing of bacteriophage lambda DNA during its assembly into heads, *J. Mol. Biol.* **91**:165–174.

Syvanen, M., and Yin, J., 1978, Studies of DNA packaging into the heads of bacteriophage lambda, *J. Mol. Biol.* **126**:333–346.

Thomas, J. O., 1974, Chemical linkage of the tail to the right-hand end of bacteriophage lambda DNA, *J. Mol. Biol.* **87**:1–9.

Tikchonenko, T. I., 1975, Structure of viral nucleic acids *in situ*, in: *Comprehensive Virology*, Vol. 5 (H. Fraenkel-Conrat and R. R. Wagner, eds.), pp. 1–117, Plenum Press, New York.

Tye, B., Huberman, J., and Botstein, D., 1974, Non random circular permutation of phage P22 DNA, *J. Mol. Biol.* **85**:501–527.

Uhlenhopp, E. L., Zimm, B. H., and Cummings, D. J., 1974, Structural aberrations in T-even bacteriophage. VI. Molecular weight of DNA from giant heads, *J. Mol. Biol.* **89**:689–702.

Virrankoski-Castrodeza, V., and Parish, J. H., 1980, Evidence for supercoiling in the DNA of bacteriophage heads, *Arch. Microbiol.* **126**:277–283.

Virrankoski-Castrodeza, V., Fraser, M. J., and Parish, J. H., 1982, Condensed DNA structures derived from bacteriophage heads, *J. Gen. Virol.* **58**:181–190.

Weil, J., Cunningham, R., Martin, R. III, Mitchell, E., and Bolling, B., 1972, Characteristics of λp4, a λ derivative containing 9% excess DNA, *Virology* **50**:373–380.

Weil, J., DeWein, N., and Casale, A., 1974, Morphogenesis of λ with genomes containing excess DNA: Functional particles containing 12 and 15% excess DNA, *Virology* **63**:352–366.

Welsh, J., and Cantor, C. R., 1986, in: *Bacterial Chromatin* (C. O. Gualerzi and C. L. Pon, eds.), pp. 30–44, Springer-Verlag, Berlin.

Widom, J., and Baldwin, R. L., 1980, Cation-induced toroidal condensation of DNA: Studies with $Co^{3+}(NH_3)_6$, *J. Mol. Biol.* **144**:431–453.

Widom, J., and Baldwin, R. L., 1983, Tests of spool models for DNA packaging in phage lambda, *J. Mol. Biol.* **171**:419–437.

Wilson, G. G., Neve, R. L., Edlin, G. J., and Konigsberg, W. H., 1979, The *Bam*H1 restriction site in the bacteriophage T4 chromosome is located in or near gene 8, *Genetics* **93**:285–296.

Witkiewicz, H., and Schweiger, M., 1982, The head protein D of bacterial virus λ is related to eukaryotic chromosomal proteins, *EMBO J.* **12**:1559–1564.

Wolfson, J. S., McHugh, G. L., Hooper, D. C., and Swartz, M. N., 1985, Knotting of DNA molecules isolated from deletion mutants of intact bacteriophage P4, *Nucleic Acids Res.* **13**:6695–6702.

Wood, W. B., and King, J., 1979, Genetic control of complex bacteriophage assembly, in:

Comprehensive Virology, Vol. 13 (H. Fraenkel-Conrat and R. R. Wagner, eds.), pp. 581–633, Plenum Press, New York.

Wunderli, H., vd Broeck, J., and Kellenberger, E., 1977, Studies related to the head-maturation pathway of bacteriophages T4 and T2. I. Morphology and kinetics of intracellular particles produced by mutants in the maturation genes, *J. Supramol. Struct.* **7:**135–161.

Yamada, M., Fujisawa, H., Kato, H., Hamada, K., and Minagawa, T., 1986, Cloning and sequencing of the genetic right end of bacteriophage T3 DNA, *Virology* **151:**350–361.

Yamagishi, H., and Okamoto, M., 1978, Visualization of the intracellular development of bacteriophage λ, with special reference to DNA packaging, *Proc. Natl. Acad. Sci. USA* **75:**3206–3210.

Yamagishi, M., Fujisawa, H., and Minagawa, T., 1985, Isolation and characterization of bacteriophage T3/T7 hybrids and their use in studies on molecular basis of DNA-packaging specificity, *Virology* **144:**502–515.

Yuan, R., Hamilton, D. L., and Burckhardt, J., 1980, DNA translocation by the restriction enzyme from *E. coli* K, *Cell* **20:**237–244.

Zachary, A. L., and Black, L. W., 1981, DNA ligase is required for encapsidation of bacteriophage T4 DNA, *J. Mol. Biol.* **149:**641–658.

Zachary, A., and Black, L. W., 1984, UV irradiation impairs *in vivo* encapsidation of bacteriophage T4 DNA, *J. Virol.* **50:**293–300.

Zachary, A., and Black, L. W., 1986, Topoisomerase II and other DNA-delay and DNA-arrest mutations impair bacteriophage T4 DNA packaging *in vivo* and *in vitro, J. Virol.* **60:**97–104.

CHAPTER 6

Filamentous Bacteriophage

PETER MODEL AND MARJORIE RUSSEL

I. INTRODUCTION

As their name implies, filamentous phages are long, thin bacteriophages (Fig. 1) ranging from about 1 to 2 μm in length and about 6–7 nm in diameter, which gives them an axial ratio of about 140–330. Those that infect male (F⁺) strains of *Escherichia coli* are the best studied from a physiological and genetic point of view, and much is known about them. Ike, which can infect *E. coli* that elaborate N pili, is similar to the F pili-specific phage in many respects, although it has substantially diverged from them at the DNA and protein sequence levels. Other filamentous phages that infect several different bacterial species have been isolated; they are often assumed to be similar.* Phage Pf1, whose biology is not well understood, has proved to the most tractable for X-ray crystallographic studies, and its structure has been the subject of much work; unfortunately, its structure differs in important respects from that of the F specific phages. In this chapter, statements made without reference to a

*The list of filamentous phages is much larger than those mentioned explicitly in this review. They include the F-specific phages (other than fd, M13, and f1) ZJ/2 (Bradley, 1964), Ec9 (Dettori and Neri, 1965), AE2 (Panter and Symons, 1966), HR (Hsu, 1968), and δA (Nishihara and Watanabe, 1967). There are also three *Salmonella* phages, If1, If2 (Lawn *et al.*, 1967), and X (Bradley *et al.*, 1981); and a *Vibrio* phage, v6 (Nakanishi *et al.*, 1966). In addition to Pf3, there is *Pseudomonas* phage Pf2 (Minamishima *et al.*, 1968). A filamentous phage specific to *Xanthomonas citri* has been isolated and characterized (Dai *et al.*, 1980), and a restriction map of its DNA has been prepared (Yang and Kuo, 1984). Two other phages closely related to Cf have been described, both of which appear, unlike any of the other filamentous phages, to enter a lysogenic state in which they integrate into the host genome (Kuo *et al.*, 1987; Dai *et al.*, 1987; see Genetics).

PETER MODEL AND MARJORIE RUSSEL • The Rockefeller University, New York, New York 10021.

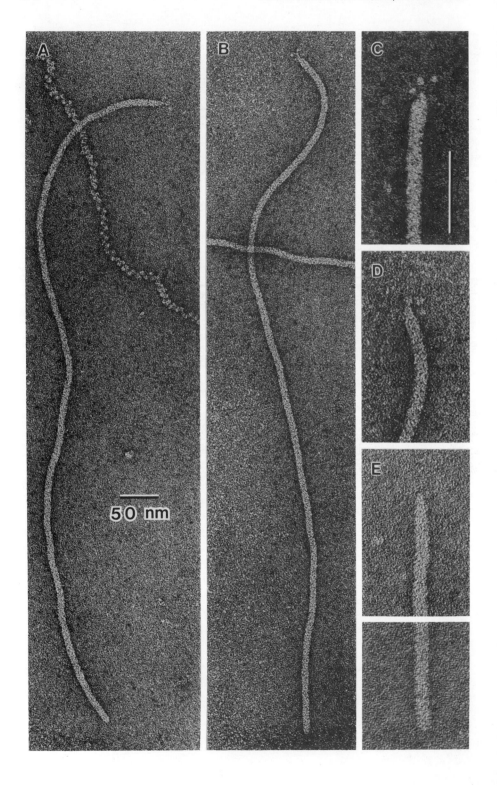

50 nm

particular organism will be assumed to refer to the intensively studied F-specific phages f1, fd, and M13, which are very similar to one another, differing at few nucleotide positions.

Among the distinguishing characteristics of the filamentous phages is that they contain single-stranded DNA, that their length is determined by the size of the DNA they encapsidate, and that they are continually extruded from their host without lysis and without markedly affecting it.

Structurally, the phages consist of a circular, single-stranded DNA genome encapsidated as a loop in what is essentially a protein tube. The walls of this protein tube are comprised of about 2700 copies of one small protein, the product of gene VIII, and the ends bear minor proteins specific to each end; thus the ends are differentiable from each other, morphologically in the electron microscope, biochemically, and by function. Although the DNA may be stacked within the particle, it need not be regularly arranged. The stoichiometry between major coat protein and phosphate residues varies from phage to phage and can be nonintegral, and, at least for the F-specific phages, there appears to be no simple symmetry relationship between the DNA and the coat. For the time being, it seems simplest to consider the DNA as packed inside a tube in an essentially random fashion. The particles are resistant to most proteases, to salt, and to heating, but they are sensitive to chaotropic agents, detergents, and to chloroform.

The phage genome encodes 10 proteins, of which five are virion structural proteins, three are required for phage DNA synthesis, and two serve assembly functions. In addition, there is an "intergenic region" which does not code for proteins but contains signals for the initiation of synthesis of both the (+) and the (−) strand of DNA, the initiation of capsid formation, and the termination of RNA synthesis. Parts of this intergenic region are dispensable, but all of the phage-encoded proteins are required for progeny phage synthesis.

Infection proceeds by attachment of the end of the phage particle that

---

FIGURE 1. Electron micrograph of fd phage, adsorption complex, and gene V protein–DNA complex. Panels A and B show whole virions, with adsorption complexes faintly visiable as knobs attached to the tapered end of each virus particle. Panel A includes a segment of the helical complex of fd gene 5 protein with fd viral DNA; the adsorption apparatus is fainter and more difficult to resolve than are the turns of the fd gene 5 protein complex. Panels C and D are enlargements, showing that the adsorption-complex knobs are apparently connected to the virion tip by stems that are too thin to be seen. Th protease subtilisin removes the viral A protein (gene III protein) as shown by electrophoretic analysis; the subtilisin treatment also removes the knobs from the virion tip, leaving denuded virions still displaying the characteristic tapered and blunt ends (panel E). The size of the knobs suggests that each is principally a monomer of the gene III protein, although other minor virion proteins may be involved. Up to three knobs per virion are resolved in the micrographs, but it is possible that one or more additional knobs remain hidden behind the virion. Bars = 50 nm. Panels A and B, 205,000×; panels C and E, 434,000×. Micrographs courtesy of Dr. Carla W. Gray, University of Texas at Dallas; reprinted with permission from Gray et al. (1981).

contains the gene III protein to the tip of the F, or sex, pilus of the host. This requirement for F$^+$ cells is entirely for adsorption. If the phage DNA is introduced into the host by some other route (transfection, or encapsidation in the coat of an unrelated phage), the need for the F factor in the host is bypassed. The phage is subsequently brought to the surface of the cell to be infected and enters. The entering coat protein monomers are deposited in the inner (cytoplasmic) membrane of the infected cell and can be reutilized as such by progeny virions. The single-stranded DNA (the + strand) enters the cell and is converted to a double-stranded (RF) form by the combined action of the host RNA polymerase and the host DNA synthesis apparatus; this step does not require the participation of any phage-encoded protein. The initial double-stranded RF molecule serves as the template for transcription and protein synthesis, and all genes are expressed immediately. One of the phage-encoded products, the gene II protein, then makes a specific break in the (+) strand of the RF, and the resulting 3' terminus is elongated by the host's DNA synthesis apparatus until it is twice the unit length. The displaced strand is then cut and circularized in a concerted fashion to give a free circular single strand and an RF molecule. Early in infection, the newly formed single strand has a high probability of undergoing the same reaction as the incoming single strand—e.g., it enters the doubling up cycle and becomes new RF. As infection proceeds, the concentration of phage-encoded proteins increases. One of these, the product of gene V, is a single-stranded DNA binding protein that can sequester the newly synthesized single strands. DNA–gene V protein complexes do not serve as templates for DNA synthesis, and so these single strands remain available for assembly into virions. These reactions are illustrated in Fig. 2.

While DNA synthesis goes on, there is a concomitant synthesis of the phage-encoded proteins. Two of the phage structural proteins have been shown to be transmembrane proteins, and the other three are believed to be membrane-associated. Since no completed virus particles can be detected within the cells, assembly of progeny virus must take place at the membrane. All of the single-stranded DNA binding (gene V) protein is removed from the single-stranded DNA and is replaced by the virion structural proteins as the phage particles are extruded through the cell envelope, without apparent damage to the host. If not stressed by conditions that disturb the optimal balance between synthesis and assembly, the host can continue to synthesize and export phages for as many generations as one can measure; the rate of curing is low, and the capacity for synthesis is high. In consequence of this, very high phage titers (up to 10^{13} particles per milliliter) are achievable.

Like other small phages, filamentous phages are heavily dependent on host functions for all macromolecular synthesis and for assembly. Thus, the study of the phage necessarily involves study of the host functions with which it interacts.

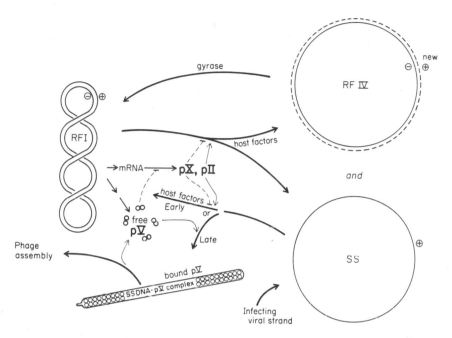

FIGURE 2. F-specific phage replication. The thickest arrows represent the DNA interconversions. Infecting single strands (SS) are converted to RFI, which produces a relaxed RF (RFIV) and a viral (+) strand (SS). This strand can either be converted to the double strand or be sequestered by gene V protein to make the V protein–DNA complex. Medium arrows coming from RFI represent the synthesis of proteins (pX, pII, pV). Thin solid arrows indicate a stimulatory role for the proteins; broken lines ending in a bar indicate inhibitory activities. pV is shown recycling into and out of the complex.

II. GENES AND PROTEINS

The complete DNA sequence of three of the F-specific phages fd (Beck *et al.*, 1978; Schaller *et al.*, 1978), M13 (Van Wezenbeek *et al.*, 1980), and f1 (Beck and Zink, 1981; Hill and Petersen, 1982) has been determined, in some cases more than once. Hence the sequence of all of the proteins they encode is known. In addition, the sequences of the DNA of Ike (Peeters *et al.*, 1985) and of Pf3 (Luiten *et al.*, 1985) have been established. The sequences of f1, fd, and M13, all of which are specific for male (F$^+$) *E. coli*, are sufficiently similar that comparisons are not especially informative, whereas that of Pf3, which infects *Pseudomonas aeruginosa*, is so far removed from that of the others that comparisons are only possible if the identity of the Pf3 gene product is clear. Ike infects *E. coli* but uses the pilus specified by plasmids of the N and I$_2$ incompatibility groups as its receptor (Bradley *et al.*, 1983). Its DNA sequence shows about 55% homology with those of the F-specific phages, and its genome organization is very similar (Peeters *et al.*, 1985). Comparisons between the F phages and Ike, therefore, are likely to be informative.

A. General

The genome of the filamentous phages is shown in Fig. 3. The genes are tightly packed but interrupted by an intergenic region between genes IV and II, which contains the (+) and (−) origins of DNA replication and

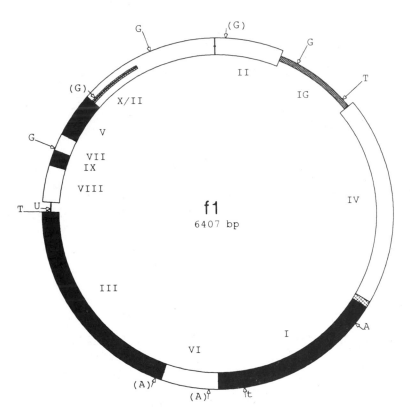

FIGURE 3. Genome of f1 showing genes (Roman numerals), the intergenic region (IG), promoters, and terminators. Promoters that are strongly active *in vivo* are shown with long arrows; weaker promoters are shown as shorter arrows. All transcription proceeds counterclockwise on the map shown. Promoters that are active *in vitro*, but for which there is some doubt as to their *in vivo* function, are shown in parentheses. The initiating nucleotide is shown at the base of the arrow. Arrows marked with a T show terminators; the long arrows mark the strong, rho-independent central terminator after gene VIII and the strong, rho-dependent terminator after gene IV. This is a composite figure, incorporating data from many laboratories. The small hatched area between genes I and IV represents gene overlap. The small arrow marked t in gene I marks a weaker, rho-dependent terminator. For references see text.

the packaging or morphogenetic signal which is in the same hairpin that contains the rho-dependent terminator for transcription. The 3' end of gene I overlaps the 5' end of gene IV, but they are read in different phases. Gene X is contained entirely within gene II and is in phase with it; hence, gene X has the same amino acid sequence as the terminal third of gene II (Yen and Webster, 1981). There is a small intergenic region between genes VIII and III; this contains a very strong, rho-independent terminator, and the promoter for gene III (Sugimoto et al., 1977; Chan et al., 1975; Edens et al., 1975; Smits et al., 1984). The genes and the proteins they encode can be grouped into those that comprise the virion (products of genes VIII, III, VI, VII, and IX), those required for DNA synthesis (genes II, V, and X), and those that serve a morphogenetic function (genes I and IV). Many of the genes (I, II, III, IV, V, VI, VII) were defined by standard genetic analysis: conditionally lethal mutants (amber or temperature-sensitive) were isolated from mutagenized phage and tested for complementation by mixed infection of the nonpermissive host with two mutants (Pratt et al., 1966). No mutants in the major coat protein gene were found in this way; isolation of a gene VIII amber mutant followed a two-step mutagenesis, in which virions were screened for altered buoyant density in CsCl gradients, and those that showed such an altered density were subjected to a second round of mutagenesis, from which an amber mutant was obtained (Pratt et al., 1969). These genes were ordered genetically by Lyons and Zinder (1972) and mapped to their cognate proteins by subjecting lysates of infected cells to electrophoresis (Henry and Pratt, 1969) or by analyzing the product of in vitro protein synthesis reactions directed by wild-type or mutant phage DNAs (Konings, 1973; Konings et al., 1973, 1975; Model and Zinder, 1974).

As a test of the sensitivity of the f1 genome to localized changes, Boeke (1981) has inserted one or two codons (in frame) at various restriction sites. Mutants could be detected by altered restriction patterns. Surprisingly, 35% of the available sites could be mutagenized in the way, and about half of these mutants had no detectable phenotype; the remainder were unable to form plaques at 42°. Thus the gene I, III, and IV proteins can tolerate the insertion of one or two amino acids, at least at certain positions, without seriously impairing their function.

The existence of gene IX was inferred from an open reading frame revealed by the DNA sequence, and its product was detected in the virion (Grant et al., 1981; Simons et al., 1979, 1981a,b), but it was not until 1982 that a mutation was created by oligonucleotide mutagenesis and used to show that the gene product is essential (Simons et al., 1982). In similar fashion, the product of gene X was detected in vitro (Model and Zinder, 1974; Konings et al., 1975) and in vivo (Yen and Webster, 1981), but not until an oligonucleotide-directed mutation changed its initiation codon from AUG to UAG was it found to be essential for the synthesis of progeny single-stranded DNA (Fulford and Model, 1984a).

B. Structural Genes and Proteins

1. Gene VIII

The gene VIII protein is the major coat protein, comprising the sides of the viral filament. The mature protein, 50 amino acids in length, has an acidic N-terminal domain, an extremely hydrophobic central region, and a basic C-terminal domain. The protein from fd was sequenced by Asbeck *et al.* (1969), and the sequence was corrected by Nakashima and Konigsberg (1974) and is shown in Fig. 4. Comparison of these sequences with those of the RNA encoding the protein showed that it is synthesized as a precursor, containing a 23-amino acid signal sequence (Sugimoto *et al.*, 1977). f1, fd, and M13 have between them only one different amino acid, in that residue 12 is asp in f1 and fd and asn in M13. This difference is sufficient to differentiate them with antisera raised against M13 (Pratt *et al.*, 1969). A mutant generated by Pratt *et al.* (1969), in which pro_6 is replaced by ser (Boeke and Model, 1979), gives rise to a phage with altered buoyant density in CsCl. When glu_2 is replaced with leu in this altered coat protein, assembly of the phage can take place if residue 12 is asp (found naturally in fd and f1), but not if it is asn as in M13 (Boeke *et al.*, 1980).

Gene VIII protein is soluble in alkali or detergents, but not in salt solutions. In deoxycholate or SDS, it exists as well-defined dimers (Makino *et al.*, 1975; Cavalieri *et al.*, 1976a). Spectral and NMR studies of the protein in various environments show that it is never as highly α helical in detergents or lipids as when part of the virion; consequently the protein must undergo a substantial conformational change upon virion formation (Nozaki *et al.*, 1976, 1978; Cross and Opella, 1980; Opella *et al.*, 1980). The protein can easily be inserted into phospholipid vesicles if present while they are formed, and it assumes an assymetric orientation, N terminus toward the outside with the central region in contact with the lipid (Wickner, 1975, 1976; Chamberlain and Webster, 1978). Since it is such a prototypic integral membrane protein, and because it can be

```
                          N
fd         A E G D D P A K A A F D S L Q A S A T E Y I G Y A W A M V V V I V G A T I G I K L F K K F T S K A S
If1      A D D A T S Q A K A A F D S L T A Q A T E M S G Y A W A L V V L V V G A T V G I K L F K K F V S R A S
Ike  A E P N A A T N Y A T E A M D S L K T Q A I D L I S Q T W P V V T T V V V A G L V I R L F K K F S S R A V
Pf1      G V I D T S A V Q S A I T D G Q G D M K A I G G Y I V G A L V I L A V A G L I Y S M L R K A
Xf     S G V G D G V D V V S A I E G A A G P I A A I G G A V L T V M V G I K V Y K W V R R A M
Pf3      M Q S V I T D V T G Q L T A V Q A D I T T I G G A I I V L A A V V L G I R W I K A Q F F
```

FIGURE 4. Sequences of filamentous phage coat proteins. The single-letter amino acid code is used. Negatively charged residues are marked with a (−), positively charged residues with a (+). The broken line represents the hydrophobic regions. The (N) above the fd sequence represents the asp → asn difference between fd and fl and M13. Sequences were aligned as by Makowski (1984). References can be found in the text.

obtained in large amounts, it has been used as a model system for the study of lipid-protein interactions (for citations see Rasched and Oberer, 1986; Webster and Lopez, 1985).

The sequences of the coat proteins of If1, Ike (Nakashima et al., 1981), Pf1 (Nakashima et al., 1975), Xf (Frangione et al., 1978), and Pf3 (Luiten et al., 1983; Putterman et al., 1984) all have an acidic N-terminal domain, hydrophobic central region, and basic C-terminal domain, but they differ in the particular residues used rather markedly from the F-specific phages (Fig. 4). As might be expected on the basis of the DNA homology, Ike most closely resembles the F phages. The sequence of the coat protein of Pf3 differs strongly from that of the other phages, and Luiten et al. (1983) and Putterman et al. (1984) have presented strong evidence that it is not synthesized with a cleavable signal sequence. It is not known whether Pf3 coat protein assumes a transmembrane disposition before phage assembly; if it does, it must either insert spontaneously or contain residues that act as an internal, uncleaved signal.

2. Gene III

Gene III encodes a protein of approximately 42,000 molecular weight, synthesized with an 18-amino acid signal peptide (Goldsmith and Konigsberg, 1977; Schaller et al., 1978). The gene product is required for termination of the virion (see Morphogenesis) and stabilization of the phage particle (see Structure) and is essential for infectivity. Chain-terminating mutations in the gene are polar on the expression of genes VI and I, so amber mutants in the gene will also show some of the phenotypes of VI and I mutants (Pratt et al., 1966, 1969). The protein forms a knob on one end of the phage (Fig. 1) (Gray et al., 1981), which can be removed with subtilisin to leave a noninfectious particle. The knob portion represents the N-terminal two-thirds of the protein (Armstrong et al., 1981) and is soluble [whereas the intact protein is extremely insoluble except in detergent solutions (Goldsmith and Konigsberg, 1977; Lin et al., 1980)]. The knob fragment can inhibit the binding of phage to their target E. coli (Armstrong et al., 1981).

In vitro manipulation of the gene (Boeke and Model, 1982) shows that the C-terminal portion, which encodes a 23-amino acid stretch of hydrophobic amino acids, serves as a membrane anchor, to hold the protein in the inner membrane of the infected cell (Boeke et al., 1982) and, in the light of the results of Armstrong et al. (1981), in the end of the phage particle as well. For the purpose of holding the gene III protein in the infected cell membrane, the natural anchor can be replaced by one derived from the hydrophobic region of gene VIII (Boeke and Model, 1982) or by entirely synthetic sequences (Davis and Model, 1985). The membrane anchor domain has been systematically changed, and the requirements for membrane anchorage have been determined (Davis et al., 1985). The efficiency with which the protein is retained in the membrane seems to be related principally to the calculated hydrophobicity, using scales such as those developed by Von Heijne (1981) and Engelman and Steitz (1981). Relocation of the membrane anchor domain to the interior of the protein halts transfer through the membrane at that point.

None of the constructs in which the amino acid sequence of the gene III protein was altered were capable of complementing gene III mutants of phage f1 (Davis, unpublished); hence the specificity of function, as part of the phage particle, is greater than that needed to retain the protein in the membrane.

Cells expressing gene III protein, whether from phage infection or from a plasmid, exhibit a variety of phenotypes (sensitivity to deoxycholate, leakage of periplasmic proteins from the cell, resistance to infection by F-specific phages, resistance to a variety of colicins, inability to form mating pairs) indicative of changes in the *E. coli* outer membrane (Zinder, 1973; Smilowitz, 1974b; Boeke *et al.*, 1982) and in particular resemble the *tolA* phenotype (Davies and Reeves, 1975; see Entry). Gene III need not be anchored in the membrane to produce these effects; the N-terminal half or two-thirds suffices (Boeke *et al.*, 1982). The protein contains two glycine-rich domains, each consisting of several repeats (with permutations) of the sequence glu gly gly gly ser. A deletion mutant, in which the first of these domains, together with some flanking sequence, is removed, no longer has any of these phenotypes (Boeke *et al.*, 1982). Nelson *et al.* (1981) have constructed a phage mutant in which a substantial part of the center of the N-terminal region of the protein has been deleted, including the first glycine-rich domain; this phage makes noninfectious particles and does not cause the membrane perturbations. Smith (1985) has shown that DNA inserted in the correct reading frame within gene III results in the formation of phage particles that can present the antigen encoded by the insert to the immune system, and he has used such phage to raise antisera to the peptides specified by the insert. Gene III of phage Ike does not contain the first glycine-rich domain (Peeters *et al.*, 1985); infection with this phage also does not perturb the membrane. Since the repeated sequence is found again further downstream in mutants or phages that do not perturb the membrane, the glycine-rich domain alone is not sufficient to cause the observed effects. Davis (unpublished), moreover, has isolated mutants that are outside but close to this region, and in which membrane perturbation is altered or absent.

3. Genes VI, VII, and IX

Genes VI, VII, and IX encode polypeptides found at the ends of the virion, the gene VI protein located at the gene III end, the other two at the opposite end. Gene VII and IX proteins are very small, consisting of 33 and 32 amino acid residues, respectively. All three are synthesized without signal sequences and are found in the capsid still containing the formyl group on the initiating formylmethionine (Simons *et al.*, 1981).

All three contain hydrophobic sequences long enough to make association with or integration into membranes plausible. Simons et al. (1981) made the reasonable suggestion that the hydrophobic stretches may encode membrane insertion domains and that it is the rapid association with the membrane that prevents removal of the formyl group from the proteins, but as yet this hypothesis has not been proved. Mutations in gene IX that map in the C-terminal, basic domain have been found that can partially suppress defects in the phage packaging signal; other such mutations map in gene I (Russel, unpublished).

C. DNA Metabolism Genes and Proteins

1. Genes II and X

Gene II is required for all phage-specific DNA synthesis other than the formation of the complementary strand of the infecting phage. Cells infected by gene II mutants behave as though they were uninfected by most assays (Pratt et al., 1966; Marvin and Hohn, 1969), and the parental RF is ultimately lost by dilution. In particular, although infection with amber mutants in all other genes results in cell death, the growth of cells is not impaired by infection with gene II mutant phage. Gene II mutants, even under permissive conditions, form turbid plaques (Pratt et al., 1966) and can often be identified by this property alone. The protein is synthesized from two initiating codons, three codons apart. Most synthesis starts at the upstream AUG (Meyer et al., 1980); it is not clear whether this has any physiological significance. The synthesis of gene II protein is negatively regulated by gene V protein (see Control of Gene Expression); very clear plaques are often a symptom of failure of this regulation (Farber and Ray, 1980; Horiuchi, Fulford, and Model, unpublished).

Gene II encodes a specific nuclease-topoisomerase which, in the presence of Mg^{2+}, either introduces a specific nick into supercoiled RF or relaxes it so as to leave a covalently closed circle without supercoils. The sequence of gene II from Ike has about 50% homology with that from the F-specific phages, but the two proteins are not interchangeable, in spite of the fact that the region required for nicking, the (+) strand origin, is highly conserved between these phages (Peeters et al., 1986). The enzymatic functions are discussed in DNA Synthesis.

Cells that contain a relatively large amount of gene II protein, induced by inactivation of gene V by temperature or mutation, or the consequence of synthesis from a multicopy plasmid, accumulate the protein in membrane-associated form or as a dense complex (Lin and Pratt, 1974; Meyer and Geider, 1979a; Webster and Rementer, 1980). Active enzyme can be isolated from such complexes by treatment with guanidine HCl (Greenstein and Horiuchi, 1987). High-level expression of gene II protein can render cells relatively uninfectible by male-specific phages (Dotto et *al.*, 1981b; Meyer and Geider, 1981); the basis of this phenomenon is not clear, but passage of cells carrying clones leads to the selection of variants that produce less gene II protein and that do plate male-specific phages (Meyer and Geider, 1981).

Gene X is encoded entirely within gene II starting at an internal AUG (codon 300) that is in phase with the initiating gene II AUG. Hence gene X has the same amino acid sequence as the C-terminal third of gene II (Yen and Webster, 1981). It is not a proteolytic product; rather, it is initiated with N-formyl methionine both *in vivo* (Yen and Webster, 1981) and *in vitro* (Model and Zinder, 1974). Like gene II, its translation is negatively regulated by gene V protein (Yen and Webster, 1982; Model *et al.*, 1982). Replacement of the initiating AUG with a UAG (amber) codon prevents the expression of gene X but permits the expression of gene II in a suppressing strain; phages containing this mutation form plaques poorly or not at all on amber suppressors unless the cells carry a plasmid capable of expressing gene X (Fulford and Model, 1984a). The helper plasmid does not express full-length gene II protein. Thus, X is an essential gene in its own right. From the *in vivo* data, X protein is needed for single-stranded DNA synthesis (see DNA Synthesis); it probably acts as an inhibitor of a gene II function. X protein has been partially purified; thus far an *in vitro* role for it has not been demonstrated.

2. Gene V

Gene V encodes a single-stranded DNA binding protein (Alberts *et al.*, 1972; Oey and Knippers, 1972). Amber mutants in the gene have a polar effect on the expression of genes VII (Lyons, 1971) and on gene IX (Simons *et al.*, 1982). It is required for single-stranded DNA synthesis (Pratt *et al.*, 1968; Salstrom and Pratt, 1971), and it acts by forming a complex with single-stranded DNA and preventing the synthesis of the complementary strand.

The protein from the F-specific phages M13, fd, and f1 is identical; it is 87 amino acids in length (Nakashima *et al.*, 1974). It forms a dimer in solution at physiological salt concentrations (Cavalieri *et al.*, 1976b; Pretorius *et al.*, 1975) and binds tightly and cooperatively to single-stranded but not double-stranded DNA (Alberts *et al.*, 1972; Oey and Knippers, 1972; Pratt *et al.*, 1974). In the absence of Mg^{2+} and in moderate salt, its affinity for single-stranded DNA is high enough to lower the T_m as much as 40°C; it can therefore "melt" DNA (or at least dAT) at room temperature. There is no indication that it will do so at conditions prevailing in the infected cell. Since the protein complexed any single-stranded DNA presented, it was described as binding to DNA nonspecifically. More detailed investigation (see below) has shown that in fact it does have some specificity; this can be masked by its generally high affinity and cooperativity. The protein is available in large quantities from filamentous phage-infected cells, and its properties have been studied intensively. Residues involved in binding, and the binding mechanism, have been studied by chemical modification, by DNA protection, and by a variety of spectral methods including NMR and fluorescence depolorization. Treatment of the protein with tetranitromethane results in the nitration of three of the five tyrosines (26, 41, 56) and greatly reduced affinity for DNA. Two-dimensional NMR suggests that only tyrosine 26 interacts strongly with DNA (King and Coleman, 1987). All three can be protected by prior binding with DNA. Reaction of the lysine residues with N-acetylimidizole abolishes the ability of the protein to bind to DNA, but these residues are not protected by DNA binding. Reaction of the single cysteine with mercury also abolishes the binding (Anderson *et al.*, 1975a). Extensive NMR analysis of the protein and its binding modes has been carried out. Both F^{19} and proton NMR confirm the involvement of tyrosines in DNA binding, probably by intercalation, and there are data suggesting that phenylalanine is also involved. The lysines show little evidence of rigid binding, indicating that they probably do not form salt bridges with the nucleotide phosphates (reviewed in Kowalczykowski *et al.*, 1981; Alma *et al.*, 1982; McPherson and Brayer, 1985). The CD data of Pretorius *et al.* (1975) also suggest that tyrosyl groups stack with DNA bases rather than interacting with other protein residues.

Alma *et al.* (1982, 1983) and Bulsink *et al.* (1985, 1986) have carried out extensive NMR and fluorescence depolarization studies of the binding properties of the protein. Some of the important conclusions from these studies are that the affinity of gene V protein for homopolymers differs markedly from one homopolymer to another, such that the binding to polydA is 2 orders of magnitude lower than to polydT, and that the affinity for RNA, although lower than for the deoxypolymers, is by no means negligible. The authors have also found that there are two different binding modes—one to oligonucleotides, with three nucleotides bound per monomer, and one for DNA, with four nucleotides per monomer. The cooperativity of binding was found to be much lower for binding to oligonucleotides, in agreement with earlier work from the Hilbers' laboratory. Shimamoto and Utiyama (1983) find that the cooperativity of gene V protein binding is related to the slower release of monomers from a bound cluster, rather than a higher rate of binding adjacent to already bound clusters.

Gene V protein has been crystalized, and a structure has been proposed at high resolution (McPherson *et al.*, 1980a,b). A refined structure has been presented by Brayer and McPherson (1983), and based on this a model for the DNA-protein complex has been proposed by these authors (see below). The protein is found as the dimer in the crystal, related about a perfect dyad axis. The two faces of the dimer are hydrophobic, and probably interact so as to prevent solvent access. The monomers are composed entirely of β structure, three β loops that project outward from a common hydrophobic core such that they form a three-stranded β sheet across the midportion of the molecule. Each monomer contains a DNA-binding cleft (discussed below). Most of the residues previously determined to be of significance in the binding are exposed to the DNA in the models proposed. An excellent detailed description of the molecule can be found in McPherson and Brayer (1985).

The complex isolated from the infected cells contains one molecule of DNA and about 1300 copies of the gene V protein, and it forms a filamentous structure which, at first glance, rather resembles the phage (Fig. 1) (Alberts et al., 1972; Oey and Knippers, 1972; Webster and Cashman, 1973; Pratt et al., 1974; Paradiso and Konigsberg, 1982). It may differ substantially in morphology from that prepared by the addition of purified gene V protein to single-stranded DNA (Pratt et al., 1974); as they pointed out, gene V protein probably binds to a short length of displaced single-stranded DNA as (+) strand synthesis occurs (see DNA Synthesis). It probably does so in the presence of other single-stranded DNA binding proteins (the E. coli SSB being the most likely), and it would thus not be unreasonable for the in vivo complex to differ from the one produced in vitro by mixing the two purified components under conditions that may not closely resemble those in the infected cell.

The in vivo complex is 1.1 μm long, 20 nm wide, and about 8 nm high, and thus is a ribbon slightly longer than the virus and a good deal wider (Pratt et al., 1974). It is structured and has a repeat of 16 nm, which has subsequently been interpreted (see below) as representing a helix. The original authors were cautious in the interpretation of their results and concerned lest the structure be an artifact of isolation; Lica and Ray (1977) cross-linked the protein to the DNA in vivo, thereby confirming the association in situ. The in vitro complex showed branching, was denser, did not show the 16-nm repeats, and had a knobbed structure (Alberts et al., 1972). The in vivo complex dissociated in NaCl concentrations higher than 0.1 M. Addition of DNA to the complex in the cell lysate occasioned a redistribution, so that some of the added DNA became coated with the protein; when a small amount of radioactive DNA was added, it acquired protein from the complex (although it still separated from the complex on sedimentation), whereas if a sixfold excess of DNA was added, the complex was demonstrably depleted of protein (Pratt et al., 1974).

Torbet et al. (1981) have directly compared the in vivo and in vitro complexes; they made the in vitro complex using 4.5 molecules of gene V protein per nucleotide of f1 DNA and found little if any difference between it and the in vivo complex. In their study, the complexes generated in vitro had helical repeats. Their complexes were shorter (0.9 μm) and narrower (10 nM) than those described by Pratt et al. (1974). From small-angle neutron scattering, they propose that the most reasonable ratio of nucleotides/protein monomer is 5, and that the DNA must lie close to the center of the complex, which is open and solvated. Gray et al. (1982a) extended and repeated these experiments using deuterated phage DNA, which they state allowed them to better define the radius of the shells occupied by the DNA and protein. They propose that the DNA is contained in a shell with a radius of gyration of 1.18–2.18 nm, while the protein is in a shell extending from 1.49 to 4.49 nm. Hence, according to Gray et al. (1982b), the DNA is clearly in the center of the complex. This study was carried out at a nucleotide/protein ratio of 3 (Materials and Methods) or 4 (Discussion).

Brayer and McPherson (1984a,b, 1985a,b) have based a model for the gene V complex on the refined high-resolution structure of the protein (Brayer and McPherson, 1983, 1984a,b). They propose that the protein dimer binds DNA in two clefts located on the outside of the dimer pair. Because of the observed twofold symmetry of the dimer, each binding cleft has the same relationship to the DNA, even though of course the two strands of the DNA loop have opposite absolute polarities. They also propose that initial binding of the DNA causes a movement of tyr_{41} away from the position it occupies in the protein crystal structure. Tyr_{41} has previously been implicated in DNA binding (Coleman and Oakley, 1980; Hilbers et al., 1978). More recent work, however, suggests that tyr_{41} is not involved in DNA interactions (King and Coleman, 1987). The structure proposed for the protein alone would have a region (a β turn created by residues 38–42) that would block side-to-side dimer formation; the movement of tyr_{41} into DNA would relieve this inhibition, and lateral association of dimers would be permitted. Thus, DNA binding itself would act as a "switch" to permit the higher-order association of dimer subunits along the DNA and could account for the cooperativity phenomena that have been observed.

The binding cleft can accomodate four nucleotides easily but a fifth less well; when, however, the position of tyr_{41} is changed, a binding site is created if two adjacent dimers are bound to the DNA. Brayer and McPherson (1984a) find that their model is consistent with the description of the complex derived from the electron microscopic images of Torbet et al. (1981). The authors also find that this structure predicts the formation of a right-handed helix consisting of five nucleotides per protein monomer, 0.91 μm long, with a diameter of 9.3 nm, a helical pitch of 9.0 nm, and 100 helical turns containing 6.4 dimers per turn, all in good agreement with many of the observed properties of the complex (Alberts et al., 1972; Pratt et al., 1974; Cavalieri et al., 1976b; Day, 1973; Anderson et al., 1975a,b; Oey and Knippers, 1972; Torbet et al., 1981). Although this model is both aesthetically and functionally very pleasing, its predictions do not seem to us to be reconcilable with the conclusions of Gray et al. (1982a). The nucleotide/protein stoichiometry reported by Bulsink et al. (1985, 1986), which is four nucleotides per protein with DNA and three with oligonucleotides, in agreement with previous reports from their laboratory (Alma et al., 1982, 1983), also does not agree with the predictions of the detailed Brayer and McPherson models. A recent CD study reports a stoichiometry of three or four nucleotides for the two binding modes, and in particular no evidence for any stoichiometry of five; the binding to DNA, at rather low salt, had a stoichiometry of 3.1 (Kansy *et al.*, 1986).

The complexes formed by the Pf1 and Pf3 DNA binding proteins and nucleic acids have also been studied, although not in nearly so exhaustive a fashion as that formed by the F-specific phages. Although quite different in detail, the general properties of the Pf1 complex are quite similar to those of the fd complex; in particular, the lengths of the two complexes are similar. Since the length of the Pf1 virion is much greater than that of the F-specific phages, the DNA in the complex is much less extended than in the assembled virion (Gray *et al.*, 1982b). The Pf3 complex contains 6 nucleotides/protein subunit and is, like the Pf1 complex, shorter than the virion. Its general properties resemble those of the others, although in almost every specific detail it differs. A curious aspect is that the complex is stable only in the presence of a reducing agent; in the absence of 2-mercaptoethanol, the complex forms aggregates (Casadevall and Day, 1985).

The DNA-binding protein of Ike is clearly related to that of the F-specific filamentous phages (Peeters *et al.*, 1983). It is 1 amino acid longer and has diverged a good deal from the identical F-specific gene V proteins, but it contains a number of the residues found to be important in the DNA binding of fd gene V at cognate locations. However, it does not contain a cysteine (which, in the F-specific phages, cannot be modified without losing DNA binding capacity; see above).

Pf1 encodes a single-stranded DNA binding protein that is almost twice as long as that of the filamentous phages and has rather little homology with other gene V proteins (Maeda *et al.*, 1982). Tsugita and Kneale (1985) have shown that in binding either to oligonucleotides or to DNA, a single lysine is protected from reagent attack—but surprisingly, different lysine residues are protected in the two cases. Pf1 may also, then, have two binding modes. The Pf3 single-stranded DNA-binding protein is 78 residues in length and has little obvious homology with any of the others (Putterman *et al.*, 1984; Luiten *et al.*, 1985). The sequences of the single-stranded DNA binding proteins currently available are shown in Fig. 5.

D. Morphogenetic Genes and Proteins

Genes I and IV encode products not found in the virion and not required for DNA synthesis (Pratt and Erdahl, 1968) or for the synthesis of any other phage proteins. When temperature-sensitive mutants in either gene are shifted to the nonpermissive temperature, virion assembly stops rapidly. The converse is true on shift-down (Pratt *et al.*, 1968; Mazur and Zinder, 1975); noninfectious particles are not produced upon I or IV infections under nonpermissive conditions (Pratt, 1969).

Gene I is a major target for mutagenesis (Pratt *et al.*, 1966; Lyons and Zinder, 1972; Boeke, 1981), and temperature-sensitive alleles are com-

```
fl    M I K V E I K P S Q A Q F T T R S G V S R - Q G K P Y S L N E Q L C Y V D L G N E Y P V L V K I T L
Ike   M L T V E I H D S Q V S V K E R S G V S Q K S G K P Y T I R E Q E A Y I D L G G V Y P A L F N F N L

fl    D E G Q P A Y A P G L Y T V H L S S F K V G Q F G S L M I D R L R L V P A K
Ike   E D G Q Q P Y P A G K Y R L H P A S F K I N N F G Q V A V G R V L L E S V K


Pf3   M N I Q I T F T D S V R Q G T S A K G N P Y T F Q E G F L H L E D K P F P L Q C Q F F V E S V I P A
      G S Y Q V P Y R I N V N N G R P E L A F D F K A M K R A

Pf1   M N M F A T Q G G V V E L W V T K T D T Y T S T K T G E I Y A S V Q S I A P I P E G A R G N A K G F
      E I S E Y N I E P T L L D A I V F E G Q P V L C K F A S V V R P T Q D R F G R I T N T Q V L V D L L
      A V G G K P M A P T A Q A P A R P Q A Q A Q A P R P A Q Q P Q G Q D K Q D K S P D A K A
```

FIGURE 5. Sequences of filamentous phage ssDNA binding proteins. The fl (fd, M13) sequence has been aligned according to Peeters *et al.* (1985). No alignment has been attempted between the Pf1 and Pf3 sequences and each other or the F-specific phages. References can be found in the text.

mon in the gene. Host thioredoxin is required for phage assembly (see Morphogenesis). It is possible to select for phage mutants that can grow on cells carrying certain mutant thioredoxin genes (under conditions such that wild-type phages will not assemble); these map to the N-terminal region of gene I and cause a change from asn_{142} to tyr. Other gene I mutants, temperature-sensitives, and even some that have no obvious phenotype are unable to grow on thioredoxin mutant strains under conditions permissive for assembly of wild-type phages. These observations suggest an interaction between gene I and host thioredoxin in assembly (Russel and Model, 1983). Gene I mutations can also be selected that partially compensate for defective packaging signals (see Morphogenesis); these also map to the N-terminal portion of gene I (Russel, unpublished).

Gene I has been cloned under the control of λ PL (Horabin and Webster, 1986). Full expression of the gene is immediately lethal to the cell carrying the plasmid. The cells stop all macromolecular synthesis, and Horabin and Webster (1986 and unpublished data) have evidence that strongly suggests that gene I protein affects energy metabolism, perhaps by acting to permeabilize the membrane to ions. Gene I expression in this construct is regulated by a thermolabile λ repressor; shift of the culture to intermediate temperatures, which gives rise to low-level expression of pI, allowed sufficient synthesis that the product could be detected; it was found to be associated with the cell envelope (Horabin and Webster, 1986). No processing was evident, and the gene does not encode a sequence that resembles a typical N-terminal signal sequence. The lethal effect was localized to the C-terminal portion of the protein, since a plasmid construction bearing an amber termination codon positioned two-thirds of the way through the gene is not inhibitory to cell growth. The longest uninterrupted run of hydrophobic amino acids is beyond the position of this amber mutation and is 20 residues long (Hill and Peterson, 1982). It may be a membrane insertion sequence. In the filamentous phage-infected cell, gene I is expressed at very low levels (see Translation), which may explain how such a cell can avoid the inhibitory effects of the gene I protein. It is also possible that the act of phage assembly prevents the lethal effect.

The function of gene IV is as little understood as that of gene I. It is made as a precursor with a cleaved signal sequence, and processing is sensitive to the ionophore CCCP (Brissette and Russel, unpublished). The mature protein fractionates to the periplasm and membrane components. It too has been cloned; very high level expression is probably lethal, since multicopy plasmids bearing gene IV under control of the strong tac promoter cannot be maintained, even in the absence of inducer; under control of the weaker *lac* UV5 promoter, the plasmids are stable (Brissette, unpublished). Expression of gene IV protein induces the synthesis of a very large amount of a host-encoded protein, whose synthesis can also be stimulated by an extreme heat shock (37 → 50°C) but which does not appear to be any of the previously described heat shock proteins (Brissette, unpublished). The identity of this *E. coli* product has not been established, nor has its role in filamentous phage assembly, if any, been established.

III. VIRION STRUCTURE

A. Composition

The virion consists of a circular, single-stranded DNA, about 6500 nucleotides in length, encapsidated in a protein sheath. The bulk of the protein comprising the protein tube is the product of a single gene, gene VIII. In the case of the F-specific phages, the mature protein contains 50 amino acid residues and is made up of three domains—an N-terminal, acidic region; a central region, which is very hydrophobic; and a C-terminal, basic region. Chemical modification studies of the intact virion (reviewed in Makowski, 1984; see also Armstrong *et al.*, 1983), the low pI (4.1 for fd; Hobom and Braunitzer, 1967), and the observation that mutations that alter the charges at the N terminus of the protein lead to altered mobility of the intact virion in agarose gels (Boeke *et al.*, 1980), all suggest that the N-terminal region is on the outside of the virion, exposed to the solvent. Wickner (1976) has shown, moreover, that antibody purified by reaction with intact phages recognizes only the amino-terminal portion of the major coat protein. The basic C terminus is not exposed (Armstrong *et al.*, 1983; Tsugita and Kneale, 1985). As might be expected, residues in the central, very hydrophobic domain are not exposed to the solvent; the extreme susceptibility of the phage to disruption by detergents and chloroform (Marvin and Hohn, 1969) is consistent with the proposal that the central hydrophobic domains interact in forming the protein tube. Structural models for the phage have suggested that the C-terminal basic residues interact with the DNA phosphates on the interior

(Marvin and Hohn, 1960; Marvin, 1978; Makowski, 1984); these models have received strong support from a recent mutagenic study of the C terminus (Hunter *et al.*, 1987), as described below. All of the filamentous phages so far studied in sufficient detail show the same structural motif—an acidic N-terminal domain, a hydrophobic center, and a basic C-terminal region—though they vary a great deal in the particulars of the sequence and in the number of charged residues comprising each region (reviewed in Makowski, 1984).

In addition to the DNA and the major coat protein, the phages contain four other proteins, two at each end. One end contains about five copies each of the gene III (Goldsmith and Konigsberg, 1977; Woolford *et al.*, 1977) and gene VI (Lin *et al.*, 1980; Grant *et al.*, 1981) proteins. This is the end with the knobs shown in Fig. 1. The knobs consist of the N-terminal portion of gene III, and they are involved in attaching to the F pilus to initiate infection (Pratt *et al.*, 1969; Gray *et al.*, 1981; Grant *et al.*, 1981; Nelson *et al.*, 1981; Armstrong *et al.*, 1981). In addition to conferring infectivity upon the phage, the gene III and VI proteins stabilize the phage particle to dissociating agents (Rossomando and Zinder, 1968; Pratt *et al.*, 1969; Lopez and Webster, 1983; Crissman and Smith, 1984). The other end of the phage contains about five molecules each of the small proteins encoded by genes VII and IX (Grant *et al.*, 1981; Simons *et al.*, 1981). This is also the end at which a hairpin that can be cross-linked within the phage by psoralen derivatives (Ikoku and Hearst, 1981) is located. This hairpin is the packaging signal, required for phage assembly (Dotto and Zinder, 1983; see Morphogenesis).

B. Properties

In the electron microscope the entire group of filamentous phages are seen as flexible, relatively undifferentiated filaments. They range in length from 720 nm (Pf3) to 1940 nm (Pf1). This variation in length is much greater than the variation in the size of the genome and reflects the fact that the number of nucleotides per coat protein varies from 1 (Pf1) to 2.4 (Pf3). The F-specific phages are 890 nm long and contain 2.3 nucleotides per coat protein (data from Thomas *et al.*, 1983; Marzec and Day, 1983).

The length of the F-specific phages (and presumably the others) is determined by the length of the DNA they contain. Cloning DNA into the phages results in the formation of longer particles (Vovis and Ohsumi, 1978; Herrmann *et al.*, 1980); deletion mutants of the phages (which require helper phage; see Defective Interfering Particles) are encapsidated into particles much shorter than unit length (Griffith and Kornberg, 1974; Hewitt, 1975; Enea and Zinder, 1975). Wild-type phages are found as double-length or higher particles at reasonably high (1–5%) frequencies; such multilength particles contain several unit-length DNA molecules, presumably packed end to end in the protein tube. This tendency toward the formation of multilength particles is enhanced in phages containing mutations in gene III, even if the gene III defect is only partial. When the host has been infected with phages of more than one genotype, representatives of both parents are found in such multilength particles at frequencies that approximate the binomial expectation (Scott and Zinder, 1967; Beaudoin and Pratt, 1974).

Although none of the filamentous phages form crystals, it has proved possible to obtain a good deal of information about them from the X-ray diffraction of oriented fibers. The phages can be divided into two classes on the basis of their helical symmetry; class I (f1, fd, M13, Ike, If1) has a fivefold screw axis, whereas class II (Pf1, Xf, Pf3) does not (Marvin, 1978). The diffraction pattern of Pf1 gives the most information; however, studies of the class I phages, when combined with other physical-chemical information, have permitted a structure for these better-studied phages to be postulated.

Both classes are made up of a protein sheath, consisting of a double layer of α helical coat protein subunits. Pf1 is about 6 nm in diameter, with a central core of about 2 nm that contains the DNA. The rods of electron density are approximately parallel with the axis of the filament, and it has been suggested that the basic C terminus lies toward the DNA, with the N terminus in the outer layer (Makowski, 1984). Although the DNA structure is not interpretable from the diffraction pattern, solid-state NMR shows that all of the phosphodiester groups have the O–P–O plane of the nonesterified oxygens perpendicular to the virion axis, which suggests that the DNA chain must be fully extended (Cross et al., 1983) and that the bases may be nearly parallel to the protein sheath. Magnetic birefringence data are in accord with these results (Torbet and Maret, 1981). Pf1 is the longest of the phages, and its DNA has a rise per nucleotide almost about twice that of the other viruses (Thomas et al., 1983). It might then be expected that the packing of DNA in Pf1 will differ from that in the F-specific phages. In these, no particular orientation of DNA can be discerned from the solid-state NMR (Cross et al., 1983). The orientation of the protein helices is slightly less parallel to the filament axis, and the two layers can be less clearly distinguished (Cross et al., 1983). The DNA in the F-specific phages occupies somewhat more of the central volume than is the case for Pf1 (Makowski, 1984).

Aside from the difference between the class I and class II symmetries, the phages within each class show structural variation and undergo structural transitions which are affected by salt, relative humidity, and temperature (Makowski, 1984). A further example of the plasticity of the structure has come from experiments carried out in Perham's laboratory; the fd (f1 and M13) major coat protein contains four lysine residues near its C terminus, only one of which, lysine 48, can be changed by mutagenesis without loss of phage viability. Hunter et al. (1987) have replaced lysine 48 with arginine, glutamine, threonine, or alanine. The three replacements with uncharged amino acids resulted in the formation of phages about 1.33 times as long as the parental phage, as determined by electron microscopy; the length of the mutant in which arginine had replaced lysine 48 was the same as the parental. The size of the DNA encapsidated in each phage was the same. Although neither the protein/DNA ratio nor the symmetry of the coat protein tube of these mutant phages has been determined, these observations strongly suggest that the packing of DNA within the phage particle is determined principally by the charge interactions between the positively charged C-terminal portion of the coat protein and the DNA phosphates. It may be relevant that the coat protein of Pf1, the longest (both in an absolute sense and per nucleotide) of the naturally occurring phages, contains only two positively charged residues near its C terminus, and its ratio of coat protein/nucleotide is about twice that of the F-specific phages or Xf, whose coat proteins contain four. However the coat protein of phage Pf3, which shows about the same axial translation per nucleotide as the F-specific phages and also contains 2.4 nucleotides per coat protein, has only two basic residues near its C terminus. Putterman et al. (1984) have pointed out that there are not enough basic residues in Pf3 to neutralize the phosphate charges in the DNA. They have suggested that its structure may, in consequence, differ radically from that of the other phages.

Boeke et al. (1980) noted that the mobility of whole virions in agarose gels was noticeably affected by single amino acid substitutions in the major coat protein that did not change its charge. The same has been observed by Hunter et al. (1987). These observations are strongly suggestive of marked conformational changes in the virion and may reflect the plasticity of its structure.

C. Dissociation

The F-specific filamentous phages are quite resistant to trypsin and Pronase, but infectivity is sensitive to Nagarse, ficin, subtilisin, and papain. The virion is sensitive to heating above 80°C, to shear and ultrasonic treatment, and to chloroform and sodium dodecyl sulfate. The stability of the particle to extremes of pH, temperature, and salt is dependent on the presence of the gene III (Pratt et al., 1969; Rossomando and Zinder, 1968; Lopez and Webster, 1983; Crissman and Smith, 1984) and gene VI protein (Lopez and Webster, 1983). Scott and Zinder (1967) showed that the target for subtilisin is the end of the particle, since diploid, genetically heterozygous particles were inactivated with the same kinetics as single-length particles. Rossomando and Zinder (1968) studied the kinetics of dissociation of the phage at alkaline pH, showing that the process involved a two-step reaction and that the rate of the initial (rate determining) step was increased when the phage particle contained a mutant (but still functional) gene III protein. They also presented evidence for the presence of gene III protein in the particle. These results were extended by Rossomando and Bladen (1969) and Rossomando (1970), who heated virions under various conditions; disassembly could be halted, and it showed a marked polarity. One end (only) of the phage could be seen as having turned into a "blob" or "flower," and on the basis of the reduced stability of gene III mutants, this was postulated to be the gene III protein-containing end. Recent experiments have shown that at least some of the N-terminal domain (comprising the "knob" in the electron micrographs) of pIII is dispensable for morphogenesis and particle stability, but if the C-terminal portion is perturbed, the particles are of multiple length and very unstable (Crissman and Smith, 1984).

Griffith *et al.* (1981) have shown that filamentous phages contract into hollow spherical particles on exposure to a water-chloroform interface, and Manning *et al.* (1981) have modified this reaction so as to obtain intermediates (I forms) between the filaments and spheroids. The I forms closely resemble filaments opened at one end, the "flowers" seen by Rossomando (1970), and it has been suggested that they may mimic intermediates that occur normally during the infection process. Lopez and Webster (1982) have examined these structures for the presence of minor capsid proteins and found that they contain the same complement of III, VI, VII, and IX proteins as do intact phages. When decorated with ferritin-conjugated antibodies to pIII, the I forms show reaction only at their open end, indicating again that it is the gene III protein end at which disassembly starts.

IV. INFECTION

A. Adsorption

The F-specific phages require the F pilus for adsorption (Loeb, 1960; Marvin and Hoffman-Berling, 1963; Zinder *et al.*, 1963) and attach to its tip (Caro and Schnos, 1966). Since the phage is morphologically quite similar to the pilus, they are often distinguished in the electron microscope by adding one of the pilus-specific RNA phages, which adsorb to the side of the pilus but not to the attached filamentous phage. F pilus formation is a complex process, which requires the direct participation of at least 12 gene products (Willets and Skurray, 1980) as well as a number of control genes, all encoded by the F factor. In addition, several host genes have been implicated in the control of pilus formation (Beutin and Achtmman, 1979; Lerner and Zinder, 1979, 1982; McEwen and Silverman, 1980a,b). Filamentous phage infectability, then, presents a large mutagenic target, and most mutants have lost all measurable F function. Some mutants of *traA*, the structural gene for the major pilus protein, F pilin (Ippen-Ihler and Minkley, 1986), are transfer-proficient but no longer susceptible to infection by RNA phages (Willets *et al.*, 1980; Minkley *et al.*, 1976). By specific selection, a number of mutants that have not been classified have been isolated in which only partial F function is lost (Meynell and Aufreieter, 1969; Tomoeda *et al.*, 1972; Orosz and Wooton, 1977; Burke *et al.*, 1979). In particular, Silverman *et al.* (1968) have isolated mutants that do not adsorb the RNA phage f2 but that can be infected by filamentous phage. Schandel *et al.* (1987) have described a mutant in *traC* that is defective in the elaboration of pili (although it contains a normal amount of pilin protein) and does not conjugate well but can still adsorb filamentous phages well enough to enable them to plaque. The authors postulate that the F-specific attachment site is formed but remains at the cell surface.

Adsorption is independent of an energy source for the cell and can occur at 0°C or in the presence of respiration inhibitors. Subsequent penetration, deencapsidation, and eclipse all require active metabolism (Marvin and Hohn, 1969). Adsorption is by way of the gene III protein, one of the minor end proteins of the phage (Henry and Pratt, 1969). The protein actually forms an adsorption structure that can be visualized in the electron microscope (Gray *et al.*, 1979, 1981); it has a sort of lollipop structure consisting of what appears to a globular domain attached to a short rod (see Fig. 1). The globular domain can be removed by subtilisin, and the resulting phages are rendered noninfectious (Rossomando and Zinder, 1968; Gray *et al.*, 1981). Examination of the residue shows that the globular domain constitutes the N-terminal domain of the gene III protein (Gray *et al.*, 1981; Armstrong *et al.*, 1981). The adsorption end of the phage also contains the gene VI protein, but the role of this protein in the visualizable structure is obscure. Mutations in gene VI confer the same phenotype as those in gene III protein (Pratt *et al.*, 1969; Lopez and Webster, 1983); particles are formed, but they are not infectious (Scott and Zinder, 1967; Salivar *et al.*, 1967; Pratt *et al.*, 1969; Lopez and Webster, 1983).

Three models have been proposed for entry of the phage DNA into the cell. The first was the "pilus conduction" model, in which the nucleic acid was proposed to enter the pilus and be transported through a central pore into the target cell (Brinton, 1965; Brinton and Beer, 1967). Marvin and Hohn (1969) have commented that it is hard to imagine a pilus conduction mechanism that could cause DNA to move in two directions (away from the cell in conjugation, toward it during infection) and that could also accommodate the entry of RNA through the side of the pilus. The observation that not only the phage DNA but also the coat protein becomes associated with the infected cell (Smilowitz, 1974a; Trenkner *et al.*, 1967; Armstrong *et al.*, 1983) also makes the conduction model unlikely. In its stead, Marvin and Hohn (1969) proposed a "pilus retraction model" in which the function of the pilus is to retract upon infection, thus drawing the phage to the surface of the cell where it can enter. Jacobson (1972) has taken electron micrographs of phage-infected cells at fixed intervals after synchronized infection and has reported that the pili appear to be shorter as infection proceeds. Novotny and Fives-Taylor (1974) have presented evidence for retraction of F pili after cyanide treatment. This retraction can be blocked by absorbtion of RNA phages (which attach to the sides of the pilus) or antipilin serum. They suggest that pili may go through cycles of retraction and regrowth and that the regrowth is inhibited by cyanide or phage infection. J. Griffith (personal communication) has suggested that pili neither conduct nor retract. He proposes that they serve as a target for the phage and that the phage can then slide or corkscrew around the pilus in what is effectively a one-dimensional diffusion process, until the tip of the phage reaches the surface of the cell. No entirely satisfactory experiment that can definitively discriminate between these various models has been carried out, and the precise role of the pili remains obscure. It seems highly unlikely that the DNA passes through the pilus, first of all because the pilus cavity is barely large enough to contain a strand of DNA, and second because the entity that enters is the entire phage, not just the DNA. Although the evidence for the retraction model seems quite persuasive, one complication should be kept in mind: the gene III protein (whether expressed from the phage or from a gene carried on a plasmid) prevents the expression of F pili (Boeke et al., 1982; Davis and Model, unpublished). Thus the absence of pili from an infected cell could be a consequence of gene III protein expression as well as, or instead of, the infection process.

B. Entry

Several proteins of E. coli other than the F-specific, pilus-related ones are required for successful phage infection, and some of these are candidates for a cell surface receptor (Smilowitz, 1974b; Sun and Webster, 1986). Some of these proteins are also needed for the action of colicins, entry of which resembles entry of filamentous phages in that they bind to a primary receptor (analogous to the pilus) but can be internalized only if certain other proteins are functional (Nagel De Zwaig and Luria, 1967). Those mutant E. coli that are defective in the import of colicins are called tol, to distinguish them from mutants that have lost the primary receptor, which are called resistant. tolA mutants, which are not sensitive to the E colicins or to colicin K, are also not infectible by filamentous phage (Smilowitz, 1974b). Phage infection requires intact tolA but also makes E. coli tolerant to these colicins and thus phenotypically mimics a tolA mutation (Zinder, 1973; Smilowitz, 1974b). As part of a detailed examination of the tol locus, Sun and Webster (1986, 1987) have found that there are actually three proteins required for the entry of either E colicins or of filamentous phage, specified by the tolQ, tolR, and tolA genes. A fourth gene in the same cluster (tolB) is required for the action of colicins E2 and E3 but not for the entry of filamentous phages (Smilowitz, 1974b) or for the action of colicin E1 (Bernstein et al., 1972; Nagel de Swaig and Luria,

1967). The phenotypes of mutations in *tolQ* and *tolR* are indistinguishable from those of a *tolA* mutation (Sun and Webster, 1987). Thus, aside from the pilus itself, which, while apparently composed of a single type of protein, is the product of at least 12 genes, there exists a fairly complex array of proteins that are needed for entry.

Filamentous phages as such are not templates for DNA synthesis, but of course removal of the protein coat makes the DNA available for use as a template. Marco *et al.* (1974) reported that broken cell preparations of both male and female cells can carry out a reaction that makes the DNA available. At the same time, the phage is rendered noninfectious. We have found that exposure of phage particles to cell extracts prepared by lysozyme treatment and freezing and thawing in the absence of detergent did not lead to any loss of viability (Model, unpublished). The experiments reported by Marco *et al.* were carried out in the presence of the nonionic detergent, Brij; since nonionic detergents can liberate phospholipids (which are themselves detergents) from the cell lipids, and since filamentous phages are quite sensitive to detergents, the physiological significance of the "eclipse" reaction is uncertain.

Infection by filamentous phages results in the association of phage protein, as well as of the DNA, with the infected cell. This was first shown by Trenkner *et al.* (1967), who also observed that labeled coat protein on heavy (5-bromodeoxyuridine containing) phages reemerged on light (presumably progeny) phages. These results were challenged by Henry and Brinton (1971), who found that they could remove much of the phage-carried protein label from the infected cells with Nagarse, a protease. They confirmed the observation of Trenkner *et al.* (1967) that the protein label can be incorporated into progeny phage but attributed this to breakdown of the phage coat and reincorporation. Smilowitz (1974a), who had previously shown that newly synthesized coat protein is associated with the inner membrane of the infected cell (Smilowitz *et al.*, 1972), repeated many of these experiments. He found that 50–60% of the major coat protein of the infecting phage becomes associated with the inner membrane of the host, and that as much as 55% of the associated label can then be recovered as phage coat on progeny particles. Similar experiments, in which infecting and progeny particles could be distinguished by size and in which incoming coat protein had been chemically modified, later confirmed the reutilization of coat protein (Armstrong *et al.*, 1983). When the experiment was conducted so that replication of the infecting phages was blocked genetically, only 2.5% of the input phage coat was exported (Smilowitz, 1974a). Two of Smilowitz's observations are particularly interesting: first, that the kinetics of reutilization of "old" coat are much slower than the export of newly synthesized coat, with a half time of 1.5 h for the "used" coat vs. 3.5 min for the "new" coat, and second, that labeled coat protein from an infecting phage can become associated with the inner membrane even in a mutant (*tolA*) host blocked for f1 DNA penetration. This suggests that uncoating precedes DNA penetration, and implies that the TolA, Q, and R proteins function in DNA uptake. It should be noted that while F-specific RNA phages go through an RNAse-sensitive step as part of the entry into the host, filamentous phage infection is not sensitive to DNAse at any stage (Tzagoloff and Pratt, 1964).

There has been a good deal of discussion in the literature on the form of the parental single strand. Forsheit and Ray (cited in Ray, 1977), Brutlag et al. (1971), and Marco et al. (1974) have been unable to detect free single-stranded DNA in the infected cell when infections are carried out after thymidine starvation or in the presence of rifampicin, both of which treatments block the synthesis of the parental double-stranded molecule. This led Marco et al. (1974) to propose that uncoating is tightly coupled to replication. We now know that the phage DNA is oriented in the particle (Shen et al., 1979; Webster et al., 1981) and, moreover, that the end at which the origin of (−) strand synthesis is located is opposite to the end that contains gene III protein, the adsorption protein (Webster et al., 1981). It is thus highly unlikely that the replication origin would be the first bit of DNA to be exposed to the interior of the cell. Kaguni and Ray (1979), moreover, have cloned a DNA synthesis origin derived from phage G4 into M13. This G4 origin, which, unlike the filamentous phage (−) strand origin, does not require initiation by RNA polymerase, functioned to permit synthesis of the parental replicative form even when the host cells were pretreated with rifampicin; since this origin is located about 1000 bases away from the M13 origin, much of the phage single-stranded DNA must have been accessible to the replication enzymes that initiate at the G4 origin. Kaguni and Ray (1979) suggested that the DNA may be free to move within the particle, with only a small region exposed at any one time. This suggestion seems a bit forced. It is possible that in the earlier experiments, the uncoated parental single strands were simply not detected. Single-stranded DNA can bind quite well to a number of cell membrane components, and some may have been lost to the pellet on subsequent centrifugation, leaving only the labeled input phages that had not infected their host. A variety of other explanations are possible, but none are entirely satisfactory.

Many of the experiments in which phage adsorption and penetration were studied used plaque formation as an assay to determine whether an infection had been initiated. If the probability of infecting a cell is less than about 0.1, no plaques, or very unsatisfactory plaques, will be formed, because multiple rounds of infection are required to generate a plaque. By the nature of the assay, then, only efficient infection will be scored. Recent developments have made it possible to generate filamentous phage transducing particles—phagelike entities that carry both phage and plasmid origins and some marker gene (usually a selectable antibiotic resistance gene) encapsidated in phage proteins (Dotto et al., 1981a). Such transducing particles can carry the plasmid into the usual F+ hosts at high efficiency, approaching unity. Successful transduction (infection) is indicated by the acquisition of antibiotic resistance by the recipient cell. Because only a single infection event is required, such an assay can be used to detect infections that occur at very low efficiency. Several recent reports (F. Stahl, W. Barnes, and K. Geider, personal communication) suggest that female (F$^-$) cells can be infected, although at vastly lower (10^{-5} to 10^{-7}) efficiency than male (F$^+$) cells. Although the filamentous particles can bypass adsorption to the pilus to a certain extent, transduction of F$^-$ cells is still dependent on *tolA*, *Q*, and *R* function (M. Russel and R. E. Webster, unpublished). These results strongly support the idea that the pilus itself is not the entry point for the phage, but rather facilitates its approach to the cell surface.

V. DNA REPLICATION

The basic outlines of filamentous phage DNA synthesis are established, although many details are still under investigation. The entering single-stranded phage DNA (the + strand) is converted to a double-stranded form by the combined actions of RNA polymerase, which synthesizes a specific primer, and DNA polymerase III holoenzyme in the presence of the *E. coli* single-stranded DNA binding protein (SSB). The phage-encoded gene II protein makes a nick in (+) strand of the resulting duplex, and synthesis proceeds by elongation at the 3' hydroxyl of the discontinuity until a complete new (+) strand is formed. This represents modified "rolling-circle" replication, proposed by Gilbert and Dressler (1968) and found for M13 by Ray (1969). The reaction requires pol III holoenzyme, SSB, and the *rep* helicase. When gene II protein is present, the new single strand is cleaved from the old, and closure of the displaced strand occurs. The parental double-stranded molecule is closed, supercoiled by gyrase, and becomes a substrate for cleavage by gene II protein. The newly formed single strand either acts as a template for complementary strand synthesis (as did the incoming strand) or is coated by the phage-encoded single-stranded DNA binding protein (gene V protein) to generate an intermediate in the assembly of progeny phage.

DNA synthesis was first studied in the icosahedral single-stranded phages (mainly φX174 and S13). In the life cycle of φX, synthesis of daughter RF molecules precedes synthesis of single strands, and once single-strand synthesis starts, synthesis of daughter RFs seems to be completely ended. For a variety of reasons, the operative paradigm for those working on φX replication was that double-strand synthesis occurred as such—i.e., the two strands were replicated simultaneously. This has, in fact, been shown to be the way plasmids such as ColEI replicate. It was even proposed at one point that for φX during single-strand synthesis both strands were made, but one was preferentially degraded. Initial work on filamentous phage replication accepted, almost unconsciously, this paradigm. In point of fact, filamentous phage replication seems to proceed one strand at a time, both on initial infection, during the period of intensive RF replication, and later for the production of single strands. As this became clearer [largely through the work of Horiuchi and Zinder (1976) and Horiuchi *et al.* (1979)], the dominant ideology governing the interpretation of φX174-based observations was also changed, and the current view is that even for this phage the dominant mode of replication is one strand at a time (Eisenberg *et al.*, 1976a,b). Very recently, and often to the surprise of the investigators (though not to confirmed filamentous phageologists), this mechanism of DNA replication has been extended to explain the replication of a number of plasmids (te Riele *et al.*, 1986).

A. Complementary Strand Synthesis

The initial step in phage-specific DNA synthesis is the synthesis of the parental complementary strand. This process does not require phage-encoded proteins; it occurs in the presence of high concentrations of chloramphenicol, and after infection by all known conditional lethal mutants under nonpermissive conditions (Pratt and Erdahl, 1968; Tadakuma and Watanabe, 1968). This reaction, then, is carried out entirely by host functions. Brutlag *et al.* (1971) demonstrated that the conversion from single-stranded to double-stranded molecules is sensitive to the antibiotic rifampicin, which inhibits RNA polymerase. These authors inferred from this sensitivity that RNA polymerase generates the primer for the synthesis of the complementary strand, and this inference has been borne out by a large number of studies, principally in the Kornberg, Hurwitz, and Schaller laboratories (Geider and Kornberg, 1974; reviewed by Kornberg, 1980; Kornberg, 1982; Wickner *et al.*, 1972; McMacken *et al.*, 1978). *In vitro*, RNA polymerase binds to the single-stranded fd DNA and initiates synthesis of a primer at a specific T residue (5757 in fd). In the absence of DNA polymerase III holoenzyme, the primer is about 30 nucleotides long; in its presence, the RNA is somewhat shorter. The specificity of initiation depends on the presence of the *E. coli* single-stranded DNA binding protein (SSB)* and requires that the RNA polymerase be saturated with sigma factor (Kaguni and Kornberg, 1982). In the absence of SSB, the *in vitro* reaction is relatively nonspecific and will occur at many places on single-stranded templates, giving rise to fairly long RNAs. Even with SSB present, templates that do not initiate *in vivo* by the action of RNA polymerase do initiate *in vitro*.

This led to a search for "specificity factors" (Vicuna *et al.*, 1977) or altered RNA polymerases (Wickner and Kornberg, 1974). Kaguni and

---

*The *E. coli* single-stranded DNA binding protein, SSB, should be carefully distinguished from the single-stranded DNA binding protein encoded by the phage, the gene V protein. The *E. coli* protein *facilitates* many reactions; the principal function of gene V protein seems to be to *inhibit* polymerization reactions (Geider and Kornberg, 1974).

Kornberg (1982) showed conclusively that sigma factor is both necessary and sufficient to render the reaction highly specific. DNA polymerase III holoenzyme then extends the RNA primer, leaving a single-stranded gap in the newly formed double strand. Removal of the RNA primer, and its replacement with DNA, requires the action of the $5' \rightarrow 3'$ exonuclease activity of DNA polymerase I; the discontinuity can then be ligated by the host DNA ligase.

There is a great deal of support for this model of complementary strand synthesis. In the presence of SSB, RNA polymerase protects a specific fragment of the (+) strand DNA from nuclease digestion (Gray et al., 1978); the sequence of "ori" RNA corresponds to that expected from RNA synthesis starting at the (−) strand origin (Geider et al., 1978), and synthesis of the complementary strand leads to the formation of the duplex containing a specific gap (Tabak et al., 1974). Results from in vivo experiments closely complement the in vitro results. By pulse labeling followed by restriction mapping, Horiuchi and Zinder (1976) showed that the in vivo (−) strand origin is within the region that contains the gap identified by Tabak et al. (1974). Kim et al. (1981) constructed deletions within the (−) strand origin and showed that formation of the parental replicative form DNA was greatly delayed in most of the constructs. Surprisingly, the phages were viable, although delayed significantly in producing progeny, and formed very turbid plaques. These constructs were reported to be relatively inactive in acting as templates for complementary strand synthesis in vitro. These observations point to an "escape" or backup route to the formation of the complementary strand. Such a backup system was also suggested by Bayne and Dumas (1979), who observed that complementary strands (purified from replicative form DNA) were moderately infectious in a spheroplast assay even though they do not serve as effective templates for DNA synthesis in vitro. Growth of filamentous phages in hosts defective for the exonuclease activity of DNA polymerase I leads to the formation of defective RF molecules, many of which contain RNA or gaps (Chen and Ray, 1976, 1978).

It has been observed (Jazwinski et al., 1973) that when cells infected by phages are labeled with histidine [absent from the major coat protein, but present in the gene III (absorption) protein], the label is found with the infected cell and sediments with RF. Infection with ts gene III mutants at the nonpermissive temperature does not lead to the formation of parental RF. These observations led to the proposal that gene III acts as a "pilot protein," leading the infecting DNA to the replication machinery (Jazwinski et al., 1973; Marco et al., 1974). This proposal has been widely disseminated. Since gene III mutants are not infectious, and since filamentous phages enter the cell together with their coat protein, these observations can be explained as a failure of the ts III mutant to infect, and by the adventitious transfer of label. There is no evident requirement for gene III protein in the in vitro formation of double strands from single strands, or in the transfection of spheroplasts or Ca^{2+}-treated *E. coli*. Thus, most workers in the field do not consider that the "pilot protein" hypothesis has been adequately supported.

B. Synthesis of the (+) Strand

Other than for the initial "doubling-up" reaction forming the parental RF, DNA synthesis in filamentous phages is entirely dependent on the presence of the gene II protein. For the synthesis of progeny single-stranded DNA, the product of gene V, a single-stranded DNA-binding protein (Alberts *et al.*, 1972; Oey and Knippers, 1972) is also required (Pratt and Erdahl, 1968). The general features of filamentous phage DNA synthesis were established initially by *in vivo* experiments (for review see Ray, 1977, 1978). These experiments suggested that the initial stages of phage-specific DNA replication consisted of the conversion of the infecting single strand into a parental double-stranded circle, followed by extensive synthesis of daughter double-stranded molecules, followed by a stage in which the predominant synthesis is of single-stranded DNA, which becomes the genome of progeny phages. Because infections carried out in the presence of chloramphenicol accumulate closed, but not nicked, double-stranded, circular molecules, Fidanian and Ray (1972) proposed that gene II introduces a specific cut into one strand of the double-stranded molecules. Ray (1969), Tseng and Marvin (1972), and Forsheit and Ray (1971) showed that isolated replication intermediates contained unit-length (−) strands and greater-than-unit-length (+) strands. This strongly suggested that this phage, like φX174, used the rolling-circle mechanism of replication proposed by Gilbert and Dressler (1969). Analysis of pulse-labeled replicating molecules suggested that there is one origin of replication for (+) strand synthesis and one for (−) strand synthesis located very nearby, and that synthesis is unidirectional and opposite from each origin (Horiuchi and Zinder, 1976). From these and other data, they proposed that the synthesis of phage DNA could be accounted for by synthesis of a (−) strand on the (+) strand template to form a double strand, followed by rolling-circle synthesis of a new (+) strand which could then either be sequestered or act again as the template for (−) strand synthesis. Ray (1969), Forsheit *et al.* (1971), and Horiuchi and Zinder (1976) also showed that although pulse labeling very quickly labels the (+) strand of double-stranded replicating DNA, label appears in free single strands only much later. They showed by pulse labeling that radioactive precursors flow first into double-stranded DNA containing a discontinuity, then into an unsupercoiled, covalently closed species, and finally into supercoiled DNA. Inhibitors of gyrase increased the level of the unsupercoiled DNA and reduced the flow of label into supercoiled DNA (Horiuchi and Zinder, 1976; Horiuchi *et al.*, 1978). The most reasonable interpretation of these results is that synthesis results in the displacement of an (originally) unlabeled single strand from a double-stranded replicative intermediate, with replacement of the viral strand by newly synthesized material, followed by covalent closure of the double-stranded form, which is acted upon by gyrase to regenerate a supercoiled, covalently closed molecule. Thus, *in vivo* the filamentous phage rolling circle rolls only once.

C. *In Vitro* DNA Synthesis

Meyer, Geider, and colleagues have carried out extensive studies of filamentous phage replication *in vitro*. They purified gene II protein (Meyer and Geider, 1979a), showed that it was specific for filamentous phage RF DNA (Meyer and Geider, 1979b), and used it to reconstitute phage DNA synthesis *in vitro* (Meyer and Geider, 1982; Geider *et al.*, 1982). Gene II protein is a highly specific enzyme, which makes a single cut between nucleotides 5781 and 5782 of phage fd RFI (Meyer *et al.*, 1979). The enzyme requires Mg^{2+} and that the substrate DNA be supercoiled, but no other cofactors. The products of the reaction are the nicked circle together with covalently closed, relaxed double-stranded DNA. If Mn^{2+} replaces Mg^{2+} in the buffer, the product of the reaction is linear DNA; this has been interpreted as indicating that gene II protein binds as a dimer (Meyer and Geider, 1979b). In the presence of DNA polymerase III holoenzyme, *rep* helicase, and *E. coli* DNA-binding protein I (SSB), the reaction generates circular single strands and nicked double-stranded DNA (RF II). In addition, a good deal of RF IV (covalently closed, relaxed circular DNA) is produced, presumably as a consequence of gene II action. A fraction of the molecules in such an experiment undergo more than one round of replication. With the use of density-labeled (heavy) input DNA, it was possible to show that early in replication the newly labeled material is of hybrid density but that the released single strands ultimately are heavy, consistent with the postulated rolling-circle replication (Meyer and Geider, 1982). Most of the product DNA is circular; little linear DNA is produced. If, however, the 5' phosphate is removed from the nicked template RF, the newly displaced single strand remains linear rather than being circularized (Meyer and Geider, 1982; Geider *et al.*, 1982).

Meyer and Geider (1982) noted that the synthesis reaction can utilize RF previously nicked by gene II protein (which they call RF II$_0$) but that this does not bypass the requirement for gene II protein in the synthesis reaction. Thus gene II protein has at least two functions: first, to cleave supercoiled RFI at a specific site, and second, to participate in the synthesis reaction. For the nicking, the substrate DNA must be supercoiled, but synthesis can occur on the appropriately cleaved RF (RF II$_0$). Control experiments showed that randomly nicked RF is not a substrate under these conditions, whether or not gene II protein is present in the reactions.

When DNA polymerase is omitted from these reactions, the remaining proteins (gene II protein, SSB, and the *rep* helicase) catalyze an ATP-dependent unwinding of the nicked DNA in a reaction similar to one previously described for the replication of ϕX174 (Scott *et al.*, 1977; Langeveld *et al.*, 1978). The *rep* helicase does not initiate unwinding on a template containing only a single-strand break (Yarranton and Gefter, 1979). The gene II protein requirement is generally assumed to reflect its interaction with the helicase to facilitate the start of unwinding, but this has not been proved. Meyer and Geider (1980) have reported that helicases I and II of *E. coli* cannot replace the *rep* helicase in either the unwinding or the synthesis reactions.

Harth *et al.* (1981) and Myer *et al.* (1981) have studied the replication of fd RF in systems composed of phage T7- and T4-specific enzymes. The T7 gene 4 protein (a helicase) and T7 DNA polymerase can utilize nicked fd RF to synthesize a single strand by rolling-circle replication. Thus, when DNA nicked with gene II protein was incubated with the two T7 enzymes, incorporation of label occurred, but free single strands were not produced. If gene II protein was present during the synthesis reaction, unit-length molecules, circular and linear in a ratio of 3 : 1, were produced, as well as some multiple-length linear molecules and a variety of replication intermediates.

A complication of the T7 system is the tendency of the T7 polymerase to "switch strands" during synthesis. In the T4 system, which consists of seven purified T4 replication proteins (Alberts *et al.*, 1980), RF that has been nicked by gene II protein is an extremely effective template for rolling-circle synthesis. If gene II product is not present in the reaction the principal products are replicating intermediates, rolling circles with longer-than-unit-length single-stranded "tails." Gene II protein added after synthesis has ended does not cleave the tails. Adding gene II protein to the reaction mixtures yields substantial amounts of linear, single-stranded molecules of unit length. The presence of the gene II protein also depresses synthesis twofold, and it increases the fraction of replication intermediates containing single-stranded tails. It would appear, then, that some component of the T4 system (possibly the gene 32-encoded single-stranded DNA-binding protein) inhibits gene II-catalyzed circularization, but not cleavage, of the rolling-circle intermediates. The T4 and T7 experiments show that gene II, without the participation of host factors, is responsible for both cleavage and circularization of the displaced (+) strands, and that cleavage and circularization appear to be linked processes which can only occur while synthesis is in progress. Although a number of explanations have been proposed for this coupling between synthesis and gene II action, a mechanistic analysis has, as yet, not been carried out.

For the most part, the *in vivo* and *in vitro* studies are consistent. Replication does occur as a rolling circle, and circular products are obtained only when the cleavage has occurred at the unique site specified by the gene II protein. *In vitro* replication can initiate on RF II$_o$ molecules— that is to say, molecules nicked at the unique site—so that several cycles of replication can result from one nick. *In vivo* this appears not to occur with any frequency; most likely the presence of ligase (which is not included in the *in vitro* reactions) seals the nicks and therefore requires that the covalently closed, double-stranded, relaxed circle be converted back into supercoils before a second round of synthesis can occur. This hypothesis is consistent with Horiuchi and Zinder's (1976) pulse-labeling data and with the observation of Fidanian and Ray (1972, 1974) that filamentous phage DNA synthesis is extremely sensitive to nalidixic acid, an inhibitor of gyrase.

In vitro single-strand synthesis has been carried out in the presence of gene V protein only in a relatively crude system (Van Dorp *et al.*, 1979). In the absence of gene V protein, the principal product was replicative form DNA, while in its presence appreciable amounts of single-strands were produced, although the overall incorporation was somewhat reduced. Gene V protein binds DNA with higher affinity than SSB, and *in vitro*, in aqueous buffers, it can displace it from single strands. It remains to be explained, then, why it does not do so at the phage or the host growing fork. Shimamoto and Utiyama (1983) have studied the binding of gene V protein kinetically and found that the cooperativity can be accounted for by the stabilization of bound gene V protein clusters to dissociation, rather than to an increase in the rate of binding to the DNA. This might account for its inability to displace SSB *in vivo*.

Although one would like to stress the concordance between the *in vivo* and *in vitro* results, there are a number of observations that cannot be reconciled with our current scheme of DNA replication. Several laboratories have reported that the products of *dnaB* and *dnaG* are required for filamentous phage synthesis *in vivo* (Dasgupta and Mitra, 1976; Olsen *et al.*, 1972; Ray *et al.*, 1975). Bouvier and Zinder (1974) reported that viable phages are not produced in a *dnaA* mutant at the nonpermissive temperature and that in such a host many of the progeny single strands are linear rather than circular. There are a number of reasons to believe that inhibition of phage production in these mutant strains is a secondary, rather than a primary, effect of the respective lesions. The biochemical roles of *dnaA*, *-B*, and *-G* proteins are now much clearer than when these reports first appeared: *dnaA* protein binds at certain origins and facilitates the helicase activity of *dnaB* protein, and *dnaG* protein is involved in primer generation on the exposed single strands (see, e.g., Kornberg *et al.*, 1987). It would appear from the results of rifampicin experiments that priming of filamentous phage complementary strand synthesis late in infection is catalyzed by RNA polymerase (Fidanian and Ray, 1974), in the same fashion as the synthesis of the complement of the infecting viral strand. Bayne and Dumas (1979) used isolated complementary (−) strands in an *in vitro* system that contained functional *dnaB* and *dnaG* activity in an effort to see whether synthesis (and thus priming) could be observed; it was not. It is difficult, therefore, to envisage a suitable direct role for *dnaA*, *-B*, or *-G* proteins in filamentous phage replication. Nonetheless, the observations are well documented; it is their interpretation that poses a problem.

D. Single-Strand Synthesis

Gene II protein is required for the synthesis of the (+) strand of filamentous phage DNA, but both gene II protein and gene V protein (a phage-encoded, single-stranded DNA-binding protein) are needed for the successful synthesis of *single* (+) strands (Pratt and Erdahl, 1968). Cells infected with phages bearing amber mutations in gene V make double-stranded (RF) DNA but no single strands (Pratt and Erdahl, 1968); treating cells infected with wild-type phages with chloramphenicol also results in the appearance of new (+) strand DNA only in RF (Ray, 1970; Salstrom and Pratt, 1971). Salstrom and Pratt (1971) also made the crucial observation that when a cell infected with phages bearing a *ts* allele in gene V were shifted to the nonpermissive temperature, *existing* single-stranded DNA was converted to double-stranded. These results suggested that gene V protein acts in an inhibitory fashion by blocking the conversion of single strands into RF, a hypothesis first put forward by Marvin and Hohn (1969). In a normal infection by wild-type phage, a period in which RF → RF synthesis predominates precedes the synthesis of single-stranded DNA. Mazur and Model (1973) showed that when gene V protein synthesis is allowed to proceed in the absence of DNA replication (so that V protein accumulates) and DNA synthesis is subsequently permitted to resume, single strands are produced almost immediately, confirming the suggestion that it is the accumulation of gene V protein that triggers the switch from RF to single-strand production. These results were interpreted as indicating that gene V protein is both necessary and sufficient for this switch in the nature of the DNA product.

Further work has shown that the situation is somewhat more complicated. Gene II protein contains within it a second open reading frame, in phase with the first, and encoding the C-terminal two-thirds of the amino acids encoded by the whole gene (Yen and Webster, 1981). Fulford and Model (1984a) have shown that this C-terminal portion of gene II protein, called the gene X protein, is essential for single-strand synthesis; if the C-terminal polypeptide is not synthesized (by mutating its initiation codon so as to retain a functional gene II), single-strand synthesis and yield of progeny phage are severely depressed. Further work (Fulford and Model, 1988a) has shown that this same effect can be obtained if gene II protein is expressed at high levels from a plasmid. When II protein is expressed under the direction of an inducible promoter, induction leads to a cessation of single-stranded DNA synthesis and an enhanced synthesis of double strands (RF). If a plasmid is present that codes only for gene X protein (and not the full-length gene II protein), its induction leads to a cessation of all phage-specific synthesis, both double- and single-stranded. Thus, it appears that in the presence of gene II protein, both the X protein and gene V protein are needed for single-stranded DNA synthesis to occur; gene II protein by itself facilitates the synthesis of double strands even in the presence of gene V protein, perhaps by blocking V protein binding at the (−) strand origin.

It is likely that the function of the gene X protein is to down-modulate this activity of the gene II protein, although this has not yet been demonstrated in an *in vitro* system. The current model, then, is that there is a tripartite tug-of-war involved in determining the nature of the product of DNA synthesis. Gene V protein pulls toward single strands; gene II protein pulls toward RF and wins, unless the X protein is also present. One prediction of this model, that gene II protein might not only facilitate doubling up of the (+) strand but be required for it if gene V protein is present, was tested with a plasmid construction which could express both gene V protein and gene II protein. The gene II also contained an amber mutation, and transcription of both genes was under control of the *lac* promoter. When this construct was placed in a cell that did not contain a suppressor (so that intact gene II protein was not made) and induced with isopropyl-β-D-thiogalactopyranoside (IPTG), the cell was rendered resistant to filamentous phage infection, and conversion of the infecting DNA from single to double strands was inefficient. If the cell contained a suppressor, so that synthesis of gene II protein was possible, plaques were obtained and the conversion from single to double strand was normal (Fulford and Model, 1988b). Since gene V regulates the synthesis of both gene II and gene X protein (see Control of Gene Expression) and its level is responsive to gene dosage (i.e., the number of RF molecules), the control of DNA synthesis in these phages is extremely complex (see Fig. 2).

E. Structure and Function of the (−) Strand Origin

The minus strand origin can be defined as the region of the f1 single strand protected by RNA polymerase (in the presence of *E. coli* SSB) against nuclease digestion, extended on the 3′ side to the position at which the RNA primer is initiated. The protected region extends, approximately, from nucleotide 5609 to 5738 (Gray *et al.*, 1978), and the first nucleotide of the RNA primer, at nucleotide 5756, is downstream from the protected region, and it extends about 30 bases, to nucleotide 5728. Much of this region can be drawn as two stable hairpins separated by an unstructured region (Fig. 6). The initiation point for primer RNA syn-

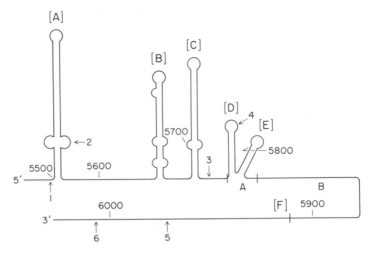

FIGURE 6. Schematic drawing of the intergenic region drawn as a single strand. Hairpinlike structures (A–E) are proposed; direct evidence is available only for the structure of hairpin A. Hairpin A, which starts at the end of gene IV(1), contains the packaging signal and rho-dependent terminator at the end of gene IV(2). Hairpins (B) and (C) constitute the (−) strand origin; RNA synthesis starts at (3) and runs to the left. (D) and (E) contain regions needed for nicking of the RF and the initiation and termination of (+) strand synthesis. The location of the gene II–catalyzed nick is shown (4). Regions A and B (no square brackets) and the vertical bars surrounding them depict the region absolutely required for (+) strand synthesis (A) and the region required by wild-type phages (B), which is dispensable if a suitably mutant phage provides the gene II protein (see text). The RNA start site for gene II is marked (5), as is the beginning of gene II (6). From Zinder and Horiuchi (1985).

thesis is outside the structured regions. Biochemical probes have shown that these regions have double-stranded character (Gray *et al.*, 1978; Shen and Hearst, 1976; Shen *et al.*, 1979). It is not obvious what is recognized in this sequence by RNA polymerase; it does not resemble any of the consensus sequences of promoters.

Kim *et al.* (1981) have made a number of *Bal31*-mediated deletions both in the protected region and in that of the primer RNA. Surprisingly, phages containing deletions were viable, but defective. All sizes of deletions had much the same phenotype; they formed very turbid plaques and showed a delayed onset (up to 30 min) of synthesis of complementary strands after infection. Kim *et al.* (1981) stated that DNA isolated from these mutants was severely impaired in its ability to direct the synthesis of complementary strands in an *in vitro* reaction. Moses *et al.* (1980) and Moses and Horiuchi (1982) have inserted foreign DNA into this same region and have also noted a serious inhibition of DNA synthesis. Thus the (−) strand origin comprises hairpins B and C in Fig. 6, together with some nucleotides 3′ to hairpin C. Perturbations in this region depress DNA synthesis, but it is not absolutely required. It is not yet known whether the primer RNA initiation site itself is required for (−) strand synthesis or whether the region drawn as hairpin B is required. It is also not known whether RNA polymerase is involved in the "bypass" reaction, and if so what is used as the binding site.

F. Structure and Function of the (+) Strand Origin

The viral strand origin was shown to be in the intergenic region by Horiuchi and Zinder (1976) and was located to (f1) restriction fragment *Hae*III-G. It was more precisely located by Meyer *et al.* (1979), who determined the position of the nick introduced by the gene II protein to be between nucleotide 5781 and 5782 in fd (Fig. 7). Horiuchi (1980) cloned a fragment that contained this cleavage site (together with surrounding sequences) into the phages, thereby duplicating the origin; when this construct was transformed into cells, the progeny had all lost one of the two origins together with all the sequences between them. This showed that the origin also contains the signal for termination of synthesis and that this termination function is active even if initiation did not occur there. Analysis of (+) strand origin function was straightforward once it was found that chimeric plasmids that contained the filamentous phage origin could be activated by infecting with filamentous phages. Activation can be measured by three consequences: (1) Replication of the resident, origin-containing plasmid is stimulated, causing an increase in plasmid copy number. (2) Replication of the infecting phage is inhibited, resulting in lower RF levels and fewer progeny phage. (3) Single-stranded plasmid DNA is packaged into phagelike transducing particles, provided that the phage packaging signal (see assembly) is also present. Since the phage origin is active only when the cells are infected with filamentous phages, and since the plasmid normally replicates from origins other than the phage origin, mutations that inactivate the origin function can be preserved and analyzed. Using this approach, Cleary and Ray (1980, 1981), Dotto and Horiuchi (1981), and Dotto *et al.* (1981a, 1982a,b, 1984) have carried out detailed mutagenic analysis of the (+) strand origin. The assays for functional origins were those described above, plus one other. In an extension of the finding by Horiuchi (1980) that filamentous phages do not maintain two origins, Dotto and Horiuchi (1981) showed that if two fully functional origins are cloned at different positions in a plasmid,

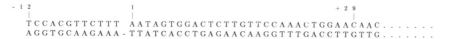

```
  -12                            1                              +29
   |                             |                               |
   TCCACGTTCTTT  AATAGTGGACTCTTGTTCCAAACTGGAACAAC.......
   AGGTGCAAGAAA-TTATCACCTGAGAACAAGGTTTGACCTTGTTG.......
```

FIGURE 7. DNA sequences immediately around the nicking site of gene II. Shown is the region absolutely essential for proper initiation and termination, although about 100 bases downstream (represented by the string of dots) are needed for efficient initiation of wild-type (+) synthesis. See text for details.

infection by filamentous phages causes the circle to resolve into two smaller circles, the relative sizes of which reflect the distance between the two phage origins. If one of the origins is defective either in initiating or terminating DNA synthesis, this resolution is perturbed, and the products differ from those obtained with unmutated origins (Dotto et al., 1982a). The Ike and fd origins, though similar, are not interchangeable (Peeters et al., 1986b). Peeters et al. (1987) have shown, however, that the Ike origin will act as a terminator for synthesis initiated at the fd origin at which gene II protein makes the nick.

In addition to these in vivo assays, it is possible to determine whether a mutated origin can be nicked in vitro with purified gene II protein. More recently, binding assays have been developed to determine which mutants can bind gene II protein (Horiuchi, 1986; Greenstein and Horiuchi, 1987). In addition, protection assays can determine the regions of the substrate DNA protected from nuclease or methylation attack by the gene II protein (Greenstein and Horiuchi, 1987). With these assays in hand, the following description of the origin has been obtained. The origin can be divided into domains centered about the nicking site (called position 0 here for convenience, since the absolute numbering differs a little in the various filamentous phages). Termination of DNA synthesis requires the leftmost sequences shown in Fig. 7, nucleotides -12 to $+(11-29)$. Initiation of DNA synthesis requires, under normal circumstances, nucleotides -4 to $\geq +100$, whereas nicking requires -4 to $+(11-29)$. The sequences required for gene II binding are somewhat less extensive than for nicking, extending from $+2$ to $+28$ (note that the nicking site itself is not required for binding). This gene II binding region is also essential for inhibition of replication of wild-type infecting phage, supporting the suggestion that the mechanism for this inhibition is the binding and sequestration of gene II protein by the origin carried on the resident high-copy-number plasmid.

Binding of gene II protein is a two-step process (as determined with gel shift assays). Initial binding is to the region from $+6$ to $+20$, which consists of two repeats in inverted orientation (see Fig. 7). The second binding complex requires, in addition, nucleotides $+21$ to $+30$ (Greenstein and Horiuchi, 1987). Although gene II nicking requires that the substrate be supercoiled, binding occurs on relaxed or linear DNA with the same specificity as on supercoils.

The functions of the sequences between $+30$ and $+130$ are obscure. Phages or plasmids that lack this region are very poor substrates for gene II-activated replication, and in vivo they are propagated about 10^{-2} as efficiently as those that contain this segment. Plasmids containing such a truncated origin also do not interfere with the replication of infecting phage (Cleary and Ray, 1981; Dotto et al., 1981a,b, 1982a, 1984; Johnston and Ray, 1984). Nonetheless, this region contains the site frequently used for the cloning of foreign DNA (Messing et al., 1977; Boeke et al., 1979), and phages containing such inserts grow well. Analysis of phages that contain such cloning sites show that they have all acquired secondary mutations that suppress the origin defect (Zinder and Horiuchi, 1985). These are of three kinds. One maps in the region upstream of the gene II initiation codon, and another is in gene V, causing an arg_{21} to cys change in the protein (Dotto and Zinder, 1984). Both of these mutations increase the level of gene II protein in the infected cell five- to 10-fold (Dotto and Zinder, 1984), presumably by altering gene V protein so that it no longer represses the translation of gene II protein (see Control), or by altering the gene II "translational operator" so that gene II expression is not affected by gene V protein. The third kind of mutation affects the coding region of gene II, causing a met_{40} to ile change in M13 MP1 (Dotto and Zinder, 1984) or Gly_{73} to any of ala, cys, arg, or ser in the M13 UK phages (Kim and Ray, 1985). Enhanced levels of gene II protein are not found in cells infected with phages that contain this mutation.

The three types of mutations can all be mimicked by growing phage mutant in this segment of the origin on host cells that contain a plasmid that hyperproduces gene II protein (Dotto and Zinder, 1984). Thus the last 100 or so nucleotides of the origin can be rendered dispensable by either increasing the quantity of gene II protein or changing its structure. The mechanism by which this occurs is not clear, since gene II protein does not bind to this region of the origin (Greenstein and Horiuchi, 1987, and unpublished). None of these suppressors are permissive for nucleotide changes in the left end of the origin (from -15 to $+30$), and no suppressors have been isolated that can compensate for mutations in this segment.

VI. EXPRESSION OF THE f1 GENES

The level of expression of the filamentous phage genes is highly skewed. As many as 10^5 to 10^6 molecules of gene VIII and gene V proteins are made per cell per generation, whereas other proteins, such as the products of genes I, VI, VII, and IX, are made in very small amounts— probably only a few hundred copies per cell per generation. The challenge, then, is to account for these widely different levels of gene expression.

A. Transcription

The RNA metabolism of the filamentous phage is extraordinarily complex. There are many promoters scattered throughout the genome, and fewer terminators, so that a number of overlapping transcripts are produced. Many of these are then processed, resulting in a large number of messenger RNAs. Analysis is further complicated because only a fraction of the promoters detected *in vitro* by RNA polymerase binding or by transcription studies seem to be active *in vivo*, as measured by detectable *in vivo* transcription during short pulses. A transcriptional map of the phage is shown in Fig. 3.

Promoters have been described on the basis of sequence analysis (Sugiura *et al.*, 1969, Schaller *et al.*, 1978; Van Wezenbeek *et al.*, 1980; Beck *et al.*, 1978; Beck and Zink, 1981; Hill and Peterson, 1982), promoter binding studies (Schaller *et al.*, 1975, Sugimoto *et al.*, 1975; Seeburg and Schaller, 1975; Takanami *et al.*, 1976; Seeburg *et al.*, 1977), and studies of transcription *in vitro* (Okamoto *et al.*, 1969; Seeburg and Schaller, 1975; Okamoto *et al.*, 1975; Konings and Schoenmakers, 1978; Chan *et al.*, 1975; Edens *et al.*, 1975, 1976) and *in vivo* (Cashman and Webster, 1979; Cashman *et al.*, 1980; Smits *et al.*, 1978, 1980; La Farina and Model, 1978, 1983; Blumer and Steege, 1984). The promoters that have been shown to give rise to RNAs *in vivo* are indicated by solid lines in Fig. 3, and the others are shown with bracketed arrows. From a transcriptional point of view, the virion circle can be divided into two parts, separated by the intergenic space and the strong terminator following gene VIII. All transcription uses the (−) or complementary strand as template (Jacob and Hofschneider, 1969; Smits *et al.*, 1978; Pieczenik *et al.*, 1975) and is shown going counterclockwise in Fig. 3. In the region extending from the intergenic region (IG) counterclockwise toward (and including) gene VIII, all transcripts appear to start with G residues, and the promoters range from moderately to very strong (reviewed by Konings and Schoenmakers, 1978). The region extending from the terminator at the beginning of gene III toward the intergenic region is transcribed much less efficiently, and the transcripts appear to start with U or A residues. No terminators have been identified within the frequently transcribed region, so all of the transcripts from this region overlap.

No transcription, either *in vivo* or *in vitro*, crosses the terminator located just distal to gene VIII (the central terminator) (Edens *et al.*, 1975; Sugimoto *et al.*, 1977; Rivera *et al.*, 1978; Cashman *et al.*, 1980). *In vivo*, transcription also does not cross the intergenic region (Smits *et al.*, 1980; La Farina and Model, 1983; Moses and Model, 1984), but *in vitro*, elongated products that do traverse the intergeneic region are observed in simple transcription experiments in which the *E. coli* termination factor rho is omitted (Okamoto *et al.*, 1975; Seeburg and Schaller, 1975; Edens *et al.*, 1975; Chan *et al.*, 1975). Unlike many other phages, all the promoters in the filamentous phage appear to be active at all times after infection. The RNAs produced, however, have different stabilities, so that the messenger spectrum changes with time after infection. The RNAs that come from the frequently transcribed part of the genome have been best characterized. There is a gradient of stability in this region, such that as one proceeds counterclockwise on the map, the RNAs become more stable (La Farina and Model, 1978, 1983; Cashman and Webster, 1979; Smits *et al.*, 1980). Processing is indicated for many of them, because pulse labeling *in vivo* shows that some (presumed primary) transcripts appear

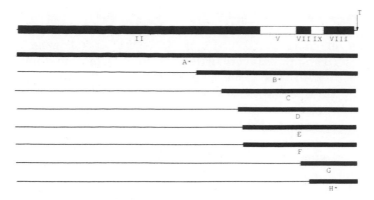

FIGURE 8. Representation of the *in vivo* messenger RNA population-encoding genes (II, X, V, VII, IX, VIII) located in the frequently transcribed portion of the genome. This is a composite, drawing on the work of many authors. See text for details.

faster than others, only to disappear and give rise to several new, smaller species, shown in Fig. 8.

Only the 3' ends of the processed RNAs are sufficiently stable to be detected; the 5' portions disappear rapidly, and their fate is unknown (Cashman and Webster, 1979; La Farina and Model, 1983; Cashman *et al.*, 1980; Blumer and Steege, 1984). The consequence of the gradient of stability, the variable strength of the promoters, and the preservation of the 3' segments of the processed messages is that there is an enormous amount of RNA that can code for gene VIII protein in cells in which the infection has been under way for some time. As much as 2% of the *total* RNA of infected *E. coli* can be accounted for as gene VIII message. Gene V encoding message is also made at very high levels. The need for such large amounts of message is clear, since some 2700 copies of the gene VIII protein are required per virion, and some 200–2000 virions are produced/cell/generation (depending on conditions and observer), which means that 5×10^5 to 5×10^6 molecules must be produced per cell per generation. A similar need exists for high levels of gene V protein. About 1300–1600 molecules are needed to cover each single strand, and there is a pool of some 100–200 single strands per cell, all in the form of single-stranded DNA–gene V protein complex. Gene V protein from this complex is efficiently reutilized (Pratt *et al.*, 1974; Webster and Cashman, 1973; Mazur and Zinder, 1975), but the continued growth and division of the infected cells requires that new gene V protein be continually synthesized.

This transcriptional arrangement seems well suited for providing the huge amounts of gene V and VIII proteins needed by the phage, and it has been formalized as the "cascade" model (Edens *et al.*, 1978) for the transcriptional amplification of gene products needed in large quantities. Although the cascade model has elegance and economy to recommend it, it may not, at the current state of the evolution of the phage, be a central regulatory mechanism. All of the messages that encode gene V also encode genes VII and IX, but very little gene VII or IX protein is made, either *in vivo* or *in vitro*. The expression of these proteins must therefore be limited by translation. Moses and Horiuchi (1982), moreover, transplanted a copy of gene VIII into the intergenic region of a phage that carried an amber mutation in the normal copy of this gene. Expression of coat protein from this transplanted gene was very strong, almost as high as wild type, when allowance was made for the somewhat lower RF DNA copy number achieved by this construct. Expression of this gene was exclusively from its own promoter and could not have been enhanced by the effects of a cascade. It is of course possible that the cascade is the remnant of some more primitive means of regulation of RNA quantity, or else may have evolved as a fine-tuning mechanism.

The processing of the primary transcripts (Cashman and Webster, 1979; Cashman *et al.*, 1980; LaFarina and Model, 1983; Smits *et al.*, 1984; Blumer and Steege, 1984) to make smaller messages is intriguing. A detailed study has been carried out by Blumer and Steege (1984), who defined the exact processing sites carefully, showed that the processing sites could function in other RNA contexts (cloned into a λ vector), and confirmed that the 5′ portion of the original transcript did not survive long enough to be detected. The nature of the processing activity remains an enigma; in particular, a role for RNAse III (which acts to cleave some messenger RNAs of other phage) has been ruled out with the use of RNAse III mutants (Cashman and Webster, 1979). It is not inconceivable that these mRNAs are self-cleaving, but no experiments bearing on the point have been reported.

Transcription on the infrequently transcribed region of the genome does not conform to a cascade model. The promoter responsible for the transcription of gene III overlaps the "central terminator," through which no transcription occurs. An RNA has been described *in vivo* that could encode genes III, VI, and I (and possibly part or all of gene IV) (La Farina and Model, 1983; La Farina, 1983) but which was present in very small amounts. Smits *et al.* (1984), using a minicell system, did not find this large RNA but did find RNA that started just upstream of gene III and terminated within gene I. Both groups found good expression of RNA capable of encoding gene IV. Taking the data as a whole, and considering the strong III-VI-I polarity, which does not extend to gene IV (Pratt *et al.*, 1966; Lyons and Zinder, 1972), it seems highly likely that this region is transcribed to give rise to an RNA that starts upstream of gene III (at position 1544; Smits *et al.*, 1984) and terminates inefficiently at a rho-dependent terminator in gene I. The proposal that a terminator is located within the beginning of gene I is strongly supported by data from Horabin and Webster (1986) on the effects of λ N protein antitermination on gene I transcription from an appropriate construct. They estimated that this terminator is about 60–70% efficient in the absence of N protein. A second promoter is located before gene IV (position 4105; Smits *et al.*, 1984). Synthesis stops at the rho-dependent terminator following gene IV or, in the absence of rho factor, within the intergenic region (Smits *et al.*, 1984; Moses and Model, 1984). These RNAs could account for the strong polarity of proximal amber mutations in gene III on genes VI and I, although translational coupling as a source of the polarity cannot be excluded.

It is by no means clear whether the complexity of RNA metabolism exhibited by the filamentous phages is necessary or even useful to them, or whether it arose because it was not selected against. Phage yields are not notably worse, for example, in a *rho* mutant host than they are in *rho*+ (Moses and Model, 1984), and the gene VIII transplantation experiment is also suggestive. By a combination of DNA manipulation and oligonucleotide mutagenesis, it might be possible to attack this question.

Early experiments on filamentous phage protein synthesis *in vivo* were carried out in mitomycin-treated or heavily UV-irradiated cells, in order to suppress the background of continuing host synthesis (Henry and Pratt, 1969). Under these conditions, cells infected by phages carrying amber mutations in gene II (which contain only a single, parental RF DNA) synthesize as much coat protein as do wild-type phages (which contain 30–50 copies of RF; Lerner and Model, 1981). These results have sometimes been interpreted as indicating a "master" RF, from which all transcription occurs, with the role of daughter RFs confined to DNA replication. When a host is used that has not been pretreated with UV or a drug, it is clear that there is substantially more phage-specific protein synthesis from wild-type than from gene II-infected cells, although the increase may not be linear (see, e.g., Model *et al.*, 1982). There is a reasonably good correlation between RF copy number and the extent of phage-specific protein synthesis *in vivo*, and thus no need to invoke a "master template" hypothesis.

B. Translation

In vivo, only the products of genes V and VIII are readily detectable on SDS polyacrylamide gels. A band corresponding to gene II becomes detectable in certain II protein-overproducing mutants, a band corresponding to gene IV has been observed (but not reproducibly), and gene III protein can be identified only by antiserum precipitation. *In vitro*, the products of coupled transcription-translation of genes III, IV, II, X, V, and VIII are readily detectable, but the product of gene I can be seen on good days, and then only when the products of an incorporation programmed with DNA from an amber mutant of gene I is run alongside as a control (Model and Zinder, 1974; Konings, 1975). Synthesis of gene II protein *in vitro* is somewhat problematic. No two synthesis extracts (even though made in much the same way) give rise to the same relative amount of this protein. This suggests that some factor required for, or inhibitory to, gene II synthesis is not recovered uniformly in these protein-synthesizing extracts (Model, unpublished; Konings, unpublished). The asymmetry of protein synthesis *in vitro* is much less than that *in vivo*, probably because an infected cell that has reached the steady state contains an enormous amount of RNA coding for genes VIII and V.

Filamentous phage protein synthesis can also be studied in minicells. These are small cells that contain little or no host DNA, formed by abnormal division of certain mutant *E. coli* (Adler *et al.*, 1967). If the parent is infected with phages, double-stranded phage-specific DNA, together with RNA polymerase, segregates into these small cells. Since there is little synthesis of host proteins in these cells, phage products can be readily detected. Filamentous phage-specific protein synthesis in minicells shows the asymmetry of synthesis observed in normal cells, but more proteins are detected (Smits *et al.*, 1978). The products of genes V and VIII are made abundantly; gene III protein is made at a lower amount, corresponding to the *in vitro* amount, but, in contrast to the *in vitro* system, very little gene II, IV, or X protein product is made. Furthermore, minicells produce a readily detectable protein of MW about 3000 (the product of gene VII, IX, or both), which is not detected in the *in vitro* reactions. The pattern of protein synthesis in minicells can be accounted for at the level of RNA metabolism. Minicells show the promoter specificity of normal cells, and the RNA made is processed as in normal cells. This leads to the accumulation of large amounts of RNA encoding the gene V, VII, IX, and VIII region and, presumably, to the destruction the message that can encode the gene II protein.

The efficiency of translation initiation can be estimated from the ratio of the products made on the longest (presumably unit length) RNA synthesized *in vitro*. Such estimates show that genes V and VIII protein are initiated more effectively than genes III, IV, or II but by less than an order of magnitude (Chan *et al.*, 1975). Thus, for these proteins differential expression must be principally due to different levels of the mRNAs encoding them. The situation is quite different with regard to genes VI, I, VII, and IX. Very little of these proteins is made *in vitro* from any size message. One must conclude, therefore, that the efficiency of translation initiation of these four genes is markedly less than that of the better-expressed genes.

Ribosome-binding and protection experiments, in which ribosomes in the presence of the appropriate initiation factors are bound to messenger RNA, the complexes are digested with an appropriate nuclease, and the messenger fragments are isolated and sequenced (Steitz, 1979), show that the RNA encoding the starts of genes V, VIII, and IV can form stable complexes with these ribosomes (Pieczenik *et al.*, 1974; Ravetch *et al.*, 1977; Blumer *et al.*, 1987). The initiation regions of the genes VIII and V are recognized even by eukaryotic (rabbit reticulocyte) ribosomes

(Legon et al., 1977). Binding stability, under these conditions, is probably not exactly a reflection of initiation efficiency, but the two must certainly be related. Those ribosome-binding sites that have been detected by binding experiments are the ones that give rise to high levels of expression in vitro. The converse is not true; gene X protein is quite strongly expressed in the in vitro system, but its ribosome-binding site is not a significant product in the messenger RNA fragment-binding assay. The translation initiation regions of each phage gene are shown in Fig. 9, together with an indication of their relative strength.

Our current understanding of translation initiation is not sufficient to allow us to explain or predict the behavior of these protein initiation regions. As Gold et al. (1981) have pointed out, frequency of initiation is certainly not a direct consequence of the degree of homology of the relevant initiation region with the 3' end of 16S ribosomal RNA. The algorithm proposed by Stormo et al. (1982), when applied to the f1 sequence, detects the correct initiation site for genes I, II, IV, V, VI, VIII, IX, and X. It does not detect the initiation site for gene III, and it reports initiations at nucleotides 3737 and 4467, where, as best we know, no gene starts. Experimental studies by Blumer et al. (1987) show that the gene IX sequences can be made to bind efficiently to ribosomes if an upstream RNA region, which could fold into a hairpin, is removed. Thus the inefficiency of gene IX translation could normally be due to steric hindrance resulting from the structure of the RNA encoding this gene. By contrast, gene VII cannot be expressed without translation of the immediately preceding region, and indeed, Blumer et al. (1987) express some doubt as to whether this sequence can bind ribosomes de novo. It may be that only ribosomes that have traversed the immediately upstream gene can initiate translation at the beginning of gene VII. In very general terms, then,

							Strength
				6006			
Gene II	TTTCT	GATTATCAAC	CGGGGTACAT	ATG	ATTGACATGC	TAGTTTTACG	S[*]
				6015			
Gene II'	ATCAA	CCGGGGTACA	TATGATTGAC	ATG	CTAGTTTTAC	GATTACCGTT	W-M
				496			
Gene X	GTTTA	AAGCATTTGA	GGGGGATTCA	ATG	AATATTTATG	ACGATTCCGC	S
				843			
Gene V	TTAAA	ATCGCATAAG	GTAATTCACA	ATG	ATTAAAGTTG	AAAATTAAACC	S
				1108			
Gene VII	CTGCG	CCTCGTTCCG	GCTAAGTAAC	ATG	GAGCAGGTCG	CGGATTTCGA	?
				1206			
Gene IX	TTGGT	ATAATCGCTG	GGGGTCAAAG	ATG	AGTGTTTTAG	TGTATTCTTT	M
				1301			
Gene VIII	TTACC	CGTTTAATGG	AAACTTCCTC	ATG	AAAAAGTCTT	TAGTCCTCAA	S
				1579			
Gene III	GCCTT	TTTTTTTGGA	GATTTTCAAC	GTG	AAAAAATTAT	TATTCGCAAT	W-M
				2856			
Gene VI	TACTG	CGTAATAAGG	AGTCTTAATC	ATG	CCAGTTCTTT	TGGGTATTCC	W
				3196			
Gene I	TCTTA	TTTGGATTGG	GATAAATAAT	ATG	GCTGTTTATT	TTGTAACTGG	W
				4220			
Gene IV	GTTTC	CATTAAAAAA	GGTAATTCAA	ATG	AAATTGTTAA	ATGTAATTAA	S

FIGURE 9. Sequences surrounding the initiation codons of the filamentous phage genes. The relative strength (strong, S; moderate, M; weak, W) is an estimate derived from the work of several authors; see text for details. Gene II is expressed strongly in vitro only in certain extracts. Gene VII binding site may not be independent of upstream translation.

the asymmetric synthesis of most of the filamentous phage proteins can be accounted for by the following:

1. Overlapping promoters in the frequently transcribed region of the genome, such that the regions near the central terminator, are transcribed into more RNA species than are those that are distal.
2. RNA processing, which results in the accumulation of stable 3′ fragments of the primary transcripts from the frequently transcribed region and the rapid loss of the 5′ fragments. This contributes to a gradient of stability in the frequently transcribed region, such that the half-life of any particular species is inversely related to its length.
3. Fairly weak transcription of genes III, VI, and I, with a fairly effective rho-dependent terminator located in the beginning of gene I.
4. A moderately strong promoter just upstream of gene IV.
5. Strong ribosome binding and initiation at genes IV, V, and VIII.
6. Inefficient initiation at genes VII and IX (and probably at VI and I).
7. Regulated translation of gene II (see Section VIII.A).

VII. MORPHOGENESIS

The filamentous phages are unique among known bacterial viruses in their mechanism of morphogenesis and dispersal. No phage particles exist within the cell; rather, they assemble at or within the membrane and are extruded into the culture medium without disrupting the membrane or compromising the viability of the infected cell. In this mechanism they are more akin to certain animal viruses that "bud" from their host, again without compromising their host.

The cytoplasmic single-stranded DNA–gene V protein complex is the virion precursor. The virion proteins encoded by genes III and VIII are synthesized as precursors, and their signal peptides are cleaved as they are inserted into the cytoplasmic membrane. Along with the other structural proteins, products of genes VI, VII, and IX, which are probably membrane-associated, they replace gene V protein along the single strand. Assembling phage particles are extruded outside the cell in a reaction that requires a cis-active signal on the single strand (the morphogenetic or packaging signal), two phage-encoded proteins (the products of genes I and IV), and probably several host proteins. The participation of one of these, thioredoxin, has been studied in some detail.

A. The Single-Stranded DNA–Gene V Protein Complex

Phage-specific single-stranded DNA appears as a DNA–gene V protein complex (Salstrom and Pratt, 1971) (see DNA Replication, and Genes and Proteins). This complex forms a filamentous, virionlike structure, but it differs in many respects from the mature virion. The gene V complex is sensitive to dissociation by high salt, and the DNA within it is digestible by added DNAse I. In the electron microscope (Fig. 1), it resembles beads on a string and is much more flexible than the assembled virion (Alberts et al., 1972; Oey and Knippers, 1972; Gray et al., 1982b; Torbet et al., 1981). The complex forms a linear, rather than a circular, structure, because the gene V protein exists as a dimer at physiological salt concentrations (Pretorius et al., 1975; Cavalieri et al., 1976b). Presumably, each dimer binds the single strand at two separate positions. Between three and five nucleotides are bound by each gene V protein molecule; the range in these estimates may reflect real differences between the complexes that were examined as well as scatter in the measurements. The stoichiometry is discussed in Genes and Proteins. Detailed examination shows that each complex contains, in addition to about 1300–1600 molecules of gene V protein, 1–3 molecules of the E. coli single-stranded DNA binding protein (SSB) and a variable number (0–65) of a protein of MW 11,000 which does not correspond to any of the phage-encoded proteins (Grant and Webster, 1984a). Thus, none of the phage products (other than V protein) are present in the complex. Released gene V protein is reutilized (Webster and Cashman, 1983; Pratt et al., 1974; Mazur and Zinder, 1975).

Plasmids that contain a filamentous phage origin of replication undergo rolling-circle replication in f1-infected cells (Dotto et al., 1981a). The resulting plasmid single strands are encapsidated by gene V protein, and this encapsidation is independent of whether the plasmid single strands also carry a morphogenetic or packaging signal (see below) (Grant and Webster, 1984b). The orientation of the DNA, or indeed whether the DNA is oriented in the gene V complex, is not known. Contact between the DNA and the gene V protein is very close, as reflected by the observation that the DNA and protein can be cross-linked at high yields in vivo (Lica and Ray, 1977) and in vitro (Anderson et al., 1975b) by UV irradiation.

No mature virions are found in the cytoplasm of the infected cell (Hoffmann-Berling et al., 1963; Hoffmann-Berling and Mazé, 1964; see also Marvin and Hohn, 1969). Smilowitz et al. (1972) have found that virtually all of the newly synthesized major coat protein is associated with the cell membrane prior to its appearance in the medium (in phage), and the same has been shown for the gene III protein (Boeke et al., 1982; Boeke and Model, 1982; Davis et al., 1985). Lopez and Webster (1983) have actually visualized assembling phage at the cell surface. Thus, morphogenesis occurs at or within the cell membrane. An idealized diagram illustrating this process is shown in Fig. 10.

B. Membrane Association of Virion Proteins

Considerable research has been done on the insertion of the major filamentous coat protein (gene VIII protein) into the cell membrane. In-

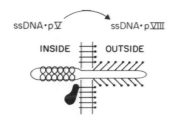

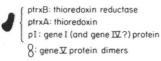

ptrxB: thioredoxin reductase
ptrxA: thioredoxin
pI: gene I (and gene IV?) protein
8: gene V protein dimers
———: major coatprotein (pVIII)
⊂⊃: phage ssDNA

FIGURE 10. A speculative cartoon showing assembly of the phage, in which gene V protein is replaced with gene VIII protein already lodged in the membrane. The dark blob represents the assembly machine, proposed to contain the proteins encoded by genes I and IV and the host protein thioredoxin. Other host proteins could easily also be involved.

deed, it was recognized as a prototypic membrane protein before it was clear that it was synthesized as a precursor, and insertion of the mature protein into detergent micelles (Makino *et al.*, 1975) and phospholipid vesicles (Wickner, 1976) has been studied. Wickner (1976) has reported that it assumes a homogeneous orientation in artificial vesicles, with all the N termini outside.

A variety of experiments have shown that the major coat protein is synthesized as a precursor with a 23 amino acid signal peptide at its N terminus (Pieczenik *et al.*, 1974; Konings *et al.*, 1975; Sugimoto *et al.*, 1977; Chang *et al.*, 1978). The cleavage activity is associated with the membrane of uninfected *E. coli* (Chang *et al.*, 1978; Wickner *et al.*, 1978) and has been purified and characterized by Zwizinski and Wickner (1980) and Wolfe *et al.* (1982).

Studies of the insertion of filamentous phage coat protein into the cell membrane have generated much data, but also much controversy. We will attempt to reflect the specific findings relevant to the phage. Ito *et al.* (1979) have reported that the coat precusor, termed either procoat or precoat, it synthesized by cytoplasmic polysomes and not on membrane-attached polysomes, and that the precoat can initially be found in soluble (= slowly sedimenting) form *in vivo*. Russel and Model (1982) reported that both precoat and coat protein very rapidly become associated with the cell membrane in a form resistant to extraction by NaOH, so rapidly that even nascent chains are attached. When signal peptide cleavage is delayed by mutation in the mature portion of the protein, the membrane association of precoat is not delayed (Russel and Model, 1981, 1982). Each group has technical criticisms of the other's experiments.

Both groups agree that insertion of precoat into the membrane is normally associated with cleavage of the signal peptide (Russel and Model, 1981, 1982; Date *et al.*, 1980a,b), leaving the mature protein spanning the membrane with its N terminus outside the cytoplasm and susceptible to externally added protease (Wickner, 1975, 1976; Ohkawa and Webster, 1981) and its C terminus exposed and accessible on the cytoplasmic side (Ohkawa and Webster, 1981). Under normal circumstances, processing is so rapid that the wild-type precursor is not detected, except in a very short pulse (Russel and Model, 1981). Certain mutant precoat proteins that are at least partially resistant to signal peptidase cleavage can be accessed by external protease (Russel and Model, 1981, 1982; Zimmermann et al., 1982; Kuhn and Wickner, 1985a,b). Date et al. (1980a,b) have demonstrated that the processing of precoat protein is strongly inhibited by energy poisons, particularly the ionophore CCCP, and that at the concentrations used, these poisons do not inhibit the action of the signal (leader) peptidase. Precursor found in CCCP-treated cells is not accessible to protease added to the outside of the cell, indicating that it has not assumed a transmembrane conformation (Date et al., 1980a,b; Russel and Model, 1982).

Precoat protein can be inserted into inverted E. coli membrane vesicles in vitro, and this insertion protects the N-terminal and central domains and leaves only the C-terminal portion accessible to protease (Wickner et al., 1978; Chang et al., 1979). The protein as synthesized in vitro rapidly loses the capacity to be inserted into membranes under the usual in vitro conditions, which may be due to aggregation; the half-life of the process is on the order of 1–2 min (Goodman et al., 1981). The precursor can be treated so as to restore its capacity to be inserted into membranes (Silver et al., 1981; Zwizinski and Wickner, 1982), and it will insert in the absence of ribosomes or soluble proteins (Silver et al., 1981). Precursor synthesized in vitro can also insert into liposomes that contain only leader (signal) peptidase (Watts et al., 1981; Ohno-Iwashita and Wickner, 1983) and into liposomes that contain no membrane-associated proteins (Geller and Wickner, 1985). The in vitro insertion reactions into liposomes are much slower, by 1–2 orders of magnitude, than insertion in vivo.

Several E. coli mutants have been isolated that affect the efficiency of protein export into the periplasm or into the membrane. Among them are secA (Oliver and Beckwith, 1981) and secY (Ito et al., 1983) mutations, which reduce export of many (but not all) proteins. Membrane insertion of the gene VIII protein is unaffected by the secA or secY lesions (Wolfe et al., 1985). Kuhn et al. (1987) have substituted the signal peptide of the coat precursor with that of an E. coli outer membrane protein (OmpA protein), which does require the function of the secY allele, and found that the independence of secY function is maintained. Thus it is a property of the mature portion of the precoat protein that renders it sec-independent.

A number of mutagenic studies have been carried out on the coat gene itself. Mutations in the signal peptide, near the cleavage site, had strong effects on the cleavage reaction but did not seem to alter the ability of the coat protein to insert into the membrane and assume a transmembrane conformation, as tested by protease accessibility (Kuhn and Wickner, 1985b). Mutations that seriously reduced the basic character of the C-terminal domain (Kuhn et al., 1986a) or that interrupted the hydrophobic nature of the signal peptide or the central stretch of the mature protein with polar residues (Kuhn et al., 1986a,b) impaired the capacity of the altered coat protein for membrane insertion. These results suggest strongly that the entire protein, from signal sequence to C-terminal region, participates in the insertion process which appears to be independent of the best characterized of the *E. coli*-encoded functions involved in protein export.

Interesting questions are whether this behavior of coat protein, which is very hydrophobic and can, under certain circumstances be induced to enter lipid bilayers even without a signal sequence (Wickner, 1976), is typical of other membrane-spanning or exported proteins, and to what extent it is a remnant of some earlier form of membrane protein. It should be noted that the major coat protein of filamentous phage Pf3 is not synthesized with a signal peptide (Luiten *et al.*, 1983; Putterman *et al.*, 1984). Unfortunately, it is not known whether this protein ever exists as a transmembrane protein, although by analogy with the proteins of the F-specific phages it should.

Although it is clear that the insertion of precoat protein is not coupled obligately to translation, wild-type coat protein inserts very rapidly. In all probability, even the nascent, uncompleted chain is inserted into the membrane, based on its resistance to extraction by sodium hydroxide (Russel and Model, 1982). Thus as proposed in a model presented by Kuhn *et al.* (1986a), precoat membrane association is probably a two-step process in which the first (associative) step is a membrane insertion which renders the protein unextractable by sodium hydroxide (but does not expose it on the *trans* side of the membrane), and the second is the energy-dependent translocation that exposes a portion of the protein to the outside (Fig. 11).

Much less is known about the membrane insertion of the other coat proteins. The adsorption (gene III) protein, synthesized as a precursor containing an 18-residue signal peptide (Beck *et al.*, 1978), is also found as a transmembrane species in the cell inner membrane (Boeke *et al.*, 1982; Davis *et al.*, 1985). The protein is held in the membrane by a membrane-spanning domain near its C terminus, leaving the N terminus and most of the rest of the protein in the periplasm, susceptible to externally added protease (Davis *et al.*, 1985).

The remaining structural proteins (gene VI, VII, and IX proteins) are not made as precursors. They all, however, have sufficient hydrophobic character to make membrane association (or insertion) a reasonable presumption. Many *E. coli* integral membrane proteins are synthesized without a cleavable signal sequence.

C. Assembly

Assembly of the virion occurs at adhesion zones, sometimes called Bayer's patches (Bayer, 1968), sites in the membrane at which the outer and inner membranes are closely apposed (Lopez and Webster, 1985a). The number of adhesion zones is increased in f1-infected cells, which

FIGURE 11. Scheme for the insertion of precoat protein into the membrane. In A, the hydrophic portions of the precoat have partially inserted, and the positively charged regions are held to the phospholipid on the membrane surface by ionic interactions. In B, the negatively charged N-terminal region of what will be the mature coat has been everted. This is postulated to require a membrane potential and is inhibited by treatment with CCCP. The signal (leader) peptidase, located on the outer face of the inner membrane, then cleaves the signal (leader) peptide, leading to mature protein oriented in the membrane as shown in C. Other host proteins that may be involved are not shown; nor is the means by which the protein got from the ribosome to the membrane.

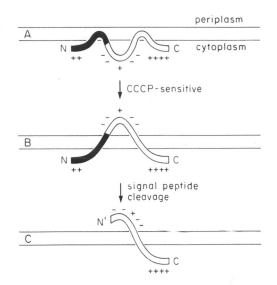

suggests that their association with assembly is functional and not merely coincidental; significantly, if the infecting phages are mutant in gene I, one of the nonstructural genes required for morphogenesis, the number of these patches is not increased (Lopez and Webster, 1985a). Thus, phages are assembled and released directly to the cell exterior, without passing through the periplasm, and the gene I protein is involved in the formation of an assembly site or port.

The assembly of particles requires the major coat (gene VIII) protein (Pratt et al., 1969), the minor coat proteins at one end of the particle (pVII and pIX), the participation of two phage-encoded nonstructural proteins (products of gene I and gene IV), and several host functions, including the host protein thioredoxin (Russel and Model, 1983, 1985, 1986). In addition, assembly is severely hindered if the DNA does not contain a filamentous phage morphogenetic signal. If either gene III or gene VI is mutant, particles are formed, but they are longer than unit length, noninfectious (Pratt et al., 1969; Lopez and Webster, 1983), and for VI mutants, unstable to CsCl (Lopez and Webster, 1983). Infection with phages mutant in genes VII and IX, which encode small proteins found at the end of the particle opposite to that at which pIII and pVI are located, also result in the formation of some multiple-length particles, but far fewer (1–3 per infected cell) are found than in gene III or VI mutant infections (Lopez and Webster, 1983; Webster and Lopez, 1985). The particles emerging from cells infected with phages mutant in gene VII are infectious, which has led Webster and Lopez (1985) to propose that the few emergent phages have simply reutilized the gene VII protein present in the infecting particles.

The packaging signal in the DNA was identified when chimeric plasmids were constructed that contained a filamentous phage origin of replication. When such constructs are infected with phages, single strands of the chimeric plasmid are packaged into virionlike particles, capable of transducing plasmid markers to a new host (Cleary and Ray, 1980; Dotto et al., 1981a; Dotto and Zinder, 1983; Zinder and Horiuchi, 1985). The chimeric plasmids made by Cleary and Ray (1980) formed transducing particles inefficiently compared to those made by Dotto et al. (1981a). The difference lay in the origin-containing fragment cloned by the two groups; a region between nucleotides 5500 and 5600 (shown as hairpin A in Fig. 6) is required for efficient formation of transducing particles but not for phage-specific DNA synthesis (Dotto et al., 1981a; Dotto and Zinder, 1983; Grant and Webster, 1984b). Dotto and Zinder (1983) showed further that this segment, which has marked dyad symmetry, will function when cloned at a distance from the origin-containing fragment, but that it must be in the same orientation relative to the origin as found in the wild-type phage; this suggests strongly that the packaging signal is functional in its single-stranded form and that it is the (+) strand that is recognized. Schaller (1979) had noted that insertion of the transposon Tn5 into this same region markedly depressed phage yields, and had proposed that this segment was involved in morphogenesis. Shen et al. (1979) and Ikoku and Hearst (1981) have shown that the region identified biologically as the packaging signal can be found as a hairpin by reaction with a psoralen derivative, and that the hairpin is located at one end of the assembled phage particle. In their studies of the orientation of the DNA in the particle, Webster et al. (1981) found that the packaging signal is located at the end opposite that at which the attachment (III) protein resides. Lopez and Webster (1983), moreover, have shown that during morphogenesis it is the end that contains the packaging signal that emerges from the cell first. Thus the packaging signal is needed at the initiation of packaging. The packaging signal of Ike can be utilized by the F-specific phages, though not as efficiently as the homologous sequence (Peeters et al., 1987).

Simons et al. (1979) and Lin et al. (1980) described the "C" protein, isolated from phage and subsequently found to consist of two very small proteins, products of genes VII and IX (Simons et al., 1981). Grant et al. (1981) showed that, like the packaging signal, the C protein is located at the end of the phage opposite to that at which the attachment protein is found. Thus these two proteins, 33 and 32 residues long, respectively, are located at the end of the particle at which assembly is initiated. Since the efficiency of formation of the single-stranded DNA–gene V protein complex is not affected by the absence of a packaging signal (Grant and Webster, 1984b), and since these two proteins are not part of this complex (Grant and Webster, 1984a), their role is probably related to the initiation of assembly of the mature particle. Recently Russel (unpublished) has isolated phage mutants that compensate for packaging region defects; some of these map in gene IX, suggesting an interaction between this protein and the packaging hairpin. Nonpermissive cells infected by gene

VII or IX amber mutant phages can make a few infectious particles, so few that they may have simply reutilized the incoming gene VII (or IX) protein (Lopez and Webster, 1983; Webster and Lopez, 1985).

The orientation of extruding phages suggests that the gene III and VI proteins act at a termination step in assembly, since that end comes out last (Lopez and Webster, 1983). Consistent with this are the high yields of noninfectious, multiple-length phage particles from cells infected by gene III or VI mutant phages (Salivar et al., 1967; Scott and Zinder, 1967; Pratt et al., 1969; Lopez and Webster, 1983). These polyphages contain many copies of unit-length DNA. Both kinds of particles are less stable than normal virions; those that lack gene VI protein are unstable to salt and cannot be isolated on CsCl gradients (Lopez and Webster, 1983). Nelson et al. (1981) have constructed a phage with an internal, in-phase deletion in gene III; this genome can direct the formation of a normal yield of noninfectious particles that contain the altered gene III protein, and these are as stable as wild-type phages (Crissman and Smith, 1984).

The actual process of assembling the phages is very rapid. Lopez and Webster (1983), in their electron microscopic study of the process, were able to detect intermediates only if the infected cells were treated with glutaraldehyde or protein cross-linkers; other methods, including quick cooling or addition of metabolic poisons such as arsenate, cyanide, or dinitrophenol, did not interrupt assembly fast enough (Webster and Lopez, 1985). Assembly involves, at the very minimum, the removal of the gene V protein from the DNA and its replacement by the major coat (gene VIII) protein. Since the gene V protein has a very high affinity for DNA (Bulsink et al., 1985), this dissociation is likely to be an energy-requiring process. The coat protein (at least as isolated from phages) can associate with DNA spontaneously to form amorphous aggregates (Rossomando, 1969), so there is no a priori reason to think energy is required for that step. The F-specific phages have a fivefold rotational symmetry; based on this, and using the assembly of tobacco mosaic virus as a model, it has been proposed that growth of the virus involves the addition of a pentamer of protein to the growing filament (Makowski, 1984). Although this is a plausible suggestion, there is at present no evidence to support it. The coat protein probably undergoes substantial conformational change in moving from the membrane to the phage, since in the membrane form it probably has no more than 50% α helix (Nozaki et al., 1978; Fodor et al., 1981), whereas in the phage the α helical content is greater than 80% (Makowski, 1984). What the energetic implications of this change are is not clear. Rowitch and Perham (1987) have shown that Pf1 coat protein is processed and inserted into the membrane correctly when expressed in E. coli rather than in its usual host, Pseudomonas aeruginosa. It cannot, however, replace a defective M13 coat protein in phage assembly. This supports the hypothesis that specific interactions between phage-encoded proteins are likely to be important in the assembly process.

In addition to its constituent proteins and DNA, assembly of the virion requires the activity of the two phage-encoded "morphogenetic proteins," pI and pIV (Pratt *et al.*, 1966), a source of energy (Ng and Dunker, 1981), the host-encoded thioredoxin, and the proper functioning of several other host genes whose products have as yet not been identified. The most likely function for gene I is to assist in the creation of an exit port for the phage (Horabin and Webster, 1986). Not much more is known about the function of the gene IV protein than was clear some 20 years ago. Pratt *et al.* (1966) reported that shifting a culture of cells infected with a temperature-sensitive gene IV mutant to the nonpermissive temperature interrupted phage synthesis very quickly, and that a downshift had the opposite effect. We now know that gene IV protein is most probably membrane-associated and contains a cleaved signal sequence (see Genes and Proteins; Brissette and Russel, unpublished) and that it induces very high levels of synthesis of another, unknown host protein (Brissette and Russel, unpublished), but we understand no more about its role in phage assembly than did Pratt.

To explore the role of host proteins in assembly, Russel and Model (1983) screened mutagenized cells to find mutants in which filamentous phage assembly could not take place. Two such mutants were isolated: one (called B27) that was temperature-sensitive for phage assembly and showed pleiotropic membrane defects at the high temperature (Model *et al.*, 1981), and a second, more genetically tractable mutant, in a gene originally called *fip*, that failed to assemble phage at high temperature but showed no other phenotype or growth defect at any temperature. During transfer of the *fip*+ gene, Lopez and Webster (1985b) isolated an additional host mutant blocked in phage morphogenesis and showed that the mutant phenotype was due to two mutations which they termed *fipB* and *fipC*. Both loci must be mutant to obtain a *fip* phenotype. The original mutation, *fip*, was found to encode the *E. coli* thioredoxin (Russel and Model, 1984, 1985; Lim *et al.*, 1985). Thioredoxin was originally identified as a cofactor in the reduction of ribonucleotides by ribonucleotide reductase (Moore *et al.*, 1964), has been shown to be a constituent of the phage T7 DNA polymerase (Modrich and Richardson, 1975; Mark and Richardson, 1976), and has been shown to have a variety of oxidation-reduction functions (Holmgren, 1985). It is widely distributed throughout the phyla.

Thioredoxin reductase, the enzyme that reduces thioredoxin at the expense of the oxidation of NADPH, was also necessary for efficient phage production (Russel and Model, 1985a,b). Although the original *fip* (or thioredoxin) mutation, which consisted of a proline-to-serine change immediately adjacent to one of the two active-site cysteine residues of thioredoxin, and the requirement for thioredoxin reductase suggested that an oxidation-reduction cycle might be required for filamentous phage assembly, this turned out not to be the case. Specific mutation of the cysteine codons, converting them to serine or alanine or both, did not markedly affect the ability of cells expressing only the mutant protein to support phage growth (Russel and Model, 1986). Indeed, these cells were able to assemble phages efficiently even in the absence of thioredoxin reductase, under conditions where wild-type thioredoxin is inadequate. This suggested that normally the requirement for thioredoxin reductase in assembly is to ensure that thioredoxin is in the reduced conformation, rather than for reducing power *per se*. The reduced and the oxidized forms of thioredoxin do, in fact, differ in conformation (see Holmgren, 1985, for review). It follows that the active-site mutants must be in the reduced conformation. Inactivation of the thioredoxin gene by deletion or by the insertion of extraneous DNA does not permit the assembly of any virions (Russel and Model, 1984).

Phage mutants that can assemble at the nonpermissive temperature on the original thioredoxin mutant host were selected, and their mutations were mapped to a single site in gene I (Russel and Model, 1983), one of the two nonstructural genes involved in assembly. The mutant phage, *gtrxA2*, compensates for a number of other thioredoxin missense mutations (Russel and Model, 1986), as does a second *gtrxA* mutant with a mutation elsewhere in gene I (Russel, unpublished). Other phage mutants in which the gene I protein is temperature-sensitive cannot assemble on the original (temperature-sensitive) thioredoxin mutant even at a temperature permissive for either mutation alone (Russel and Model, 1983). This genetic interconnection between thioredoxin and gene I protein suggests that the two proteins interact, although direct biochemical evidence for this has not been found.

Like filamentous phage, phage T7 can utilize thioredoxins lacking one or both sulfydryl groups of the active site (Huber *et al.*, 1986), but it cannot grow on strains in which the thioredoxin gene is deleted. The maximal activity of the T7 DNA polymerase is comparable between wild-type and cysteine-mutant thioredoxins, although the affinity of the T7-encoded subunit for the mutant thioredoxins is lower. Tabor *et al.* (1986) have found that the T7-encoded constituent of the polymerase is, by itself, capable of polymerization, but that it has lost its processivity. If one is permitted to extrapolate from T7 DNA synthesis to filamentous phage morphogenesis, it may be that this protein confers a similar property on the assembly of the virion; clearly, in order for the rapid and sequential addition of so many coat protein molecules, a high degree of processivity in the enzymatic reactions is required.

VIII. GENETICS AND PHYSIOLOGY

A. Control of Gene Expression

Filamentous phages can begin to extrude progeny about 10 min after infection, under ideal conditions, yet they can reach a steady state about 30 min postinfection and will remain persistent parasites for as many generations as can be measured (Marvin and Hohn, 1969). This very rapid onset and subsequent stabilization implies the action of controlling elements. The continued presence of the phages over generations is not due to the segregation of uninfected cells followed by reinfection; studies with female cells, into which phage DNA can be transfected, but in which phage infection is extremely inefficient, shows that the curing rate is quite low (Merriam, 1977; Lerner and Model, 1981).

Pratt *et al.* (1966) and many workers after him (e.g., Marvin and Hohn, 1969) observed that infection of cells with phage mutants was usually lethal to the host. The exceptions were mutant in gene II. The initial inference was that the gene II product is lethal; this is not correct. Gene II is required for the formation of progeny RF and single strands (see DNA synthesis). In its absence, the parental RF is the only template for the transcription of the phage-encoded products, so the proteins encoded by all the genes are held to a relatively low level. Since the parental RF cannot replicate, it is diluted out by cell growth, and the culture therefore soon consists primarily of uninfected cells. Gene II, moreover, has been cloned (Meyer and Geider, 1981; Dotto *et al.*, 1981b), and its overexpression is not, by itself, lethal to the host. A number of phage gene products can be lethal: pI and pIV expressed from the cloned genes (see Morphogenetic Genes) appear to be lethal in small amounts; the major coat protein (gene VIII) cannot be cloned under its own promoter unless an amber mutation is present in the gene (Boeke, unpublished); and gene V may also be detrimental when fully expressed from a strong promoter (Fulford, unpublished). If, however, gene II protein is expressed at high levels in cells that also contain a filamentous phage origin in a second or on the same plasmid, the combination is lethal. In general, it has been observed (Zinder, unpublished) that phages with amber mutations in genes that permit the assembly of (uninfectious) particles at reasonably high efficiency, such as those in genes III or VI, kill the infected host more slowly and less efficiently than do phages with amber mutations that block particle formation (such as those in genes I, IV, V, VII, or VIII). These observations all suggest that balanced phage growth is needed to ensure host survival. Cell survival is reduced in infections by phages with a partial defect in assembly, infections in which all phage proteins are present in functional form; this again suggests that the precise balance between the supply of components and assembly is important. Many of the phage-encoded elements that help to adjust the level of gene products to one another are static; they are not known, or expected, to be sensitive to feedback (dynamic) signals resulting from phage gene expression or the environment. These include promoters, which may be strong or weak, terminators, ribosome binding sites, etc. (see Genes and Proteins).

Phage-specific DNA synthesis does show characteristics that suggest a dynamic control mechanism. Normal infection goes through three more or less well-defined stages: an initial stage, in which RF increases rapidly but phages are not yet produced; an intermediate stage, in which

RF replication continues but phages are being extruded, and a third stage (the steady state), in which phages are produced but RF replication is barely detectable. Since the phage infection continues indefinitely, and the infected cells grow and divide, RF synthesis must continue at some level if the infection is not to be cured by simple dilution of the RF pool.

These stages are reflected in phage production. As reviewed in Marvin and Hohn (1969), the initial phase in which no progeny are produced is followed by a burst of phage, and then by a prolonged period in which 200–2000 phages per cell per generation (depending on conditions) are made. DNA synthesis reflects these stages. For the first few minutes of infection, RF synthesis is the exclusive product of replication (Ray et al., 1966; Pratt and Erdahl, 1968; Forsheit et al., 1971); after this, most of the label added during a pulse flows into the (+) strand of RF and thence into the single strand (Ray, 1969; Horiuchi and Zinder, 1976; Lerner and Model, 1981).

It is clear that at least one locus for regulation is the switch from RF to single-strand synthesis. Gene V protein is required for the synthesis of single strands (Pratt and Erdahl, 1968; Pratt et al., 1974); Salstrom and Pratt (1971) showed that it acts by inhibiting the formation of RF, and the details of the complex that it forms are now well understood (see Sections II.C and VII.A). Mazur and Model (1973) showed that in normal infections the onset of single-strand synthesis can be advanced if gene V protein is allowed to accumulate in the absence of DNA synthesis; this suggested that under normal conditions the accumulation of gene V protein is necessary and sufficient to initiate the synthesis of single strands. In addition to sequestering single strands, gene V protein can inhibit the translation of the messenger RNA encoding gene II and gene X (Yen and Webster, 1982; Model et al., 1982; Fulford and Model, 1984b).

There appear to be two sites at which repression can occur, one affecting the translation of gene II, and the other that of gene X, since alteration of the gene II site still leaves gene X repressible by gene V protein (W. D. Fulford and P. Model, 1988b). Some homology between these two regions has recently been detected (B. Michel, unpublished data). Quite high concentrations of *free* gene V protein are needed for this translational repression, and added single-stranded f1 DNA relieves it (Model et al., 1982; Fulford and Model, 1984b). The repression of gene II mRNA translation is specific. T4 gene 32 protein is autogenously controlled (Russel et al., 1976) and its *in vitro* synthesis can be inhibited by the addition of p32 (Lemaire et al., 1978). Gene 32 protein does not, however, inhibit the translation of gene II mRNA, nor does pV affect the translation of gene 32 mRNA (Fulford and Model, 1984b). Inhibition of gene II expression can be expected to occur only when the amount of gene V protein exceeds that used to form the single-stranded DNA-gene V protein complexes. We have thus the beginnings of a feed-back loop. An increase in the number of RF molecules represents an increased number of transcription templates, which will lead to the synthesis of more gene

V protein. This will trigger a switch to single-stranded DNA synthesis, and, since the single-stranded DNA-gene V complex is not a template for replication or transcription, will prevent the accumulation of yet more RF. An excess of RF will lead to the synthesis of more gene V protein than can be complexed to single-stranded DNA, which in turn leads to a repression of gene II synthesis. A shortage of gene V protein (relative to single strands) will stimulate RF synthesis both because single strands will not be made, and because the repression of gene II protein will be lifted. Two more recent observations also have regulatory significance. The C-terminal 2/3 of gene II protein is expressed separately (as X protein) and is required if synthesis of single strands is to occur (see Section II.C). It has also been noted (W. D. Fulford and P. Model, unpublished data) that in the presence of gene V protein, some gene II protein is needed for the (−) strand component of the RF to be made. When gene II protein is made in excess, on the other hand, it so strongly stimulates the synthesis of the (−) strand (e.g., RF) that single-strand synthesis is seriously inhibited (Fulford and Model, unpublished).

The entities involved in this regulation and the control points are depicted in Fig. 2. There is an insufficiency of data, particularly quantitative data, to allow the formulation of a quantitative model to account for the observed accumulation of RF and the initiation of the steady state, but these are being sought.

B. Restriction and Modification

Any discussion of recombination in the filamentous phage necessarily involves the *E. coli* B restriction system, as the procedures used to study recombination relied extensively on the sensitivity of the phage to B restriction and on the genetic markers that their two B-sensitive sites provided.

E. coli K and *E. coli* B specify related class I restriction systems. Unlike the class II restriction systems, in which the restriction (cleavage) occurs within the recognition site, class I enzymes recognize a specific site, then migrate along the DNA in an ATP-dependent fashion, cleaving at some essentially random location (Horiuchi and Zinder, 1972; Horiuchi *et al.*, 1974). In both systems, modification enzymes modify (often by methylation) bases within the recognition site, thereby blocking recognition and subsequent cleavage by their cognate restriction enzymes. The F-specific filamentous phages are sensitive to EcoB restriction but not EcoK (Arber, 1966), and K-grown phages plate with an efficiency of about 10^{-3} on B cells. Repeated cycling of survivors of EcoB restriction between K and B strains results in the selection of phage mutants that have lost one or both of their B sites; the former plate with an efficiency of about 0.03 and the latter at unit efficiency (Arber and Kuhnlein, 1967; Boon and Zinder, 1970). It is with the use of these phages that Arber and co-workers showed that the susceptibility to restriction-modification is a defined genetic trait (Arber and Kuhnlein, 1967).

Modification can be used as a test of the fate of infecting DNA. When phages grown on *E. coli* K are used to infect *E. coli* K, and the infected cells are plated on *E. coli* B, plaques form at low efficiency, 10^{-3}. By contrast, when phages grown on B cells are used to infect K, and these infected cells are plated on *E. coli* B, the efficiency is much higher, 0.2 (Boon and Zinder, 1970; Zinder, 1974). This phenomenon represents repackaging of the input DNA which, since it was originally grown on B, was modified and hence able to plaque on B cells; phages containing DNA molecules that had been replicated in K cells cannot plaque on B, because they lack B modification. The ability to distinguish input from progeny DNA molecules has proved useful in sorting out what goes on during filamentous phage recombination.

C. Recombination

Recombination frequencies among the filamentous phages are low, whereas the frequency of double-length phage particles is high (1–5%; see Morphogenesis). Thus if cells are mixedly infected by complementing mutants, progeny will form, and the fraction that plaques on a nonpermissive host reflects the diploid phage, not true recombinants. The propensity of f1 to form such diploids required genetic mapping to be carried out with double mutants, each mutant in gene II and another (different) gene (Lyons and Zinder, 1971). Recombination, by necessity, has thus been studied using noncomplementing mutants, usually different gene II ambers; under nonpermissive conditions, no replication beyond the initial conversion from single- to double-stranded DNA occurs (see DNA Replication) in such mixedly infected cells, so only when the input DNAs have recombined to generate a wild-type template will gene II protein be synthesized, replication occur, and progeny phages to be produced. If the infecting phages are, in addition, B-modified, the plating properties of the recombinant products can be used to distinguish unreplicated from replicated recombinants. Experiments of this sort showed that recombination can occur between unreplicated (but doubled-up) molecules and thus that some sort of breaking and joining occurs (Boon and Zinder, 1970). Recombination is dependent on host *rec* functions (cited in Enea *et al.*, 1975).

Filamentous phage recombination is asymmetric. In a modified single-burst procedure, which allows for the isolation and analysis of products from individual recombination events, Boon and Zinder (1971) showed that a large fraction of the bursts include wild-type recombinants and only one of the parental genotypes; the remaining bursts produce only the wild-type recombinant. The reciprocal recombinant (double amber) is almost never detected. This is presumably not due to selection, since double gene II ambers have been constructed and are complemented efficiently with wild-type phages. Asymmetric recombination of this sort between closely spaced genes has been widely observed, and it has been especially well studied in the fungi, where it is called "gene conversion" (Fogel and Mortimer, 1969).

Two basic models were originally proposed to account for the asymmetry of parental and recombinant products—an asymmetric hetero-duplex model and a breakage and copying model (Boon and Zinder, 1971). The results of subsequent crosses in which only one of the gene II amber mutant parents was sensitive to B restriction (Hartman and Zinder, 1974a,b) supported the former. This model for recombination in the fila-mentous phages proposes that one parental RF acts as recipient and is invaded by a single strand from the other (donor) RF; the donor RF is apparently lost in this process, but the mechanism by which this occurs has not been established. If the invasion is incomplete (the recipient is heteroduplex for part of its genome but remains homoduplex for the rest), replication will result in the formation of one homoduplex recombinant and one parental molecule. Heteroduplex repair processes could compli-cate this process, but this has been measured by introducing hetero-duplex molecules constructed in vitro; the frequency of such repair was found to be quite low compared with the frequency of "homogenotiza-tion" by replication (Enea et al., 1975). In other words, the heteroduplex molecules segregate via replication much faster than they do via mis-match repair.

Gene conversion events have recently been the subject of much in-terest, since they are believed to be involved in a variety of programmed genomic changes in bacterial pathogens, yeast (mating types), and try-panosome surface antigen switching (reviewed by Borst and Greaves, 1987). Many of these may follow, formally at least, the pattern of filamen-tous phage recombination.

D. Defective Interfering Particles

When filamentous phages are passaged at high multiplicity (by trans-ferring phages grown on one set of cells onto fresh cells without plaque purification), defective interfering (DI) particles accumulate. This was first observed by Griffith and Kornberg (1974) and by Hewitt (1975), and the evolution of these particles was carefully studied by Enea and Zinder (1975) and later by Horiuchi (1983). DI particles manifest themselves in three ways: first, the titer of infectious particles produced in a single passage cycle decreases; second, short phage particles accumulate in large amounts (easily seen by electron microscopy, by electrophoresis of whole phages, or on sucrose gradients); and third, plaques have a peculiar, mot-tled appearance.

The short particles (or "mini" phages) contain circular DNA much smaller than unit length. Analysis of the corresponding double-stranded RF mini-DNA shows that they have all suffered a large deletion that removes almost the entire coding region of the phage genome, leaving the intergenic region and beginning of gene II joined to the end of gene IV (see Fig. 3 for the phage genetic map). Since they do not contain any intact genes, they are completely parasitic on the coinfecting phage, which acts as helper. Most of these particles have also undergone a duplication of part of the intergenic space, in which the origins of both (+) and (−) strand DNA synthesis are located. None contain more than one fully functional (+) strand origin (Chen and Ray, 1978), which is reasonable, since a DNA molecule with two functional (+) strand origins resolves into two components during rolling-circle replication (Horiuchi, 1980; Dotto and Horiuchi, 1981; see DNA Replication). These miniphages do contain several (−) strand origins. Since they are made in large amounts, eventually accounting for half or more of the particles of a mixed infection, they must have a replication advantage over the wild-type helper phages. It is presumably some combination of the large deletion and the multiple (−) strand origins that gives them this advantage; the poor growth of a miniphage that lacks reiterated origins (Enea et al., 1977) points to the importance of the latter.

Using heavily mutagenized phages and exposing them to fresh DI particles during serial transfer, Enea and Zinder (1982) were able to select mutants resistant to interference by miniphages. These mutants, called IR (for interference-resistant), do not show the peculiar mottled plaques made by wild-type phages in the presence of the DI particles. They contain gene II mutations—one in the coding region, which changes amino acid 182 from threonine to isoleucine ($C_{143}{\rightarrow}T$), and one in the upstream, untranslated region, $G_{5986}{\rightarrow}A$. The coding change alone confers a partial IR phenotype; the second change does not itself confer a clear phenotype but enhances the effect of the coding region change. The effect of these mutations on DNA synthesis reflects their growth properties; whereas in cells mixedly infected with DI particles and wild-type helper phage, synthesis of replicative form DNA is heavily biased toward the DI particles, in cells coinfected with the IR mutant helper and DI particles, the balance is skewed in favor of the IR helper. Phenomenologically, then, the effect of the IR mutation(s) is to make gene II protein more cis acting; the biochemical basis for this has not been determined.

A related approach to the genesis of DI particles and IR helpers was taken by Horiuchi (1983), who carried out mass transfer experiments without mutagenesis, with close monitoring of the phage yields and the structure of the phages as they evolved. DI interfering particles accumulated starting at about the 13th mass transfer. Again, these had deleted much of the genome and had no complete genes, and they contained duplications within the intergenic space. After further mass transfers, the yield of plaque formers began to rise again; these now contained various duplications of the (−) strand origin of DNA synthesis, as well as the normal complement of genes. These new phages (called maxiphages) grew better in the presence of DI particles than their unduplicated progenitors; however, they were less interference-resistant than the gene II mutants isolated by Enea and Zinder (1982). In the absence of DI particles, the maxiphages grew about as well as wild-type phages. When such maxiphages were propagated in mass transfer experiments, they, too, gave rise to DI particles, and the duplications in the DI particles were the same as those in their maxiphage parent. These experiments were carried out in both $recA^+$ and $recA^-$ hosts; although the absolute number of phage was reduced in $recA^-$ hosts, the mini- and maxiphages appeared at the same points in the cycle of transfers.

Continued mass transfer of these phage products led to a diminution of the size of the reiterated segment together with an increase in the number of reiterations. Some of the miniphages eventually contained a 51-base quintuplication of a region derived from the intergenic space. In any single-transfer series, the miniphage and its associated maxi helper ended up with very much the same tandem reiterations, indicating that recombination between them was quite common.

E. Lysogeny

Although "carrier states" have been reported, none of the F-specific filamentous phages form true lysogens. Most of the carrier states can be accounted for by host or phage mutants (or conditions such as temperature) which render phage replication or infection inefficient. Cultures containing infected cells will not appear to be infected, but phages can be rescued at low levels. Two phages related to Cf (which infects the plant pathogen *Xanthomonas citri*) do seem to exhibit true lysogeny. Phage Cflt undergoes a more or less standard lysogenic cycle; it plates to give turbid plaques, does not gravely affect the growth of cells, has a low phage yield, and renders its host immune to superinfection. Southern blot analysis shows that the phage integrates at a specific site on the host genome (Kuo *et al.*, 1987). Cells infected with phage Cf16 produce a large number of phage progeny; when the cells are plated, and large yellow colonies are repeatedly chosen, lysogens are eventually found (Dai *et al.*, 1987). In many of these cells, free RF is no longer found, but Cf16 DNA has been integrated into the host DNA. The lysogenic state is not cured by agents such as acridine orange, antiphage serum, or ethidium bromide. The lysogens, upon further cultivation, can give rise to mature phage particles. Although Cf16 has a restriction map similar to that of CF and is serologically indistinguishable, CF16 lysogens are immune to superinfection with Cf16 but not Cf. The relationship between Cf16 and Cflt is not completely clear, but they are not believed to be the same phage (Dai *et al.*, 1987).

F. Filamentous Phages as Cloning Vectors

Filamentous phages make useful cloning vectors for several reasons. First, there is no *a priori* constraint on the size of the DNA that can be cloned in them, since the particle length simply increases in proportion to the increased DNA (see Morphogenesis) (in practice, plaque size diminishes with inserts of 6 kb or more). Second, very high yields of pure single-stranded DNA can be obtained easily, because the phage contains single-stranded DNA and phage accumulates to high levels (up to around 10^{13} phages per milliliter in liquid culture), and high yields of double-stranded DNA can be obtained because of the high copy number of intracellular, replicative form DNA. Third, as with other phage vectors, they can be easily transferred between bacterial strains, and they are well suited for cloning genes whose products are deleterious to the host because of the rapidity at which progeny phages are produced (phage production begins about 10 min after infection at 37°C).

Two principal series of filamentous phage vectors are generally used, and they have been widely described (see Zinder and Boeke, 1982; Geider, 1986; Smith, 1987, for reviews). In brief, the M13 vectors constructed by Messing and co-workers (see Yanisch-Perron *et al.*, 1985) are useful because they contain multiple cloning sites and a visible marker for scoring insertion of DNA. Their disadvantage has been the reported (anecdotal) instability of some inserts, especially those larger than about 5 kb; this may occur because the cloning sites are located within the (+) strand origin of replication (see DNA Replication), at position 5865, which was once the *HaeIII*G-D border. Although compensating mutations have arisen that restore origin function, these phages may still be somewhat impaired. The cloning sites in the f1 vectors (Zinder and Boeke, 1982) are at position 5614, originally the *HpaII*A-H border, between the packaging signal and the origin of (−) strand synthesis. Insertion at this position does not disrupt any functional regions, and some inserts that were unstable in an M13 vector were reportedly more stable in f1. The disadvantage of the f1 vectors is that no fragment permitting a color test for successful insertion has been introduced, and the widely used vectors each contain a single cloning site; derivatives with a polylinker insertion have been constructed (Russel, unpublished).

Plasmids that contain the filamentous phage intergenic region (Dente *et al.*, 1983), which includes their origins of DNA synthesis and packaging or morphogenetic signal, combine useful features of the plasmid and the phage, making it possible to maintain the cloned DNA within the cell or to convert it to single-stranded form; upon infection by a suitable helper phage, the phage origin of replication is activated, and single-stranded "transducing" particles are produced (as well as progeny helper phages). Which strand of the cloned DNA is packaged depends on its orientation with respect to the phage origin and packaging signal. If the plasmid contains, in addition to an f1/M13 intergenic region, the intergenic region from the filamentous phage Ike cloned in an orientation opposite to the other intergenic region, either strand of the cloned DNA can be packaged into transducing particles (Peeters *et al.*, 1986a; Konings *et al.*, 1986). Because the gene II proteins of these phages are not interchangeable (Peeters *et al.*, 1986b), infection by an Ike helper phage activates only the Ike origin, whereas an f1/M13 helper activates only its cognate origin. Phages carrying an IR mutation (Enea and Zinder, 1982; see Defective Interfering Particles) provide the best yields of transducing particles, and an improved IR helper phage that has had its packaging signal deleted, which produces a higher ratio of transducing particles to helper phages, has recently been developed (Russel *et al.*, 1986).

A useful chimeric vector with parts of λ, f1, and pBR322 that can be packaged by the λ *in vitro* packaging system has been constructed (Stratagene; Fernandez *et al.*, unpublished results). It contains two f1 origins of DNA replication, so that when cells carrying it are infected with helper phages, the region between the two origins resolves into a circle (see DNA Replication) containing the pBR322 portion of the construct, one filamentous phage origin, and the cloned DNA. Since the construct also contains appropriately located T7 and SP6 promoters, it can be used to generate almost any kind of recombinant nucleic acid desired.

Several very useful reviews that contain more detailed information on the use of the filamentous phages as vectors are available (Zinder and Boeke, 1982; Geider, 1986).

IX. OTHER REVIEWS AND CONCLUSIONS

A. Other Reviews

A number of very useful reviews of the filamentous phages have been published. Of the general reviews, that by Rasched and Oberer (1986) is the most recent and, since it takes a slightly different point of view from this review, is very useful. The early review by Hohn and Marvin (1969) is dated but is a gold mine of information available before 1969, and is surprisingly prescient in many of its suggestions and ideas. Other general reviews are by Ray (1977), an entire book which is the outgrowth of a Cold Spring Harbor meeting (Denhardt *et al.*, 1978), and a review by Denhardt (1975). Some of the more specialized topics are covered by reviews or long articles that are quasi reviews. They include genetics and recombination (Zinder, 1974, 1978; Pratt, 1969); DNA synthesis (Baas, 1985; Zinder and Horiuchi 1985; Meyer and Geider, 1980; Kornberg, 1980, 1982; Horiuchi *et al.*, 1979; Schaller, 1979); virion structure (Makowski, 1984); gene V protein and the gene V protein–single-stranded DNA complex structure (McPherson and Brayer, 1984; Brayer and McPherson, 1984a); cloning (Geider, 1986; Zinder and Boeke, 1982); phage assembly (Webster and Lopez, 1985); and regulation (Fulford *et al.*, 1986).

B. Conclusions

Filamentous phages are fascinating for themselves, in part because they so little resemble other phages, in part because of their intimate relationship to their host. The close association of the phage with the host membrane makes the biochemistry of entry and assembly particularly challenging; this is an area that needs, and is receiving, a good deal of research attention.

It is always surprising how complex an entity that contains only 10 genes can be. Although we do have a basic understanding of transcription, translation, and DNA synthesis, we still don't have very good ideas of what genes IV and I do, and we don't have very good ideas about how VI, VII, and IX function or what the exact role of each is. We don't have a quantitative model of control. One or more of these subjects will soon be solved but will probably give rise to new questions.

The phages have been excellent model systems with which to study DNA synthesis, recombination, transcription-translation, and the insertion of proteins into the membrane. They may yet have a role as models of simple biological control and for the process of "facilitated assembly," which seems to require far more factors than the constituent parts.

ACKNOWLEDGMENTS. We thank our colleagues, Norton Zinder and Kensuke Horiuchi, for reading some of this chapter and making corrections and helpful suggestions. We also appreciate interesting and helpful discussions with R. E. Webster. They have not had an opportunity to read all of the material, so we must take responsibility for errors of omission and commission. Our work has been supported by grants from the National Science Foundation and the National Institutes of Health.

REFERENCES

Adler, H. L., Fisher, W. D., Cohen, A., and Hardigree, A. A., 1967, Miniature *Escherichia coli* deficient in DNA. *Proc. Natl. Acad. Sci. USA* **57:**321–326.

Alberts, B., Frey, L., and Delius, H., 1972, Isolation and characterization of gene 5 protein of filamentous bacterial viruses, *J. Mol. Biol.* **68:**139–152.

Alberts, B. M., Barry, J., Bedinger, P., Burke, R. E., Hibner, U., Liu, C.-C., and Sheridan, R., 1980, Studies of replication mechanisms with the T4 bacteriophage *in vitro* system, in: *Mechanistic Studies of DNA Replication and Genetic Recombination: ICN–UCLA Symposium on Molecular and Cellular Biology* (B. M. Alberts, ed.), pp. 449–473, Academic Press, New York.

Alma, N. C. M., Harmsen, B. J. M., VanBoom, J. H., Van der Marel, G., and Hilbers, C. W., 1982, ^{1}H NMR studies of the binding of bacteriophage-M13-encoded gene 5 protein to oligo(deoxyadenylic acid)s of varying length, *Eur. J. Biochem.* **122:**319–326.

Alma, N. C. M., Harmsen, B. J. M., DeJong, E. A. M., Vanderven, J., and Hilbers, C. W., 1983, Fluorescence studies of the complex formation between the gene 5 protein of bacteriophage M13 and polynucleotides, *J. Mol. Biol.* **163:**47–62.

Anderson, E., Nakashima, Y., and Coleman, J. E., 1975a, Chemical modifications of functional residues of a gene 5 DNA-binding protein, *Biochemistry* **14:**907–917.

Anderson, E., Nakashima, Y., and Konigsberg, W., 1975b, Photo-induced cross-linkage of gene 5 protein and bacteriophage fd DNA$^+$, *Nucleic Acids Res.* **2:**361–371.

Arber, W., 1966, Host specificity of DNA produced by *Escherichia coli*. 9. Host controlled modification of bacteriophage fd, *J. Mol. Biol.* **20:**483–496.

Arber, W., and Kuhnlein, U., 1967, Mutationeller verlust B-spezifischer restriktion des bakteriophagen fd, *Pathol. Microbiol.* **30:**946–952.

Armstrong, J., Perham, R. N., and Walker, J. E., 1981, Domain-structure of bacteriophage fd adsorption protein, *FEBS Lett.* **135:**167–172.

Armstrong, J., Hewitt, J. A., and Perham, R. N., 1983, Chemical modification of the coat protein in bacteriophage-fd and orientation of the virion during assembly and disassembly, *EMBO J.* **2:**1641–1646.

Asbeck, V. F., Beyreuther, K., Kohler, H., Von Wettstein, G., and Braunitzer, G., 1969, Die kostitution des hullproteins des phagen fd, *Hoppe-Seyler's Z. Physiol. Chem.* **350:** 1047–1066.

Baas, P. D., 1985, DNA replication of single-stranded *Escherichia coli* DNA phages, *Biochim. Biophys. Acta* **825:**111–139.

Banner, D. W., Nave, C., and Marvin, D. A., 1981, Structure of the protein and DNA in fd filamentous bacterial virus, *Nature* **289:**814–816.

Bayer, M. E., 1968, Areas of adhesion between wall and membrane of *Escherichia coli*, *J. Gen. Microbiol.* **53:**395–404.

Bayne, M. L., and Dumas, L. B., 1979, Initiation of DNA synthesis on the isolated strands of bacteriophage f1 replicative-form DNA, *J. Virol.* **29:**1014–1022.

Beaudoin, J., and Pratt, D., 1974, Antiserum inactivation of electrophoretically purified M13 diploid virions: Model for the F-specific filamentous bacteriophages, *J. Virol.* **13:**466–469.

Beck, E., and Zink, B., 1981, Nucleotide sequence and genome organization of filamentous bacteriophages f1 and fd, *Gene* **16:**35–58.

Beck, E., Sommer, R., Auerswald, E. A., Kurz, C., Zink, B., Osterburg, G., Schaller, H., Sugimoto, K., Sugisaki, H., Okamoto, T., and Takanami, M., 1978, Nucleotide sequence of bacteriophage fd DNA, *Nucleic Acids Res.* **5:**4495–4503.

Bernstein, A., Rolfe, B., and Onodera, K., 1972, Pleiotropic properties and genetic organization of the *tolA,B* locus of *Escherichia coli* K-12, *J. Bacteriol.* **112:**74–83.

Beutin, L., and Achtman, M., 1979, Two *Escherichia coli* chromosomal cistrons, *sfrA* and *sfrB*, which are needed for expression of F factor *tra* functions. *J. Bacteriol.* **139:**730–737.

Blumer, K. J., and Steege, D. A., 1984, mRNA processing in *Escherchia coli:* An activity encoded by the host processes bacteriophage f1 mRNAs, *Nucleic Acids Res.* **12:**1847–1861.

Blumer, K. J., Ivey, M. R., and Steege, D. A., 1987, Translational control of phage f1 gene expression by differential activities of the gene V, VII, IX, and VIII initiation sites, *J. Mol. Biol.* **197:**439–456.

Boeke, J. D., 1981, One and two codon insertion mutants of bacteriophage f1, *Mol. Gen. Genet.* **181:**288–291.

Boeke, J. D., and Model, P., 1979, Molecular basis of the am8h1 lesion in bacteriophage M13, *Virology* **96:**299–301.

Boeke, J. D., and Model, P., 1982, A prokaryotic membrane anchor sequence: Carboxyl terminus of bacteriophage f1 gene III protein retains it in the membrane, *Proc. Natl. Acad. Sci. USA* **79:**5200–5204.

Boeke, J. D., Vovis, G. F., and Zinder, N. D., 1979, Insertion mutant of bacteriophage f1 sensitive to EcoRI, *Proc. Natl. Acad. Sci. USA* **76:**2699–2702.

Boeke, J. D., Russel, M., and Model, P., 1980, Processing of filamentous phage pre-coat protein: Effect of sequence variations near the signal peptidase cleavage site, *J. Mol. Biol.* **144**:103–116.

Boeke, J. D., Model, P., and Zinder, N. D., 1982, Effects of bacteriophage f1 gene III protein on the host cell membrane, *Mol. Gen. Genet.* **186**:185–192.

Boon, T., and Zinder, N. D., 1970, Genetic recombination in bacteriophage f1: Transfer of parental DNA to the recombinant, *Virology* **41**:444–452.

Boon, T., and Zinder, N. D., 1971, Genotypes produced by individual recombination events involving bacteriophage f1, *J. Mol. Biol.* **58**:133–151.

Borst, P., and Greaves, D. R., 1987, Programmed gene rearrangements altering gene expression, *Science* **235**:658–667.

Bouvier, F., and Zinder, N. D., 1974, Effects of *dnaA* thermosensitive mutation of *Escherichia coli* on bacteriophage f1 growth and DNA synthesis, *Virology* **60**:139–150.

Bradley, D. E., 1964, Some preliminary observations on filamentous and RNA bacteriophages, *J. Ultrastruct. Res.* **10**:385–389.

Bradley, D. E., Coetzee, J. N., Bothma, T., and Hedges, R. W., 1981, Phage-X: A plasmid-dependent, broad host range, filamentous bacterial virus, *J. Gen. Microbiol.* **126**:389–396.

Bradley, D. E., Coetzee, J. N., and Hedges, R. W., 1983, Inci2 plasmids specify sensitivity to filamentous bacteriophage IKe, *J. Bacteriol.* **154**:505–507.

Brayer, G. D., and McPherson, A., 1983, Refined structure of the gene-5 DNA-binding protein from bacteriophage-fd, *J. Mol. Biol.* **169**:565–596.

Brayer, G., and McPherson, A., 1984a, Cooperative interactions of the gene 5 protein, *J. Biomol. Struct. Dynam.* **2**:495–510.

Brayer, G. D., and McPherson, A., 1984b, Mechanism of DNA binding to the gene 5 protein of bacteriophage-fd, *Biochemistry* **23**:340–349.

Brayer, G. D., and McPherson, A., 1985a, A model for intracellular complexation between gene-5 protein and bacteriophage fd DNA, *Eur. J. Biochem.* **150**:287–296.

Brayer, G. D., and McPherson, A., 1985b, Topological comparison of 2 helix destabilizing proteins—ribonuclease-a and the gene-5 DNA-binding protein, *J. Biomol. Struct. Dynam.* **3**:173–183.

Brinton, C., 1965, The structure, function, synthesis and genetic control of bacterial pili and a molecular model for DNA and RNA transport in gram negative bacteria, *Trans. NY Acad. Sci.* **27**:1003–1054.

Brinton, C., and Beer, H., 1967, The interaction of male-specific bacteriophages with F-pili, in: *The Molecular Biology of Viruses* (J. S. Colter and W. Paranchych, eds.), pp. 251–289, Academic Press, New York.

Brutlag, D., Schekman, R., and Kornberg, A., 1971, A possible role for RNA polymerase in the initiation of M13 DNA synthesis, *Proc. Natl. Acad. Sci. USA* **68**:2826–2829.

Bulsink, H., Harmsen, B. J. M., and Hilbers, C. W., 1985, Specificity of the binding of bacteriophage M13 encoded gene-5 protein to DNA and RNA studied by means of fluorescence titrations, *J. Biomol. Struct. Dynam.* **3**:227–247.

Bulsink, H., Vanresandt, R. W. W., Harmsen, B. J. M., and Hilbers, C. W., 1986, Different DNA-binding modes and cooperativities for bacteriophage M13 gene-5 protein revealed by means of fluorescence depolarisation studies, *Eur. J. Biochem.* **157**:329–334.

Burke, J. M., Novotny, C. P., and Fives-Taylor, P., 1979, Defective F pili and other characteristics of F *lac* and Hfr *Escherichia coli* mutants resistant to bacteriophage R17, *J. Bacteriol.* **140**:525–531.

Caro, L. G., and Schnos, M., 1966, The attachment of the male-specific bacteriophage f1 to sensitive strains of *Escherichia coli*, *Proc. Natl. Acad. Sci. USA* **48**:532–546.

Casadevall, A., and Day, L. A., 1985, The precursor complex of Pf3 bacteriophage, *Virology* **145**:260–272.

Cashman, J. S., and Webster, R. E., 1979, Bacteriophage f1 infection of *Escherichia coli*: Identification and possible processing of f1-specific *in vivo* mRNAs, *Proc. Natl. Acad. Sci. USA* **76**:1169–1173.

Cashman, J. S., Webster, R. E., and Steege, D. A., 1980, Transcription of bacteriophage fl: The major *in vivo* RNAs, *J. Biol. Chem.* **255:**2554–2562.

Cavalieri, S., Goldthwait, D., and Neet, K., 1976a, The isolation of a dimer of gene 8 protein of bacteriophage fd, *J. Mol. Biol.* **102:**713–772.

Cavalieri, S. J., Neet, K. E., and Goldthwait, D. A., 1976b, Gene 5 protein of bacteriophage fd: A dimer which interacts cooperatively with DNA, *J. Mol. Biol.* **102:**697–711.

Chamberlain, B. K., and Webster, R. E., 1978, Effect of membrane-associated fl bacteriophage coat protein upon activity of *Escherichia coli* phosphatidylserine synthetase, *J. Bacteriol.* **135:**883–887.

Chan, T. S., Model, P., and Zinder, N. D., 1975, *In vitro* protein synthesis directed by separated transcripts of bacteriophage fl DNA, *J. Mol. Biol.* **99:**369–382.

Chang, C. N., Blobel, G., and Model, P., 1978, Detection of prokaryotic signal peptidase in an *Escherichia coli* membrane fraction: Endoproteolytic cleavage of nascent fl pre-coat protein, *Proc. Natl. Acad. Sci. USA* **75:**361–365.

Chang, C. N., Model, P., and Blobel, G., 1979, Membrane biogenesis: Cotranslational integration of the bacteriophage fl coat protein into an *Escherichia coli* membrane fraction, *Proc. Natl. Acad. Sci. USA* **76:**1251–1255.

Chen, T. C., and Ray, D. S., 1976, Replication of bacteriophage M13. X. M13 replication in a mutant of *Escherichia coli* defective in the 5′ → 3′ exonuclease associated with DNA polymerase I, *J. Mol. Biol.* **106:**589–604.

Chen, T. C., and Ray, D. S., 1978, Replication of bacteriophage M13. XIII. Structure and replication of cloned M13 miniphage, *J. Mol. Biol.* **125:**107–121.

Cleary, J. M., and Ray, D. S., 1980, Replication of the plasmid pBR322 under the control of a cloned replication origin from the single-stranded DNA phage M13, *Proc. Natl. Acad. Sci. USA* **77:**4638–4642.

Cleary, J. M., and Ray, D. S., 1981, Deletion analysis of the cloned replication origin region from bacteriophage M13, *J. Virol.* **40:**197–203.

Coleman, J. E., and Oakley, J. L., 1980, Physical chemical studies of the structure and function of DNA binding (helix-destabilizing) proteins, *Crit. Rev. Biochem.* **7:**247–289.

Crissman, J. W., and Smith, G. P., 1984, Gene-III protein of filamentous phages: Evidence for a carboxyl-terminal domain with a role in morphogenesis, *Virology* **132:**445–455.

Cross, T. A., and Opella, S. J., 1980, Structural properties of fd coat protein in sodium dodecyl sulfate micelles, *Biochem. Biophys. Res. Commun.* **92:**478–484.

Cross, T. A., Tsang, P., and Opella, S. J., 1983, Comparison of protein and deoxyribonucleic-acid backbone structures in bacteriophage fd and bacteriophage Pf1, *Biochemistry* **22:**721–726.

Dai, H., Chiang, K. S., and Kuo, T. T., 1980, Characterization of a new filamentous phage Cf from *Xanthomonas citri*, *J. Gen. Virol.* **46:**277–289.

Dai, H., Tsay, S.-H., Kuo, T.-T., Lin, Y.-H., and Wu, W.-C., 1987, Neolysogenization of *Xanthomonas campestris* pv. *citri* infected with filamentous phage Cf16, *Virology* **156:**313–320.

Dasgupta, S., and Mitra, S., 1976, The role of *Escherichia coli* dnaG function in coliphage M13 DNA synthesis, *Eur. J. Biochem.* **67:**47–51.

Date, T., Zwizinski, C., Ludmerer, S., and Wickner, W., 1980a, Mechanisms of membrane assembly: Effects of energy poisons on the conversion of soluble M13 coli phage procoat to membrane-bound coat protein, *Proc. Natl. Acad. Sci. USA* **77:**827–831.

Date, T., Goodman, J. M., and Wickner, W. T., 1980b, Procoat, the precursor of M13 coat protein, requires an electrochemical potential for membrane insertion, *Proc. Natl. Acad. Sci. USA* **77:**4669–4673.

Davies, J. K., and Reeves, P., 1975, Genetics of resistance to colicins in *Escherchia coli* K-12: Cross-resistance among colicins of group A, *J. Bacteriol.* **123:**102–117.

Davis, N. G., and Model, P., 1985, An artificial anchor domain: Hydrophobicity suffices to stop transfer, *Cell* **41:**607–614.

Davis, N. G., Boeke, J. D., and Model, P., 1985, Fine structure of a membrane anchor domain, *J. Mol. Biol.* **181:**111–121.

Day, L. A., 1973, Circular dichroism and ultraviolet absorption of a deoxyribonucleic acid binding protein of filamentous bacteriophage, *Biochemistry* **12**:5329–5339.

Denhardt, D. T., 1975, The single stranded DNA phages, *CRC Crit. Rev. Microbiol.* **4**:161–223.

Denhardt, D. G., Dresseler, D., and Ray, D. S., *The Single-Stranded DNA Phages,* Cold Spring Harbor Laboratory, Cold Spring Harbor, NY.

Dente, L., Cesareni, G., and Cortese, R., 1983, pEMBL: A new family of single stranded plasmids, *Nucleic Acids Res.* **11**:1645–1655.

Dettori, R., and Neri, M. F., 1965, Batteriofago filamentoso specifico per cellule Hfr ed F$^+$ di *E. coli* K12, *G. Microbiol.* **13**:111–121.

Dotto, G. P., and Horiuchi, K., 1981, Replication of a plasmid containing two origins of bacteriophage f1, *J. Mol. Biol.* **153**:169–176.

Dotto, G. P., and Zinder, N. D., 1983, The morphogenetic signal of bacteriophage f1, *Virology* **130**:252–256.

Dotto, G. P., and Zinder, N. D., 1984, Reduction of the minimal sequence for initiation of DNA synthesis by qualitative or quantitative changes of an initiator protein, *Nature* **311**:279–280.

Dotto, G. P., Enea, V., and Zinder, N. D., 1981a, Functional analysis of bacteriophage f1 intergenic region, *Virology* **114**:463–473.

Dotto, G. P., Enea, V., and Zinder, N. D., 1981b, Gene II of phage f1: Its functions and its products, *Proc. Natl. Acad. Sci. USA* **78**:5421–5424.

Dotto, G. P., Horiuchi, K., and Zinder, N. D., 1982a, Initiation and termination of phage f1 plus-strand synthesis, *Proc. Natl. Acad. Sci. USA* **79**:7122–7126.

Dotto, G. P., Horiuchi, K., Jakes, K. S., and Zinder, N. D., 1982b, Replication origin of bacteriophage f1: Two signals required for its function, *J. Mol. Biol.* **162**:335–343.

Dotto, G. P., Horiuchi, K., Jakes, K. S., and Zinder, N. D., 1983, Signals for the initiation and termination of synthesis of the viral strand of bacteriophage f1, *Cold Spring Harbor Symp. Quant. Biol.* **47**:717–722.

Dotto, G. P., Horiuchi, K., and Zinder, N. D., 1984, The functional origin of bacteriophage f1 DNA replication: Its signal and domains, *J. Mol. Biol.* **172**:507–521.

Edens, L., Konings, R. N. H., and Schoenmakers, J. G. G., 1975, Physical mapping of central terminator for transcription on bacteriophage M13 genome, *Nucleic Acids Res.* **2**:1811–1820.

Edens, L., Vanwezenbeek, P., Konings, R. N. H., and Schoenmakers, J. G. G., 1976, Mapping of promoter sites on genome of bacteriophage M13, *Eur. J. Biochem.* **70**:577–587.

Edens, L., Konings, R. N. H., and Schoenmakers, J. G. G., 1978, Cascade mechanism of transcription in bacteriophage M13 DNA, *Virology* **86**:354–367.

Eisenberg, S., Scott, J. F., and Kornberg, A., 1976a, Enzymatic replication of viral and complementary strands of duplex DNA of phage ϕX174 proceeds by separate mechanisms, *Proc. Natl. Acad. Sci. USA* **73**:3151–3155.

Eisenberg, S., Scott, J. F., and Kornberg, A., 1976b, Enzyme system for replication of duplex circular DNA: Replicative form of phage ϕX174, *Proc. Natl. Acad. Sci. USA* **73**:1594–1597.

Enea, V., and Zinder, N. D., 1975, A deletion mutant of bacteriophage f1 containing no intact cistrons, *Virology* **68**:105–114.

Enea, V., and Zinder, N. D., 1982, Interference resistant mutants of phage f1, *Virology* **122**:222–226.

Enea, V., Vovis, G. F., and Zinder, N. D., 1975, Genetic studies with heteroduplex DNA of bacteriophage f1. Asymmetric segregation, base correction and implications for the mechanisms of genetic recombination, *J. Mol. Biol.* **96**:495–509.

Enea, V., Horiuchi, K., Turgeon, B. G., and Zinder, N. D., 1977, Physical map of defective interfering particles of bacteriophage f1, *J. Mol. Biol.* **111**:395–414.

Engelman, D. M., and Steitz, T., 1984, On the folding and insertion of globular membrane proteins, in: *The Protein Folding Problem* (D. B. Wetlaufer, ed.), pp. 87–113, Westview Press, Boulder, CO.

Farber, M. B., and Ray, D. S., 1980, Clear-plaque mutation of bacteriophage M13 affects the regulation of viral DNA synthesis, *J. Virol.* **33:**1106–1110.

Fidanian, H. M., and Ray, D. S., 1972, Replication of bacteriophage M13. VII. Requirement of gene 2 protein for the accumulation of a specific RFII species, *J. Mol. Biol.* **72:**51–63.

Fidanian, H. M., and Ray, D. S., 1974, Replication of bacteriophage M13. VIII. Differential effects of rifampicin and nalidixic acid on the synthesis of the two strands of M13 duplex DNA, *J. Mol. Biol.* **83:**63–82.

Fodor, S. P. A., Dunker, A. K., Ng, Y. C., Carstern, D., and Williams, R. W., 1981, Lipid-tail group dependent structure of the fd gene 8 protein, in: *Bacteriophage Assembly* (M. DuBow, ed.), pp. 441–445, Alan R. Liss, New York.

Fogel, S., and Mortimer, R. K., 1969, Informational transfer in meiotic gene conversion, *Proc. Natl. Acad. Sci. USA* **62:**96–103.

Forsheit, A. B., and Ray, D. S., 1971, Replication of bacteriophage M13. VI. Attachment of M13 DNA to a fast-sedimenting host cell component, *Virology* **43:**647–664.

Forsheit, A. B., Ray, D. S., and Lica, L., 1971, Replication of bacteriophage M13. V. Single-strand synthesis during M13 infection, *J. Mol. Biol.* **57:**117–127.

Frangione, B., Nakashima, Y., Konigsberg, W., and Wiseman, R. L., 1978, The amino acid sequence of the major coat protein subunit of the filamentous virus Xf, *FEBS Lett.* **96:**381–384.

Fulford, W. D., 1986, The regulation of bacteriophage f1 DNA replication, Ph.D. Thesis, Rockefeller University, New York.

Fulford, W., and Model, P., 1984a, Gene X of bacteriophage f1 is required for phage DNA synthesis. Mutagenesis of in-frame overlapping genes, *J. Mol. Biol.* **178:**137–153.

Fulford, W., and Model, P., 1984b, Specificity of translational regulation by two DNA binding proteins, *J. Mol. Biol.* **173:**211–226.

Fulford, W., Russel, M., and Model, P., 1986, Aspects of the growth and regulation of the filamentous phages, *Prog. Nucleic Acid Res. Mol. Biol.* **33:**141–168.

Fulford, W., and Model, P., 1988a, Regulation of bacteriophage f1 DNA replication. I. New functions for genes II and X, *J. Mol. Biol.* (in press).

Fulford, W., and Model, P., 1988b, The bacteriophage f1 DNA replication genes. II. The roles of gene V protein and gene II protein in complementary strand synthesis, *J. Mol. Biol.* (in press).

Geider, K., 1978, Interaction of DNA with DNA-binding proteins. Protein exchange and complex stability, *Eur. J. Biochem.* **87:**617–622.

Geider, K., 1986, DNA cloning vectors utilizing replication functions of the filamentous phages of *Escherichia coli*, *J. Gen. Virol.* **67:**2287–2303.

Geider, K., and Kornberg, A., 1974, Conversion of M13 viral single strand to double-stranded replicative forms by purified proteins, *J. Biol. Chem.* **249:**3999–4005.

Geider, K., Beck, E., and Schaller, H., 1978, An RNA transcribed from DNA at the origin of phage fd single strand to replicative form conversion, *Proc. Natl. Acad. Sci. USA* **75:**645–649.

Geider, K., Baumel, I., and Meyer, T. F., 1982, Intermediate stages in enzymatic replication of bacteriophage fd duplex DNA, *J. Biol. Chem.* **257:**6488–6493.

Geller, B. L., and Wickner, W., 1985, Membrane assembly from purified components. 8. M13 procoat inserts into liposomes in the absence of other membrane proteins, *J. Biol. Chem.* **260:**13281–13285.

Gilbert, W., and Dressler, D., 1968, DNA replication: The rolling circle model. *Cold Spring Harbor Symp. Quant. Biol.* **32:**473–484.

Gold, L., Pribnow, D., Schneider, T., Shinedling, S., Singer, B. S., and Stormo, G., 1981, Translational initiation in prokaryotes, *Annu. Rev. Microbiol.* **35:**365–403.

Goldsmith, M. E., and Konigsberg, W. H., 1977, Adsorption protein of bacteriophage fd: Isolation, molecular properties, and location in virus, *Biochemistry* **16:**2686–2694.

Goodman, J. M., Watts, C., and Wickner, W., 1981, Membrane assembly: Post translational insertion of M13 procoat protein into *Escherichia coli* membranes and its proteolytic conversion to coat protein *in vitro*, *Cell* **24:**437–441.

Grant, R. A., and Webster, R. E., 1984a, Minor protein content of the gene V protein/phage single-stranded DNA complex of the filamentous bacteriophage f1, *Virology* **133:**315–328.

Grant, R. A., and Webster, R. E., 1984b, The bacteriophage f1 morphogenetic signal and the gene V protein/phage single-stranded DNA complex, *Virology* **133:**329–340.

Grant, R. A., Lin, T. C., Konigsberg, W., and Webster, R. E., 1981, Structure of the filamentous bacteriophage f1. Location of the A, C and D minor coat proteins, *J. Biol. Chem.* **256:**539–546.

Gray, C. P., Sommer, R., Polke, C., Beck, E., and Schaller, H., 1978, Structure of the origin of DNA replication of bacteriophage fd, *Proc. Natl. Acad. Sci. USA* **75:**50–53.

Gray, C. W., 1987, Electron microscopy of the single strand DNA binding protein of Ike virus complexed with DNA, *Biophys. J.* **51:**150.

Gray, C. W., Brown, R. S., and Marvin, D. A., 1979, Direct visualization of adsorption protein of fd phage, *J. Supramol. Struct.* **S3:**91.

Gray, C. W., Brown, R. S., and Marvin, D. A., 1981, Adsorption complex of filamentous fd virus, *J. Mol. Biol.* **146:**621–627.

Gray, C. W., Kneale, G. G., Leonard, K. R., Siegrist, H., and Marvin, D. A., 1982b, A nucleoprotein complex in bacteria infected with Pf1 filamentous virus: Identification and electron microscopic analysis, *Virology* **116:**40–52.

Gray, D. M., Gray, C. W., and Carlson, R. D., 1982a, Neutron scattering data on reconstituted complexes of fd deoxyribonucleic acid and gene 5 protein show that the deoxyribonucleic acid is near the center, *Biochemistry* **21:**2702–2713.

Griffith, J., and Kornberg, A., 1974, Mini M13 bacteriophage: Circular fragments of M13 DNA are replicated and packaged during normal infections, *Virology* **59:**139–152.

Griffith, J., Manning, M., and Dunn, K., 1981, Filamentous bacteriophage contract into hollow spherical particles upon exposure to a chloroform-water interface, *Cell* **23:**747–753.

Harth, G., Baumel, I., Meyer, T. F., and Geider, K., 1981, Bacteriophage fd gene-2 protein. Processing of phage fd viral strands replicated by phage T7 enzymes, *Eur. J. Biochem.* **119:**663–668.

Hartman, N., and Zinder, N. D., 1974a, Effect of B specific restriction and modification of DNA on linkage relationships in f1 bacteriophage. I. Studies on mechanism of B restriction *in vivo*, *J. Mol. Biol.* **85:**345–356.

Hartman, N., and Zinder, N. D., 1974b, Effect of B specific restriction and modification of DNA on linkage relationships in f1 bacteriophage. II. Evidence for a heteroduplex intermediate in f1 recombination, *J. Mol. Biol.* **85:**357–369.

Henry, T. J., and Brinton, C. C., 1971, Removal of the coat protein of bacteriophage M13 or fd from the exterior of the host after infection, *Virology* **46:**754–763.

Henry, T. J., and Pratt, D., 1969, The proteins of bacteriophage M13, *Proc. Natl. Acad. Sci. USA* **62:**800–807.

Herrmann, R., Neugebauer, K., Pirkl, E., Zentgraf, H., and Schaller, H., 1980, Conversion of bacteriophage fd into an efficient single-stranded DNA vector system, *Mol. Gen. Genet.* **177:**231–242.

Hewitt, J. A., 1975, Miniphage: Class of satellite phage to M13, *J. Gen. Virol.* **26:**87–94.

Hill, D. F., and Petersen, G. B., 1982, Nucleotide sequence of bacteriophage f1 DNA, *J. Virol.* **44:**32–46.

Hobom, G., and Braunitzer, G., 1967, Virusproteine. II. Untersuchung polycyclischer aromatischer amine auf ihre mutagene wirkung am phagen fd, *Hoppe-Seyler's Z. Physiol. Chem.* **348:**804–807.

Hoffmann-Berling, H., and Mazé, R., 1964, Release of male-specific bacteriophages from surviving host bacteria, *Virology* **22:**305–313.

Hoffmann-Berling, H., Durwald, H., and Beulke, I., 1963, Ein fadiger DNA-S phage (fd) und ein spharischer RNS-phage (fr) wirtsspezifisch fur mannliche stamme von *E. coli* III. Biologisches Verhalten von fd und fr, *Z. Naturforsch.* **18b:**893–898.

Holmgren, A., 1985, Thioredoxin, *Annu. Rev. Biochem.* **54:**237–271.

Horabin, J. I., and Webster, R. E., 1986, Morphogenesis of f1 filamentous bacteriophage: Increased expression of gene I inhibits bacterial growth, *J. Mol. Biol.* **188**:403–413.

Horiuchi, K., 1980, Origin of DNA replication of bacteriophage f1 as the signal for termination, *Proc. Natl. Acad. Sci. USA* **77**:5226–5229.

Horiuchi, K., 1983, Co-evolution of a filamentous bacteriophage and its defective interfering particles, *J. Mol. Biol.* **169**:389–407.

Horiuchi, K., 1986, Interaction between gene II protein and the DNA replication origin of bacteriophage f1, *J. Mol. Biol.* **188**:215–223.

Horiuchi, K., and Zinder, N. D., 1972, Cleavage of bacteriophage f1 DNA by the restriction enzyme of *Escherichia coli* B, *Proc. Natl. Acad. Sci. USA* **69**:3220–3224.

Horiuchi, K., and Zinder, N. D., 1976, Origin and direction of synthesis of bacteriophage f1 DNA, *Proc. Natl. Acad. Sci. USA* **73**:2341–2345.

Horiuchi, K., Vovis, G. F., and Zinder, N. D., 1974, Effect of deoxyribonucleic acid length on the adenosine triphophatase activity of *Escherichia coli* restriction endonuclease B, *J. Biol. Chem.* **249**:543–552.

Horiuchi, K., Ravetch, J. V., and Zinder, N. D., 1979, DNA replication of bacteriophage f1 *in vivo*, *Cold Spring Harbor Symp. Quant. Biol.* **43**(P1):389–399.

Hsu, Y.-C., 1968, Propagation or elimination of viral infection in carrier cells, *Bacteriol. Rev.* **32**:387–399.

Huber, H. E., Russel, M., Model, P., and Richardson, C. C., 1986, Interaction of mutant thioredoxins of *Escherichia coli* with the gene 5 protein of phage T7, *J. Biol. Chem.* **261**:15006–15012.

Hunter, G. J., Rowitch, D. H., and Perham, R. N., 1987, Interactions between DNA and coat protein in the structure and assembly of filamentous bacteriophage fd, *Nature* **327**:252–254.

Ikoku, A. S., and Hearst, J. E., 1981, Identification of a structural hairpin in the filamentous chimeric phage M13 Gori1, *J. Mol. Biol.* **151**:245–259.

Ippen-Ihler, K. A., and Minkley, E. G., 1986, The conjugation system of F, the fertility factor of *Escherichia coli*, *Annu. Rev. Genet.* **20**:593–624.

Ito, K., Mandel, G., and Wickner, W., 1979, Soluble precursor of an integral membrane protein: Synthesis of procoat protein in *Escherichia coli* infected with bacteriophage M13, *Proc. Natl. Acad. Sci. USA* **76**:1199–1203.

Ito, K., Wittekind, M., Nomura, M., Shiba, K., Yura, T., Miura, A., and Nashimoto, H., 1983, A temperature-sensitive mutant of *E. coli* exhibiting slow processing of exported proteins, *Cell* **32**:789–797.

Jacob, E., and Hofschneider, P. H., 1969, Replication of the single-stranded DNA bacteriophage M13: Messenger RNA synthesis directed by replicative form DNA, *J. Mol. Biol.* **46**:359–363.

Jacobson, A., 1972, Role of F pili in the penetration of bacteriophage f1, *J. Virol.* **10**:835–843.

Jazwinski, S. M., Marco, R., and Kornberg, A., 1973, A coat protein of the bacteriophage M13 virion participates in membrane-oriented synthesis of DNA, *Proc. Natl. Acad. Sci. USA* **70**:205–209.

Johnston, S., and Ray, D. S., 1984, Interference between M13 and ori M13 plasmids is mediated by a replication enhancer sequence near the viral strand origin, *J. Mol. Biol.* **177**:685–700.

Kaguni, J., and Ray, D. S., 1979, Cloning of a functional replication origin of phage G4 into the genome of phage M13, *J. Mol. Biol.* **135**:863–878.

Kaguni, J. M., and Kornberg, A., 1982, The sigma subunit of RNA polymerase holoenzyme confers specificity in priming M13 viral DNA replication, *J. Biol. Chem.* **257**:5437–5443.

Kansy, J. W., Clack, B. A., and Gray, D. M., 1986, The binding of fd gene 5 protein to polydeoxynucleotides: Evidence from CD measurements for two binding modes, *J. Supramol. Struct.* **3**:1079–1110.

Kim, M. H., and Ray, D. S., 1985, Mutational mechanisms by which an inactive replication origin of bacteriophage M13 is turned on are similar to mechanisms of activation of *ras* proto-oncogenes, *J. Virol.* **53**:871–878.

Kim, M. H., Hines, J. C., and Ray, D. S., 1981, Viable deletions of the M13 complementary strand origin, *Proc. Natl. Acad. Sci. USA* **78**:6784–6788.

King, G. C., and Coleman, J. E., 1987, Two dimensional ^{1}H NMR of gene 5 protein indicates that only two aromatic rings interact significantly with oligodeoxynucleotide bases, *Biochemistry* **26**:2929–2937.

Konings, R. N. H., 1973, Synthesis of phage M13-specific proteins in a DNA-dependent cell-free system, *FEBS Lett.* **35**:155–160.

Konings, R. N. H., and Schoenmakers, J. G. G., 1978, Transcription of the filamentous phage genome, in: *The Single-Stranded DNA Phages* (D. T. Denhardt, D. Dressler, and D. S. Ray, eds.), pp. 507–530, Cold Spring Harbor Laboratory, Cold Spring Harbor, NY.

Konings, R. N. H., Jansen, J., Cuypers, T., and Schoenmakers, J., 1973, Synthesis of bacteriophage M13-specific proteins in a DNA dependent cell-free system. II. *In vitro* synthesis of biologically active gene 5 protein, *J. Virol.* **12**:1466–1472.

Konings, R. N. H., Hulsebos, T., and Vandenhondel, C. A., 1975, Identification and characterization of *in vitro* synthesized gene products of bacteriophage M13, *J. Virol.* **15**:570–584.

Konings, R. N. H., Luiten, R. G. M., and Peeters, B. P. H., 1986, Mike, a chimeric filamentous phage designed for the separate production of either DNA strand of pKUN vector plasmids by F[+] cells, *Gene* **46**:269–276.

Kornberg, A., 1980, *DNA Replication*, W. H. Freeman, San Francisco.

Kornberg, A., 1982, *DNA Replication: 1982 Supplement*, W. H. Freeman, San Francisco.

Kornberg, A., Baker, T. A., Bertsch, L. L., Bramhill, D., Funnell, B. E., Lasken, R. S., Make, H., Maki, S., Kuzuhisa, S., and Wahle, E., 1987, Enzymatic studies of replication of *oriC* plasmids, in: *DNA Replication and Recombination* (R. McMacken and T. J. Kelly, eds.), pp. 137–149, Alan R. Liss, New York.

Kowalczykowski, S. C., Bear, D. G., and Von Hippel, P. H., 1981, Single-stranded DNA binding proteins, in: *The Enzymes*, Vol. 14 (P. D. Boyer, ed.), pp. 373–444, Academic Press, New York.

Kuhn, A., and Wickner, W., 1985a, Isolation of mutants in M13 coat protein that affect its synthesis, processing, and assembly into phage, *J. Biol. Chem.* **260**:15907–15913.

Kuhn, A., and Wickner, W., 1985b, Conserved residues of the leader peptide are essential for cleavage by leader peptidase, *J. Biol. Chem.* **260**:15914–15918.

Kuhn, A., Wickner, W., and Kreil, G., 1986a, The cytoplasmic carboxy terminus of M13 procoat is required for the membrane insertion of its central domain, *Nature* **322**:335–339.

Kuhn, A., Kreil, G., and Wickner, W., 1986b, Both hydrophobic domains of M13 procoat are required to initiate membrane insertion, *EMBO J.* **5**:3681–3685.

Kuhn, A., Kreil, G., and Wickner, W., 1987, Recombinant forms of M13 procoat with an OmpA leader sequence or a large carboxy-terminal extension retain their independence of *secY* function, *EMBO J.* **6**:501–505.

Kuo, T.-T., Lin, Y.-H., Huang, C.-M., Chang, S.-F., Dai, H., and Feng, T.-Y., 1987, The lysogenic cycle of the filamentous phage Cflt from *Xanthomonas campestris* pv. *citri*, *Virology* **156**:305–312.

La Farina, M., 1983, Transcription in bacteriophage f1-infected *Escherichia coli:* Very large RNA species are synthesized on the phage DNA, *Mol. Gen. Genet.* **191**:22–25.

La Farina, M., and Model, P., 1978, Transcription in bacteriophage f1-infected *Escherichia coli.* I. Translation of RNA *in vitro*, *Virology* **86**:368–375.

La Farina, M., and Model, P., 1983, Transcription in bacteriophage f1-infected *Escherichia coli* messenger populations in the infected cell, *J. Mol. Biol.* **164**:377–393.

Langeveld, S. A., Van Mansfeld, A. D. M., Baas, P. D., Jansz, H. S., Van Arkel, G. A., and Weisbeek, P. J., 1978, Nucleotide sequence of the origin of replication in bacteriophage phiX174 RF DNA, *Nature* **271**:417–420.

Lawn, A. M., Meynell, E., Meynell, G. G., and Datta, N., 1967, Sex pili and the classification of sex factors in the enterobacteriaccae, *Nature* **216**:343–346.

Legon, S., Model, P., and Robertson, H. D., 1977, Interaction of rabbit reticulocyte ribosomes with bacteriophage fl messenger RNA and of *Escherichia coli* ribosomes with rabbit globin messenger RNA, *Proc. Natl. Acad. Sci. USA* **74**:2692–2696.

Lemaire, G., Gold, L., and Yarus, M., 1978, Autogenous translational repression of bacteriophage T4 gene 32 expression *in vitro*, *J. Mol. Biol.* **126**:73–90.

Lerner, T. J., and Model, P., 1981, The "steady state" of coliphage fl: DNA synthesis late in infection, *Virology* **115**:282–294.

Lerner, T. J., and Zinder, N. D., 1979, Chromosomal regulation of sexual expression in *Escherichia coli*, *J. Bacteriol.* **137**:1063–1065.

Lerner, T. J., and Zinder, N. D., 1982, Another gene affecting sexual expression of *Escherichia coli*, *J. Bacteriol.* **150**:156–160.

Lica, L., and Ray, D. S., 1977, Replication of bacteriophage M13. XII. *In vivo* cross-linking of a phage-specific DNA binding protein to the single-stranded DNA of bacteriophage M13 by ultraviolet irradiation, *J. Mol. Biol.* **115**:45–59.

Lim, C. J., Haller, B., and Fuchs, J. A., 1985, Thioredoxin is the bacterial protein encoded by fip that is required for filamentous bacteriophage fl assembly, *J. Bacteriol.* **161**:799–802.

Lin, N. S. C., and Pratt, D., 1974, Bacteriophage M13 gene-2 protein; increasing its yield in infected cells, and identification and localization, *Virology* **61**:334–342.

Lin, T. C., Webster, R. E., and Konigsberg, W., 1980, Isolation and characterization of the C and D proteins coded by gene IX and gene VI in the filamentous bacteriophage fl and fd, *J. Biol. Chem.* **255**:10331–10337.

Loeb, T., 1960, Isolation of a bacteriophage specific for the F^+ and Hfr mating types of *Escherichia coli* K12, *Science* **131**:932–933.

Lopez, J., and Webster, R. E., 1982, Minor coat protein composition and location of the A protein in bacteriophage fl spheroids and I forms, *J. Virol.* **42**:1099–1107.

Lopez, J., and Webster, R. E., 1983, Morphogenesis of filamentous bacteriophage fl: Orientation of extrusion and production of polyphage, *Virology* **127**:177–193.

Lopez, J., and Webster, R. E., 1985a, Assembly site of bacteriophage fl corresponds to adhesion zones between the inner and outer membranes of the host cell, *J. Bacteriol.* **163**:1270–1274.

Lopez, J., and Webster, R. E., 1985b, fipB and fipC: Two bacterial loci required for morphogenesis of the filamentous bacteriophage fl, *J. Bacteriol.* **163**:900–905.

Luiten, R. G. M., Schoenmakers, J. G. G., and Konings, R. N. H., 1983, The major coat protein gene of the filamentous *Pseudomonas aeruginosa* phage Pf3: Absence of an N-terminal leader signal sequence, *Nucleic Acids Res.* **11**:8073–8085.

Luiten, R. G. M., Putterman, D. G., Schoenmakers, J. G. G., Konings, R. N. H., and Day, L. A., 1985, Nucleotide sequence of the genome of Pf3, an IncP-1 plasmid-specific filamentous bacteriophage of *Pseudomonas aeruginosa*, *J. Virol.* **56**:268–276.

Lyons, L. B., 1971, Genetic studies of bacteriophage fl, Ph.D. Thesis, Rockefeller University, New York.

Lyons, L. B., and Zinder, N. D., 1972, The genetic map of the filamentous bacteriophage fl, *Virology* **49**:45–60.

Maeda, K., Kneale, G. G., Tsugita, A., Short, N. J., Perham, R. N., Hill, D. F., and Petersen, G. F., 1982, The DNA binding protein of Pf1 filamentous bacteriophage: Amino acid sequence and structure of the gene, *EMBO J.* **1**:255–261.

Makino, S., Woolford, J. L., Tanford, C., and Webster, R. E., 1975, Interaction of deoxycholate and of detergents with coat protein of bacteriophage fl, *J. Biol. Chem.* **250**:4327–4332.

Makowski, L., 1984, Structural diversity in filamentous bacteriophages, in: *The Structures of Biological Macromolecules and Assemblies*, Vol. 1: *The Viruses* (A. McPherson and F. Jurnak, eds.), pp. 203–253, Wiley, New York.

Manning, M., Chrysolgelos, S., and Griffith, J., 1981, Mechanism of coliphage M13 contraction: Intermediate structures trapped at low temperatures, *J. Virol.* **40:**912–919.

Marco, R., Jazwinski, S. M., and Kornberg, A., 1974, Binding, eclipse and penetration of the filamentous bacteriophage M13 in intact and disrupted cells, *Virology* **62:**209–223.

Mark, D. F., and Richardson, C. C., 1976, *Escherichia coli* thioredoxin: A subunit of bacteriophage T7 DNA polymerase, *Proc. Natl. Acad. Sci. USA* **73:**780–784.

Marvin, D. A., 1978, Structure of the filamentous phage virion, in: *The Single-Stranded DNA Phages* (D. T. Denhardt, D. Dressler, and D. S. Ray, eds.), pp. 583–603, Cold Spring Harbor Laboratory, Cold Spring Harbor, NY.

Marvin, D. A., and Hoffmann-Berling, H., 1963, Physical and chemical properties of two new small bacteriophages, *Nature* **219:**485–486.

Marvin, D. A., and Hohn, B., 1969, Filamentous bacterial viruses, *Bacteriol. Rev.* **33:**172–209.

Mazur, B. J., and Model, P., 1973, Regulation of coliphage f1 single-stranded DNA synthesis by a DNA-binding protein, *J. Mol. Biol.* **78:**285–300.

Mazur, B. J., and Zinder, N. D., 1975, The role of gene V protein in f1 single-strand synthesis, *Virology* **68:**490–502.

McEwen, J., and Silverman, P., 1980a, Chromosomal mutations of *Escherichia coli* that alter expression of conjugative plasmid functions, *Proc. Natl. Acad. Sci. USA* **77:**513–517.

McEwen, J., and Silverman, P., 1980b, Genetic analysis of *Escherichia coli* K-12 chromosomal mutants defective in expression of F-plasmid functions. Identification of genes cpxA and cpxB, *J. Bacteriol.* **144:**60–67.

McMacken, R., and Kornberg, A., 1978, Multi-enzyme system for priming replication of φX174 viralDNA, *J. Biol. Chem.* **253:**3313–3319.

McMacken, R., Ueda, K., and Kornberg, A., 1977, Migration of *Escherichia coli* DNA B protein on template DNA strand as a mechanism in initiating DNA replication, *Proc. Natl. Acad. Sci. USA* **74:**4190–4194.

McPherson, A., and Brayer, G. D., 1985, The gene 5 protein and its molecular complexes, in: *Biological Molecules and Assemblies*, Vol. II: *Nucleic Acids and Interactive Proteins* (F. A. Jurnak and A. McPherson, eds.), pp. 325–392, Wiley, New York.

McPherson, A., Jurnak, F. A., Wang, A. H. J., Kolpak, F., Rich, A., Molineux, I., and Fitzgerald, P. M. D., 1980a, The structure of a DNA unwinding protein and its complexes with oligodeoxynucleotides by X-ray diffraction, *Biophys. J.* **32:**155–173.

McPherson, A., Wang, A. H. J., Jurnak, F. A., Molineux, I., Kolpak, F., and Rich, A., 1980b, X-ray diffraction studies on crystalline complexes of the gene 5 DNA-unwinding protein with deoxyoligonucleotides, *J. Biol. Chem.* **255:**3174–3177.

Merriam, V., 1977, Stability of carrier state in bacteriophage M13-infected cells, *J. Virol.* **21:**880–888.

Messing, J., Gronenborn, B., Mullerhill, B., and Hofschneider, P. H., 1977, Filamentous coliphage M13 as a cloning vehicle: Insertion of a *Hind*II fragment of *lac* regulatory region in M13 replicative form *in vitro*, *Proc. Natl. Acad. Sci. USA* **74:**3642–3646.

Meyer, T. F., and Geider, K., 1979a, Bacteriophage fd gene-II protein. I. Purification, involvement in RF replication, and the expression of gene II, *J. Biol. Chem.* **254:**12636–12641.

Meyer, T. F., and Geider, K., 1979b, Bacteriophage fd gene-II protein. II. Specific cleavage and relaxation of supercoiled RF from filamentous phages, *J. Biol. Chem.* **254:**12642–12646.

Meyer, T. F., and Geider, K., 1980, Replication of phage fd with purified proteins, in: *Mechanistic Studies of DNA Replication and Genetic Recombination*, ICN-UCLA Symposium on Molecular and Cellular Biology (B. M. Alberts, ed.), pp. 579–588, Academic Press, New York.

Meyer, T. F., and Geider, K., 1981, Cloning of bacteriophage fd gene 2 and construction of a plasmid dependent on fd gene 2 protein, *Proc. Natl. Acad. Sci. USA* **78:**5416–5420.

Meyer, T. F., and Geider, K., 1982, Enzymatic synthesis of bacteriophage fd viral DNA, *Nature* **296:**828–832.

Meyer, T. F., Geider, K., Kurz, C., and Schaller, H., 1979, Cleavage site of bacteriophage fd gene-II protein in the origin of viral strand replication, *Nature* **278:**365–367.

Meyer, T. F., Beyreuther, K., and Geider, K., 1980, Recognition of two initiation codons for the synthesis of phage fd gene-2 protein, *Mol. Gen. Genet.* **180:**489–494.

Meyer, T. F., Baumel, I., Geider, K., and Bedinger, P., 1981, Replication of phage fd RF with fd gene 2 protein and phage T4 enzymes, *J. Biol. Chem.* **256:**5810–5813.

Meynell, G. G., and Aufreiter, E., 1969, Selection of mutant bacterial sex factors determining altered sex pili, *J. Gen. Microbiol.* **59:**429–430.

Minamishima, Y., Takeya, K., Ohnishi, Y., and Amako, K., 1968, Physicochemical and biological properties of fibrous *Pseudomonas* bacteriophages, *J. Virol.* **2:**208–213.

Minkley, E. G. Jr., Polen, S., Brinton, C. C., and Ippen-Ihler, K., 1976, Identification of the structural gene for F-pilin, *J. Mol. Biol.* **108:**111–121.

Model, P., and Zinder, N. D., 1974, *In vitro* synthesis of bacteriophage f1 proteins, *J. Mol. Biol.* **83:**231–251.

Model, P., Russel, M., and Boeke, J. D., 1981, Filamentous phage assembly: Membrane insertion of the major coat protein, in: *Bacteriophage Assembly* (M. S. DuBow, ed.), pp. 389–400, Alan R. Liss, New York.

Model, P., McGill, C., Mazur, B., and Fulford, W. D., 1982, The replication of bacteriophage f1: Gene V protein regulates the synthesis of gene II protein, *Cell* **29:**329–335.

Modrich, P., and Richardson, C. C., 1975, Bacteriophage T7 deoxyribonucleic acid replication *in vitro*, *J. Biol. Chem.* **250:**5508–5514.

Moore, E. C., Reichard, P., and Thelander, L., 1964, Enzymatic synthesis of deoxyribonucleotides. V. Purification and properties of thioredoxin reductase from *Escherichia coli*, *J. Biol. Chem.* **239:**3445–3452.

Moses, P. B., and Horiuchi, K., 1982, Effects of transposition and deletion upon coat protein gene expression in bacteriophage f1, *Virology* **119:**231–244.

Moses, P. B., and Model, P., 1984, A rho-dependent transcription termination signal in bacteriophage f1, *J. Mol. Biol.* **172:**1–22.

Moses, P. B., Boeke, J. D., Horiuchi, K., and Zinder, N. D., 1980, Restructuring the bacteriophage f1 genome: Expression of gene VIII in the intergenic space, *Virology* **104:**267–278.

Nagel De Zwaig, R., and Luria, S. E., 1967, Genetics and physiology of colicin-tolerant mutants of *Escherichia coli*, *J. Bacteriol.* **94:**1112–1123.

Nakanishi, H., Iida, Y., Maeshima, K., Teramoto, T., Hosaka, Y., and Ozaki, M., 1966, Isolation and properties of bacteriophages of *Vibrio parahaemolyticus*, *Biken J.* **9:**149–157.

Nakashima, Y., and Konigsberg, W., 1974, Reinvestigation of a region of the fd bacteriophage coat protein, *J. Mol. Biol.* **88:**598–600.

Nakashima, Y., Dunker, A. K., Marvin, D. A., and Konigsberg, W., 1974, Amino-acid sequence of a DNA binding-protein, gene 5 product of fd filamentous bacteriophage, *FEBS Lett.* **40:**290–292.

Nakashima, Y., Wiseman, R., Konigsberg, W., and Marvin, D. A., 1975, Primary structure and sidechain interactions of Pf1 filamentous bacterial virus coat protein, *Nature* **253:**68–71.

Nakashima, Y., Frangione, B., Wiseman, R., and Konigsberg, W., 1981, Primary structure of the major coat protein of the filamentous bacterial viruses If1 and IKe, *J. Biol. Chem.* **256:**5792–5797.

Nelson, F. K., Friedman, S. M., and Smith, G. P., 1981, Filamentous phage DNA cloning vectors: A non-infective mutant with a non-polar deletion in gene III, *Virology* **108:**338–350.

Ng, Y. C., and Dunker, A. K., 1981, Effects of metabolic inhibitors on the assembly of fd phage, in: *Bacteriophage Assembly* (M. S. DuBow, ed.), pp. 467–474, Alan R. Liss, New York.

Nishihara, T., and Watanabe, I., 1967, Purification and properties of fibrous DNA phage δA, *Virus* **17:**118–124.

Novotny, C. P., and Fives-Taylor, P., 1974, Retraction of F pili, *J. Bacteriol.* **117:**1306–1311.

Nozaki, Y., Chamberlain, B. K., Webster, R. E., and Tanford, C., 1976, Evidence for a major conformational change of coat protein in assembly of fl bacteriophage, *Nature* **259:**335–337.

Nozaki, Y., Reynolds, J. A., and Tanford, C., 1978, Conformational states of a hydrophobic protein. The coat protein of fd bacteriophage, *Biochemistry* **17:**1239–1246.

Oey, J. L., and Knippers, R., 1972, Properties of the isolated gene 5 protein of bacteriophage fd, *J. Mol. Biol.* **68:**125–138.

Ohkawa, I., and Webster, R. E., 1981, The orientation of the major coat protein of bacteriophage fl in the cytoplasmic membrane of *Escherichia coli*, *J. Biol. Chem.* **256:**9951–9958.

Ohno-Iwashita, Y., and Wickner, W., 1983, Membrane assembly from purified components. 5. Reconstitution of rapid and asymmetric assembly of M13 procoat protein into liposomes which have bacterial leader peptidase, *J. Biol. Chem.* **258:**1895–1900.

Okamoto, T., Sugiura, M., and Takanami, M., 1969, Length of the RNA transcribed on the replicative form DNA of coliphage fd, *J. Mol. Biol.* **45:**101–111.

Okamoto, T., Sugimoto, K., Sugisaki, H., and Takanami, M., 1975, Studies on bacteriophage fd DNA. 2. Localization of RNA initiation sites on cleavage map of fd genome, *J. Mol. Biol.* **95:**33–44.

Oliver, D. B., and Beckwith, J., 1981, *E. coli* mutant pleiotropically defective in the export of secreted proteins, *Cell* **25:**765–772.

Olsen, W. L., Staudenbauer, W. L., and Hofschneider, P. H., 1972, Replication of bacteriophage M13: Specificity of the *Escherichia coli* dnaB function for replication of double-stranded M13 DNA, *Proc. Natl. Acad. Sci USA* **69:**2570–2573.

Opella, S. J., Cross, T. A., Diverdi, J. A., and Sturm, C. F., 1980, Nuclear magnetic resonance of the filamentous bacteriophage fd, *Biophys. J.* **32:**531–548.

Orosz, L., and Wooton, J. C., 1977, Isolation of four phenotypic classes of transfer proficient, pilus-specific-bacteriophage-resistant mutants of an F-like plasmid of *Escherichia coli* K12, *Mol. Gen. Genet.* **157:**223–230.

Panter, R. A., and Symons, R. H., 1966, Isolation and properties of a DNA-containing rod-shaped bacteriophage, *Aust. J. Biol. Sci.* **19:**565–573.

Paradiso, P., and Konigsberg, W., 1982, Photochemical cross linking of protein–nucleic acid complexes. The attachment of the fd gene 5 protein to fd DNA, *J. Biol. Chem.* **257:**1462–1467.

Peeters, B. P. H., Konings, R. N. H., and Schoenmakers, J. G. G., 1983, Characterization of the DNA binding protein encoded by the N-specific filamentous *Escherichia coli* phage IKe. Binding properties of the protein and nucleotide sequence of the gene, *J. Mol. Biol.* **169:**197–215.

Peeters, B. P. H., Peters, R. M., Schoenmakers, J. G. G., and Konings, R. N. H., 1985, Nucleotide sequence and genetic organization of the genome of the N-specific filamentous bacteriophage IKe: Comparison with the genome of the F-specific filamentous phage M13, fd and fl, *J. Mol. Biol.* **181:**27–39.

Peeters, B. P. H., Schoenmakers, J. G. G., and Konings, R. N. H., 1986a, Plasmid pKUN9, a versatile vector for the selective packaging of both DNA strands into single-stranded DNA-containing phage-like particles, *Gene* **41:**39–46.

Peeters, B. P. H., Schoenmakers, J. G. G., and Konings, R. N. H., 1986b, The gene II proteins of the filamentous phages Ike and Ff (M13, fd and fl) are not functionally interchangeable during viral strand replication, *Nucleic Acids Res.* **14:**5067–5080.

Peeters, B. P. H., Schoenmakers, J. G. G., and Konings, R. N. H., 1987, Comparison of the DNA sequences involved in replication and packaging of the filamentous phages IKe and Ff (M13, fd, and fl), *DNA* **6:**139–147.

Pieczenik, G., Model, P., and Robertson, H. D., 1974, Sequence and symmetry in ribosome binding sites of bacteriophage fl RNA, *J. Mol. Biol.* **90:**191–214.

Pieczenik, G., Horiuchi, K., Model, P., McGill, C., Mazur, B. J., Vovis, G. F., and Zinder, N. D., 1975, Is mRNA transcribed from the strand complementary to it in a DNA duplex? *Nature* **253:**131–132.

Pratt, D., 1969, Genetics of single-stranded DNA bacteriophages, *Annu. Rev. Genet.* **3**:343–362.

Pratt, D., and Erdahl, W. S., 1968, Genetic control of bacteriophage M13 DNA synthesis, *J. Mol. Biol.* **37**:181–200.

Pratt, D., Tzagoloff, H., and Erdahl, W. S., 1966, Conditional lethal mutants of the small filamentous coliphage M13. I. Isolation, complementation, cell killing, time of cistron action, *Virology* **30**:397–410.

Pratt, D., Tzagoloff, H., and Beaudoin, J., 1969, Conditional lethal mutants of the small filamentous coliphage M13. II. Two genes for coat proteins, *Virology* **39**:42–53.

Pratt, D., Laws, P., and Griffith, J., 1974, Complex of bacteriophage M13 single-stranded DNA and gene 5 protein, *J. Mol. Biol.* **82**:425–439.

Pretorius, H. T., Klein, M., and Day, L. A., 1975, Gene V protein of fd bacteriophage. Dimer formation and role of tyrosyl groups in DNA binding, *J. Biol. Chem.* **250**:9262–9269.

Putterman, D. G., Casadevall, A., Boyle, P. D., Yang, H. L., Frangione, B., and Day, L. A., 1984, Major coat protein and single-stranded DNA-binding protein of filamentous virus Pf3, *Proc. Natl. Acad. Sci. USA* **81**:699–703.

Rasched, I., and Oberer, E., 1986, Ff coliphages: Structural and functional relationships, *Microbiol. Rev.* **50**:401–427.

Ravetch, J., Horiuchi, K., and Model, P., 1977, Mapping of bacteriophage f1 ribosome binding sites to their cognate genes, *Virology* **81**:341–351.

Ray, D. S., 1969, Replication of bacteriophage M13. II. The role of replicative forms in single-strand synthesis, *J. Mol. Biol.* **43**:631–643.

Ray, D. S., 1970, Replication of bacteriophage M13. VI. Synthesis of M13-specific DNA in the presence of chloramphenical, *J. Mol. Biol.* **53**:239–250.

Ray, D. S., 1977, Replication of filamentous bacteriophages, in: *Comprehensive Virology* (H. Fraenkel-Conrat and R. R. Wagner, eds.), pp. 105–175, Plenum Press, New York.

Ray, D. S., 1978, *In vivo* replication of filamentous phage DNA, in: *The Single-Stranded DNA Phages* (D. T. Denhardt, D. Dressler, and D. S. Ray, eds.), pp. 325–339, Cold Spring Harbor Laboratory, Cold Spring Harbor, NY.

Ray, D. S., Bscheider, H. P., and Hofschneider, P., 1966, Replication of the single-stranded DNA of the male-specific bacteriophage M13. Isolation of intracellular forms of phage-specific DNA, *J. Mol. Biol.* **21**:473–483.

Ray, D. S., Dueber, J., and Suggs, S., 1975, Replication of bacteriophage M13. IX. Requirement of the *Escherichia coli* dnaG function for M13 duplex DNA replication, *J. Virol.* **16**:348–355.

Rivera, M. J., Smits, M. A., Quint, W., Schoenmakers, J. G. G., and Konings, R. N. H., 1978, Expression of bacteriophage M13 DNA *in vivo:* Localization of transcription initiation and termination signal of messenger RNA coding for major capsid protein, *Nucleic Acids Res.* **5**:2895–2912.

Rossomando, E. F., 1969, Studies on the structure of the bacteriophage f1, Ph.D. Thesis, Rockefeller University, New York.

Rossomando, E. F., 1970, Studies on the structural polarity of bacteriophage f1, *Virology* **42**:681–687.

Rossomando, E. F., and Bladen, H. A., 1969, Physical changes associated with heating bacteriophage f1, *Virology* **39**:921–924.

Rossomando, E. F., and Zinder, N. D., 1968, Studies on the bacteriophage f1. I. Alkali-induced disassembly of the phage into DNA and protein, *J. Mol. Biol.* **36**:387–399.

Rowitch, D. H., and Perham, R. N., 1987, Cloning and expression of the filamentous bacteriophage Pf1 major coat protein gene in *Escherichia coli.* Membrane protein processing and virus assembly, *J. Mol. Biol.* **195**:873–884.

Russel, M., and Model, P., 1981, A mutation downstream from the signal peptidase cleavage site affects cleavage but not membrane insertion of phage coat protein, *Proc. Natl. Acad. Sci. USA* **78**:1717–1721.

Russel, M., and Model, P., 1982, Filamentous phage precoat is an integral membrane protein. Analysis by a new method of membrane preparation, *Cell* **28**:177–184.

Russel, M., and Model, P., 1983, A bacterial gene, fip, required for filamentous bacteriophage f1 assembly, *J. Bacteriol.* **154:**1064–1076.

Russel, M., and Model, P., 1984, Replacement of the *fip* gene of *Escherichia coli* by an inactive gene cloned on a plasmid, *J. Bacteriol.* **159:**1034–1039.

Russel, M., and Model, P., 1985a, Thioredoxin is required for filamentous phage assembly, *Proc. Natl. Acad. Sci. USA* **82:**29–33.

Russel, M., and Model, P., 1985b, Direct cloning of the *trxB* gene that encodes thioredoxin reductase, *J. Bacteriol.* **163:**238–242.

Russel, M., and Model, P., 1986, The role of thioredoxin in filamentous phage assembly. Construction, isolation, and characterization of mutant thioredoxins, *J. Biol. Chem.* **261:**14997–15005.

Russel, M., Gold, L., Morrissett, H., and O'Farrell, P. Z., 1976, Translational, autogenous regulation of gene 32 expression during bacteriophage T4 infection, *J. Biol. Chem.* **251:**7263–7270.

Russel, M., Kidd, S., and Kelley, M. R., 1986, An improved filamentous helper phage for generating single-stranded plasmid DNA, *Gene* **45:**333–338.

Salivar, W. O., Tzagoloff, H., and Pratt, D., 1964, Some physico-chemical and biological properties of the rod-shaped coliphage M13, *Virology* **24:**359–371.

Salivar, W. O., Henry, T. J., and Pratt, D., 1967, Purification and properties of diploid particles of coliphage M13, *Virology* **32:**41–51.

Salstrom, J. S., and Pratt, D., 1971, Role of coliphage M13 gene V in single-stranded DNA production, *J. Mol. Biol.* **61:**489–501.

Schaller, H., 1979, The intergenic region and the origins for filamentous phage DNA replication, *Cold Spring Harbor Symp. Quant. Biol.* **43:**401–408.

Schaller, H., Gray, C., and Herrmann, K., 1975, Nucleotide sequence of an RNA polymerase binding site from DNA of bacteriophage fd, *Proc. Natl. Acad. Sci. USA* **72:**737–741.

Schaller, H., Beck, E., and Takanami, M., 1978, Sequence and regulatory signals of the filamentous phage genome, in: *The Single-Stranded DNA Phages* (D. T. Denhardt, D. Dressler, and D. S. Ray, eds.), pp. 139–163, Cold Spring Harbor Laboratory, Cold Spring Harbor, NY.

Schandel, K. A., Maneewannakul, S., Ippen-Ihler, K., and Webster, R. E., 1987, A *traC* mutant that retains sensitivity to f1 bacteriophage but lacks F pili, *J. Bacteriol.* **169:**3151.

Scott, J. F., Eisenberg, S., Bertsch, L. L., and Kornberg, A., 1977, Enzyme system for replication of duplex circular DNA-replicative form of phage πX174. 3. Mechanism of duplex DNA replication revealed by enzymatic studies of phage πX174 catalytic strand separation in advance of replication, *Proc. Natl. Acad. Sci. USA* **74:**193–197.

Scott, J. R., and Zinder, N. D., 1967, Heterozygotes of phage f1, in: *The Molecular Biology of Viruses* (J. S. Colter and W. Paranchych, eds.), pp. 212–218, Academic Press, New York.

Seeburg, H. P., 1975, Analysis of transcriptional control on genome of *Escherichia coli* bacteriophage fd, *Hoppe-Seyler's Z. Physiol. Chem.* **356:**277.

Seeburg, H. P., and Schaller, H., 1975, Mapping and characterization of promoters in bacteriophage fd, f1 and M13, *J. Mol. Biol.* **92:**261–277.

Seeburg, H. P., Nusslein, C., and Schaller, H., 1977, Interaction of RNA polymerase with promoters from bacteriophage fd, *Eur. J. Biochem.* **74:**107–113.

Shen, C. K. J., and Hearst, J. E., 1976, Psoralen-crosslinked secondary structure map of single-stranded virus DNA, *Proc. Natl. Acad. Sci. USA* **73:**2649–2653.

Shen, C. K. J., Ikoku, A., and Hearst, J. E., 1979, Specific DNA orientation in the filamentous bacteriophage fd as probed by psoralen crosslinking and electron-microscopy, *J. Mol. Biol.* **127:**163–175.

Shimamoto, N., and Utiyama, H., 1983, Mechanism and role of cooperative binding of bacteriophage fd gene 5 protein to single-stranded deoxyribonucleic-acid, *Biochemistry* **22:**5869–5878.

Silver, P., Watts, C., and Wickner, W., 1981, Membrane assembly from purified components. 1. Isolated M13 procoat does not require ribosomes or soluble proteins for processing by membranes, *Cell* **25:**341–345.

Silverman, P. M., Rosenthal, S., Mobach, H., and Valentine, R. C., 1968, Two new classes of F-pili mutants of *Escherichia coli* resistant to infection by the male-specific bacteriophage f2, *Virology* **36**:142–146.

Simons, G. F. M., Konings, R. N. H., and Schoenmakers, J. G. G., 1979, Identification of two new capsid proteins in bacteriophage M13, *FEBS Lett.* **106**:8–12.

Simons, G. F. M., Beinterma, J., Duisterwinkel, F. J., Konings, R. N. N., and Schoenmakers, J. G. G., 1981a, Genes VI, VII and IX of bacteriophage M13: Identification of their products as minor capsid proteins, in: *Bacteriophage Assembly* (M. Dubow, ed.), pp. 401–411, Alan R. Liss, New York.

Simons, G. F. M., Konings, R. N. H., and Schoenmakers, J. G. G., 1981b, Genes VI, genes VII, and genes IX of phage M13 code for minor capsid proteins of the virion, *Proc. Natl. Acad. Sci. USA* **78**:4194–4198.

Simons, G. F. M., Veeneman, G. H., Konings, R. N. H., Van Boom, J. H., and Schoenmakers, J. G. G., 1982, Oligonucleotide-directed mutagenesis of gene IX of bacteriophage M13, *Nucleic Acids Res.* **10**:821–832.

Smilowitz, H., 1974a, Bacteriophage f1 infection: Fate of the parental coat protein, *J. Virol.* **13**:94–99.

Smilowitz, H., 1974b, Bacteriophage f1 infection and colicin tolerance, *J. Virol.* **13**:100–106.

Smilowitz, H., Carson, P., and Robbins, P., 1972, Association of newly synthesized f1 major coat protein with infected host cell inner membrane, *J. Supramol. Struct.* **1**:8–18.

Smith, G. P., 1985, Filamentous fusion phage. Novel expression vectors that display cloned antigens on the virion surface, *Science* **228**:1315–1317.

Smith, G. P., 1987, Filamentous phage as cloning vectors, in: *Vectors: A Survey of Molecular Cloning Vectors and Their Uses* (R. L. Rodriguez and D. T. Denhardt, eds.), pp. 61–84.

Smits, M. A., Simons, G., Konings, R. N. H., and Schoenmakers, J. G. G., 1978, Expressions of bacteriophage M13 DNA *in vivo*. 1. Synthesis of phage-specific RNA and protein in minicells, *Biochim. Biophys. Acta* **521**:27–44.

Smits, M. A., Schoenmakers, J. G. G., and Konings, R. N. H., 1980, Expression of bacteriophage M13 DNA *in vivo*. Isolation, identification and characterizations of phage-specific messenger RNA species, *Eur. J. Biochem.* **112**:309–321.

Smits, M. A., Jansen, J., Konings, R. N. H., and Schoenmakers, J. G. G., 1984, Initiation and termination signals for transcription in bacteriophage M13, *Nucleic Acids Res.* **12**:4071–4081.

Steitz, J. A., 1979, Prokaryotic ribosome binding sites, *Methods Enzymol.* **60**:311–321.

Stormo, G. D., Schneider, T. D., Gold, L., and Ehrenfeucht, A., 1982, Use of the perceptron algorithm to distinguish translational initiation sites in *Escherichia coli, Nucleic Acids Res.* **10**:2997–3011.

Sugimoto, K., Okamoto, T., Sugisaki, H., and Takanami, M., 1975, Nucleotide sequence of an RNA polymerase binding site on bacteriophage fd DNA, *Nature* **253**:410–414.

Sugimoto, K., Sugisaki, H., Okamoto, T., and Takanami, M., 1977, Studies on bacteriophage fd DNA. 4. Sequence of messenger RNA for major coat protein gene, *J. Mol. Biol.* **111**:487–507.

Sugiura, M., Okamoto, T., and Takanami, M., 1969, Starting nucleotide sequences of RNA synthesized on the replicative form DNA of coliphage fd, *J. Mol. Biol.* **43**:299–315.

Sun, T.-P., and Webster, R. E., 1986, *fii*, a bacterial locus required for filamentous phage infection and its relation to colicin-tolerant *tolA* and *tolB, J. Bacteriol.* **165**:107–115.

Sun, T.-P., and Webster, R. E., 1987, Nucleotide sequence of a gene cluster involved in the entry of the E colicins and the single-stranded DNA of infecting filaentous phage into *Escherichia coli, J. Bacteriol.* **169**:2667–2674.

Tabak, H. F., Griffith, J., Geider, K., Schaller, H., and Kornberg, A., 1974, Initiation of deoxyribonucleic acid synthesis. VII. A unique location of gap in the M13 replicative duplex synthesized *in vitro, J. Biol. Chem.* **249**:3049–3054.

Tabor, S., Huber, H. E., and Richardson, C. C., 1986, *Escherichia coli* thioredoxin: An accessory protein for bacteriophage T7 DNA polymerase, in: *Thioredoxin and Glu-*

taredoxin Systems: Structure and Function (A. Holmgren, C.-I. Branden, H. Jornvall, and B.-M. Sjoberg, eds.), pp. 285–300, Raven Press, New York.

Tadakuma, T., and Watanabe, I., 1968, Formation of fibrous bacteriophage δA. II. Effects of Cm on DNA replication, Jpn. J. Bacteriol. 23:478–479.

te Riele, H., Michel, B., and Ehrlich, S. D., 1986, Are single-stranded circles intermediates in plasmid DNA replication? EMBO J. 5:631–637.

Thomas, G. J. Jr., Prescott, B., and Day, L. A., 1983, Structure similarity, difference and variability in the filamentous viruses fd, If1, IKe, Pf1 and Xf. Investigation by laser Raman spectroscopy, J. Mol. Biol. 165:321–356.

Tomoeda, M., Inuzuka, M., and Date, T., 1975, Bacterial sex pili, Prog. Biophys. Mol. Biol. 30:23–56.

Torbet, J., and Maret, G., 1981, High-field magnetic birefringence study of the structure of rod-like phages Pf1 and fd in solution, Biopolymers 20:2657–2669.

Torbet, J., Gray, D. M., Gray, C. W., Marvin, D. A., and Siegrist, H., 1981, Structure of the fd DNA–gene 5 protein complex in solution. A neutron small-angle scattering study, J. Mol. Biol. 146:305–320.

Trenkner, E., Bonhoeffer, F., and Gierer, A., 1967, The fate of the protein component of bacteriophage fd during infection, Biochem. Biophys. Res. Commun. 28:932–939.

Tseng, B. Y., and Marvin, D. A., 1972, Filamentous bacterial viruses. V. Asymmetric replication of fd duplex deoxyribonucleic acid, Virology 10:371–383.

Tsugita, A., and Kneale, G. G., 1985, Identification of lysine residues at the binding site of bacteriophage Pf1 DNA-binding protein, Biochem. J. 228:193–199.

Tzagoloff, H., and Pratt, D., 1964, The initial steps in infection with coliphage M13, Virology 24:372–380.

Van Dorp, B., Schneck, P. K., and Staudenbauer, W. L., 1979, Replication of M13 duplex DNA in soluble extracts of Escherichia coli, Eur. J. Biochem. 94:445–450.

Van Wezenbeek, P. M. G. F., Hulsebos, T. J. M., and Schoenmakers, J. G. G., 1980, Nucleotide sequence of the filamentous bacteriophage M13 DNA genome; comparison with phage fd, Gene 11:129–148.

Vicuna, R., Hurwitz, J., Wallace, S., and Girard, M., 1977, Selective inhibition of in vitro DNA synthesis dependent on πX174 compared with fd DNA, J. Biol. Chem. 252:2524–2533.

Von Heijne, G., 1981, On the hydrophobic nature of signal sequences, Eur. J. Biochem. 116:419–422.

Vovis, G. F., and Ohsumi, M., 1978, The filamentous phages as transducing particle, in: The Single-Stranded DNA Phages (D. T. Denhardt, D. Dressler, and D. S. Ray, eds.), pp. 445–448, Cold Spring Harbor Laboratory, Cold Spring Harbor, NY.

Watts, C., Silver, P., and Wickner, W., 1981, Membrane assembly from purified components. 2. Assembly of M13 procoat into liposomes reconstituted with purified leader peptidase, Cell 25:347–353.

Webster, R. E., and Cashman, J. S., 1973, Abortive infection of Escherichia coli with the bacteriophage f1: Cytoplasmic membrane proteins and the f1 DNA-gene 5 protein complex, Virology 55:20–38.

Webster, R. E., and Lopez, J., 1985, Structure and assembly of the class I filamentous bacteriophage, in: Virus Structure and Assembly (S. Casjens, ed.), pp. 235–268, Jones and Bartlett, Boston.

Webster, R. E., and Rementer, M., 1980, Replication of bacteriophage f1—a complex containing gene II protein in gene V mutant-infected bacteria, J. Mol. Biol. 139:393–405.

Webster, R. E., Grant, R. A., and Hamilton, L. A. W., 1981, Orientation of the DNA in the filamentous bacteriophage f1, J. Mol. Biol. 152:357–374.

Wickner, W., 1975, Asymmetric orientation of a phage coat protein in cytoplasmic membrane of Escherichia coli, Proc. Natl. Acad. Sci. USA 72:4749–4753.

Wickner, W., 1976, Assymetric orientation of phage M13 coat protein in Escherichia coli cytoplasmic membranes and in synthetic vesicles, Proc. Natl. Acad. Sci. USA 73:1159–1163.

Wickner, W., and Kornberg, A., 1974, Novel form of RNA-polymerase from *Escherichia coli*, *Proc. Natl. Acad. Sci. USA* **71**:4425–4428.

Wickner, W., Brutlag, D., Schekman, R., and Kornberg, A., 1972, RNA synthesis initiates *in vitro* converson of M13 DNA to its replicative form, *Proc. Natl. Acad. Sci. USA* **69**:965–969.

Wickner, W., Mandel, G., Zwizinski, C., Bates, M., and Killick, T., 1978, Synthesis of phage M13 coat protein and its assembly into membranes *in vitro*, *Proc. Natl. Acad. Sci. USA* **75**:1754–1758.

Willets, N., and Skurray, R., 1980, The conjugation system of F-like plasmids, *Annu. Rev. Genet.* **14**:41–76.

Willetts, N. S., Moore, P. M., and Pranchcych, W., 1980, Variant pili produced by mutants of the F*lac* plasmid, *J. Gen. Microbiol.* **117**:455–464.

Wolfe, P. B., Silver, P., and Wickner, W., 1982, The isolation of homogeneous leader peptidase from a strain of *Escherichia coli* which overproduces the enzyme, *J. Biol. Chem.* **257**:7898–7902.

Wolfe, P. B., Rice, M., and Wickner, W., 1985, Effects of two sec genes on protein assembly into the plasma membrane of *Escherichia coli*, *J. Biol. Chem.* **260**:1836–1841.

Woolford, J. L., 1976, The interaction of the major coat protein of bacteriophage f1 with the membranes of *E. coli* and with detergents, Ph.D. Thesis, Duke University, Durham, NC.

Woolford, J. L., Steinman, H. M., and Webster, R. E., 1977, Adsorption protein of bacteriophage f1: Solubilization in deoxycholate and localization in f1 virion, *Biochemistry* **16**:2694–2700.

Yang, M.-K., and Kuo, T.-T., 1984, A physical map of the filamentous bacteriophage Cf genome, *J. Gen. Virol.* **65**:1173–1181.

Yanisch-Perron, C., Vieira, J., and Messing, J., 1985, Improved M13 phage cloning vectors and host strains: Nucleotide sequences of the M13mp18 and pUC19 vectors, *Gene* **33**:103–119.

Yarranton, G. T., and Gefter, M. L., 1979, Enzyme-catalyzed DNA unwinding: Studies on *Escherichia coli* rep protein, *Proc. Natl. Acad. Sci. USA* **76**:1658–1662.

Yen, T. S. B., and Webster, R. E., 1981, Bacteriophage f1 gene II and X proteins. Isolation and characterization of the products of two overlapping genes, *J. Biol. Chem.* **256**:11259–11265.

Yen, T. S. B., and Webster, R. E., 1982, Translational control of bacteriophage f1 gene II and gene X proteins by gene V protein, *Cell* **29**:337–345.

Zimmermann, R., Watts, C., and Wickner, W., 1982, The biosynthesis of membrane-bound M13 coat protein; energetics and assembly intermediates, *J. Biol. Chem.* **257**:6529–6536.

Zinder, N. D., 1973, Resistance to colicins E3 and K induced by infection with bacteriophage f1, *Proc. Natl. Acad. Sci. USA* **70**:3160–3164.

Zinder, N. D., 1974, Recombination in bacteriophage f1, in: *Mechanisms in Recombination* (R. F. Grell, ed.), pp. 19–28, Plenum, New York.

Zinder, N. D., 1978, Genetic recombination, in: *The Single-Stranded DNA Phages* (D. T. Denhardt, D. Dressler, and D. S. Ray, eds.), pp. 403–415, Cold Spring Harbor Laboratory, Cold Spring Harbor, NY.

Zinder, N. D., and Boeke, J. D., 1982, The filamentous phage (Ff) as vectors for recombinant DNA—A review, *Gene* **19**:1–10.

Zinder, N. D., and Horiuchi, K., 1985, Multiregulatory element of filamentous bacteriophages, *Microbiol. Rev.* **49**:101–106.

Zinder, N. D., Valentine, R. C., Roger, M., and Stoekenius, W., 1963, f1, a rod-shaped male-specific bacteriophage that contains DNA, *Virology* **20**:638–640.

Zwizinski, C., and Wickner, W., 1980, Purification and characterization of leader (signal) peptidase from *Escherichia coli*, *J. Biol. Chem.* **255**:7973–7977.

Zwizinski, C., and Wickner, W., 1982, The purification of m13 procoat, a membrane-protein precursor, *EMBO J.* **1**:573–578.

CHAPTER 7

Bacteriophage N4

Diane R. Kiino and Lucia B. Rothman-Denes

I. INTRODUCTION

Coliphage N4 is a lytic phage specific for *Escherichia coli* K12 with a linear double-stranded genome 72 kbp in length. The phage, originally isolated from the sewers of Genoa (Schito *et al.*, 1965), presents several unique features including the use of three different DNA-dependent RNA polymerases to transcribe its genome, a virion-encapsulated RNA polymerase which is injected along with the phage DNA upon infection, and the presence of 3' extensions at each end of its linear genome.

II. THE VIRION

Electron microscopy of negatively stained N4 virions shows a hexagonally shaped head approximately 700 Å in diameter, a base plate, a small noncontractile tail, and a number of short tail fibers originating from the junction between the head and the tail (Fig. 1A). The particle weight is about 83×10^6, with 47–50% of that weight being DNA (Schito *et al.*, 1966a). Virions are composed of at least 11 proteins ranging in denatured molecular weight from 16,500 to 350,000 as determined by SDS-PAGE (Falco *et al.*, 1980). The major capsid protein, which makes up 65% of the total protein of the virion, is MW 48,000.

DIANE R. KIINO AND LUCIA B. ROTHMAN-DENES • Departments of Biochemistry and Molecular Biology, and Molecular Genetics and Cell Biology, University of Chicago, Chicago, Illinois 60637.

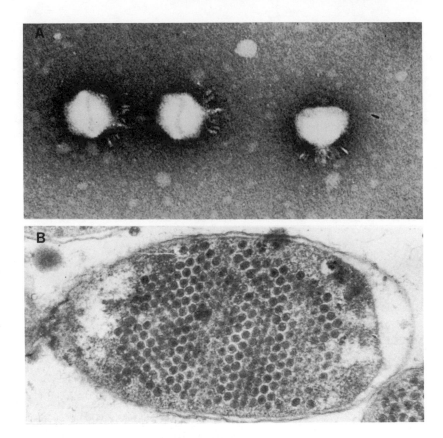

FIGURE 1. (A) Electron micrograph of bacteriophage N4 virions stained with 2% phosphotungstic acid. ×175,000. (Courtesy of M. Ohtsuki, University of Chicago.) (B) Electron micrograph of an ultrathin section of *E. coli* K12S 4 h after N4 infection. ×44,000. Courtesy of Dr. G. C. Schito, Institute of Microbiology, University of Genoa.

III. THE GENOME

The genome is a linear double-stranded DNA molecule approximately 72 kbp in length (Sinha *et al.*, 1973; Zivin *et al.*, 1980) with a G+C content of 44 moles% (Schito *et al.*, 1966b). Direct repeats of variable length, 390–440 bp, and 3′ extensions are present at the ends of the genome (Zivin *et al.*, 1980; Ohmori *et al.*, 1988). The left end is relatively unique, with microheterogeneity at the 3′ terminus yielding primarily 5- or 6-base 3′ protruding sequences: 3′-CATAA or 3′-CATAAA. In contrast, at least six discrete families of the right end exist, differing in length by 10 bp and giving rise to the variability in the length of the terminal repeats. Each of these families of ends has a microheterogeneity of length with 1- to 3-base 3′ extensions (Fig. 2) (Ohmori *et al.*, 1988).

Surprisingly, the N4 genome is resistant to cleavage by a wide range

Left ends

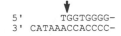

```
5'          TGGTGGGG-
3' CATAAACCACCCC-
```

Right ends

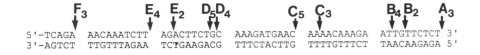

```
      F₃              E₄ E₂  D₅D₄              C₅ C₃            B₄ B₂    A₃
5'-TCAGA   AACAAATCTT  AGACTTCTGC  AAAGATGAAC  AAAACAAAGA  ATTGTTCTCT 3'
3'-AGTCT   TTGTTTAGAA  TCTGAAGACG  TTTCTACTTG  TTTTGTTTCT  TAACAAGAGA 5'
```

FIGURE 2. Structure of the ends of the N4 genome. Arrows indicate ends. A_n to F_n indicate specific ends for some members of each of the six families, A to F.

of restriction endonucleases including *Ava*I, *Bam*HI, *Ban*I, *Ban*II, *Cla*I, *Eco*RI, *Eco*RV, *Hind*III, *Kpn*I, *Nae*I, *Nar*I, *Nco*I, *Pst*I, *Pvu*I, *Pvu*II, *Sal*I, *Sma*I, *Sph*I, *Sst*I, *Sst*II, and *Xho*II. *Hae*II, *Mlu*I, and *Nru*I cleave the 72-kb genome only once (Ohmori *et al.*, 1988; Zivin *et al.*, 1980). Fragments of N4 cloned into *E. coli* vectors remain resistant to these restriction enzymes, indicating that resistance is due to the absence of enzyme recognition sequences and not to phage-induced base modifications or an N4-encoded antirestriction activity (Malone *et al.*, 1988; Krüger and Bickle, 1983). This finding is not unprecedented. The genome of T7 is notorious for lacking recognition sequences for restriction enzymes present in enterobacteria, and the sequenced fraction of the φ29 genome lacks *Bacillus* restriction sites (Rosenberg *et al.*, 1979; Ito and Roberts, 1979; Sharp, 1986). The N4 genome is also resistant to those restriction enzymes present in enterobacteria. We speculate that this reflects the host range of N4 in nature.

IV. N4 ADSORPTION

N4 infection is initiated by the attachment of the phage to at most five sites per bacterium. To characterize the N4 receptor, we have isolated *E. coli* mutants unable to adsorb phage N4 (D. Kiino, unpublished). Unexpectedly, the mutations map to three loci on the *E. coli* chromosome. Most of these independent mutations map to a locus approximately 15% linked to *purE* by P1 cotransduction. It is likely that this locus defines the structural gene for the N4 receptor. Although the genes for two previously characterized outer-membrane proteins, *fepA* and *ompT*, map within this region (McIntosh *et al.*, 1979; Rupprecht *et al.*, 1983), neither is the N4 receptor gene. A strain containing a *fepA* deletion remains N4-sensitive, and plasmids carrying *ompT* do not complement our mutations. Therefore, we conclude that the N4 receptor is encoded by a previously undescribed gene: *nfrA*. Screening of an *E. coli* DNA library has yielded a clone that complements all of the mutations that map to *nfrA*.

Two adsorption mutants do not map to *nfrA* and are not complemented by the clone described above. These mutations may define genes involved in the regulation of expression of the N4 receptor. Alternatively, the N4 receptor may be composed of multiple components, and these genes encode some of these other components. Further genetic analysis should distinguish between these possibilities. The characterization of the N4 receptor protein will provide insights into injection of the viral genome and RNA polymerase.

V. N4 GROWTH CYCLE

A. Early Events

The first detectable event after N4 infection is early transcription, which is catalyzed by the virion-encapsulated RNA polymerase. Soon thereafter, host replication stops. This requires an early gene product, since infection in the presence of chloramphenicol or by UV-attenuated phages fails to inhibit host DNA replication (Rothman-Denes *et al.*, 1972; Schito, 1973). The host chromosome remains intact, however, differing from infections by other lytic bacteriophages, which generally degrade the host DNA (Luria and Human, 1950; Mathews, 1977; Snustad *et al.*, 1983). Transcription of host cAMP-dependent operons is also inhibited after N4 infection, but, in general, host RNA transcription continues unaffected (Rothman-Denes *et al.*, 1972).

B. Intermediate Events

Three products of N4 early transcription, proteins of MW 30,000, 40,000, and 15,000, are required for the synthesis of N4 middle transcripts which begin to appear 3 min after infection. These transcripts encode, in part, proteins required for N4 DNA replication. N4-specific DNA synthesis begins approximately 10 min after infection (Rothman-Denes and Schito, 1974).

C. Late Events

Late RNA synthesis requires the activity of the *E. coli* RNA polymerase and begins 13–15 min after infection. Approximately 30 min after infection, the first progeny appear (Schito, 1974). Rather than actively lysing the host cell like some other bacteriophages, up to 3000 N4 particles per infected cell accumulate intracellularly over a 3-h period (Pesce *et al.*, 1969). At this time, phase contrast microscopy shows refractive polar regions, and electron microscopy reveals enlarged cells filled with paracrystalline arrays of virions (Fig. 1B) (Schito, 1967, 1974). It is therefore easy to obtain high-titer lysates of N4 in a situation analogous to obtaining high-titer lysates of phage lambda defective in the lysis gene, S (Adhya *et al.*, 1971).

VI. N4 TRANSCRIPTION

Transcription of the N4 genome can be divided into three temporal stages referred to as early, middle, and late (Zivin *et al.*, 1981). RNA synthesis during each of these three stages is catalyzed by a different RNA polymerase, two of which are N4-coded, and the third being the *E. coli* RNA polymerase (Rothman-Denes and Schito, 1974; Vander Laan *et al.*, 1977; Falco and Rothman-Denes, 1979; Zivin *et al.*, 1981). DNA–RNA hybridization analysis shows that early and middle transcription occur at the left end of the genome and proceed with a rightward polarity, whereas late transcription occurs at the right end of the genome with a leftward polarity (see Fig. 3) (Zivin *et al.*, 1981). We will now discuss each stage of N4 transcription in greater detail.

A. Early Transcription

Most bacterial DNA viruses, such as lambda, the T-even, and T-odd phages, exploit the host RNA polymerase to carry out transcription of their early genes (Rabussay and Geiduschek, 1977; Weisberg *et al.*, 1977). N4 is unique, however, because it carries its own phage-encoded RNA polymerase which is injected along with the phage genome upon infection. This rifampicin-resistant RNA polymerase transcribes the early genes during the first 5 min of infection. The activity, first described as a rifampicin- and chloramphenicol-resistant activity, has since been purified to homogeneity from N4 virions (Rothman-Denes and Schito, 1974; Falco *et al.*, 1977, 1980). The purified enzyme consists of a single polypeptide with a native molecular weight of 320,000, making it one of the largest polypeptides known. The enzyme is purified from virions where it is present in 1–2 copies (Falco *et al.*, 1980). N4 temperature-sensitive mutations conferring defects in early transcription map in the N4 virion RNA polymerase, demonstrating unequivocally its role in N4 early transcription (Falco *et al.*, 1977). *In vitro*, this RNA polymerase strongly prefers denatured N4 DNA as a template, having little activity on native N4 DNA or heterologous denatured or native DNAs (Falco *et*

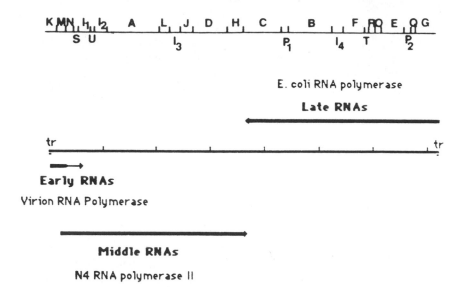

FIGURE 3. Top: *Hpa*I restriction endonuclease map of N4 DNA (Zivin *et al.*, 1980). Bottom: Transcriptional map of the N4 genome (Zivin *et al.*, 1981). Arrows indicate direction of transcription of each RNA class. The thickness of the arrow represents the relative amount of transcription through the region. The identity of the enzyme responsible for each transcription is shown. Terminal repeats (tr) are indicated.

al., 1978). Transcription of denatured N4 DNA by the purified enzyme is asymmetric and restricted to the early region of the N4 genome. Moreover, initiation occurs at unique sites which coincide with the sites of *in vivo* early transcription initiation (Haynes and Rothman-Denes, 1985).

The DNA sequences flanking the sites of early N4 transcription initiation, aligned with respect to the initiating nucleotide (+1), are shown in Fig. 4 (Haynes and Rothman-Denes, 1985). The first initiation site, P1, is located 116 bp from the left end of the genome and, because it lies in the terminal redundancy, is also present at the right end. P2 and P3 are located approximately 580 bp and 3 kbp from the left end of the genome, respectively. The sequences share homology between −18 and +1, with the longest region being a GC-rich heptamer centered at −12. The activity of the N4 virion RNA polymerase on these sites, when present on single-stranded vectors (M13mp7), has shown unequivocally that the determinants of promoter-RNA polymerase interaction are present on the template DNA strand (P. Markiewicz and A. Glucksmann, unpublished; Rothman-Denes *et al.*, 1985). Deletion analysis indicates that this region is important for promoter activity (P. Markiewicz, unpublished). Nucleotide changes at the conserved positions reduce *in vitro* activity, demonstrating that these bases are required for RNA polymerase recognition (A. Glucksmann, unpublished; Rothman-Denes *et al.*, 1987). Finally, sev-

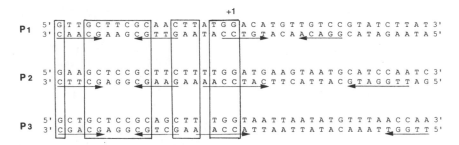

FIGURE 4. Sequence of the N4 virion RNA polymerase promoters. Conserved sequences are boxed. Arrows indicate the inverted repeats. +1 indicates the site of transcription initiation. From Haynes and Rothman-Denes (1985).

eral heterologous denatured DNAs support, although at a low level, virion RNA polymerase transcription at specific sites. Inspection of these sites has revealed that they show weak homology to N4 virion RNA polymerase promoters (Rothman-Denes *et al.*, 1985; Markiewicz *et al.*, 1988).

Each N4 virion RNA polymerase initiation site also contains two sets of inverted repeats, the first of which is centered around the conserved heptamer. The second set of inverted repeats is less well conserved, differing in the length of and the distance between the repeats. Oligonucleotide-directed, site-specific mutagenesis of both sets of inverted repeats has shown that only the upstream one is necessary for promoter activity on a single-stranded template (Rothman-Denes *et al.*, 1987). It is tempting to speculate that the formation of a stem-loop structure at this set of inverted repeats is required for productive RNA polymerase-promoter recognition.

It is unlikely, however, that denatured DNA serves as the *in vivo* template for this RNA polymerase, so we thought that our *in vitro* assay may lack host factors which allow transcription from a native N4 DNA template. In characterizing the N4 RNA polymerase, Falco *et al.* (1978) found that the DNA gyrase inhibitor coumermycin blocked early N4 transcription in drug-sensitive but not drug-resistant cells. This suggested that negative supercoiling of the DNA template was necessary for early transcription. The virion RNA polymerase does not bind to promoter-containing, double-stranded DNAs (Haynes and Rothman-Denes, 1985). Transient opening of the DNA helix induced by negative supercoiling might facilitate productive interaction between the template and RNA polymerase. However, supercoiled template alone is not sufficient for transcriptional activity *in vitro*.

Since single-stranded DNA-binding proteins shift the helix-coil equilibrium toward an open DNA conformation, we tested the ability of cells carrying the *ssb1* mutation in the *E. coli* single-stranded DNA-binding protein (SSB) to support N4 growth. We found that *E. coli* SSB is required for N4 early RNA synthesis (Rothman-Denes *et al.*, 1985). Furthermore, *E. coli* SSB activates transcription on double-stranded supercoiled template *in vitro* (Rothman-Denes *et al.*, 1985). SSB does not activate transcription on a linear double-stranded or relaxed circular DNA template. Transcriptional activation by SSB is specific. Other single-stranded DNA-binding proteins tested cannot substitute for *E. coli* SSB (i.e., T7 gene 2.5 protein, T4 gene 32 protein, and N4 DBP), and antibodies to *E. coli* SSB abolish SSB transcriptional activation (P. Markiewicz, unpublished). Optimal activity on supercoiled templates occurs at a low SSB : DNA ratio, and transcription initiation occurs specifically at early N4 promoters.

We have considered three possibilities to explain the role of supercoiling and SSB in N4 virion RNA polymerase promoter activation (Rothman-Denes *et al.*, 1985). SSB binding to single-stranded regions on supercoiled DNA could allow virion RNA polymerase to bind and then migrate along the DNA to a promoter. Alternatively, SSB might bind specifically at the promoter, at single-stranded regions created by supercoiling. Virion RNA polymerase would recognize the promoter's sequence and structural elements in the same manner that it does on single-stranded DNA. Finally, SSB might interact specifically with RNA polymerase to provide it with the ability to interact productively with the promoter on a double-stranded, supercoiled template. We do not currently know whether activation occurs through SSB-RNA polymerase interactions, SSB-template interactions, or a combination of these. The inability of other single-stranded DNA-binding proteins to substitute for SSB indicates that SSB is not merely stabilizing single-stranded regions on the template and might argue for SSB-RNA polymerase interactions. Footprinting analysis on denatured N4 DNA has revealed that *E. coli* SSB, but not other single-stranded DNA-binding proteins, is able to interact specifically with templates carrying early N4 promoters (Glucksmann and Rothman-Denes, 1986). It may therefore not be necessary to invoke protein-protein interaction between N4 RNA polymerase and SSB, but a sequence-specific interaction between SSB and the N4 early promoters.

The availability of an *in vitro* transcription system that recognizes the promoters on a double-stranded template allowed us to define the determinants of termination for the N4 virion RNA polymerase. Preliminary mapping of *in vivo* transcripts suggested the existence of a defined termination site in *Hpa*I fragment K approximately 1300 bp from the left end of the genome (L. Haynes, unpublished) (Fig. 3). Cloning of that region downstream from a virion RNA polymerase promoter leads to specific termination. Sequencing of the template at the site of termination revealed a nine-base palindrome separated by five bases, followed by a row of five thymidines (C. Malone, unpublished). These results suggest that the sequence determinants for termination by the N4 virion RNA polymerase may be similar to eubacterial factor-independent termination sequences (Platt, 1986).

B. Middle Transcription

N4 middle transcripts appear by 3 min after infection (Zivin et al., 1981) and are synthesized by a second phage-encoded RNA polymerase (N4 RNA polymerase II). Middle transcription differs from early transcription in that it is rifampicin-resistant but chloramphenicol-sensitive (Rothman-Denes and Schito, 1974; Vander Laan et al., 1977; Falco and Rothman-Denes, 1979a). N4 middle RNA synthesis requires the activity of three N4 early gene products (Rothman-Denes and Schito, 1974; Zehring et al., 1983). Two of these gene products, p4 and p7, are soluble and have been purified to homogeneity using an in vitro complementation assay (Zehring and Rothman-Denes, 1983; Zehring et al., 1983). The native molecular weight of p4 is 40,000, and that of p7 is 30,000. These two proteins constitute a heterodimeric rifampicin-resistant RNA polymerase, N4 RNA polymerase II.

Affinity-labeling experiments (Grachev et al., 1986) have shown that the 30,000-MW subunit contains the nucleoside triphosphate binding site (A. Schaffner and K. Abrevaya, unpublished). The preferred template for N4 RNA polymerase II is denatured DNA with little or no activity on N4 or heterologous native DNAs. Transcription on denatured N4 DNA occurs in a random fashion, however, and is not specific for in vivo sites of middle-transcription initiation. The third protein required for N4 middle RNA synthesis, p17, is a DNA-inner membrane–associated peptide of MW 15,000 (Zehring et al., 1983). We have not been able to purify this protein owing to its very hydrophobic nature and its tight association with the bacterial inner membrane. Preliminary in vitro evidence indicates that p17 may be the factor that confers specificity for N4 middle promoters and allows transcription from a native N4 DNA template (K. Abrevaya, personal communication).

Middle transcription spans 30 kb of the N4 genome, the leftmost region being transcribed in both the early and middle modes (see Fig. 3). Several approaches were required to determine the sites of middle-transcription initiation. Initially, plasmids carrying cloned N4 fragments from the middle region were tested in vivo for their ability to support rifampicin-resistant, plasmid-specific RNA synthesis dependent on N4 infection and more specifically on p4, p7, and p17 functions (Zehring et al., 1983; K. Abrevaya, unpublished). Fragments imparting that property were analyzed for the ability to hybridize to N4 RNAs that had been radiolabeled in vitro with [α-^{32}P]GTP and vaccinia guanylyl transferase.

Finally, in vivo sites of middle-transcription initiation were mapped by S1-nuclease analysis. Fragments yielding defined S1 products were also totally protected from S1 digestion, suggesting extensive overlapping transcription in this region of the genome (K. Abrevaya, unpublished). Conserved regions at seven sites of middle-transcription initiation are presented in Fig. 5. The sequence 3'–t/aAAAT–5' is present at the +1 region, and the sequence 3'–Tt/aCTGGACa/t–5' is present 14–21 nu-

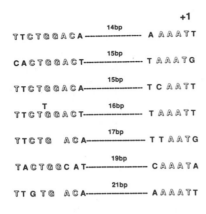

FIGURE 5. Conserved sequences at *in vivo* middle N4 RNA synthesis transcription initiation sites. The template strand sequence is shown. A consensus sequence is shown at the bottom. From K. Abrevaya (personal communication).

cleotides upstream (K. Abrevaya, personal communication; Rothman-Denes *et al.*, 1987).

The identification of sites of N4 middle-transcription initiation has permitted us to develop an *in vitro* system where utilization of these sites is dependent on purified N4 RNA polymerase II and DNA-membrane salt-wash complex from N4-infected cells containing p17 (K. Abrevaya, unpublished). This system will allow a genetic analysis of the N4 middle promoters and the purification of p17 to establish its role in N4 middle transcription.

C. Late Transcription

N4 late transcription is rifampicin-sensitive in rifampicin-sensitive strains of *E. coli* but resistant in resistant hosts, indicating that it is catalyzed by the host RNA polymerase. Indeed, temperature-sensitive *E. coli* mutants in the β or β′ subunits of RNA polymerase are able to support N4 growth at the permissive but not the restrictive temperature (Zivin *et al.*, 1981). Late N4 transcripts begin to appear about 12 min after infection, originating from the right half of the genome and proceeding with a leftward polarity. Although these transcripts appear after N4 DNA replication has started, their appearance is not dependent on concurrent or previous N4 DNA replication. N4 mutants defective in the N4-coded DNA polymerase (*dnp*) or in *dns*, another N4 gene required for replication, are able to produce late transcripts (N. Y. Baek, unpublished). Interestingly, N4 mutants defective in the N4-coded, single-stranded DNA-binding protein are defective not only in N4 DNA replication but also in late transcription (N. Y. Baek, unpublished). The implication of these results is under investigation.

Sites of late N4 transcription initiation have been identified by S1-nuclease mapping (N. Y. Baek, unpublished). Sequencing of five such regions shows weak homology to the *E. coli* promoter consensus sequence at the −10 and −35 regions (Fig. 6). In addition, there is no strong sequence homology shared by the late promoters at the −10 or −35 regions. A conserved sequence (5'AGTCGGTT3') is present, however, around the site of transcription initiation.

As mentioned previously, transcription of cellular genes by host RNA polymerase continues after N4 infection (Rothman-Denes *et al.*, 1972), indicating that the enzyme remains active. The rate of host transcription is reduced to half that in uninfected cells only after the onset of N4 DNA replication (Rothman-Denes *et al.*, 1972). Why is the onset of late transcription delayed? An attractive possibility is the physical inaccessibility of the late region of the genome early after infection due to the nature of the injection process itself. Indeed, polar injection of the DNA starting at the left (early) end would preclude the utilization of the right half of the genome as a template by the *E. coli* transcriptional machinery. This cannot be the case, however, since replication of the genome precedes late transcription. Alternatively, late promoter activation may occur through the phage-induced appearance of an activating factor which allows recognition of late N4 promoters by the host RNA polymerase either through a modification of the polymerase or by interaction with the DNA template. N4 late promoters, when present on linear DNAs, are

+1

AGACGTTTGGTTGAAGAACTCAGGGCGGCTGTTAGACTCCGTGATAAC

TGAAGTCGTTATTGATTCTATTACTAACCAGTACAATAGTCGGTTGC

GCAAAGACTACCCTAAAATACAAGTTGATGGTAAAGTCGGTTCTGG

ACCGAGTTTGCACTGACCTTTGCTAACTTTATTAAGCTGGTTAATG

TTAACCTCGTGGTTCCCTGGTTCAAAGCTGGTAAGATGTATTTTCCT

-35		-10
TCTTGACA	17 bp	TATAAT 6-7bp A/G

FIGURE 6. Sequences surrounding *in vivo* sites of N4 late-transcription initiation. The approximate site of transcription initiation is marked by a bracket above each sequence. Sequences −10 and −35 are presented in boldface. A conserved sequence present at all sites is underlined. The *E. coli* promoter consensus sequence is presented below. From N. Y. Baek (personal communication).

poor templates for purified *E. coli* RNA polymerase (N. Y. Baek, unpublished). On a supercoiled template, however, they are very active. A change in the topology of the DNA late in infection or the help of an accessory protein might be required for late transcription to occur.

VII. N4 REPLICATION

As previously mentioned, the N4 genome is a linear double-stranded DNA molecule containing direct terminal repeats with noncomplementary 3′ extensions. Upon N4 infection, replication of the host genome stops in a manner that is dependent on transcription of early N4 genes (Rothman-Denes and Schito, 1974). N4 replication can be detected 7–10 min after infection.

To determine what host functions are required for N4 replication, *E. coli* temperature-sensitive mutants defective in a number of replicative genes were tested for their ability to support N4 growth and to permit incorporation of [³H]thymidine into N4 DNA at the nonpermissive temperature (Rist *et al.*, 1983; Guinta *et al.*, 1986b). The functions of three host genes, *dnaF*, *lig*, and *gyrB*, were found to be required for N4 replication (Table I). These encode ribonucleotide reductase, DNA ligase, and DNA gyrase, respectively. Cells defective in the DNA polymerase activity of DNA polymerase I (*polA1*) were able to support N4 growth. The 5′–3′ exonuclease activity of DNA polymerase I, however, is required for N4 replication, because cells defective in this activity (*polAex1*) did not support N4 growth even though they did incorporate [³H]thymidine into N4 DNA. Guinta *et al.* (1986b) explained this discrepancy by showing that the 5′–3′ exonuclease activity is required for processing of N4 Okazaki fragments. The functions of the *dnaA*, *dnaB*, *dnaC*, *dnaE*, and *dnaG* genes of *E. coli* are not required for N4 DNA synthesis, suggesting

TABLE I. Host and Phage Functions Required for
N4 DNA Replication

Gene	Source	Function and properties
dnaF	*E. coli*	Ribonucleotide reductase
gyr A and B	*E. coli*	DNA gyrase
lig	*E. coli*	Ligase
polA	*E. coli*	5′–3′ exonuclease
dnp	N4	DNA polymerase with 3′–5′ exonuclease, 87,000 MW
dbp	N4	Single-stranded DNA-binding protein, 30,000 MW
exo	N4	5′–3′ exonuclease, 45,000 MW
dns	N4	Unknown function, 78,000 MW
vrp	N4	Virion RNA polymerase

that the phage must code for functions required for initiation, priming, polymerization, and strand displacement during replication.

Five phage-encoded functions directly involved in N4 replication have been identified through the isolation of phage containing amber and temperature-sensitive mutations in each of these genes (Table I) (Rist et al., 1983; Guinta et al., 1986b). These functions are an N4 DNA polymerase (dnp), a single-stranded DNA binding protein (dbp), a 5'–3' exonuclease (exo), the virion-encapsulated RNA polymerase (vrp), and an unknown function (dns). Besides the virion-encapsulated RNA polymerase (see section on early transcription), the N4 DNA polymerase (Lindberg et al., 1988), the single-stranded DNA binding protein (Rist and Lindberg, unpublished), and the 5'–3' exonuclease (Guinta et al., 1986a) have been purified to apparent homogeneity. The DNA polymerase, a 87,000-MW polypeptide, catalyzes accurate DNA synthesis due to an active 3'–5' exonuclease activity. As with other replicative polymerases, the N4 enzyme lacks 5'–3' exonuclease activity, cannot strand-displace, and is nonprocessive (Lindberg et al., 1988). These results suggest that a processivity factor(s) and helicase activities must be N4 encoded.

N4 DNA polymerase activity is greatly stimulated by the N4 single-stranded DNA-binding protein which binds with moderate cooperativity to single-stranded DNA covering 11 bp per protein monomer (G. Lindberg, unpublished). The 5'–3' N4-coded exonuclease has a denatured molecular weight of 45,000 and exists as a dimer. Its preferred substrate is duplex DNA containing 3' extensions (i.e., N4 DNA), which it degrades by a distributive mechanism. It is inactive on nicks or gaps (Guinta et al., 1986a). These properties suggest that it might play a role in recombination or replication of the ends of the N4 genome.

We have developed an in vitro replication system which shows a marked preference for double-stranded N4 DNA as a template with little activity on heterologous or denatured templates. The system uses extracts from N4-infected polA1 cells. Extracts from mutant-N4 infections demonstrated that the dnp, dbp, and exo gene products, but not the dns gene product, are required in the in vitro replication system. The in vitro system, therefore, does not express all the properties of in vivo N4 replication.

Replication in the in vitro system initiates at two specific sites at each end of the N4 genome and proceeds toward the center (Rist et al., 1983, 1986). This is in agreement with electron microscopic analysis of in vivo-replicating N4 DNA molecules, which shows Y-shaped molecules and molecules with single-stranded tails rather than replication bubbles (J. K. Rist and M. Pearle, unpublished), suggesting origins of replication near the ends of the genome. Two-dimensional gel electrophoresis of the terminal restriction fragments from in vitro-replicating N4 DNA molecules suggests that initiation occurs through hairpin priming of the single-stranded ends (Rist et al., 1986). Since the in vivo origin of N4 replication is not yet known, the relevance of the in vitro mode of initiation remains to be determined. The utilization of an RNA primer has not been ruled out, and indeed the role that the N4 virion RNA polymerase plays in replication has not been elucidated. The accumulation of Okazaki-like fragments after infection of *polAex1* or *lig* mutants suggests discontinuous DNA synthesis, and it is possible that the virion RNA polymerase synthesizes primers for this process as well.

The 3' extensions of the N4 genome are unusual, and since all known DNA polymerases synthesize in a 5' → 3' direction, N4 must have a novel mechanism for replicating these sequences. Analysis of restriction products of intracelluar N4 DNA detects a restriction fragment containing one copy of the terminal redundancy flanked by the right and left ends of the genome (joint fragment). Furthermore, *in vivo* pulse-chase experiments show that label accumulates in the joint fragment and chases into both the right and left genome ends. We have not yet identified the *in vivo* structure that contains the joint fragment, but it is likely that the joint fragment originates through homologous recombination at the terminal redundancy. Analysis of replicating N4 DNA by electron microscopy reveals longer-than-unit-length molecules, suggesting concatemer formation (M. Pearle, unpublished). What enzyme or enzymes are responsible for the generation of the N4 DNA ends from processing of concatemers? Simple site-specific cleavage of the concatemer during packaging to yield the correct 3' extensions at each end will result in a net loss of half of the replicated DNA. Concatemer formation followed by staggered cleavage at the terminal redundancy has been proposed for the generation of the mature ends of T7 DNA (Watson, 1972). This model, when applied to N4, could result in blunt-ended molecules that may or may not contain the sequences present in the extension. If the sequences are present, generation of the extensions would require very controlled exonuclease digestion or endonucleolytic cleavage during packaging. On the other hand, if the sequences are absent at one end, they could be copied from joint fragment sequences by strand invasion as proposed by Wamsley *et al.* (1984) for the generation of the ends of yeast chromosomes. Recent cloning of the joint fragment will permit us to answer some of these questions (G. Lindberg, unpublished).

VIII. N4 GENETICS

The analysis of N4 development has been hindered by the lack of a genetic map. Schito (1973) isolated a collection of suppressor sensitive mutants. Very high levels of recombination, however, have prevented the generation of a linkage map. We have cloned all but two of the *Hpa*I fragments of the N4 genome (Fig. 3) into pBR322 (Malone *et al.*, 1988). Two regions of the genome amounting to 3.7 kb and originating from *Hpa*I fragments M and D have not been cloned. These may encode N4 functions lethal to the host. *Hpa*I M is transcribed early in infection and could encode the function inhibiting host DNA replication. We suspect that *Hpa*I fragment D encodes a function involved in DNA replication (*dbp*, *exo*, or *dns*), since other replication functions map nearby.

The cloned N4 fragments have allowed us to map a large collection of suppressor-sensitive and temperature-sensitive mutants by marker rescue. Mutations in genes coding for the 15,000-, 40,000-, and 30,000-MW proteins required for middle transcription map to *Hpa*I fragments K, N, and I1, respectively. The gene for the N4 DNA polymerase spans the *Hpa*I I3-J fragment junction. Mutations in the N4 virion RNA polymerase map to *Hpa*I fragments B and I4 in the late region of the genome (Fig. 3) (Malone *et al.*, 1988). These results demonstrate that the N4 virion RNA polymerase, which is part of the phage particle, is synthesized with other morphogenetic proteins.

Heat- and citrate-induced deletions defined nonessential regions of the N4 genome (Malone *et al.*, 1988). Deletions were obtained with high frequency in *Hpa*I fragment A, which is part of the middle transcriptional region (Fig. 3). The largest deletion spans 6 kb of DNA. The ability to isolate heat- and citrate-resistant N4 phages implies that N4 does not encapsidate its DNA by full-head packaging, but rather through the recognition of specific sequences at both ends of the genome (Parkinson and Huskey, 1971). That is indeed the case, since deleted phages have wild-type terminal sequences (D. Hyman, unpublished; Malone *et al.*, 1988).

IX. PROSPECTS

We have presented our current understanding of bacteriophage N4. What little we have learned already shows that N4 is unique among the lytic phages. The study of its transcription and replication has provided us with a miriad of unanswered questions.

The reason for N4's complicated transcriptional strategy remains unknown. Although originally thought to be transcriptionally autarchic (Rabussay and Geiduschek, 1977), N4 depends on the host for transcriptional regulation in more than just the use of the host RNA polymerase for late transcription. The use of three different RNA polymerases to catalyze transcription during the life cycle provides a valuable resource to study structure-function relationships in DNA-dependent RNA polymerases. Our present understanding of the mechanism of promoter recognition by both N4-coded RNA polymerases has already shown that they use novel mechanisms of RNA polymerase-promoter recognition. Present results already suggest that productive N4 virion RNA polymerase-promoter interaction requires the recognition of specific sequences and DNA secondary structure. Future experiments will concentrate on the elucidation of the role of *E. coli* single-stranded DNA-binding protein and supercoiling in this process. N4 RNA polymerase II is the smallest RNA polymerase thus far characterized. Its promoters have two sets of conserved sequences positioned at variable distances, resulting in their location at variable sides of the DNA helix from each other. We expect that the purification of the 15,000-MW protein also required for N4 middle transcription and its eventual characterization will shed light on the mechanism of recognition of N4 middle promoters. Finally, we expect that genetic analysis of sequences required for N4 late transcription will aid in elucidating the mechanism of late-transcription activation.

Little is known about the injection of proteins into bacterial cells. The study of the localization of the virion RNA polymerase in the virion and its injection into the host will provide clues as to the mechanism. The recent cloning of the *nfrA* gene and its future characterization is the first step in that direction. The availability of the cloned N4 receptor will facilitate the isolation of *E. coli* mutants unable to support N4 growth (Toni and Schito, 1975). This approach will allow the characterization of *E. coli* gene products required for N4 development.

The generation of the 3′ single-stranded ends present on mature N4 DNA cannot be explained easily using known mechanisms of replication of linear genomes. Identification of the *in vivo* origin of N4 DNA replication and further characterization of *in vivo* replication intermediates will allow delineation of what could be a novel pathway for replicating linear genomes.

ACKNOWLEDGMENTS. We thank Dr. Helen Revel and all of the members of our laboratory for comments on the manuscript. L.B.R.-D. thanks Dr. G. C. Schito for introducing her to bacteriophage N4. Work in our laboratory was supported by NIH grants AI 12575 and GM 35170. D.R.K. was supported partially by NIH Training Postdoctoral Program in Human and Biochemical Genetics GM 05743.

REFERENCES

Adhya, S., Sen, A., and Mitra, S., 1971, The role of gene S, in: *The Bacteriophage Lambda* (A. D. Hershey, ed.), pp. 743–746, Cold Spring Harbor Laboratory, Cold Spring Harbor, NY.

Falco, S. C., and Rothman-Denes, L. B., 1979a, Bacteriophage N4-induced transcribing activities in *Escherichia coli*. I. Detection and characterization in cell extracts, *Virology* **95**:454.

Falco, S. C., and Rothman-Denes, L. B., 1979b, Bacteriophage N4-induced transcribing activities in *Escherichia coli*. II. Association of the N4 transcriptional apparatus with the cytoplasmic membrane, *Virology* **95**:466.

Falco, S. C., VanderLaan, K., and Rothman-Denes, L. B., 1977, Virion-associated RNA polymerase required for bacteriophage N4 development, *Proc. Natl. Acad. Sci. USA* **74**:520.

Falco, S. C., Zivin, R., and Rothman-Denes, L. B., 1978, Novel template requirements of N4 virion RNA polymerase, *Proc. Natl. Acad. Sci. USA* **75**:3220.

Falco, S. C., Zehring, W., and Rothman-Denes, L. B., 1980, DNA-dependent RNA polymerase from bacteriophage N4 virions. Purification and characterization, *J. Biol. Chem.* **255**:4339.

Glucksmann, A., and Rothman-Denes, L. B., 1987, N4 virion RNA polymerase-promoter interaction, in: *DNA-Protein Interactions* (E. B. Thompson and J. Papaconstantinou, eds.), pp. 67–76, University of Texas Press, Austin.

Grachev, M. A., Hartmann, G. R., Maximova, T. G., Mustaev, A. A., Schaffner, A. R., Sieber, H., and Zaychikov, E. F., 1986, High selective affinity labelling of RNA polymerase B (II) from wheat germ, *FEBS Lett.* **200**:287.

Guinta, D., Stambouly, J., Falco, S. C., Rist, J. K., and Rothman-Denes, L. B., 1986a, Host and phage-coded functions required for coliphage N4 DNA replication, *Virology* **150**:33.

Guinta, D., Lindberg, G., and Rothman-Denes, L. B., 1986b, Bacteriophage N4 coded 5'–3' exonuclease: Purification and characterization, *J. Biol. Chem.* **261**:10736.

Haynes, L. L., and Rothman-Denes, L. B., 1985, N4 virion RNA polymerase sites of transcription initiation, *Cell* **41**:597.

Ito, J., and Roberts, R. J., 1979. Unusual base sequence arrangement in phage φ29 DNA, *Gene* **5**:1.

Krüger, D. H., and Bickle, T. A., 1983, Bacteriophage survival: Multiple mechanisms for avoiding the deoxyribonucleic acid restriction systems of their hosts, *Microbiol. Rev.* **47**:345.

Lindberg, G., Rist, J. K., Kunkel, T., Sugino, A., and Rothman-Denes, L. B., 1988, Purification and characterization of bacteriophage N4-coded DNA polymerase, *J. Biol. Chem.* (in press).

Luria, S., and Human, M. L., 1950, Chromatin staining of bacteria during bacteriophage infection, *J. Bacteriol.* **59**:551.

Malone, C., Spellman, S., Hyman, D., and Rothman-Denes, L. B., 1988, Cloning and generation of a genetic map of bacteriophage N4, *Virology* **162**:328.

Markiewicz, P., Glucksmann, A., and Rothman-Denes, L. B., 1988, N4 virion DNA-dependent RNA polymerase: Initiation sequences utilized by the enzyme on heterologous templates, *Nucleic Acids Res.* **16**:1011.

Mathews, C. K., 1977, Reproduction of large virulent bacteriophages, in: *Comprehensive Virology*, Vol. 7 (H. Fraenkel-Conrat and R. R. Wagner, eds.), pp. 179–294, Plenum Press, New York.

McIntosh, M. A., Chenault, S. S., and Earhart, C. F., 1979, Genetic and physiological studies on the relationship between colicin B resistance and ferricntcrochelin uptake in *Escherichia coli* K-12. *J. Bacteriol.* **137**:653.

Ohmori, H., Haynes, L. L., and Rothman-Denes, L. B., 1988, Terminally repeated sequences of the coliphage N4 genome, *J. Mol. Biol.* (in press).

Parkinson, J. S., and Huskey, R. J., 1971, Deletion mutants of bacteriophage lambda. I. Isolation and initial characterization, *J. Mol. Biol.* **56**:369.

Pesce, A., Satta, G., and Schito, G. C., 1969, Factors in lysis-inhibition by N4 coliphage, *G. Microbiol.* **17**:119.

Platt, T., 1986, Transcription termination and the regulation of gene expression, *Annu. Rev. Biochem.* **55**:339.

Rabussay, D., and Geiduschek, E. P., 1977, Regulation of gene action in the development of lytic bacteriophages, in: *Comprehensive Virology*, Vol. 8 (H. Fraenkel-Conrat and R. R. Wagner, eds.), pp. 1–196, Plenum Press, New York.

Rist, J. K., Guinta, D. R., Sugino, A., Stambouly, J., Falco, S. C., and Rothman-Denes, L. B., 1983, Bacteriophage N4 DNA replication, in: *Mechanisms of DNA Replication and Recombination* (N. R. Cozzarelli, ed.), pp. 245–254, Alan R. Liss, New York.

Rist, J. K., Pearle, M., Sugino, A., and Rothman-Denes, L. B., 1986, Development of an *in vitro* bacteriophage N4 DNA replication system, *J. Biol. Chem.* **261**:10506.

Rosenberg, A. H., Simon, M. N., and Studier, F. W., 1979. Survey and mapping of restriction cleavage sites in bacteriophage T7 DNA, *J. Mol. Biol.* **135**:907.

Rothman-Denes, L. B., and Schito, G. C., 1974, Novel transcribing activities in N4-infected *Escherichia coli*, *Virology* **60**:65.

Rothman-Denes, L. B., Haselkorn, R., and Schito, G. C., 1972, Selective shut-off of catabolite-sensitive host RNA synthesis by bacteriophage N4, *Virology* **50**:95.

Rothman-Denes, L. B., Haynes, L., Markiewicz, P. M., Glucksmann, A., Malone, C., and Chase, J., 1985, Bacteriophage N4 virion RNA polymerase promoters, in: *Sequence Specificity in Transcription and Translation* (R. Calendar and L. Gold, eds.), pp. 41–53, Alan R. Liss, New York.

Rothman-Denes, L. B., Abravaya, K., Glucksmann, A., Malone, C., and Markiewicz, P. M., 1987, Bacteriophage N4-coded RNA polymerases, in: *RNA Polymerase and the Regulation of Transcription* (W. S. Reznikoff, R. R. Burgess, J. E. Dahlberg, C. A. Gross, M. T. Record, and M. P. Wickens, eds.), pp. 37–46, Elsevier, New York.

Rupprecht, K. R., Gordon, G., Lundigran, M., Gayda, R. C., Markovitz, A., and Earhart, C., 1983, *ompT: Escherichia coli* K-12 structural gene for protein a (3b), *J. Bacteriol.* **153:**1104.

Schito, G. C., 1973, The genetics and physiology of coliphage N4, *Virology* **55:**254.

Schito, G. C., 1974, Development of coliphage N4: Ultrastructural studies, *J. Virol.* **13:**186.

Schito, G. C., Molina, A. M., and Pesce, A., 1965, Un nuovo batteriofago attivo sul ceppo K12 di *E. coli.* I. Caractteristiche biologiche, *Boll. Inst. Sieroter. Milanese* **44:**329.

Schito, G. C., Rialdi, G., and Pesce, A., 1966a, Biophysical properties of N4 coliphage, *Biochim. Biophys. Acta* **129:**482.

Schito, G. C., Rialdi, G., and Pesce, A., 1966b, The physical properties of the deoxyribonucleic acid of N4 coliphage, *Biochim. Biophys. Acta* **129:**491.

Sharp, P. M., 1986, Molecular evolution of bacteriophages: Evidence of selection against the recognition sites of host restriction enzymes, *Mol. Biol. Evol.* **3:**75.

Snustadt, D. P., Snyder, L., and Kutter, E., 1983, Effects on host genome structure and expression, in: *Bacteriophage T4* (C. K. Mathews, E. M. Kutter, G. Mosig, and P. Berget, eds.), American Society for Microbiology, Washington.

Toni, M., and Schito, G. C., 1975, Aspetti della replicazione del batteriofago N4 in ceppi di *Escherischia coli* isolati da materiale patologico, *Atti XVII Congresso Nazional. Soc. Ital. Microbiol.*, pp. 579–586.

Vander Laan, K., Falco, S. C., and Rothman-Denes, L. B., 1977, The program of RNA synthesis in N4-infected *Escherichia coli, Virology* **76:**596.

Wamsley, R. W., Chan, C. S. M., Tye, B.-K., and Petes, T. D., 1984, Unusual DNA sequences associated with the ends of yeast chromosomes, *Nature* **310:**157.

Watson, J. D., 1972, Origin of concatemeric T7 DNA, *Nature New Biol.* **239:**197.

Weisberg, R. A., Gottesman, S., and Gottesman, M. E., 1977, Bacteriophage λ: The lysogenic pathway, in: *Comprehensive Virology*, Vol. 8 (H. Fraenkel-Conrat and R. R. Wagner, eds.), pp. 197–258, Plenum Press, New York.

Zehring, W. A., and Rothman-Denes, L. B., 1983, Purification and characterization of coliphage N4 RNA polymerase II activity from infected cell extracts, *J. Biol. Chem.* **258:**8074.

Zehring, W. A., Falco, S. C., Malone, C., and Rothman-Denes, L. B., 1983, Bacteriophage N4-induced transcribing activities in *E. coli.* III. A third cistron required for N4 RNA polymerase II activity, *Virology* **126:**678.

Zivin, R., Malone, C., and Rothman-Denes, L. B., 1980, Physical map of coliphage N4 DNA, *Virology* **104:**205.

Zivin, R., Zehring, W., and Rothman-Denes, L. B., 1981, Transcriptional map of bacteriophage N4. Location and polarity of N4 RNAs, *J. Mol. Biol.* **152:**335.

CHAPTER 8

Lipid-Containing Bacteriophages

Leonard Mindich and Dennis H. Bamford

I. INTRODUCTION

Bacteriophages that contain lipid are not a true taxonomic class, in that the various subgroups are not clearly related to each other in terms of evolution. The lipid-containing structures of the various groups differ in complexity of composition as well as in location within the virion. However, these viruses can be considered together, because much of the interest in them has stemmed from their utility as model systems for the study of membrane structure, assembly, and translocation. In the two cases where intensive genetic analysis of structure and assembly has been possible, bacteriophages $\phi6$ and PRD1/PR4, it has been found that the virus specifies one or more proteins that play a morphogenetic role in the formation or placement of the membrane structure without having a permanent structural role in the virion. The mechanism of action of these proteins is under investigation.

Lipid-containing bacteriophages can be separated into three distinct groups on the basis of morphology. $\phi6$ has a polyhedral nucleocapsid that is covered by the membrane; whereas virtually all the other lipid-containing phages have the membrane structure inside of the polyhedral capsid. A phage designated MVL2 which infects mycoplasmas and appears to bud from the surface of infected cells represents a third type of structure that is lacking a polyhedral capsid; however, this phage has not been well characterized structurally. The genomic RNA of $\phi6$ is found

LEONARD MINDICH • Department of Microbiology, Public Health Research Institute, New York, New York 10016.   DENNIS H. BAMFORD • Department of Genetics, University of Helsinki, Helsinki SF-00100, Finland.

TABLE I. Some Characteristics of Lipid Phages

Phage	Nucleic acid	Lipids	Buoyant density in CsCl (g/ml)	Diameter	Host	Reference
PM2	DNA circle	10%	1.28	60 nm	Altermonas espejiano	Espejo and Canelo, 1968
φ6	dsRNA 3pc	20%	1.27	80 nm	P. phaseolicola	Vidaver et al., 1973
PR4, PRD1	DNA, linear	13%	1.265	65 nm	Gram-negative with plasmids of P, N or W compatability groups	Bradley and Rutherford, 1975 Davis et al., 1982
AP50	DNA	14.3%	1.307	80 nm	B. anthracis	Nagy et al., 1982
DS6A	n.d.	11.7%	n.d.	n.d.	M. tuberculosis H37RV	Bowman et al., 1973
I3	DNA	15%	n.d.	90 nm	M. smegmatis SN2	Gope and Gopinathan, 1982
φNS11	DNA, linear	12%	1.25	75 nm	B. acidocardarius TA6	Sakaki et al., 1977
Dp-1	DNA	8.5%	1.47		S. pneumoniae R36A	Lopez et al., 1977
MVL2	DNA circle	10–12%		52–125 nm	A. laidlawii	Gourlay et al., 1973

inside a polyhedral nucleocapsid. In the case of the other phages, all have DNA that is found inside the membrane vesicle.

The group of lipid-containing phages is extremely diverse in terms of the genera of host bacteria (Table I). Lipid-containing phages have been described for gram-positive and gram-negative bacteria as well as for mycoplasma. Phage φNS11 infects an acidophilic thermophile. Most of the phages do not have conventional tails. The exceptions are DS6A, which infects *Mycobacterium tuberculosis*, and Dp-1, which is a pneumococcal phage. Several of the phages seem related, at least morphologically, to the PRD1 group. Dp-1, φNS11, and AP50 all have linear DNA genomes, which in the case of the PRD1 group has been shown to have protein at the termini, and in the case of the others there are hints that they too may be derivatized. Most of these phages also show a taillike extension of the membrane vesicle that might be involved in attachment. Although φ6 is very sensitive to detergents and nonpolar solvents such as chloroform, most of the other lipid-containing phages are not very sensitive. On the other hand, many phages that do not contain lipid are sensitive to these treatments. Consequently, solvent sensitivity is not a valid criterion for indicating the presence or absence of lipid (see Mindich, 1978).

In this chapter, we will be discussing φ6 and the PRD1 family in detail. Our discussion will not be limited to the lipid or membrane-specific aspects of these phage systems. Since these phages are not widely known, we will attempt to present as full a treatment as possible of their structures, life cycles, and areas of special interest. We will not be dealing with several phages that are similar to the PRD1 family, that have not been studied extensively, or that have been adequately reviewed. DNA replication in PRD1 will be discussed in Chapter 9 of this volume along with φ29 and other phages with genome-associated proteins. PM2 has been covered in several reviews (Brewer, 1980; Mindich, 1978). Although a considerable amount of work has been done on the structure of PM2, relatively little has been done on its genetics. The mycoplasma budding phage MLV2 has been thoroughly reviewed (Razin, 1985).

II. BACTERIOPHAGE φ6

A. Life Cycle

Bacteriophage φ6 was discovered by Vidaver *et al.* (1973). Its normal host is *Pseudomonas syringae* and many of its pathovars, especially *P. syringae pv phaseolicola* (Cuppels *et al.*, 1981). We will designate this organism as *P. phaseolicola*. Mutants of φ6 will infect *P. pseudoalcaligenes* (Mindich *et al.*, 1976b). The φ6 virion is composed of an outer lipid-protein membrane which envelopes a nucleocapsid composed of five proteins and the segmented dsRNA genome (Sinclair *et al.*, 1975; Van Etten *et al.*, 1976) (Fig. 1). The receptor for this virus is a chro-

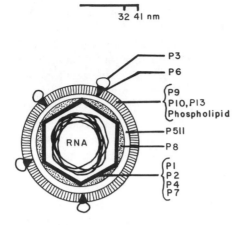

FIGURE 1. Diagram of the structure of φ6. The three pieces of genomic dsRNA are found in a toroidal coil inside a dodecahedral structure composed of P1, P2, P4, and P7. This is enclosed by a shell of P8. Protein P5 is found associated with the P8 surface. Outside of this is the membrane composed of phospholipids and proteins P9, P10, P13, P6, and P3. The first three are probably associated with the inner face of the membrane, and P6 is probably embedded in the membrane but accessible to the outside, where P3 attaches to it.

mosomally coded pilus by which the host bacterium adheres to the leaf surfaces of bean plants (Romantschuk and Bamford, 1986). The pilus apparently retracts to bring the virus particle into contact with the host cell outer membrane (Romantschuk and Bamford, 1985) (Figs. 2,3). The viral membrane fuses with the host outer membrane through an interaction mediated by a membrane-associated hydrophobic phage protein, P6 (Romantschuk et al., unpublished). The fusion results in the nucleocapsid being located in the periplasmic space of the host cell (Fig. 4).

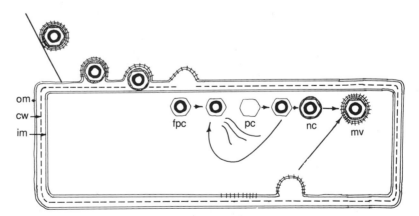

FIGURE 2. The life cycle of φ6. The virion attaches to a pilus and is brought into contact with the outer membrane (om). The viral membrane fuses with the outer membrane to place the nucleocapsid in the periplasmic space. The murein (cw) is digested by viral lysozyme P5, and the filled procapsid (fpc) enters the cell, leaving P8 behind. The procapsid transcriptase synthesizes complete copies of the three genomic segments. The L message is translated to produce P1, P2, P4, and P7, which constitute the procapsid (pc). This is filled with dsRNA and continues transcription until it is covered by P8 to form nucleocapsids (nc). Membrane proteins are placed in the host membrane and then transfer to the virion (mv) along with host lipids. The membrane formation or translocation is dependent upon protein P12.

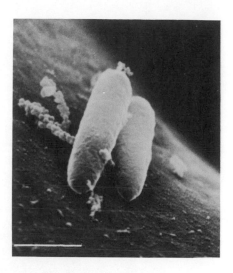

FIGURE 3. A scanning electron micrograph of *P. phaseolicola* with a single pilus that is covered with virions of φ6. Scale bar: 1 μm. From Romantschuk and Bamford (1986).

Digestion of the peptidoglycan with virion-associated lytic enzyme, P5 (Mindich and Lehman, 1979), leads to a closer association of the particle with the inner membrane of the host. Part of the nucleocapsid penetrates the host cytoplasmic membrane (Bamford *et al.*, 1987), and the nucleocapsid-associated RNA polymerase is activated. Although equimolar amounts of transcripts of the three genomic segments are synthesized, only the message of segment *L* is translated (Sinclair *et al.*, 1975). Later in infection, the transcription of the *S* and *M* genomic segments increases to about 10 times that of the *L* segment, and the proteins coded for by those segments are synthesized (Coplin *et al.*, 1975).

The first assembled particle observed in the cells is a procapsid (Mindich and Davidoff Abelson, 1980) (Fig. 5). The procapsid is filled with

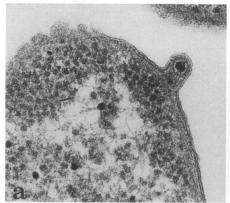
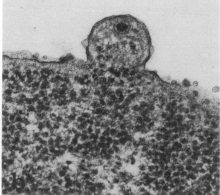

FIGURE 4. Electron micrograph of sections of cells infected with φ6 showing the infecting nucleocapsids in the periplasmic space. From Bamford *et al.* (1976).

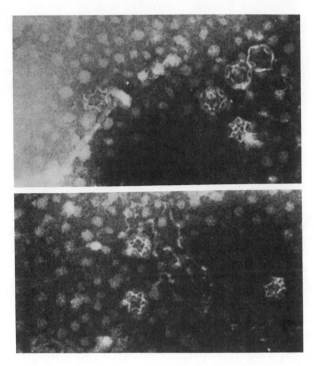

FIGURE 5. Electron micrograph of procapsids stained with uranyl acetate. From Mindich and Davidoff Abelson (1980).

RNA. The filled procapsid is then covered by a shell of protein P8 to form the nucleocapsid which is enveloped by the phage membrane inside of the host cell (Bamford and Mindich, 1980). This takes place with the aid of a nonstructural assembly factor, P12 (Mindich and Lehman, 1983). Following membrane assembly, the adsorption protein P3 is attached to the virion surface (Mindich and Lehman, 1983). About 90 min postinfection, the mature virions are released by lysis of the host cell caused by the virus-coded lytic enzyme together with an additional virus-coded lysis factor (Kakitani et al., 1978; Mindich and Lehman, 1979). A schematic drawing of the φ6 life cycle is presented in Fig. 2.

B. Structure of the Virion

1. The Composition of φ6

The virion of φ6 has a mass of 99×10^6 daltons (Day and Mindich, 1980). The chemical composition has been determined by Vidaver et al. (1973) and by Day and Mindich (1980). The values agree and are approximately 10% RNA, 20% phospholipid, and 70% protein. The genome consists of three pieces of double-stranded RNAs (Semancik *et al.*, 1973), which have been subjected to cDNA cloning (Mindich *et al.*, 1985; Revel *et al.*, 1986) and sequencing (McGraw *et al.*, 1986). On the basis of sequence analysis, the genomic pieces are 2948 bp for segment *S* (McGraw *et al.*, 1986), 4057 bp for segment *M* (Gottlieb *et al.*, unpublished results), and 6374 bp for segment *L* (Mindich *et al.*, unpublished results). The base compositions of the segments are 55.2%, 56.7%, and 55.5% guanine and cytosine, respectively. These values agree well with the chemical determinations of Semancik *et al.* (1973).

The phospholipid analysis of the phage lipids revealed 8% cardiolipin, 35% phosphatidyl ethanolamine, and 57% phosphatidyl glycerol (Sands, 1973). The fatty-acid composition of the virion was reported to be similar to that of host bacterium *P. phaseolicola* (Vidaver *et al.*, 1973). The relatively high proportion of phosphatidyl glycerol in the virion as compared to the host lipids is a general characteristic of phages PM2 and ϕ6 and the PRD1 family. It is not known how the lipid composition of any of these viruses is determined, although in the case of PR4, there is a close association between the major capsid protein and phophatidyl glycerol in the virion (Davis and Cronan, 1985).

The amount of phospholipid per virion of ϕ6 is not enough to construct a complete lipid bilayer at the radius of the membrane (Day and Mindich, 1980). There is enough lipid to cover about half of the necessary surface area. Similar results have been obtained for PM2 (Schneider *et al.*, 1978), PR4 (Davis *et al.*, 1982), and ϕNS11 (Sakaki *et al.*, 1979). It seems that the viral membranes must have large proportions of their surface areas occupied by protein.

The first ϕ6 protein analysis (Sinclair *et al.*, 1975) showed that the virion contains 10 proteins. The protein molecular weights were analyzed using SDS-PAGE. The molecular weight estimates for the virion proteins were from 93,000 to 6000. The proteins were designated by their mobilities in electrophoresis so that the slowest moving protein was P1 and the fastest, P10. The infected cells produced two additional proteins, designated P11 and P12. Proteins P1, P2, P4, and P7 were synthesized early in the infection, and the rest of the proteins late. It was possible to locate the genes for proteins P1, P2, and P7 in one linkage group, those for proteins P3, P6, and P10 in another, and those for proteins P5, P8, P9, P11, and P12 in the last linkage group (Lehman and Mindich, 1979; Mindich *et al.*, 1976a).

The sum of the molecular weight of proteins P1, P2, P4, and P7 is such that only the largest genome segment (*L*) can code for them (Sinclair *et al.*, 1975). The *in vitro* translation studies of the separated ϕ6 genome fragments showed that proteins P1, P2, P4, and P7 are coded from the large (*L*) fragment; proteins P3, P6, and P10 from the medium (*M*) fragment; and proteins P5, P8, and P9 from the small (*S*) genome fragment (Cuppels *et al.*, 1980). Similar but not as complete results were also obtained by Emori *et al.* (1980).

TABLE II. Amino Acid Composition of φ6 Proteins

Protein	P1	P2	P3	P4	P5	P6	P7	P8	P9	P10	P12	P13
Mol. wt. (kD)	85.0	74.8	69.2	35.0	23.2	17.2	17.3	16.0	9.5	4.3	20.3	7.7
Ala	88	58	86	37	33	22	20	21	12	8	24	10
Arg	51	43	24	17	16	0	4	7	5	0	5	6
Asn	33	25	23	10	10	0	8	5	1	1	3	0
Asp	37	42	40	24	5	2	8	7	4	2	12	1
Cys	3	7	9	4	0	0	0	0	0	0	4	0
Gln	29	19	36	5	14	3	3	7	4	0	8	3
Glu	45	41	19	11	14	4	11	10	5	1	5	3
Gly	43	49	61	26	16	19	8	11	8	3	14	3
His	18	14	7	5	3	0	5	1	1	0	5	0
Ile	45	26	27	21	7	19	8	10	6	2	6	2
Leu	73	63	52	30	19	16	24	19	7	7	17	14
Lys	25	37	24	13	10	10	5	6	5	4	9	3
Met	20	24	18	10	0	1	5	5	0	1	7	1
Phe	28	30	17	8	11	10	2	3	5	1	7	0
Pro	31	36	32	16	7	6	12	7	5	2	14	4
Ser	58	45	39	27	16	18	13	10	6	2	14	9
Thr	49	29	41	22	8	16	7	3	5	3	11	5
Trp	11	12	17	2	2	7	3	0	1	0	0	0
Tyr	23	28	22	7	10	2	3	6	1	1	2	2
Val	59	36	54	36	18	12	12	11	8	4	28	6
Total	769	664	648	331	219	167	161	149	89	42	195	72
N-met	+	−	+	−	−	−	+/−	+	−	+	?	+
Net ch.	+12	+11	−4	0	+10	+4	−5	−3	+2	+1	+2	+5

The nucleotide sequence analysis combined with the amino acid sequencing of the N termini of all the structural proteins has located the genes in the cDNA genome fragments allowing the calculation of the exact molecular weights for the φ6 proteins (McGraw et al., 1986; Mindich et al., unpublished) (Table II). The sequence analysis revealed a new φ6 protein migrating at the same position as P10. This protein was designated P13 (Table II). The stoichiometry of the protein composition of φ6 was calculated on the basis of the distribution of radioactive label in the viral proteins and the mass of the virion (Table III).

2. Protein Localization

Treatment of φ6 particles with nonionic detergent Triton X-100 removes proteins P3, P6, P9, P10, and P13 (Sinclair et al., 1975; Van Etten et al., 1976). The isolated nucleocapsid contains proteins P1, P2, P4, P7, and P8 (Van Etten et al., 1976). P5, the viral lysin, is partly found in the membrane fraction and partly in the nucleocapsid fraction when the nucleocapsids and membranes are separated, using Triton X-100 (Bamford and Palva, 1980; Mindich and Lehman, 1979). In Triton X-114 partition purification of nucleocapsids, protein P5 is found in the water phase with the nucleocapsid but not associated with it (Olkkonen and Bamford, 1987). In controlled Triton X-100 disruption studies, it was possible to isolate φ6 membrane vesicles (Bamford and Palva, 1980) (Fig. 6). The isolated φ6 membranes contained proteins P6, P9, and P10 and reduced amounts of P3 (Bamford and Palva, 1980). The consensus opinion is that P5 is associated loosely with the nucleocapsid and that proteins P3, P6, P9, P10, and P13 are associated with the membrane.

Proteins P6, P9, and P10 are 100% associated with the Triton phase in a Triton X-114 phase partition experiment, whereas protein P3 appears predominantly in the water phase (Bamford et al., 1987). This suggests that although P3 is a membrane constituent, it is not an integral mem-

Table III. Protein Content of φ6 Virions

Protein	Mol. wt. (kD)	Mass/virion (Md)	Molecules/ virion (calculated)	Molecules/ virion (proposed)	Location
P1	85.0	8.7	102	120	Procapsid
P2	74.8	1.0	13	20	Procapsid
P3	69.2	5.1	74		Membrane
P4	35.0	3.9	112	120	Procapsid
P5	23.2	2.1	91		Nucleocapsid
P6	17.2	2.3	134		Membrane
P7	17.3	1.6	92	100	Procapsid
P8	16.0	16.9	1056		Nucleocapsid
P9	9.5	20.0	2109		Membrane
P10	4.3	7.4	1720		Membrane

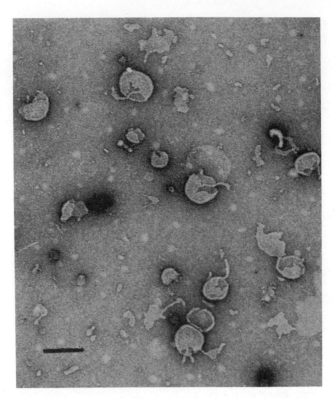

FIGURE 6. Electron micrograph of membrane vesicles removed from φ6 virions by treatment with low concentrations of Triton X-100. Scale bar: 200 nm. From Bamford and Palva (1980).

brane protein. Mutant viruses that do not synthesize protein P6 do not assemble P3 on the virion (Mindich *et al.*, 1976c). Retinoids and butylated hydroxytoluene (BHT) remove P3 from the virion (Bamford, 1981; Reinhardt *et al.*, 1980), and φ6 mutants resistant to BHT have altered protein P6 (Bamford *et al.*, 1987). The only protein located on the virus surface on the basis of iodination with lactoperoxidase was P3 (Van Etten *et al.*, 1976). Proteolytic cleavage experiments of intact viruses showed that P3 was readily accessible and P6 was somewhat less accessible (Stitt and Mindich, 1983a). These experiments suggest that P6 is anchored in the membrane and somewhat accessible to the outside. P3 is attached to P6. Proteins P9, P10, and P13 are either within the membrane or associated with its inner face.

3. Disruption Studies of φ6 Nucleocapsids

Isolated nucleocapsids contain proteins P1, P2, P4, P7, and P8. Genetic studies showed that mutants that do not synthesize P8 accumulate a particle composed of P1, P2, P4, and P7 (Mindich and Davidoff Abelson, 1980). This particle was called the procapsid. Nucleocapsid disruption studies showed that there is an internal dodecahedral protein skeleton composed of protein P1 inside the nucleocapsid (Ktistakis and Lang, 1987; Olkkonen and Bamford, 1987).

Nucleocapsids can be disrupted by several different treatments. Guanidine hydrochloride (0.5 M) partially removes P8 (Olkkonen and Bamford, 1987), but higher concentrations lead to the stripping of the remainder of the proteins from the P1 cage. EDTA also strips P8 from the nucleocapsid, but it removes much of the other proteins as well, leaving intact a cage structure of P1 (Ktistakis and Lang, 1987; Olkkonen and Bamford, 1987). Protease treatment also removes P8 first and the other proteins subsequently. It appears that the association of P7 to the procapsid is less tenacious than those of P2 and P4.

Complexes of procapsid proteins can be isolated after disruption treatments. The composition of these complexes may have bearing on the associations in the virion. The following subviral complexes could be isolated by chemical treatment of the nucleocapsid (Olkkonen and Bamford, 1987). EDTA treatment of the nucleocapsid released a P1 cage, a tetramer of P4, and monomers of P2, P7, and P8. Urea treatment (5 M) released a structure sedimenting as ~ 550-kD particle composed of proteins P1, P2, and P4 and a smaller complex consisting of proteins P1 and P4 (150 kD). The ratio of P1 to P4 in these particles remained the same as in the intact virion. Taking into account the dodecahedral symmetry and the calculated numbers of proteins in the nucleocapsid (102 for P1 and 112 for P4; see Table III), the dodecahedron is composed, most probably, of 120 molecules of P1.

A dodecahedral structure has the same symmetries as an icosahedron and might be expected to follow the rules of Caspar and Klug (1962). However, 120 subunits would correspond to a triangulation number of 2, which was considered to be a forbidden structure. The subunits might form asymmetric dimers arranged as a T=1 structure (Day and Mindich, 1980). The dodecahedral symmetry of the procapsid and the constant P1/P4 ratio in the intact virion and in the P1, P4– and the P1, P4, P2– containing particles obtained with urea suggest that the actual number of P4 molecules in the virion would also be 120 and that they would be associated with the 30 edges of the dodecahedron as tetramers. The location of P2 in the structure remains unknown, but it would be tempting to position it on the vertices of the dodecahedron, leading to a predicted number of 20 molecules per virion.

4. Physical Properties and Visualization of φ6 and Its Nucleocapsid

The diameters of intact viruses and nucleocapsids were found by turbidity measurements to be 82 and 64 nm, respectively (Day and Mindich, 1980). Similar values were obtained by low-angle X-ray diffraction

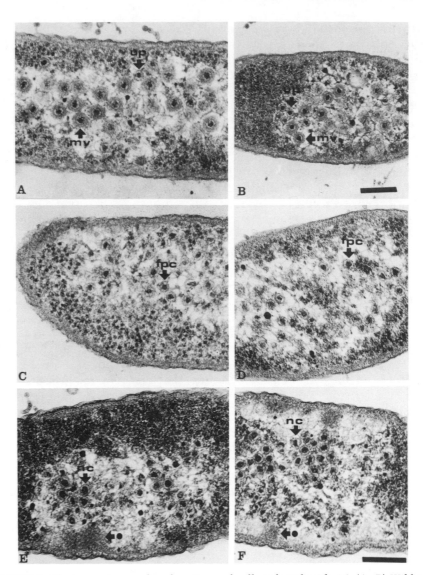

FIGURE 7. Electron micrographs of sections of cells infected with φ6. (A, B) Wild-type infection showing mature virions (mv) and unenveloped particles (up). (C, D) Infection with class 812 mutant showing filled procapsids (fpc). (E, F) Infection with class 12 mutant showing nucleocapsids (nc). From Bamford and Mindich (1980).

(Berger and Kennedy, 1980). The sedimentation coefficient for virions was found to be 406S, and for nucleocapsids it was 298S. The masses of the particles were determined to be 99×10^6 and 40×10^6 daltons. The refractive index increment of 0.152 g^{-1} cm^3 (Day and Mindich, 1980) and the diffusion coefficient of D_{20w} $2.66 \cdot 10^{-8}$ $cm^2 sec^{-1}$ (Berger and Kennedy, 1980) were also determined. The density of the virion in CsCl is

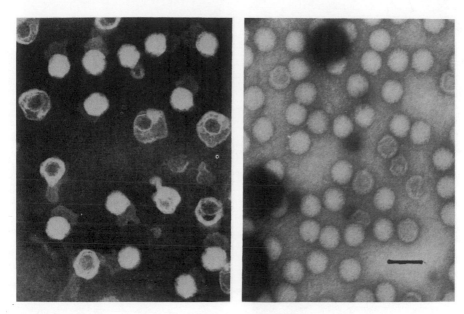

FIGURE 8. Electron micrographs of φ6 virions stained with phosphotungstate (left). Note the distortion of the membrane on the particles and the appearance of the procapsid shell inside some particles (Vidaver *et al.*, 1973). Electron micrograph of nucleocapsids (right) stained with ammonium molybdate (Olkkonen and Bamford, 1987). Scale bar: 100 nm.

1.27 g/cm³ (Vidaver *et al.*, 1973) and in sucrose 1.24 g/cm³ (Bamford and Palva, 1980).

Electron microscopy has been used to visualize both the virus and its nucleocapsid. Thin sectioning of the virus revealed an electron-dense core of about 30 nm in diameter, obviously containing the nucleic acid. The core is surrounded by a spherical capsid structure at 50 nm diameter. This nucleocapsid is surrounded by a membranous layer giving the virus a diameter of about 75 nm with this technique (Bamford *et al.*, 1976) (Fig. 7). Sectioned nucleocapsids obtained by Triton X-100 treatment corresponded to the spherical capsid structure with nucleic acid core, as seen in intact virus preparations (Bamford *et al.*, 1976).

Negative staining with uranyl oxalate indicated a diameter of 80 nm for the virion and 65 nm for the nucleocapsid (Bamford and Lounatmaa, 1978) (Fig. 8). Uranyl acetate staining of the nucleocapsid showed a double-layer capsid with about 60 nm diameter (Mindich and Davidoff Abelson, 1980) and similarly with phosphotungstate at pH 4.5 (Ktistakis and Lang, 1987). Staining with phosphotungstate at pH 6.5 or 7.0 revealed a complex, cagelike structure for the nucleocapsid having an average diameter of 45 nm. Two- and three-dimensional analysis of these structures showed that the various images obtained by tungstic acid staining were different projections of a dodecahedral cage structure (Steely and Lang, 1984; Yang and Lang, 1984) (Fig. 9).

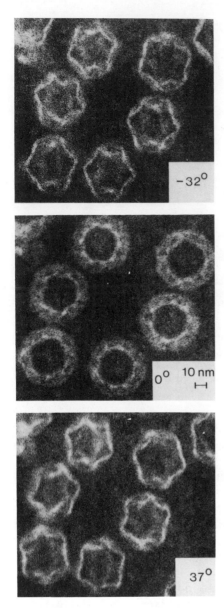

FIGURE 9. A group of φ6 nucleocapsids negatively stained with neutralized PTA generated
different images when tilted through several
values of the tilt angle. The tilt angle is defined
as the angle between the plane of the specimen
grid and a plane normal to the electron beam.
Tilt axis vertical. From Yang and Lang (1984).

When the stability of the nucleocapsid was tested using potassium
tungstate at pH 6.5 in concentrations used in negative staining, it was
observed that the nucleocapsid was completely disrupted, whereas another stain, ammonium molybdate, did not have any effect on the nucleocapsid (Olkkonen and Bamford, 1987). It could be shown that the
dodecahedral cage was present after tungstate staining, but it contained
only a single protein species, namely P1, all other nucleocapsid proteins
being released. This shows that the image of tungstate-stained nucleocap-

sid represents a much simpler structure than the entire nucleocapsid and should be interpreted with great caution.

Virus mutants incapable of synthesizing nucleocapsid protein P8 form particles (procapsids) that are indistinguishable from nucleocapsids in sectioned material (Bamford and Mindich, 1980) (Fig. 9). These particles resemble the dodecahedral cages when stained with tungstate or uranyl acetate (Mindich and Davidoff Abelson, 1980) (Fig. 5).

The electron microscopic measurements of nucleocapsids using tungstic acid differ greatly from the values obtained by other staining or physical methods. This is caused by the degradative effect of the stain to the particle. The diameter values obtained by ammonium molybdate or uranyl salts (60–65 nm) agree well with the physical measurements (64–66 nm). For the whole virion, both uranyl oxalate staining and freeze-fracturing gave 80 nm as the diameter, which agrees with the physical measurements (74–82 nm). In both cases, sectioned material gave lower values, obviously owing to the dehydration of the particles. The dodecahedral P1 cage located in the nucleocapsid interior and obtained by tungstate treatment has an average diameter of 46 nm. The approximate 60-nm diameter of the nucleocapsid and the suggested outer radius of 29 nm for the RNA is not in agreement with the 45- or 46-nm dodecahedral core if it is supposed to contain the nucleic acid. The suggested 29 nm might contain additional components, but it is more likely that the observed dodecahedral cage is somewhat collapsed. Figure 7 shows electron microscopic images of $\phi6$ and $\phi6$ nucleocapsids.

Using different fixation methods, images of the nucleic acid in the virion suggested that it is located as a ring along the nucleocapsid inner surface (Gonzalez et al., 1977; Langerberg and Sharpee, 1978). The data of low-angle X-ray scattering had their best fit with a model in which the RNA forms five concentric shells spaced 30 Å apart between the radii 14 and 29 nm (Berger and Kennedy, 1980). The calculated RNA volume is sufficient to fill less than half of a sphere at 29 nm radius.

Freeze-fracturing studies of the virion revealed both concave and convex fracture faces of the phage membrane, indicating that the two membrane leaflets can be separated (Bamford and Lounatamaa, 1978). The convex surface associated with the nucleocapsid appeared smooth, whereas the concave membrane leaflet representing the outer membrane surface was composed of 10-nm particles. The fractured virus diameter was about 80 nm.

C. Genetics and Molecular Cloning of the $\phi6$ Genome

1. Mutations

$\phi6$ has a rather high rate of mutation. Temperature-sensitive mutants are found at a frequency of 0.5% in the absence of mutagenesis. Treatment of whole virions with nitrosoguanidine increases this frequency to 5% (Sinclair et al., 1976).

To isolate nonsense mutants of φ6, it was necessary to develop nonsense suppressor host strains. This was done by introducing a plasmid containing amber mutations in the genes for ampicillin resistance and tetracycline resistance into the host strain and selecting for mutants that were simultaneously resistant to both antibiotics and screening the resistant cells for the ability to support the growth of amber mutant phages of another type that had been developed in E. coli (Mindich et al., 1976b). This selection did not work for the natural host of φ6, P. phaseolicola. Fortunately, it was possible to isolate an alternate host for φ6, which is designated P. pseudoalcaligenes ERA. This strain was able to yield nonsense suppressor mutants. The suppressor strain used for most of the genetic studies with φ6 is called S4.

Wild-type φ6 does not infect P. pseudoalcaligenes; however, host range mutants appear at a frequency of about 5×10^{-6}, and these propagate on both P. pseudoalcaligenes and the original host P. phaseolicola. The phage with the host range mutation is designated φ6hl. In addition, the growth of the hl mutant is restricted somewhat in strain S4. An additional mutation was selected that gives acceptable growth on S4, and the phage that is used for all genetic studies is called φ6hls (Mindich et al., 1976b).

Approximately 250 nonsense mutants of φ6hls have been isolated (Lehman and Mindich, 1979). The mutants were classified by analyzing the patterns of phage-directed protein synthesis in the nonsuppressor hots. Mutants were obtained that affected the appearance of all proteins except P4, P10, and P13. The mutants could be placed in three linkage groups, consistent with the observation of three genomic segments of dsRNA (Lehman and Mindich, 1979). Missense mutations in P10 allowed its placement as well. A temperature-sensitive mutation in gene 4 has recently been isolated by H. Revel (Revel et al., 1986).

A striking observation in the gel patterns of the nonsense mutants was the strong polarity exhibited by some of the mutations. Mutations in gene 8 always prevented the synthesis of P12, mutations in P9 prevented the synthesis of P5, and P7 mutations abolished P2 synthesis. The mechanism of this polarity will be discussed later on in this chapter. A more moderate polarity was seen in the synthesis of proteins P3 and P6, in which nonsense mutants of either inhibited but did not abolish the synthesis of the other (Sinclair et al., 1976).

Although the genes of φ6 could be assigned to consistent linkage groups and these groups could be assigned to particular genomic segments on the basis of their specific coding requirements, a more secure placement was effected by the study of in vitro translation of phage-derived mRNA (Cuppels et al., 1980) and ultimately by the cloning and sequencing of the genomic segments (McGraw et al., 1986; Mindich et al., 1985; Revel et al., 1986; Mindich et al., unpublished). No recombination has been observed between mutations within a particular linkage group. This does not mean that it cannot occur, since the sensitivity of recombination experiments is not great owing to the high reversion frequencies of the mutations (about 10^{-4}) (Sinclair et al., 1976).

2. Molecular Cloning of the φ6 Genome

The virion of φ6 contains transcriptase activity that is activated by treatment with nonionic detergents and that is capable of synthesizing full-length transcripts of the three genomic segments (Partridge et al., 1979). These transcripts were shown to have the same ends as the double-stranded genomic segments (Iba et al., 1982).

In vitro transcripts were tailed with polyA polymerase and used as templates for cDNA synthesis using AMV reverse transcriptase, the cDNA was tailed with polydC, and the second strand was synthesized using an oligodG primer. The cDNA was then tailed with polydC and annealed to plasmid pBR322 that had been cut with Pst1 and tailed with polydG. Cloned fragments of all the φ6 genomic fragments have been isolated, and the entire genome has been represented in a few large clones (Mindich et al., 1985). Each of the segments has been reproduced in two fragments. Alternatively, denatured dsRNA was tailed with polyA and used as template for cDNA synthesis. RNA was digested, and strands of opposite polarity were annealed and extended before insertion into a tailed pBR322 vector (Revel et al., 1986).

The cloned fragments have been sequenced by both chemical (Maxam and Gilbert, 1980) and chain termination methods (Sanger et al., 1977). Figure 10 shows the arrangement of the genes in the three segments as well as the major restriction endonuclease sites and the larger cloned fragments. The assignments of all genes with the exception of those for P12 were confirmed by comparison with amino acid sequence data from the N termini of isolated viral proteins (McGraw et al., 1986; Mindich et al., unpublished). In addition, the open reading frames were consistent with the sizes of the proteins expected from PAGE analysis, with the grouping expected from genetic studies and the polarity relationships observed with nonsense mutants (Lehman and Mindich, 1979). In addition, cloned cDNA fragments were capable of directing in vitro synthesis of φ6 proteins (Mindich et al., 1985) or in vivo synthesis under T7 polymerase control (Revel et al., 1986).

Most of the genes were found to have well-defined ribosome-binding (SD) sequences preceding them (Fig. 11). Three of the genes had either poorly spaced or nonexisting SD sequences; these were genes 2, 5, and 12 (McGraw et al., 1986; Mindich et al., unpublished). These genes were previously found to be subject to strong polarity when adjacent genes suffered nonsense mutations (Lehman and Mindich, 1979). It appears that φ6 uses a novel means of controlling the expression of its genes. In these cases, the upstream genes are expressed at a high level, and the downstream genes are expressed at about 10% of that level. The ribosomes are loaded on at the SD region of the upstream protein, translate that gene,

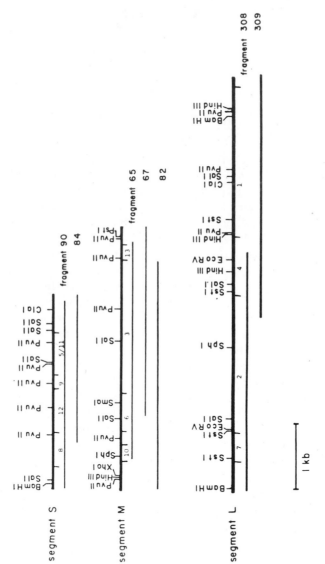

FIGURE 10. Map of the ϕ6 genome. The three segments are shown with the cleavage sites for several restriction endonucleases. The arrangement of the numbered genes is also shown. Several large cDNA copies of the segments are also presented. From Mindich et al. (1985) and Revel et al. (1986).

Nucleotide Sequences of the 5′ Regions of the φ6 Genes

```
                                    *
                          UAAGGAGGUGAUC              Rev Comp of 16S RNA
                                8
        GUUCCCACUAAUAAUAAAGGAAUACGCACAUGUUG           P8
                              9
        CAGAUGGUCCACCGUAAGGAUGUUCCGUAAUGCCA           P9
                              7
        GGCCGUCAUCUGACAGUAAGGAGUAGCAAAUGCGC           P3
                             8
        GGAGACGCGGCCGAUGGUGGAGGUGCUCAGUGAGU           P6
                            9
        UCCUCAACCCAUAAUAAGAGAUCCAUUCAAUGGAC           P10
                          7
        GUCGUCCUCAAUCUCAUCGGGAAGUGACCAUGGUA           P13
                            6
        GUGCUAACUUCUCUCUGUAAGGGUAUAAGAUGUUC           P1
                          7
        UUUCUCCGUUCUGUAAUGCCGAGGUAAUCAUGCCG           P4
                         8 or 9
        GUAUCCGACUUUUAUAAGGACGGUGUGUAAUGACU           P7

                           11
        CAGCUGAAUGACAUGGGAUACCGCUCGUAAUGGUU           P12
                           11
        CCAACAUCCCUUUUCUGGCCUAACUCCUCGUGUCC           P5
                          12
        CCGUUCGAUGUCGAUGAGGUAAGCGCCUGAUGCCG           P2
```

FIGURE 11. The nucleotide sequence around the initiating codons for each of the φ6 proteins. The initiating codon AUG or GUG is underlined, as are sequences showing homology to the reverse complement of the terminus of 16S RNA. The numbers refer to the distance between the first base of the initiating codon and the A residue indicated by the asterisk. From McGraw et al. (1986) and Mindich et al. (unpublished).

then most fall off, and the residual number are left to synthesize proteins P2, P5, or P12. This mechanism seems to work rather well in that the relative quantity of proteins synthesized in infected cells is rather close to that found in virions (Fig. 12). Nonsense mutations in the upstream genes would then be expected to result in the complete elimination of synthesis of the downstream gene products.

The downstream genes, in the three cases, begin close to the termination codons of the preceding ones (McGraw et al., 1986). The initiating AUG of gene 12 shares the A of the terminating codon UAA for gene 8. In the case of gene 5, there is a gap of six nucleotides, and in the case of gene 2, there is an overlap between the initiation codon and the termination codon of the preceding gene.

3. Expression of φ6 Genes from Plasmids Containing cDNA

The cDNA copies of the φ6 genome were originally isolated as inserts into the ampicillin resistance gene of pBR322 (Mindich et al., 1985), some in the direction of the amp transcription, others in reverse. In general, those fragments that were inserted in the correct direction

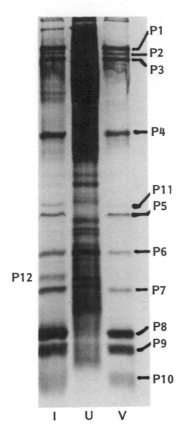

FIGURE 12. Autoradiogram of polyacrylamide gel of φ6 proteins. Purified virions (V); uninfected cells (U); infected cells labeled in the presence of rifampin (I). From Sinclair *et al.* (1975).

yielded transcripts that resulted in *in vitro* synthesis of peptides corresponding to the proper φ6 gene products. Fragments or parts of fragments could also be inserted into expression vectors such as pUC8 and pUC9 with the resulting synthesis of mRNA controlled by the *Lac* promoter of the plasmid. The cDNA material would not be expected to contain natural promoter sequences, since mRNA in phage infection is derived from viral transcription of entire genomic segments (Coplin *et al.*, 1975).

To study the expression of the DNA material in the host of φ6, *P. phaseolicola*, it was necessary to construct expression vectors that would propagate in pseudomonads. Several chimeric plasmids have been used that combine pBR322 derivatives such as pUC8 or pKK223-3 (a tac promotor plasmid) with derivatives of RSF1010 (a broad-host-range plasmid). In the earliest studies, a plasmid designated pLM235 was used (Mindich *et al.*, 1985). This plasmid contains the entire pUC8 and part of RSF1010. cDNA fragments were ligated into the Pst 1 site, and the transcripts were controlled by the *Lac* promoter. Because the *Lac* promoter is poorly expressed in pseudomonads, this plasmid was modified by mutation to yield pLM254, which has a promoter mutation in the −9 position G → A

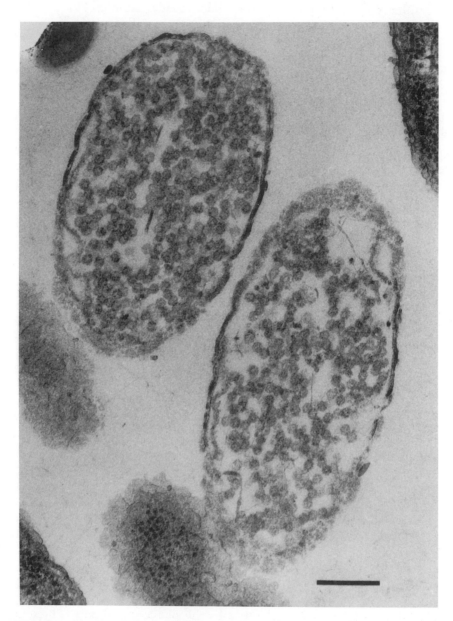

FIGURE 13. Electron micrograph of sections of *E. coli* carrying plasmids with the complete cDNA copy of genomic segment *L*. Particles have the same composition as procapsids. The cells have lost most of their ribosomes, thereby facilitating visualization of the particles. Scale bar: 200 nm. From Gottlieb *et al.* (1988).

and results in higher expression in pseudomonads (Mindich *et al.*, 1985). Using pLM254, we have found that cDNA material results in complementation of nonsense mutants in genes 1, 2, 3, 5, 6, 7, 8, 9, and 12. H. Revel has found complementation of a *ts* mutation in gene 4 (Revel *et al.*, 1986). This means that complementation has worked for all mutation classes that could be tested, since there are no present nonsense mutants in gene 4 and no nonsense or *ts* mutants in genes 10 and 13.

Another set of plasmids represented by pLM372 are derivatives of RSF1010 and a tac promoter plasmid. These plasmids yield very high expression in both *E. coli* and *P. phaseolicola*. Plasmid pLM372 contains the *LacI*^{q} gene as well, so that expression can be controlled in both *E. coli* and *P. phaseolicola*. A derivative of pLM372 containing a cDNA copy of the entire *L* segment promotes the synthesis in *E. coli* of large amounts of the four gene products expected—P1, P2, P4, and P7 (Gottlieb *et al.*, 1988)—with P1 constituting about 5–10% of the total cell protein. These proteins assemble to form a structure of the appearance and composition of the φ6 procapsid (Fig. 13).

4. Organization of the φ6 Genome

φ6 has three genomic segments of double-stranded RNA (Semancik *et al.*, 1973). The segments are designated *L*, *M*, and *S* and contain 6374, 4057, and 2948 bp, respectively. The segments have a base composition of 55%, 57%, and 55% G plus C. The arrangement of the genes is shown in Fig. 10. It is shown that the genes are clustered together and that each segment has noncoding regions of several hundred base pairs at each end. Segment *M* has a region between genes 10 and 6 that may be untranslated. There is a high degree of homology between the ends of the three segments (Iba *et al.*, 1982). The homology is perfect for 17 bp at the 3' end (with respect to the mRNA) and then falls off gradually until homology disappears at about position 80 (Fig. 14). At the 5' end, the homology is perfect for 18 bp and then ends abruptly. There is a single base difference in the second base position between the *L* segment and the other two.

The *L* segment contains the genes that are expressed early. These are the genes that code for the proteins of the procapsid P1, P2, P4, and P7. Three of the genes have discernible Shine-Dalgarno sequences, but gene 2 does not.

The *M* segment contains genes 10, 6, 3, and 13. All the proteins produced by this segment are found in the phage membrane. P6 is the most hydrophobic and is the anchor for P3 which is hydrophilic and contains the host attachment specificity. P10 is involved in lysis but is not a lysozyme. Either or both proteins P10 and P13 play an important role in membrane formation. There is a strange polarity relationship between genes 6 and 3 in that nonsense mutations in either diminish the expression of the other, but not completely (Sinclair *et al.*, 1976). It is not

Nucleotide Sequence at the 5' Termini of the Ø6 Segments

L   GUAAAAAAACUUUAUAUAGUCUUUUACCUGGAUUCUCUGUG
       | |||||||||||||
       GGAAAAAAACUUUAUAUAUAUUUCUACGUUGAGCUCCGUAUA

M ||||||||||||
       GGAAAAAAACUUUAUAUAUAACUCUUAUAUAAGUGCCCUUAGC

S

Nucleotide Sequence at the 3' Termini of the Ø6 Segments

L   UCCAUAAGUCCUUAGAUUUCUAAGGCGGAGACUCGCUUUGCGAGCGUCCAAUAGGACGGCCCCUCGGGGGCUCUCUCUCU
      | |||||||||||||||||||||||||||||||||| |||||||| | ||||||| |||||||||||||
      UAAAUAAGUCCUUAGAUUUCUAAGGCGAGACUCGCUUUGCGAUCCAAUAGGAUGGCCCCUUCGGGGGCUCUCUCUCU

M ||||||||| |||| |||||||| ||||||||||||||||| |||||||||||||||||||||
      UAAACAAGUCCUUGUAUAAC–AAGGCGAGACUCACUAUGUGAGCGUCCAAUAGGACGGCCCCUUCGGGGGCUCUCUCUCU

S

FIGURE 14. Nucleotide sequences at the termini of the three genomic segments of φ6. Vertical lines denote homology. Only the plus strand is presented, and the sequences read left to right from 5' to 3'. From McGraw et al. (1986) and Mindich et al. (unpublished).

known whether this is actually an effect of expression or stability of the proteins or something else.

The S segment contains genes 8, 12, 9, and 5. P8 forms a shell over the RNA-filled procapsid to form the nucleocapsid. P12 is the only viral protein that is not a component of the virion. It is necessary for the envelopment of the nucleocapsid by the phage membrane (Mindich and Lehman, 1983). P9 is the major membrane protein, and P5 is the lysozyme that is necessary for both entry of the virus into the cell and lysis of the cell at the end of infection (Mindich and Lehman, 1979). P11 forms a band that migrates slightly slower than P5 in SDS gels. Missense mutations that change the migration of P5 also change that of P11. Both proteins lack methionine. Since the amino terminus of P5 is consistent with the earliest possible start for gene 5, we believe that P11 is either a modified form of P5 or somewhat larger owing to "read-through" of gene 5. In any case, P11 does not seem to be necessary, as it is not made in *P. pseudoalcaligenes* or at low temperature in *P. phaseolicola*.

D. Entry of Bacteriophage φ6

φ6 is the only known dsRNA bacteriophage. Cells do not have enzymes to replicate dsRNA, and this type of virus has to bring its own polymerases into the cell. φ6 faces a complicated rigid gram-negative cell wall with two membranes and a peptidoglycan layer between them. Thus, the infection mechanism differs grossly from those of other bacterial viruses.

1. Adsorption

In the original description of φ6, the adsorption rate constant for the virus was measured to be about 3.5×10^{-10} ml/min, and the virus was seen associated with pili expressed by the host *P. phaseolicola* (Vidaver *et al.*, 1973). The pilus association was later confirmed. Shortly after infection, the virions were seen associated with the host pili (Fig. 2) with a variety of electron microscopic techniques (negative staining, thin sectioning, freeze fracturing, and by using scanning electron microscopy) (Bamford *et al.*, 1976; Bamford and Lounatmaa, 1978, 1982; Cuppels *et al.*, 1979; Romantschuk and Bamford, 1985). One of the major classes of φ6-resistant mutants did not adsorb phages and was found to be devoid of pili (Cuppels *et al.*, 1979; Romantschuk and Bamford, 1985).

The presence of φ6-specific pili was not associated with independently replicating plasmids in the original host or in other φ6-sensitive. *P. syringae* and *P. pseudoalcaligenes* strains. The *P. syringae* and *P. pseudoalcaligenes* pili differ in morphology (Romantschuk and Bamford, 1985).

Phage-resistant mutants have been isolated that show increased adsorption of phage and hyperextended pili. It appears that pilus retraction is needed to bring the virus closer to the surface into contact with the outer membrane (Romantschuk and Bamford, 1985). Protein P3 on the virus surface has been demonstrated to be the adsorption protein binding to the pilus (Mindich et al., 1976c). Partially purified pili from infected cells have been shown to have labeled P3 proteins associated with them (M. Romantschuk, personal communication); however, isolated protein P3 is unable to adsorb to host bacteria (Romantschuk and Bamford, 1985). The adsorption of phages to pili was shown to be independent of divalent cations and was efficient at pH 5.0–8.5 (Romantschuk and Bamford, 1985).

2. Phage Membrane Fusion with the Host Outer Membrane

When infecting virus particles reach the surface of the outer membrane, a fusion between the phage membrane and the host outer membrane occurs at the site of the pilus attachment (Bamford et al., 1976; Bamford and Lounatmaa, 1978, 1982) (Fig. 2). Biochemical studies showed that after infection, it was possible to coisolate phage lipids and phage membrane proteins P6, P9, P10, and P13 with the host outer membrane. The association of protein P3 with the fused outer membrane could not be studied (Bamford et al., 1987).

Fluorescence-quenched lipids in phage particles showed increased fluoresence due to dilution after association with host cells. This indicated that there is a continuum between the phage and host membranes. The fusion was also shown to be nonleaky, in that periplasmic alkaline phosphatase was not found in the medium (Bamford et al., 1987). An in vitro fusion assay was developed in which individual virus particles were brought together by sedimentation, and the fusion was analyzed by rate zonal centrifugation (Bamford et al., 1987). Using particles lacking proteins P3 and/or P6, it was possible to show that the in vitro fusion was dependent on the presence of protein P6 and was enhanced by the removal of protein P3. Particles lacking both of these proteins were unable to fuse either with each other or with particles that did contain proteins P6 and P3 or P6 alone, indicating that P6 is the fusogenic protein and that the fusion requires a "fusion receptor structure" on the target membrane. The fusion event was shown both in vivo and in vitro to occur at pH 5.0–8.5 and to be independent of divalent cations.

The fusion event brings the nucleocapsid inside the outer membrane but outside the peptidoglycan of the host cell. It has been shown that phage-specific protein P5 is a lytic enzyme (Iba et al., 1979; Kakitani et al., 1978; Mindich and Lehman, 1979). The location of this protein between the membrane and nucleocapsid surface facilitates the enzymatic digestion of the peptidoglycan, which is a necessary step in infection (Mindich and Lehman, 1979). Host cell variants with altered sensitivity to φ6 lysin have been isolated. They show a pseudolysogenic phenotype with slow release of viruses into the medium (Cuppels *et al.*, 1979; Romantschuk and Bamford, 1981).

3. Nucleocapsid Entry through the Cytoplasmic Membrane

Soon after infection, it is possible to isolate a particle containing proteins P1, P2, P4, and P7 of the infecting phage inside the host cells. It appeared that P8 was left outside (Kakitani *et al.*, 1980; Romantschuk *et al.*, unpublished). Nucleocapsid penetration was studied by analyzing phage components in the periplasm and cytoplasmic membrane and inside cells after infection. The success of these studies was dependent on the development of a technique for removing the unfused phages associated with ϕ6 receptors. Careful washing of the cell with concentrations of Triton X-100, which destroys the phages but does not affect the infected host cells, made the nucleocapsid entry studies possible. These studies also showed that on the average, only one virus enters each cell.

The nucleocapsid shell protein P8 dissociates into the periplasm, and the rest of the nucleocapsid penetrates the cytoplasmic membrane. The nucleocapsid can be arrested in the periplasm by addition of sodium azide and the protonophore CCCP (carbonyl cyanide m-chlorophenyl hydrozone). *In vitro* studies with nucleocapsids showed that it was possible to infect host cell spheroplasts with nucleocapsids.

In previous studies, subviral particles were isolated from infected cells 20 min postinfection. A particle containing RNA and P1, P2, P4, and P7 was isolated, as was an RNA-less particle containing proteins P1 and P2 (Kakitani *et al.*, 1980). We are somewhat dubious of these results, as we have never seen procapsids isolated with their RNA complement intact.

E. Transcription and Replication of ϕ6 RNA

The genome of ϕ6 is three pieces of double-stranded RNA. During infection, complete transcripts of these segments are found (Coplin *et al.*, 1975). Shortly after entry, there is a production of equimolar amounts of the three transcripts; however, a transition takes place midway in infection that results in the production of approximately 10 times as much of the S and M transcripts as L (Coplin *et al.*, 1975).

Nucleocapsids isolated from mature virions by detergent treatment are capable of synthesizing complete transcripts of the three segments *in vitro* (Partridge *et al.*, 1979). In the presence of magnesium ions, the production of transcripts is biased similarly to that found in late infection; however, in the presence of manganese ions, more of the L transcript is found (Emori *et al.*, 1983). The extent of L transcription is also dependent upon specific nucleotide triphosphate concentrations. The *in vitro* transcripts are capable of directing the *in vitro* synthesis of all the phage proteins (Cuppels *et al.*, 1980). This synthesis is more or less in proportion to that found in infected cells, indicating that specific factors are not necessary to control gene expression. The synthesis of transcripts involves a strand displacement mechanism (Usala *et al.*, 1980; Van Etten *et al.*, 1980). This is in contrast to the observation that reovirus transcription is conservative (Joklik, 1981).

The machinery for transcription does not involve any of the late proteins of φ6. Nonsense mutations in the late genes do not affect either transcription or replication of RNA (Sinclair and Mindich, 1976). This is also true for gene 8, which determines the protein that covers the nucleocapsid structure. Nonsuppressor cells infected with nonsense mutants in genes 1 or 2 show a low level of single-stranded RNA synthesis that results in the synthesis of early proteins, but these cells do not synthesize double-stranded RNA or single-stranded RNA at the levels found in normally infected cells (Sinclair and Mindich, 1976). This indicates that at least proteins P1 and P2 are necessary for RNA synthesis. It has not been possible to determine the role of P7 in RNA synthesis, because its mutations are polar on the production of P2, which is necessary. P4 has not yielded nonsense mutants, but a *ts* mutant has recently been found by H. Revel (Revel *et al.*, 1986), so it seems likely that all four of the early proteins are necessary for synthesis of RNA.

Mutants that cannot produce protein P8 synthesize a particle that is called the procapsid. This particle is found to be filled with RNA inside of cells (Bamford and Mindich, 1980) and to appear as cage structures (Mindich and Davidoff Abelson, 1980) similar to those seen in micrographs of viral nucleocapsids. The procapsids appear to be dodecahedral bodies (Yang and Lang, 1984). Their composition would be expected to be approximately 120 molecules of P1 and P4, about 20 molecules of P2, and about 100 molecules of P7 (Day and Mindich, 1980). Radioactive amino acid labels move from the procapsids to nucleocapsids to mature virions, indicating that they are on the normal assembly pathway (Emori *et al.*, 1982; Mindich *et al.*, 1979). No RNA synthetic competence has been found for procapsids, although one might expect them to be able to form double-stranded RNA from the single-stranded transcripts. In fact, one would expect the procapsids to be able to package the genomic segments either after or during synthesis or by first packaging the single-stranded precursors. In any case, the packaging must be very efficient, because the infectivity of φ6 is virtually one, and each particle has the same amount of RNA, which amounts to one complete genome equivalent (Day and Mindich, 1980).

A model for RNA synthesis in φ6-infected cells that relies on the information accumulated from φ6 studies and those of reovirus would have the infecting particle that enters the cytoplasm be a filled procapsid that is in some way different from the later ones. This particle would start transcription of the three pieces of single-stranded RNA. Only the *L* transcript would be translated and would form the procapsid proteins, and these would assemble to form empty procapsids. These would pick up single-stranded RNA. The double-stranded RNA would be synthesized either during this process or afterward. These filled procapsids should be capable of initiating new transcription, and this would likely be of the late type with larger amounts of the S and M transcripts. Ultimately, the particles would be coated by protein P8, which would convert them to nucleocapsids, and they would then stop RNA synthesis. There must be a mechanism to prevent P8 from covering empty procapsids; however, one can imagine a structural change in the procapsid when it becomes filled.

1. Protein Synthesis in φ6-Infected Cells

Early in infection, the proteins of the procapsids P1, P2, P4, and P7 are synthesized (Sinclair *et al.*, 1975). Later on, the remainder of the proteins are made, and the relative proportion of the proteins is very similar to that found in the mature virion. Since the messenger transcripts are complete, it appears that the regulation of gene expression must be posttranscriptional. The observation that *in vitro* synthesis of the proteins has approximately the same relative proportions strengthens this point.

It has been found that the means of control is in the nature of the initiation or rate of synthesis of some proteins, perhaps through the strength of association with SD sequences in some cases, and in others, where low production is desired, there is no SD sequence, and the protein synthesis is initiated by ribosomes that were involved in the synthesis of the upstream neighboring gene product (McGraw *et al.*, 1986) (Fig. 11).

It is not known why late proteins are not synthesized early in infection. At that time, there is synthesis of transcripts of the S and M segments in about equal proportions to that of L, but only the L genes are expressed (Sinclair *et al.*, 1975). In an alternate host, *P. pseudoalcaligenes*, protein P3 is expressed from segment M early in infection. This shows that the specificity of early expression is not determined simply by the particular transcript that the gene is on, since proteins P6, P10, and P13, which are on segment M, are not expressed early.

2. Assembly of the φ6 Membrane

In the late part of the infection, all phage proteins are made. Protein P8 forms a shell around the filled procapsids. This structure, called the nucleocapsid, acquires a lipid-containing membrane inside the host cell, in the absence of budding. The proteins of the membrane are P3, P6, P9, P10, and P13. Mutants with nonsense mutations in gene 3 produce virions that lack P3; mutants in gene 6 produce virions that lack both P3 and P6, which is consistent with our model that hydrophilic P3 binds to hydrophobic P6 in the viral membrane. The presence of neither P3 nor P6 is necessary for the formation of the viral membrane. Mutants that cannot make P9 produce particles that have no membrane, indicating that P9 plays a vital role in the formation or attachment of the membrane (Mindich *et al.*, 1976c). No nonsense mutants in genes 10 or 13 have been isolated yet. It is therefore not clear whether they play necessary roles in the formation of the membrane.

Protein P12 is the only viral protein that is not a component of the virion. Mutants that do not synthesize P12 do not produce enveloped particles; only nucleocapsids accumulate. P12 therefore plays a vital role in membrane formation. Temperature-sensitive mutants of P12 have been isolated, and at restrictive temperatures infected cells produce nucleocapsids but not enveloped particles. If cells infected with a *ts* mutant of P12 are pulse-labeled with radioactive amino acids at the restrictive temperature (28°C), all viral proteins are labeled; if the label is chased and the cells are placed at the permissive temperature (18°C), complete viral particles are formed. The hydrophobic proteins P6, P9, P10, and P13 in the complete particles are not labeled, indicating that active P12 is necessary at the time of synthesis of the hydrophobic proteins in order for them to be placed in the membrane. It is of interest that protein P3 does appear with label in such particles, suggesting that it is incorporated into the viral membrane after the membrane is placed on the virion and that P3 attachment does not depend on active P12 at the time of its synthesis (Mindich and Lehman, 1983).

When infected cells are pulse-labeled for less than a few minutes, lysed, and fractionated on sucrose gradients, it is found that a particle sedimenting at somewhat less than 100S is labeled. The radioactivity in this particle is in proteins P9, P6, and P10/P13. P13 was not distinguished from P10. The particle can be observed with greater ease in fractions of CsCl gradients, where it has a density of 1.18 g/cm^3 (Stitt and Mindich, 1983b). The density of the particle suggests that it contains lipid, and indeed the particle density is increased by treatment with phospholipases. Proteins P9 and P10 in the particle are not accessible to protease, suggesting that the orientation of the proteins in the particle is the same as in the virion (Stitt and Mindich, 1983b). The formation of this particle is dependent on the activity of P12. Nonsense mutants in gene 12 or *ts* mutants at restrictive temperature do not produce it (Stitt and Mindich, 1983b).

This particle would appear to be a precursor of the viral membrane. However, it is not clear whether it is an actual membrane precursor or a by-product of one. It is possible that there is a free membrane vesicle precursor, but it may also be that a patch of viral proteins in the host-membrane is released when the cells are lysed with lysozyme or sonication. It is also possible that the true precursor structure is a vesiclelike body that is attached to the host membrane and released upon rupture of the cell.

The particle can be formed in cells that do not assemble nucleocapsids. This is accomplished by infecting cells carrying plasmids able to direct the synthesis of P12, with phage mutants unable to direct the synthesis of P8 and P12. Under these circumstances procapsids accumulate, and the membrane "particle" can be labeled, but the label does not chase into virions. This experiment excludes the possibility that the membrane precursor particle is simply a partially completed structure that was assembled on the nucleocapsid surface (Fig. 15, III) (McGraw and Mindich, unpublished). The particle can also be labeled in cells infected with a mutant unable to produce P9. In this case, the particle contains P6 and P10/P13 (McGraw and Mindich, unpublished).

A model that would rationalize the information we have collected for membrane assembly would have P12 interacting with the nascent hydrophobic viral proteins so as to guide them to the host membrane and perhaps to facilitate their proper insertion. With the exception of P6, the other hydrophobic proteins have considerable total charge (Table II) and could very well be soluble when synthesized. It is also possible that P12 interacts with all the phage membrane proteins or just one, perhaps P10, to create a proper integration site in the membrane. It seems likely that P12 acts catalytically, since it is synthesized in lesser amounts than P9 and P10. It does not seem that P12 is involved in processing the proteins, since the mature proteins lose only the N-terminal methionine at most. P9 is necessary for the placement of the membrane on the virion; howev-

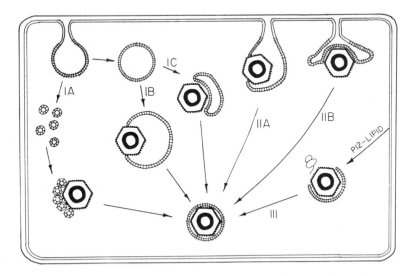

FIGURE 15. Models for the transfer of membrane material to φ6 virions. Phage proteins and host lipids are transferred from the host membrane in small vesicles (IA). A large free vesicle of normal orientation is entered by a nucleocapsid (IB), or a large free vesicle everts over a nucleocapsid (IC). Nucleocapsid enters an attached vesicle of normal orientation (IIA) or is covered by an everting, reversed-orientation, attached vesicle (IIB). The viral membrane is assembled on the surface of the nucleocapsid (III). From Stitt and Mindich (1983b).

er, it may be that P9 is not necessary for formation of the membrane complex but is necessary for its association with the nucleocapsid.

The hydrophobic proteins would be inserted into the host cytoplasmic membrane either as a patch or as an attached vesicle. This structure would be the source of the particle we have observed. A remaining puzzle is the orientation of the proteins in the patch or vesicle. The results of protease treatment suggest that the particle has the same orientation as the mature viral membrane. If this is so, it is difficult to construct a simple interaction of the nucleocapsid and membrane intermediate that would result in the placement of the nucleocapsid inside of the membrane. Several models are illustrated in Fig. 15. Alternatives IA and III have been rejected on the basis of arguments presented earlier. The models for IB and IC involve a free vesicle intermediate that is either inverted or right side out. In the case of IB, we have to postulate a mechanism of bringing the nucleocapsid into the vesicle. In the case of IC, the vesicle would interact with the nucleocapsid through P9 and evert; this model would require that the true vesicle be inside out and that the particle we isolate has changed its orientation. The models IIA and IIB are similar to IB and IC except that they propose that the vesicle is attached to the host membrane. The same considerations hold as before.

III. PRD1-TYPE PHAGES

A. Introduction

Bacteriophage PRD1 is a model virus for a family of viruses in the tectiviridae group (International Committee on Taxonomy of Viruses). This group contains viruses infecting both gram-negative and gram-positive hosts. The closely related viruses infecting gram-negative hosts (PRD1, PR3, PR4, PR5, PR722, L17) have been studied in greater detail than those members infecting gram-positive hosts (AP50, ϕNS11, Bam35). In this section we will discuss the best-characterized members of this group, PRD1 and PR4. These viruses can infect a variety of gram-negative hosts, *Escherichia coli* and *Salmonella typhimurium* among them, harboring plasmids in P, N, and W incompatibility groups (Bradley and Rutherford, 1975; Olsen et al., 1974; Stanisich, 1974). The receptor for these viruses is plasmid-coded, and pili have been implicated (Bradley, 1976; Bradley and Cohen, 1977). It has also been observed that the sensitive cells can bind a high number of virions on their surface (Bradley, 1974; Lundstrom et al., 1979; Olsen et al., 1977).

The viral DNA is found within a lipid-containing membrane vesicle (Fig. 16). The vesicle is covered by a protein capsid (Bamford and Mindich, 1982). After infection, the capsid is seen on the surface of the cell, but the lipid layer is contracted (Lundstrom et al., 1979). The phage genome replicates in a linear form (Bamford and Mindich, 1984), and genes are expressed in a regulated manner with very early, early, and late genes.

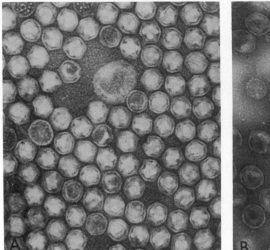
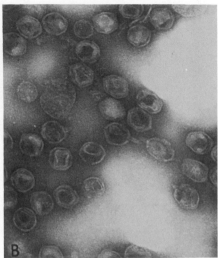

FIGURE 16. Electronmicrograph of PR4 stained with phosphotungstate. DNA-filled particles (left) and empty particles (right). Note the collapsed appearance of the membrane
vesicles in the empty particles. From Lundstrom *et al.* (1979).

The early gene products are involved in replication and transcription
control; the late ones are structural or morphogenetic proteins (Mindich
et al., 1982b).

Shortly after synthesis, phage proteins localized in the virus membrane are found in the host cytoplasmic membrane, and the capsid proteins are found soluble in the cell (Mindich *et al.*, 1982a). The virion
assembles by the encapsulation of the virus lipid membrane by the capsid
proteins (Mindich *et al.*, 1982a). The viral lipids are derived from the host
cell lipid pool (Muller and Cronan, 1983). The empty virions are found in
the nucleoplasm of the cell, and after DNA packaging they accumulate
into the ribosome-rich cell periphery (Lundstrom *et al.*, 1979). Cellular
lysis is caused by the phage-specific lytic enzyme (Davis and Cronan,
1983; Mindich *et al.*, 1982b) about 1 hr after infection, liberating a few
hundred progeny phages into the medium (Bamford *et al.*, 1981). Figure
17 depicts schematically the life cycle of PRD1-type phages.

1. Structure

The morphological, protein, and DNA comparison of PRD1 family
phages PRD1, PR3, PR4, PR5, PR722, and L17 (Bamford *et al.*, 1981;
Coetzee and Bekker, 1979) and the comparison of the nucleic acid sequences of the DNA termini (Savilahti and Bamford, 1986) show that
these viruses are very closely related, although they are isolated from
different parts of the world. Structural results obtained with one virus are

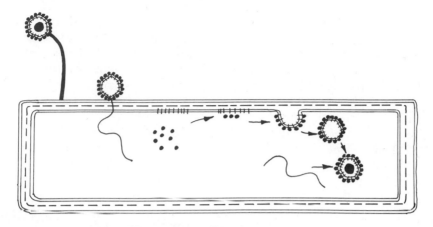

FIGURE 17. A diagram of the life cycle of PRD1/PR4. The virion attaches to the tip of a pilus, but it is not clear that this is necessary for infection. Particles are adsorbed to the surface and inject their DNA, leaving the capsid and membrane vesicle behind. Capsid proteins are found as soluble multimers shortly after synthesis. Membrane proteins are associated with the host membrane fraction. No precursors to the empty particles are found. Particle formation is dependent on several nonstructural proteins. The empty particle packages genomic DNA to become a mature virion.

relevant for the others, and they will be dealt with together in this discussion.

2. Chemical Composition and Proteins

The chemical composition for PR4 is given as 14% DNA, 73% protein, and 13% lipid (Davis et al., 1982), and for PR5, 15% DNA, 65% protein, and 20% lipid (Wong and Bryan, 1978). In two cases, the genome length has been measured with greater accuracy, giving a value of 14,500 bp with electron microscopy for PR4 (Davis et al., 1982) and, by cloning and restriction enzyme mapping, 14,700 bp for PRD1 (McGraw et al., 1983; Mindich and McGraw, 1983). The DNA replicates in a linear form with a protein-priming initiation system (Bamford et al., 1983; Bamford and Mindich, 1984; Savilahti and Bamford, 1986). The replication mechanisms used by bacteriophages that have genomic proteins are covered in detail in Chapter 9 of this volume.

The most thorough lipid analysis was done on phage PR4 (Muller and Cronan, 1983). Phage grown in wild-type E. coli contain 56% phosphatidyl ethanolamine, 37% phosphatidyl glycerol, and 4.6% cardiolipin. Two percent of the lipids are neutral lipids. The fatty-acid compositions of the viral and cellular phospholipids are identical (Davis et al., 1982). The lipid composition of PR4 was altered by growth on mutants of E. coli defective in fatty acid or phospholipid metabolism (Muller and Cronan, 1983). It was found that the level of saturation in the fatty acids could be increased from 41% to 69%. The resulting phages showed striking losses of infectivity at low temperatures in a manner that suggests that the phage membrane undergoes a phase transition that is lethal to the phage. In addition, it was possible to alter the phospholipid composition of the virus such that variations from 28% to 60% in phosphatidylethanolamine, from 22% to 39% in phosphatidylglycerol, and from 1% to 15% in cardiolipin occurred. It was also possible to form virions containing as much as 35% phosphatidylserine. PR4 normally does not contain any phosphatidylserine. These changes occurred without affecting the viability of the phage, showing that the lipid composition does not have to be maintained within narrow limits.

Both the PRD1 (Mindich et al., 1982a,b) and the PR4 systems (Davis et al., 1982; Davis and Cronan, 1983) involved structural as well as nonstructural proteins. In PRD1, eight of the 25 identified viral proteins are not components of the virion (Fig. 18).

B. Protein Localization and Particle Disruption

The structural data have accumulated simultaneously from phages PRD1 and PR4, and no separation between the organisms will be made subsequently in this paragraph. Electron microscopic observations revealed a polyhedral 65-nm-diameter particle with a rigid surface layer and a membranous inner layer. Freeze-fracturing revealed an internal cleavable fracture face, indicating the presence of an internal lipid bilayer (Bradley and Rutherford, 1975; Lundstrom et al., 1979). The occurrence of a lipid bilayer in the phage structure is also shown by the presence of half of the PE in each leaflet (Davis and Cronan, 1985) and by the cooperative nature of the melting of the lipids (Muller and Cronan, 1983). Guanidine hydrochloride treatment allows the separation of the phage protein surface as capsomers containing a major and a minor capsid protein and a membrane vesicle containing 15 viral proteins and the phage DNA (Fig. 19). A small increase in the guanidine concentration leads to the release of the DNA and to transformation of the spherical vesicle to a narrow cylinder. This transformation is a controlled event, since mutant vesicles lacking a specific membrane protein, P18, remain spherical under these conditions (Bamford and Mindich, 1982). The cylinder formation may be important in DNA injection, since empty virus particles exhibit this cylinder passing through one of the vertices.

Protease treatment of the isolated membrane vesicles led to the degradation of all but one of the membrane-associated proteins (Bamford and Mindich, 1982), showing that they are not protected by the bilayer. No discrimination of the side of the membrane could be done, since they looked open in electron microscopy. Alkyl imidate labeling showed that the proteins are in intimate contact with the bilayer and accessible from outside (Davis and Cronan, 1985).

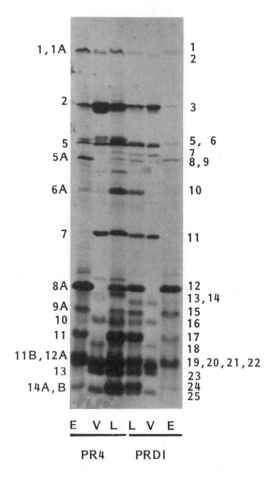

FIGURE 18. Autoradiogram of polyacrylamide gel of labeled proteins of PRD1 and PR4. Cells were infected after UV irradiation. Early pattern (E); late pattern (L); purified virions (V). Designation of proteins follows Mindich *et al.* (1982b) for PRD1 and Davis and Cronan (1983) for PR4.

The major capsid protein enclosing the membrane vesicle shows linkage only with phosphatidylglycerol in the virion, suggesting that the protein or capsomer complex composed of it is embedded in a phosphatidylglycerol annulus. This specific interaction may be the reason for the relative enrichment of the phage membrane in phosphatidylglycerol as compared to host membranes (Davis *et al.*, 1982). One additional PRD1 protein, P8, is located on the 5′ ends of the linear phage DNA and thus is inside the phage membrane vesicle (Bamford *et al.*, 1983; Bamford and Mindich, 1984). The internal location of this protein was confirmed by the finding that it was the only virion protein in PR4 that was inaccessible to imidate labeling (Davis and Cronan, 1985).

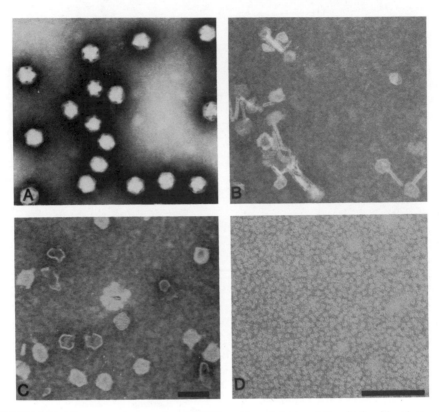

FIGURE 19. Electron micrographs of PRD1 subjected to guanidine hydrochloride treatment. (A) Intact particles. (B) Empty vesicles showing transition to tubular form. (C) Vesicles containing DNA. (D) Capsomers. Scale bar: 100 nm. From Bamford and Mindich (1982).

C. Genetics and Cloning

Restriction digests of the DNAs of the PRD1 family show some differences but in general have great similarity (Bamford *et al.*, 1981). The DNA of PRD1 is not susceptible to most restriction endonucleases of 6-base specificity, perhaps owing to its extensive host range (Bamford *et al.*, 1981; Mindich and McGraw, 1983). We have found that PRD1 and PR4 do show host restriction when plating on *P. pseudoalcaligenes*, which has a restriction system of specificity GGCC (Mindich, unpublished). All but the right end of the PRD1 genome has been cloned as partial HaeII fragments in pBR322 (Mindich and McGraw, 1983). The end that could not be cloned contains genes 12 and 19, which are expressed early and whose expression might be lethal to *E. coli*. A physical restriction map of the genome was determined with the fragments generated by HaeII cutting, MboI and MnlI (McGraw *et al.*, 1983). The anomolous behavior of two of the HaeII fragments on agarose gels suggested that the genome contained terminal proteins. This was later confirmed (Bamford *et al.*, 1983), and the nature of the bond was determined (Bamford and Mindich, 1984).

Nonsense mutants of PRD1 were isolated through the use of suppressor strains of *S. typhimurium* (Mindich *et al.*, 1982b). Nonsense mutants were also isolated from PR4 (Davis and Cronan, 1983). Although there are some differences in the protein gel patterns of the two viruses, it is possible to assign homologies between the two sets (Fig. 18, Table IV). In the case of PRD1, we found that infection led to the synthesis of at least 25 specific proteins, of which 17 were components of the virion. The program of protein synthesis could be divided into three groups designated very early, middle early, and late (Mindich *et al.*, 1982b). Nonsense mutations could be arranged in 17 groups on the basis of genetic complementation. Most of these groups could be assigned to specific proteins on the basis of a correlation with missing bands on acrylamide gels. Attempts to construct a genetic map through recombination frequencies in two-factor crosses failed, because the frequency of recombination did not vary between markers except in cases where they were later found to be very close or in the same gene. It seems likely that this is due to the special mode of replication of the PRD1 genome, although φ29, the bacillus phage with terminal genomic protein, does yield a coherent ge-

Table IV. Comparison of PRD1 and PR4 proteins

	PRD1[a]				PR4[b]		
Gene	Protein	Mol. wt. (kD)	Synthesis	Virion	Gene	Mol. wt. (kD)	Role
I	P1	68	E		1A	68	DNA synthesis
II	P2	68	L	V	1	68	Attachment to host
III	P3	42	L	V	2	42	Major capsid protein
V	P5	30	L	V	5	30	Minor capsid protein
VIII	P8	28	E	V	5A	28	Genomic protein
IX	P9	28	L	V	6	27	DNA packaging
X	P10	26	L		6A	26	Assembly
XI	P11	23	L	V	7	23	Infectivity
XII	P12	20	E		8A	20	Regulatory, DNA synthesis
XIV	P14		L	V			Infectivity
XV	P15		ME		9A		Lysin
XVI	P16	17	L	V	10	17	Infectivity
XVII	P17	15	L				Assembly
XVIII	P18	11	L	V	11	11	Infectivity
XIX	P19	9	ME		11B	9	
XX	P20		L	V			DNA packaging?
XXII	P22		L	V			DNA packaging/
XXIII	P23		L	V	13		Infectivity

[a]Mindich *et al.* (1982b).
[b]Davis *et al.* (1983).

netic map (Mellado *et al.*, 1976). The cloned fragments of the genome were capable of complementing the nonsense mutants, and it was therefore possible to construct a genetic map that was correlated with the physical map determined from the HaeII restriction pattern (McGraw *et al.*, 1983) (Fig. 20). In conjunction with Table IV, it can be seen that the distribution of genes is organized so that the early functions are at the ends of the genome, with the later ones at the center. Analysis of the consequences of nonsense mutations on viral functions allowed an assignment of the roles of many of the viral proteins (Davis and Cronan, 1983; Mindich *et al.*, 1982a).

D. Assembly of PRD1

Early after infection with PRD1, three proteins are synthesized—P1, P8, and P12 (Mindich *et al.*, 1982b). P1 is a phage-specific polymerase with four regions of extensive sequence homology with φ29 polymerase (Savilahti and Bamford, unpublished), and P8 is the terminal genomic protein. In the absence of either P1 or P8, DNA is not replicated, and only the early proteins are synthesized. In the absence of P12, the normal shutoff of the synthesis of early phase protein synthesis does not take place. The middle early class of proteins are seen rather early in infection but are not present in the absence of proteins P1 or P8. These proteins are P15 and P19. P19 appears to be dispensable, but P15 is a lysin that is responsible for the lysis of the host at the end of the infection. P15 works in conjunction with an unidentified protein coded for by gene A that acts as a lytic factor much as gene S product functions in lysis induced by phage lambda.

The late program of synthesis involves the rest of the viral-encoded proteins. At least 20 late proteins are seen, and 17 of these are components of the virion. All but two of the virion proteins are found in the membrane structure. Even the host attachment protein, P2, is a component of the membrane. In addition, protein P8 is covalently bound to the DNA.

In the absence of individual membrane proteins, the virion is assembled, although in some cases it is not filled with DNA. In the absence of the major capsid protein, P3, no subviral structures are observed either in sucrose gradients or in electron micrograph sections of infected cells (Fig. 21). Several nonstructural proteins also seem necessary for the assembly of particles. In particular, P10, which is a hydrophobic protein, and P17, which is a soluble protein, are necessary for particle formation, although neither one is a component of the virion (Mindich *et al.*, 1982a).

No evidence has been found for a membrane vesicle intermediate in the formation of the PRD1 or PR4 particles. The only particles that form have the two capsid proteins and essentially complete membranes. In the cases where individual membrane proteins are not made, the membrane

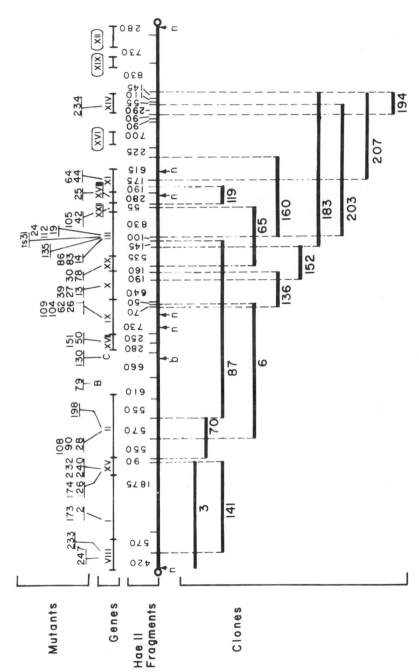

FIGURE 20. Map of the PRD1 genome. Nonsense and *ts* mutants are placed above the cloned fragments that gave complementation. The Hae2 restriction map was derived from the analysis of the sizes of partial Hae2 fragments and is consistent with the placement of sites in the cloned fragments. Restriction sites for Mnl1 (n) and Mbo1 (b) are indicated. Genes are located on the basis of marker rescue with cloned fragments or, in the case of those enclosed in boxes, on the basis of *in vitro* translation activities. From McGraw *et al.* (1983).

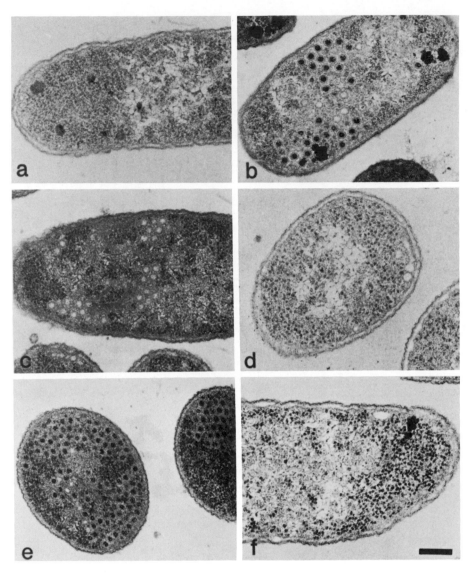

FIGURE 21. Electron micrographs of sections of *S. typhimurium* LT2(pLM2) infected with PRD1 wild type and mutants. (a) Uninfected; (b) wild-type; (c) mutant deficient in protein P9; (d) mutant deficient in protein P1; (e) mutant deficient in accessory lytic factor; and (f) mutant deficient in the major capsid protein P3. Scale bar: 200 nm. From Mindich *et al.* (1982a).

is formed without them, but if the major capsid protein is not made or if one of several nonstructural proteins is not made, then no particles are seen (Bamford and Mindich, 1982; Davis and Cronan, 1983; Mindich *et al.*, 1982a). It is interesting that the attachment protein is found on particles that have not packaged DNA. There is a particular protein P9 that is found only in particles that have packaged DNA. P9 is necessary for DNA packaging.

Pulse-chase experiments with wild-type virus infections yielded results that were consistent with those of the mutant studies. It was found that label appeared first in empty particles and then moved into filled ones. The earliest particles found contained all the virion proteins except P9, and the empty particles contained the host attachment protein P2. The capsid proteins P3 and P5 were first found as soluble proteins in multimer form before becoming associated with empty particles. When viral particles were disrupted with guanidine hydrochloride, vesicles were observed along with doughnut-shaped capsomeres composed of P3. P5 was found in the same fractions but, because of its low abundance, is probably not a component of all the P3 capsomeres.

On the basis of the mutant and labeling studies, it is possible to propose a model for the life cycle of the PRD1 family of viruses (Fig. 17). The virus attaches to the ends of pili of the host cells; however, virions are also found attached to the surface of the cells. It is not clear whether the pilus attachment is necessary for adsorption. The DNA is injected into the host cells, leaving behind the empty capsid containing the contracted membrane vesicle. The virion does not have a normal tail, but it appears that an extension of the membrane vesicle is the attachment apparatus and, as mentioned previously, the attachment protein is a component of the viral membrane. The process of infection is inhibited by the presence of fatty acids in the medium (Sands et al., 1979); this is consistent with the involvement of the membrane in the infection process.

Upon infection, the very early proteins are made, DNA synthesis begins, and the program of protein synthesis progresses through middle early to the late stage, at which time the virion and morphogenetic proteins are made. The membrane proteins of the virion are incorporated into the host cytoplasmic membrane, and the capsid proteins are soluble and in multimer form. In a process that is dependent upon the presence of capsomeres, the membrane structure is excised from the host membrane to form the empty vesicle inside of the capsid (Fig. 17). The particle is then ready for DNA packaging, which involves protein P9 as well as the empty particle and the protein-linked DNA (Fig. 17). The cells lyse at the end of infection because of the action of a lysin, P15, and an accessory lytic factor coded for by gene A.

IV. MORPHOGENETIC PROTEINS IN PHAGE MEMBRANE ASSEMBLY

In each case that has been studied, it appears that the membrane proteins of lipid-containing phages are inserted into the host membrane. The lipids of the phage membrane derive from host lipids that were synthesized both during and prior to infection. Although the lipids are qualitatively identical to those of the host membrane, it is usually found that the proportion of phosphatidylglycerol is increased in the viral membrane. The amount of lipid in the viral membrane is usually less than half the amount needed to build a bilayer at the observed radius. This suggests that the viral membranes are primarily protein. This is not exceptional in that bacterial membranes usually contain between 70% and 80% protein (Mindich, 1975).

In the case of φ6, a soluble nonstructural protein, P12, is necessary for the formation of the viral membrane. It is not yet clear whether P12 acts in the placements of the viral proteins into the host membrane or the transfer of the lipids and proteins to the virion structure. It does seem that P12 must act at the time of synthesis of the viral membrane proteins. In the case of PRD1, two nonstructural proteins, P10 and P17, have been found to be necessary for the formation of viral membrane. P10 is a membrane-bound protein, and P17 is soluble. In addition, the major capsid protein, P3, is also necessary for the formation of the viral membrane. As in the case of φ6, it is not known whether the role of the nonstructural proteins is in the placement of the viral membrane proteins into the host membrane or the excision and translocation of the structure into the virion.

ACKNOWLEDGMENTS. We are grateful to Drs. H. Revel, D. Lang, N. Ktistakis, J. Cronan, and T. Davis for valuable discussions of the material we have covered and for sending us unpublished information. We thank J. Hagenzieker for the preparation of photographs and A. Howard for manuscript preparation.

REFERENCES

Bamford, D., 1981, Lipid-containing bacterial viruses: Disruption studies on φ6, in: Bacteriophage Assembly (M. S. du Bow, ed.), pp. 477–489, Alan R. Liss, New York.

Bamford, D. H., and Lounatmaa, K., 1978, Freeze-fracturing of Pseudomonas phaseolicola infected by the lipid-containing bacteriophage φ6, J. Gen. Virol. 39:161–170.

Bamford, D. H., and Lounatmaa, K., 1982, Further electron microscopic studies on the infection process of the lipid-containing bacteriophage φ6, J. Gen. Virol. 61:149–152.

Bamford, D. H., and Mindich, L., 1980, Electron microscopy of cells infected with nonsense mutants of bacteriophage φ6, Virology 107:222–228.

Bamford, D., and Mindich, L., 1982, Structure of the lipid-containing bacteriophage PRD1: Disruption of wild-type and nonsense mutant phage particles with guanidine hydrochloride, J. Virol. 44:1031–1038.

Bamford, D. H., and Mindich, L., 1984, Characterization of the DNA-protein complex at the termini of the bacteriophage PRD1 genome, J. Virol. 50:309–315.

Bamford, D. H., and Palva, E. T., 1980, Structure of the lipid-containing bacteriophage φ6: Disruption by Triton X-100 treatment, Biochim. Biophys. Acta 601:245–259.

Bamford, D. H., Palva, E. T., and Lounatmaa, K., 1976, Ultrastructure and life cycle of the lipid-containing bacteriophage φ6, J. Gen. Virol. 32:249–259.

Bamford, D. H., Rouhiainen, L., Takkinen, K., and Soderlund, H., 1981, Comparison of the lipid-containing bacteriophages PRD1, PR3, PR4, PR5 and L17, *J. Gen. Virol.* **57**:365–373.

Bamford, D., McGraw, T., MacKenzie, G., and Mindich, L., 1983, Identification of a protein bound to the termini of bacteriophage PRD1 DNA, *J. Virol.* **47**:311–316.

Bamford, D. H., Romantschuk, M., and Somerharju, P. J., 1987, Membrane fusion in procaryotes: Bacteriophage φ6 membrane fuses with the *Pseudomonas syringae* outer membrane, *EMBO J.* **6**:1467–1473.

Berger, H., and Kennedy, K., 1980, Physical measurements on the lipid-containing bacteriophage φ6, *Biochim. Biophys. Acta* **633**:68–76.

Bowman, B. U. Jr., Newman, H. A. I., Moritz, J. M., and Koehler, R. M., 1973, Properties of mycobacteriophage DS6A. II. Lipid composition, *Am. Rev. Respir. Dis.* **107**:42–49.

Bradley, D. E., 1974, Adsorption of bacteriophages specific for *Pseudomonas aeruginosa* R factors RP1 and R1822, *Biochem. Biophys. Res. Commun.* **57**:893–900.

Bradley, D. E., 1976, Adsorption of the R-specific bacteriophage PR4 to pili determined by a drug resistance plasmid of the W compatibility group, *J. Gen. Microbiol.* **95**:181–185.

Bradley, D. E., and Cohen, D. R., 1977, Adsorption of lipid-containing bacterioiphages PR4 and PRD1 to pili determined by a P-1 incompatibility group plasmid, *J. Gen. Microbiol.* **98**:619–623.

Bradley, D. E., and Rutherford, E. L., 1975, Basic characterization of a lipid-containing bacteriophage specific for plasmids of the P, N, and W compatibility groups, *Can. J. Microbiol.* **21**:152–163.

Brewer, G. J., 1980, Control of membrane morphogenesis in bacteriophage, *Int. Rev. Cytol.* **68**:53–96.

Caspar, D., and Klug, A., 1962, Physical principles in the construction of regular viruses, *Cold Spring Harbor Symp. Quant. Biol.* **27**:1–24.

Coetzee, W. F., and Bekker, P. J., 1979, Pilus-specific, lipid-containing bacteriophages PR4 and PR772: Comparison of physical characteristics of genomes, *J. Gen. Virol.* **45**:195–200.

Coplin, D. L., Van Etten, J. L., Koski, R. K., and Vidaver, A. K., 1975, Intermediates in the biosynthesis of double-stranded ribonucleic acids of bacteriophage φ6, *Proc. Natl. Acad. Sci. U.S.A.* **72**:849–853.

Cuppels, D. A., Vidaver, A. K., and Van Etten, J. L., 1979, Resistance to bacteriophage φ6 by *Pseudomonas phaseolicola*, *J. Gen. Virol.* **44**:493–504.

Cuppels, D. A., Van Etten, J. L., Burbank, D. E., Lane, L. C., and Vidaver, A. K., 1980, *In vitro* translation of the three bacteriophage φ6 RNAs, *J. Virol.* **35**:249–251.

Cuppels, D. A., Van Etten, J. L., Lambrecht, P., and Vidaver, A. K., 1981, Survey of phytopathogenic pseudomonads for a restriction and modification system active on the double-stranded ribonucleic acid phage φ6, *Curr. Microbiol.* **5**:247–249.

Davis, T. N., and Cronan, J. E. Jr., 1983, Nonsense mutants of the lipid-containing bacteriophage PR4, *Virology* **126**:600–613.

Davis, T. N., and Cronan, J. E. Jr., 1985, An alkyl imidate labeling study of the organization of phospholipids and proteins in the lipid-containing bacteriophage PR4, *J. Biol. Chem.* **260**:663–671.

Davis, T. N., Muller, E. D., and Cronan, J. E. Jr., 1982, The virion of the lipid-containing bacteriophage PR4, *Virology* **120**:287–306.

Day, L. A., and Mindich, L. 1980, The molecular weight of bacteriophage φ6 and its nucleocapsid, *Virology* **103**:376–385.

Emori, Y., Iba, H., and Okada, Y., 1980, Assignment of viral proteins to the three double-stranded RNA segments of bacteriophage φ6 genome: Translation of φ6 messenger RNAs transcribed *in vitro*, *Mol. Gen. Genet.* **180**:385–389.

Emori, Y., Iba, H., and Okada, Y., 1982, Morphogenetic pathway of bacteriophage φ6. A flow analysis of subviral and viral particles in infected cells, *J. Mol. Biol.* **154**:287–310.

Emori, Y., Iba, H., and Okada, Y., 1983, Transcriptional regulation of three double-stranded RNA segments of bacteriophage φ6 *in vitro*, *J. Virol.* **46**:196–203.

Espejo, R. T., and Canelo, E. S., 1968, Properties of bacteriophage PM2: A lipid-containing bacterial virus, *Virology* **34:**738–747.

Gonzalez, C. F., Langenberg, W. G., Van Etten, J. L., and Vidaver, A. K., 1977, Ultrastructure of bacteriophage φ6: Arrangements of the double-stranded RNA and envelope, *J. Gen. Virol.* **35:**353–359.

Gope, M. L., and Gopinathan, K. P., 1982, Presence of lipids in mycobacteriophage 13, *J. Gen. Virol.* **59:**131–138.

Gottlieb, P., Strassman, J., Bamford, D. H., and Mindich, L., 1988, Production of a polyhedral particle in *Escherichia coli* from a cDNA copy of the large genomic segment of bacteriophage φ6, *J. Virol.* **62:**181–187.

Gourlay, R. N., Garwes, D. J., Bruce, J., and Wyld, S. G., 1973, Further studies on the morphology and composition of mycoplasmatales virus-laidlawii 2, *J. Gen. Virol.* **18:**127–133.

Iba, H., Nanno, M., and Okada, Y., 1979, Identification and partial purification of a lytic enzyme in the bacteriophage φ6 virion, *FEBS Lett.* **103:**234–237.

Iba, H., Watanabe, T., Emori, Y., and Okada, Y., 1982, Three double-stranded RNA genome segments of bacteriophage φ6 have homologous terminal sequences, *FEBS Lett.* **141:**111–115.

Joklik, W. K., 1981, Structure and function of the reovirus genome, *Microbiol. Rev.* **45:**483–501.

Kakitani, H., Emori, Y., Iba, H., and Okada, Y., 1978, Lytic enzyme activity associated with double-stranded RNA bacteriophage φ6, *Proc. Jpn. Acad.* **54:**337–340.

Kakitani, H., Iba, H., and Okada, Y., 1980, Penetration and partial uncoating of bacteriophage φ6 particle, *Virology* **101:**475–483.

Ktistakis, N. T., and Lang, D., 1987, The dodecahedral framework of the bacteriophage φ6 nucleocapsid is composed of protein P1, *J. Virol.* **61:**2621–2623.

Langenberg, W. G., and Sharpee, R. L., 1978, Chromic-acid formaldehyde fixation of nucleic acids of bacteriophage φ6 and infectious bovine rhinotracheitis virus, *J. Gen. Virol.* **39:**377–380.

Lehman, J. F., and Mindich, L., 1979, The isolation of new mutants of bacteriophage φ6, *Virology* **97:**164–170.

Lopez, R., Ronda, C., Tomasz, A., and Portoles, A., 1977, Properties of "diplophage": A lipid-containing bacteriophage, *J. Virol.* **24:**201–210.

Lundstrom, K. H., Bamford, D. H., Palva, E. T., and Lounatmaa, K., 1979, Lipid-containing bacteriophage PR4: Structure and life cycle, *J. Gen. Virol.* **43:**583–592.

Maxam, A., and Gilbert, W., 1980, Sequencing end-labeled DNA with base-specific chemical cleavages, *Methods Enzymol.* **65:**499–560.

McGraw, T., Yang, H., and Mindich, L., 1983, Establishment of a physical and genetic map for bacteriophage PRD1, *Mol. Gen. Genet.* **190:**237–244.

McGraw, T., Mindich, L., and Frangione, B., 1986, Nucleotide sequence of the small double-stranded RNA segment of bacteriophage φ6: Novel mechanism of natural translational control, *J. Virol.* **58:**142–151.

Mellado, R. P., Moreno, F., Vinuela, E., Salas, M., Reilly, B. E., and Anderson, D., 1976, Genetic analysis of bacteriophage φ29 of *Bacillus subtilis:* Integration and mapping of reference mutants of two collections, *J. Virol.* **19:**495–500.

Mindich, L., 1975, Studies on bacterial membrane biogenesis using glycerol auxotrophs, in: *Membrane Biogenesis* (A. Tzagoloff, ed.), pp. 429–454, Plenum, New York.

Mindich, L., 1978, Bacteriophages and contain lipid, in: *Comprehensive Virology,* Vol. 12 (H. Fraenkel-Conrat and R. R. Wagner, eds.), pp. 271–335, Plenum, New York.

Mindich, L., and Davidoff Abelson, R., 1980, The characterization of a 120 S particle formed during φ6 infection, *Virology* **103:**386–391.

Mindich, L., and Lehman, J., 1979, Cell wall lysin as a component of the bacteriophage φ6 virion, *J. Virol.* **30:**489–496.

Mindich, L., and Lehman, J., 1983, Characterization of φ6 mutants that are temperature sensitive in the morphogenetic protein P12, *Virology* **127:**438–445.

Mindich, L., and McGraw, T., 1983, Molecular cloning of bacteriophage PRD1 genomic fragments, *Mol. Gen. Genet.* **190**:233–236.

Mindich, L., Sinclair, J. F., Levine, D., and Cohen, J., 1976a, Genetic studies of temperature-sensitive and nonsense mutants of bacteriophage φ6, *Virology* **75**:218–223.

Mindich, L., Cohen, J., and Weisburd, M., 1976b, Isolation of nonsense suppressor mutants in *Pseudomonas*, *J. Bacteriol.* **126**:177–182.

Mindich, L., Sinclair, J. F., and Cohen, J., 1976c, The morphogenesis of bacteriophage φ6: Particles formed by nonsense mutants, *Virology* **75**:224–231.

Mindich, L., Lehman, J., and Sinclair, J. F., 1979, Biogenesis of φ6, a bacteriophage that contains lipid, in: *Microbiology 1979* (D. Schlessinger, ed.), pp. 38–41, American Society for Microbiology, Washington.

Mindich, L., Bamford, D., McGraw, T., and Mackenzie, G., 1982a, Assembly of bacteriophage PRD1: Particle formation with wild-type and mutant viruses, *J. Virol.* **44**:1021–1030.

Mindich, L., Bamford, D., Goldthwaite, C., Laverty, M., and Mackenzie, G., 1982b, Isolation of nonsense mutants of lipid-containing bacteriophage PRD1, *J. Virol.* **44**:1013–1020.

Mindich, L., MacKenzie, G., Strassman, J., McGraw, T., Metzger, S., Romantschuk, M., and Bamford, D., 1985, cDNA cloning of portions of the bacteriophage φ6 genome, *J. Bacteriol.* **162**:992–999.

Muller, E. D., and Cronan, J. E. Jr., 1983, The lipid-containing bacteriophage PR4. Effects of altered lipid composition on the virion, *J. Mol. Biol.* **165**:109–124.

Nagy, E., Herczegh, O., and Ivanovics, G., 1982, Lipid-containing anthrax phage AP50: Structural proteins and life cycle, *J. Gen. Virol.* **62**:323–329.

Olkkonen, V. M., and Bamford, D. H., 1987, The nucleocapsid of the lipid-containing dsRNA bacteriophage φ6 contains a protein skeleton consisting of a single polypeptide species, *J. Virol.* **61**:2362–2367.

Olsen, R. H., Siak, J., and Gray, R. H., 1974, Characteristics of PRD1, a plasmid-dependent broad host range DNA bacteriophage, *J. Virol.* **14**:689–699.

Olsen, R. H., Siak, J., and Shipley, P. L., 1977, *Pseudomonas* plasmid RP1-encoded surface components: A somatic receptor for phage PRD1, in: *Microbiology 1977* (D. Schlessinger, ed.), pp. 138–144, American Society for Microbiology, Washington.

Partridge, J. E., Van Etten, J. L., Burbank, D. E., and Vidaver, A. K., 1979, RNA polymerase activity associated with bacteriophage φ6 nucleocapsid, *J. Gen. Virol.* **43**:299–307.

Razin, S., 1985, Molecular biology and genetics of mycoplasmas (Mollicutes), *Microbiol. Rev.* **49**:419–455.

Reinhardt, A., Auperin, D., and Sands, J., 1980, Mechanism of virucidal activity of retinoids: Protein removal from bacteriophage φ6 envelope, *Antimicrob. Agents Chemother.* **17**:1034–1037.

Revel, H. R., Ewen, M. E., Busslan, J., and Pagratis, N., 1986, Generation of cDNA clones of the bacteriophage φ6 segmented dsRNA genome: Characterization and expression of L segment clones, *Virology* **155**:402–417.

Romantschuk, M., and Bamford, D. H., 1981, φ6-resistant phage-producing mutants of *Pseudomonas phaseolicola*, *J. Gen. Virol.* **56**:287–295.

Romantschuk, M., and Bamford, D. H., 1985, Function of pili in bacteriophage φ6 penetration, *J. Gen. Virol.* **66**:2461–2469.

Romantschuk, M., and Bamford, D. H., 1986, The causal agent of halo blight in bean, *Pseudomonas syringae* pv. *phaseolicola*, attaches to stomata via its pili, *Microbiol. Pathogenesis* **1**:139–148.

Sakaki, Y., Yamada, K., Oshima, M., and Oshima, T., 1977, Bacteriophage φNS11: A lipid-containing phage of acidophilic thermophilic bacteria. II. Purification and some properties of the phage, *J. Biochem.* **82**:1451–1456.

Sakaki, Y., Maeda, T., and Oshima, T., 1979, Bacteriophage φNS11: A lipid-containing phage of acidophilic thermophilic bacteria IV. Sedimentation coefficient, diffusion coefficient, partial specific volume, and particle weight of the phage, *J. Biochem.* **85**:1205–1211.

Sands, J. A., 1973, The phospholipid composition of bacteriophage φ6, *Biochem. Biophys. Res. Commun.* **55:**111–116.

Sands, J. A., Reinhardt, A., Auperin, D., and Landin, P., 1979, Inhibition of entry of the lipid-containing bacteriophage PR4 by fatty acid derivatives, *J. Virol.* **29:**413–416.

Sanger, F., Nicklen, S., and Coulson, A. R., 1977, DNA sequencing with chain-terminating inhibitors, *Proc. Natl. Acad. Sci. USA* **74:**5463–5467.

Savilahti, H., and Bamford, D. H., 1986, Linear DNA replication: Inverted terminal repeats of five closely related *Escherichia coli* bacteriophages, *Gene* **49:**199–205.

Schneider, D., Zulauf, M., Schafer, R., and Franklin, R. M., 1978, Neutron small angle scattering on bacteriophage PM2, *J. Mol. Biol.* **124:**97–122.

Semancik, J. S., Vidaver, A. K., and Van Etten, J. L., 1973, Characterization of a segmented double-helical RNA from bacteriophage φ6, *J. Mol. Biol.* **78:**617–625.

Sinclair, J. F., and Mindich, L., 1976, RNA synthesis during infection with bacteriophage φ6, *Virology* **75:**209–217.

Sinclair, J. F., Tzagoloff, A., Levine, D., and Mindich, L., 1975, Proteins of bacteriophage φ6, *J. Virol.* **16:**685–695.

Sinclair, J. F., Cohen, J., and Mindich, L., 1976, The isolation of suppressible nonsense mutants of bacteriophage φ6, *Virology* **75:**198–208.

Stanisich, V. A., 1974, The properties and host range of male-specific bacteriophages of *Pseudomonas aeruginosa, J. Gen. Microbiol.* **84:**332–342.

Steely, H. T. Jr., and Lang, D., 1984, Electron microscopy of bacteriophage φ6 nucleocapsid: Two-dimensional image analysis, *J. Virol.* **51:**479–483.

Stitt, B. L., and Mindich, L., 1983a, The structure of bacteriophage φ6: Protease digestion of φ6 virion, *Virology* **127:**459–462.

Stitt, B. L., and Mindich, L., 1983b, Morphogenesis of bacteriophage φ6: A presumptive viral membrane precursor, *Virology* **127:**446–458.

Usala, S. J., Brownstein, B. H., and Haselkom, R., 1980, Displacement of parental RNA strands during in vitro transcription by bacteriophage φ6 nucleocapsids, *Cell* **19:**855–862.

Van Etten, J., Lane, L., Gonzalez, C., Partridge, J., and Vidaver, A., 1976, Comparative properties of bacteriophage φ6 and φ6 nucleocapsid, *J. Virol.* **18:**652–658.

Van Etten, J. L., Burbank, D. E., Cuppels, D. A., Lane, L. C., and Vidaver, A. K., 1980, Semiconservative synthesis of single-stranded RNA by bacteriophage φ6 RNA polymerase, *J. Virol.* **33:**769–773.

Vidaver, A. K., Koski, R. K., and Van Etten, J. L., 1973, Bacteriophage φ6: A lipid-containing virus of *Pseudomonas phaseolicola, J. Virol.* **11:**799–805.

Wong, F. H., and Bryan, L. E., 1978, Characteristics of PR5, a lipid-containing plasmid-dependent phage, *Can. J. Microbiol.* **24:**875–882.

Yang, Y., and Lang, D., 1984, Electron microscopy of bacteriophage φ6 nucleocapsid: Three-dimensional image analysis, *J. Virol.* **51:**484–488.

CHAPTER 9

Phage T4 Structure and Metabolism

GISELA MOSIG AND FRED EISERLING

I. INTRODUCTION AND OVERVIEW

A. History

The development of T-even bacteriophages in infected *E. coli* cells has provided paradigms for many processes and regulatory mechanisms that now constitute a foundation of molecular biology (Cairns *et al.*, 1966). Perhaps foremost of these are the principles of virus propagation (Ellis and Delbrück, 1939) and the demonstration that the nucleic acid component of virus particles suffices to establish infection and to direct synthesis of all virion proteins (Hershey and Chase, 1952).

Analyses of various individual aspects of T-even growth led early on to the first formulations of several fundamental biological concepts: (1) genetic recombination as exchange between DNA molecules involving "heterozygous" overlaps (Hershey and Chase, 1951); (2) the concept of the gene (Benzer, 1957) and the operational differences among recon, muton, and cistron; (3) the demonstration of mRNA (Volkin and As-trachan, 1956; Brenner *et al.*, 1961); (4) the nonoverlapping triplet code (Crick *et al.*, 1961; Streisinger *et al.*, 1966), with nonsense triplets as termination signals (Benzer and Champe, 1962); (5) the colinearity of the gene with the corresponding polypeptide (Sarabhai *et al.*, 1964) (but see spliced and "skipped" introns, below); (6) repair of damages in DNA in

GISELA MOSIG • Department of Molecular Biology, Vanderbilt University, Nashville, Tennessee 37235.   FRED EISERLING • Department of Microbiology, University of California, Los Angeles, California 90024.

the light (Dulbecco, 1949) and in the dark (Harm, 1961); (7) restriction and modification of DNA (Luria, 1953); and (8) defined pathways leading to the assembly of complex macromolecular structures (Edgar and Wood, 1966).

The significance of more details of the infectious process is most profitably evaluated by comparisons with other systems. Of all phages discussed in this volume, the T-even phages are among the most successful molecular parasites. They depend for their propagation on many vital functions of their host—energy metabolism, membranes, transcriptional and translational machines—but they manage to subvert these functions gradually to their own purpose in an exquisitely timed choreography. This subversion is accomplished at several levels:

1. A cascade of phage-induced transcription factors and DNA-binding proteins modifies the host's RNA polymerase. Together, these phage-encoded proteins ultimately allow precisely timed expression of certain classes of differentially regulated phage genes. At the same time, these modifications interfere with and turn off expression of host genes.
2. RNA processing, phage-encoded translational repressors, and poorly understood modifications of ribosomes modulate translation from the primary phage transcripts.
3. The host genome and host mRNA, present at the time of infection, are rapidly degraded, and the breakdown products are reutilized for phage propagation.

In contrast, DNA replication and recombination of the T-even phages are largely autonomous. These processes require almost exclusively phage-encoded proteins which are assembled to protein machines (Nossal and Alberts, 1983; Alberts, 1984; Mosig et al., 1984). An exception is the first, or "primary," initiation of DNA replication. Primary initiation has components of host control, since it requires host RNA polymerase and depends on the state of that RNA polymerase at the time of infection. Subsequent initiations depend entirely on phage-encoded recombination proteins. We believe (see below) that this switch in the modes of DNA replication is a most critical component in the strategy of T-even phages to escape the controls of their host.

Most recent work on the T-even phages has concentrated on bacteriophage T4, mainly because of isolation and characterization of a large collection of conditional lethal (temperature-sensitive and nonsense) mutants, pioneered by Edgar and Epstein and their colleagues (Epstein et al., 1964). Their work has provided a most powerful impetus for molecular analyses of this phage. Mutations now define approximately 130 genes (Table I). Sequencing thus far has revealed an additional 70 unidentified open reading frames in search of a function. This information is continuously being updated, most recently by Kutter et al. (1987).

TABLE I. Genes of Bacteriophage T4

Gene	Mutant phenotype	Restrictive host	Function or product	Mol. wt. of product (× 1000)	References[a]
rIIA	Rapid lysis, suppressor of lig⁻ and some 32⁻, nonessential	rex⁺ lysogens, tab R	Membrane protein affects membrane ATPase of *E. coli*	72,74,83,95	16,61,92a
(m=sum)	Suppressor of lig⁻ nonessential				61
(rc)	Acriflavine resistance				61
60	DNA delay	S/6, 25°	Membrane protein, DNA topoisomerase subunit	16,18, **18.6**	42,61,41a
39	DNA delay	S/6, 25°	Membrane protein, DNA topoisomerase subunit, DNA-dependent ATPase	63→22, **58.5**	41,42,61
pla CTr5x	Nonessential	CTr5x			61
(goF=go9H =comCα =mot C?)	Nonessential		Mutations overcome block in HDF (rho) hosts		61,80,99
cef=mb=M1 =mot C?	Nonessential	roc⁻ CT439	Modifier of suppressor tRNAs and of species 1, 2, and 3 RNA	18	61,78,80
(del[39–56] segment 4 =mot B?)	Nonessential		Modifier of transcription?	12	61,80

(continued)

TABLE I. (Continued)

Gene	Mutant phenotype	Restrictive host	Function or product	Mol. wt. of product (× 1000)	References[a]
(pseF)	Nonessential		5' phosphatase	56	61
(dda)	Nonessential		DNA-dependent ATPase, DNA helicase		27,44,56,61
dexA = sud?	Nonessential suppressor of 32−	opt A	Exonuclease A	**26.0**	27,56,61
(mod)	Nonessential		Adenylribosylation of RNA polymerase	27	61,93a
soc	Nonessential		Small outer capsid protein	9	7,57,58,61
69	DNA-negative	S/6, 25°	dCTPase dUTPase	**46, 26**	57,61,69,70
56 overlaps 69			dCDPase dUDPase	19	57,61,70
dam	Nonessential		DNA adenine methylase	**30**	57,61,88
58–61 (uvsZ)	DNA delay DNA arrest UV-sensitive	S/6, 25°	Primase subunit	40, **39.5**	10,12,61,72,90 61
41	DNA arrest, single-stranded DNA, UV-sensitive		GTP-, dGTP-, ATP-, dATPase, helicase, primase subunit	58,60,63,66, **53.8**	37,38,61,72,90
40	Polyheads		Helper of head vertex assembly	14,18	37,61,64,111
(sp=rIV) in gene 40	Suppressor of e−, rapid lysis			**13.4**	61,72a
uvsX = fdsA	UV-sensitive, recombination-deficient, suppressor of 49−		RecA-like recombination protein	40, **43.8**	17,37,26,31,61,116,116a

βgt	no β-glucosylation of HMC-DNA	β-glucosyltransferase	46	61,103
42	DNA-negative	dCMP-hydroxymethylase	25	53,61,101,103
(imm)	Immunity to superinfection exclusion		77,45	61
43	DNA-negative	DNA polymerase	112, **103.6**	61,98
(dsd)	DNA delay	DNA polymerase		18
regA		Translational regulation of (early) protein synthesis	**14.6**	1,2,21,61,67,104
62	DNA-negative	DNA polymerase accessory protein, ssDNA-dependent rATPase, dATPase	**21.4**	61
44	DNA-negative, no late mRNA		**35.9**	61
45		Accessory protein of DNA and RNA polymerases	**24.7**	61,59
rpbA	Nonessential	RNA polymerase binding, "15K," protein	**11.4**	39,113
46	DNA arrest, recombination-deficient, reduced host degradation	Control of recombination nuclease	**63.5**	30,61
47			**39.1**	30,61
αgt	No α-glucosylation of HMC-DNA	α-glucosyl transferase	**46.6**	30,61,102
(gor)	Suppressor of RNA polymerase defect			61
55	No late RNA synthesis	RNA polymerase sigma factor for late T4 promoters	**21.5**	25,30,61

(continued)

TABLE I. (*Continued*)

Gene	Mutant phenotype	Restrictive host	Function or product	Mol. wt. of product (× 1000)	References[a]
uvsU	UV-sensitive				110,111
49	Partially filled heads, highly branched DNA		Endonuclease VII, cleaves recombinational junctions	**18.1**	6,48a,61,103
(pin)	Nonessential		Inhibitor of *E. coli* protease		89,91,94
nrdC	Nonessential		Thioredoxin	**10.0**	54,61,103
arn	DNA degradation under certain conditions		Antirestriction nuclease (vs. *E. coli* rgl B)		61
(Su30)	Nonessential, suppressor of lig⁻				61
rI	Nonessential, rapid lysis				61
tk	Nonessential		Thymidine kinase	28, **21.6**	61,66,108
vs	Nonessential		Modifier of valyl-tRNA synthetase	**13.1**	60,61,66,73,74,108
regB	Nonessential, folate analogue-resistant		Regulation of gene expression		61
(stI)	Nonessential "star"				61
(stIII)	Nonessential, suppressor of e⁻ and t⁻, star				61
v=denV	UV-sensitive		Endonuclease V, N-glycosidase	**16.1**	61,82,84,106,107
ipII	Nonessential		Internal protein II	**11.7**, 10	61,106
ipIII	Semiessential		Internal (core) protein III	**23.5**, 21	61
				21.7	
e	No lysis		Endolysin	**18.7**	61,63,75

Gene/product	Phenotype	CT	Function	Map	References
(goF3.03.2)			Perhaps an ORF upstream of e (?)		61,63
Stable species 1 (=C)RNA	Grow on HDF hosts		Unknown		61,78
Stable species 2 (=D) RNA			Unknown		61,78
tRNAs arg ileu thr ser pro gly leu gln psu₄op psu_a⁺ psu_b⁺ psu_t⁺ psu₃⁺ psu₂⁺ psu SB	Nonessential (nonsense suppressors)	CT439	tRNA precursors		9,33,34,61
ipI		CT595	Internal protein I	10, **8,9**	61,112
57	Poor tail fiber assembly, by-passed in certain host mutants		Morphogenetic catalyst of long and short tail fiber assembly	18,6	9,61 9,61
(hm)			Mutator		61
1	Nonessential DNA-negative		dHMP-kinase	22, **24**, 25	9,28,61
3	Unstable tails		Tail tube, proximal tip	29	9,28,61
2=64	Inactive filled heads, noninfectious particles		Head completion, terminal DNA-protecting protein	25	9,28,61
50	Inactive filled heads, noninfectious particles		Head completion		61

(continued)

TABLE I. (Continued)

Gene	Mutant phenotype	Restrictive host	Function or product	Mol. wt. of product (× 1000)	References[a]
65	Inactive filled heads, noninfectious particles		Head completion		61
4	Inactive or empty capsids		Head completion		61
53	Defective tails		Baseplate, 1/6 arm	23	61
5	Defective tails		Baseplate, central hub, tail lysozyme	**37.4**, 44,77	61,71,104
6	Defective tails, permit fiberless plating		Baseplate, 1/6 arm	**78.8**, 78,86	61
7	Defective tails, permit fiberless plating		Baseplate, 1/6 arm	127,140	52,61
8	Defective tails		Baseplate, 1/6 arm	39,46	52,61
9	Defective tails, fiberless particles		Baseplate, long tail fiber attachment	30,34	52,61
10	Defective tails		Baseplate, 1/6 arm	88,90	61,77
11	Defective tails		Baseplate, 1/6 arm	24,25,26	61,77
12	Defective tails		Baseplate, short tail fibers	55,57,58	61
wac	Nonessential		Whisker antigen	52	61
13			Head completion	33	61
14			Head completion	30	61
15	Defective tails		Proximal tail sheath stabilizer	32,35	61
16	DNA packaging-defective, empty heads		Head filling	**18.3**	61,79
17=q	Quinacrine-resistant, DNA packaging-defective, suppressors of certain 32− or 20− mutations		Head filling	**69, 70.0** **+46**	61,79

Gene	Phenotype	Function	Molecular weight	References
18	Defective tails	Tail sheath monomer	70,80, **71.4**	3,4,61
19	Defective tails	Tail tube monomer	20,21, **18.5**	3,4,61
20	Polyheads	Head plug protein (connector to neck)	63,65,67	61
67=pip	Head defect		**9.1**	61
68	Isometric heads	Prohead core protein	**17**	48
21	Faulty heads	Maturation protease, head assembly core	27.5→18.5→ small peptides	61
22	Faulty heads	Head assembly core (later degraded)	**29.8**→2.5	61,76
23	No or faulty heads, grow on *lit*− hosts(CTr5x)	Major head subunit (*cis*-acting)	**56.0**→48.7	61,76
gol(in 23)		One of the products of genes 20–24 is cleaved to a packaging-related, DNA-dependent ATPase endonuclease	43	11,61 61
24=os	Faulty heads, osmotic shock resistance	Vertex head subunit	**48.4**→46	61,115
hoc=eph	Nonessential	Minor capsid protein	**39.1**, 40	12,61,115
inh		Inhibitor of gene 21 protease	**35**	61
dar=uvsW	Suppressor of 59−, 46−, UV-sensitive, recombination-deficient			19,55,61,114,117
uvsY=fdsB	UV-sensitive, DNA synthesis-reduced, recom-	Recombination protein	**15.8**	17,19,21,32,55,61,100,117

(continued)

TABLE I. (Continued)

Gene	Mutant phenotype	Function or product	Mol. wt. of product (× 1000)	References[a]
	bination-deficient, suppressor of 49−			
25	Tail defects	Baseplate, 1/6 arm tail lysozyme	15	32,55,61,71,117
26	Tail defects	Baseplate, central hub	41	61
51	Tail defects	Baseplate, central hub	**16.5**	49,61,117
27	Tail defects, permit fiberless plating	Baseplate, central hub	48,49	61,117
28	Tail defects	Baseplate, distal surface of central hub, gamma glutamyl hydrolase	24,25, **20.1**	61,117
29	Tail defects	Baseplate, tail "bulge," "folyl polyglutamyl synthetase	77, **64.5**	22,43,61
48	Tail defects	Baseplate, tail tube fiber, length "measure"(?)	37,44, **39.7**	22,23,43,61
54	Tail defects	Baseplate, tail tube polymerization initiator(?)	36, **35.0**	22,23,43,61
alt	Nonessential	Adenylribosylation of RNA polymerase, (packaged wtih DNA)	75→67	61

Gene	Defect/phenotype	Host	Function	Map position	References
30=lig	DNA arrest, hyper-rec		DNA ligase	55.2	5,6
rIII	Nonessential, rapid lysis				61
(Stable species 3 RNA)	Unknown				78
31	Capsid protein lumps, suppressor of mutations in host-defective (groE and 2 others) E. coli genes		Organizer of head protein assembly and DNA replication	16	20,61,92
cd	Nonessential		dCMP deaminase		61
pseT	Nonessential	CTr5x (lit−)	Deoxyribonucleotide 3' phosphatase-5' polynucleotide kinase	30, **34**	4,46,47,61,65
alc=unf	Allows late transcription of cytosine-containing DNA	E. coli (pR 386)	Unfolding of host DNA, RNA polymerase-DNA-binding protein	**19.1**	3,36,50,61,83,97
63	Poor tail fiber attachment		RNA ligase, helper of tail fiber attachment	**43.5**	6,83
denA	Nonessential, defective in host DNA degradation		Endonuclease II	**15.8**	1,83
nrdB	Nonessential		Ribonucleotide reductase β subunit (split gene)	35,40, **45.3**	9,61,93
nrdA	Nonessential		Ribonucleotide reductase α subunit	80,85	5,61,62
td	Nonessential	Thymidylate synthase−	Thymidylate synthase, baseplate central hub component, (split gene)	32, **33.0**	3,14,24,61,81
frd			Dihydrofolate reductase, baseplate wedge component (1/6 arm)	**21.6**	81

TABLE I. (Continued)

Gene	Mutant phenotype	Restrictive host	Function or product	Mol. wt. of product (× 1000)	References[a]
32	DNA arrest, recombination and excision-repair-deficient, UV-sensitive	(Tab 32)	Single-stranded DNA-binding, helix-destabilizing protein	33.5	5,16
59	DNA arrest			26.0	45
33	No late RNA synthesis		RNA polymerase-binding protein	12.8	45
ORF	goF026c2?		RNA polymerase-binding protein?	10.4	40a
das=suα (sur)	Suppressor of 46− and 47− / Suppressor of 46−, 47−, uvsX−				34,51 / 19,20
34	Fiberless particles		Proximal tail fiber subunit (A antigen)	145	22,46
35	Fiberless particles		Hinge tail fiber subunit	39,40	2,41
36	Fiberless particles		Small distal tail fiber subunit	24.3	61
37	Fiberless particles, host range		Large distal tail fiber subunit	112.8	61,85
38	Fiberless particles		Assembly catalyst of gp37	26,27,28	61,85
t=stII	Lysis defective, suppressor of gene 63 and rII mutations			25.2	61,6−,8−a
motA=sip	Regulation of middle gene expression, suppressor of rII− in K(λ)		Activator of middle promoters	24	8,4,15
(rV)	Temperature-dependent rapid lysis				61

Gene	Phenotype	Conditions	Function	Molecular weight	References
52	DNA delay	S/6, 25°	Membrane protein, DNA topoisomerase subunit	52, **50.6**	40,61,87
ac	Nonessential, acriflavine-resistant			5.0	61,11a
(ama)(rs)	Nonessential, acriflavine-resistant			5.4	61,11a
stp	Nonessential		Suppressor of pseT mutation, anticodon nuclease	5.3 or 3.2	61,11a
ndd=D2b	Nuclear disruption defective	CT447		15,11.1	11a,61,95,96
pla262	Nonessential	CT262			61
denB	Nonessential		Endonuclease IV	22	51,61
D1	Nonessential				61
rIIB	Nonessential, rapid lysis, suppressor of 30$^-$ and some 32$^-$ mutations	rex$^+$ lysogens, Tab R	Membrane protein, affector of membrane ATPase of E. coli	33,41, **35.5**	16,40,61,92a

[a]References: 1. Adari et al. (1985). 2. Adari and Spicer (1986). 3. Arisaka et al. (1987). 4. Arisaka et al. (1986). 5. Armstrong et al. (1983). 6. Barth et al. (1986). 7. Bijlenga et al. (1978). 8. E. Brody [personal communication]. 9. Broida and Abelson (1985). 10. Burke et al. (1985). 11. Champness and Snyder (1984). 11a. Chapman et al. (1988). 12. Childs and Pilon (1983). 13. Chu et al. (1984). 14. Chu et al. (1986). 15. Chu F, personal communication. 16. Colowick and Colowick (1983). 17. Conkling and Drake (1984). 18. Cunningham and Berger (1977a). 19. DeVries and Wallace (1983). 20. Doermann and Simon (1984). 21. Drake (1985). 22. Duda et al. (1986). 23. Duda et al. (1985). 24. Ehrenman et al. (1986). 25. Elliot and Geiduschek (1984). 26. Fujisawa et al. (1985). 27. Gauss et al. (1987). 28. E. Goldberg [personal communication]. 29. Gott et al. (1986 and personal communication, 1986). 30. Gram and Rüger (1985). 31. Griffith and Formosa (1985). 32. Gruidl and Mosig (1986). 33. Guerrier-Takada et al. (1984). 34. Hahn et al. (1986). 35. Herman et al. (1984). 36. Herman and Snustad (1985). 37. Hinton and Nossal (1986). 38. Hinton et al. (1985). 39. Hsu et al. (1987). 40. Huang (1986a). 41. Huang (1986b). 41a. Huang et al. (1988). 42. Huang et al. (1985). 43. L. Ishimoto and F. Eiserling [personal communication]. 44. Jongeneel et al. (1984). 45. Jabbar and Snyder (1984). 46. Kaufmann and Amitsur (1986). 47. Kaufmann et al. (1986). 48. Keller et al. (1984). 48a. Kemper et al. (1984). 49. Kozloff and Lute (1984). 50. Kutter et al. (1984). 51. Kutter (unpublished). 52. Kuz'min et al. (1983). 53. Lamm (in preparation). 54. Le Master (1986). 55. T. C. Lin and W. Konigsberg [personal communication]. 56. Macdonald and Mosig (1984a). 57. Macdonald and Mosig (1984b). 58. Macdonald et al. (1984). 59. Malik et al. (1985). 60. G. Marchin [personal communication]. 61. Mathews et al. (1983). 62. C. Mathews and J. Booth [personal communication]. 63. McPheeters et al. (1986). 64. G. Michaud, L. Black, and D. Hinton [personal communication]. 65. Midgley and Murray (1985). 66. Mileham et al. (1984). 67. Miller et al. (1985). 67a. Montag et al. (1987). 68. Mosig (1985). 69. Mosig and Macdonald (1986). 70. Mosig (1987). 71. Nakagawa et al. (1985). 72. M. Nakanishi and B. Alberts [personal communication]. 72a. Obringer et al. (1988). 73. Olson and Marchin (1984). 74. Olson and Marchin (1985). 75. Owen et al. (1983). 76. Parker et al. (1984). 77. Plishker and Berget (1984). 78. Plunkett and McClain (in preparation). 79. Powell (in preparation). 80. Pulitzer et al. (1985). 81. Purohit and Mathews (1984). 82. Radany et al. (1984). 83. Rand and Gait (1984, and personal communication). 84. Recinos et al. (1986). 84a. Riede (1987). 85. Riede et al. (1985). 86. Riede et al. (1986). 87. Rowe et al. (1984). 88. Schlagman and Hattman (1983). 89. Schoemaker (1983). 90. Selick et al. (1987). 91. Simon et al. (1983). 92. Simon and Randolph (1984). 92a. Singer et al. (1983). 93. Sjoberg et al. (1986). 93a. Skorko et al. (1977). 94. K. Skorupski and L. Simon [personal communication]. 95. D. P. Snustad and D. Oppenheimer [personal communication]. 96. Snustad et al. (1985). 97. Snustad et al. (1986). 98. E. Spicer et al. (1988). 98a. Stitt (1978). 99. Stitt and Mosig (in preparation). 100. Takahashi et al. (1985). 101. C. Thylen [personal communication]. 102. Tomaschewski et al. (1985). 103. Tomaschewski and Rüger (1987). 104. Trojanowska et al. (1984). 105. Uzan et al. (1983). 106. Valerie et al. (1984). 107. Valerie et al. (1985). 108. Valerie et al. (1986). 109. Wakem and Ebisuzaki (1984a). 110. Wakem and Ebisuzaki (1984b). 111. Wakem et al. (1984). 112. J. Wiberg and M. Murtha [personal communication, 1984]. 113. Williams et al. (1987). 114. Wu et al. (1984). 115. Yasuda et al. (1987). 116. Yonesaki and Minagawa (1985). 116a. Yonesaki et al. (1985). 117. Zograf et al. (1985).

[b]Molecular weights deduced from DNA sequences are boldfaced.

The work until 1983 has been summarized by the combined effort of the entire T4 community (Mathews et al., 1983). Here we will largely refer to individual chapters of that book for details, and concentrate on an overview and on new results and insights gained since those chapters were written. To avoid repetition, we refer the reader to the information in Table I whenever a protein or gene product is being discussed. When appropriate, we will draw comparisons with the other T-even phages.

B. The Genome

The genome of T4 contains about 166,000 bp of DNA whose cytosine residues are hydroxymethylated and glucosylated. (The chromosome contains about 171,000 base pairs; see below.) This modification makes T4 DNA refractory to T4 enzymes that are designed to destroy the host's DNA, and to most restriction enzymes. Using genetic tricks, T4 can be grown with nonglucosylated HMC DNA or with unmodified cytosine in its DNA (Kutter and Snyder, 1983). This DNA has been instrumental in cloning and sequencing large parts of the T4 genome (Kutter and Rüger, 1983; Kutter et al., 1987).

Mature DNA molecules, packaged in the virions, are linear. They are cut to fill a preformed head from highly branched, "concatemeric" intracellular DNA (see below) with 3–5% terminal redundancy so that individual chromosomes are almost randomly permuted (Streisinger et al., 1964, 1967; Kim and Davidson, 1974) over the circular genetic map (Fig. 1).

C. The Life Cycle

A simplified overview of T4's life cycle follows (Fig. 2). Adsorption of phage particles, with or without DNA (particles without DNA are known as "ghosts"), kills the host cells by largely unknown mechanisms—i.e., shuts off their protein synthesis and prevents them from replicating. Injection of the phage DNA initiates phage propagation. It causes three major, independent changes in the host chromosome, none of them essential for T4 development: (1) a disruption of the nucleoid into smaller segments that appear to migrate toward the cell envelope; (2) unfolding of the host chromosome; and (3) degradation of the host DNA.

Gradually, transcription switches from host to various classes of phage genes by a cascade of phage-coded transcription factors and RNA polymerase modifications. The classes are distinguished by a variety of criteria, and the nomenclature can appear bewildering to the uninitiated. As a first approximation, "early," or "prereplicative," genes are expressed before the onset of replication, whereas expression of "late" genes requires comcomitant DNA replication. "Early" genes are, however, fur-

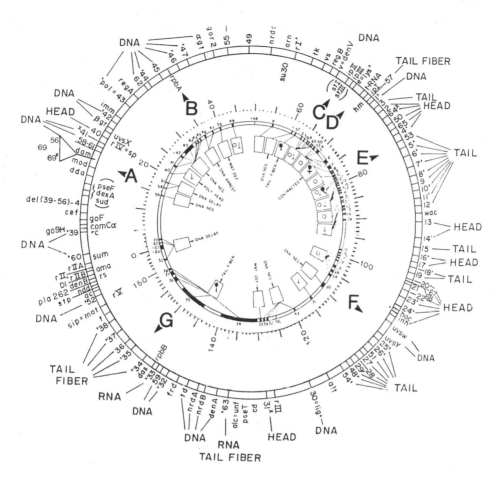

FIGURE 1. A map of the known T4 genes (Table I). Distances are based on recombination frequencies (inner circle; Edgar and Wood, 1966), on electronmicroscopy and restriction enzyme analysis (middle circle; Kutter *et al.*, 1987), and on the probability of packaging cuts (outer circle; Mosig, 1968). The arrowheads labeled with large capital letters point to origins of DNA replication.

ther subdivided into several classes. Immediately after infection, the host RNA polymerase holoenzyme recognizes a set of early T4 promoters that resemble the consensus sequence of *E. coli* promoters. The corresponding genes are called "immediate early," since their transcription requires no prior expression of any phage genes. Some of these early T4 genes code for proteins that alter the specificity of the host RNA polymerase by a variety of mechanisms: (1) by adenylribosylation of the RNA polymerase; (2) by binding to specific DNA sequences to allow transcription from so-called "middle" mode promoters; or (3) by allowing antitermination of transcription at what would otherwise be stop signals for RNA polymerase. Whereas adenylribosylation is still in search of a function, one or

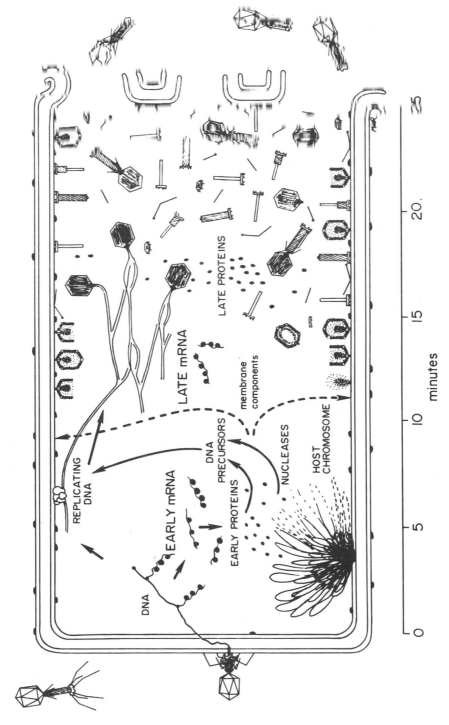

FIGURE 2. Overview of the T4 life cycle (see text for description). Modified from Mathews et al. 1983.

both of the other two mechanisms are required for expression of so-called "delayed early" genes. No T4-encoded sigma factor has been found to be required for transcription of delayed early genes. Most importantly, in many cases there is no clear distinction between "immediate early," "middle," and "delayed early" modes of transcription, since most early T4 genes can be transcribed from several promoters.

Collectively, early genes code for (1) nucleases that degrade the host DNA, (2) enzymes in the deoxyribonucleotide biosynthesis complex, (3) proteins of the replication and recombination machines, (4) proteins that modify the host membrane, (5) proteins that modify the T4 DNA to protect it from restriction, (6) several tRNAs, and (7) at least one sigma factor required for transcription of late genes. In addition, some early transcripts are used as primers to initiate DNA replication at specific origins.

Once the required T4 replication proteins have been made, DNA replication starts. At that time, T4 gene expression switches from the prereplicative, early mode to the so-called "late" mode. The late genes code for components of the viral particles and for enzymes that cut and package the complex vegetative DNA into capsids or that are involved in ultimately lysing the host cell.

D. "Unnecessary" Complexities?

This simplified scheme should mainly serve as a guide through the complexities discussed below. T4 codes for many more genes than the number that would appear necessary to accomplish lytic infection. Many of the T4 genes appear to be nonessential, because alternative pathways, phage- or host-encoded, duplicate their functions, or because they code for accessory helper proteins that are not absolutely required but facilitate individual steps in the infectious process.

There is a long list of redundancies. The number of different proteins in the virion far exceeds the number that suffices in other viruses. As already mentioned, many early genes are expressed in different modes. Similarly, some genes, the so-called "quasi-late," are expressed both early and late, and as a rule they have several different promoters. There are at least three distinct strategies to initiate DNA replication. There are at least three separate modes of DNA repair. There are several restriction-modification systems.

What is the meaning of these complexities? Are they adaptations to different environments and growth conditions in which their hosts grow? Are they remnants of the ongoing evolutionary struggle between this parasite and its host? Regardless of the answers to these questions, it is useful to think about them in terms of the rules about phage evolution discussed by Campbell (1988). The T4 genome is assembled by mixing and matching different components, entire genes or gene segments, from the genomes of other phages, plasmids or host genomes, and evolutionary pressure is still at work to coordinate these various components into a functional unit. In support of this view, a quick glance at T4's genome (Fig. 1) tells us that genes of related functions are clustered, but only to a limited extent. Early and late genes are neither spatially nor temporally clearly separated. Whereas it was originally thought that early genes are transcribed in one direction, from one strand of the DNA, and late genes are transcribed in the opposite direction (Guha et al., 1971), more and more exceptions to this rule are becoming apparent (Macdonald et al., 1984; McPheeters et al., 1986; Gruidl and Mosig, 1986; Barth et al., 1986, 1988), and the direction of transcription cannot be used to classify early or late transcripts. After we have described various individual steps of T4 infection, we will try to comment further on the evolutionary aspects.

II. STRUCTURE AND INITIATION OF INFECTION

Phage T4 devotes more than 40% of its total genetic information to the synthesis and assembly of structural components, and it is among the most complex of bacterial viruses. In some ways, a T4 particle is more like a cellular organelle in its structural complexity than a large virus. Figure 3 shows a drawing of T4 structure derived from electron microscope data and lists the known structural components of the phage. Twenty-four genes are involved in head morphogenesis, and the head itself contains at least 10 different polypeptide components. The tail and fibers make up another 26 structural proteins plus five other gene products needed for assembly.

The long tail fibers and whiskers near the head serve as environmental sensors to recognize the presence of a bacterial cell. The first event in the T4 infectious cycle is the release of the long tail fibers from their stored position along the sheath and whiskers, permitting the thin tips of the long fibers to interact reversibly with the cell surface at diglucosyl residues in the outer membrane in E. coli B lipopolysaccharide (Goldberg, 1980) or at the OmpC protein site in E. coli K12 (Furukawa and Mizushima, 1982). Fiber binding occurs via gp37 in T4, but also via gp38 in phage T2 and several T-even phages (Riede et al., 1987a). Fiber attachment is to the bacterial surface protein OmpF (T2) or the OmpA protein (phage K3) (Riede et al., 1987b).

While moving over the outer membrane surface, the long fibers are thought to transmit receptor-modulated binding and conformational change information to the baseplate, via the gene 9 product, which acts as an inhibitor of activation (Crowther, 1980). T4 and other phages are known to adsorb to or cause "zones of adhesions" between inner and outer membranes (Bayer, 1968), but the significance of this localization is still a mystery. The fiber-binding step activates the baseplate, which is then triggered into the hexagon-star transformation (Simon and Ander-

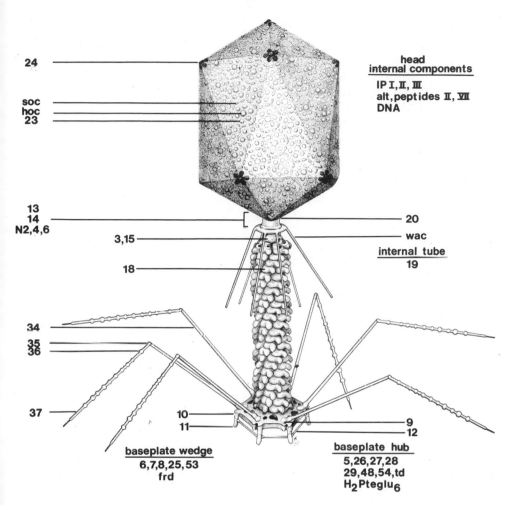

FIGURE 3. Structure of the T4 virion based on electron microscopy at 2- to 3-nm resolution. The locations of protein components are indicated by gene number except for several unknown connector proteins, called N 2, 4, and 6, and the baseplate component dihydropteroyl hexaglutamate, called $H_2Pteglu_6$. The portal vertex composed of gp20 is attached to the upper ring of the neck structure, inside the head itself. The internal tail tube is inside the sheath and itself contains a structural component in its central channel. The baseplate contains short tail fibers made of gp12; these are shown in a stored or folded conformation.

son, 1967a,b) by the contact of the gp12 short tail fibers with the cell surface receptor proteins (for review, see Berget and King, 1983). The short fibers of gp12 have been shown to bind to LPS in phage T4 (Zorzopulos *et al.*, 1982) and also for other T-even phages (Riede, 1987), where it was shown that heptose residues in the *E. coli* K12 LPS are involved in binding. Thus, for all T-even phages it appears that the short tail fibers bind to surface LPS and not to the outer membrane proteins (Riede, 1987).

The structural changes that take place during the hexagon-star transformation are the outward extension of the tail pins, in which gp11 folds
out to form the points of the star, the switch of gp9 from the outside of
the hexagon toward the inside of the star, and the switch in the position
of gp10 from a folded position in hexagons to an extended 35-nm fiber in
stars (Crowther et al., 1977; see also Fig. 12 in the chapter by Casjens and
Hendrix, 1988). The hexagon is stabilized by the presence of gp12; in its
absence, many isolated baseplates spontaneously convert from hexagon
to star. Sheath contraction is probably also regulated by the long tail
fibers, since Yamamoto and Uchida (1975) and Arscott and Goldberg
(1976) have shown that fiberless phages are more resistant to chemically
induced sheath contraction than are phages with the normal complement
of long tail fibers. The sheath contraction process begins when the connection of the annulus of sheath subunits at the surface of the baseplate
to the central tube weaken and the gp18 subunits move apart. As the ring
expands, subunits above move down into the spaces created by the baseplate expansion, setting off the contraction process and driving the tail
tube downward into the bacterial cell.

Several models have been discussed for the nature of the protein
interactions during sheath contraction (Kellenberger and Boy de la Tour,
1964; Moody, 1973; Caspar, 1980), and T4 sheath contraction is one of
the best studied of macromolecular structural protein rearrangements. In
one model (the "loaded spring"), the sheath is held in the extended form
by bonds to gp18 subunits above and below, with no significant contact
to the tail tube. Contraction can be triggered by baseplate expansion and
release of the bonds holding the tail tube to the baseplate or, artificially,
by release of the sheath-baseplate attachment by urea or detergents.
Sheath contraction normally moves the tail tube through the baseplate,
which remains attached to the sheath. In some cases, however, the contracted sheath separates from the baseplate, which remains at the end of
the tube. Various agents effect this separation (To et al., 1969; Winkler et
al., 1962). These results show that under some conditions, the bonds
connecting the baseplate to the tube are stronger than those connecting it
to the sheath subunits.

The "induced conformational change" model of Kellenberger (1980)
proposes that sheath extension is maintained by gp18–gp19 interactions
and that there is no tension along the sheath. Contraction is triggered by
a wave of conformational change through the tube, which releases the
gp18–gp19 interaction, and contraction follows this wave. This model is
consistent with Moody's (1973) observations of partially contracted
sheaths and the artificial cross-linking of sheath to tube by formaldehyde
treatment. It fits various experimental observations involving artificial
contraction and mechanisms of sheath assembly involving gp18–gp19
interactions. A combination of models, with conformational energy supplied by gp18–gp19 interactions and initiation by release of gp18–gp19
interactions, is represented in Caspar's (1980) model. Caspar constructed

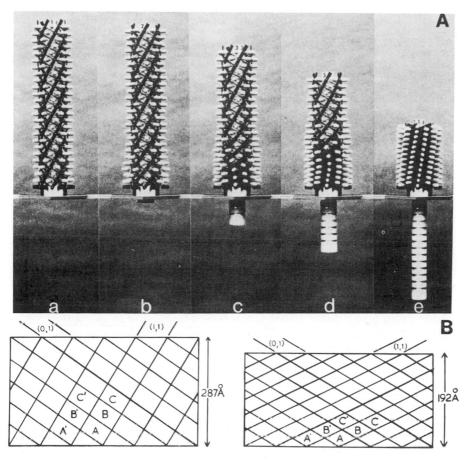

FIGURE 4. Sheath contraction. (A) Conversion of the stretched form to the relaxed form in a series of photographs of a model constructed by Caspar (1980), showing the penetration of the tail tube as a result of the rearrangement of the gp18 subunits. (B) A representation of the surface lattice of the sheath before and after contraction, based on Amos and Klug (1975) and Moody (1973). The (1,1) lines (left) give rise to prominent right-handed helical grooves, and after contraction (right) gp18 changes conformation but maintains the same bonding relationships, shown by letters A, B, C.

a working mechanical device in which energy for contraction is provided by stretched springs. Figure 4 shows in detail the steps in the contraction of this device, which illustrates clearly the structural relationships during the contraction process, based on Moody's results.

The last step in infection, DNA injection, requires additional signals and responses, but is poorly understood. Several virion proteins are injected with the DNA. Some functions of the earliest part of the life cycle may be dependent on these proteins. Goldberg (1983) has suggested that gp2 arrives with the DNA to protect the ends from exonuclease action, and that proteins at the tail tube tip play an important role in assuring DNA entrance into the cell, perhaps as pilot proteins, that prepare it for the earliest events in transcription and recombination.

III. REGULATION OF TRANSCRIPTION

T4's development is largely determined by precisely coordinated subversions of the host's RNA polymerase to permit initiation from different classes of T4-specific promoters. In addition, antitermination is thought to be important for expression of certain genes. The switch from pre-replicative, early transcription to late transcription requires both distinct alterations of the DNA template (by replication, partial nucleolytic digestion, or alterations in torsional stress by topoisomerases) and the association of at least one phage-encoded sigma factor (gp 55) with the host core RNA polymerase. In combination, these factors help the host core RNA polymerase to recognize T4 late promoters with a unique consensus sequence TATAAATA. Excellent reviews have dealt with the complexities of the T4 transcriptional program (Rabussay, 1983; Brody et al., 1983; Christensen and Young, 1983; Geiduschek et al., 1983; Geiduschek and Kassavetis, 1988). Here, we will give mainly an overview and will emphasize the contention that the complexity results from an assemblage of diverse regulatory genes, originally derived from other sources but now integrated to optimize T4 growth under a variety of conditions.

The diversion of E. coli's RNA polymerase to late T4 promoters is determined by an interplay of two mechanisms: (1) a cascade of T4-coded transcription factors, which alter the specificity of the host-coded RNA polymerase for certain promoters (Fig. 5), and (2) alterations in the structure of the DNA template, brought about mainly by interwoven DNA replication and recombination (Fig. 6) and by modification systems discussed below. Obviously, this distinction is mainly useful to put order in our minds, since, in reality, the mechanisms overlap. On the one hand, some of the transcription factors are DNA-binding proteins that could alter promoter recognition by altering the structure of the DNA. On the other hand, the usual modification of T4 DNA by hydroxymethylation of cytosine and its glucosylation, as well as methylation of adenines, is thought to influence recognition specificity even of unmodified RNA polymerase. Since most early T4 genes are under dual or triple control, most of the early transcription or antitermination factors characterized so far appear nonessential under defined laboratory conditions.

Immediately after infection, gpalt, an enzyme injected with the infecting DNA, reversibly modifies one α subunit of the RNA polymerase by ADP ribosylation of Arg 265. Irreversible ADP ribosylation of both subunits at the same Arg residue is later catalyzed by gpmod, an early enzyme. This modification reduces the affinity of core RNA polymerase for the host's major (70K) sigma factor, and it results in more efficient

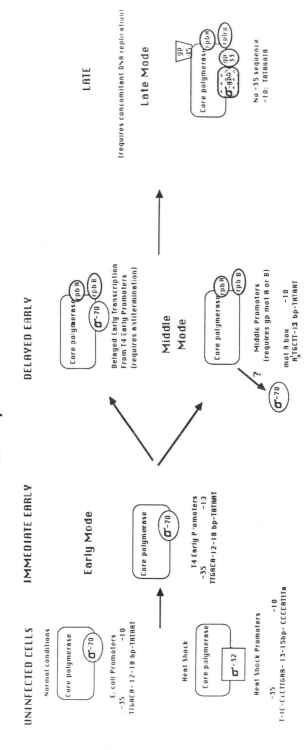

FIGURE 5. The association of various transcription factors described in the text, with the host core RNA polymerase. The "motA box" of middle promoters (Brody *et al.*, 1983; Guild *et al.*, 1988) is recognized by a specific DNA-binding protein (gpmotA; Uzan *et al.*, 1983). Another DNA-binding protein, which also binds RNA polymerase gpunf/alc (Snustad *et al.*, 1986; Snyder and Iorissen, 1988; E. Kutter, pers. commun.), prevents transcription elongation from cytosine-containing DNA (Kutter *et al.*, 1984).

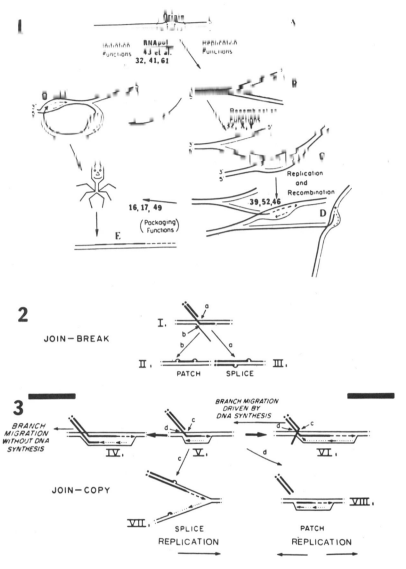

FIGURE 6. The replication-recombination-packaging pathway of T4 DNA described in the text. From Mosig (1983).

transcription termination by the host termination factor Rho than in transcripts made by unmodified RNA polymerase (Rabussay, 1983). It is nonessential for T4 growth. The RNA polymerase holoenzyme, with the *E. coli* 70K sigma factor, regardless of ADP ribosylation, recognizes T4 early promoters *in vivo* and *in vitro* (Gram *et al.*, 1984). It is becoming apparent, however, that the relative strengths of several early promoters differ *in vitro*, when the template contains normal cytosine, and *in vivo*, when the template contains glucosylated HMC (e.g., compare Gram *et al.*, 1984, and Macdonald and Mosig, 1984b). It is not yet known whether this difference is due to differences in the template or in the RNA polymerase or both.

Delayed early transcripts are distinguished operationally from immediate early transcripts by the fact that they are not made when protein synthesis is inhibited after phage infection. They can arise by different mechanisms: either by transcription from early promoters through potential terminators, facilitated by putative phage-coded antitermination functions, or by initiation from middle promoters. Many, if not most, delayed early genes are served by both of these mechanisms. This can become important when host restriction mechanisms cleave the DNA upstream of a middle promoter, thereby inactivating the immediate early but not the delayed early expression of a gene. An example is the expression of the *rIIB* gene (which is under such dual control) in nonglucosylated phage DNA in a restricting rgl^+ host (for review, see Revel, 1983).

T4 middle promoters are thought not to require phage-encoded substitute sigma factors. Instead, at least one class of middle promoters with a consensus "mot box," TAT/AGCTT, ~13 bp upstream of the −10 region (Brody *et al.*, 1988; Guild *et al.*, 1988), requires an activator protein gp*mot*, a DNA-binding protein that does not copurify with RNA polymerase (Brody *et al.*, 1983; Uzan *et al.*, 1983). Pulitzer *et al.* (1985) have postulated that there are two additional genes, *motB* and *motC*, involved in middle mode transcription. These genes map in a nonessential region between genes *39* and *56*. It is unknown whether they affect transcription from the same middle promoters mentioned above. To distinguish them, however, the original *mot* gene is now called *motA* (Fig. 5). There are conflicting reports whether these middle promoters require host sigma factors (see Rabussay, 1983; Geiduschek *et al.*, 1983). *MotA*-dependent promoters for *uvsY* and *69* function, albeit with very low activity, in *motA* mutant infections (Gruidl and Mosig, 1986) and *in vitro* with purified *E. coli* RNA polymerase, respectively (Macdonald and Mosig, 1984b). Shinedling *et al.* (1986) have reported that the *motA*-dependent *rIIB* promoter is expressed from supercoiled plasmids in uninfected cells. Supercoiling is not absolutely required, however, since Macdonald and Mosig (1984b) obtained some transcripts from a *mot*-dependent promoter on linearized templates *in vitro* without gp*motA*.

Transcription through potential termination signals is thought to require T4-encoded antitermination function(s). It has also been proposed that coupled translation might be responsible for antitermination (Brody *et al.*, 1983). One of the most compelling arguments for T4-coded antitermination factors comes from the work of Revel *et al.* (1980) and Stitt *et al.* (1980). Starting with a host mutant defective in propagating T4 (with a mutationally altered transcription termination factor Rho that is insensitive to the phage lambda antiterminator gpN), Stitt (1978) isolated T4 mutants that overcome the block and grow in this host. One of them, goF 1, maps in the nonessential region near gene 39. Pulitzer et al. (1979) have described a similar mutation (comCα). Another one of Stitt's mutations, goF 303.2, maps immediately upstream of the lysozyme gene e, probably in an open reading frame described by McPheeters et al. (1986). Two more goF mutations were tentatively mapped between genes 55 and 5 and between genes 55 and 51, respectively. This suggests not one but several T4 encoded antiterminators. Any one of these four mutations might alter an antiterminator function in a similar way as lambda N or Q mutations. It is also possible that some of the goF mutations affect T4-encoded termination functions.

During the delayed early time, two phage-encoded proteins, now called gprpbA and gprpbB, associate with the host RNA polymerase (Stevens, 1972, 1977). The gene for the former maps near gene 55 and codes for a nonessential 11.4-kD protein (Hsu et al., 1987; Williams et al., 1987). This protein was formerly called the "15K" protein. Association of the RNA polymerase with gprpbA, like the adenylribosylation mentioned above, reduces the affinity for host sigma factor. GprpbA is, however, dispensable (Williams et al., 1987). An open reading frame, coding for a 10.4-kD protein adjacent to gene 33, was thought to code for a second RNA polymerase binding protein, gprpoB, formerly called the 10K protein. Hahn et al. (1986) suggest that their 10.4-kD protein might have an antitermination function. It would be interesting to see whether one of Stitt's goF mutations, mentioned above, maps in this gene. More recently, however, Orsini and Brody (1988) found two 10-kD proteins at different map positions.

The most dramatic change in transcription specificity occurs during the switch from early to late transcription. The late promoter consensus box, TATAAATA, located a few bases upstream of the transcript start, can direct late transcription without requiring a "−35" region (Elliott and Geiduschek, 1984; Volker et al., 1984). Whereas this sequence was at first considered invariant, promoters in which this sequence is modified can initiate transcription in vitro (Kassavetis et al., 1987) with gp55-containing RNA polymerase as well as in vivo (McPheeters et al., 1986; Montag et al., 1987; Barth et al., 1988; Powell et al., in preparation). In phage-infected cells, transcription of late genes requires genes 33 and 55, which code for two proteins that associate with host core RNA polymerase in vivo and in vitro. Late transcription in vivo is also known to require the 24.7-kD bifunctional gp45, which is a component both of the T4 DNA replication machine (see below) and of RNA polymerase (Malik et al., 1985). Late transcription also requires a competent DNA template. Competence is usually achieved by concomitant DNA replication. In the absence of DNA replication, conditions that cut, nick, or partially digest the DNA can substitute: a combination of ligase and nuclease mutations (Geiduschek et al., 1983) or the restriction cleavage of nonglucosylated DNA by the host's Rgl system (Dharmalingam and Goldberg, 1976). Interestingly, all of these conditions also promote recombination even in the absence of DNA replication (Broker and Doermann, 1975). Perhaps, recombination or the intermediates generated by this process can activate late promoters. *In vitro*, some T4 late genes (e.g., *23*) are transcribed from supercoiled templates without requiring concomitant DNA replication (Albright *et al.*, 1988). It remains to be seen whether this is true for all late genes. *In vivo*, there is a dramatic difference in expression of different late T4 genes when both phage and host type II topoisomerases are inhibited by mutations or by drugs or by both. For example, gp23 is greatly reduced, but gp*e* (lysozyme) is elevated (Mosig *et al.*, 1983; Lin and Mosig, 1987), when both phage and host topoisomerases are inactive.

Overproduction of gp55 from expression vectors (Gram and Rüger, 1985) has allowed the demonstration that this protein is the long-sought T4 sigma factor for late transcription which does not require host sigma 70 (Kassavetis *et al.*, 1986). Interestingly, gp55 shares one similar domain with all other sigma factors sequenced thus far, i.e., the domain thought to recognize the core polymerase (Gribskov and Burgess, 1986).

Normal T4 late transcription requires that the template contain HMC, not cytosine; otherwise, T4's gp*alc/unf* prevents late transcription. This gene product, recently shown to be a DNA-binding protein, to interact with RNA polymerase, and to interfere with elongation (Snustad *et al.*, 1986; Snyder and Jorissen, 1988; R. Drivdahl and E. Kutter, personal communication), is involved in the unfolding of the host chromosome (hence its name *unf*) and, to some extent, in turning off transcription from the host genome. This turnoff mechanism works independently of the host genome degradation by T4-coded nucleases. How gp*alc* accomplishes its function is still a mystery, partly because it is nonessential except in strains containing the plasmid pR386 (Herman and Snustad, 1982). The last observation can serve as an example for the premise that the complexity of T4's transcriptional program cannot be understood solely in terms of T4's interaction with its host, but that it has evolved in response to other components that may reside in the same host.

During transition times, the RNA polymerases present in T4-infected cells must be a mixture of different species, containing different T4-coded factors (Rabussay, 1983). Geiduschek and his colleagues (see Geiduschek and Kassavetis, 1987) and Goldfarb and his colleagues (Malik *et al.*, 1985; A. Goldfarb, personal communication) have made thorough analyses of these different polymerase species. Malik *et al.* (1985) have demonstrated that ratios of the T4-coded accessory proteins can vary in different mutants, even when the structural genes for the accessory proteins are unaffected. Specifically, mutations in DNA replication genes alter the RNA polymerase composition. To some extent, this can be interpreted in terms of competition of RNA polymerase and replisomes for gp45, which is a component of both complexes. The results may, however, hint at some closer association between the two protein complexes. Goldfarb's and Geiduschek's groups have also provided complementary evidence that wild-type gp55 cannot displace the host's sigma 70 factor under normal conditions. A. Goldfarb (personal communication) has isolated mutants in which RNA polymerase accessory proteins show different association properties. These results and considerations imply that T4's transcriptional program does not resemble a hard wired circuit, even though it is ultimately geared toward lytic development. At least during transition states, the competition between various accessory proteins makes the RNA polymerase flexible to adapt to changing conditions during infection and to various mutations (Kahmaay, 1983), often to the chagrin of its investigators.

The presence of minor sigma factors in uninfected *E. coli* (for review, see Reznikoff *et al.*, 1985) suggests that the T4-induced transcription factors, specifically the sigma factor gp55, have to compete with these factors for access to RNA polymerase. This is probably of minor consequence under normal laboratory conditions, except when, during infections with temperature-sensitive mutants, heat shock conditions exist. Results from Wiberg's and from our lab show that, at high temperatures (Wiberg *et al.*, 1987; Frazier and Mosig, 1988) the *E. coli* heat shock sigma factor (sigma 32) is required for T4 growth. This largely reflects the requirement for sigma 70 in transcription from early T4 promoters, because at high temperatures, sigma 32 is required to replenish sigma 70 and for efficient synthesis of other heat shock proteins; e.g., gp*groEL* is required for T4 morphogenesis (Black and Showe, 1983; Chapter 5, this volume). Overproduction of the *groE* proteins can, for example, suppress defective *E. coli* dnaA mutations (Chapter 3, this volume). We suspect additional roles of the heat shock sigma factor in T4 growth.

Many differences in results with the same *ts* mutant under different conditions of infection can be explained by differences in induction of the heat shock response at the time of infection. For example, many gene *32* mutants, which had been classified as being completely defective in DNA replication at 42°C (Epstein *et al.*, 1964), undergo at least one round of DNA replication (see below) when cells have been adapted to the high temperature prior to infection (Mosig and Breschkin, 1975; Breschkin and Mosig, 1977a,b; Dannenberg and Mosig, 1981).

IV. POSTTRANSCRIPTIONAL CONTROLS

As with other eubacterial phages, posttranscriptional mechanisms modulate expression of T4 genes in a variety of ways: (1) by proteins affecting ribosome structure and function; (2) by translational repressors; (3) by modulating translational initiation via potential secondary RNA structures; (4) by processing of primary transcripts; and (5) by the rate of degradation. In addition, and so far unique among eubacterial phages, expression of certain T4 genes requires splicing or skipping of segments of primary transcripts.

It should be emphasized that expression of any specific gene depends ultimately on the effects of several of these components interwoven with each other and with the transcriptional controls discussed above. The efficient translation of a coding sequence may, in turn, affect mRNA stability and, via translational coupling, alter translational initiation of a downstream ORF. At each of these levels, there is a chance for regulatory modulation. Several mechanisms are known; others are inferred (Wiberg and Karam, 1983; Von Hippel et al., 1983; Schmidt and Apirion, 1983). We now discuss them separately.

A. T4-Evoked Modifications of Ribosomes

Turning off translation of host messages is the first step in the switch from host to phage metabolism. In contrast to the gradual transition of transcription from host genes to consecutive classes of T4 genes, translation of host messages ceases immediately after T4 infection. Apparently such translation is inhibited by infection with DNA-free particles, so-called ghosts (for review, see Duckworth, 1970). It is thought that some cells can recover from this immediate turnoff, but in successfully infected cells, by that time, ribosomes have been programmed to translate T4 messages exclusively. A few host membrane proteins are the notable exceptions. There is an extensive controversial literature, reviewed with great fairness by Wiberg and Karam (1983), concerning to what extent T4 infection alters the host's ribosomes. On balance, it appears that ribosomes from T4-infected cells differ in the content of the host-coded S1 protein and that they acquire a few phage-coded proteins. These changes are thought to be responsible for preferential translation of T4 versus host or coinfecting phage messages. Few if any of these T4-coded proteins have been identified, owing to lack of conditional lethal mutations. One possible candidate is the nonessential regB gene (Chace and Hall, 1975).

B. Translational Repressors

Two T4-encoded translational repressors of different specificity have served as paradigms for analyzing regulation of specific genes at the translational level (Gold et al., 1984): (1) the product of gene 32 (Alberts and Frey, 1970), the single-stranded DNA binding protein (alias helix-destabilizing protein), the prototype of an autoregulatory protein; and (2) the RegA protein (Wiberg and Karam, 1983), which regulates expression of several prereplicative T4 genes, including its own. It prevents translation from a number of early T4 messages when T4 has switched to the late mode of transcription.

Gene 32 protein binds cooperatively to single-stranded DNA and is a major scaffolding protein for protein machines involved in DNA replication, recombination, and repair (see Section VI). The autoregulation of gene 32 protein (Krisch and Allet, 1982; Von Hippel et al., 1983) is designed to establish and maintain physiological levels of this protein. The protein binds both to single-stranded DNA and RNA, but with slightly higher affinity to the former. Thus, when more protein is around than is needed to cover all single-stranded DNA, the excess will bind to RNA, preferentially to unstructured RNA. The gene 32 transcripts contain several repeats of a sequence that is particularly unlikely to fold into secondary structure (Fig. 7). This sequence is the preferred target of excess gene 32 protein, which, when bound, obliterates the ribosome-binding site and thus represses translation. Translation of other mRNAs is affected only at much higher gene 32 protein concentrations. Consistent with the model, overproduction of gene 32 protein in an expression vector system was achieved only after most of the proposed target sequences were deleted (Shamoo et al., 1986). The exquisite mathematical formulation of this theory is consistent with the actual concentrations of gene 32 protein found in the cell. A recent observation suggested, however, that gene 32 protein recognizes not only the unstructured nature but some sequence specificity in the RNA target, since there is no mutual competition with a single-stranded DNA-binding protein from single-stranded DNA phages (Fulford and Model, 1984). The 5' hairpin in Fig. 7 has recently been found to participate in additional base-pairing, generating a "pseudo-knot" that is thought to nucleate specific binding of gene 32 protein to this sequence (L. Gold, personal communication).

It has been observed that gene 32 mutants, even under permissive conditions for growth, overproduce the corresponding protein. This effect is readily explained if the altered protein has a generally reduced affinity for single-stranded nucleic acids, or if it has reduced affinity for its specific target, or both. The unusual stability of gene 32 message, which greatly facilitated the discovery of the translational regulatory circuit, is itself due to a specific sequence in that RNA that can confer resistance to degradation to other transcripts when it is present in cis configuration (Gorski et al., 1985). Apparently, the early transcripts are less stable than late ones. There is also a possible role of antisense RNA in gene 32 autoregulation (Belin et al., 1987).

Translational regulation by the regA gene product has been studied by an exquisite combination of biochemical and genetic analyses. Karam et al. (1981) showed that a target for RegA protein overlaps the initiation region of the rIIB gene. A comparison with initiation regions of several other regA-controlled T4 genes suggested, at first, a consensus target site (Spicer and Konigsberg, 1983). As more T4 genes are sequenced, the significance of that consensus becomes less certain. For example, there is a sequence similar to the "consensus" sequence upstream of the late gene soc (Macdonald and Mosig, 1984b) that does not fit into the regA regulation pattern, and there is no such consensus around the ribosome-binding site of regA, which itself is under regA control. Replacing the ribosome-binding site of regA with a different one removes autoregulatory repres-

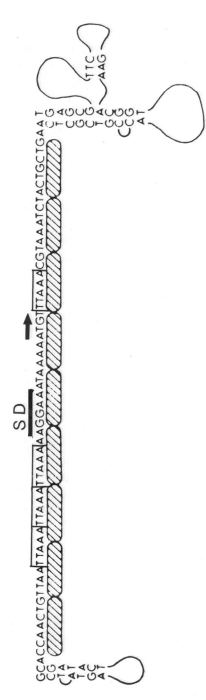

FIGURE 7. The AT-rich DNA sequence preceding the coding region of gene 32 containing the regulating signals. The Shine–Dalgarno sequence (bar), the initiation codor (arrow) of gene 32, and the multiple repeats indicated by Krisch and Allet (1982) (boxed) are marked. Modified from von Hippel *et al.* (1983) and Krisch and Allet (1982).

sion of regA (Adari and Spicer, 1986). It now appears that RegA protein recognizes unique-rich sequences (Miller et al., 1985, 1987).

It has been proposed that regA regulation is important for controlling synthesis of replisome components in appropriate amounts and ratios. Part of the argument derives from the map position of regA in the middle of replication genes. For evaluating this argument, it should be kept in mind that functionally related genes are clustered far less in T4 than in other phages (see Fig. 1). RegA mutants are not defective in DNA replication (Wiberg and Karam, 1983). Recently, it has been shown that regA inhibits the synthesis of some E. coli proteins and enhances synthesis of others (Miller et al., 1987).

C. Sequestering the Ribosome-Binding Site in Double-Stranded RNA

It is well established that translational initiation can be prevented by sequestering the ribosome-binding site in double-stranded RNA (Iserentant and Fiers, 1980; Gold et al., 1981). T4 uses this mechanism to prevent or reduce the early translation of at least three late genes—soc (Macdonald et al., 1984), e (McPheeters et al., 1986), and 49 (Barth et al., 1988)—from early transcripts that are initiated from early promoters upstream of these genes. In all three cases, the long early RNA can form a hairpin that sequesters the ribosome-binding site in a double-stranded region. The shorter late transcripts, initiated from true late promoters closer to the ribosome-binding site, cannot form the potential stem-loop structures and are therefore more efficiently translated (Fig. 8). The significance of this interplay of transcriptional and translational controls may well relate to the frequent alternation of early and late genes on the T4 genome. Transcripts designed for early genes may fail to terminate and accidentally traverse through late genes, thus potentially disrupting the developmental program. Sequestering the ribosome-binding sites of such transcripts in a hairpin would counteract this potential hazard (Reznikoff et al., 1985). RNA processing at specific sites may play an additional role in controlling translation of gene 49 (Barth et al., 1988).

D. RNA Processing

The activation of primary transcripts by RNA processing is of utmost importance in the final activity of T4-coded tRNAs. The complex processing pathway, summarized in the review by Schmidt and Apirion (1983), has been worked out in exquisite detail by the combined efforts of several laboratories. It serves as a model for understanding function and interactions of processing RNases and the relationship of tRNA structure and function (Broida and Abelson, 1985; McClain et al., 1987).

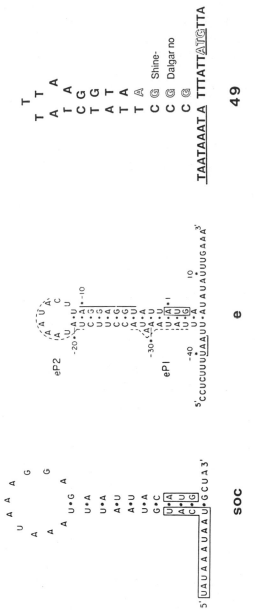

FIGURE 8. Probable folding of early transcripts from three genes that are predominantly expressed late. In each case, transcripts initiated from the late promoter shown cannot form this structure.

T4 codes for eight tRNAs and two tRNA-like structures of unknown function. The entire tRNA region (Fig. 9) is not essential under most laboratory conditions but is thought to be advantageous, because the T4 tRNAs supplement host tRNAs for those codons that are rare in the host but frequent in T4 messages. (T4 DNA has only 33% GC compared with 50% in E. coli DNA.) The GUA recognizing E. coli tRNA^Arg is rapidly cleaved after T4 infection (Yudelevich, 1971; Kano-Sueoka and Sueoka, 1969), and this codon is avoided in T4 (Hattman et al., 1985) In addition, the T4 tRNA^Ile becomes important in certain host strains in which the anticodon loop of the isoaccepting host tRNA is cleaved by T4-coded enzymes and not resealed (Snyder, 1983). Five of the T4-coded tRNAs can mutate to become nonsense suppressors (McClain et al., 1987). Such mutations readily accumulate in T4 strains containing multiple nonsense mutations.

The T4 tRNA region can be transcribed from several promoters (Broida and Abelson, 1985) as a large transcript containing all genes and, most likely, from one or more additional internal promoters. There are two putative transcription terminators—one within the tRNA^ile, and one after the species 1 region (Fig. 9). Transcription through the latter terminator is probably responsible for the nontranslated early transcripts that traverse the lysozyme gene e, discussed above.

The primary transcripts are processed in several steps, via tRNA dimer intermediates, to the final active tRNAs and the two additional tRNA-like species (1 and 2) mentioned above. This stepwise processing is accomplished by several host RNases, to some extent by autocatalysis, and by a nucleotidyltransferase that adds CAA to some of the products (Deutscher et al., 1974). At least one T4-coded gene, called mb, M1, or cef by different investigators (Wilson and Abelson, 1972; Pulitzer et al., 1985; Rodriguez, 1976; Plunkett and McClain, in preparation), is involved in synthesis or processing of three tRNAs. Mb/cef maps in a nonessential region of the T4 genome. Its function is unknown, but there is a host mutant in which the T4 gene is essential (Rodriguez, 1976). Inactivation of any one of the processing enzymes does not arrest processing, but channels the precursors into a different pathway.

These results can be interpreted to mean that the RNA processing enzymes interact in a loose complex that coordinates the various steps in the processing sequence, while the primary transcripts are still being synthesized (Schmidt and Apirion, 1983). An alternative interpretation, discussed by Apirion and his collaborators, is that different processing pathways are dictated by different folding patterns of the RNA, which had been cleaved at different sites. Gurevitz and Apirion (1985) have shown that the tRNA precursors can fold into different alternative structures. The presumed RNaseF cleavage site in Fig. 9 is subject to auto-cleavage when, and only when, this RNA segment is folded in a certain configuration. RNaseF (Watson et al., 1984) is now thought to be a factor

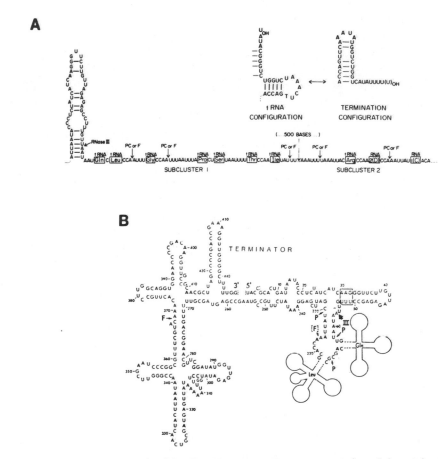

FIGURE 9. (A) Organization of the T4 tRNA genes. Transcription is from left to right. The tRNA sequences are identified by boxes, and the interstitial sequences are shown, arranged in a probable secondary structure. Sites of nuclease cleavage on the primary transcript are indicated. The tRNA^{ile} can assume the two possible configurations indicated. Modified from Schmidt and Apirion (1983). (B) An alternative secondary structure near the RNase III cleavage site shown in A. In this structure, the 5' and 3' ends of the precursor RNA are in close proximity. From Gurevitz and Apirion (1985).

facilitating such autocleavage. RNaseP set a precedent for the facilitating role of proteins, whose catalysis is determined by an RNA component (for review, see Cech and Bass, 1986).

Gurevitz and Apirion (1985) have also shown that RNaseIII affects not only RNA processing, but also termination of transcription. They discuss that the unprocessed precursor RNA can fold in such a way that the 3' and 5' ends are close together, but that in the most stable structure of the processed RNA these ends are far apart.

E. RNA Degradation

Most T4 RNAs are rapidly degraded, albeit with different speed. Clearly, relative transcript stabilities must contribute to the relative abundance of T4 gene products that finally accumulate. Some transcript degradation is thought to start at 5' ends and to proceed until the responsible enzymes are stopped by secondary structures. For example, the 5' end of the tRNA precursor RNA mentioned above is thought to be generated by a nuclease that stopped at the hairpin drawn in Fig. 9 (Schmidt and Apirion, 1983). As mentioned above, Gorski et al. (1985) have shown that the DNA corresponding to the 5' region of the very stable gene 32 message, when transferred to other genes, confers stability to messages of these genes. It is thought that nucleolytic nibbling from the 3' ends might be even more prevalent and that it also can be stopped by secondary structures in the transcripts (Kennell, 1986). In addition, some of the host enzymes that successfully process precursors to useful tRNAs probably degrade other transcripts to trash. Except for the role of hairpins in stopping degradation, little is known about the rules governing stability of T4 messages. Analysis of the gene 32 transcripts suggests that some degradation is temporally regulated by phage-determined factors (Belin et al., 1987). A role for REP sequences (Newbury et al., 1987) is not known.

F. Introns in T4 Transcripts

Introns in pre-mRNA have been the biggest recent surprises in T4 biology. The genes td (thymidylate synthase) (Chu et al., 1984, 1986; Belfort et al., 1985, 1986) sunY (Shub et al., 1988), nrdB (nucleotide reductase) (Sjöberg et al., 1986; Gott et al., 1986), and 60 (T4 topoisomerase subunit) (Huang et al., 1988) are interrupted by intervening sequences. The first three of these introns can self-excise, like the type I intervening sequences of Tetrahymena ribosomal precursor RNA or of fungal mitochondrial RNA (Ehrenman et al., 1986; for review of RNA-catalyzed splicing, see Cech and Bass, 1986). These three introns contain an open reading frame, of yet unknown function. Like other type I introns, they have certain conserved sequence elements. Prior to splicing, these elements can fold into complex tertiary structures, which are thought to constitute the active centers of "ribozymes." Analysis of nondirected mutations has shown that changes in at least two different conserved elements, forming stem-loop structures (Fig. 10A), result in defective splicing of the td RNA (Hall et al., 1987). The use of these and other mutations combined with the ease of genetic manipulations in T4 will undoubtedly enhance the understanding of such RNA-catalyzed reactions.

Most surprising is the recent finding that the intron in gene 60 is not excised but simply skipped during translation, probably because it can fold into a superstable hairpin (Fig. 10B) (Huang et al., 1988). Hairpins of

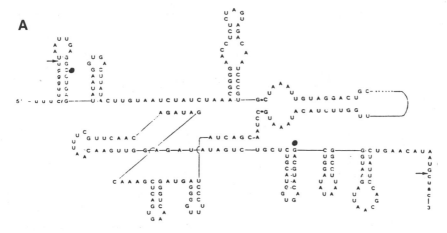

FIGURE 10. (A) Mutations (dots) in the *td*-intron that prevent self-splicing of the transcript. From Hall *et al.* (1987). The intron is drawn according to a model proposed by F. Michel; arrows indicate the splice junctions. (B) The RNA segment whose translation is skipped in the gene *60* transcript and the folding that is likely to cause the skipping. From Huang *et al.* (1988).

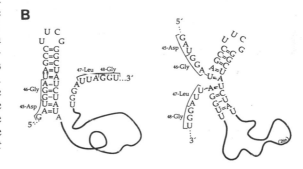

similar structure and stability occur frequently elsewhere in intercistronic regions (Tuerk *et al.*, 1988).

One or two more spliceable intervening sequences have been detected by labeling the splicing intermediate with [^{32}P]-GTP *in vitro* (Gott *et al.*, 1986; Chu *et al.*, 1987). The *td*, but not the *nrd*B, intron is also found in the closely related T2 and T6 phages (Chu *et al.*, 1987; Pedersen-Lane and Belfort, 1987).

V. MODIFICATION AND RESTRICTION OF T4 DNA

T-even phage DNA is modified at several levels: cytosine residues are replaced by 5-hydroxymethylcytosine (HMC), which is glucosylated to different extents in the different phages. These modifications have at least three consequences: (1) They protect the phage DNA from phage-encoded nucleases that are meant to degrade host DNA so that it can be scavenged for phage DNA synthesis. (2) They afford protection against restriction enzymes of the host or of resident plasmids or prophages. (3) They alter the structure of the DNA so that it can readily flip into a conformation similar to D-DNA (Saenger, 1984). These structural altera-

tions might alter recognition of DNA by several proteins and thus affect
different processes: transcription initiation (Macdonald and Mosig,
1984b; Gram et al., 1984), recombination (Mosig, 1966, 1968; Levy and
Goldberg, 1980), recognition by primase (Hinton et al., 1987; Selick et al.,
1987), and cleavage by T4 DNA topoisomerase (Kreuzer and Huang, 1983;
Kreuzer and Alberts, 1984) and by certain nucleases (Warner and Snustad,
1983; Carlson and Wiberg, 1983).

The roles of cytosine modification by hydroxymethylation and
glucosylation and of adenine methylation in T4 growth are well reviewed
by Revel (1983) and Hattman (1983), respectively. Warner and Snustad
(1983) have summarized the known and putative roles of T4-coded and
host-coded nucleases in T4 growth, and Snustad et al. (1983) have re-
corded the remarkable events that accompany unfolding and eventual
degradation of the host DNA. What follows is only an attempt to discuss
the mechanisms of modification in terms of the phage's strategy to remain a true parasite: to gradually degrade the host's DNA while saving its
own. Understanding the complexities of this strategy was the basis of the
successful attempts to construct phage strains whose DNA contains normal cytosine and can therefore be cleaved by ordinary restriction enzymes (for review, see Kutter and Snyder, 1983). These phages grow,
albeit poorly, but only in hosts lacking host-specific restriction mechanisms (hsp).

In normal T4 development, hydroxymethylcytosine (HMC) substitution occurs at the level of precursor biosynthesis. The two enzymes most
important for this substitution are dCTPase, the product of gene 56,
which degrades dCTP (as well as dUTP and the corresponding diphos-
phates), and dCMP hydroxymethylase, the product of gene 42, which
modifies the cytosine mononucleotides. When these enzymes are defective, cytosine is incorporated into phage DNA, albeit at a reduced rate,
but no progeny particles are produced, because the DNA is rapidly degraded. Even if that DNA escapes degradation (as in certain mutants
discussed below), it does not serve as a template for late transcription,
because the T4-coded gpalc/unf, a DNA-binding and RNA-polymerase-
binding protein responsible for the unfolding of host DNA (Snustad et al.,
1986; R. Drivdahl and E. Kutter, personal communication), prevents transcription from cytosine-containing DNA.

The phage-encoded nucleases responsible for degradation of cytosine
DNA are endoII (gpdenA), which produces single-strand nicks in double-
stranded DNA, and endoIV (gpdenB), which cuts single-stranded DNA to
fragments with some sequence preference (Carlson and Wiberg, 1983;
Carlson and Øvervatn, 1986). These fragments are further degraded to
nucleotides by the gene 46/47-controlled exonuclease. The degradation
products are reutilized for T4 DNA replication. Neither endoII nor endo-
IV is essential under laboratory conditions. If these two endonucleases
are mutationally inactivated, cytosine-containing T4 DNA can survive.
Whereas it was thought that endoII plays a major role in host DNA
degradation, and endoIV in degradation of T4 cytosine-containing DNA

(for review, see Warner and Snustad, 1983), recent results of Carlson and Øvervatn (1986) show that endoII is also the principal enzyme initiating degradation of T4 cytosine-containing DNA. The enzyme is, however, inhibited by very small amounts of HMC in the DNA. This observation explains why this function of endoII was not apparent in the earlier experiments.

In the absence of a functional *alc* gene, T4 late genes are transcribed from C-DNA, and functional phage particles are produced. In this case, however, T4 growth becomes sensitive to host-specific restriction mechanisms, to which it is normally resistant.

In HMC-containing DNA, glucosylation provides another level of protection against host restriction mechanisms (RglA and RglB), originally thought to be specifically directed against HMC DNA (Revel and Luria, 1970). It has become apparent, however, that the Rgl systems are identical with the Mcr systems that restrict DNA containing methylcytosine in specific sequences (Raleigh and Wilson, 1986; Raleigh *et al.*, 1988). The T4 early *arn* (antirestriction nuclease) gene product inactivates one of these host restriction systems, (RglB = McrB), by an unknown mechanism (Dharmalingam and Goldberg, 1979; Dharmalingam *et al.*, 1982).

T-even DNA is glucosylated by α- and β-glucosyltransferases that modify HMC residues in DNA. In T4 DNA, all HMC residues are modified, 70% with α- and 30% with β-glucosyl linkages. In contrast, in T2 and in T6 DNA, 25% of the HMC residues are not glucosylated. In T6, however, many glucose residues are further glucosylated by an additional β-glucosyl linkage.

The differences in the glucosylation patterns are dictated by the differences in the corresponding enzymes of the different phages. Gram and Rüger (1986) have compared the nucleotide sequences of the corresponding genes. Interestingly, these genes are related to each other with patches of homology separated by nonhomologous regions.

T2 and T4 DNA, but not T6 DNA, are further modified by adenine methylation. From 0.5% to 1.5% of the adenine residues is methylated to give N^6 methyladenine, mainly, but not exclusively, in the sequence GATC. Methylation occurs in completed DNA chains by phage-encoded deoxyadenosine methylases ("dam"). T6 lacks such an enzyme. Even though T4 and *E. coli* methylate adenines in the same target sequences, the host enzymes do not substitute for mutated T-even enzymes. The failure of the host enzyme to methylate T-even DNA may be due to the presence of HMC at the last position of the target sequence. The T4 *dam* gene has been mapped (Schlagman and Hattman, 1983) and sequenced (Macdonald and Mosig, 1984b). There is little if any homology at the DNA level between the phage and host *dam* methylases. There is, however, considerable homology at the protein level. This homology is concentrated in four patches with similar predicted hydropathicity profiles, separated by patches of unrelated amino acids. Interestingly, three of the homologous regions can also be aligned with the DNA modification methylase of *D. pneumonia, Dpn*II. These comparisons suggest an evolutionary relationship between these related enzymes. The divergence of the DNA sequence is readily explained by selection for those codon changes that conform to the average codon usage and base composition of the organism in which the corresponding *dam* gene resides (Hattman *et al.*, 1985).

The only proven physiological role of adenine methylation is protection against the phage P1 restriction system. This role becomes apparent only when the HMC-glucosylation system is inactivated. It is intriguing to find (Macdonald and Mosig, 1984b) that the *dam* gene maps adjacent to an origin of DNA replication (see Section VI). The search for a possible role of *dam* methylation in DNA replication has, however, been fruitless.

VI. DNA REPLICATION AND RECOMBINATION

A. Overview of Replication *in Vivo*

The potential of a virus to produce many copies in a short time requires the capacity for rapid replication of its own DNA. Again, T4 DNA replication shows complexities that, in isolation, could appear unnecessary for viral propagation. To make sense, they should be considered in the context of the total viral developmental program and evolutionary history. DNA replication competes with transcription, DNA repair, recombination, and packaging and uses a multitude of overlapping strategies that can respond to many different circumstances and growth conditions.

1. Many of the complex prereplicative transcriptional and posttranscriptional controls discussed above are designed to ensure that replication proteins and recombination proteins, which are also essential for most of T4 DNA replication (see below), as well as enzymes that degrade host DNA and those that provide precursors for phage DNA, are synthesized in sufficient amounts and in optimal proportions.

2. Like many other viruses, T4 initiates its DNA replication by different mechanisms during different stages of its life cycle. The early mode can be considered in terms of the replicon model (Jacob *et al.*, 1963; Pritchard, 1978); i.e., interactions of positive and negative control elements with specific origin sequences regulate replication at the level of initiation. It requires RNA polymerase and is subject to host-determined and, later, phage-determined modulations of that enzyme.

3. Different replication modes are necessary to ultimately escape the host's controls. In T4, most subsequent initiations depend on phage encoded replication and recombination proteins and use recombinational intermediates as DNA primers. Except for the synthesis of the participating proteins, this mode is uncontrolled.

We shall first give an overview of T4's general strategy (Kozinski, 1983; Mosig, 1983), then discuss its details, and finally relate it to the function of T4 replication and recombination proteins (Nossal and Alberts, 1983; Kreuzer and Huang, 1983; Huang, 1983; Williams and Konigsberg, 1983) and genes (Bernstein and Wallace, 1983; Drake and Ripley, 1983; Mosig, 1983; Hinton *et al.*, 1987; Selick *et al.*, 1987; Kreuzer and Menkens, 1987). In addition, enzymes involved in precursor biosynthesis have been shown to interact *in vivo* and *in vitro* with each other and with the replication complex (Mathews and Allen, 1983). Both genetic (Mosig *et al.*, 1979) and biochemical experiments (Formosa *et al.*, 1983; Formosa and Alberts, 1984) support the interaction of replication and recombination proteins (Fig. 11). The interactions of these proteins serve as paradigms for the concept of protein machines (Alberts, 1984).

The general model we have proposed for T4 DNA metabolism is

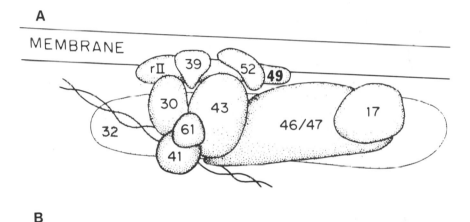

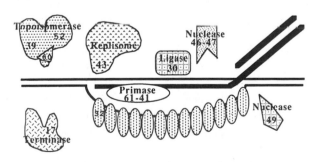

FIGURE 11. (A) Cartoon of interactions of T4 proteins with gp32 deduced from genetic interactions. From Mosig *et al.* (1984). The numbers refer to genes in Table I. (B) Different proteins are thought to interact in different complexes.

shown in Fig. 6. The first round of replication is initiated *de novo* at specific origin sequences (Fig. 6A). When the first growing point reaches one end of the chromosome (Fig. 6B), the 3' OH end of the template for the lagging strand remains single-stranded, because it is unlikely that there is an initiation sequence for an Okazaki piece precisely at the end (Watson, 1972). Starting with its 3' OH end, this single-stranded segment invades a homologous DNA segment. In cells infected with several T4 chromosomes, the end will most likely invade the interior of another chromosome (Fig. 6C), because, as mentioned above, T4 chromosomes are circularly permuted. In cells infected with a single T4 chromosome, the single-stranded end can only find homology within the terminal redundancy (which is several thousand base pairs long) at the other end. In this case, invasion generates a circle with a tail (Fig. 6C'). Note, however, that the tail protruding from the circle was initiated neither from a single-strand nick nor from an end. It is one of the two tails generated after a replisome that had initiated replication *de novo* at an internal origin reached an end (Dannenberg and Mosig, 1983). The other tail is engaged in the invasion. The most important intermediates for continued DNA replication are the displacement loops (D loops) with attached double-stranded branches (see rectangular insert in Fig. 6C). For simplicity, this insert shows an invasion into an unreplicated homologous region, although invasions into replicated chromosomes are more frequent (Dannenberg and Mosig, 1983). When all proteins of the replication machines are available and functional, the invading 3' OH end can prime leading strands of new replication forks and initiate a new replisome (Fig. 6D,D'). When such a replisome reaches the end of its template, it generates another single-stranded end that can reiterate the process by another invasion. Ultimately, this reiteration of recombination-initiated replication generates a branched DNA network in which individual chromosomes are no longer distinguishable by electron microscopy (Huberman, 1969; Kemper and Brown, 1976; Dannenberg and Mosig, 1983).

In the direction opposite to that of replication, branch migration might extend the original heteroduplex regions. Alternatively, the intermediates can be cut once to allow bidirectional replication, or they are cut and joined to give patch or splice recombinants according to conventional pathways of recombination (Stahl, 1979; Whitehouse, 1982; Broker and Lehman, 1971; Broker, 1973). Finally, the branched structures generated by a combination of these pathways have to be trimmed and cut to linear chromosomes that fit into preformed heads (Steisinger *et al.*, 1967; Luftig *et al.*, 1971; Mosig *et al.*, 1972; for review, see Black and Showe, 1983; Black, this volume).

Recombination-initiated DNA replication is not only advantageous but also essential for T4 growth. Since initiation from primary origins requires recognition of early, *E. coli*–like, origin promoters (Macdonald *et al.*, 1983; Mosig *et al.*, 1987) by the host's RNA polymerase (Luder and Mosig, 1982), the association of T4-encoded peptides with that RNA polymerase during T4 development, discussed above, also shuts off DNA replication from primary origins. Therefore, T4 depends on other initiation mechanisms. Under most conditions, the predominant one is secondary initiation from recombinational intermediates. This initiation is insensitive to inhibitors of RNA polymerase but sensitive to inactivation of recombination proteins (Luder and Mosig, 1982). When the RNA polymerase is inactivated by rifampicin and the gene 46/47 recombination nuclease is inactivated by mutations, a tertiary mode of DNA replication becomes apparent (Kreuzer and Alberts, 1985, 1986) in a plasmid replication system originally developed by Mattson et al. (1983).

We shall now discuss in more detail some aspects and requirements of the different processes that interface with DNA replication.

B. Genetics of "Primary" Origin Initiation

There are a number of primary origins in the T4 genome (arrowheads in Fig. 1) (for reviews, see Kozinski, 1983; Mosig, 1983; King and Huang, 1982; Yee and Marsh, 1985), but at least in E. coli B, under conditions of single infection, most individual simple chromosomes that are not yet branched or longer than unity contain only one replication eye (Fig. 12) (Dannenberg and Mosig, 1983; Yee and Marsh, 1985). Two factors may limit the number of growing points at that time: (1) the amount of T4 replication proteins (Werner, 1968), and (2) control of T4 primary origins by positive and/or negative elements, requiring activation or derepression. Host RNA polymerase is most likely required to make primers for leading-strand DNA synthesis during primary initiation (Luder and Mosig, 1982; Mosig et al., 1987). Leading strands are initiated even when both T4 primase (gene 58/61) and E. coli primase (dnaG) are inactivated by mutations (Luder, 1981). The first nascent T4 DNA is not covalently linked to parental DNA; this demonstrates that it is not initiated from a nick or from an end (Kozinski, 1983). T4 primase is, however required to initiate lagging-strand Okazaki pieces. When the T4 primase gene 58/61 is mutated, T4 chromosomes continue to replicate by displacement synthesis. The displacement loops can be seen in the electron microscope (Luder, 1981; Mosig et al., 1981b). This displacement synthesis explains the earlier observations that gene 58/61 mutants (Hamlett and Berger, 1975) accumulate large single-stranded regions after infection of restrictive hosts. DNA replication then slows down, presumably, as origin initiation is inactivated.

Eventually, the displaced strand must be copied, because the mutants, after some delay, synthesize DNA (at about half of the normal rate) and the proportion of single-stranded regions declines (Yegian et al., 1971; Hamlett and Berger, 1975; Mufti and Bernstein, 1974; Luder, 1981). This late DNA synthesis in the gene 58/61 mutants depends on functional recombination proteins and on T4 topoisomerase (Mosig et al., 1980; Luder, 1981). Since it generates double-stranded DNA, even though primase is inactive, we have proposed (Luder, 1981; Mosig et al., 1980)

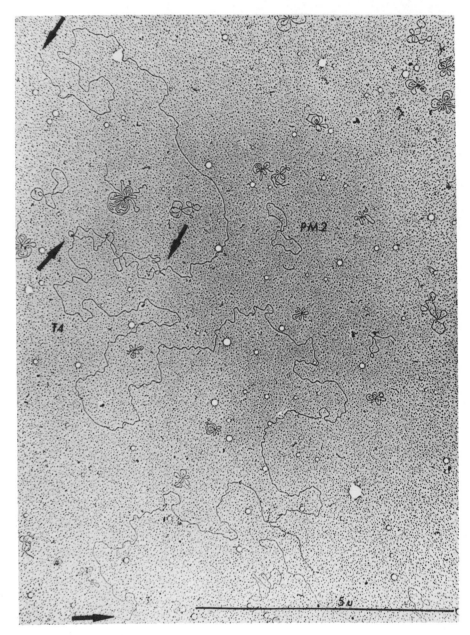

FIGURE 12. An early replicating T4 chromosome. From Dannenberg and Mosig (1983).

that, in this case, breaks or ends in the chromosomes that are invaded during recombination can prime lagging-strand synthesis (see recombination-dependent replication, discussed below). The infecting gene *58/61* mutant chromosomes are initially replicated by displacement synthesis with near wild-type speed (Luder, 1981). This finding is somewhat surprising, since coupling of leading- and lagging-strand synthesis accelerates DNA synthesis *in vitro* (Hinton *et al.*, 1987; Selick *et al.*, 1987).

Single-stranded DNA also accumulates in mutants that lack the other T4 primase/helicase subunit, gp41 (Oishi, 1968). The pattern of primary replication is at first similar to that of gene *58/61* mutants (Mosig, unpublished). In contrast to the gene *58/61* mutants, the gene *41* mutants do not resume DNA replication, most likely because the helicase activity of gp41 is required to unwind the DNA at the replication fork (Hinton *et al.*, 1987; Selick *et al.*, 1987).

Under different conditions of infection, incidentally used in most cases by different investigators, one or a few of the origins shown in Fig. 1 seem to predominate. Instead of considering these results as controversial, we prefer to think that primary initiation, because of its requirement for host RNA polymerase, is subject to many aspects of transcriptional control of the host, related to its physiological state at the time of infection (discussed in Section II, above). In this view, host-encoded transcription factors can determine which origin is used at first. Since the required T4 replication proteins (Werner, 1969) are synthesized concomitantly with the T4 proteins that modify the RNA polymerase and ultimately turn off origin initiation, any origin first selected by the host RNA polymerase will appear as the predominant T4 origin. All electron microscopic analyses agree that reinitiation from the same origin, although it occurs, is rare (Delius *et al.*, 1971; Dannenberg and Mosig, 1983; Yee and Marsh, 1985).

As a first step toward characterizing factors that influence origin selection, G. Lin in our laboratory has shown that different primary origins are preferred in the presence or absence of functional host gyrase. Since prior to initiation the T4 chromosomes are still linear and unbranched, it is unlikely that gyrase at that time works via altering global torsional stress in the T4 chromosomes. It can introduce localized torsional stress, if DNA segments are topologically constrained (Liu *et al.*, 1979; Sinden and Pettijohn, 1982). We consider the additional and not mutually exclusive possibility that the host gyrase affects the synthesis and delicate balance of host transcription factors, which in turn affect origin utilization.

Mutants in genes *39, 52,* and *60,* which are now known to code for a type II DNA topoisomerase (Huang, 1986a,b; Stetler *et al.*, 1979; Liu *et al.*, 1979), like primase mutants mentioned above, have a so-called DNA delay phenotype. They start the first round of replication at the same time as wild-type T4, then show a lag period, and, after that delay, resume DNA replication at approximately half the normal rate (Yegian *et al.*, 1971). The defect is worse at lower than at higher temperatures (Mufti and Bernstein, 1974). These mutants are deficient in initiation, not in elongation (McCarthy *et al.*, 1976). McCarthy (1979) has reported that *E. coli* gyrase and T4 topoisomerase can substitute for each other in T4 growth. Based on these results, Liu *et al.* (1979) proposed that the T4 topoisomerase is an origin-specific gyrase and that it is required for the unwinding of origins prior to initiation. We found that in these mutants initiation of leading strands occurs in the direction of transcription from two of the primary origins that we have tested (Mosig et al., 1983). Initiation in the other direction, however, is defective regardless of host gyrase activity or the growth temperature (Mosig et al., 1983; M. Gruidl and G. Mosig, in preparation). We conclude that host gyrase cannot substitute for defective T4 topoisomerase in this aspect of origin initiation. Genetic analyses of primase-topoisomerase double mutants (Luder, 1981; Mosig et al., 1980) suggest that the T4 topoisomerase interacts with T4 primase during primary DNA replication.

As discussed below, the T4 DNA topoisomerase has additional roles in recombination-dependent DNA replication and in late transcription. It is in late transcription that host gyrase can substitute for defective T4 topoisomerase (Lin and Mosig, 1987).

Thus far, only one primary T4 origin, oriA in Fig. 1, has been sequenced and analyzed in some detail (Fig. 13A). This origin maps within the coding region of gene 69 (Macdonald and Mosig, 1984b). Three in-frame overlapping proteins are made from this region. The largest is a membrane protein involved in DNA replication (Mosig and Macdonald, 1986; Mosig et al., 1987). A shorter peptide, gp69*, is initiated from an internal ribosome-binding site on a short transcript, initiated from an internal promoter. Gp69* shares the C-terminal portion with gp69. In addition, gene 56 (dCTPase) mutations overlap with gene 69 (Mosig et al., 1987). We recently found that the dCTPase and the predicted gp69 have the same amino terminal end (T. Gary et al., in preparation). Since the molecular mass of the dCTPase is only 19 kD, as compared with 46 kD of gp69, and since there is no internal stop codon in gene 69, we believe that the dCTPase is translated from a truncated transcript (see Fig. 13A) or, less likely, proteolytically processed from gp69. The significance of this overlap of two replication proteins with the dCTPase, which is a member of the precursor synthesizing complex (Mathews et al., 1983), will be further discussed below.

In gene 69 mutants, oriA is not used, and overall DNA replication is drastically reduced at low growth temperatures (Macdonald and Mosig, 1984b). Since it is now evident that all dCTPase (gene 56) mutations also alter the coding sequence of gene 69, it should not be surprising that the gene 56 mutants are deficient in using oriA and thus are deficient in DNA replication under certain conditions (for review, see Mathews and Allen, 1983). We hypothesize that these are conditions that require oriA function. All T4 strains produce T4 DNA containing cytosine, instead of the glucosylated hydroxymethylcytosine characteristic of wild-type T4 (Kutter and Snyder, 1983), have a dCTPase mutation and thus do not produce gp69. In these strains or in clones derived from them, oriA functions poorly if at all (Yee and Marsh, 1985; Kreuzer and Alberts, 1986).

The important signals and replicative intermediates found in oriA (Fig. 13A) (Macdonald, 1983; Mosig et al., 1987) are E. coli–like promot-

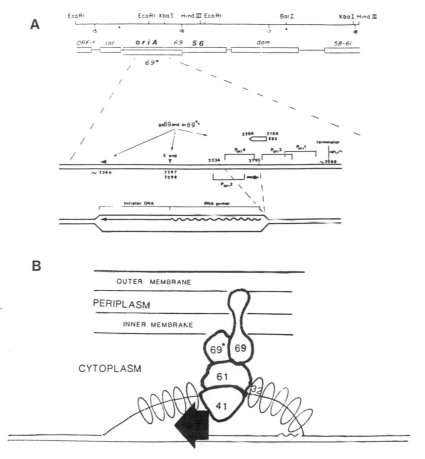

FIGURE 13. (A) Organization of the *oriA* region. The upper line is a restriction map of the entire region. Numbers below that line are distances in kb from the rIIA/B junction. The second line shows genes and open reading frames in that region. The third line shows an expanded map of the positions of *oriA* promoters, RNA start sites, RNA–DNA transition and the major DNA arrest site, the Shine–Dalgarno sequence (RBS), and the end of the putative pentapeptide coded there, numbered as in the DNA sequence in Macdonald and Mosig (1984b). (B) A scheme of the postulated anchoring of an initiation-replication complex to the membrane by gp69. The arrow represents the leading strand replisome, gps 61 and 41 are the T4 primase-helicase, and gp32 is the T4 single-stranded DNA-binding protein. From Mosig *et al.* (1987).

ers upstream of an RNA-DNA copolymer and a unique 5′ end of the nascent DNA. These findings support earlier evidence (Luder, 1981; Luder and Mosig, 1982) that leading-strand synthesis is primed by RNA, initiated by host RNA polymerase from early promoters. These promoters are expected to be neglected after the RNA polymerase has acquired the T4-encoded sigma factor gp55 (Elliott and Geiduschek, 1984) and other less well-characterized factors. There are four potential primer promoters for initiation in the counterclockwise direction in the *oriA* region: three weak overlapping promoters inside the coding region of gp69*, and a stronger promoter that initiates the 69* message. It is not known whether one of these is preferred as a primer promoter. The transition to DNA synthesis occurs at one of two adjacent nucleotides (Mosig *et al.*, 1987; P. Macdonald and G. Mosig, in preparation). In addition, we have shown that leading-strand synthesis can be prematurely terminated after approximately 70 nucleotides have been polymerized to yield a short "initiator DNA" (Macdonald *et al.*, 1983). Interestingly, there are potential priming sites for lagging-strand synthesis on the opposite DNA strand.

As discussed below, there is considerable evidence that the five proteins that constitute a T4 replisome interact with the primase-helicase complex, thereby coupling leading- and lagging-strand synthesis, and that the helicase activity of the primase complex helps to unwind the DNA ahead of the fork (Hinton *et al.*, 1987; Selick *et al.*, 1987). Possibly, the association of a replisome with the primase-helicase (gp61 and gp41) at these sites facilitates extension of the "initiator DNA." Interestingly, a gene *69* mutation arose spontaneously as a partial suppressor of a primase mutation (Macdonald and Mosig, 1984b). Extension of the initiator DNA may also be helped by attachment of the DNA associated with replisomes to the membrane via the large gp69 (Fig. 13B) (Mosig and Macdonald, 1986). This idea is speculative and requires testing and probably revisions, but it is consistent with earlier observations that replicating T4 DNA is associated with the cell envelope (Miller, 1972; Siegel and Schaechter, 1973) and that the *oriA* region of parental DNA strands is preferentially membrane-bound (Marsh *et al.*, 1971).

This idea also provides a rationale for the temporal regulation of the two proteins made from the *oriA* region, gp69 and gp69*. The smaller peptide, gp69*, can be translated from an immediate early transcript. It could engage other replication proteins in the formation of a prereplicative complex that assembles on free DNA (Miller and Kozinski, 1970), whereas the larger, gp69, which contains the hydrophobic domain, made later from a delayed early transcript, could anchor this complex to the cell envelope. There are several plausible advantages of origin associations with the membrane, e.g., energy supply to the replisome and to the precursor-synthesizing complex. Two laboratories have demonstrated the existence of a complex synthesizing DNA precursors (Chiu and Greenberg, 1968; Reddy *et al.*, 1977; for review, see Mathews and Allen, 1983), and there is considerable genetic and biochemical evidence that this complex associates with replication and priming proteins (Flanegan and Greenberg, 1977; Chiu and Greenberg, 1973; Drake, 1973; Chao *et al.*, 1977; Karam *et al.*, 1983; Macdonald and Hall, 1984). The dCTPase is part of this precursor-synthase complex. The overlap of the dCTPase gene *56* with the *oriA* region and with gene *69* may be significant for the regulation and correct assembly of this multicomponent macromolecular synthesis machine.

Another origin, *oriF*, is contained within the sequence encompassing T4 gene *uvsY* (Takahashi *et al.*, 1985; Gruidl and Mosig, 1986; Gruidl and Mosig, unpublished). This origin is active in primary initiation (Halpern *et al.*, 1979; Macdonald *et al.*, 1983; M. Gruidl, personal communication) as well as in "tertiary initiation" (Kreuzer and Alberts, 1986; Kreuzer and Menkens, 1987; and see below). That it is located within a hot spot of recombination (Womack, 1965; Rottlander *et al.*, 1967) suggests that there is also preferential recombination-directed, "secondary" initiation (discussed below) in this region.

As in origins of other replicons (Chapter 3, this volume), there is an unusually AT-rich region, and there are overlapping repeats near the *uvsY* promoter. The *uvsY* protein shows a patch of similarity (Gruidl and Mosig, 1986) with the replication initiation protein of plasmid R6K (Germino and Bastia, 1982). It remains to be shown whether, in the primary and tertiary modes, DNA chains are initiated at the same site in the *oriF* region, and whether all domains of this origin region are shared by several different initiation mechanisms or if some domains are specific for only one of them.

Compared with the recombinational hot spot between genes *34* and *35* (see below), the hot spot near *uvsY* results in less distortion of the overall T4 map (Mosig, 1966, 1968). The difference between the two hot spots might be explained if in the *uvsY* region short, single-stranded DNA segments, generated during origin initiation and displaced from the template, invade homologous DNA and generate specifically patch-type recombinants from the D loops.

C. Physiology of Tertiary Initiation

The "tertiary mode" is defined by its independence of the gene 46/47 recombination nuclease, by the lack of a homology requirement, and by stimulation when the host RNA polymerase is inhibited by rifampicin (Kreuzer and Alberts, 1986; Kreuzer and Menkens, 1987). *UvsY* is transcribed from a *motA*-dependent promoter (Gruidl and Mosig, 1986; Guild *et al.*, 1988), and Kreuzer and Menkens (1987) have shown, by extensive deletion analysis, that this *motA*-dependent promoter, but not the *uvsY* coding sequence, is required for "tertiary" initiation. The requirement for middle-mode, *motA*-dependent promoters appears to present a paradox, since all T4 transcription is inhibited by rifampicin. Possibly, gp*motA* activates tertiary initiation from *oriF* in the absence of RNA polymerase. Alternatively, short oligonucleotides, synthesized in the presence of rifampicin, could be important for this type of initiation, either as primers or to facilitate opening of the origin.

D. Genetics of Recombination-Dependent (Secondary) Initiation

In contrast to origin initiation, recombination-dependent (secondary) initiation uses DNA primers—i.e., the invading strand of a recombinational D loop (Fig. 6). It is thus independent of RNA polymerase (insensitive to rifampicin). It can also circumvent the requirement for primase in copying the strand that is, at first, displaced during synthesis of the leading strand. Gene 58/61 (primase) mutants can produce double-stranded DNA and package it, though with some delay (Epstein et al., 1964; Yegian et al., 1971; Mufti and Bernstein, 1974; Mosig et al., 1981b), even when the host primase gene is mutated. They require functional recombination genes to do this (Luder, 1981).

The secondary recombination-dependent initiation mode does not depend on specific sequences except for hot spots of recombination, and it is not regulated. This mode does not require origin-specific proteins such as gp69, but it requires the recombination genes 46/47 (recombination exonuclease), uvsX (RecA-like synapsis protein), uvsY (function unknown), and 59 (function unknown). In addition, gene 32 (single-stranded DNA binding protein) mutants can initiate from primary origins but are defective in the recombination-dependent mode (Mosig and Breschkin, 1975; Breschkin and Mosig, 1977a,b; Dannenberg and Mosig, 1981). Host functions appear not to substitute for defective T4 recombination functions in recombination-dependent replication, because they do not recognize the modified T4 DNA, because the host enzymes do not fit into T4's replication machines, or both. All recombination-deficient mutants initiate origin replication like wild-type T4, but arrest it when accessory proteins associate with RNA polymerase.

Even if all primary origin initiation is abolished, T4 can apparently initiate DNA replication from recombinational intermediates when all proteins of the replication elongation machine are functional. Tomizawa (1967) and Broker and Lehman (1971) have shown that recombination between parental infecting T4 chromosomes can occur in the absence of DNA replication. As expected, in this situation, replication starts much later and is less efficient than when origin initiation is functioning, and all T4 DNA sequences are replicated equally (M. Gruidl, personal communication).

Except for mutations in gene 32, which is the scaffolding protein of several different protein complexes that act on DNA, single mutants in T4 recombination genes are somewhat leaky; i.e., they produce some progeny and some recombinants, even though the mutational defect appears to inactivate the corresponding protein. It is therefore thought that T4 has alternative pathways of recombination that can substitute for each other to some extent. In support of several pathways, Cunningham and Berger (1977a,b) have constructed various multiple mutants that now appear almost totally defective in recombination. Extensive studies on recombination-dependent DNA repair in multiple mutants (Bernstein and Wallace, 1983; Wakem and Ebisuzaki, 1984a,b; Wakem et al., 1984; Wachsman and Drake, 1987) also support this view.

In addition to the recombination genes, which are needed to initiate formation of D loops, the T4 topoisomerase (genes 39, 52, and 60; Kreuzer and Huang, 1983; Huang, 1986a,b) is required for recombination-dependent replication but not for recombination itself. The topoisomerase mutants had originally been described as being somewhat defective in DNA replication ("DNA delay" phenotype; Epstein et al., 1964; Yegian et al., 1971). If any of the T4 topoisomerase genes are mutationally altered, the frequency of recombinants among the (reduced) viable progeny is higher than in wild-type T4, and the intracellular DNA appears broken and less complex than the highly branched concatemers seen in wild-type infections (Mufti and Bernstein, 1974; Naot and Shalitin, 1972; Yegian et al., 1971). Most likely, packaging selects for those molecules that have recombined the fragments into longer structures.

Obviously, hot spots of recombination are expected to be preferred initiation sites in this secondary mode, and the best-known recombinational hot spot between genes 34 and 35 (see Fig. 1) is indeed a preferred replication initiation site (Kozinski, 1983). As discussed above, this may also be true for the recombinational hot spot near uvsY.

According to Kozinski (1983), covalently linked recombinants appear only very late after infection. Dannenberg and Mosig (1983), however, have clearly demonstrated that initiation of recombination, and thus the primers required for secondary replication forks occur before all parental DNA has been replicated once. Under wild-type conditions, recombination-dependent initiation generates the vast majority of T4 replication forks. By the time sufficient T4 replication proteins have been synthesized, sufficient amounts of T4-encoded sigma factor (gp55) and other transcription factors have also accumulated to turn off transcription initiation from early promoters and turn on late promoters. This is the reason (Luder and Mosig, 1982) that all recombination-deficient T4 mutants arrest DNA replication prematurely (DNA arrest = DA phenotype) (Hosoda et al., 1971; Shah and Berger, 1971; Wu et al., 1972; Shah, 1976) and that this arrest is circumvented by additional gene 55 mutations or by inhibitors of protein synthesis (for review, see Mosig, 1983). It also explains why reinitiation bubbles from primary origins are rare (Delius et al., 1971; Dannenberg and Mosig, 1983; Yee and Marsh, 1985). Since primary origin initiation requires RNA polymerase, the flexibility of transcriptional controls, discussed above, implies that distortions of the transcriptional program (e.g., using inhibitors of protein or RNA synthesis or certain mutations) can also, directly and indirectly, alter the relative contributions of different origins and of primary-origin-directed versus recombination-directed versus tertiary modes of DNA replication. Thus, different experimental results should not necessarily be considered controversial.

Recombination-directed initiation of DNA replication provides the simplest explanation for the early observation that in T-even phages the number of recombinational pairings during one infectious cycle ("rounds of mating") equals the rounds of replication (Levinthal and Visconti, 1953; Visconti and Delbruck, 1953) and for other observations that had suggested a copy-choice mechanism of recombination (for review, see Hershey, 1958).

E. Biochemistry of Replication Proteins

The virtuoso biochemical characterization of replication proteins, singly and in combination (reviewed in Nossal and Alberts, 1983; Hinton *et al.*, 1987; Selick *et al.*, 1987), together with the genetic experiments discussed above, has led to understanding precise functions and interactions of proteins that constitute a T4 replication machine (Alberts, 1984). The functions of these proteins are discussed in detail in Chapter 3 of this volume, and will be reviewed only briefly here.

Seven proteins, corresponding to seven of the 30 genes that are known to be involved in *in vivo* DNA replication, form an active replication complex that moves with near *in vivo* speed and fidelity on appropriate templates. The T4 DNA polymerase (gp43), together with its accessory proteins gp44/62 and gp45, form the DNA polymerase holoenzyme. This holoenzyme interacts with and is helped by gp32, which covers all single-stranded DNA regions and may act as a scaffolding protein for the replisome. The five proteins together can replicate properly primed single-stranded templates. In double-stranded templates, the DNA ahead of the fork is unwound by the helicase activity of gp41, which has a dual role. In addition to its helicase activity, it interacts with gp58/61 to form an active primase complex on the lagging strand. The two holoenzyme complexes (on the leading strand and lagging strand, respectively) are thought to interact, thereby folding the template of the lagging strand (see Keppel *et al.*, this volume), so that the primase-helicase complex is properly positioned to unwind the helix ahead of the fork. When this seven-protein complex has copied the gap in the lagging strand, it releases the template and initiates the next Okazaki piece. Additional proteins are probably required to sweep other proteins from the template. For example, the *dda* helicase is required to release RNA polymerase from the DNA template in *in vitro* reactions and, by inference, *in vivo* (Jongeneel *et al.*, 1984). The gene *41* helicase cannot substitute for *dda* helicase in that capacity.

In contrast to *E. coli*, whose DNA polymerase holoenzyme can be isolated as a complex, the T4 holoenzyme seems to fall apart during purification. C. McHenry (personal communication) has suggested a plausible explanation for this difference. Since there are many replication complexes in T4-infected cells but only a few in uninfected *E. coli*, evolution has selected for weaker interactions between T4 replication proteins than for the corresponding *E. coli* proteins. This argument can be expanded. Since T4 DNA polymerase participates in DNA replication, recombination, and repair, and each of these processes requires T4 DNA polymerase interacting with different proteins (Alberts, 1984), strong interactions of the T4 DNA polymerase with proteins in one of these complexes might inhibit its participation in other complexes.

Initiation from primary T4 origins has not yet been accomplished *in vitro*, perhaps because we do not know all of the required proteins. By analogy with other systems (see Chapter 3, this volume), initiation of replication is thought to require many more proteins, e.g., for priming and prepriming DNA synthesis. One candidate is an ORF between genes *41* and *61* (Selick *et al.*, 1987). Since there are several primary origins and several replication modes in T4, and since at least some of the initiation proteins might be origin-specific (as discussed above, gene *69* is required at *oriA*), genetic inactivation of any one origin is unlikely to be lethal for T4.

Recent elegant experiments of Formosa and Alberts (1986) have succeeded in reconstituting recombination-dependent initiation *in vitro*. This reaction requires a double-stranded template and a homologous single-stranded fragment that, after invasion, provides the primer from which very long strands can be synthesized, if the template is circular. The reaction depends on UvsX protein to promote strand invasion, the five proteins (DNA holoenzyme and gp32) that can perform the partial reaction, discussed above, and *dda* helicase to unwind the template ahead of the fork (the gene *41* helicase cannot substitute).

Surprisingly, the reaction leads to conservative DNA replication. The priming polynucleotide and the nascent DNA strand are extruded from the template as a D-loop bubble migrates along the template. Formosa and Alberts (1986) suggest that this conservative DNA synthesis mimics the *in vivo* recombination-dependent replication, and they discuss how this reaction can explain T4 DNA repair (for review, see Bernstein and Wallace, 1983). This suggestion may be true, but at this time several caveats have to be kept in mind with respect to the details of the conservative bubble migration mechanism. First, there are major differences in the substrates: *in vitro*, single-stranded fragments are made to invade, whereas *in vivo*, these single-stranded segments lie at the tips of large double-stranded segments (Fig. 6). Second, the extrusion of the single strands may occur because some components are missing in the *in vitro* reaction; e.g., the products of genes *46*, *47*, and *59* are required *in vivo*. Both *in vivo* and in the cellophane disk system (Huang, 1979, 1983), T4 topoisomerase stimulates DNA replication, but it is not required in the reaction described by Formosa and Alberts (1986). Addition of purified gp39 to lysates made from gene *39* mutants stimulates DNA replication in the cellophane disk lysate system. This system does not initiate DNA replication from exogenously added T4 DNA, but it will sustain DNA replication when it is made from infected cells that had started T4 replication. One plausible interpretation of Huang's results is that recombination-dependent initiation is stimulated by T4 topoisomerase *in vitro*.

Neither electron micrographs nor S1 sensitivity of intracellular T4 DNA (Delius *et al.*, 1971; Dannenberg and Mosig, 1983; Hamlett and Berger, 1975; Luder, 1981) indicates that there are extensive single-stranded regions in late-replicating wild-type T4 DNA. Even in primase-deficient (gene *58/61*) mutants, the proportion of single-stranded regions detected by these methods declines later after infection, when recombination-dependent replication accelerates (Hamlett and Berger, 1975; Luder, 1981; Mosig *et al.*, 1981b).

Be that as it may, it is extremely promising for understanding details of the mechanism that the most prevalent mode of initiation of DNA synthesis in T4 can work *in vitro*. Since there are apparently several recombination pathways operating *in vivo*, one might expect different recombination-dependent modes of DNA synthesis *in vitro* as well.

VII. DNA PACKAGING

The final stage in DNA metabolism is packaging of the actively replicating and recombining molecules into a single double helix about 171 kb long by a competent packaging machine composed of a mature prohead and specialized packaging proteins. This topic is discussed in detail in Chapter 5 of this volume, and only an outline is presented here. Figure 14 shows the steps in the maturation of the T4 prohead. The mature prohead contains a procapsid made of gp23 assembled around the scaffolding proteins, and contains the initiator portal protein gp20. Packaging begins following removal of the scaffolding proteins and processing of all the structural proteins by proteolysis and expansion of the prohead. Packaging proteins (gp16, gp17, and a fragment of gp23) are transiently associated with the complex and introduce DNA into the head via the portal structure. These proteins, and gp49, trim the DNA free of any remaining branches and cut the molecule once the head has been filled, preparing it for oriented attachment to the tail. Since a number of defective DNA-related functions interrupt packaging, these must be required at specific stages, including DNA ligase (gp30), endonucleaseVII (gp49), endoV (*den*V), and T4 topoisomerase (Chapter 5, this volume).

VIII. VIRION STRUCTURE AND ASSEMBLY

It is now clear that in all phage assembly systems studied, obligatory pathways of morphogenesis are determined at the level of protein-protein interactions and not at the level of sequential transcription of the structural genes (Kellenberger, 1980). However, the complex regulation of T4 transcription and translation, discussed above, could help to adjust the final levels of structural gene products late in infection (Wiberg and Karam, 1983). These regulated levels in turn are important in controlling successful assembly of the phage structures. It is interesting that there are multiple transcription initiation sites for many genes encoding struc-

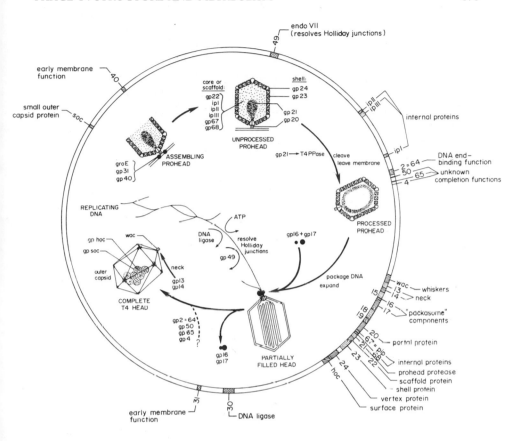

FIGURE 14. Assembly and maturation of the T4 prohead (modified from Black and Showe, 1983) and location of genes that control these processes. Interspersed tail genes are indicated on the inside of the circle.

tural proteins: the gene *23* region (Kassavetis and Geiduschek, 1982), the gene *18–19* region, the tail sheath and tube genes (Arisaka *et al.*, 1988), and the gene *16–17* region (Powell, Franklin, Arisaka, and Mosig, in preparation).

A. Head Structure and Assembly

The completed T4 head has an icosahedral surface lattice of $T = 13$, elongated along a fivefold axis (Moody, 1965; Aebi *et al.*, 1974; Branton and Klug, 1975). The length of the T4 head is defined by a number, Q, related to the icosahedral T-number. An illustration of Q-numbers is shown in Fig. 15, on models of the T4 head. The evidence for the structure of normal T4 is based on the ability to count capsomeres between fivefold vertices along the elongated head axis and, to some extent, on the length-to-width ratio. This was defined by Branton and Klug (1975) in their freeze-fracture studies as $l/w = 1.35$, based on those occasional, favorable cleavage planes which exposed the maximum length of the phage, and they concluded that Q = 17. However, this method could lead to an underestimate of l/w and thus of Q (see below). Studies of head length variants of T4 demonstrated that functional heads can be assembled that contain shorter and longer DNA (Eiserling *et al.*, 1970; Mosig, 1963, 1966, 1968; Mosig *et al.*, 1971, 1972; Cummings *et al.*, 1973; Doermann *et al.*, 1973a,b). The petite T4 variant containing 0.70 normal DNA length appears isometric (T = 13, Q = 13). Intermediate-length particles have also been described (Mosig *et al.*, 1971, 1972; Doermann *et al.*, 1973a,b). Under certain growth conditions using *ptg* mutants (Doermann *et al.*, 1973a,b), normal, intermediate, and petite phages are produced. Electron microscopy shows that there are different lengths, falling into three main classes, whereas all widths are similar. These data with three classes of head length fit to Q-numbers of 13 for petite phages, 17 for intermediates, and 21 for normal-length phages (illustrated in Fig. 6). Fractional genome lengths can be measured by biological methods (Mosig, 1963, 1968; Mosig *et al.*, 1971). Results of Mosig *et al.* (1972) gave DNA lengths of 0.67, 0.76, 0.90, and 1.00 and led to a slightly different model (Walker *et al.*, 1972). Measurements by Doermann *et al.* (1973a,b), using different growth conditions, gave values of 0.71, 0.86, and 1.03. The discrepancy remains to be resolved.

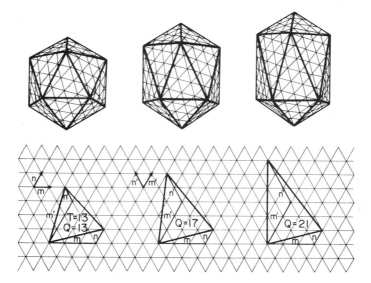

FIGURE 15. Surface lattice arrangements predicted for petite isometric, intermediate, and normal-length T4 heads (above). The definitions of the lattice parameters are shown below. For the isometric phage, the surface lattice is defined completely by the triangulation number (T), given as $T(m,n) = m^2 + mn + n^2$; in the drawing m = 3, n = 1, and T = 13. For an icosahedron elongated along a fivefold axis, another number, Q, is used to define the extent of elongation. The Q number can be any integer greater than T and is defined by the coordinates m' and n'. For the intermediate phage shown, m' = 3, n' = 2, and Q = 17. The normal-length head shown has m' = 3, n' = 3, and Q = 21.

The diameter of particles in solution measured using X-ray diffraction (Earnshaw et al., 1976, 1978) gives the width of T4 as 85 nm, measured on both giant and petite phages. The agreement of the solution-determined and electron microscope values of 85 nm is satisfying. For a curved structure such as the T4 head, the inner radius of the protein shell is compressed with respect to the outer radius. Assuming that the lattice constant at the inner radius is 12.5 nm, calculations by M. Wurtz and E. Kellenberger (personal communication) show that the lattice constant at the outer radius would be 14.7 nm, a value consistent with a diameter from the head of 85 nm. Also, measurements on electron micrographs of thin sections of T4 heads, where some shrinkage is expected, give outer-dimension values of 82 nm by 105 nm (Wunderli et al., 1977). Thus, the consensus value for normal T4 head size is 85 nm by 115 nm, and $T = 13$, $Q = 21$. The inner volume of the head is estimated at 4×10^{-16} ml, and the chromosome of approximately 171,000 bp is packaged at a density of 0.5 g/ml, neglecting water (Earnshaw et al., 1978). It should be kept in mind, however, that if there are different length distributions under different physiological growth conditions, the consensus length value might be different.

The surface lattice design was determined directly by freeze-fracture techniques on phage T2 (Branton and Klug, 1975), which lacks the T4 minor proteins Hoc and Soc. The presence of these additional proteins in T4 makes the detailed structural determination difficult, because the normal phage head appears very smooth. The discovery of "giant" phages, elongated to various degrees along the fivefold axis (Cummings et al., 1973; Doermann et al., 1973a,b), permitted detailed optical diffraction analysis of the electron micrographs because of the larger number of repeats, resulting in a higher signal-to-noise ratio.

The location of the proteins Soc and Hoc was determined by Ishii and Yanagida (1977) and by Aebi et al. (1977) using giant T4 phage (see Fig. 3). The Hoc protein lies at the center of a ring (capsomer) of cleaved gp23, and there are six copies of gpsoc around each six-membered capsomer of cleaved gp23. The location of a protein directly on a local sixfold axis of symmetry is interesting and unusual, implying some symmetric interaction with gp23. Although Soc and Hoc proteins may confer some additional capsid stability, osmotic shock resistance is controlled by the gp24 vertex protein (Leibo et al., 1979). It is still a mystery how the vertex protein controls the entry and exit of small molecules through the capsid. Gp24 was localized to the vertices of the head (Müller-Salamin et al., 1977) by using antibody directed against purified gp24. Differential extraction of T4 capsids (in 7M urea, pH 11) removes all the cleaved gp24 as seen by SDS gel electrophoresis, and gaps appear at the vertices, confirming this location. It has been postulated that the fivefold vertices are replaced by cleaved gp23 in certain gene 23 missense mutants that bypass the requirement for gp24 (McNicol et al., 1977). A direct test of this interesting and attractive idea has not yet been made.

The T4 prohead expands during maturation. Although the function of this expansion is unknown, it may "lock" the capsid into a stable structure. The early prohead lacks the minor proteins described above, and, like the phage lambda *D* protein, Hoc and Soc proteins are added later, after expansion of the capsid lattice from 11.2 nm (Aebi *et al.*, 1974) to 12.9 nm (Aebi *et al.*, 1976), followed by the cleavages of gp23 and gp24. Most of the T4 head proteins have now been localized in the head structure, but some protein components have not yet been correlated with genetic lesions. The products of three genes known to be involved with head morphogenesis (genes *4, 50,* and *65*) have not yet been identified as protein bands on gels, and the product of gene *2* is thought to bind to chromosomal ends during assembly.

The neck and portal vertex of T4 is a complex structure that includes gp13, gp*wac* (whiskers), gp14, gp20, and possibly two or three other proteins (Coombs and Eiserling, 1977). The upper knob of the neck is the site of the portal vertex, made of gp20, that binds to the neck and to the capsid (Driedonks and Caldentey, 1983). This structure, which has six- or 12-fold symmetry, consists of a disk of 12 copies of gp20. The role of the portal vertex structure in DNA packaging and ejection is discussed elsewhere in this volume by Black, and by Casjens and Hendrix in Volume 1. The six whiskers made up from 18 gp*wac* molecules are attached to the lower of the two knobs protruding from the connector structure. These whiskers promote long tail fiber attachment, extension, and retraction (Conley and Wood, 1975; Wood and Crowther, 1983), and serve as part of the environmental sensing system of the phage that maintains the long fibers in a retracted and protected configuration until needed.

B. Size Determination

T4 head length determination permits substantial variations. It is apparently regulated primarily by some kind of protein–protein interactive vernier mechanism (described below). However, head length is also affected by varying the relative intracellular concentrations of the head proteins. Models for regulation of the length of phage structures include the following:

1. *Ruler, template, or scaffold.* The length of the structure is determined by the length of another molecule or structure that forms by self-assembly. Examples are TMV and M13, where length is determined by a nucleic acid ruler. Tail length in phage lambda and T4 is probably determined by a protein ruler. The size of the lambda and P22 icosahedral head is determined by self-assembling protein scaffold (King *et al.*, 1978). It has been proposed that the length of the elongated T4 head could also be determined by a preassembled core or scaffold (Kellenberger, 1980).
2. *Vernier.* This model functions like a mechanical vernier used in measuring micrometers. An example is two linear structures made of protein subunits of differing size. During copolymeriza-

tion, the ends will only be in register after a certain number of subunits have been added, and polymerization would then stop. Such a model was proposed by Paulson and Laemmli (1977) as an explanation for the regulation of T4 head length, based on differing structural repeats between the scaffold or core protein and the coat protein.

3. *Cumulated strain.* As protein subunits assemble into a structure, they are progressively distorted as a result of their bonding interactions. Ultimately, this distortion results in a switch of the entire structure into a lower energy conformation where no further subunit addition is possible (Kellenberger, 1980; Caspar, 1980).

4. *Kinetic.* The relative rates of assembly of an elongating, multisubunit scaffold and a surrounding multisubunit shell determine the length of the final structure. The velocity of assembly depends on the relative concentrations of the two components. The outer shell is assumed to have an intrinsic curvature that will close off the growing structure at a point determined by the relative subunit concentrations (Showe and Onorato, 1978).

Figure 14 summarizes the assembly pathway and the structure of the T4 phage head and shows the relative map positions of the genes coding for morphopoietic components. Head length is determined at a very early stage, prior to the formation of the unprocessed prohead.

One of the early demonstrations that mutations in the head gene region could affect head length was the discovery that a mutant, E920g, produced large numbers of short-headed phages (Eiserling *et al.*, 1970). Subsequently, more mutations were isolated (Doermann *et al.*, 1973a,b), all of which, including E920g, map in gene *23*, the major head protein gene. Recently, Doermann and collaborators have characterized this region in more detail (Doermann *et al.*, 1987; Mooney *et al.*, 1987; Yasuda *et al.*, 1987; Doermann and Pao, 1987) and have established the following: (1) the complete nucleotide sequence of gene *23* (head protein), gene *24* (vertex protein), and the 814 bp intergenic region, (2) the nucleotide positions of nine *amber* mutants in gene *23* and three in gene *24*; (3) the nucleotide positions of 26 missense mutants in gene *23* that produce head-length variants (*petite* and *giant*, *ptg* mutants); (4) the positions of 7 *byp*ass 24 (*byp* 24) mutations that eliminate the need for the normally essential vertex protein gp24 (all these mutations are located in gene *23*); (5) the locations of a number of mutations that modify the cold sensitivity of *byp* 24 mutations, called *trb* mutants (temperature range of *byp*ass; these are also located in gene *23*); and (6) the existence of two regions of protein sequence homology between gp23 and gp24.

The story that emerges from these findings is as follows. Certain missense mutations in gene *23* result in specifically altered head lengths. By selecting for such mutants based on sedimentation properties, no new mutants other than those at existing sites could be isolated. The mutations are located at 12 sites clustered in three locations in gene *23*. The total span of the three clusters is 155 bp, which is less than 10% of the total gene 23 sequence. The idea proposed is that these tightly clustered mutations signal those segments of gp23 that interact with the other proteins that regulate head length. Based on studies of second-site suppressors, Doherty (1982a,b) showed that at least the mutant site *ptg* BU1980 in gp23 specifically interacts with *both* the gp22 core protein and the gp24 vertex protein.

The phenotypes of the *ptg* mutants are reproducible: a given mutant has a characteristic head length distribution. An important observation is that predominantly one class of intermediate head length is found between the isometric petite head and the normal-length T4 head. This implies that a specific length-determining mechanism operates, because in theory there could be numerous intermediate stop points between the icosahedral (T = 13, Q = 13) petite head and the (T = 13, Q = 21) normal-length head. The number Q represents the extent of elongation of the head along a fivefold icosahedral axis, and can be any integer. Each integer represents the addition of one more gp23 hexamer to the elongating head before the pentameric cap is closed (see Fig. 15). This in turn implies that there is an important length-determining role for gp23 and that it is not passively dependent on the prior assembly of a form-determining scaffold. Based on the bypass 24 mutations and the regions of protein homology between gp23 and gp24, it makes a stronger argument that the gene 23 head protein may itself form the vertex pentamers under certain conditions.

C. *In Vitro* Assembly

Studies conducted on the *in vitro* assembly and disassembly of gp23 have been done by Kellenberger's group in Basel (Caldentey and Kellenberger, 1986). Mutants of T4 defective in head assembly (genes *20, 22,* and *40*), when examined by electron microscopy, accumulate large numbers of tubular assemblies of uncleaved (M_r 56,000) gp23 called "polyheads." Mutants in genes *20* and *40* are defective in prohead initiation. Mutant-infected cells accumulate large quantities of unassembled gp23 until late in infection, when initiation of assembly of the tubular structures begins (Laemmli and Eiserling, 1968). These mutant-infected cells still make the internal scaffolding protein (gp22), and the polyheads are mostly the same diameter, although the cylindrical structure parameters (pitch angles) vary from tube to tube (Yanagida *et al.*, 1970). However, in gene *22* mutants that lack the scaffold (core) protein, multilayered cylinders form around those tubes that assemble spontaneously, giving rise to tubes of different diameters.

In vitro, the uncleaved gp23 shell protein (derived from dissociated polyheads) can be reversibly assembled into polyheads and dissociated, like numerous other entropy-driven assembly systems such as flagella, microtubules, and tobacco mosaic virus (Caldentey and Kellenberger,

1986): assembly is favored by high salt and temperatures and takes place rapidly above 1 mg/ml, pH 6.8–7.0, 20°C, about 0.2 M ionic strength. Dissociation is strongly favored at low ionic strength (0.01 M), high pH (up to 9.0), and low temperature (below 6°C). Protein that is denatured in urea as measured by a very different CD spectrum can be reassembled into a form with the native CD spectrum and polyhead structure, showing that the information needed to form tubes from single chains of gp23 is contained in the primary amino acid sequence of the protein.

Polyhead tubes are made of hexamers of gp23, with a diameter of 7.6 nm (Steven et al., 1976). Above pH 8, at low ionic strength in the cold, sedimentation analysis shows only monomers. As the pH is lowered, mixtures of monomers, dimers, and higher oligomers up to hexamers are formed, making it likely that the hexamer is a true intermediate in polyhead formation (Caldentey and Kellenberger, 1986). Thus, much of the head assembly information is contained in the coat protein subunit. The mutants with known amino acid changes leading to altered head length (ptg mutants) will permit future tests of whether the width or other assembly properties of the tubular polyheads formed in vitro from these proteins are also changed. If so, it would suggest that a great deal of shape information is in this subunit and that further studies on gp23 mutants with different amino acid substitutions could produce recognizably different types of polyhead structures in vitro.

D. Tail Structure and Assembly

Phage tails are attached to the specialized vertex used to initiate capsid assembly and are designed to bind to cell surfaces and initiate nucleic acid transfer to the host cell (Fig. 16). Phages with contractile sheaths, such as T4, have the most complex arrangement of viral proteins yet studied in detail. Each tail has an intricate baseplate and tail fibers composed of many parts that change conformation during infection, resulting in sheath contraction and DNA injection. Detailed studies of the T4 sheath (Moody, 1973; Krimm and Anderson, 1967; Amos and Klug, 1975; Smith et al., 1976; Lepault and Leonard, 1985) and the baseplate (Crowther et al., 1977; Berget and King, 1983) have given the most complete structure analysis for any bacteriophage. Because of the large number of repeating units in the extended sheath and the fact that they are arranged with helical symmetry, a single electron micrograph presents many different views of the same subunit, which has permitted a three-dimensional analysis of its structure. The T4 tail sheath is composed of a single protein, gp18 (King and Mykolajewycz, 1973; Dickson, 1974). Hexose amine is present as about 3% by weight or 10 residues per subunit (Tschopp et al., 1979). The DNA sequence of gene 18 has been correlated with the amino acid analysis (Arisaka et al., 1987) to give a fairly complete picture of gp18.

The 144 copies of gp18 are arranged in 24 rings of six subunits each.

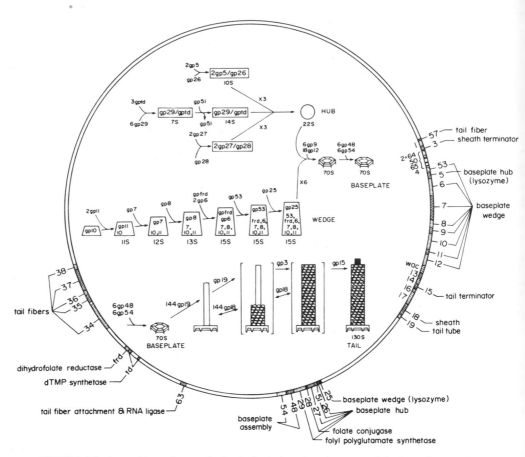

FIGURE 16. Assembly pathways for both the hub and wedge parts of the baseplate, and the steps in tail assembly, showing the positions of genes for tail and tail fiber synthesis and assembly. Head genes interspersed among tail genes are shown inside the circle.

The rings are spaced 4.1 nm apart, and the sheath is 22 nm across in the extended configuration. The distal row of subunits is in contact with the baseplate proteins, and the row of gp18 nearest the head binds to the terminator made of gp15 and possibly gp3. All subunits are in close contact with those of the central tube, made of gp19. The subunits in each ring are rotated by about 17° to the right with respect to those below, giving rise to the helical lines visible in electron micrographs. The stacked-disk structure is reoriented in the original viewing direction every 7 stacks of disks, giving 42 subunits in each repeat. This represents 21 distinct views of the subunit in a single electron micrograph, since half the views are the same. The main features of the structure are six helical "tunnels" and two sets of grooves on the surface. The deepest grooves give rise to the prominent right-handed helix seen on the surface (Fig. 3). The gp18 subunit has protruding knobs at the tips, which are likely to fit into corresponding holes in the baseplate at the terminal annulus. Amos and Klug (1975) portray each gp18 in the extended sheath as sloping downward from inner to outer radius, and this is also visible in the reconstructions of frozen-hydrated tails (Lepault and Leonard, 1985; see Fig. 5 of Casjens and Hendrix, Vol. 1), although it should be noted that there is less downward slope in the model presented by Smith *et al.* (1976).

Sheath contraction was described earlier, and shown by Moody (1973) to be a displacive transition in which the axial repeat decreases from 4.1 nm to 1.5 nm and the twist angle changes from 17° to 32°. From detailed structural studies of polysheath (Kellenberger and Boy de la Tour, 1964) and three-dimensional reconstructions (Amos and Klug, 1975), the dramatic change in the shape of the sheath upon contraction was shown to be related to relatively small changes in the overall conformation of gp18. The gp18 conformational change occurs before sheath contraction itself is completed.

E. The Baseplate and Tube: Structure and Assembly

T4 baseplates consist of a central hub, six outer wedges, and six tail spikes (King, 1980; Berget and King, 1983). Using rotational filtering to improve the signal-to-noise ratio of electron micrographs of isolated baseplates, Crowther *et al.* (1977) determined the architecture of the hexagonal and star-shaped baseplates to about 3.0 nm resolution. For an illustration, see Fig. 12 of the chapter by Casjens and Hendrix, Volume 1 of this title. Having described the complete structures, they examined mutants lacking various protein components to locate them in the structure. Three of the proteins studied, gp9, gp11, and gp12, account for a considerable fraction (40%) of the total mass of the baseplate, and they can all be added after the hexagonal structure is completed. This permitted relatively unambiguous determination of their locations. Since gp9 is needed for tail fiber attachment and is located near the site where tail fibers join to the baseplate, and since antiserum directed at gp9 determinants blocks fiber attachment, it is concluded that the gp9 structure is the site of tail fiber binding.

The gene *11* product has been shown to be the distal portion of the tail pin. If gp11 is missing, gp12 cannot bind; thus gp11 must supply the gp12 binding site. Kells and Haselkorn (1974) showed that gp12 forms the six 35-nm short fibers. In some wild-type phage and in isolated tails, these 35-nm fibers are not always visibly extended from the baseplate, suggesting that they occupy a stored or folded position.

The earliest step in baseplate wedge assembly is the binding of gp10 to gp11, but if gp11 is missing, then gp10 binds to gp7 and gp8. Thus, gp11 can add late in assembly and could be a more recently developed T4 protein. In this regard, it is interesting that gp11 has been found to be immunologically related to gp10 (Berget and King, 1983) and may have evolved from it by gene duplication. Confirmation of this notion awaits the DNA sequence analysis.

The baseplate contains structural proteins that are known to have enzymatic activities (reviewed by Kozloff, 1983). These include dihydrofolate reductase, thymidylate synthetase, gp28 (γ-glutamyl hydrolase), gp29 (folyl polyglutamate synthase), gp5 and gp25 (lysozymelike cell wall breakdown enzymes), and possibly gp12 (unknown catalysis related to zinc metalloproteins). Of these, the role of gp5 (Kao and McClain, 1980a,b) and gp25 (Szewczyk et al., 1986) seems to be clear, in that infection would be aided by baseplate murolytic enzymes (Nakagawa et al., 1985). The function of the other enzyme components in the infectious cycle is obscure.

Contractile sheaths of phage tails, as pointed out by Bradley (1967), have remarkably constant structural design: an inner tubular part assembled from identical subunits of a roughly 20-kD protein, arranged in 4.0-nm stacked disks, surrounded by a sheath with the same periodicity, made of an assembly of a larger, roughly 60-kD protein. Such structures are thought to represent an evolutionary increase in complexity over the phages such as lambda, where conformational changes in a simpler basal structure are sufficient to permit DNA to be transferred from the phage head to the bacterial cell through a tube made of a single protein species. T4 presumably gains both increased adsorption and injection efficiency and ability to adapt to varying cell surface environments by such increased complexity.

Tail tube structure has been studied in detail by Moody and Makowski (1981). Using low-angle X-ray diffraction on oriented gels of T2 polytubes, they found the annular repeat of the stacked disks of gp19 to be 4.06 nm. The tube has an average diameter of 9.0 nm and an inner hole of 3.5 nm. The symmetry of the tube matches that of the sheath in that the tube is polar and the annuli have C6 symmetry. Mass determination by scanning transmission electron microscopy has shown that the central hole in the T4 tube baseplate is occupied by mass that is absent in tube baseplate partially emptied by treatment with guanidine HCl (Duda et al., 1985). This is probably due to the "tape measure" protein that determines tail length. In phage lambda, the tape measure is the gene H protein, but its location is unknown within the tail structure (Casjens and Hendrix, Vol. 1, this book). Three T4 proteins (TAPs; tube-associated proteins) are found after guanidine HCl treatment, the products of genes 48, 54, and 29. Of these, only gp29 is long enough to form a "ruler" protein in an alpha-helical conformation similar to that proposed for lambda gpH (Katsura and Hendrix, 1984). It seems much to ask of gp29 that it (1) initiate baseplate hub assembly, (2) perform its enzymatic function as a folyl polyglutamate synthase, (3) position itself such that, after gp48 and gp54 have acted, it is in the center of a ring of gp19 tube protein subunits, and (4) elongate along with gp19 to limit tail length during tube assembly. Although, as Michael Faraday said, "Nothing is too wonderful to be true," alternative candidates for the tape measure are an extended form of TAP gp48 (Pryciak et al., 1986) or some combination of multimers of gp48 and gp54 or gp29.

F. Tail Fiber Structure and Assembly

The six long tail fibers of T4 are oriented for assembly onto the baseplate via the whiskers (see Fig. 9, Casjens and Hendrix, 1988) although some other structure must serve this function in T2, which lacks whiskers. Fibers about 3.0–4.0 nm thick and 150 nm long are made by the joining of two half-fibers (King, 1980). The half-fiber bound to the baseplate is constructed from two molecules of gp34 that have a terminal thickening near the attachment site. The half-fiber that binds to the cell surface is more complex and is made of one gp35 and two copies each of gp36 and gp37. The thin tip of gp37 contacts the cell surface. The two gp37 molecules are oriented in the same direction, colinear with the fibers and with the C terminus near the distal tip (Beckendorf, 1973).

In phage T2, gp37 is proteolytically processed to remove about 120 residues (Drexler et al., 1986). This cleavage is probably at the C terminus, since phages T2 and T4 share an identical 50–amino acid sequence at the N terminus (Riede et al., 1986). It is noteworthy that T4 gene 37 is inactivated by a terminal cleavage in gene 36–defective extracts (reviewed in Wood and Crowther, 1983).

From combined X-ray diffraction and electron microscopic studies, it has been proposed that the distal half-fiber is composed of a set of globular domains at specific regions along the half-fiber and that much of the polypeptide chains are in a cross-beta conformation with face-to-face packing of both gp36 and gp37 (Earnshaw et al., 1979; Oliver and Crowther, 1981). The globular domains are indicated as bumps on the fibers in Fig. 17 and in the review by Wood and Crowther (1983).

Fiber assembly requires the function of gp38, and it is thought to act catalytically in phage T4 by action upon the C-terminal end of gp37 (reviewed in Wood and Crowther, 1983). Recent work has shown that gp38 also participates with gp37 in host range determination in phage T2 and several T-even-like phages (Riede et al., 1985). These workers suggest that gp38 forms a structural component of the tail fiber during assembly of these phages. This has now been directly demonstrated by immunoelectron microscopy (Riede et al., 1986) that shows gp38 localized at the distal tip of the fiber. The protein is involved in receptor recognition and thus functions as an adhesin, or cell-surface-binding protein similar to those found in the pili of bacterial pathogens.

Throughout the assembly process, host cell functions are required for proper construction of many parts of the virus. Tail fiber assembly depends on the proper interaction of gp57 with some component of the host cell, possibly a membrane structure, since gene 57 mutant infections accumulate half-fibers bound to the cell envelope fractions, and host mutants of E. coli have been isolated that do not require gene 57 function (Revel et al., 1976). Other steps in tail assembly and especially head assembly require host functions (groE). These are discussed in detail by Casjens and Hendrix (1988).

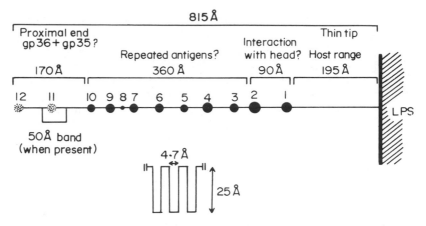

FIGURE 17. Model for the organization of protein domains in the distal half of the T4 tail fiber, modified from Wood and Crowther (1983). The bottom portion shows the orientation of the polypeptide chain in the proposed cross-beta configuration.

IX. OUTLOOK

As suggested in the beginning, many complexities and redundancies of T4 can perhaps best be understood in terms of its evolutionary history. We have mentioned some relevant aspects throughout this chapter. Two considerations stand out: (1) The concept of protein machines, first developed to describe the exquisite structures formed during virion assembly, and their conformational changes during the process of infection has been extended to the smaller, more fragile macromolecular assemblies that drive, among others, DNA replication, DNA precursor biosynthesis, recombination, repair, packaging, and transcription. (2) The processes that are driven by these protein machines are tightly interrelated by physiological connections as well as by sharing of certain proteins. Thus, neither functioning nor evolution of mechanisms and processes can be understood in isolation.

DNA sequences and deduced protein sequences, advancing rapidly through the joint efforts of the T4 community, can now be correlated with these findings to evaluate possible general principles. Three aspects learned from such studies are as follows: (1) As might have been expected, T4 proteins share certain similarities with proteins of similar function in other systems. In most cases, the similarities are patchy, and they are not apparent at the DNA level. (2) Some T4 proteins, seemingly unrelated, share patches of homology, even at the DNA level. (3) It is becoming increasingly apparent that many T4 genes produce more than one in-frame protein, probably because multiple forms are important in the proper assembly and function of the corresponding protein machines.

Some examples of patchy protein similarities that suggest evolutionary relationships are summarized below:

1. The gene 23 head protein shares a region of homology near the middle of its sequence with that of gene 24 (Yasuda et al., 1987) and may substitute for it in gene 23 mutations that bypass the gene 24 requirement.

2. Sequence relationship between the region coding for the thin tip of the tail fiber gene 37 and the gin region of bacteriophage Mu; also gp38 of phage K3 is homologous to E. coli cell surface OmpA protein (Riede et al., 1987b). There is also a remarkable amino acid sequence similarity between the gp37 tip and the phage lambda tail operon sequence ORF 314 and for gene 38 and lambda ORF 194. These presumably reflect related functions in viral cell recognition proteins (George et al., 1983; Michel et al., 1986).

3. A protein (gp69), encoded by the oriA region and required for initiation at oriA, with the E. coli DnaA initiation protein (Mosig and Macdonald, 1986).

4. A protein encoded by the oriF region (gpuvsY), with an initiator protein of plasmid R6K (Gruidl and Mosig, 1986), suggesting that different origins of T4 might have been derived from different replicons.

5. The T4 Dam methylase, with the isomodifying enzymes E. coli Dam methylase and DpnII methylase of Diplococcus pneumoniae (Hattman et al., 1985).

6. Two T4 DNA topoisomerase subunits, gp39 and gp52, with other topoisomerases of both prokaryotic and eukaryotic origin (Huang, 1986a,b).

7. The T4 endonuclease VII (gp49), which cleaves recombinational intermediates with the equivalent endonucleaseI of phage T7. Another segment of this protein resembles the T4 thioredoxin (Barth et al., 1988).

8. The T4 DNA ligase (gp 30) with the T7 DNA ligase (Armstrong et al., 1983).

9. The T4 UvsX protein, with the equivalent RecA protein of E. coli (Fujisawa et al., 1985).

10. The sigma factor for late T4 transcription, gp55, with other sigma factors (Gram and Rüger, 1985; Gribskov and Burgess, 1986).

11. The ribonucleotide reductase of T4 with E. coli ribonucleotide reductase (Sjöberg et al., 1986).

12. A protein encoded downstream of gene 49, with phage lambda's RexA protein, which restricts growth of T4 rII mutants (Barth et al., 1987), and with T7 gp5.5, which is required for growth on lambda lysogens.

13. Gp17, part of the ATP-dependent DNA packaging complex (Chapter 5, this volume), has two regions of homology with ATP-binding packaging proteins of other phages (Powell et al., in preparation).

14. The T4 lysozyme (gpe) with lysozymes of phages P22 and φ29 (Weaver et al., 1985; Garvey et al., 1986).

Interestingly, most similarities (except for those within T4) are not seen at the DNA level, perhaps because silent codon changes are rapidly selected that correspond to T4 tRNA anticodons and that change the base composition such that it resembles the high AT content of T4 DNA. A comparison of the T4 and E. coli Dam methylases (Hattman et al., 1986) illustrates this view. CUG is the most frequently used E. coli leucine codon, and 13 of the 26 leucine codons are CUG. In contrast, none of the 29 T4 leucine codons is CUG, in keeping with the fact that E. coli leucyl tRNA is rapidly cleaved after T4 infection. The total number of lysine + arginine codons is almost identical in the two proteins, but E. coli uses 18 lysine and 19 arginine residues, whereas T4 uses 31 lysine (A-rich) and 7 arginine (GC-rich) codons. Examples for other codons are also consistent with the idea that AT-rich codons are selected in T4.

It appears that partial duplications and gene fusions might contribute to the evolutionary adaptation of genes that might have originally been derived from other systems. Interestingly, in several such genes (69, 49, and 17 are known), two or more in-frame overlapping peptides are encoded by the same DNA sequence, but some are translated from different transcripts, initiated from different promoters. Perhaps such overlapping proteins are particularly well suited for proper assembly of protein complexes (Casjens and Hendrix, 1988; Chapter 3, this volume; Smith and Parkinson, 1980). For example, gene 49 (endonuclease VII) codes for two such peptides that share the C-terminal segment. The N-terminal segment of the longer peptide is homologous, even at the DNA level, with the T4 thioredoxin. By analogy with assembly of single-stranded filamentous phages (Chapter 6, this volume) or with the T7 DNA polymerase (Chapter 3, this volume), this "thioredoxin domain" might be used in assembly of a macromolecular machine (Barth et al., 1988). Gene 17, mentioned above, also codes for two proteins. The unique domain of the longer protein has homology (also at the DNA level) to the DNA binding domain of gene 32 (Powell et al., in preparation), consistent with genetic results indicating that these two proteins interact or compete (Mosig et al., 1981a).

Gene 69, required for initiation at oriA and spanning this origin, codes for three overlapping proteins, gp69, gp69* (Macdonald and Mosig, 1984b; Mosig and Macdonald, 1986), and T4 dCTPase, encoded by the N-terminal portion (Gary, Lukas, Trupin, and Mosig, in preparation). Perhaps this overlap facilitates the interaction of the replication complex with the precursor synthesizing complex (Keppel et al., this volume).

We have discussed elsewhere (Mosig, 1987) how the original strategy of T4 DNA replication together with the strategy of the transcriptional program provides a most powerful selection for efficient recombination. Recombination between partially homologous sequences, in turn, might generate gene fusions and different proteins. Many homologies, unexpected at first, of T4 sequences with sequences of its host, other phages or plasmids (George *et al.*, 1983; Riede *et al.*, 1985, 1986; Gruidl and Mosig, 1986; Huang, 1986a,b; Michel *et al.*, 1986; Mosig and Macdonald, 1986; Prasad and Chiu, 1987; Barth *et al.*, 1988; Powell *et al.*, in preparation), and, in the case of introns, with fungi (Michel and Dujon, 1986; Pederson-Lane and Belfort, 1987), could provide the substrate for "mix-and-match" evolution. The sharing of protein segments among replication, transcription, and packaging components, and recombination between the corresponding DNA, might facilitate the rapid coevolution of these components and their integration into the complex T4 system.

ACKNOWLEDGMENTS. We thank Nancy Canan and Cindy Young for their help and patience in editing and processing this review, and the members of our laboratories for many stimulating discussions and comments. G.M. thanks Ruth Ehring, Helen Revel, Betty Kutter, and Lavonne Batalden for critical readings of her contribution; Mark Frazier for drawing Fig. 5; and NIH (GM13221) for financial support. F.E. is grateful to M. Carmen Rayner for drawing Figs. 2, 14, 15, and 16 and to NIH for support (AI14092).

REFERENCES

Adari, H. Y., and Spicer, E. K., 1986, Translational repression *in vitro* by the bacteriophage T4 RegA protein, *Proteins Struct. Function Genet.* **1**:116.

Adari, H. Y., Rose, K., Williams, K. R., Konigsberg, W. H., Lin, T. C., and Spicer, E. K., 1985, Cloning, nucleotide sequence, and overexpression of the bacteriophage T4 *regA* gene, *Proc. Natl. Acad. Sci. USA* **82**:1901.

Aebi, U., Bijlenga, R., Van der Broek, J., Van der Broek, R., Eiserling, F., Kellenberger, C., Kellenberger, E., Mesyanzihinov, V., Muller, L., Showe, M., Smith, R., and Steven, A., 1974, The transformation of tau-particles into T4 heads. II. Transformations of the surface lattice and related observations on form determination, *J. Supramol. Struct.* **2**:253.

Aebi, U., Bijlenga, R., ten Heggeler, B., Kistler, J., Steven, A. C., and Smith, P. R., 1976, Comparison of the structural and chemical composition of giant T-even phage heads, *J. Supramol. Struct.* **5**:475.

Aebi, U. R., Van Driel, R., Bijlenga, R. K. L., ten Heggeler, B., Van der Broek, R., Steven, A., and Smith, P. R., 1977, Capsid fine structure of T-even bacteriophages. Binding and localization of two dispensable capsid proteins into P23 surface lattice, *J. Mol. Biol.* **110**:687.

Alberts, B. M., 1984, The DNA enzymology of protein machines, *Cold Spring Harbor Symp. Quant. Biol.* **49**:1.

Alberts, B. M., and Frey, L., 1970, T4 bacteriophage gene *32:* A structural protein in the replication and recombination of DNA, *Nature* **227**:1313.

Albright, L. M., Kassavetis, G. A., and Geiduschek, E. P., 1988, Bacteriophage T4 late transcription from plasmid templates is enhanced by negative supercoiling, *J. Bacteriol.* **170**:1279.

Amos, L. A., and Klug, A., 1975, Three dimensional image reconstructions of the contractile tail of the T4 bacteriophage, *J. Mol. Biol.* **99**:51.

Arisaka, F., Ishimoto, L., Kassavetis, G., Kumazaki, T., Ishii, S., and Eiserling, F. A., 1988, The nucleotide sequence of the tail tube structural gene of bacteriophage T4, *J. Virol.* **62**:882.

Armstrong, J., Brown, R. S., and Tsugita, A., 1983, Primary structure and genetic organization of phage T4 DNA ligase, *Nucleic Acids Res.* **11:**7145.

Arscott, P. G., and Goldberg, E. B., 1976, Cooperative action of the T4 tail fibers and baseplate in triggering conformational changes and in determining host range, *Virology* **69:**15.

Barth, K. A., Mosig, G., Trupin, M., and Powell, D., 1986, Phage T4 gene *49* (endonuclease VII) is transcribed early and late, Cold Spring Harbor Meeting on Molecular Genetics of Bacteria and Phage, p. 24.

Barth, K. A., Powell, D., Trupin, M., and Mosig, G., 1988, Regulation of two nested proteins from gene *49* (recombination endonuclease VII) and of λ Rex A-like protein of bacteriophage T4, *Genetics* (submitted).

Bayer, M. E., 1968, Adsorption of bacteriophage to adhesions between cell wall and membrane of *Escherichia coli, J. Virol.* **2:**346.

Beckendorf, S. K., 1973, Structure of the distal half of the bacteriophage T4 tail fiber, *J. Mol. Biol.* **73:**37.

Belfort, M., Pedersen-Lane, J., West, D., Ehrenman, K., Maley, G., Chu, F., and Maley, F., 1985, Processing of the intron-containing thymidylate synthase (*td*) gene of phage T4 is at the RNA level, *Cell* **41:**375.

Belfort, M., Pedersen-Lane, J., Ehrenman, K., Chu, F. K., Maley, G. F., Maley, F., McPheeters, D. S., and Gold, L., 1986, RNA splicing and *in vivo* expression of the intron-containing *td* gene of bacteriophage T4, *Gene* **41:**93.

Belin, D., Mudd, E. A., Prentki, P., Yu, Y.-Y., and Krisch, H. M., 1987, Sense and antisense transcription of bacteriophage T4 gene *32*. Processing and stability of the mRNAs, *J. Mol. Biol.* **194:**231.

Benzer, S., 1957, The elementary units of heredity, in: *The Chemical Basis of Heredity* (B. Glass, ed.), pp. 70–93, John Hopkins University Press, Baltimore.

Benzer, S., and Champe, S. P., 1962, A change from nonsense to sense in the genetic code, *Proc. Natl. Acad. Sci. USA* **48:**1114.

Berget, P. B., and King, J., 1983, T4 tail morphogenesis, in: *Bacteriophage T4* (C. Mathews, E. Kutter, G. Mosig, and P. Berget, eds.), pp. 246–258, American Society for Microbiology, Washington.

Bernstein, C., and Wallace, S. S., 1983, DNA repair, in: *Bacteriophage T4* (C. K. Mathews, E. M. Kutter, G. Mosig, and P. B. Berget, eds.), pp. 138–151, American Society for Microbiology, Washington.

Bijlenga, R. K. L., Ishii, T., and Tsugita, A., 1978, Complete primary structure of the small outer capsid (soc) protein of bacteriophage T4, *J. Mol. Biol.* **120:**249.

Black, L. W., and Showe, M. K., 1983, Morphogenesis of the T4 head, in: *Bacteriophage T4* (C. K. Mathews, E. M. Kutter, G. Mosig, and P. B. Berget, eds.), pp. 219–245, American Society for Microbiology, Washington.

Bradley, D. E., 1967, Ultrastructure of bacteriophages and bacteriocins, *Bacteriol. Rev.* **31:**230.

Branton, D., and Klug, A., 1975, Capsid geometry of bacteriophage T2: Freeze-etching study, *J. Mol. Biol.* **92:**559.

Brenner, S., Barnett, L., Crick, F. H. C., and Orgel, A., 1961, The theory of mutagenesis, *J. Mol. Biol.* **3:**121.

Breschkin, A. M., and Mosig, G., 1977a, Multiple interactions of a DNA-binding protein *in vivo*. I. Gene *32* mutations of phage T4 inactivate different steps in DNA replication and recombination, *J. Mol. Biol.* **112:**279.

Breschkin, A. M., and Mosig, G., 1977b, Multiple interactions of a DNA-binding protein *in vivo*. II. Effects of host mutations on DNA replication of phage T4 gene *32* mutants, *J. Mol. Biol.* **112:**295.

Brody, E., Rabussay, D., and Hall, D. H., 1983, Regulation of transcription of prereplicative genes, in: *Bacteriophage T4* (C. K. Mathews, E. M. Kutter, G. Mosig, and P. B. Berget, eds.), pp. 174–183, American Society for Microbiology, Washington.

Broida, J., and Abelson, J., 1985, Sequence organization and control of transcription in the bacteriophage T4 tRNA region, *J. Mol. Biol.* **185:**545.

Broker, T. R., 1973, An electron microscopic analysis of pathways for bacteriophage T4 DNA recombination, *J. Mol. Biol.* **81:**1.

Broker, T. R., and Doermann, A. H., 1975, Molecular and genetic recombination of bacteriophage T4, *Annu. Rev. Genet.* **9:**213.

Broker, T. R., and Lehman, I. R., 1971, Branched DNA molecules: Intermediates in T4 recombination, *J. Mol. Biol.* **60:**131.

Burke, R. L., Munn, M., Barry, J., and Alberts, B. M., 1985, Purification and properties of the bacteriophage T4 gene *61* RNA priming protein, *J. Biol. Chem.* **260:**1711.

Cairns, J., Stent, G. S., and Watson, J. D., eds., 1966, *Phage and the Origins of Molecular Biology*, Cold Spring Harbor Laboratory, Cold Spring Harbor, NY.

Caldentey, J., and Kellenberger, E., 1986, Assembly and disassembly of bacteriophage T4 polyheads, *J. Mol. Biol.* **188:**39.

Campbell, A., 1984, Types of recombination: Common problems and common strategies, *Cold Spring Harbor Symp. Quant. Biol.* **49:**839.

Campbell, A., 1988, Phage evolution and speciation, in: *The Bacteriophages*, Vol. 1 (R. Calender, ed.), pp. 1–14, Plenum Press, New York.

Carlson, K., and Øvervatn, A., 1986, Bacteriophage T4 endonucleases II and IV, oppositely affected by dCMP hydroxymethylase activity, have different roles in the degradation and in the RNA polymerase dependent replication of T4 cytosine-containing DNA, *Genetics* **114:**669.

Carlson, K., and Wiberg, J. S., 1983, In vivo cleavage of cytosine-containing bacteriophage T4 DNA to genetically distinct, discretely sized fragments, *J. Virol.* **48:**18.

Casjens, S., and Hendrix, R., 1988, Control mechanisms in dsDNA bacteriophage assembly, in: *The Bacteriophages*, Vol. 1 (R. Calender, ed.), pp. 15–92, Plenum Press, New York.

Caspar, D. L. D., 1980, Movement and self-control in protein assemblies. Quasi-equivalence revisited, *Biophys. J.* **32:**103.

Cech, T. R., and Bass, B. L., 1986, Biological catalysis by RNA, *Annu. Rev. Biochem.* **55:**599.

Chace, K. V., and Hall, D. H., 1975, Characterization of new regulatory mutants of bacteriophage T4. II. New class of mutants, *J. Virol.* **15:**929.

Champness, W. C., and Snyder, L., 1984, Bacteriophage T4 *goL* site: Sequence analysis and effects of the site on plasmid transformation, *J. Virol.* **50:**555.

Chapman, D., Morad, I., Kaufmann, G., Gait, M. J., Jorissen, L., and Snyder, L., 1988, Nucleotide and deduced amino acid sequence of *stp:* The bacteriophage T4 anticodon nuclease gene, *J. Mol. Biol.* **199:**373.

Chao, J., Leach, M., and Karam, J., 1977, In vivo functional interaction between DNA polymerase and dCMP-hydroxymethylase of bacteriophage T4, *J. Virol.* **24:**557.

Childs, J. D., and Pilon, R., 1983, Evidence that bacteriophage T4 *ephl* is a missense *hoc* mutation, *J. Virol.* **46:**629.

Chiu, C.-S., and Greenberg, G. R., 1968, Evidence for a possible direct role of dCMP hydroxymethylase in T4 phage DNA synthesis, *Cold Spring Harbor Symp. Quant. Biol.* **33:**351.

Chiu, C.-S., and Greenberg, G. R., 1973, Mutagenic effects of temperature-sensitive mutants of gene *42* of bacteriophage T4. *J. Virol.* **12:**199.

Christensen, A. C., and Young, E. T., 1983, Characterization of T4 transcripts, in: *Bacteriophage T4* (C. K. Mathews, E. M. Kutter, G. Mosig, and P. B. Berget, eds.), pp. 184–188, American Society for Microbiology, Washington.

Chu, F. K., Maley, G. F., Maley, F., and Belfort, M., 1984, Intervening sequence in the thymidylate synthase gene of bacteriophage T4, *Proc. Natl. Acad. Sci. USA* **81:**3049.

Chu, F. K., Maley, G. F., West, D. K., Belfort, M., and Maley, F., 1986, Characterization of the intron in the phage T4 thymidylate synthase gene and evidence for its self-excision from the primary transcript, *Cell* **45:**157.

Chu, F. K., Maley, F., Martinez, J., and Maley, G. F., 1987, Interrupted thymidylate synthase gene of bacteriophages T2 and T6 and other potential self-splicing introns in the T-even bacteriophages, *J. Bacteriol.* **169:**4368.

Colowick, M. S., and Colowick, S. P., 1983, Membrane ATPase activation on infection of E. coli K (λ) cells with phage T4 rII mutants, *Trans. N.Y. Acad. Sci.* **41:**35.

Conkling, M. A., and Drake, J. W., 1984, Isolation and characterization of conditional alleles of bacteriophage T4 genes *uvsX* and *uvsY*, *Genetics* **107**:505.

Conley, M. P., and Wood, W. B., 1975, Bacteriophage T4 whiskers: A rudimentary environment-sensing device, *Proc. Natl. Acad. Sci. USA* **72**:3701.

Coombs, D., and Eiserling, F. A., 1977, Studies on the structure, protein composition, and assembly of the neck of bacteriophage T4, *J. Mol. Biol.* **116**:375.

Crick, F. H. C., Barnett, L., Brenner, S., and Watts-Tobin, R. J., 1961, General nature of the genetic code for proteins, *Nature* **192**:1227.

Crowther, R. A., 1980, Mutants of bacteriophage T4 that produce infective fiberless particles, *J. Mol. Biol.* **137**:159.

Crowther, R. A., Lenk, E. V., Kikuchi, Y., and King, J., 1977, Molecular reorganization in the hexagon to star transition of the baseplate of bacteriophage T4, *J. Mol. Biol.* **116**: 489.

Cummings, D. J., Chapman, V. A., Delong, S. S., and Couse, M. L., 1973, Structural aberrations in T-even bacteriophage. III. Induction of "lollipops" and their partial characterizations, *Virology* **54**:245.

Cunningham, R. P., and Berger, H., 1977a, A new DNA-delay mutation in bacteriophage T4D, *Virology* **79**:320.

Cunningham, R. P., and Berger, H., 1977b, Mutations affecting genetic recombination in bacteriophage T4D. I. Pathway analysis, *Virology* **80**:67.

Dannenberg, R., and Mosig, G., 1981, Semi-conservative DNA replication is initiated at a single site in recombination-deficient gene *32* mutants of bacteriophage T4, *J. Virol.* **40**:890.

Dannenberg, R., and Mosig, G., 1983, Early intermediates in bacteriophage T4 DNA replication and recombination, *J. Virol.* **45**:813.

Delius, H., Howe, C., and Kozinski, A. W., 1971, Structure of the replicating DNA from bacteriophage T4, *Proc. Natl. Acad. Sci. USA* **68**:3049.

Deutscher, M. P., Foulds, J., and McClain, W. H., 1974, Transfer ribonucleic acid nucleotidyltransferase plays an essential role in the normal growth of *Escherichia coli* and in the biosynthesis of some bacteriophage transfer ribonucleic acids, *J. Biol. Chem.* **249**:6696.

DeVries, J. K., and Wallace, S. S., 1983, Expression of cloned bacteriophage T4 *uvsW* and *uvsY* genes in Rec$^+$ and Rec$^-$ *Escherichia coli*, *J. Virol.* **47**:406.

Dharmalingam, K., and Goldberg, E. B., 1976, Phage-coded protein prevents restriction of unmodified progeny T4 DNA, *Nature* **260**:454.

Dharmalingam, K., and Goldberg, E. B., 1979, Restriction *in vivo*. IV. Effect of restriction of parental DNA on the expression of restriction alleviation systems in phage T4, *Virology* **96**:404.

Dharmalingam, K., Revel, H. R., and Goldberg, E. B., 1982, Physical mapping and cloning of bacteriophage T4 antirestriction endonuclease gene, *J. Bacteriol.* **149**:694.

Dickson, R. C., 1974, Protein composition of the tail and contracted sheath of bacteriophage T4, *Virology* **59**:123.

Doermann, A. H., and Pao, A., 1987, Genetic control of capsid length in bacteriophage T4. IV. Phenotypes displayed by *ptg* mutants, *J. Virol.* **61**:2835.

Doermann, A. H., and Simon, L. D., 1984, Bacteriophage T4 bypass 31 mutations that make gene *31* nonessential for bacteriophage T4 replication: Mapping bypass 31 mutations by UV rescue experiments, *J. Virol.* **51**:315.

Doermann, A. H., Eiserling, F. A., and Boehner, L., 1973a, Capsid length in bacteriophage T4 and its genetic control, in: *Virus Research* (C. F. Fox and W. S. Robinson, eds.), pp. 243–258, Academic Press, New York.

Doermann, A. H., Eiserling, F. A., and Boehner, L., 1973b, Genetic control of capsid length in bacteriophage T4. I. Isolation and preliminary description of four new mutants, *J. Virol.* **12**:374.

Doermann, A. H., Pao, A., and Jackson, P., 1987, Genetic control of capsid length in bacteriophage T4: Clustering of *ptg* mutants in gene *23*, *J. Virol.* **61**:2823.

Doherty, D. H., 1982a, Genetic studies on capsid-length determination in bacteriophage T4.

I. Isolation and partial characterization of second-site revertants of a gene *32* mutation affecting capsid length, *J. Virol.* **43**:641.

Doherty, D. H., 1982b, Genetic studies on capsid-length determination in bacteriophage T4. II. Genetic evidence that specific protein-protein interactions are involved, *J. Virol.* **43**:655.

Donelli, G., Guglielmi, F., and Pauletti, L., 1972, Structure and physiochemical properties of bacteriophage G. I. Arrangement of protein subunits and contraction process of tail sheath, *J. Mol. Biol.* **71**:113.

Drake, J. W., 1973, The genetic control of spontaneous and induced mutation rates in bacteriophage T4, *Genetics* **73**(Suppl.):45.

Drake, J. W., 1985, Photodynamic inactivation and mutagenesis by angelicin (isopsoralen) or thiopyronin (methylene red) in wild-type and repair-deficient strains of bacteriophage T4, *J. Bacteriol.* **162**:1311.

Drake, J. W., and Ripley, L. S., 1983, The analysis of mutation in bacteriophage T4: Delights, dilemmas, and disasters, in: *Bacteriophage T4* (C. Mathews, E. Kutter, G. Mosig, and P. Berget, eds.), pp. 312–320, American Society for Microbiology, Washington.

Drexler, K., Riede, I., and Henning, U., 1986, Morphogenesis of the long tail fibers of bacteriophage T2 involves proteolytic processing of the polypeptide (gene product 37) constituting the distal part of the fiber, *J. Mol. Biol.* **191**:267.

Driedonks, R. A., and Caldentey, J., 1983, Gene *20* product of bacteriophage T4. 2. Its structural organization in prehead and bacteriophage, *J. Mol. Biol.* **166**:341.

Duckworth, D. H., 1970a, Biological activity of bacteriophage ghosts and "take-over" of host functions by bacteriophage, *Bacteriol. Rev.* **34**:344.

Duckworth, D. H., 1970b, The metabolism of T4 phage ghost-infected cells. I. Macromolecular synthesis and transport of nucleic acid and protein precursors, *Virology* **40**:673.

Duda, R. L., Wall, J. S., Hainfeld, J. F., Sweet, R. M., and Eiserling, F. A., 1985, Mass distribution of a probable tail-length-determining protein in bacteriophage T4, *Proc. Natl. Acad. Sci. USA* **82**:5550.

Duda, R. L., Gingery, M., and Eiserling, F. A., 1986, Potential length determiner and DNA injection protein is extruded from bacteriophage T4 tail tubes *in vitro*, *Virology* **151**:296.

Dulbecco, R., 1949, Reactivation of ultraviolet-inactivated bacteriophage by visible light, *Nature* **163**:949.

Earnshaw, W. C., Casjens, S., and Harrison, S. C., 1976, Assembly of the head of bacteriophage P22: X-ray diffraction from heads, proheads, and related structures, *J. Mol. Biol.* **104**:387.

Earnshaw, W. C., King, J., Harrison, S. C., and Eiserling, F. A., 1978, The structural organization of DNA packaged within the heads of T4 wild-type, isometric, and giant bacteriophages, *Cell* **14**:559.

Earnshaw, W. C., Goldberg, E. B., and Crowther, R. A., 1979, The distal half of the tail fiber of bacteriophage T4, *J. Mol. Biol.* **132**:101.

Edgar, R. S., and Wood, W. B., 1966, Morphogenesis of bacteriophage T4 in extracts of mutant-infected cells, *Proc. Natl. Acad. Sci. USA* **55**:498.

Ehrenman, K., Pedersen-Lane, J., West, D., Herman, R., Maley, F., and Belfort, M., 1986, Processing of phage T4 *td*-encoded RNA is analogous to the eukaryotic group I splicing pathway, *Proc. Natl. Acad. Sci. USA* **83**:5875.

Eiserling, F. A., Geiduschek, E. P., Epstein, R. H., and Metter, E. J., 1970, Capsid size and deoxyribonucleic acid length: The petite variant of bacteriophage T4, *J. Virol.* **6**:865.

Elliot, T., and Geiduschek, E. P., 1984, Defining a bacteriophage T4 late promoter: Absence of a "−35" region, *Cell* **36**:211.

Ellis, E. L., and Delbrück, M., 1939, The growth of bacteriophage, *J. Gen. Physiol.* **22**:365.

Epstein, R. H., Bolle, A., Steinberg, C. M., Kellenberger, E., Boy de la Tour, E., Chevallay, R., Edgar, R. S., Susman, M., Denhardt, G. H., and Lielausis, A., 1964, Physiological studies of conditional lethal mutants of bacteriophage T4D, *Cold Spring Harbor Symp. Quant. Biol.* **28**:375.

Flanegan, J. B., and Greenberg, G. R., 1977, Regulation of deoxyribonucleotide biosynthesis during *in vivo* bacteriophage T4 replication, *J. Biol. Chem.* **252**:3019.

Formosa, T., and Alberts, B. M., 1984, The use of affinity chromatography to study proteins involved in bacteriophage T4 genetic recombination, *Cold Spring Harbor Symp. Quant. Biol.* **49**:363.

Formosa, T., and Alberts, B. M., 1986, DNA synthesis dependent on genetic recombination: Characterization of a reaction catalyzed by purified bacteriophage T4 proteins, *Cell* **47**:793.

Formosa, T., Burke, R. L., and Alberts, B. M., 1983, Affinity purification of bacteriophage T4 proteins essential for DNA replication and genetic recombination, *Proc. Natl. Acad. Sci. USA* **80**:2442.

Frazier, M., and Mosig, G., 1988, Roles of the *Escherichia coli* heat shock sigma factor-32 in early and late gene expression of bacteriophage T4, *J. Bacteriol.* **170**:1384.

Fujisawa, H., Yonesaki, T., and Minagawa, T., 1985, Sequence of the T4 recombination gene, *uvsX*, and its comparison with that of the *recA* gene of *Escherichia coli*, *Nucleic Acids Res.* **13**:7473.

Fulford, W., and Model, P., 1984, Specificity of translational regulation by two DNA-binding proteins, *J. Mol. Biol.* **173**:211.

Furukawa, H., and Mizushima, S., 1982, Roles of cell surface components of *Escherichia coli* K12 in bacteriophage T4 infection: Interaction of tail core with phospholipids, *J. Bacteriol.* **150**:916.

Gauss, P., Gayle, M., Winter, R., and Gold, L., 1987, The bacteriophage T4 *dexA* gene: Sequence and analysis of a gene conditionally required for DNA replication, *Mol. Gen. Genet.* **206**:24.

Geiduschek, E. P., and Kassavetis, G., 1988, Changes in RNA polymerase, in: *The Bacteriophages*, Vol. 1 (R. Calendar, ed.), pp. 93–116, Plenum Press, New York.

George, D. G., Yeh, L.-S. L., and Barker, W. C., 1983, Unexpected relationships between bacteriophage lambda hypothetical proteins and bacteriophage T4 tail-fiber proteins, *Biochem. Biophys. Res. Commun.* **115**:1061.

Germino, J., and Bastia, D., 1982, Primary structure of the replication initiation protein of plasmid R6K, *Proc. Natl. Acad. Sci. USA* **79**:5475.

Gold, L., Pribnow, D., Schneider, T., Shinedling, S., Singer, B. S., and Stormo, G., 1981, Translational initiation in prokaryotes, *Annu. Rev. Microbiol.* **35**:365.

Gold, L., Inman, M., Miller, E., Pribnow, D., Schneider, T. D., Shinedling, S., and Stormo, G., 1984, Translational regulation during bacteriophage T4 development, in: *Gene Expression: The Translational Step and Its Control* (B. F. C. Clark and H. U. Petersen, eds.), pp. 379–394, Munksgaard, Copenhagen.

Goldberg, E. B., 1980, Bacteriophage nucleic acid penetration, in: *Receptors and Recognition*, Series B, Vol. 7: *Virus Receptors*, Part 1: *Bacterial Viruses* (L. L. Randall and L. Phillipson, eds.), pp. 115–141, Chapman and Hall, London.

Goldberg, E. B., 1983, Recognition, attachment, and injection, in: *Bacteriophage T4* (C. Mathews, E. Kutter, G. Mosig, and P. Berget, eds.), pp. 32–39, American Society for Microbiology, Washington.

Gorski, K., Roch, J.-M., Prentki, P., and Krisch, H. M., 1985, The stability of bacteriophage T4 gene *32* mRNA: A 5′ leader sequence that can stabilize mRNA transcripts, *Cell* **43**:461.

Gott, J., Shub, D., and Belfort, M., 1986, Multiple self-splicing introns in bacteriophage T4: Evidence from autocatalytic GTP, *Cell* **47**:81.

Gram, H., and Rüger, W., 1985, Genes *55*, α*gt*, *47* and *46* of bacteriophage T4: The genomic organization as deduced by sequence analysis, *EMBO J.* **4**:257.

Gram, H., and Rüger, W., 1986, The α-glucosyltransferases of bacteriophages T2, T4 and T6: A comparison of their primary structures, *Mol. Gen. Genet.* **202**:467.

Gram, H., Liebig, H.-D., Hack, A., Niggemann, E., and Rüger, W., 1984, A physical map of bacteriophage T4 including the positions of strong promoters and terminators recognized *in vitro*, *Mol. Gen. Genet.* **194**:232.

Gribskov, M., and Burgess, R. R., 1986, Sigma factors from *E. coli*, *B. subtilis*, phage SP01, and phage T4 are homologous proteins, *Nucleic Acids Res.* **14**:6745.

Griffith, J., and Formosa, T., 1985, The UvsX protein of bacteriophage T4 arranges single-stranded and double-stranded DNA into similar helical nucleoprotein filaments, *J. Biol. Chem.* **260**:4484.

Gruidl, M. E., and Mosig, G., 1986, Sequence and transcripts of the bacteriophage T4 DNA repair gene *uvsY*, *Genetics* **114**:1061.

Guerrier-Takada, C., McClain, W. H., and Altman, S., 1984, Cleavage of tRNA precursors by the RNA subunit of *E. coli* ribonuclease P (M1 RNA) is influenced by 3'-proximal CCA in the substrates, *Cell* **38**:219.

Guha, A., Szybalski, W., Salser, W., Bolle, A., Geiduschek, E. P., and Pulitzer, J. F., 1971, Controls and polarity of transcription during bacteriophage T4 development, *J. Mol. Biol.* **59**:329.

Guild, N., Gayle, M., Sweeney, R., Hollingsworth, T., Modeer, T., and Gold, L., 1988, Transcriptional activation of bacteriophage T4 middle promoters by the *motA* protein, *J. Mol. Biol.* **199**:241.

Gurevitz, M., and Apirion, D., 1985, The RNase III (EC 3.1.26.3) processing site near the 5' end of an RNA precursor of bacteriophage T4 and its effect on termination, *Eur. J. Biochem.* **147**:581.

Hahn, S., Kruse, U., and Rüger, W., 1986, The region of phage T4 genes *34, 33* and *59:* Primary structures and organization on the genome, *Nucleic Acids Res.* **14**:9311.

Hall, D. H., Povinelli, C. M., Ehrenman, K., Pedersen-Lane, J., Chu, F., and Belfort, M., 1987, Two domains for splicing in the intron of the phage T4 thymidylate synthase (*td*) gene established by nondirected mutagenesis, *Cell* **48**:63.

Halpern, M. E., Mattson, T., and Kozinski, A. W., 1979, Origins of phage T4 DNA replication as revealed by hybridization to cloned genes, *Proc. Natl. Acad. Sci. USA* **76**:6137.

Hamlett, N. V., and Berger, H., 1975, Mutations altering genetic recombination and repair of DNA in bacteriophage T4, *Virology* **63**:539.

Harm, W., 1961, Gene-controlled reactivation of ultraviolet-inactivated bacteriophage, *J. Cell. Comp. Physiol.* **58**:69.

Hattman, S., 1983, DNA modification: Methylation, in: *Bacteriophage T4* (C. K. Mathews, E. M. Kutter, G. Mosig, and P. B. Berget, eds.), pp. 152–155, American Society for Microbiology, Washington.

Hattman, S., Wilkinson, J., Swinton, D., Schlagman, S., Macdonald, P. M., and Mosig, G., 1985, Common evolutionary origin of the phage T4 *dam* and host *Escherichia coli dam* DNA-adenine methyltransferase genes, *J. Bacteriol.* **164**:932.

Herman, R. E., and Snustad, D. P., 1982, Plasmid pR386 renders *Escherichia coli* cells restrictive to the growth of bacteriophage T4 *unf* mutants, *J. Virol.* **41**:330.

Herman, R. E., Haas, N., and Snustad, D. P., 1984, Identification of the bacteriophage T4 *unf* (=*alc*) gene product, a protein involved in the shutoff of host transcription, *Genetics* **108**:305.

Hershey, A. D., 1958, The production of recombinants in phage crosses, *Cold Spring Harbor Symp. Quant. Biol.* **23**:19.

Hershey, A. D., and Chase, M., 1951, Genetic recombination and heterozygosis in bacteriophage, *Cold Spring Harbor Symp. Quant. Biol.* **16**:471.

Hershey, A. D., and Chase, M., 1952, Independent functions of viral protein and nucleic acid in growth of bacteriophage, *J. Gen. Physiol.* **36**:39.

Hinton, D. M., and Nossal, N. G., 1986, Cloning of the bacteriophage T4 *uvsX* gene and purification and characterization of the T4 uvsX recombination protein, *J. Biol. Chem.* **261**:5663.

Hinton, D. M., Silver, L. L., and Nossal, N. G., 1985, Bacteriophage T4 DNA replication protein 41, *J. Biol. Chem.* **260**:12851.

Hinton, D. M., Richardson, R. W., and Nossal, N. G., 1987, Bacteriophage T4 DNA replication: Role of the T4 41 and 61 protein primase-helicase and the T4 *uvsX* recombination protein, in: *DNA Replication and Recombination* (R. McMacken and T. J. Kelly, eds.), pp. 173–182, Alan R. Liss, New York.

Hosoda, J., Mathews, E., and Jansen, B., 1971, Role of genes 46 and 47 in bacteriophage T4 replication. I. *In vivo* deoxyribonucleic acid replication, *J. Virol.* **8**:372.

Hsu, T., Wei, R., Dawson, M., and Karam, J. D., 1987, Identification of two new bacterio-

    phage T4 genes that may have roles in transcription and DNA replication, *J. Virol.*
    61:366.
Huang, W. M., 1979, Positive regulation of T-even phage DNA replication by the DNA
    delay protein of gene *39*, *Cold Spring Harbor Symp. Quant. Biol.* **48**:495.
Huang, W. M., 1983, Appendix: T4 DNA replication on cellophane disks, in: *Bacteriophage
    T4* (C. Mathews, E. Kutter, G. Mosig, and P. Berget, eds.), pp. 97–102, American Society
    for Microbiology, Washington.
Huang, W. M., 1986a, The 52-protein subunit of T4 DNA topoisomerase is homologous to
    the gyrA-protein of gyrase, *Nucleic Acids Res.* **14**:7379.
Huang, W. M., 1986b, Nucleotide sequence of a type II DNA topoisomerase gene: Bacterio-
    phage T4 gene *39*, *Nucleic Acids Res.* **14**:7751.
Huang, W. M., Wei, L. S., and Casjens, S., 1985, Relationship between bacteriophage T4 and
    T6 DNA topoisomerase, *J. Biol. Chem.* **260**:8973.
Huang, W. M., Ao, S.-Z., Casjens, S., Orlandi, R., Zeikus, R., Weiss, R., Winge, D., and Fang,
    M., 1988, A persistent untranslated sequence within bacteriophage T4 DNA to-
    poisomerase gene *60*, *Science* **239**:1005.
Huberman, J. A., 1969, Visualization of replicating mammalian and T4 bacteriophage DNA,
    Cold Spring Harbor Symp. Quant. Biol. **33**:509.
Iserentant, D., and Fiers, W., 1980, Secondary structure of messenger RNA efficiency of
    translation initiation, *Gene* **9**:1.
Ishii, T., and Yanagida, M., 1977, The two dispensable structural proteins (*soc* and *hoc*) of
    the T4 phage capsid: Their properties, isolation and characterization of defective mu-
    tants, and their binding with the defective heads *in vitro*, *J. Mol. Biol.* **109**:487.
Jabbar, M. A., and Snyder, L., 1984, Genetic and physiological studies of an *Escherichia coli*
    locus that restricts polynucleotide kinase- and RNA ligase-deficient mutants of bacte-
    riophage T4, *J. Virol.* **51**:522.
Jacob, F., Brenner, S., and Cuzin, F., 1963, On the regulation of DNA replication in bacteria,
    Cold Spring Harbor Symp. Quant. Biol. **28**:329.
Jongeneel, C. V., Formosa, T., and Alberts, B. M., 1984, Purification and characterization of
    the bacteriophage T4 *dda* protein: A DNA helicase that associates with the viral helix-
    destabilizing protein, *J. Biol. Chem.* **259**:12925.
Kano-Sueoka, T., and Sueoka, N., 1969, Leucine tRNA and cessation of *Escherichia coli*
    protein synthesis upon phage T2 infection, *Proc. Natl. Acad. Sci. USA* **62**:1229.
Kao, S. H., and McClain, W. H., 1980a, Baseplate protein of bacteriophage T4 with both
    structural and lytic functions, *J. Virol.* **34**:95.
Kao, S. H., and McClain, W. H., 1980b, Roles of T4 gene *5* and gene *S* in cell lysis, *J. Virol.*
    34:104.
Karam, J. D., Gold, L., Singer, B. S., and Dawson, M., 1981, Translational regulation: Identi-
    fication of the site on bacteriophage T4 *r*IIB and mRNA recognized by the *regA* gene
    function, *Proc. Natl. Acad. Sci. USA* **78**:4669.
Karam, J. D., Trojanowska, M., and Baucom, M., 1983, Interactions of T4-induced enzymes
    in vivo: Inferences from intergenic suppression, in: *Bacteriophage T4* (C. K. Mathews,
    E. M. Kutter, G. Mosig, and P. B. Berget, eds.), pp. 334–341, American Society for
    Microbiology, Washington.
Kassavetis, G. A., and Geiduschek, E. P., 1982, Bacteriophage T4 late promoters: Mapping 5′
    ends of T4 gene *23* messenger RNA, *EMBO J.* **1**:107.
Kassavetis, G. A., Zentner, P. G., and Geiduschek, E. P., 1986, Transcription at bacterio-
    phage T4 variant late promoters: An application of a newly devised promoter-mapping
    method involving RNA chain retraction, *J. Biol. Chem.* **261**:14256.
Kassavetis, G. A., Zentner, P. G., and Geiduschek, E. P., 1987, Lock-step transcription:
    Application to promoter mapping, in: *RNA Polymerase and the Regulation of Tran-
    scription* (W. S. Reznikoff, R. R. Burgess, J. E. Dahlberg, C. A. Gross, M. T. Record Jr.,
    and M. P. Wickens, eds.), pp. 471–478, Elsevier, New York.
Katsura, I., and Hendrix, R. W., 1984, Length regulation in bacteriophage lambda tails, *Cell*
    39:691.

Kaufmann, G., and Amitsur, M., 1985, Host transfer RNA cleavage and reunion in T4-infected *Escherichia coli* CTR5X, *Nucleic Acids Res.* **13:**4333.

Kaufmann, G., David, M., Borasio, G. D., Teichmann, A., Paz, A., and Amitsur, M., 1986, Phage and host genetic determinants of the specific anticodon loop cleavages in bacteriophage T4-infected *Escherichia coli* CTR5X, *J. Mol. Biol.* **188:**15.

Kellenberger, E., 1980, Control mechanisms in the morphogenesis of bacteriophage heads, *Biosystems* **12:**201.

Kellenberger, E., and Boy de la Tour, E., 1964, On the fine structure of normal and "polymerized" tail sheath of phage T4, *J. Ultrastruct. Res.* **11:**545.

Keller, B., Sengstag, C., Kellenberger, E., and Bickle, T. A., 1984, Gene *68*, a new bacteriophage T4 gene which codes for the 17K prohead core protein, is involved in head size determination, *J. Mol. Biol.* **179:**415.

Kells, S. S., and Haselkorn, R., 1974, Bacteriophage T4 short tail fibers are the product of gene *12*, *J. Mol. Biol.* **83:**473.

Kemper, B., and Brown, D. T., 1976, Function of gene *49* of bacteriophage T4. II. Analysis of intracellular development and the structure of very fast-sedimentating DNA, *J. Virol.* **18:**1000.

Kemper, B., Jensch, F., Depka-Prondzynski, M. V., Fritz, H.-J., Borgmeyer, U., and Mizuuchi, K., 1984, Resolution of Holliday structures by endonuclease VII as observed in interactions with cruciform DNA, *Cold Spring Harbor Symp. Quant. Biol.* **49:**815.

Kennell, D., 1986, The instability of messenger RNA in bacteria, in: *Maximizing Gene Expression* (W. Reznikoff and L. Gold, eds.), pp. 101–142, Butterworths, Boston.

Kim, J.-S., and Davidson, N., 1974, Electron microscope heteroduplex studies of sequence relations of T2, T4, and T6 bacteriophage DNAs, *Virology* **57:**93.

King, G. J., and Huang, W. M., 1982, Identification of the origins of phage T4 DNA replication, *Proc. Natl. Acad. Sci. USA* **79:**7248.

King, J., 1980, Regulation of protein interactions as revealed in phage morphogenesis, in: *Biological Regulation and Development*, Vol. 2 (R. Goldberg, ed.), pp. 101–134, Plenum, New York.

King, J., and Mykolajewycz, N., 1973, Bacteriophage T4 tail assembly: Proteins of sheath, core, and baseplate, *J. Mol. Biol.* **75:**339.

King, J., Hall, C., and Casjens, S., 1978, Control of the synthesis of phage P22 scaffolding protein is coupled to capsid assembly, *Cell* **15:**551.

Klar, A. J. S., and Strathern, J. N., eds., 1984, *Cold Spring Harbor Symposia on Quantitative Biology*, Vol. 49, Cold Spring Harbor Laboratory, Cold Spring Harbor, NY

Kozinski, A. W., 1983, DNA metabolism *in vivo*, in: *Bacteriophage T4* (C. K. Mathews, E. M. Kutter, G. Mosig, and P. B. Berget, eds.), pp. 111–119, American Society for Microbiology, Washington.

Kozloff, L. M., 1983, The T4 particle: Low-molecular-weight compounds and associated enzymes, in: *Bacteriophage T4* (C. Mathews, E. Kutter, G. Mosig, and P. Berget, eds.), pp. 25–31, American Society for Microbiology, Washington.

Kozloff, L. M., and Lute, M., 1984, Identification of bacteriophage T4D gene products 26 and 51 as baseplate hub structural components, *J. Virol.* **52:**344.

Kreuzer, K. N., and Alberts, B. M., 1984, Site-specific recognition of bacteriophage T4 DNA by T4 type II DNA topoisomerase and *Escherichia coli* DNA gyrase, *J. Biol. Chem.* **259:**5339.

Kreuzer, K. N., and Alberts, B. M., 1985, A defective phage system reveals bacteriophage T4 replication origins that coincide with recombination hotspots, *Proc. Natl. Acad. Sci. USA* **82:**3345.

Kreuzer, K. N., and Alberts, B. M., 1986, Characterization of a defective phage system for the analysis of bacteriophage T4 DNA replication origins, *J. Mol. Biol.* **188:**185.

Kreuzer, K. N., and Huang, W. M., 1983, T4 DNA topoisomerase, in: *Bacteriophage T4* (C. K. Mathews, E. M. Kutter, G. Mosig, and P. B. Berget, eds.), pp. 90–96, American Society for Microbiology, Washington.

Kreuzer, K. N., and Menkens, A. E., 1987, Plasmid model systems for the initiation of bacteriophage T4 DNA replication, in: *DNA Replication and Recombination* (R. McMacken and T. J. Kelley, eds.), pp. 451–471, Alan R. Liss, New York.

Krimm, S., and Anderson, T. F., 1967, Structure of normal and contracted tail sheaths of T4 bacteriophage, *J. Mol. Biol.* **27**:197.

Krisch, H. M., and Allet, B., 1982, Nucleotide sequences involved in bacteriophage T4 gene *32* translational self-regulation, *Proc. Natl. Acad. Sci. USA* **79**:4937.

Kutter, E., and Rüger, W., 1983, Map of the T4 genome and its transcription control sites, in: *Bacteriophage T4* (C. Mathews, E. Kutter, G. Mosig, and P. B. Berget, eds.), pp. 277–290, American Society for Microbiology, Washington.

Kutter, E., and Snyder, L., 1983, Appendix: Production of cytosine-containing T4 phage, in: *Bacteriophage T4* (C. K. Mathews, E. M. Kutter, G. Mosig, and P. B. Berget, eds.), pp. 56–57, American Society for Microbiology, Washington.

Kutter, E., Drivdahl, R., and Rand, K., 1984, Identification and characterization of the *alc* gene product of bacteriophage T4, *Genetics* **108**:291.

Kutter, E., Guttman, B., Rüger, W., Tomaschewski, J., and Mosig, G., 1987, Bacteriophage T4, in: *Genetic Maps 1987*, Vol. 4 (S. J. O'Brien, ed.), p. 22, Cold Spring Harbor Laboratory, Cold Spring Harbor, NY.

Kuz'min, N. P., Kryukov, V. M., Tanyashin, V. I., and Baev, A. A., 1983, Mapping of phage T4 DNA cleavage sites by endonuclease EcoRV, *Dokl. Acad. Sci. USSR* **269**:995.

Laemmli, U. K., and Eiserling, F. A., 1968, Studies on the morphopoiesis of the head of phage T-even. IV. The formation of polyheads, *Mol. Gen. Genet.* **101**:333.

Leibo, S. P., Kellenberger, E., Kellenberger–Van der Kamp, C., Frey, T. G., and Steinberg, C. M., 1979, Gene *24*-controlled osmotic shock resistance in bacteriophage T4: Probable multiple gene functions, *J. Virol.* **30**:327.

LeMaster, D. M., 1986, Nucleotide sequence and protein overproduction of bacteriophage T4 thioredoxin, *J. Virol.* **59**:759.

Lepault, J., and Leonard, K., 1985, 3-Dimensional structure of unstained frozen-hydrated extended tails of bacteriophage T4, *J. Mol. Biol.* **182**:431.

Levinthal, C., and Visconti, N., 1953, Growth and recombination of bacterial viruses, *Genetics* **38**:500.

Levy, J. N., and Goldberg, E. B., 1980, Region-specific recombination in phage T4. I. A special glucosyl-dependent recombination system, *Genetics* **94**:519.

Lin, G., and Mosig, G., 1987, Differential regulation of phage T4 late promoters by T4 DNA topoisomerase and *E. coli* DNA gyrase, American Society for Microbiology, 87th annual meeting, abstracts, M-8:238.

Liu, L. F., Liu, C.-C., and Alberts, B. M., 1979, T4 DNA topoisomerase: A new ATP dependent enzyme essential for initiation of T4 bacteriophage DNA replication, *Nature* **281**:456.

Luder, A., 1981, Mechanisms of DNA chain initiation in the primase-defective gene *58-61* mutants of bacteriophage T4, Ph.D. Thesis, Vanderbilt University, Nashville, TN.

Luder, A., and Mosig, G., 1982, Two alternative mechanisms for initiation of DNA replication forks in bacteriophage T4: Priming by RNA polymerase and by recombination, *Proc. Natl. Acad. Sci. USA* **79**:1101.

Luftig, R. B., Wood, W. B., and Okinaka, R., 1971, Bacteriophage T4 head morphogenesis. On the nature of gene *49* defective heads and their role as intermediates, *J. Mol. Biol.* **57**:555.

Luria, S. E., 1953, Host-induced modification of viruses, *Cold Spring Harbor Symp. Quant. Biol.* **18**:237.

Macdonald, P. M., 1983, Structural and functional analyses of a DNA replication origin in the bacteriophage T4, Ph.D. Thesis, Vanderbilt University, Nashville, TN.

Macdonald, P. M., and Hall, D. H., 1984, Genetic evidence for physical interactions between enzymes of nucleotide synthesis and proteins involved in DNA replication in bacteriophage T4, *Genetics* **107**:343.

Macdonald, P. M., and Mosig, G., 1984a, Cloning and physical mapping of an early region of the bacteriophage T4 genome, *Genetics* **106**:1.

Macdonald, P. M., and Mosig, G., 1984b, Regulation of a new bacteriophage T4 gene, 69, that spans an origin of DNA replication, *EMBO J.* **3**:2863.

Macdonald, P. M., Seaby, R. M., Brown, W., and Mosig, G., 1983, Initiator DNA from a primary origin and induction of a secondary origin of bacteriophage T4 DNA replication, in: *Microbiology—1983* (D. Schlessinger, ed.), pp. 111–116, American Society for Microbiology, Washington.

Macdonald, P. M., Kutter, E., and Mosig, G., 1984, Regulation of a bacteriophage T4 late gene, *soc*, which maps in an early region, *Genetics* **106**:17.

Malik, S., Dimitrov, M., and Goldfarb, A., 1985, Initiation of transcription by bacteriophage T4–modified RNA polymerase independently of host sigma factor, *J. Mol. Biol.* **185**:83.

Marsh, R. C., Breschkin, A. M., and Mosig, G., 1971, Origin and direction of bacteriophage T4 DNA replication. II. A gradient of marker frequencies in partially replicated T4 DNA as assayed by transformation, *J. Mol. Biol.* **60**:213.

Mathews, C. K., and Allen, J. R., 1983, DNA precursor biosynthesis, in: *Bacteriophage T4* (C. K. Mathews, E. M. Kutter, G. Mosig, and P. B. Berget, eds.), pp. 59–70, American Society for Microbiology, Washington.

Mathews, C. K., Kutter, E. M., Mosig, G., and Berget, P. B., eds., 1983, *Bacteriophage T4*, American Society for Microbiology, Washington.

Mattson, T., Van Houwe, G. V., and Epstein, R., 1983, Recombination between bacteriophage T4 and plasmid pBR322 molecules containing cloned T4 DNA, *J. Mol. Biol.* **170**:357.

McCarthy, D., 1979, Gyrase-dependent initiation of bacteriophage T4 DNA replication: Interaction of *Escherichia coli* gyrase with novobiocin, coumermycin and phage DNA-delay gene products, *J. Mol. Biol.* **127**:265.

McCarthy, D., Minner, C., Bernstein, H., and Bernstein, C., 1976, DNA elongation rates and growing point distributions of wild-type T4 and DNA-delay amber mutant, *J. Mol. Biol.* **106**:963.

McClain, W. H., Foss, K., Schneider, J., Guerrier-Takada, C., and Altman, S., 1987, Suppressor and novel mutants of bacteriophage T4 tRNA^{Gly}, *J. Mol. Biol.* **193**:223.

McNicol, L. A., Simon, L. D., and Black, L. W., 1977, A mutation which bypasses the requirement for p24 in bacteriophage T4 capsid morphogenesis, *J. Mol. Biol.* **116**:261.

McPheeters, D. S., Christensen, A., Young, E. T., Stormo, G., and Gold, L., 1986, Translational regulation of expression of the bacteriophage T4 lysozyme gene, *Nucleic Acids Res.* **14**:5813.

Michel, C. J., Jacq, B., Arques, D. G., and Bickle, T. A., 1986, A remarkable amino acid sequence homology between a phage T4 tail fibre protein and ORF314 of phage lambda located in the tail opcron, *Gene* **44**:147.

Michel, F., and Dujon, B., 1986, Genetic exchanges between bacteriophage T4 and filamentous fungi? *Cell* **46**:323.

Midgley, C., and Murray, N., 1985, T4 polynucleotide kinase: Cloning of the gene (*pseT*) and amplification of its product, *EMBO J.* **4**:2695.

Mileham, A. J., Murray, N. E., and Revel, H. R., 1984, λ-T4 hybrid bacteriophage carrying the thymidine kinase gene of bacteriophage T4, *J. Virol.* **50**:619.

Miller, E. S., Winter, R. B., Campbell, K. M., Power, S. D., and Gold, L. 1985, Bacteriophage T4 RegA protein: Purification of a translational repressor, *J. Biol. Chem.* **260**:13053.

Miller, E. S., Karam, J., Dawson, M., Trojanowska, M., Gauss, P., and Gold, L., 1987, Translational repression: Biological activity of plasmid-encoded bacteriophage T4 *regA* protein, *Mol. Biol.* **194**:307.

Miller, R. C. Jr., 1972, Association of replicative T4 deoxyribonucleic acid and bacterial membranes, *J. Virol.* **10**:920.

Miller, R. C. Jr., and Kozinski, A. W., 1970, Early intracellular events in the replication of bacteriophage T4 deoxyribonucleic acid. V. Further studies on the T4 protein–deoxyribonucleic acid complex, *J. Virol.* **5**:490.

Montag, D., Degen, M., and Henning, U., 1987, Nucleotide sequence of gene *t* (lysis gene) of the *E. coli* phage T4, *Nucleic Acids Res.* **15**:6736.

Moody, M. F., 1965, The shape of the T-even bacteriophage head, *Virology* **26**:567.

Moody, M. F., 1973, Sheath of bacteriophage T4. III. Contraction mechanism deduced from partially contracted sheaths, *J. Mol. Biol.* **60:**613.

Moody, M. F., and Makowski, L., 1981, X-ray diffraction study of tail tubes from bacteriophage T2L, *J. Mol. Biol.* **150:**217.

Mooney, D. T., Stockard, J., Parker, M. L., and Doermann, A. H., 1987, Genetic control of capsid length in bacteriophage T4: DNA sequence analysis of petite and petite/giant mutants, *J. Virol.* **61:**2828.

Mosig, G., 1963, Genetic recombination in bacteriophage T4 during replication of DNA fragments, *Cold Spring Harbor Symp. Quant. Biol.* **28:**35.

Mosig, G., 1966, Distances separating genetic markers in T4 DNA, *Proc. Natl. Acad. Sci. USA* **56:**1177.

Mosig, G., 1968, A map of distances along the DNA molecule of phage T4, *Genetics* **59:**137.

Mosig, G., 1983, Relationship of T4 DNA replication and recombination, in: *Bacteriophage T4* (C. K. Mathews, E. M. Kutter, G. Mosig, and P. B. Berget, eds.), pp. 120–130, American Society for Microbiology, Washington.

Mosig, G., 1985, Bacteriophage T4 gene *32* participates in excision repair as well as recombinational repair of UV damages, *Genetics* **110:**159.

Mosig, G., 1987, The essential role of recombination in phage T4 growth, *Annu. Rev. Genet.* **21:**347.

Mosig, G., and Breschkin, A. M., 1975, Genetic evidence for an additional function of phage T4 gene *32* protein: Interaction with ligase, *Proc. Natl. Acad. Sci. USA* **72:**1226.

Mosig, G., and Macdonald, P., 1986, A new membrane-associated DNA replication protein, the gene *69* product of bacteriophage T4, shares a patch of homology with the *Escherichia coli dnaA* protein, *J. Mol. Biol.* **189:**243.

Mosig, G., and Powell, D., 1985, Heteroduplex loops are packaged in gene *49* (endonuclease VII) mutants of bacteriophage T4, American Society for Microbiology, 85th annual meeting, M4:209 (abstract).

Mosig, G., Ehring, R., Schliewen, W., and Bock, S., 1971, The patterns of recombination and segregation in terminal regions of T4 DNA molecules, *Mol. Gen. Genet.* **113:**51.

Mosig, G., Carnigan, J. R., Bibring, J. B., Cole, R., Bock, H.-G. O., and Bock, S., 1972, Coordinate variation in lengths of DNA molecules and head lengths in morphological variants of bacteriophage T4, *J. Virol.* **9:**857.

Mosig, G., Luder, A., Garcia, G., Dannenberg, R., and Bock, S., 1979, *In vivo* interactions of genes and proteins in DNA replication and recombination of phage T4, *Cold Spring Harbor Symp. Quant. Biol.* **43:**501.

Mosig, G., Benedict, S., Ghosal, D., Luder, A., Dannenberg, R., and Bock, S., 1980, Genetic analysis of DNA replication in bacteriophage T4, in: *Mechanistic Studies of DNA Replication and Genetic Recombination* (B. Alberts, ed.), pp. 527–543, Alan R. Liss, New York.

Mosig, G., Ghosal, D., and Bock, S., 1981a, Interactions between the maturation protein gp17 and the single-stranded DNA binding protein gp32 initiate DNA packaging and compete with initiation of secondary DNA replication forks in phage T4, in: *Bacteriophage Assembly* (M. DuBow, ed.), pp. 139–150, Alan R. Liss, New York.

Mosig, G., Luder, A., Rowen, L., Macdonald, P., and Bock, S., 1981b, On the role of recombination and topoisomerase in primary and secondary initiation of T4 DNA replication, in: *The Initiation of Replication* (D. Ray, ed.), pp. 277–295, Academic Press, New York.

Mosig, G., Macdonald, P., Lin, G., Levin, M., and Seaby, R., 1983, Gene expression and initiation of DNA replication of bacteriophage T4 in phage and host topoisomerase mutants, in: *Mechanisms of DNA Replication and Recombination* (N. R. Cozzarelli, ed.), pp. 173–186, Alan R. Liss, New York.

Mosig, G., Shaw, M., and Garcia, G. M., 1984, On the role of DNA replication, endonuclease VII, and *r*II proteins in processing of recombinational intermediates in phage T4, *Cold Spring Harbor Symp. Quant. Biol.* **49:**371.

Mosig, G., Macdonald, P. M., Powell, D., Trupin, M., and Gary, T., 1987, A membrane protein involved in initiation of DNA replication from the *oriA* region of phage T4, in: *DNA Replication and Recombination* (R. McMacken and T. J. Kelly, eds.), pp. 403–414, Alan R. Liss, New York.

Mufti, S., and Bernstein, H., 1974, The DNA-delay mutants of bacteriophage T4, *J. Virol.* **14:**860.

Müller-Salamin, L., Onorato, L., and Showe, M. K., 1977, Localization of minor protein components of the head of bacteriophage T4, *J. Virol.* **24:**121.

Nakagawa, H., Arisaka, F., and Ishii, S.-I., 1985, Isolation and characterization of the bacteriophage T4 tail-associated lysozyme, *J. Virol.* **54:**460.

Naot, Y., and Shalitin, C., 1972, Defective concatemer formation in cells infected with deoxyribonucleic acid–delay mutants of bacteriophage T4, *J. Virol.* **10:**858.

Newbury, S. F., Smith, N. H., Robinson, E. C., Hiles, I. D., and Higgins, C. F., 1987, Stabilization of translationally active mRNA by prokaryotic REP sequences, *Cell* **48:**297.

Nossal, N. G., and Alberts, B. M., 1983, Mechanism of DNA replication catalyzed by purified T4 replication proteins, in: *Bacteriophage T4* (C. K. Mathews, E. M. Kutter, G. Mosig, and P. B. Berget, eds.), pp. 71–81, American Society for Microbiology, Washington.

Obringer, J., McCreary, P., and Bernstein, H., 1988, Bacteriophage T4 genes *sp* and *40* are the same gene, *J. Virol.* (submitted).

Oishi, M., 1968, Studies of DNA replication *in vivo.* III. Accumulation of single-stranded isolation product of DNA replication by conditional mutant strains of T4, *Proc. Natl. Acad. Sci. USA* **60:**1000.

Oliver, D. B., and Crowther, R. A., 1981, DNA sequence of the tail fiber genes 36 and 37 of bacteriophage T4, *J. Mol. Biol.* **153:**545.

Olson, N. J., and Marchin, G. L., 1984, Valyl-tRNA synthetase modification-dependent restriction of bacteriophage T4, *J. Virol.* **51:**42.

Olson, N. J., and Marchin, G. L., 1985, Response of a phage modification factor to enhanced production of its target molecule, *J. Virol.* **53:**702.

Orsini, G., and Brody, E. N., 1988, Phage T4 DNA codes for two distinct 10-kD proteins which strongly bind to RNA polymerase, *Virology* **162:**397.

Owen, J. E., Schultz, D. W., Taylor, A., and Smith, G. R., 1983, Nucleotide sequence of the lysozyme gene of bacteriophage T4: Analysis of mutations involving repeated sequences, *J. Mol. Biol.* **165:**229.

Parker, M. L., Christensen, A. C., Boosman, A., Stockard, J., Young, E. T., and Doermann, A. H., 1984, Nucleotide sequence of bacteriophage T4 gene *23* and the amino acid sequence of its product, *J. Mol. Biol.* **180:**399.

Paulson, J. R., and Laemmli, U. K., 1977, Morphogenetic core of the bacteriophage T4 head. Structure of the core in polyheads, *J. Mol. Biol.* **111:**459.

Pedersen-Lane, J., and Belfort, M., 1987, Variable occurrence of the *nrdB* intron in the T-even phages suggests intron mobility, *Science* **237:**182.

Plishker, M. F., and Berget, P. B., 1984, Isolation and characterization of precursors in bacteriophage T4 baseplate assembly. III. The carboxyl termini of protein P11 are required for assembly activity, *J. Mol. Biol.* **178:**699.

Prasad, B. V. V., and Chiu, W., 1987, Sequence comparison of single-stranded DNA binding proteins and its structural implications, *J. Mol. Biol.* **193:**579.

Pritchard, R. H., 1978, Control of DNA replication in bacteria, in: *DNA Synthesis, Present and Future* (I. Molineux and M. Kohiyama, eds.), pp. 1–26, Plenum, New York.

Pryciak, P. M., Conway, J. D., Eiserling, F. A., and Isenberg, D., 1986, Cylindrical beta structure: A hypothetical protein structure, in: *Protein Structure, Folding, and Design* (D. Oxender and C. F. Fox, eds.), pp. 243–246, Alan R. Liss, New York.

Pulitzer, J. F., Coppo, A., and Caruso, M., 1979, Host-virus interactions in the control of T4 prereplicative transcription. II. Interaction between *tabC(rho)* mutants and T4 *mot* mutants, *J. Mol. Biol.* **135:**979.

Pulitzer, J. F., Colombo, M., and Ciaramella, M., 1985, New control elements of bacteriophage T4 pre-replicative transcription, *J. Mol. Biol.* **182:**249.

Purohit, S., and Mathews, C. K., 1984, Nucleotide sequence reveals overlap between T4 phage genes encoding dihydrofolate reductase and thymidylate synthase, *J. Biol. Chem.* **259:**6261.

Rabussay, D., 1983, Phage-evoked changes in RNA polymerase, in: *Bacteriophage T4* (C. K.

Mathews, E. M. Kutter, G. Mosig, and P. B. Berget, eds.), pp. 167–173, American Society for Microbiology, Washington.

Radany, E. H., Naumovski, L., Love, J. D., Gutekunst, K. A., Hall, D. H., and Friedberg, E. C., 1984, Physical mapping of the phage T4 denV gene reveals apparent genetic map distortion near an origin of DNA replication, J. Virol. **52**:846.

Raleigh, E. A., and Wilson, G., 1986, Escherichia coli K-12 restricts DNA containing 5-methylcytosine, Proc. Natl. Acad. Sci. USA **83**:9070.

Rand, K. N., and Gait, M. J., 1984, Sequence and cloning of bacteriophage T4 gene 63 encoding RNA ligase and tail fibre attachment activities, EMBO J. **3**:397.

Recinos, A. III, Augustine, M. L., Higgins, K. M., and Lloyd, R. S., 1986, Expression of the bacteriophage T4 denV structural gene in Escherichia coli, J. Bacteriol. **168**: 1014.

Reddy, G. P. V., Singh, A., Stafford, M. E., and Mathews, C. K., 1977, Enzyme associations in T4 phage DNA precursor synthesis, Proc. Natl. Acad. Sci. USA **74**:3152.

Revel, H. R., 1983, DNA modification: Glucosylation, in: Bacteriophage T4 (C. K. Mathews, E. M. Kutter, G. Mosig, and P. B. Berget, eds.), pp. 156–165, American Society for Microbiology, Washington.

Revel, H. R., and Luria, S., 1970, DNA-glucosylation in T-even phage: Genetic determination and role in phage-host interaction, Annu. Rev. Genet. **4**:177.

Revel, H. R., Herrmann, R., and Bishop, R. J., 1976, Genetic analysis of T4 tail fiber assembly. II. Bacterial host mutants that allow bypass of T4 gene 57 function, Virology **72**:255.

Revel, H. R., Stitt, B. R., Lielausis, I., and Wood, W. B., 1980, Role of the host cell in bacteriophage T4 development. I. Characterization of host mutants that block T4 head assembly, J. Virol. **33**:366.

Reznikoff, W. S., Siegele, D. A., Cowing, D. W., and Gross, C. A., 1985, The regulation of transcription initiation in bacteria, Annu. Rev. Genet. **19**:355.

Riede, I., 1986, T-even type phages can change their host range by recombination with gene 34 (tail fibre) or gene 23 (head), Mol. Gen. Genet. **205**:160.

Riede, I., 1987a, Receptor specificity of the short tail fibers (gp 12) of T-even type Escherichia coli phages, Mol. Gen. Genet. **206**:110.

Riede, I., 1987b, Lysis gene t of T-even bacteriophages: Evidence that colicins and bacteriophage genes have common ancestors, J. Bacteriol. **169**:2956.

Riede, I., Degen, M., and Henning, U., 1985, The receptor specificity of bacteriophages can be determined by a tail fiber modifying protein, EMBO J. **4**:2343.

Riede, I., Drexler, K., Eschbach, M.-L., and Henning, U., 1986, DNA sequence of the tail fiber genes 37, encoding the receptor recognizing part of the fiber, of bacteriophages T2 and K3, J. Mol. Biol. **191**:255.

Riede, I., Drexler, K., Schwarz, H., and Henning, U., 1987a, T-even type bacteriophages use an adhesin for recognition of cellular receptors, J. Mol. Biol. **194**:23.

Riede, I., Drexler, K., Eschbach, M.-L., and Henning, U., 1987b, DNA sequence of genes 38 encoding a receptor-recognizing protein of bacteriophages T2, K3 and of K3 host range mutants, J. Mol. Biol. **194**:31.

Rodriguez Prieto, A., 1976, Isolation and characterization of mutants in a pair of Escherichia coli and T4 genes whose interaction is essential for phage development, Ph.D. Thesis, Vanderbilt University, Nashville, TN.

Rottlander, E., Hermann, K. O., and Hertel, R., 1967, Increased heterozygote frequency in certain regions of the T4 chromosome, Mol. Gen. Genet. **99**:34.

Rowe, T. C., Tewey, K. M., and Lui, L. F., 1984, Identification of the breakage-reunion subunit of T4 DNA topoisomerase, J. Biol. Chem. **259**:9177.

Saenger, W., 1984, Principles of Nucleic Acid Structure, Springer-Verlag, New York.

Sarabhai, A. S., Stretton, A. O. W., and Brenner, S., 1964, Co-linearity of the gene with the polypeptide chain, Nature **201**:13.

Schlagman, S., and Hattman, S., 1983, Molecular cloning of a functional dam$^+$ gene coding for T4 DNA-adenine methylase, Gene **22**:139.

Schmidt, F. J., and Apirion, D., 1983, T4 transfer RNAs: Paradigmatic system for the study of RNA processing, in: *Bacteriophage T4* (C. Mathews, E. Kutter, G. Mosig, and P. Berget, eds.), pp. 208–217, American Society for Microbiology, Washington.

Schoemaker, J., 1983, A T4 function which stabilizes proteins in *E. coli*, *Trends Biotechnol.* **1**:99.

Selick, H. E., Barry, J., Cha, T.-A., Munn, M., Nakanishi, M., Wong, M. L., and Alberts, B. M., 1987, Studies on the T4 bacteriophage DNA replication system, in: *DNA Replication and Recombination* (R. McMacken and T. J. Kelly, eds.), pp. 183–214, Alan R. Liss, New York.

Shah, D. B., 1976, Replication and recombination of gene *59* mutant of bacteriophage T4D, *J. Virol.* **17**:175.

Shah, D. B., and Berger, H., 1971, Replication of gene *46–47* amber mutants of bacteriophage T4D, *J. Mol. Biol.* **57**:17.

Shamoo, Y., Adari, H., Konigsberg, W. H., Williams, K. R., and Chase, J. W., 1986, Cloning of T4 gene *32* and expression of the wild-type protein under lambda promoter P_L regulation in *Escherichia coli*, *Proc. Natl. Acad. Sci. USA* **83**:8844.

Shinedling, S., Walker, L. T., and Gold, L., 1986, Cloning the complete *rIIB* gene of bacteriophage T4 and some observations concerning its middle promoters, *J. Virol.* **60**:787.

Showe, M. K., and Onorato, L., 1978, A kinetic model for form determination of the head of bacteriophage T4, *Proc. Natl. Acad. Sci. USA* **75**:4165.

Shub, D. A., Gott, J. M., Xu, M.-Q., Lang, B. F., Michel, F., Tomaschewski, J., Pedersen-Lane, J., and Belfort, M., 1988, Structural conservation among three homologous introns of bacteriophage T4 and the group I introns of eukaryotes, *Proc. Natl. Acad. Sci. USA* **85**:1151.

Siegel, P. J., and Schaechter, M., 1973, Bacteriophage T4 head maturation: Release of progeny DNA from the host cell membrane, *J. Virol.* **11**:359.

Simon, L. D., and Anderson, T. F., 1967a, The infection of *Escherichia coli* by T2 and T4 bacteriophage as seen in the electron microscope. I. Attachment and penetration, *Virology* **32**:279.

Simon, L. D., and Anderson, T. F., 1967b, The infection of *Escherichia coli* by T2 and T4 bacteriophage as seen in the electron microscope. II. Structure and function of the baseplate, *Virology* **32**:298.

Simon, L. D., and Randolph, B., 1984, Bacteriophage T4 bypass 31 mutations that make gene *31* nonessential for bacteriophage T4 replication: Isolation and characterization, *J. Virol.* **51**:321.

Simon, L. D., Randolph, B., Irwin, N., and Binkowski, G., 1983, Stabilization of proteins by a bacteriophage T4 gene cloned in *Escherichia coli*, *Proc. Natl. Acad. Sci. USA* **80**:2059.

Sinden, R. R., and Pettijohn, D. E., 1982, Torsional tension in intracellular bacteriophage T4 DNA: Evidence that a linear DNA duplex can be supercoiled *in vivo*, *J. Mol. Biol.* **162**:659.

Singer, B. S., Shinedling, S. T., and Gold, L., 1983, The *rII* genes: A history and a prospectus, in: *Bacteriophage T4* (C. Mathews, E. Kutter, G. Mosig, and P. Berget, eds.), pp. 327–333, American Society for Microbiology, Washington.

Sjöberg, B.-M., Hahne, S., Mathews, C. Z., Mathews, C. K., Rand, K. N., and Gait, M. J., 1986, The bacteriophage T4 gene for the small subunit of ribonucleotide reductase contains an intron, *EMBO J.* **5**:2031.

Skorko, R., Zillig, W., Rohrer, H., Fujiki, H., and Mailhammer, R., 1977, Purification and properties of the NAD^+: protein ADP-ribosyltransferase responsible for the T4 phage-induced modification of the subunit of the DNA-dependent RNA polymerase of *Escherichia coli*, *Eur. J. Biochem.* **79**:55.

Smith, P. R., Aebi, U., Josephs, R., and Kessel, M., 1976, Studies of the structure of the T4 bacteriophage tail sheath, *J. Mol. Biol.* **106**:243.

Smith, R. A., and Parkinson, J. S., 1980, Overlapping genes at the *cheA* locus of *Escherichia coli*, *Proc. Natl. Acad. Sci. USA* **77**:5370.

Snustad, D. P., Snyder, L., and Kutter, E., 1983, Effects on host genome structure and expression, in: *Bacteriophage T4* (C. Mathews, E. Kutter, G. Mosig, and P. Berget, eds.), pp. 40–55, American Society for Microbiology, Washington.

Snustad, D. P., Casey, A. C., and Herman, R. E., 1985, Plasmid-dependent inhibition of growth of bacteriophage T4 *ndd* mutants, *J. Bacteriol.* **163:**1290.

Snustad, D. P., Haas, N., and Oppenheimer, D. G., 1986, The bacteriophage T4 regulatory protein gp*unf/alc* binds to DNA in the absence of RNA polymerase, *J. Virol.* **60:**1145.

Snyder, L., 1983, T4 polynucleotide kinase and RNA ligase, in: *Bacteriophage T4* (C. Mathews, E. Kutter, G. Mosig, and P. Berget, eds.), pp. 351–355, American Society for Microbiology, Washington.

Snyder, L., and Jorissen, L., 1988, *E. coli* mutations which prevent the action of the T4 *unf/alc* protein map in RNA polymerase, *Genetics* **118:**173.

Spicer, E. K., and Konigsberg, W. H., 1983, Organization and structure of four T4 genes coding for DNA replication proteins, in: *Bacteriophage T4* (C. Mathews, E. Kutter, G. Mosig, and P. Berget, eds.), pp. 291–301, American Society for Microbiology, Washington.

Spicer, E. K., Rush, J., Fung, C., Reha-Krantz, L. J., Karam, J. D., and Konigsberg, W. H., 1988, Primary structure of T4 DNA polymerase: Evolutionary relatedness to eucaryotic and other procaryotic DNA polymerases, *J. Biol. Chem.* (in press).

Stahl, F. W., 1979, *Genetic Recombination: Thinking about It in Phage and Fungi*, W. H. Freeman, San Francisco.

Stetler, G. L., King, G. J., and Huang, W. M., 1979, T4 DNA-delay proteins, required for specific DNA replication, form a complex that has ATP-dependent DNA topoisomerase activity, *Proc. Natl. Acad. Sci. USA* **76:**3737.

Steven, A. C., Aebi, U., and Showe, M. K., 1976, Folding and capsomere morphology of the P23 surface shell of bacteriophage T4 polyheads from mutants in five different head genes, *J. Mol. Biol.* **102:**373.

Stevens, A., 1972, New small polypeptides associated with DNA-dependent RNA polymerase of *Escherichia coli* after infection with bacteriophage T4, *Proc. Natl. Acad. Sci. USA* **69:**603.

Stevens, A., 1977, Inhibition of DNA-enzyme binding by an RNA polymerase inhibitor from T4 phage-infected *Escherichia coli*, *Biochim. Biophys. Acta* **475:**193.

Stitt, B. L., 1978, Role of the host cell in bacteriophage T4 development, Ph.D. Thesis, California Institute of Technology, Pasadena.

Stitt, B., Revel, H., Lielausis, I., and Wood, W. B., 1980, Role of the host cell in bacteriophage T4 development. II. Characterization of host mutants that have pleiotropic effects on T4 growth, *J. Virol.* **35:**775.

Streisinger, G., Edgar, R. S., and Denhardt, G. H., 1964, Chromosome structure in phage T4. I. Circularity of the linkage map, *Proc. Natl. Acad. Sci. USA* **51:**775.

Streisinger, G., Okada, Y., Emrich, J., Newton, J., Tsugita, A., Terzaghi, E., and Inouye, M., 1966, Frameshift mutations and the genetic code, *Cold Spring Harbor Symp. Quant. Biol.* **31:**77.

Streisinger, G., Emrich, J., and Stahl, M. M., 1967, Chromosome structure in phage T4. III. Terminal redundancy and length determination, *Proc. Natl. Acad. Sci. USA* **57:**292.

Szewczyk, B., Bienkowska-Szewczyk, K., and Kozloff, L. M., 1986, Identification of T4 gene 25 product, a component of the tail baseplate, as a 15K lysozyme, *Mol. Gen. Genet.* **202:**363.

Takahashi, H. M., Kobayashi, M., Noguchi, T., and Saito, H., 1985, Nucleotide sequence of bacteriophage T4 *uvsY* gene, *Virology* **147:**349.

To, C. M., Kellenberger, E., and Eisenstark, A., 1969, Disassembly of T-even bacteriophage into structural parts and subunits, *J. Mol. Biol.* **46:**493.

Tomaschewski, J., and Rüger, W., 1987, Nucleotide sequence and primary structures of gene products coded for by the T4 genome between map positions 48.266 Kb and 39.166 Kb, *Nucleic Acids Res.* **15:**3632.

Tomaschewski, J., Gram, H., Crabb, J., and Rüger, W., 1985, T4-induced alpha- and beta-glucosyltransferase: Cloning of the genes and a comparison of their products based on sequencing data, *Nucleic Acids Res.* **13:**7551.

Tomizawa, I., 1967, Molecular mechanisms of genetic recombination in bacteriophage:

Joint molecules and their conversion to recombinant molecules, *J. Cell. Physiol.* **70** (Suppl. 1):201.

Trojanowska, M., Miller, E.S., Karam, J., Stormo, G., and Gold, L., 1984, The bacteriophage T4 *regA* gene: Primary sequence of a translational repressor, *Nucleic Acids Res.* **12**:5979.

Tschopp, J., Arisaka, F., Van Driel, R., and Engel, J., 1979, Purification, characterization and reassembly of the bacteriophage T4D tail sheath protein P18, *J. Mol. Biol.* **128**:247.

Tuerk, C., Gauss, P., Thermes, C., Groebe, D. R., Gayle, M., Guild, N., Stormo, G., D'Aubenton-Carafa, Y., Uhlenbeck, O. C., Tinoco, Jr., I., Brody, E. N., and Gold, L., 1988, CUUCGG hairpins: Extraordinarily stable RNA secondary structures associated with various biochemical processes, *Proc. Natl. Acad. Sci. USA* **85**:1364.

Uzan, M., Leautey, J., D'Aubenton-Carafa, Y., and Brody, E., 1983, Identification and biosynthesis of the bacteriophage T4 mot regulatory protein, *EMBO J.* **2**:1207.

Valerie, K., Henderson, E. E., and DeRiel, J. K., 1984, Identification, physical map location and sequence of the *denV* gene from bacteriophage T4, *Nucleic Acids Res.* **12**:8085.

Valerie, K., Henderson, E. E., and DeRiel, J. K., 1985, Expression of a cloned *denV* gene of bacteriophage T4 in *Escherichia coli*, *Proc. Natl. Acad. Sci. USA* **82**:4763.

Valerie, K., Stevens, J., Lynch, M., Henderson, E., and DeRiel, J., 1986, Nucleotide sequence and analysis of the 58.3- to 65.5-kb early region of bacteriophage T4, *Nucleic Acids Res.* **14**:8637.

Visconti, N., and Delbrück, M., 1953, The mechanism of genetic recombination in phage, *Genetics* **38**:5.

Volker, T. A., Keller, B., and Bickle, T. A., 1984, Deletion analysis of a bacteriophage T4 late promoter, *Gene* **33**:207.

Volkin, E., and Astrachan, L., 1956, Phosphorus incorporation *Escherichia coli* ribonucleic acid after infection with bacteriophage T2, *Virology* **2**:149.

Von Hippel, P. H., Kowalczykowski, S. C., Lonberg, N., Newport, J. W., Paul, L. S., Stormo, G. D., and Gold, L., 1983, Autoregulation of expression of T4 gene *32:* A quantitative analysis, in: *Bacteriophage T4* (C. Mathews, E. Kutter, G. Mosig, and P. Berget, eds.), pp. 202–207, American Society for Microbiology, Washington.

Wachsman, J. T., and Drake, J. W., 1987, A new epistasis group for the repair of DNA damage in bacteriophage T4: Replication repair, *Genetics* **115**:405.

Walker, Jr., D. H., Mosig, G., and Bayer, M. E., 1972, Bacteriophage T4 head models based on icosahedral symmetry, *J. Virol.* **9**:872.

Wakem, L. P., and Ebisuzaki, K., 1984a, An analysis of DNA repair and recombination functions of bacteriophage T4 by means of suppressors: The role of *das*, *Virology* **137**:324.

Wakem, L. P., and Ebisuzaki, K., 1984b, A new suppressor of mutations in the DNA repair-recombination genes of bacteriophage T4: *sur*, *Virology* **137**:331.

Wakem, L. P., Zahradka, C. L., and Ebisuzaki, K., 1984, The coupling of DNA repair-recombination functions with DNA replication in bacteriophage T4: A new DNA repair mutant, *Virology* **137**:338.

Warner, H. R., and Snustad, D. P., 1983, T4 DNA nucleases, in: *Bacteriophage T4* (C. K. Mathews, E. M. Kutter, G. Mosig, and P. B. Berget, eds.), pp. 103–109, American Society for Microbiology, Washington.

Watson, J. D., 1972, Origin of concatemeric T7 DNA, *Nature New Biol.* **239**:197.

Watson, N., Gurevitz, M., Ford, J., and Apirion, D., 1984, Self cleavage of a precursor RNA from bacteriophage T4, *J. Mol. Biol.* **172**:301.

Weaver, L. H., Rennell, D., Poteete, A. R., and Mathews, B. W., 1985, Structure of phage P22 gene *19* lysozyme inferred from its homology with phage T4 lysozyme, *J. Mol. Biol.* **184**:739.

Werner, R., 1968, Distribution of growing points in DNA of bacteriophage T4, *J. Mol. Biol.* **33**:679.

Werner, R., 1969, Initiation and propagation of growing points on the DNA of phage T4, *Cold Spring Harbor Symp. Quant. Biol.* **33**:501.

Whitehouse, H. L. K., 1982, *Genetic Recombination: Understanding the Mechanisms*, John Wiley, New York.

Wiberg, J. S., and Karam, J. D., 1983, Translational regulation in T4 phage development, in: *Bacteriophage T4* (C. Mathews, E. Kutter, G. Mosig, and P. Berget, eds.), pp. 193–201, American Society for Microbiology, Washington.

Wiberg, J. S., Mowrey-McKee, M. F., and Stevens, E. J., 1987, Induction of heat-shock regulon of *Escherichia coli* markedly increases production of bacterial viruses at high temperature, *J. Virol.* **62:**234.

Williams, K. P., Kassavetis, G. A., Esch, F. S., and Geiduschek, E. P., 1987, Identification of the gene encoding an RNA polymerase-binding protein of bacteriophage T4, *J. Virol.* **61:**597.

Williams, K. R., and Konigsberg, W. H., 1983, Structure-function relationships in the T4 single-stranded DNA binding protein, in: *Bacteriophage T4* (C. K. Mathews, E. M. Kutter, G. Mosig, and P. B. Berget, eds.), pp. 82–89, American Society for Microbiology, Washington.

Wilson, J. H., and Abelson, J. N., 1972, Bacteriophage T4 transfer RNA. II. Mutants of T4 defective in the formation of functional suppressor transfer RNA, *J. Mol. Biol.* **69:**57.

Winkler, U., Johns, H. E., and Kellenberger, E., 1962, Comparative study of some properties of bacteriophage T4D irradiated with monochromatic ultraviolet light, *Virology* **18:**343.

Womack, F. C., 1965, Cross reactivation differences in bacteriophage T4D, *Virology* **26:**758.

Wood, W. B., and Crowther, R. A., 1983, Long tail fibers: Genes, proteins, assembly, and structure, in: *Bacteriophage T4* (C. Mathews, E. Kutter, G. Mosig, and P. Berget, eds.), pp. 259–269, American Society for Microbiology, Washington.

Wu, J.-R., Yeh, Y.-C., and Ebisuzaki, K., 1984, Genetic analysis of *dar, uvsW* and *uvsY* in bacteriophage T4: *dar* and *uvsW* are alleles, *J. Virol.* **52:**1028.

Wu, R., Ma, F., and Yeh, Y.-C., 1972, Suppression of DNA-arrested synthesis in mutants defective in gene *59* of bacteriophage T4, *Virology* **47:**147.

Wunderli, H., Van der Broek, J., and Kellenberger, E., 1977, Studies related to the head-maturation pathway of bacteriophages T4 and T2. I. Morphology and kinetics of intracellular particles produced by mutants in the maturation genes, *J. Supramol. Struct.* **7:**135.

Yamamoto, M., and Uchida, H., 1975, Organization and function of the tail of bacteriophage T4. II. Structural control of the tail contraction, *J. Mol. Biol.* **92:**207.

Yanagida, M., Boy de la Tour, E., Alff-Steinberger, C., and Kellenberger, E., 1970, Studies on the morphopoiesis of the head of bacteriophage T-even. VIII. Multilayered polyheads, *J. Mol. Biol.* **50:**35.

Yasuda, G. K., Parker, M. L., and Mooney, D. T., 1988, The nucleotide sequence of bacteriophage T4 gene *24* and the gene *23-24* intergenic region, *J. Virol.* (in press).

Yee, J.-K., and Marsh, R. C., 1985, Locations of bacteriophage T4 origins of replication, *J. Virol.* **54:**271.

Yegian, C. D., Mueller, M., Selzer, G., Russo, V., and Stahl, F. W., 1971, Properties of DNA-delay mutants of bacteriophage T4, *Virology* **46:**900.

Yonesaki, T., and Minagawa, T., 1985, T4 phage gene *uvsX* product catalyzes homologous DNA pairing, *EMBO J.* **4:**3321.

Yonesaki, T., Ryo, Y., Minagawa, T., and Takahashi, H., 1985, Purification and some of the functions of the products of bacteriophage T4 recombination genes, *uvsX* and *uvsY*, *Eur. J. Biochem.* **148:**127.

Yudelevich, A., 1971, Specific cleavage of an *Escherichia coli* leucine transfer RNA following bacteriophage T4 infection, *J. Mol. Biol.* **60:**21.

Zograf, Y. N., Ogryz'ko, V. V., Bass, I. A., and Chernyi, D. I., 1985, Region of W-29 genes in T4 phage: Cloning and expression, *Mol. Biol. (Mosk.)* **19:**818.

Zorzopulos, J., DeLong, S., Chapman, V., and Kozloff, L. M., 1982, Host receptor site for the short tail fibers of bacteriophage T4D, *Virology* **120:**33.

CHAPTER 10

Phages of Cyanobacteria

EUGENE MARTIN AND RANDALL BENSON

I. INTRODUCTION

The cyanobacteria hold an unusually well-defined but anomalous position in the biologic world. For many years, the taxonomic position of these microorganisms was in doubt. With the advent of the electron microscope, it was determined that the cyanobacteria were prokaryotic and not eukaryotic in nature (Stanier and Van Neil, 1962). Like other prokaryotic cells (bacteria), they exhibit a homogeneous protoplasm owing to the absence of common membrane-bound organelles, such as nuclei and chloroplasts. However, the cyanobacteria also exhibit several nonbacterial characteristics. Unlike other bacteria, some cyanobacteria can be found in multicellular forms with protoplasmic connections, and all cyanobacteria contain chlorophyll and biliproteins, which are used for photosynthesis with the production of molecular oxygen.

The outstanding similarity between the cyanobacteria and other bacteria can be found in the nature of their respective cell walls. In 1965, Jost described the multilayered cyanobacterial cell wall. It closely resembles the gram-negative bacterial cell wall with respect to the major mucopeptide component. Cyanobacterial cell walls, however, are surrounded by mucilagenous sheath (Fogg *et al.*, 1973). Internal to the cell wall, the protoplasm is surrounded by a thin plasma membrane. The outer regions of the protoplasm exhibit an extensive network of flattened vesicles, the photosynthetic lamellae or thylakoids (Menke, 1961). The thylakoids and associated photosynthetic pigments are the site of cellular photosynthesis (Calvin and Lynch, 1952). Among the prominent protoplasmic inclusions identifiable in cyanobacteria are polyphosphate bodies, poly-

---

EUGENE MARTIN AND RANDALL BENSON • Department of Biological Sciences, University of Nebraska, Lincoln, Nebraska 68588-0118.

glycan bodies, polyhedral bodies, cyanophycin granules, and often gas vesicles. DNA fibrils and ribosomes are found within the nucleoplasmic region of the protoplasm.

The widespread abundance of cyanobacteria in freshwater can create a multifaceted nuisance. Cyanobacteria commonly grow to such dense populations, especially in eutrophic lakes, that they become destructive. Cyanobacterial blooms can clog the filters of reservoirs, impart musty tastes to drinking water, and produce offensive odors in recreational lakes. Their death and decay can often cause deoxygenation of water, resulting in the death of many aquatic heterotrophs including fish (Fig. 1). Some cyanobacteria, while alive, produce toxins that can kill or sicken

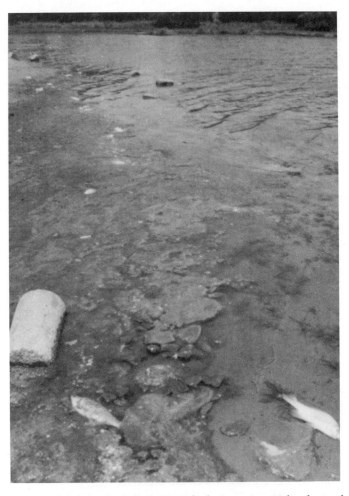

FIGURE 1. Lake within the Salt Valley Watershed in eastern Nebraska undergoing a cyanobacterial bloom with a concomitant fish kill in the summer of 1981.

fowl and cattle that drink the water (Gorham, 1960; Shilo, 1971; Fogg *et al.*, 1973). Attempts to regulate the growth of nuisance cyanobacteria have, in the past 20 years, shifted from the manipulations of physical and chemical conditions to the use of biologic agents. It was during this search for natural control agents of cyanobacterial blooms that numerous viruses lytic for both unicellular and filamentous cyanobacteria were isolated. These viruses, called algophages (Goryushin and Chaplinskaya, 1968), cyanophages (Luftig and Haselkorn, 1968; Padan *et al.*, 1967), or phycoviruses (Schneider *et al.*, 1964), were first reported with the isolation of cyanophage LPP-1 by Safferman and Morris (1963).

The cyanophages lytic for unicellular cyanobacteria are shown in Table I. SM-1, the first isolated cyanophage specific for unicellular cyanobacteria, forms clear 1- to 2-mm plaques on its hosts *S. elongatus* UTEX 563 and *Microcystis aeruginosa* NRC-1 (*Synechococcus* NRC-1 UTEX 1937) (Safferman *et al.*, 1969b). The virus possesses an icosahedral head, a very short collar, and protruding from the collar, a thin appendage that could be a tail (Safferman *et al.*, 1969b; Mackenzie and Hasselkorn, 1972a). The DNA of SM-1 has a buoyant density of 1.725 g/cm³ and a guanine + cytosine (G + C) content of 66–67% (Mackenzie and Haselkorn, 1972b). Infectious SM-1 virions contain at least 12 proteins. The two major ones have molecular weights of 40,000 and 25,000, respectively, and are considered to be the major capsid proteins (Mackenzie and Haselkorn, 1972b). Safferman *et al.* (1969b) demonstrated that cyanophage SM-1 did not require Mg^{2+} or other cations for the maintenance of viral stability.

Cyanophage AS-1 and AS-1M form clear plaques of 1–2 mm in 3–4 days or 1–2 days, respectively, at 20°C on their hosts *Anacystis nidulans* UTEX 625 or *Synechococcus cedrorum* UTEX 1191. These viruses are morphologically identical. They possess an icosahedral head, relatively rigid tail, contractile sheath, and baseplate with tail pins. The DNAs of AS-1 and AS-1M have a buoyant density of 1.714 g/cm³ and a G + C content of 52–55% (Safferman *et al.*, 1972; Sherman and Connelly, 1976). Purified infectious AS-1M virions contain about 30 distinct bands on SDS-acrylamide gels (Sherman and Connelly, 1976). The four major bands have molecular weights of 77,000, 33,000, 17,000, and 16,000, respectively. It is believed that the major head protein is probably found in the 33,000-MW band (Sherman and Pauw, 1976). AS-1 and AS-1M were also shown not to require Mg^{2+} or other cations for the maintenance of viral stability (Safferman *et al.*, 1972; Sherman and Connelly, 1976).

Cyanophage S-1 is specifically lytic for *Synechococcus* sp. NRC-1 (*Microcystis aeruginosa* NRC-1) (Adolph and Haselkorn, 1973). S-1 forms large turbid plaques only after several weeks of incubation. The virus possesses an icosahedral head, long flexible tail, and baseplate. The DNA of S-1 has a buoyant density of 1.739 g/cm³ and a G + C content of 70–74%. SDS-acrylamide gels of dissociated S-1 virions revealed at least 13 bands (Adolph and Haselkorn, 1973). Three of these bands (39,000,

Table I. Comparison of Cyanophages Specific for Unicellular Cyanobacteria

Cyanophage	Host range	Head diameter (nm)	Tail morphology	Reference
SM-1	*Synechococcus elongatus* UTEX 563 *Microcystis aeruginosa* NRC-1	67	Collar, 6 nm long	Safferman *et al.*, 1969b
AS-1	*Anacystis nidulans* UTEX 625 *Synechococcus cedrorum* UTEX 1191	90	Contractile, 250 nm long	Safferman *et al.*, 1972
S-1	*Microcystis aeruginosa* NRC-1	50	Noncontractile, 140 nm long	Adolph and Haselkorn, 1973
SM-2	*Synechococcus elongatus* UTEX 563 *Microcystis aeruginosa* NRC-1	50-55	Noncontractile, 130–140 nm long	Fox *et al.*, 1976
AS-2	*Anacystis nidulans* *Synechococcus cedrorum* *Synechococcus* sp. NRC-1	Not known	Not known	Stewart and Daft, 1976
AS-1M	*Anacystis nidulans* *Synechococcus cedrorum*	90	Contractile, 240 nm long	Sherman and Connelly, 1976
S-2L	*Synechococcus* sp. 698	56	Noncontractile, 120 nm long	Khudyakov, 1977
S-3L	*Synechococcus schmidlea*	81	Contractile, 161 nm long	Kozyakov, 1981
S-4L	*Synechococcus* sp. 698	75	Noncontractile, 300 nm long	Khudyakov and Mat-veev, 1982
S-5L	*Synechococcus* sp. 698	80	Collar, 16 nm long	Khudyakov and Mat-veev, 1982

11,000, and 10,000 MW) are considered the major structural proteins. The stabilizing effects of Mg^{2+} or other cations on cyanophage S-1 are not known.

Cyanophage SM-2 was isolated in 1976 by Fox *et al.* and has been shown to produce 0.5- to 2.0 mm plaques on lawns of either host, *Microcystis aeruginosa* NRC-1 UTEX 1937 (*Synechococcus* NRC-1) or *Synechococcus elongatus* UTEX 563, in 4–7 days. The virus possesses a

polyhedral head, narrow noncontractile flexible tail, and barlike tail plate
(Fox *et al.*, 1976) (Fig. 2). The DNA of SM-2 has buoyant density of 1.729
g/cm^3 and a G + C content 69–70%. SDS-acrylamide gels of dissociated
SM-2 virions revealed at least 11 bands. Two of these bands (with molecular weights of 39,000 and 24,000) are considered to be the major
structural proteins (Benson and Martin, 1984). Cyanophage SM-2 has
been shown to require Mg^{2+} or other cations for the maintenance of viral
stability (Benson and Martin, 1981).

Cyanophage S-2L was isolated in 1977 by Khudyakov and has been
shown to be specifically lytic for *Synechococcus* sp. 698 (Leningrad). The
virus possesses a polyhedral head; narrow, noncontractile, flexible tail;
and a connector (barlike tail plate) (Khudyakov, 1977). Cyanophage S-3L,
isolated in 1981 by Kozyakov, is lytic for *Synechococcus schmidlea* and
has a polyhedral head and contractile tail with baseplate. Cyanophages
S-4L and S-5L were isolated in 1981 by Khudyakov and Matveev. Both
lyse *Synechococcus* sp. 698 (Leningrad) and possess polyhedral heads.
S-4L has a long, noncontractile tail with connector (barlike tail plate).
S-5L possesses a short collar and no tail. A summary of the physicochemical characteristics of the unicellular cyanobacterial cyanophage
can be found in Table II.

The cyanophages lytic for filamentous cyanobacteria are shown in

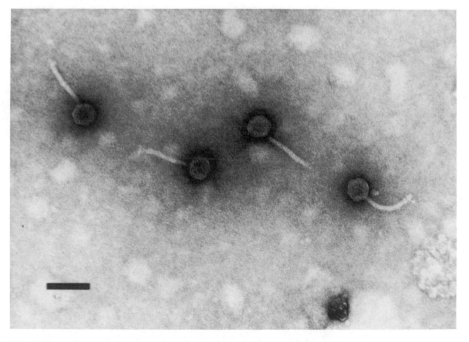

FIGURE 2. Electron micrograph of cyanophage SM-2. The intact virion is shown to possess
a polyhedral head and a long flexible tail with a barlike tail plate. Scale bar: 100 nm.

Table II. Physicochemical Characteristics of Unicellular Cyanobacterial Cyanophage Particles

	SM-1	AS-1[c]	S-1[d]	SM-2	AS-1M[g]	S-2L[h]	S-3L[i]	S-4L[i]	S-5L[i]
Type of nucleic acid	DNA	DNA	DNA	DNA[g]	DNA	DNA	DNA	DNA	DNA
Buoyant density of DNA (g/cm³)	1.725[a]	1.714	1.739	1.729[e]	1.714	—	1.80	—	—
Buoyant density in CsCl (g/cm³)	1.480[b]	—	1.501	1.483[e]	1.490	—	—	—	—
G + C content	66–67%[a]	52–55%	70–74%	69–70%[e]	52–55%	—	67.3%	46%	66%
Mg²⁺ requirement	NR	NR	—	Yes[f]	NR	—	Yes	NR	NR
Temperature of inactivation (°C)	55[a]	60	—	60[f]	50	65	57.5	70	70
Temperature range of greatest stability	4–40[a]	—	—	4–40[f]	4–45	0–60	0–45	0–60	0–60
pH range of greatest stability	5–11[a]	4–10	—	5–11[f]	4–10	4–11	6–11	5–11	5–11

[a]Safferman et al., 1969b.
[b]Mackenzie and Haselkorn, 1972b.
[c]Safferman et al., 1972.
[d]Adolph and Haselkorn, 1973.
[e]Benson and Martin, 1981.
[f]Fox et al., 1976.
[g]Sherman and Connelly, 1976.
[h]Khudyakov, 1977.
[i]Kozyakov, 1981.
[j]Khudyakov and Matveev, 1982.
NR = Not required.

TABLE III. Comparison of Cyanophages Specific
for Filamentous Cyanobacteria

Cyanophage	Host range (members of genera)	Head diameter (nm)	Tail morphology	Reference
LPP-1	Lyngbya, Plectonema, and Phormidium	60	Short, contractile	Safferman and Morris, 1963
LPP-2	Lyngbya, Plectonema, and Phormidium	60	Short, contractile	Safferman et al., 1969a
LPP-3A	Lyngbya, Plectonema, and Phormidium			Nesterova et al., 1983
A-1(L) through A-9(L)	Anabaena spp.	60–62	Long, contractile	Kozyakov, 1977
AN-11 through AN-22	Anabaena spp. Nostoc spp.	50–63	Variable	Hu et al., 1981
N-1	Nostoc muscorum	55	Long, contractile	Adolph and Haselkorn, 1971

Table III and can be divided into two groups based on the hosts lysed. These are the LPP and the A/AN/N groups. The LPP group of cyanophages have as their hosts members of the genera Lyngbya, Plectonema, and Phormidium. LPP-1, the first filamentous cyanobacterial cyanophage isolated (Safferman and Morris, 1963), has a polyhedral head and short noncontractile tail (Luftig and Haselkorn, 1968). The LPP-1 DNA has a buoyant density of 1.48 g/cm^3 and a G + C content of 53–55%. LPP-1 has 14 protein structural bands with the major bands observed at molecular weights of 39,000 and 13,000 (Sherman and Haselkorn, 1970c). LPP-1M was shown to have 13 protein structural bands with the two major bands found at molecular weights of 14,000 and 44,000 (Adolph and Haselkorn, 1972). These viruses, like other cyanophages of filamentous cyanobacteria, have an absolute requirement for divalent cations. LPP-2 (Safferman et al., 1969a) is morphologically similar to LPP-1 (polyhedral head and short noncontractile tail) but of a differing serotype (Fig. 3). Adolph and Haselkorn (1972) found that LPP-2 contains two major structural protein bands (with molecular weights of 42,000 and 11,000) among the 13 or 14 bands observed. LPP-2 also requires cations for maintenance of viral stability. LPP-3A, isolated in 1983 by Nesterova et al., belongs to the same group. It has a buoyant density of 1.706 g/cm^3. No further characterization of the virus has been done.

The second group of cyanophages specific for filamentous cyanobacteria are those that have as their host members of the genera Anabaena and Nostoc. These cyanophages are identified as A-1(L) through A-9(L) (Kozyakov, 1977) and AN-11 through AN-22 (Hu et al., 1981). All cyanophages of this group have polyhedral heads but vary in tail pres-

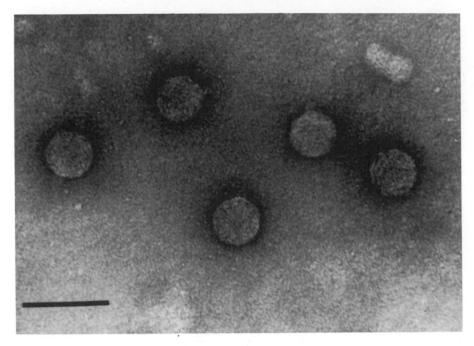

FIGURE 3. Electron micrograph of cyanophage LPP-2N, a Nebraskan isolate. The intact virion is shown to possess a polyhedral head and a short, noncontractile tail. Scale bar: 100 nm. Unpublished micrograph courtesy of S. J. Booth.

ence/length and other morphologic aspects (Table III). One of the most completely characterized cyanophages of this group is N-1 (Adolph and Haselkorn, 1971), which has as its sole host *Nostoc muscorum*. It possesses a hexagonal head and a long contractile tail with beaded fibers on the neck. The DNA of N-1 has a buoyant density of 1.696 g/cm³ and a G + C content of 37% (Adolph and Haselkorn, 1971). The major structural proteins of N-1 have molecular weights of 37,000 and 14,000, respectively. A summary of the physicochemical characteristics of cyanophages specific for filamentous cyanobacteria can be found in Table IV. The protein profiles of the cyanophages (for both unicellular and filamentous cyanobacterial hosts) mentioned throughout the foregoing text have been used as an important characteristic for cyanophage identification and comparison.

Cyanophages can be separated into groups based on their need for monovalent or divalent cations to maintain viral stability. Viruses specific for filamentous cyanobacteria (LPP-1, LPP-2, N-1) have demonstrated an absolute requirement for Mg^{2+} or similar cations. Without these cations present in the environment, viral tails separate and heads burst (Goldstein *et al.*, 1967; Luftig and Haselkorn, 1968; Safferman and Morris, 1964; Schneider *et al.*, 1964; Adolph and Haselkorn, 1971). Uni-

TABLE IV. Physicochemical Characteristics of Filamentous Cyanobacterial Cyanophage Particles

Cyanophage	Nucleic acid type	Buoyant density in CaCl (g/cm³)	G + C content	Mg²⁺ requirement	Temp. of inactivation (°C)	Temp. range of stability	pH range of stability
LPP-1[a]	DNA	1.48	53–55	Yes	55	4–40	5–11
LPP-2[b]	DNA	1.48	53–55	Yes	55	4–40	5–11
LPP-3A[c]	DNA	1.706	—	Yes	—	—	—
A-1(L)[d] through A-9(L)	DNA	—	—	—	—	—	—
AN-11[e] through AN-22	DNA	—	—	—	—	—	—
N-1[f]	DNA	1.498	37	Yes	—	—	—

[a]Luftig and Haselkorn, 1967.
[b]Safferman et al., 1969a.
[c]Nesterova et al., 1983.
[d]Kozyakov, 1977.
[e]Hu et al., 1981.
[f]Adolph and Haselkorn, 1971.

cellular cyanobacterial viruses have shown a lesser requirement for cations. SM-1 (Safferman *et al.*, 1969b), AS-1 (Safferman *et al.*, 1972), and
AS-1M (Sherman and Connelly, 1976) maintain high percentages of infectivity even after dialysis against distilled water for 10–24 h. SM-2 has
demonstrated a degree of cation sensitivity similar to that of the filamentous cyanobacterial viruses (Benson and Martin, 1984).

The action of various cyanophages on their cyanobacterial hosts has
long been of interest to researchers. The focal point of much attention has
been on alterations, or the lack thereof, to the photosynthetic lamellae of
infected host cells. It has been demonstrated that cyanophages specific
for filamentous cyanobacteria (LPP-1, LPP-1G, and N-1) cause rapid invagination and destruction of photosynthetic membranes (Sherman and
Haselkorn, 1970a; Padan *et al.*, 1970; Adolph and Haselkorn, 1972). Unicellular cyanobacterial cyanophage (SM-1, AS-1, AS-1M, and SM-2) infection of host cells, on the other hand, does not cause photosynthetic membrane invagination and destruction until late in the infection cycle
(Padan *et al.*, 1967; Pearson *et al.*, 1975; Sherman *et al.*, 1976; Leach *et
al.*, 1980) (Fig. 4).

The significance of intact or disrupted photosynthetic lamellae in
the replication of cyanophage is important. It is generally agreed that

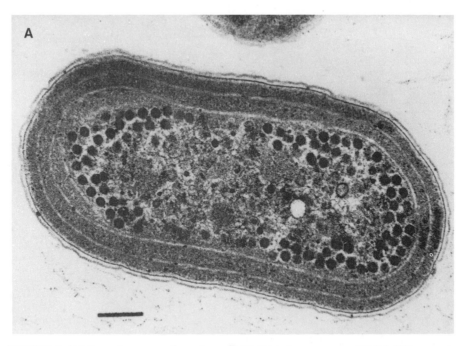

FIGURE 4. (A) *Synechococcus elongatus* and (B) *Synechococcus* sp. NRC-1 (*Microcystis
aeruginosa* NRC-1). Both electron micrographs show cells 22 h after infection with
cyanophage SM-2. In both cells, the photosynthetic lamellae remain intact, and the new
virions are predominantly found in the polar peripheries of the nucleoplasm.

viruses get the energy needed for replication from host cells. In photoautotrophic organisms, this energy would be generated by photosynthesis. To determine the role of photosynthetically derived energy in the replication of cyanophages, photosynthetic inhibition and dark incubation have been used. Examination of a filamentous cyanobacterial-cyanophage system found that the use of DCMU [3-(3,4-dichlorophenyl)-1,1-dimethylurea] caused no reduction of virus titer in LPP-1 infections, but CCCP (carbonyl-cyanide m-chlorophenyl hydrazone) completely eliminated virus replication (Sherman and Haselkorn, 1971). This suggested that the dependence of cyanophages of filamentous cyanobacteria on photophosphorylation was not complete.

The effect of photosynthetic inhibitors on the replication of unicellular cyanobacterial cyanophage differs. SM-1 infection of *Synechococcus cedrorum*, AS-1 infection of *Anacystis nidulans*, and SM-2 infection of *Synechococcus elongatus* are very dependent on the host photosynthetic mechanism (Mackenzie and Haselkorn, 1972c; Allen and Hutchinson, 1976; Benson and Martin, 1981). In these cases, viral synthesis could be completely inhibited by the use of DCMU or CCCP in the light.

In many cyanophage systems (LPP-1, N-1, SM-2), dark incubation of infected host cells for varying periods of time has been used to further elucidate the role of host cell photophosphorylation in supporting viral

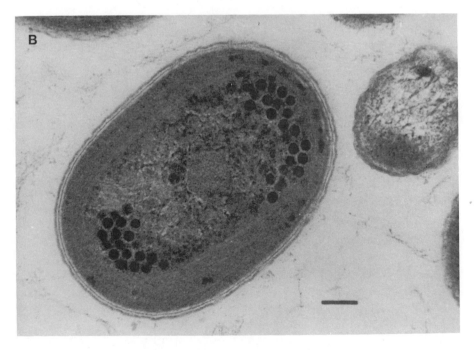

FIGURE 4. (*Continued*)

replication. In all systems examined, both unicellular and filamentous, extended dark incubation of host cells reduced or eliminated viral replication (Padan *et al.*, 1970; Adolph and Haselkorn, 1972; Benson and Martin, 1981).

Much evidence exists to demonstrate the effect of light on cyanophage replication and virus adsorption. Research (Cseke and Farkas, 1979) has suggested that light plays a stimulatory role in the adsorption of cyanophages. Cseke and Farkas (1979) demonstrated that adsorption of AS-1 to host cells in the light was double that of virus adsorption in the dark. Of equal importance was the fact that upon a 10-fold increase in Na^+ concentration in the medium, dark adsorption of AS-1 increased to the level of light-mediated adsorption found in low Na^+ medium. Since light, or the lack thereof, affects virus adsorption by decreasing the amounts of energy needed to maintain adsorption, a lack of photosynthetically derived energy would cause premature release of virus particles. This was demonstrated in the SM-2 cyanophage system.

The ensuing portions of this article will emphasize major lines of cyanophage research that have occurred since this topic was thoroughly reviewed by Brown (1972), Padan and Shilo (1973), Safferman (1973), Stewart and Daft (1976), and Sherman and Brown (1978). Possibly because the cyanobacteria occupy such a unique position among living organisms, there has occurred tremendous diversity among the lines of research pursued. This experimentation will be examined in genetic, physiological, and ecological aspects.

II. GENETICS

A. Nucleic Acids and Their Synthesis in Cyanophage-Infected Cells

Linear double-stranded DNA has been found for all the cyanophages analyzed to date. Sherman and Brown (1978) compared the DNA of three viruses that attack unicellular hosts. The molecular weight and the G + C content (%) of their DNA are respectively: SM-1, $56-62 \times 10^6$ and 66; S-1, $23-26 \times 10^6$ and 70–74; AS-1M, 57×10^6 and 52–55. Also described were three cyanophages that parasitize filamentous hosts. The DNA of these viruses had the following molecular weights and G + C contents (%): LPP-1, 27×10^6 and 53; LPP-2, 28×10^6 and 52; N-1, $41-45 \times 10^6$ and 37–41. Sherman and Brown (1978) further noted that the above-mentioned cyanophage genomes have the capacity to code for between 40 and 100 proteins.

After this brief description of cyanophage DNA, incorporation of nucleic acid precursors and viral DNA synthesis will be examined. The incorporation of nucleic acid precursors into uninfected cyanobacteria was examined by Pigott and Carr (1971). When ^{14}C-labeled purine and pyrmidine bases were included in the growth medium of A. nidulans, minimal amounts were taken up and incorporated as measured by the TCA-precipitable material. With the exception of uracil, only a very small proportion of the total exogenous material was assimilated by the cyanobacterium. Sherman and Pauw (1976) demonstrated that uninfected cells of S. cedrorum were relatively impermeable to ^{3}H-adenine and ^{3}H-uracil. However, upon infection with AS-1M, a rise in the uptake of these materials occurred at 3 h postinfection and continued throughout the remainder of the 12-h lytic cycle. The ^{3}H-adenine was then found incorporated into the newly synthesized AS-1M DNA. Blashka et al. (1982) found increased uptake of ^{3}H-adenine, ^{3}H-thymidine, ^{3}H-uracil, and ^{14}C-uridine in AS-1-infected cells of A. nidulans. For all of these nucleic acid precursor substrates, over 50% of the total incorporation occurred prior to the fourth hour of the 14-h replication cycle. Both ^{3}H-adenine and ^{3}H-thymidine were implicated as direct precursors for DNA synthesis in the phage-infected cells. Additional experimentation showed that an increase in the multiplicity of infection to above 5–6 did not substantially increase the uptake and incorporation of ^{14}C-adenine. Blashka et al. (1982) proposed that the altered increased incorporation of DNA precursors in AS-1-infected cells was not due to a hole-punching phenomenon generated during phage injection of its DNA, but rather occurred as a result of a single or a few phage particles causing an alteration of host permeability. Increased use of these DNA precursors would then occur via phage biosynthetic pathways.

For cyanophages that infect filamentous hosts, both Sherman and Haselkorn (1970b) with LPP-1 and its 14-h replication cycle and Nesterova et al. (1983) with LPP-3A and its 5.5-h lytic cycle found that increased levels of ^{3}H-adenine were taken up and incorporated in virus-infected cells. In both cases, ^{3}H-adenine incorporation into viral DNA began within about 1 h and continued throughout the replicative cycle.

Over the past 5 years, Blashka and Hwang-Lee and their associates have undertaken the task of unraveling the molecular mechanisms taking place in the synthesis of viral DNA in the AS-1/A. nidulans infective cycle. The cyanophage AS-1 was initially isolated by Safferman et al. (1972). Because cyanophage AS-1 and its host A. nidulans both have DNA that has a buoyant density of 1.714 g/ml, this has constrained a thorough analysis of viral DNA synthesis in this system. Hwang-Lee et al. (1982a) have found a unique type of viral DNA in A. nidulans infected with AS-1. Figure 5 shows the banding profile of AS-1 DNA and E. coli DNA in a CsCl density gradient; whereas Fig. 6 denotes the banding profile of DNA purified from A. nidulans infected with AS-1 for 5 h plus the E. coli control DNA. A new species of DNA was observed and termed phage-induced light DNA (PIL-DNA). Hwang-Lee et al. (1982a) further determined that "PIL-DNA had three distinctive characteristics: (1) buoyant density (1.701 g/ml, viz. host and phage DNA of 1.714 g/ml); (2) temporal synthesis; PIL-DNA appears during the latent hours of infection and is

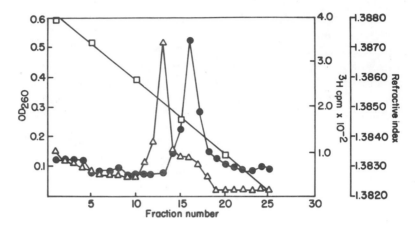

FIGURE 5. The banding profile of purified AS-1 DNA and *E. coli* DNA in a CsCl density gradient. The preparation of DNAs from cyanophage AS-1 and ^{3}H-adenine-labeled *E. coli* are described in Hwang-Lee *et al.* (1982a). The purified DNAs were then subjected to a CsCl preparative ultracentrifugation as delineated in Hwang-Lee *et al.* (1982a). The linearity of the CsCl gradient was checked by monitoring the refractive index of every fifth fraction. The fractions were monitored spectrophotmetrically for UV-absorbing material at OD_{260} nm, and 20-µl aliquots of each fraction were used to assay for alkaline-stable, acid-precipitable radioactivity. □—□, Refractive index; △—△, absorbance at 260 nm of AS-1; ●—●, [3]H– *E. coli* DNA. From Hwang-Lee *et al.* (1982a).

observed at about 5 h postinfection but is not present during the later hours (9 h postinfection); and (3) fate, no PIL-DNA has yet been detected in phage particles or uninfected host cells." However, PIL-DNA represented up to 50% of the total DNA at 5 h postinfection.

Hwang-Lee *et al.* (1982b) continued their characterization of PIL-DNA and found that ^{3}H-adenine following infection was taken up and incorporated almost exclusively into newly synthesized AS-1 DNA, with minimal amounts being associated with the PIL-DNA. This was followed through 0–9 h of the 14-h replicative cycle. In contrast, with $NaH^{14}CO_3$, the PIL-DNA was preferentially made radioactive for the period 0–5 h. For the period 6–9 h of the lytic cycle, the $^{14}CO_3$ label was found for both AS-1 DNA and PIL-DNA. Both Pearson *et al.* (1975) and Sherman *et al.* (1976) have determined that photosynthesis essentially continues up to lysis in virus-infected unicellular cyanobacteria. Blashka *et al.* (1983) further postulated that the biosynthesis of AS-1 DNA involves considerable use of precursors (e.g., ^{3}H-adenine) taken either from cellular pools directly and/or from the breakdown products of host DNA. The *de novo* biosynthesis of new precursors via photosynthesis using recently fixed CO_2 (via $NaH^{14}CO_3$) would not be a major source of AS-1 nucleotides until the later stages of the viral replicative cycle.

Blashka *et al.* (1983) extended this line of research in using cyanophages AS-1, their own laboratory strain of AS-1, and AS-1M with cyanobacterial hosts *A. nidulans* and *S. cedrorum.* In all of these com-

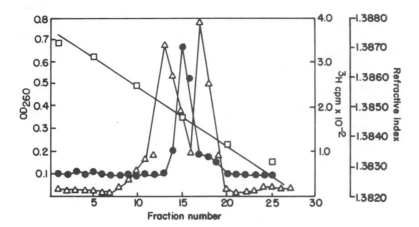

FIGURE 6. Banding profile of DNA purified from *Anacystis nidulans* infected with AS-1 for 5 h in a CsCl density gradient. An exponential growing synchronized culture of *A. nidulans* was infected with AS-1 for 5 h. The preparation of DNAs from infected cells and ^{3}H-adenine-labeled *E. coli* were described in Hwang-Lee *et al.* (1982a). The purified DNAs were then subjected to a CsCl preparative ultracentrifugation as delineated in Hwang-Lee *et al.* (1982a). The linearity of the CsCl gradient was checked by monitoring the refractive index of every fifth fraction. The fractions were monitored spectrophotometrically for UV-absorbing material at OD_{260} nm, and 20-µl aliquots of each fraction were used to assay for alkaline-stable, acid-precipitable radioactivity. □—□, Refractive index; △—△, absorbance at 260 nm of infected *A. nidulans*; ●—● ^{3}H–*E. coli* DNA. From Hwang-Lee *et al.* (1982a).

binations, PIL-DNA was formed with label from $NaH^{14}CO_3$, whereas newly synthesized viral DNA contained label from ^{3}H-adenine. Later in the replicative cycle, label from $NaH^{14}CO_3$ was also noted in the viral DNA. Use of other precursors such as ^{3}H-thymidine, ^{3}H-uracil, and ^{14}C-glucose-6-phosphate in place of the ^{3}H-adenine all resulted in the radioactivity's being rapidly associated with phage DNA and not the PIL-DNA.

Hwang-Lee *et al.* (1983a) continued their research to help more fully elucidate the nature of PIL-DNA. They concluded that both preexisting host DNA and preexisting AS-1 DNA are involved in the synthesis of PIL-DNA. When Sherman and Pauw (1976) examined the fate of labeled host DNA of *S. cedrorum* infected by AS-1M, the breakdown of the *S. cedrorum* DNA began almost immediately after infection and was optimal by 3 h of the 12-h replicative cycle. This DNA degradation occurred in response to the formation of a phage-dependent early protein with nuclease activity.

Szekeres (1981) and Szekeres *et al.* (1983) have described a restriction-modification system in *A. nidulans* infected by cyanophage AS-1. AS-1-infected cells were found to contain an endonuclease that split host DNA but not AS-1 DNA. This could be the same or similar enzyme to that described above by Sherman and Pauw (1976).

Returning to both the AS-1 and the AS-1M systems, the early breakdown of the host DNA and the subsequent incorporation of its nucleotides are apparent. A further conclusion for the AS-1 work was that the production of PIL-DNA was dependent on the integrity of the cyano-phage DNA. Hwang-Lee et al. (1983a) further postulated:

> Perhaps the PIL-DNA is an intermediate in the production of new viral DNA which utilizes the intact phage DNA genomes or stretches of phage DNA, along with degraded host DNA and newly synthesized components derived from freshly photoreduced carbon (^{14}C). If this is true, the remaining un-answered question is why this PIL-DNA is banding at a different buoyant density to that of the host/phage DNA.

Previously, Hwang-Lee et al. (1982a) had determined that upon den-sity-gradient centrifugation, PIL-DNA had a much lighter density than AS-1 DNA. In a later paper, Hwang-Lee et al. (1983a) reported that AS-1 DNA and PIL-DNA have many characteristics in common: fractionating properties on polylysine Kieselguhr chromatography, equal base com-positions when calculated from thermal denaturation data, and almost identical restriction fragments. Such a discrepancy between density-gra-dient centrifugation properties and thermal denaturation could involve the presence of a modified base. The authors postulated that since PIL-DNA has a lighter buoyant density and a T_M identical to the phage (and host) DNA, the existence of a methylated purine or pyrimidine might be expected. Thin-layer chromatography of the hydrolyzed bases from PIL-DNA suggested that the modified base present was 5-methylcytosine. When the PIL-DNA was formed in the presence of $NaH^{14}CO_3$, the ^{14}C label upon autoradiography of the separated bases was found for all the bases (including the modified base). It was therefore determined that only a portion of the cytosine found for the PIL-DNA was converted to the methylated form.

As mentioned previously, Szekeres et al. (1983) have described a restriction-modification system in AS-1-infected A. nidulans. Although the host cell DNA was readily degraded by the AS-1 endonuclease, the AS-1 viral DNA proved to be resistant to both the AS-1 endonuclease and other restriction endonucleases that all had a recognition site with a central dG-dC nucleotide. Both the work described here (Szekeres et al., 1983) and that by Hwang-Lee et al. (1982a) suggest that some form of cytosine appears to be the base affected by the modification system. At the time of these two papers, both groups indicated that further investiga-tion was necessary to completely elucidate the form of cytosine involved and when its modification actually occurred.

In addition to the modified cytosine found for AS-1, another unusual base for cyanophage S-2L has been previously reported by Kirnos et al. (1977) and Khudyakov et al. (1978). S-2L, which infects three strains of Synechococcus, has been found to have DNA that contains 2,6-di-aminopurine (2-amino-adenine) completely substituted for adenine. The 2,6-diaminopurine was found to stabilize the secondary structure of the S-2L DNA, thereby causing a somewhat higher melting temperature than that of the usual adenine-containing DNA of equivalent base composition. The authors projected that in S-2L-infected cyanobacteria, 2,6-di-aminopurine deoxyribonucleoside triphosphate is synthesized and then incorporated by DNA polymerase into newly formed S-2L DNA.

Hwang-Lee et al. (1985a) then investigated the effect that the DNA inhibitors hydroxyurea and nalidixic acid had on the AS-1 infected A. nidulans cells. These inhibitor studies were found to affect the infective system as a whole and therefore could not be utilized to distinguish specific cessation of cell DNA synthesis from cyanophage DNA synthesis. Hwang-Lee et al. (1985a) also observed that (1) the burst size of AS-1 was drastically reduced by both inhibitors, (2) release of the viruses formed occurred prematurely, and (3) nalidixic acid blocked the formation of the PIL-DNA, whereas hydroxyurea had no effect on PIL-DNA formation.

Before leaving cyanophages that infect unicellular cyanobacteria and particularly the AS-1/Anacystis system, we will examine the work of Farkas and his associates on virus-induced nucleases. Udvardy et al. (1976) found that in AS-1-infected cells exposed to light, the level of deoxyribonuclease (DNase) activity increased 15- to 20-fold 1–5 h after infection. In contrast, ribonuclease (RNase) increased 15- to 20-fold 4–5 h into the infective cycle. In complete darkness, the levels of DNase and RNase levels remained unaltered. The dramatic increase of DNase also occurred when the infected cells were exposed initially to light for 2 h and then kept in darkness for the rest of the experiment. These results will be more specifically examined in Section III of this chapter. Lehmann et al. (1979) further characterized the RNase and found it to have a molecular weight of 12,000 and a pH optimum of 7.5, to degrade RNA to short-chain oligonucleotides, and to have a relative specificity for uridylic acid. Additional work of Borbely et al. (1976) determined that AS-1 upon infecting its host interfered with the ribosomal RNA (rRNA) metabolism of A. nidulans. This interference caused an inhibition of the postmaturational cleavage of the 23S rRNA.

Sherman and Brown (1978) thoroughly reviewed the subject of viral DNA synthesis in filamentous, cyanobacterial host systems. Because host P. boryanum DNA and viral LPP-1 DNA can readily be separated on CsCl equilibrium gradients, a more complete analysis of DNA synthesis in these systems was obtained earlier than for the unicellar AS-1/Anacystis infective system.

Nesterova et al. (1983) have reported a new cyanophage (LPP-3A) for the filamentous cyanobacterial host P. boryanum. The replication cycle of 5.5 h is much shorter than the 14- to 18-h replication cycles reported for LPP-1, LPP-1A, and LPP-2. The synthesis of LPP-3A DNA begins 1.5–2 h after infection and increases up to 5 h, when the viral specific DNA accounts for 81% of the total DNA of the infected cells. Incorporation of ^{3}H-adenine into the newly synthesized viral DNA occurred rapidly at 2 h and continued throughout the infective cycle.

Mendzhul et al. (1980) examined the DNA composition of the

cyanophages A-2, LPP-1A, and N-2. All of these viruses attack filamentous cyanobacteria. Whereas A-2 and LPP-1A contained the four standard nitrogenous bases, the N-2 virus that infects *Nostoc linckia* was found to contain an anomaly in the primary structure which is manifested by the replacement of thymine with a base with different structural properties. Even with this report, most of the work concerning unusual purine and pyrimidine bases, special cyanophage restriction/modification systems, and unusual DNA (e.g., PIL-DNA) has occurred not with virus-infected filamentous sytems, but with virus-infected unicellular systems.

B. Lysogeny with Emphasis on Filamentous Cyanobacteria

This topic was extensively reviewed by Sherman and Brown in 1978. As mentioned by these authors, a great deal of energy was being expended in this area to help elucidate the processes of lysogeny and transduction in the hope that the cyanobacteria and their viruses could then be used for sophisticated genetic mapping. Most of the early reports of lysogeny involved the host *P. boryanum* and the following cyanophages: LPP-1D (Cannon *et al.*, 1971); LPP-1D and LPP-2 (Cannon and Shane, 1972); P-2 (Singh and Singh, 1972; Singh *et al.*, 1969); LPP-2SPI (Padan *et al.* 1972); and N-1 (Singh, 1975). Singh and Singh (1972) and Singh *et al.*, (1969) also worked with AR-1 and *Anabaenopsis raciborskii*.

The LPP-2SPI with its host *P. boryanum* became the definitive system for the study of lysogeny in the cyanobacteria. The important papers of Padan *et al.* (1972) and Rimon and Oppenheim (1975, 1976) will be only briefly critiqued here, since they are thoroughly reviewed by Sherman and Brown (1978).

Padan *et al.* (1972) worked with a strain of *P. boryanum* referred to as "SPI" that continually liberated phages and that, although immune to superinfection of LPP-2 viruses, was attacked by LPP-1 viruses. Whereas ultraviolet light, X-rays, and mitomycin C were unable to cause induction, SPI seemed to contain the temperate virus now referred to as LPP-2SPI. Rimon and Oppenheim (1975) were then able to isolate a temperature-sensitive mutant of LPP-2SPI that lysogenizes *Plectonema*; this virus was termed LPP-2SPI cts 1. This new virus lysogenized its host in a stable fashion at 26°C, but when the cells were heated at 40°C in the light, the provirus was induced. The concomitant dual requirement of induction on both temperature and photosynthesis makes this a very complex system to unravel.

Cocito and Goldstein (1977) provided experimentation that continued to elucidate the lysogenic strain SPI cts 1 of the cyanobacterium *P. boryanum*. Inhibitors of transcription (actinomycin D and rifampin), translation (chloramphenicol and virginiamycin, which contains 2 components, VM and VS), and photosynthesis (DCMU and CCCP) were all employed to test their capacity to block the multiplication of phage in induced lysogens. Their findings can be summarized as follows: (1) All of the inhibitors but VS inhibit phage production. (2) VS, although inactive *per se*, increases the inhibitory action of VM. (3) All of the inhibitors produce a larger effect when added before induction than if added soon after induction. (4) The inhibition by actinomycin, rifampin, DCMU, and CCCP is higher at 26°C in the dark than at 40°C in the light.

The effect that the transcriptional inhibitor actinomycin D has when added at various phases of the lytic cycle is shown in Fig. 7. Actinomycin D greatly reduced the virus yield when added immediately after induction. This effect continued with its addition up to 2 h, but if added at 3 or 4 h, little inhibition occurred. Rifampin produced the same inhibition pattern as actinomycin D. The lytic cycle was irreversibly blocked by protein synthesis inhibitors only during the induction period. After the induction period, the protein synthesis antibiotics lost their effect quickly, showing no activity if added at about 1 h. The photosynthetic inhibitors DCMU and CCCP were also more active when added before induction than when they were added after induction, whereas DCMU and CCCP allowed no virus in the former situation; in the latter situation, either a delay in virus production or no effect at all occurred. A further experiment showed that a block of protein synthesis during induction prevents a lytic cycle development at a nonpermissive temperature.

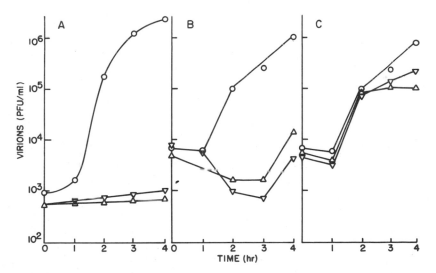

FIGURE 7. Action of transcriptional inhibitors. (A) Lysogens were induced (40°C, light, 10 min) in the absence (O) or in the presence of either rifampin (∇) or actinomycin D (△) (50 µg/ml), harvested, and transferred to antibiotic-free medium for virus multiplication. (B and C) Portions of cell cultures, which were induced in the absence of antibiotics, were incubated for 1 h with actinomycin (50 µg/ml, 26°C, dark) (control = no actinomycin) and growth further in antibiotic-free medium. (B) Control (O) and actinomycin during the 1st (△) or 2d (∇) hour after induction. (C) Control (O) and actinomycin during the 3d (△) or 4th (∇) hour after induction. From Cocito and Goldstein (1977).

Cocito and Goldstein (1977) postulated that their data indicated that (1) prophage induction in the lysogenic strain SPI cts 1 relies on the synthesis of early viral proteins; (2) induction of the viral mRNA is unstable, and it becomes rapidly inactivated when its translation is prevented; (3) inhibition of photosynthesis prevents the induction message from being expressed; and (4) it is therefore suggested that the SPI cts 1 prophage codes for a mutated repressor. This mutated repressor is reversibly inactivated at a nonpermissive temperature, and this inactivation must occur at the same time that the message coded for by the very early genes is translated for a successful induction of the lytic cycle. Cocito and Goldstein (1977) also concluded that the requirement of photosynthetic reactions for induction and not subsequent virus development suggests that lysogenic cyanobacterial processes of genetic recombination and provirus excision may require some coenzymes that are made by the photosynthetic apparatus.

With the excellent early studies of Safferman et al. (1969a) and Padan et al. (1972), followed by the definitive work of Rimon and Oppenheim (1975) and Cocito and Goldstein (1977), the lysogenic system of the SPI cts 1 strain P. boryanum has been extremely well elucidated. Before leaving the topic of lysogeny, we will examine some other reports. Padhy and Singh (1978) reported a lysogenic system involving the N-1 cyanophage and Nostoc muscorum. In contrast to the LPP-2SPI cts 1 system, heat treatment (45°C for 14 h) of the lysogenic strain failed to induce lysis, but mitomycin C (1–2μg/ml) was effective in causing lysis. Kraus (1974, 1980) has made an important contribution in focusing on the significance of the isolation and maintenance of pure strains. Through the use of host-range, plaque-morphology studies of archetype LPP-1, it was shown that certain derivatives were identical to the temperate cyanophage S-3. Kraus further suggested that with the similarities between cyanobacterial and other gram-negative bacterial cell walls, lysogeny and transduction may be a primary means of genetic exchange within the cyanobacteria and possibly to other types of bacteria.

Although all of work discussed so far has concerned filamentous cyanobacterial hosts, there have been a few preliminary reports of lysogeny with unicellular cyanobacterial systems. Bisen et al. (1985) described lysogeny in the AS-1/A. nidulans system. Vance (1977) also reported such an occurrence for a toxin-producing strain of Microcystis aeruginosa NRC-1 (this strain has now been included within the genus Synechococcus). Mitomycin C was shown to induce prophage in the toxic strains but not in the nontoxic strains. The possibility that toxigenicity was the result of the lysogenization was suggested.

C. Mutagenic Agents

Sherman and Brown (1978) have previously reviewed the major early work in this area of Rimon and Oppenheim. Therefore, this research will be only briefly summarized here. Rimon and Oppenheim (1974), through a systematic search, reported the induction and isolation of 23 N-methyl-N'-nitro-N-nitrosoguanidine (MNNG)-induced, temperature-sensitive (ts) mutants in cyanophage LPP2-SPI. They found that the mutants were arranged into 14 distinct complementation groups. The genetic map for LPP2-SPI was worked out and appeared to be linear, with no evidence of being terminally redundant or circularly permuted.

Rimon and Oppenheim (1976) then utilized the technique of sodium dodecyl sulfate (SDS)-polyacrylamide slab-gel electrophoresis and auto-radiography to examine the 24 virus-induced proteins, 12 of which are present in the mature phages. Many of the virus-induced proteins could be classified into early and late proteins, and the model suggested positive regulatory functions for their activation. Some of the viral genes were specifically involved in the shutoff of host protein synthesis. The effects of the ts mutations on LPP-2SPI gene expression at the nonpermissive temperature were followed, and this allowed the mutants to be divided into different classes. This further demonstrated that some of the viral genes have complex pleiotropic effects on protein synthesis. The linear genetic map of LPP-2SPI appears to have a region at the right end, which is involved in early phage regulation, whereas the genes responsible for head and tail formation are located in the left half of the map (Rimon and Oppenheim, 1976). As mentioned by Sherman and Brown (1978), the basic framework with this LPP-2SPI system has been established, but much remains to be done in the areas of DNA synthesis, insertion, excision, and repression.

The work in this area that has occurred subsequent to that of Rimon and Oppenheim has involved various systems but has not been as definitive. Singh and Kashyap (1976) induced host-range (h), rapid-lysis (r), and temperature-sensitive (ts) markers in cyanophage LPP-1. The h and ts markers were efficiently induced by UV, MNNG, 2-aminopurine (2AP), and acriflavine, and r mutants were induced by UV and acriflavine. Mutations induced by UV were photoreactable by visible light. In 1977, Singh and Kashyap investigated the properties of two ts mutants of spontaneous origin in LPP-1. The mechanism of temperature sensitivity is postulated as a base substitution leading to a ts protein that loses its activity under nonpermissive conditions. The two ts mutants in this study were unable to grow at the nonpermissive temperature (40°C), and the temperature-sensitive phase lasted for 2–3 h during the replicative cycle as determined by shift-up and -down experiments. The two ts mutants phages differed from the wild type in being more sensitive to both EDTA shock and photodynamic inactivation. Although all of these data with the mutant strains of LPP-1 are interesting, they have done little to definitively elucidate the real genetic basis of the system.

From 1979 until the present, the majority of work concerning mutagenic agents has involved the AS-1/*Anacystis nidulans* system. Amla (1979a) showed that mutations can be induced in cyanophage AS-1 by UV, MNNG, and acriflavine. With all three mutagens, 2-h virus-infected cells were the most sensitive to the induction of viral mutations. This can be explained by the fact that the viral genome is undergoing active replication and is prone to errors even in the presence of repair systems. The effect of UV was reversed by visible light *in vivo*, suggesting the presence of a photoreactivation enzyme in the cyanobacterium which repairs both cellular and viral DNA.

Amla (1979b) found that black, blue, and white lights were able to photoreactivate the UV-irradiated, virus-infected *A. nidulans*, whereas green, yellow, and red lights were not. But when *A. nidulans* virus-infected cells were incubated for more than 2 h in black light, there was a rapid loss in viral viability that could be restored by a shift to red light. The author postulated that two types of repair systems were functioning: (1) a cyanobacterial photoreactivating enzyme, and (2) repair of UV damage to the photosynthetic apparatus. Amla (1979c) also isolated two mutants—a yellow mutant, which was phycobilin-deficient, and a blue mutant, which had more phycobilin than normal (Fig. 8). The yellow mutant was UV-sensitive and multiplied more slowly with a reduced burst size in comparison to the AS-1 parent phage. The blue mutant was UV-resistant and had similar multiplication and burst size to the parent AS-1 virus. Photosystem II contains as its main pigment phycocyanin, which absorbs around half the light quanta required by *Anacystis* for photosynthesis (Jones and Myers, 1965). Because the blue mutant contains more phycocyanin than the parent, the author suggests that is why the blue mutant was more UV-resistant than the parent strain.

Amla (1979a, 1981a) also consistently observed that a few minute

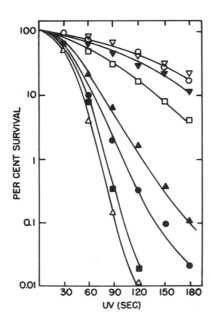

FIGURE 8. UV sensitivity (dark survival) and photoreactivation in visible light. UV sensitivity: ●, parent; ▲, blue; △, yellow mutants; ■, blue mutant + DCMU. Photoreactivation: ○, parent; ▽, blue; ▼, yellow mutants; □, blue mutant + DCMU. From Amla (1979c).

plaques appear spontaneously on plates among the normal plaques of AS-1. The frequency of these minute plaques was enhanced by mutagenic treatment. Both Amla and Singh and Kashyap (1977) in their mutagenic work with LPP-1 and ts mutants suggest that the increased sensitivity of their strains possibly reflected a phenotypic alteration in the protein coat of the respective viruses.

Kashyap and Gupta (1982) have examined the other side of the AS-1/*A. nidulans* system in their work on the pleiotrophic behavior of an AS-1-resistant mutant (AN/AS-1). AN/AS-1 was found to have a slower rate of nutrient uptake (nitrate, nitrite, ammonia, and phosphate) and an increased sensitivity to Cu^{2+}, exemplified by a higher uptake of the cation. The increased level of Cu^{2+} led in turn to a greater inhibition of acid phosphatase for the mutant strain. Previous research has elucidated the peptidoglycan, protein, and lipopolysaccharide of the gram-negative-like cell walls of *A. nidulans* (Katz et al., 1977; Samimi and Drews, 1978). Resistance to cyanophages in phage-resistant mutants is probably due to alterations in cell wall proteins and LPS that prevent AS-1 attachment. Kashyap and Gupta (1982) further suggest that the faster rate of Cu^{2+} uptake by the mutant could possibly be related to the synthesis or depression of hidden proteins (porins). This type of observation has been made by Nidaido (1979) for some mutants of *Escherichia coli* altered in their outer membrane region. Recently, Bisen et al. (1985) have also reported obtaining virus-resistant mutants of *A. nidulans* both spontaneously and by MNNG induction.

Some other recent work has involved the mutagen UV and the As-1/*A. nidulans* replicative system. Rasool (1985) studied the UV reactivation of AS-1 in host cells and has reported the existence of SOS repair for the cyanobacteria. Hwang-Lee et al. (1985b) have investigated the effect that UV irradiation prior to infection of host cells by AS-1 has on the overall replicative cycle. The results they obtained were similar to those of previous research.

III. PHYSIOLOGY

A. Cation Requirements and the Adsorption of Cyanophages to Host Cells

As mentioned previously, the LPP-1, LPP-2, and N-1 viruses, which attack filamentous hosts, and the SM-2 virus, which attacks unicellular hosts, all have an absolute requirement for Mg^{2+} or similar cations. The divalent cations are much more efficient than monovalent cations in maintaining viral infectivity. Table V illustrates the results of dialyzing cyanophage SM-2 at 4°C for 24 h against the respective solutions (Benson and Martin, unpublished data). SM-2 lost all or most of its infectivity when incubated in distilled water, deionized water, or 0.002 M EDTA.

TABLE V. Cation Stability of Cyanophage SM-2

Cation or substance	Average titer	Percent control
Dialysis vs. divalent cations		
MMH[a,b]	5.8×10^9	100
0.001 M $MgCl_2$	5.39×10^9	92.9
0.01 M $MgCl_2$	5.20×10^9	98.5
0.001 M $MnCl_2$	6.36×10^9	110
DD-H_2O	4.9×10^6	0
Dialysis vs. monovalent cations		
MMH	5.8×10^9	100
0.002 M NaCl	7.86×10^7	1.35
0.02 M NaCl	8.7×10^8	15
0.2 M NaCl	6.22×10^9	107
DD-H_2O	4.9×10^6	0
Dialysis vs. EDTA		
MMH	4.0×10^8	100
0.002 M EDTA	2.27×10^7	5.7
0.02 M EDTA	5.8×10^7	14.5
Dialysis vs. back titer		
H_2O—MMH back titer	2.1×10^7	0.4

[a]MMH, growth medium of Fox *et al.* (1976) with $2\times$ K_2HPO_4.
[b]Five milliliters of an SM-2 viral suspension was dialyzed against 2 L of each solution for 24 h with one change of solution at 12 h.

The divalent cations (Mg^{2+} or Mn^{2+}) did a better job of conferring viral stability than did the monovalent cation (Na^+). The cation requirement of SM-2 was found to be nonreversible. Infectivity could not be regained by subsequent dialysis against cation solutions.

Amla (1981b) exposed three strains of AS-1 (wild-type, a host-range mutant, and a minute plaque-forming mutant) to two chelating agents (EDTA and sodium citrate) and then diluted the respective solutions rapidly in distilled water. The free cyanophage strains were rapidly inactivated, whereas intracellular virus particles were comparatively resistant. Addition of monovalent (Na^+) and divalent cations (Mg^{2+} or Ca^{2+}) provided considerable protection to the free virus solutions. The addition of glucose or sucrose did not provide any protection for the free viral strains. From the work with both SM-2 and AS-1, it is projected that cations are involved in maintaining the integrity of phage protein subunits. Following suspension in distilled water (e.g., SM-2) or diluting the phage in the presence of a chelating agent (e.g., AS-1), the cations are removed from the phage-protein, thereby disturbing the native structure. Previous work focusing on cation requirements for LPP-1 suggested that the cations are required for DNA stabilization (Goldstein *et al.*, 1967; Luftig and Haselkorn, 1968). This was also suggested by work with the SM-2 system.

In turning to the actual adsorption of the viruses by cyanobacterial cells, Cseke and Farkas (1979) have suggested that light plays a stimulatory role in the adsorption of the cyanophage. They demonstrated that adsorption of AS-1 to host cells in the light was double that of virus adsorption in the dark. Of equal importance was that upon a 10-fold increase in Na^+ concentration in the medium, dark adsorption of AS-1 increased to the level of light-mediated adsorption found in low Na^+ medium. Since light, or the lack thereof, affects virus adsorption by decreasing the amounts of energy needed to maintain adsorption, a lack of photosynthetically derived energy would cause premature release of virus particles. This was also demonstrated in the SM-2 cyanophage system (Benson and Martin, unpublished data). Figure 9 shows that by increasing the Na^+ ion concentration to 10×, the SM-2 virus titer could be greatly increased over that of dark-incubated host cell culture virus titers. In fact, the viral titer of the dark plus 10× Na^+-incubated virus-infected cells substantially approached that of light-incubated virus-infected cells. Cseke and Farkas (1979) postulate that the effect of the cation's increasing phage adsorption and hence replication could be explained by charge neutralization permitting the phage to attach more firmly to the receptors. Light apparently exerts a similar effect on cell wall surface charges via photochemical reactions and/or light-induced changes in the immediate ionic milieu of the host cells.

Samimi and Drews (1978) report that both lipopolysaccharide and protein materials of host cells are involved as receptor materials in the adsorption of AS-1. In a proposed model system, the LPS would be responsible for the first steps of recognition, enabling the attached phage to select a position over an adhesion zone of the outer membrane and the cytoplasmic membrane. The receptor complex may also be contiguous to specific proteins that span the outer membrane and aid the phage in its injection of DNA into the host cell. Oliveira et al. (1982) further showed

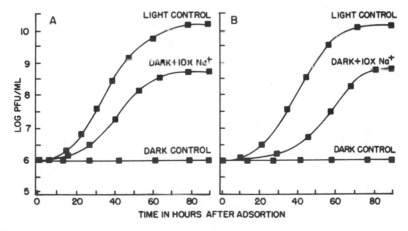

FIGURE 9. The effect of 10× Na^+ ion concentration on the replication of cyanophage SM-2 in (A) *Synechococcus elongatus* and (B) *Synechococcus* sp. NRC-1 (*Microcystis aeruginosa* NRC-1). Two-hour virus adsorption period preceded O-h virus titer.

that AS-1 adsorbed to liposomes. The results indicated that the adsorption required the presence of phosphatidylcholine (from soybean) and cholesterol, but strangely enough not algal lipids extracted from host cells of *A. nidulans.*

B. Metabolite Incorporation

In addition to their previously mentioned work on the incorporation of nucleic acid precursors in cyanophage-infected host cells, Blashka *et al.* (1982) have investigated the incorporation of labeled sugars and amino acids. Minimal amounts of glucose and glucose-6-phosphate were taken up by uninfected *A. nidulans* cells. However, substantial amounts of these sugars were taken up and incorporated by AS-1-infected cells. This uptake peaked at 6 h postinfection, after which a decrease of incorporated substrates was observed during the last 2 h of the replication cycle. The incorporation patterns for 16 amino acids by uninfected, and infected cells were examined. Although all 16 amino acids showed appreciable incorporation into uninfected cells, in the infected cells, some amino acids showed greater incorporation, some exhibited equal incorporation, and some were incorporated to a lesser level. In the case of sugars, it is possible a permease is activated in the virus-infected cells or that the sugars enter because of virus-mediated changes in the cell envelope. For the amino acids, it is more likely that the control mechanisms for transport are affected.

C. Host Metabolism and Cyanophage Replication

Farkas and his associates have conducted extensive studies on the ability of the cyanobacteria to regulate their metabolism at the level of gene expression (Udvardy *et al.*, 1984; Juhasz *et al.*, 1986). In addition, they have studied the effect that viruses have on selected aspects of the metabolism of infected cells (Udvardy *et al.*, 1976; Balogh *et al.*, 1979; Borbely *et al.*, 1980; Cseke *et al.*, 1981). Many of the cyanobacteria are obligate photoautotrophs, and the shift of their energy metabolism from light to dark conditions relies on the activation of the oxidative pentose phosphate cycle in uninfected cells. Udvardy *et al.* (1976) have attributed this shift to the "light inactivation of one of the key enzymes of the oxidative pathway (glucose-6-phosphate dehydrogenase) and light activation of a reductive pentose phosphate cycle enzyme, ribulose-5-phosphate kinase." Singer and Doolittle (1975) have also shown that there is a preferential dark *de novo* synthesis of glucose-6-phosphate dehydrogenase and glycogen phosphorylase, both of which are specifically required for the dark endogenous energy metabolism of the obligate photoautotrophs. These results indicate that obligate photoautotrophs have quite extensive synthetic processes that can be carried out in the dark.

Balogh *et al.* (1979), using *A. nidulans* cells infected with cyanophage AS-1, found that the phage-infected cells exhibited an enhanced activity for glucose-6-phosphate dehydrogenase. Thus, the inhibition of glucose-6-phosphate dehydrogenase in the light is lifted by the cyanophage attack. In the AS-1-infected cells, the total amount of DNA was shown to increase to a level four times higher than the DNA content of uninfected cells. Therefore, the authors postulated that the breakdown products of host DNA are insufficient to meet the requirements for building blocks of phage DNA synthesis. Additional materials for phage DNA synthesis could be obtained through the channeling of photosynthetic products via glucose-6-phosphate into the oxidative pentose phosphate pathway.

Cseke *et al.* (1981) compared the different responses of autotrophic and heterotrophic prokaryotes to phage infection and determined that the regulator properties of their respective glucose-6-phosphate dehydrogenases formed the basis for this difference. In the healthy cyanobacteria, glucose-6-phosphate dehydrogenase is maintained in a low-activity form by a powerful reducing system proposed to be a NADPH-linked thioredoxin reductase. The virus-induced processes provide for an increased consumption of the NADPH, creating a more oxidative milieu which in turn leads to the formation of the oxidized hyperactive form of glucose-6-phosphate dehydrogenase. This enzyme in a feedback type of process tries to produce more NADPH to offset the increased requirements caused by the phage infection. In work with *Escherichia coli* and other heterotrophic bacteria, no similar regulatory mechanism has been elucidated (Levy, 1979).

Borbely *et al.* (1980) found that *Anacystis* accumulated large amounts of guanosine 3'-diphosphate-5'-diphosphate (ppGpp) upon nutritional or energy starvation induced by a light-to-dark shift or by treatment with uncouplers (e.g., carbonylcyanide-m-chlorophenylhydrazone). In contrast, the phage-infected cells, when subjected to the light-dark shift or treatment with uncouplers, did not respond with ppGpp accumulation. Thus, the phage-infected *Anacystis* did not feel starvation under identical conditions to which the healthy cells exhibited a starving reaction (e.g., the accumulation of ppGpp). The authors suggest a possible simplistic explanation in that the ample reserve materials (glycogen, phycocyanin, polyphosphate) can be readily mobilized via the cyanophage attack, thereby reducing the need for the ppGpp emergency signal. It was also shown that the ability to synthesize ppGpp was not terminated by the AS-1 infection. In contrast, the infection with T4 phage in *Escherichia coli* does not affect the accumulation of ppGpp under treatments similar to those applied to the Anacystis work: "This difference in response of phage-infected heterotrophic and photoautotrophic cells to starvation seems to reflect differences in control of nutritional or energy metabolism rather than differences in ability to synthesize ppGpp," according to Borbely *et al.* (1980).

As mentioned in the Genetics section of this paper, Udvardy *et al.* (1976) found that in *A. nidulans* cells infected with AS-1, the very low nuclease levels increased dramatically. It was further determined that the virus-induced increase in the DNase level could be supported by dark metabolism if the dark period was preceded by a short exposure of the infected cells to light. Inhibition of photosystem II with DCMU during the early illumination period strongly decreased the subsequent, infection-dependent increase in the DNase activity in the dark. The authors further suggest that, "in spite of the obligate photoautotrophic nature of *A. nidulans*, dark metabolism is able to support fully the formation of some specific proteins if the triggering of their synthesis takes place in light."

The early increase of DNase activity in virus-infected *A. nidulans* was found to resemble the situation in virus-infected *E. coli* but was not observed for virus-infected photosynthetic eukaryotic cells (Udvardy *et al.*, 1976). However, when excessive cell damage had occurred late in the infection cycle, substantial RNase activity was noted in virus-infected cells of both *Anacystis* and higher plants.

Bisen *et al.* (1986), using cyanobacterium *Phormidium uncinatum* infected with LPP-1, have examined the cellular glycogen pool and nitrate reductase (NR) activity under both light and dark conditions. Cyan-

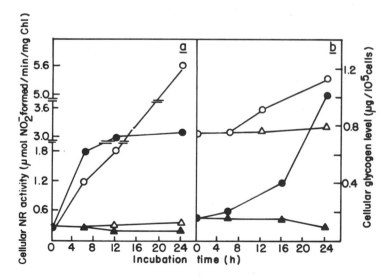

FIGURE 10. Developmental kinetics of *P. uncinatum* cellular NR activity and glycogen level after LPP-1 infection 12-h light- or dark-preincubated cultures were infected with viral lysates (infected cultures) or supplemented with equal volumes of heat-killed lysates (uninfected control cultures) and incubated under similar conditions. (a) Cellular NR activity of infected (●, ○) and uninfected (▲, △) cultures of under light (○, △) or dark (●, ▲) conditions. (b) Cellular glycogen level of infected (●, ○) and uninfected (▲, △) cultures under light (○, △) or dark (●, ▲) conditions. From Bisen *et al.* (1986).

ophage infection resulted in a steep rise in NR activity under both light and dark conditions (Fig. 10). The authors suggest that the LPP-1 enhancement of host nitrate assimilation serves to increase protein synthesis, which is required for viral multiplication. It can be seen from Fig. 10 that the cellular glycogen level for illuminated uninfected cells is about four times the glycogen level for dark-incubated uninfected cells. LPP-1 infection increased the glycogen level for both light- and dark-incubated cells. Therefore, from these observations and the earlier work of Farkas and his associates, it has been determined that glycogen is broken down via the oxidative pentose phosphate cycle in dark-incubated cyanophage-infected cells. This breakdown can then provide the energy and reductants for nitrate uptake and its reduction. For cyanophage-infected cells in the light, it is proposed that photophosphorylation and the noncyclic electron flow with its concomitant production of reducing power provide for nitrate reduction.

Further background on the effects that photosynthetic inhibitors and light-dark regimens have on cyanophage replication in both unicellular and filamentous cyanobacteria has been briefly presented in the introductory portion of this chapter and has also been thoroughly reviewed by Sherman and Brown (1978).

IV. ECOLOGY

A. Cyanophage Control of Cyanobacterial Blooms

The introduction of this chapter and the previous review articles of Padan and Shilo (1973) and Stewart and Daft (1976, 1977) have covered earlier investigations concerning the cyanophage control of cyanobacterial blooms in detail, so only some more recent work will be considered at this point.

The high specificity of cyanophages lends them to be strongly considered as ideal agents for the selective reduction or elimination of nuisance cyanobacterial species. With nuisance species being cut back or eliminated, more desirable algal species could then gain predominance. Chemical algicides often eliminate both desirable and nuisance algae. Both Desjardins and Olson (1983) in California and Martin (1982) and Martin et al. (1978) in Nebraska have made detailed studies on the cyanophage regulation of cyanobacteria in freshwater systems. The U.S. Corps of Engineers have stated that cyanobacterial blooms with the often concomitant production of toxins are among the most serious water pollution problems in freshwater bodies.

Desjardins and Olson (1983) were able to exhibit some control of bloom concentrations of *Plectonema boyanum* in outdoor pond facilities with cyanophage LPP-1. This cyanophage was most effective when present before the bloom developed. This indicated that cyanophages are more likely to be useful in preventing a cyanobacterial bloom, rather than destroying a bloom already well in progress.

Martin (1982) used a combination of cyanophage and bacterial agents to regulate cyanobacterial blooms in selected lakes of the Salt Valley Watershed of eastern Nebraska. Two substantial blooms were located and investigated from their onset. One bloom occurred in the east bay of East Twin Lake and consisted of four cyanobacterial genera: *Microcystis*, *Anabaena*, *Aphanizomenon*, and *Oscillatoria*. Barrel enclosures with open bottoms and tops were placed into the water at the edge of the lake (Fig. 11A). These enclosures each contained about 20 gal of lake water and could be set up within an hour's time. In the experiment shown, four barrel enclosures were employed. One enclosure was left alone with no biological regulatory agents added, and combinations of the various biological regulatory agents were added to the other three enclosures.

In Fig. 11B, the flask on the left was from a barrel to which no biological regulatory agents were added. Dense cyanobacterial growth was still in evidence. The flask on the right was from a barrel to which cyanophage SM-2 and several bacterial agents were added. After several

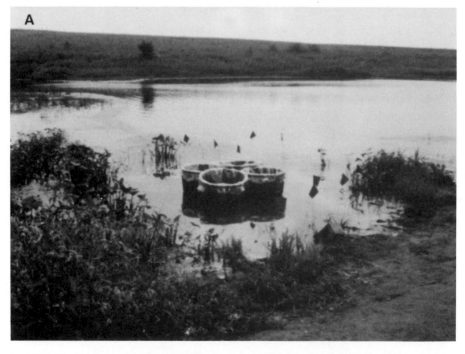

FIGURE 11. (A) Cyanobacterial bloom site in East Twin Lake, Salt Valley Watershed, in eastern Nebraska. Four-barrel enclosure placed in water at time of bloom. (B) Flasks containing samples from two of the barrels several days after initiation of the bloom. Flask on left from barrel to which no biological regulatory agents were added. Flask on right contained sample from a barrel to which a combination of biological regulatory agents was added.

days, the biological regulatory agents had greatly reduced the cyanobacterial numbers. When either the cyanophage or the bacteria were used by themselves, considerable but not optimal reduction in cyanobacteria was noted. Use of our agents in controlling certain cyanobacterial blooms in small ponds also gave some success. One outcome of these field tests was that it usually took a higher concentration of our biological regulatory agents to control the cyanobacteria in the field than in a comparable sample of a laboratory microcosm. An explanation for this is that cyanobacteria carried in the laboratory often lose the ability to produce sheath material found for the naturally occurring strains. Thus, the laboratory cyanobacteria are more susceptible to attack by biological agents.

In some related studies, Fallon and Brock (1979) have shown in Lake Mendota in Wisconsin that lytic organisms such as viruses and bacteria increase in numbers in response to the seasonal development of cyanobacteria. The peak values of plaque-forming units were in the range of 1–5 × 10³/ml. This level was about 10-fold higher than the values obtained by Daft et al. (1975) in some English reservoirs. Coulombe and Robinson (1981) investigated the collapse of Aphanizomenon flos-aquae blooms in shallow eutrophic pothole lakes in southwestern Manitoba. Although no single triggering mechanism could be determined, morphological evidence of viruslike particles within Aphanizomenon cells suggested cyanophage participation in the cell destruction. Other factors that seemed to be related to the bloom collapses were photooxidation, oxygen toxicity, and fungal and bacterial pathogens.

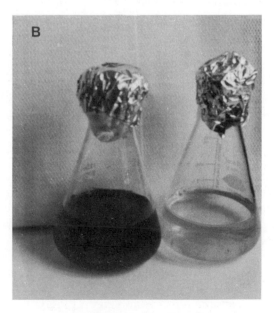

FIGURE 11. (Continued)

B. Cyanobacterial-Cyanophage Interactions in Continuous Culture

It is well documented that cyanophages are found in a wide range of freshwater bodies over considerable environmental variations. Both Safferman and Morris (1967) and Padan and Shilo (1973) have observed that the susceptible cyanobacteria were never dominant in ponds where appropriate cyanophages appeared in significant numbers. Such a population equilibrium indicates that resistant cyanobacterial strains do not develop readily and that the viruses continually lyse the sensitive cyanobacteria. Padan and Shilo (1973) noted that the foregoing scenario was indicative of the worldwide distribution of LPP-type cyanophages and their host cyanobacteria *Lyngbya*, *Phormidium*, and *Plectonema*. With other types of cyanophages, it is quite possible that virus-resistant strains of cyanobacteria could develop more readily. In this type of situation, one would expect to find larger numbers of cyanobacteria and fewer viruses. To further complicate the situation is the finding of lysogenic strains among both unicellular and filamentous cyanobacteria. Thus, under certain environmental conditions, these cyanobacterial strains themselves can serve as a source of the cyanophages.

Cannon *et al.* (1976) and Barnet *et al.* (1981) have employed continuous culture systems to investigate the long-term interactions between populations of cyanobacteria and cyanophages. When Barnet *et al.* (1981) grew the filamentous *Plectonema boryanum* 594 or the unicellular *Aphanothece stagnina* in chemostats with viruses LPP-DUN 1 and Aph-1, respectively, an initial series of reciprocal oscillations in cyanobacterial and cyanophage numbers occurred (Fig. 12). For both systems, the magnitude of these reciprocal oscillations decreased successively until an equilibrium population of the cyanobacterium and virus was established. The authors attributed the aforementioned major oscillations to the production of both mutant cyanobacteria and cyanophages. Minor fluctuations also occurred after mutant viruses appeared, probably because of the continued instability in the multicomponent system. In explaining the earlier observations of Padan and Shilo (1973) that LPP1 viruses can be continually isolated from many natural freshwater systems, Barnet *et al.* (1981) suggested that the completely resistant strains of cyanobacteria do not dominate in these systems, because they grow more slowly than the nonresistant strains. These authors summarized their work by stating that, "overall, mutant strains of both cyanobacteria and cyanophage will probably continually evolve in nature, and the use of cyanophage as an algicide will be of limited longterm value, although it may give some short-term success."

Barnet *et al.* (1984) investigated the effect that suspended particulate material had on cyanobacterial-cyanophage interactions in continuous culture. With *Plectonema* and cyanophage LPP-DUN 1, the number of

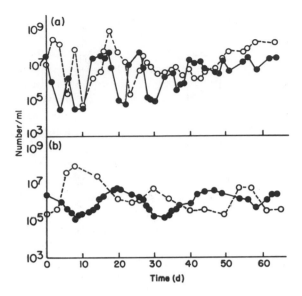

FIGURE 12. Interaction of cyanobacteria and phages in continuous cultures: (a) *Plectonema boryanum* plus LPP-DUN1, dilution rate 0–035; (b) *Aphanothece stagnina* plus Aph-1 dilution rate 0–063. ●, Cyanobacteria; ○, phages

cells and virus particles oscillated in a reciprocal manner. With the addition of the silt, the oscillation in *Plectonema* biomass was damped down without decreasing the numbers of viral particles. Although the silt could serve as a protective material and the decrease the rate of viral adsorption to the host cells, the resulting slower increase in virus titer was offset by the higher numbers of *Plectonema* cells available for viral propagation.

C. Use of Cyanobacterial-Cyanophage Systems to Bioassay Pesticides

Mallison and Cannon (1984) investigated the use of *Plectonema* and cyanophages LPP-1 and LPP-2 as an indicator system for assaying the effects of pesticides. A range of phototoxic agents had varying effects on the replication of LPP-1. In a one-step growth experiment, the following pesticides used at a concentration of 2×10 μg-ml in the medium gave a burst size (% of control) as follows: DCMV, 12; atrazine, 20; aldicarb, 32; isotox, 43; ametryn, 48; fluometeron, 86; and malathion, 103. Their work forms a promising start to the use of cyanobacterial-cyanophage assay systems to test chemical agents cheaply and quickly before testing the pesticides on plants.

V. CONCLUDING REMARKS

The prokaryotic cyanobacteria, with their characteristic of aerobic photosynthesis, comprise a position in the biologic world that closely relates them to many different types of organisms (e.g., bacteria, eukaryotic algae, and plants). With the discovery of cyanophages, this in turn provided an excellent opportunity to investigate the genetics, physiology, and ecology of virus-infected cyanobacteria. Although research in this area of virus-infected cells seemed to have peaked around 1980, the main focus of this chapter was to make a thorough appraisal of the researchers who have continued to pursue an understanding of this unique biological system: cyanobacterial cells infected with cyanophages.

REFERENCES

Adolph, K. W., and Haselkorn, R., 1971, Isolation and characterization of a virus infecting the blue-green alga *Nostoc muscorum, Virology* **46:**200.

Adolph, K. W., and Haselkorn, R., 1972, Comparison of the structure of blue-green algal viruses LPP-1M and LPP-2 and bacteriophage T7, *Virology* **47:**701.

Adolph, K. W., and Haselkorn, R., 1973, Isolation and characterization of a virus infecting a blue-green alga of the genus *Synechococcus, Virology* **54:**230.

Allen, M. M., and Hutchinson, F., 1976, Effect of some environmental factors on cyanophage AS-1 development in *Anacystis nidulans, Arch. Mikrobiol.* **110:**55.

Amla, D. V., 1979a, Mutagenesis of free and intracellular cyanophage AS-1 by ultraviolet, N-methyl-N'-nitro-N-nitrosoguanidine and acriflavine, *Mutat. Res.* **59:**147.

Amla, D. V., 1979b, Photoreactivation of ultraviolet irradiated blue-green alga *Anacystis nidulans* and cyanophage AS-1, *Arch. Virol.* **59:**173.

Amla, D. V., 1979c, Characteristics of pigment mutants of *Anacystis nidulans:* Ultraviolet sensitivity and multiplication of cyanophage AS-1, *Biochem. Physiol. Pflanzen* **174:**678.

Amla, D. V., 1981a, Isolation and characteristics of minute plaque forming mutant of cyanophage AS-1, *Biochem. Physiol. Pflanzen* **176:**83.

Amla, D. V., 1981b, Chelating agent shock of cyanophage AS-1 infecting unicellular blue-green algae, *Indian J. Exp. Biol.* **19:**209.

Balogh, A., Borbely, G., Cseke, S., Udvardy, J., and Farkas, G. L., 1979, Virus infection affects the molecular properties and activity of glucose-6-P dehydrogenase in *Anacystis nidulans,* a cyanobacterium, *FEBS Lett.* **105:**158.

Barnet, Y. M., Daft, M. J., and Stewart, W. D. P., 1981, Cyanobacteria-cyanophage interactions in continuous culture, *J. Appl. Bacteriol.* **51:**541.

Barnet, Y. M., Daft, M. J., and Stewart, W. D. P., 1984, The effect of suspended particulate material on cyanobacteria-cyanophage interactions in liquid culture, *J. Appl. Bacteriol.* **56:**109.

Benson, R. L., and Martin, E. L., 1981, Effects of photosynthetic inhibitors and light-dark regimes on the replication of cyanophage SM-2, *Arch. Microbiol.* **129**(2):165.

Benson, R. L., and Martin, E. L., 1984, Physicochemical characterization of cyanophage SM-2, *Arch. Microbiol.* **140:**212.

Bisen, P. S., Audholia, S., and Bhatnagar, A. K., 1985, Mutation to resistance for virus AS-1 in the cyanobacterium *Anacystis nidalans, Microbiol. Lett.* **29:**7.

Bisen, P. S., Bagchi, S. N., and Audholia, S., 1986, Nitrate reductase activity of a cyanobacterium *Phormidium uncinatum* after cyanophage LPP-1 infection, *Microbiol. Lett.* **33:**69.

Blashka, K. H., Hwang-Lee, L., Cohn, G., Blamire, J., and McGowan, R. E., 1982, Altered metabolite incorporation into the cyanobacteria *Anacystis nidulans* as a result of cyanophage AS-1 infection, *Microbios* 34:141.

Blashka, K. H., Hwang-Lee, L., McGowan, R. E., and Blamire, J., 1983, DNA metabolism during infection of *Anacystis nidulans* by cyanophage AS-1: 3 alternative precursors and host/phage systems for PIL-DNA, *Microbios* **36**:93.

Borbely, G., Kolcsei, M., and Farkas, G. L., 1976, The postmaturational cleavage of 23S ribosomal RNA in *Anacystis nidulans* is inhibited by infection with cyanophage AS-1, *Mol. Biol. Rep.* **3**:139.

Borbely, G., Kari, C., Gulyas, A., and Farkas, G. L., 1980, Bacteriophage infection interferes with quanosine 3'-diphosphate-5'-diphosphate accumulation induced by energy and nitrogen starvation in cyanobacterium *Anacystis nidulans*, *J. Bacteriol.* **144**:859.

Brown, R. M. Jr., 1972, Algal viruses, *Adv. Virus Res.* **17**:243.

Calvin, M., and Lynch, V., 1952, Grana-like structure of *Synechococcus cedrorum*, *Nature* **169**:455.

Cannon, R. E., and Shane, M. S., 1972, The effect of antibiotic stress on protein synthesis in the establishment of lysogeny of *Plectonema boryanum*, *Virology* **49**:130.

Cannon, R. E., Shane, M. S., and Bush, V. N., 1971, Lysogeny of a blue-green alga, *Plectonema boryanum*, *Virology* **45**:149.

Cannon, R. E., Shane, M. S., and Whitaker, J. M., 1976, Interaction of *Plectonema boryanum* (Cyanophyceae) and the LPP-cyanophages in continuous culture, *J. Phycol.* **12**:418.

Cocito, C., and Goldstein, D., 1977, Inhibition of lytic induction in lysogenic cyanophyces, *J. Virol.* **23**:483.

Coulombe, A. M., and Robinson, G. G. C., 1981, Collapsing *Aphanizomenon flos-aquae* blooms: Possible contributions of photo-oxidation, O_2 toxicity, and cyanophages, *Can. J. Bot.* **59**:1277.

Cseke, C., and Farkas, G. L., 1979, Effect of light on the attachment of cyanophage AS-1 to *Anacystis nidulans*, *J. Bacteriol.* **137**:667.

Cseke, C., Balogh, A., and Farkas, G. L., 1981, Redox modulation of glucose-6-P dehydrogenase in *Anacystis nidulans* and its "uncoupling" by phage infection, *FEBS Lett.* **126**:85.

Desjardins, P. R., and Olson, G. B., 1983, Viral control of nuisance cyanobacteria (blue-green algae), California Water Resources Center Contribution No. 185, pp. 1–35.

Fallon, R. D., and Brock, T. D., 1979, Lytic organisms and photooxidative effects: Influence on blue-green algae (cyanobacteria) in Lake Mendota, Wisconsin, *Appl. Environ. Microbiol.* **38**:499.

Fogg, G. E., Stewart, W. D. P., Fay, P., and Walsby, A. E., 1973, *The Blue-Green Algae*, Academic Press, New York.

Fox, J. A., Booth, S. J., and Martin, E. L., 1976, Cyanophage SM-2: A new blue-green algal virus, *Virology* **73**:557.

Goldstein, D. A., Bendet, I. J., Lauffer, M. A., and Smith, K. M., 1967, Some biological and physiochemical properties of blue-green algal virus LPP-1, *Virology* **32**:601.

Gorham, P. R., 1960, Toxic waterblooms of blue-green algae, *Can. Vet. J.* **1**:235.

Goryushin, V. A., and Chaplinskaya, S. M., 1968, The discovery of viruses lysing blue-green algae in the Dneprovsk reservoirs, *Mikrobiol. Zh. (Kiev)* **28**:94.

Hu, N. T., Thiel, T., Giddings, T. Jr., and Wolk, C. P., 1981, New *Anabaena* and *Nostoc* cyanophages from sewage settling ponds, *Virology* **114**:236.

Hwang-Lee, L., Blashka, K. H., Blamire, J., and McGowan, R. E., 1982a, DNA metabolism during infection of *Anacystis nidulans* by cyanophage AS-1. I. Identification of a unique species of DNA, *Microbios* **35**:49.

Hwang-Lee, L., Blashka, K. H., McGowan, R. E., and Blamire, J., 1982b, DNA metabolism during infection of *Anacystis nidulans* by cyanophage AS-1. II. Analysis of DNA synthesis patterns and discrimination of precursor utilization, *Mircobios* 35:111.

Hwang-Lee, L., Cohn, G., Blashka, K. H., Blamire, J., and McGowan, R. E., 1983a, DNA metabolism during infection of *Anacystis nidulans* by cyanophage AS-1. IV. Studies on the source of PIL-DNA, *Microbios* 36:101.

Hwang-Lee, L., Cohn, G., Blashka, K. H., McGowan, R. E., and Blamire, J., 1983b, DNA metabolism during infection of *Anacystis nidulans* by cyanophage AS-1. V. Biophysical characterization of PIL-DNA, *Microbios* **36**:191.

Hwang-Lee, L., Cohn, G., Blamire, J., and McGowan, R., 1985a, DNA metabolism during infection of *Anacystis nidulans* by cyanophage AS-1. VI. Effect of hydroxyurea and nalidixic acid on the development of cyanophage AS-1, *Microbios* **43**:245.

Hwang-Lee, L., Cohn, G., Cosowsky, L., McGowan, R., and Blamire, J., 1985b, DNA metabolism during infection of *Anacystis nidulans* by cyanophage AS-1. VII. UV-induced alterations of the AS-1/*A. nidulans* lytic cycle, *Microbios* **43**:277.

Jones, L. W., and Myers, J., 1965, Pigment variation in *Anacystis nidulans* induced by light of selected wavelength, *J. Phycol.* **1**:6.

Jost, M., 1965, Die ultrastruktur von *Oscillatoria rubescens*, D. C. *Arch. Mikrobiol.* **50**:211.

Juhasz, A., Csizmadia, V., Borbely, G., Udvardy, J., and Farkas, G. L., 1986, The pyridine nucleotide-dependent D-glucose dehydrogenase of *Nostoc* sp. strain Mac, a cyanobacterium, is subject to thioredoxin modulation, *FEBS Lett.* **194**:121.

Kashyap, A. K., and Gupta, S., 1982, Pleiotropic behavior of a cyanophage AS-1-resistant mutant of *Anacystis nidulans*, *Mol. Gen. Genet.* **185**:365.

Katz, A., Weckesser, J., Drews, G., and Mayer, H., 1977, Chemical and biological studies on the lipopolysaccharides (O-antigen) of *Anacystis nidulans*, *Arch. Microbiol.* **113**:247.

Khudyakov, I. Y., 1977, Characteristics of a new cyanophage, S-2L, lysing the unicellular cyanobacterium belonging to *Synechococcus* genus, *Mikrobiologiya* **46**:547.

Khudyakov, I. Y., and Matveev, A. V., 1982, New cyanophages S-4L and S-5L causing lysis of the cyanobacterium *Synechococcus elongatus*, *Mikrobiologiya* **51**(1):102.

Khudyakov, I. Y., Kirnos, M. D., Alexandrushkina, N. I., and Vanyushin, B. F., 1978, Cyanophage S-2L contains DNA with 2,6-diaminopurine substituted for adenine, *Virology* **88**:8.

Kirnos, M. D., Khudyakov, I. Y., Alexandrushkina, N. I., and Vanyushin, B. F., 1977, 2-Aminoadenine is an adenine substituting for a base in S-2L cyanophage DNA, *Nature* **270**:369.

Kozyakov, S. Y., 1977, Cyanophages of the series A(L) specific for the blue-green alga *Anabaena variabilis*, *Eksperimental'naya al'gologiya Trudi Petergof. Biol. Inst. (Leningrad State Univ.)* **25**:151.

Kozyakov, S. Y., 1981, Characteristics of a new cyanophage specific for the cyanobacterium *Synechococcus schmidlea*, *Mikrobiologiya* **50**(3):543.

Kraus, M. P., 1974, Host range and plaque morphology of blue-green algal viruses, Seagrant publication SG-DEL-I-74, College of Marine Studies, University of Delaware, Newark, 29 pp. (mimeographed).

Kraus, M. P., 1980, Host-range, plaque-morphology studies of cyanophage LPP-1, *J. Phycol.* **16**:186.

Leach, J. E., Lee, K. W., Martin, E. L., and Benson, R. L., 1980, Ultrastructure of the infection cycle of cyanophage SM-2 in *Synechococcus elongatus* (Cyanophyceae), *J. Phycol.* **16**:307.

Lehmann, J., Volkl, W., Udvardy, J., Borbely, G., Sivok, B., and Farkas, G. L., 1979, Characterization of a ribonuclease from *Anacystis nidulans* infected with cyanophage AS-1, *Phytochemistry* **18**:541.

Levy, H. R., 1979, Glucose-6-phosphate dehydrogenases, *Adv. Enzymol.* **48**:97.

Luftig, R., and Haselkorn, R., 1967, Morphology of a virus of blue-green algae and properties of its deoxyribonucleic acid, *J. Virol.* **1**:344.

Luftig, R., and Haselkorn, R., 1968, Studies on the structure of blue-green algae virus LPP-1, *Virology* **34**:664.

Mackenzie, J. J., and Haselkorn, R., 1972a, An electron microscope study of infection by the blue-green algal virus SM-1, *Virology* **49**:505.

Mackenzie, J. J. and Haselkorn, R., 1972b, Physical properties of blue-green algal virus SM-1 and its DNA, *Virology* **49**:497.

Mackenzie, J. J., and Haselkorn, R., 1972c, Photosynthesis and the development of blue-green algal virus SM-1, *Virology* **49**:517.

Mallison, S. M., and Cannon, R. E., 1984, Effects of pesticides on cyanobacterium *Plectonema boryanum* and cyanophage LPP-1, *Appl. Environ. Microbiol.* **47**:910.

Martin, E. L., 1982, The biological regulation of bloom-causing blue-green algae: A feasible alternative, Nebraska Water Resources Center Project Completion Report A-056, pp. 1–36.

Martin, E. L., Leach, J. E., and Kuo, K. J., 1978, Biological regulation of bloom-causing blue-green algae, in: *Microbial Ecology* (M. W. Loutit and J. A. R. Miles, eds.), pp. 62–67, Springer-Verlag, Berlin.

Mendzhul, M. I., Lysenko, T. G., and Moshkovskii, N. N., 1980, Certain peculiarities of primary DNA structure of cyanophages A-2, N-2, and LPP-1A, *Mikrobiol. Z. (Kiev)* **42**:232.

Menke, W., 1961, Uber das lamellar-system des chromatoplasms von cyanophycean, *Z. Naturf.* **16**:543.

Nesterova, N. V., Tkacheva, N. V., Sagun, T. S., and Mashkovskii, N. N., 1983, Dynamics of DNA synthesis by cyanophage LPP-3A in *Plectonema boryanum* cells, *Mikrobiologiya* **52**(3):461.

Nikaido, H., 1979, Non-specific transport through the outer membrane, in: *Bacterial Outer Membranes, Biogenesis and Functions* (M. Inouye, ed.), pp. 361–407, John Wiley, New York.

Oliveria, A. R., Mudd, J. B., Desjardins, P. R., 1982, AS-1 cyanophage adsorption to liposomes, *J. Gen. Virol.* **61**:153.

Padan, E., and Shilo, M., 1973, Cyanophages –viruses attacking blue-green algae, *Bacteriol. Rev.* **37**:343.

Padan, E., Shilo, M., and Kislev, N., 1967, Isolation of "cyanophages" from freshwater ponds and their interaction with *Plectonema boryanum, Virology* **32**:234.

Padan, E., Ginzburg, D., and Shilo, M., 1970, The reproductive cycle of cyanophage LPP-1G in *Plectonema boryanum* and its dependence on photosynthesis and respiratory systems, *Virology* **40**:514.

Padan, E., Shilo, M., and Oppenheim, A. B., 1972, Lysogeny of the blue-green alga *Plectonema boryanum* by LPP2-SPI cyanophage, *Virology* **47**:525.

Padhy, R. N., and Singh, P. K., 1978, Lysogeny in the blue-green alga *Nostoc muscorum, Arch. Microbiol.* **117**:265.

Pearson, J. J., Small, E. A., and Allen, M. M., 1975, Electron microscopic study of the infection of *Anacystis nidulans* by the cyanophage AS-1, *Virology* **65**:469.

Pigott, G. H., and Carr, N. G., 1971, The assimilation of nucleic acid precursors by intact cells and protoplasts of the blue-green alga *Anacystis nidulans, Arch. Mikrobiol.* **79**:1.

Rasool, S. A., 1985, Studies on UV reactivation of cyanophage AS-1 in the cells of cyanobacterium *Anacystis nidulans, Indian J. Exp. Biol.* **23**:38.

Rimon, A., and Oppenheim, A. B., 1974, Isolation and genetic mapping of temperature-sensitive mutants of cyanophage LPP-2SPI, *Virology* **62**:567.

Rimon, A., and Oppenheim, A. B., 1975, Heat induction of the blue-green alga *Plectonema boryanum* lysogenic for the cyanophage SPIctsI, *Virology* **64**:454.

Rimon, A., and Oppenheim, A. B., 1976, Protein synthesis following infection of the blue-green alga *Plectonema boryanum* with the temperate virus SPI and its ts mutants, *Virology* **71**:444.

Safferman, R. S., 1973, Phycoviruses, in: *The Biology of the Blue-Green Algae* (N. G. Carr and B. A. Whitton, eds.), pp. 214–237, University of California Press, Berkeley.

Safferman, R. S., and Morris, M. E., 1963, Algal virus: Isolation, *Science* 140:679.

Safferman, R. S., and Morris, M. E., 1964, Growth characteristics of the blue-green algal virus LPP-1, *J. Bacteriol.* **88**:771.

Safferman, R. S., and Morris, M. E., 1967, Observations on the occurrence, distribution and seasonal incidence of blue-green algal viruses, *Appl. Microbiol.* **15**:1219.

Safferman, R. S., Morris, M., Sherman, L. A., and Haselkorn, R., 1969a, Serological and electron microscopic characterization of a new group of blue-green algal viruses (LPP-2), *Virology* **39**:775.

Safferman, R. S., Schneider, I. R., Steere, R. L., Morris, M. E., and Diener, T. O., 1969b, Phycovirus SM-1: A virus infecting unicellular blue-green algae, *Virology* **37**:386.

Safferman, R. S., Diener, T. O., Desjardins, P. R., and Morris, M. E., 1972, Isolation and characterization of AS-1, a phycovirus infecting the blue-green algae, *Anacystis nidulans* and *Synechococcus cedrorum*, *Virology* **47**:105.

Samimi, B., and Drews, G., 1978, Adsorption of cyanophage AS-1 to unicellular cyanobacteria and isolation of receptor material from *Anacystis nidulans*, *J. Virol.* **25**:164.

Schneider, I. R., Diener, T. O., and Safferman, R. S., 1964, Blue-green algal virus LPP-1: Purification and partial characterization, *Science* **144**:1127.

Sherman, L. A., and Brown, R. M. Jr., 1978, Cyanophages and viruses of eukaryotic algae, in: *Comprehensive Virology 12* (H. Fraenkel-Conrat and R. R. Wagner eds.), pp. 145–234, Plenum Press, New York.

Sherman, L. A., and Connelly, M., 1976, Isolation and characterization of a cyanophage infecting the unicellular blue-green algae *Anacystis nidulans* and *Synechococcus cedrorum*, *Virology*, **72**:540.

Sherman, L. A., and Haselkorn, R., 1970a, LPP-1 infection of the blue-green alga *Plectonema boryanum*. I. Electron microscopy, *J. Virol.* **6**:820.

Sherman, L. A., and Haselkorn, R., 1970b, LPP-1 infection of the blue-green alga *Plectonema boryanum*. II. Viral DNA synthesis and host DNA breakdown, *J. Virol.* **6**:834.

Sherman, L. A., and Haselkorn, R., 1970c, LPP-1 infection of the blue-green alga *Plectonema boryanum*. III. Protein synthesis, *J. Virol.* **6**:841.

Sherman, L. A., and Haselkorn, R., 1971, Growth of the blue-green algae virus LPP-1 under conditions which impair photosynthesis, *Virology* **45**:739.

Sherman, L. A., and Pauw, P., 1976, Infection of *Synechococcus cedrorum* by the cyanophage AS-1M. II. Protein and DNA synthesis, *Virology* **71**:1727.

Sherman, L. A., Connelly, M., and Sherman, D., 1976, Infection of *Synechococcus cedrorum* by the cyanophage AS-1M. I. Ultrastructure of infection and phage assembly, *Virology* **71**:1.

Shilo, M., 1971, Biological agents which cause lysis of blue-green algae, *Mitt. Int. Verein. Limnol.* **19**:206.

Singer, R. A., and Doolittle, W. F., 1975, Control of gene expression in blue-green algae, *Nature* **253**:650.

Singh, P. K., 1975, Lysogeny of blue-green alga *Plectonema boryanum* by long tailed virus, *Mol. Gen. Genet.* **137**:181.

Singh, R. N., and Kashyap, A. K., 1976, Mutagenesis in cyanophage LPP-1, *Mutat. Res.* **37**:19.

Singh, R. N., and Kashyap, A. K., 1977, Isolation and characterization of temperature sensitive mutants of cyanophage LPP-1, *Mol. Gen. Genet.* **154**:31.

Singh, R. N., and Singh, P. K., 1972, Transduction and lysogeny in blue-green algae, in: *Taxonomy and Biology of Blue-Green Algae* (T. V. Desikachary, ed.), pp. 258–261, University of Madras Press, Madras, India.

Singh, R. N., Singh, P. K., and Varanasi, P. K., 1969, Lysogeny and induction of lysis in blue-green algae and their viruses, *Proc. 56th Int. Sci. Cong.* **56**:272.

Stanier, R. Y., and Van Niel, C. B., 1962, The concept of a bacterium, *Arch. Mikrobiol.* **42**:17.

Stewart, W. D. P., and Daft, M. J., 1976, Algal lysing agents of freshwater habitats, in: *Microbiology in Agriculture, Fisheries and Food* (F. A. Skinner and J. G. Carr, eds.), pp. 63–90, Academic Press, New York.

Stewart, W. D. P., and Daft, M. J., 1977, Microbial pathogens of cyanophycean blooms, in: *Advances in Aquatic Microbiology*, Vol. 1 (M. R. Droop and H. W. Jannasch, eds.), pp. 177–218, Academic Press, New York.

Szekeres, M., 1981, Phage-induced development of a site-specific endonuclease in *Anacystis nidulans*, a cyanobacterium, *Virology* **111**:1.

Szekeres, M., Szmidt, A. E., and Torok, I., 1983, Evidence for a restriction/modification-like system in *Anacystis nidulans* infected by cyanophage AS-1, *Eur. J. Biochem.* **131**:137.

Udvardy, J., Sivok, B., Borbely, G., and Farkas, G. L., 1976, Formation in the dark, of virus-induced deoxyribonuclease activity in *Anacystis nidulans*, an obligate photoautotroph, *J. Bacteriol.* **126**:630.

Udvardy, J., Borbely, G., Juhasz, A., and Farkas, G. L., 1984, Thioredoxins and the redox modulation of glucose-6-phosphate dehydrogenase in *Anabaena* sp. strain PCC 7120 vegetative cells and heterocysts, *J. Bacteriol.* **157**:681.

Vance, B. D., 1977, Prophage induction in toxic *Microcystis acruginosa* NRC-1, *Meeting of Phycology Society of America*, p. 70 (405).

CHAPTER 11

Bacteriophage P22

ANTHONY R. POTEETE

I. INTRODUCTION

P22 is a temperate phage of *Salmonella typhimurium*, in which it mediates generalized transduction (Zinder and Lederberg, 1952); its versatility in this role makes it a mainstay of *Salmonella* genetics. In the past 10 years, studies of P22 have focused primarily on three features of the phage.

1. P22 is a relative of coliphage λ. Elements of the relationship include a conserved genetic structure and small patches of DNA sequence homology. Lambda and P22 form viable hybrid phages by recombination. This relationship makes P22 the most extensively characterized of the "lambdoid" phages and affects studies of both phages. On the one hand, an enormous volume of research on λ has produced a detailed description of its life cycle, much of which is applicable in principle to P22. The predictive power of this description influences the design and interpretation of experiments involving P22, even when the process being examined is unique to P22. On the other hand, because the two phages employ fundamentally similar mechanisms in a number of processes, the description of these mechanisms in λ is enriched by comparison with P22. Comparative studies of λ- and P22-mediated transcriptional regulation have been especially fruitful.

2. P22 encodes an antirepressor. In so doing, P22 imposes an extra level of regulation on top of the mechanisms that regulate the establishment and maintenance of lysogeny—mechanisms that are otherwise fundamentally similar in P22 and λ. Antirepressor induces lytic growth by directly antagonizing the action of the phage repressor. It inactivates the

ANTHONY R. POTEETE • Department of Molecular Genetics and Microbiology, University of Massachusetts Medical School, Worcester, Massachusetts 01605.

647

repressors of a number of related phages, including that of λ. Anti-repressor synthesis is regulated at the transcriptional and translational levels by genetic elements that have no λ counterparts. Studies of P22 antirepressor's mechanism of action and its expression have made an interesting contribution to our understanding of gene regulation.

3. P22 has proved to be a particularly accessible object for morphogenetic studies. The structure and assembly of P22 capsids and baseplates, as well as aspects of DNA packaging peculiar to generalized transducing phages, are areas of ongoing interest.

The biology of P22 has been the subject of reviews by Levine (1972) and Susskind and Botstein (1978a). General methods for working with P22 have been described by Davis et al. (1980). In this chapter, few papers published before 1977 are cited. Specific earlier references can be found in the previous reviews. In particular, most of the following section is based on research reviewed by Susskind and Botstein (1978a). It is a general description of the P22 life cycle, the conceptual outline of which has not significantly changed in the past 10 years. In the past decade, however, our understanding of the molecular structures and mechanisms underlying this life cycle has grown spectacularly; this development is charted mainly in the final section, which is a description of what is known about the structures of P22 genes and the mechanisms of action of the proteins they encode.

II. LIFE CYCLE

P22 chooses between two pathways following infection of its host: lytic growth and lysogeny. Similarly, in a lysogen, prophage P22 elaborates a regulatory system that continuously chooses between maintenance of the lysogenic state and induction of lytic growth. The following description of molecular events involved in the P22 life cycle starts by considering the case of lytic growth following infection.

A. Lytic Growth

The earliest event in the infection of *Salmonella typhimurium* by P22 is binding and hydrolysis by the phage's tail of the outer polysaccharide (O antigen) portion of the bacterial lipopolysaccharide. Attachment of the virion to a secondary, more internal receptor is accompanied by ejection of a number of minor protein components of the phage. Injection of phage DNA into the cytoplasm of the host requires at least some of the ejected proteins.

The injected phage DNA serves as a template for transcription by the host cell RNA polymerase in the absence of phage-encoded factors. Three important small mRNAs are produced by this "immediate early" transcription, from three different promoters: P_L, P_R, and P_{ant} (Fig. 1). The P_L transcript encodes the gene *24* protein, which induces RNA polymerase to transcribe past terminators at the ends of the short P_L and P_R RNAs. This antitermination activity is necessary for efficient expression of downstream genes in the P_L and P_R operons. The P_R transcript encodes Cro protein, which acts as a repressor, binding to operators that overlap P_R and P_L, thus turning down the rate of transcription of the two operons (Poteete *et al.*, 1986). This turning down of P_L and P_R transcription is necessary for entry into the lytic pathway: if it does not occur, the infecting phage is channeled into lysogeny by overproduction of *c*1 protein (Winston and Botstein, 1981a; see below). The timing of these early transcriptional regulatory events must be such that gene *24* protein antiterminates a significant number of transcripts before Cro accumulates to a high enough concentration to stop their synthesis. The third significant small transcript, from P_{ant}, encodes Arc protein and antirepressor (Susskind, 1980; Susskind and Youderian, 1982; Youderian *et al.*, 1982). The function of antirepressor seems to be to induce lytic growth of any P22-related prophages that may be present in the infected cell. It is completely dispensable for both lytic growth and lysogeny by the infecting phage. Arc protein is a repressor that binds to an operator that overlaps P_{ant}, turning down transcription from it. This regulation of P_{ant} is essential: without it, antirepressor is overproduced to the point where it interferes with both lytic growth and establishment of lysogeny (Susskind, 1980).

The P22 genes that are transcribed as a result of gene *24* protein antitermination activity include those involved in homologous recombination (from P_L) as well as those involved in DNA replication and late transcriptional regulation (from P_R). Also transcribed are two regulatory genes that are involved in the establishment of lysogeny—*c*3 and *c*1. The actions of these two genes are discussed below; they will be overlooked for now in order to simplify the description of the lytic pathway.

The late transcriptional regulatory gene, *23*, encodes a protein that specifically antiterminates transcription originating from the promoter P_{LATE}. This promoter is active immediately following infection, in the absence of phage-encoded factors, but its transcripts are quite short, encoding no proteins. Under the influence of gene *23* protein, however, the P_{LATE} transcript extends through gene *9*, for a length of over 20,000 bases. The genes involved in cell lysis and phage assembly constitute a single operon (Casjens and Adams, 1985).

P22 DNA replication requires the functions of two phage genes, *18* and *12*, as well as host cell DNA replication proteins including DNA polymerase. The key product of replication is the concatemer, which is probably produced by a rolling-circle mechanism. The concatemer, containing multiple tandem repeats of the P22 genome, is the precursor of the mature phage chromosome. Packaging of DNA into virions is initiated from a specific sequence, called *pac*, and proceeds in one direction (through the head genes; see Fig. 1). The capacity of the phage head for

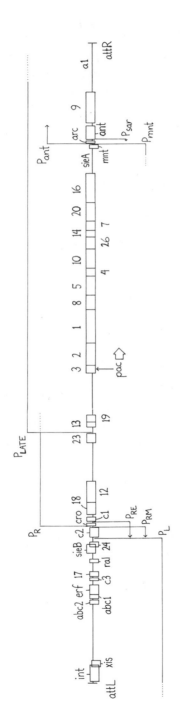

FIGURE 1. Prophage P22 genetic map. All of the genes and sites indicated, except genes 4 through sieA, and a1, are located in blocks of determined sequence (references as given in the text; S. Casjens, personal communication). Blocks of sequence are spaced according to the restriction map of Casjens et al. (1983). The map order of genes 4 through 16 is known from genetic experiments; their lengths were calculated from the molecular weights of their protein products (see Table I, 1 kD protein = 27.3 bp); it was assumed that they are closely spaced, without significant overlaps (see Susskind and Botstein, 1978; Youderian and Susskind, 1980b). The start points and extents of transcripts are shown, labeled with the names of the relevant promoters. In the cases of P_{sar} and P_{ant} the ends of the transcripts are known; P_{RM} and P_{RE} transcripts are assumed to terminate between P_L and $c2$; other 3' termini are unknown, as indicated by the dotted lines. The DNA replication origin (not shown) is thought to be located in gene 18 (see text).

DNA determines at which point in the concatemer packaging terminates with the cutting out of a mature phage chromosome. A headful of DNA (about 43,500 bp) is packaged regardless of genome size. The P22 genome size is about 41,800 bp. Thus, in the initial round, packaging begins at a *pac* site and proceeds for about 1700 bp past the next *pac* site (Casjens *et al.*, 1987). The phage chromosome produced this way has a direct sequence repeat of 1700 bp at each end. Packaging of the concatemer appears to occur in sequential steps: the second round begins where the first round ends, not at *pac*, producing a phage chromosome in which a different sequence is repeated (Fig. 2). In a population of phage particles, the sequences most often represented in the repetitious ends of the chromosomes are those immediately to the right of the *pac* site; the frequency with which a sequence element appears in the ends decreases with distance rightward from *pac*. This distribution presumably reflects the frequency with which concatemers serve as substrate for one, two, three, etc. rounds of packaging.

The limited sequence specificity of the P22 DNA packaging machinery provides a ready explanation for generalized transduction. Occasionally, packaging initiates at a *pac*-like site in the host cell chromosome, producing a sequential series of transducing particles (Schmieger, 1982).

A circular DNA molecule is needed for rolling-circle replication (as well as for prophage integration in the lysogenic pathway; see below). It is generated by homologous recombination between the heterogeneous, repetitious ends of the DNA injected by the phage. P22 can make use of either its own or the host cell's homologous recombination system for this purpose. The P22 homologous recombination system consists of Erf protein; other components, such as host-encoded factors or phage DNA replication proteins, may be involved as well. Of the two systems, that of the phage is the more active: wild-type P22 replicates well in *recA*$^+$ cells, whereas P22 *erf*$^-$ replicates poorly in wild-type cells (and, as one would expect, nonproductively in *recA*$^-$ hosts). Erf promotes a high level of intermolecular phage recombination as well. Genetic markers separated by half of the phage chromosome can segregate as if they were unlinked in phage crosses.

The assembly of P22 virions proceeds via an ordered pathway involving four steps: prohead assembly, DNA packaging, head maturation, and

FIGURE 2. Sequential headful packaging of concatemeric P22 DNA generated by rolling-circle replication.

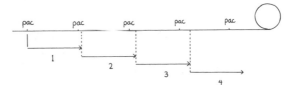

tail addition. Each step except the last involves several phage-encoded proteins. The assembly pathway is illustrated in Fig. 3.

The P22 prohead consists for the most part of a shell of the major capsid protein, the product of gene 5, assembled around a core of "scaffolding protein," the product of gene 8. In addition, four other proteins, the products of genes 1, 7, 16, and 20, are present in small amounts, possibly constituting a "portal" structure for passage of DNA. Defective proheads with normal appearance (at the level of resolution of electron microscopy) can assemble in the absence of all of the minor proteins.

In the packaging step, DNA enters the prohead, scaffolding protein leaves, and the capsid shell expands. This process requires, in addition to proheads and DNA, ATP and a protein complex with subunits encoded by phage genes 2 and 3; the 2 and 3 proteins participate in packaging without becoming permanently incorporated into the phage head. The proheads must contain gene 1 protein in order to package DNA. The other minor prohead proteins are dispensable for assembly *per se*, but the phagelike particles assembled in their absence are unable to inject DNA into the cytoplasm of the host cell in a subsequent infection. Scaffolding protein exits intact and active from the prohead and can participate in subsequent rounds of prohead assembly.

The tendency of P22 DNA packaging to initiate at the *pac* site may be conferred by gene 3 protein. Phages bearing certain mutant alleles of gene 3, designated HT, apparently package host and phage DNA at random. These high-frequency transducing strains are quite useful for *Salmonella* genetics (Sanderson and Roth, 1983).

The phage heads produced in the DNA packaging step are unstable until the protein products of genes 4, 10, and 26 are added. Heads lacking any of these proteins rapidly lose their DNA outside the cell. Phage assembly is completed by addition to the finished head of six trimers of tail protein, the product of gene 9.

Lysis of the infected cell is accomplished by two phage-encoded proteins, the products of genes 13 and 19. Gene 19 protein is a lysozyme. It gains access to the cell wall by the action of gene 13 protein, which creates channels through the cytoplasmic membrane.

B. Lysogeny

In a P22 lysogen, the phage chromosome (prophage) is integrated into the host cell chromosome. The prophage has a unique structure: it always has the same location in the host chromosome and the same gene order, as illustrated in Fig. 1. Integration is accomplished by recombination between specific sites in the phages and bacterial chromosomes, called *att*P and *att*B, respectively. Reciprocal crossing over between these two sites generates recombinant sites, *att*L and *att*R, that flank the prophage on the left and right sides, respectively, of the conventional pro-

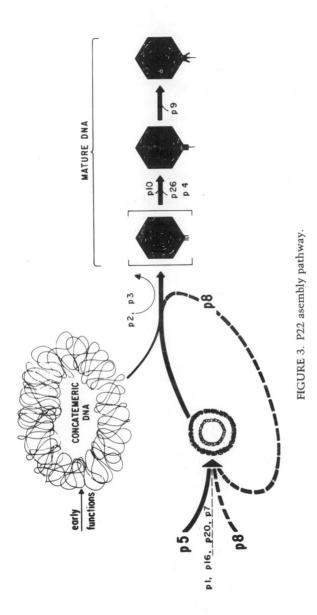

FIGURE 3. P22 asembly pathway.

phage map. This site-specific recombination requires a circular phage chromosome and integrase, the product of P22 gene *int*.

The lysogenic state is characterized by expression of a handful of phage genes involved in its maintenance and the absence of expression of genes involved in lytic growth. For the most part, this state of affairs is attributable to the action of the phage repressor, encoded by gene *c2*. Repressor binds to operators overlapping the promoters P_L and P_R, turning off transcription from them and, at the same time, turning on transcription of its own gene from P_{RM}. Maintenance of the lysogenic state also requires a second repressor, encoded by the *mnt* gene, whose sole function is to turn off expression of antirepressor by binding to an operator that overlaps P_{ant}. A P22 lysogen is "immune" to infection by P22: *c2* and *mnt* repressors in the cell bind to operator sites in the superinfecting phage's DNA, preventing expression of its lytic genes.

Three other P22 genes expressed in the lysogen impede infection by P22 or other *Salmonella* phages. The product of gene *sieB* interferes with lytic growth of a number of *Salmonella* phages; P22 itself bears a determinant called *esc* that shields it from interference by *sieB*. The *sieA* gene product interferes with DNA injection by a number of phages, including P22. The *a1* gene encodes a function that alters the structure of the bacterial O antigen, thus interfering with (but not completely eliminating) adsorption by P22.

The probability that a cell infected with P22 will become a lysogen is dependent on a number of factors, including the nutritional status of the cell and the multiplicity of infection. The availability of a preferred carbon source, such as glucose, and low multiplicity of infection promote lytic development of the phage. High-multiplicity infection in the right medium, though, can result in the conversion of nearly all the cells in a culture into lysogens. These effects on the frequency of lysogenization are probably mediated through variations in the stability and rate of synthesis of the phage's *c1* protein (Winston and Botstein, 1981b).

Gene *c1* is the first to be transcribed following antitermination of P_R transcripts. Its product is a regulatory protein that has at least two activities that promote the establishment of lysogeny. First, it induces transcription of the *c2* repressor gene from the promoter P_{RE}, which is inactive in the absence of *c1* protein (Ho *et al.*, 1986). Once repressor is made, it promotes transcription of its own gene from P_{RM}. Second, *c1* protein causes a delay in DNA replication and late gene expression. Gene *c3* protein, encoded by the P_L transcript, is thought to aid in the establishment of lysogeny by stabilizing *c1* protein.

P22 can maintain the lysogenic state indefinitely. However, exposure of the lysogen to DNA-damaging treatments can cause efficient switching into lytic growth. This process, called induction, entails reversal of repression and of prophage integration. The former is accomplished by proteolysis of *c2* repressor, promoted by activated cellular *RecA* protein. The reversal of integration, known as excision, requires expression of the phage genes *int* and *xis*. Lytic growth then ensues much as it does when P22 infects a nonlysogenic host cell, with at least two interesting differences: (1) homologous recombination is not essential for DNA replication, presumably because the necessary circular phage chromosome is generated by excisive recombination, and (2) the *mnt* repressor is probably not inactivated during induction. Its presence seems to interfere with expression of the tail gene; phages produced by induction of a lysogen are tail-deficient as a result.

C. Genetic Plasticity

It is possible to eliminate almost any P22 function by mutation and yet be left with a life form that can be propagated and that retains distinctive features of the phage's biology. As much as 40% of the P22 genome is dispensable for both lytic growth and lysogeny. Of the remainder, very little is essential for both. Moreover, any phage gene product that is normally essential for lytic growth can be made conditionally essential by propagation of the phage in host cells that have been genetically engineered to supply the gene product (or an acceptable substitute) to the infecting phage. P22 lacking its tail gene can even form plaques if it is plated with a mixture of indicator bacteria and tail protein.

Most of this genetic plasticity is not unique to P22 but rather is characteristic of bacteriophages in general. In two cases, though, particular attributes of P22 have led to the development of genetic techniques that employ phages with significantly altered genetic structures.

The first case concerns the integrative recombination system. Replacement of P22's system with that of another phage creates a hybrid that integrates at the second phage's attachment site. Its replacement with a plasmid replication origin can turn P22 into a plaque-forming plasmid like coliphage P1. Of greater practical utility, replacement of the P22 integrative recombination system with the ends of a transposon creates a hybrid that can integrate into many sites in the host chromosome when supplied with transposase. The resulting prophages are "locked in" owing to their lack of excisive recombination functions; when induced, they replicate *in situ*. DNA packaging initiated at the locked-in *pac* site proceeds in one direction along the bacterial chromosome for several sequential phage headfuls, generating a stock of defective particles that transduce nearby bacterial genes at extremely high frequencies. The construction of such P22 transposons and their use in *Salmonella* genetics have been described by Youderian *et al.* (1988).

The second case concerns the properties of P22 phages with oversize genomes. Heterologous DNA can be inserted into the P22 chromosome by genetic engineering *in vitro*, or by transposition or aberrant prophage excision *in vivo*. The headful DNA packaging mechanism of P22 gives the resulting oversize phages interesting properties. As an example, consider a P22 prophage containing a 5000-bp insertion in a gene that is not essential for lytic growth or lysogeny. Following induction, such a prophage circularizes by excisive recombination, and replicates normally. Indeed, the entire lytic pathway, including DNA packaging, proceeds normally. However, each headful of DNA that is packaged represents less than an entire genome. Even if the packaged segment contains all of the essential phage genes, it is not terminally repetitious and so will be unable to circularize by homologous recombination between its ends following infection of a subsequent host. Unable to circularize, it cannot grow lytically or form lysogens.

The defective phages can be manipulated in a number of ways, though, that make them into useful genetic tools. First, they can propagate lytically and establish lysogeny by infection at high multiplicity. Because of the permuted relationship of ends generated by packaging to sequences in the genome, two defective phages infecting the same cell are likely to have between them all of the sequences of the oversize genome. A complete, circular chromosome can be generated by intermolecular recombination and can then go on to grow lytically (as it does following induction) or to lysogenize the new host. Second, the insertion itself can serve as a counterselectable marker in genetic crosses. This property leads to a useful technique for introducing otherwise nonselectable genetic markers into P22. Insertion-bearing P22 is crossed with a hybrid plasmid that contains a segment of the P22 chromosome, a segment that includes sequences corresponding to the point at which heterologous DNA is inserted in the oversize phage. Plating of the progeny from such a cross selects for phages that have lost the insertion, and thus regained terminal repetition and plaque-forming ability, by recombination with the plasmid. Mutations in the P22 sequences borne by the plasmid, including point mutations, deletions, substitutions, and small insertions, appear at a high frequency among the recombinants. Finally, simple plating for plaque-forming revertants of oversize phages is a useful selection for phage deletion mutants. Methods for working with oversize P22 have been described by Weinstock *et al.* (1979), Fenton and Poteete (1984), and Knight *et al.* (1987).

III. GENETIC STRUCTURE AND FUNCTION

The sequence of about two-thirds of the P22 genome is known. Most of the remainder consists of structural genes encoding proteins that have been identified by SDS-PAGE. It is thus possible to draw a reasonably accurate P22 genetic map based on physical measurements rather than on recombination frequencies. In Fig. 1, the locations and boundaries of P22 structural genes with known functions are indicated, along with the origins and extents of the major transcripts. A further summary description of the structural genes, indicating functions, molecular weights of the encoded polypeptides, and the names of analogous genes in phage λ, is

TABLE I. P22 Genes and Proteins

| Gene | Function | λ Analog | Subunit mol. wt. (kD) | |
			Sequence[a]	SDS gel[b]
int	Integration, excision	*int*	44.3	42
xis	Excision	*xis*	12.8	ND[c]
abc2 ⎫	Modulation of RecBCD	*gam*	11.6	ND
abc1 ⎭	activity		10.9	ND
erf	Homologous recombination	*bet*	22.9	27.5
c3	Establishment of lysogeny	*cIII*	5.7	ND
17	Escape from Fels-2 exclusion		12.2	18.5
ral	Modulation of host restriction	*ral*	7.4	ND
sieB	Superinfection exclusion	*sieB*	22.3	ND
24	Early transcriptional control	*N*	10.6	ND
c2	Maintenance of lysogeny	*cI*	24.0	29
cro	Early transcriptional control	*cro*	6.8	ND
c1	Establishment of lysogeny	*cII*	10.1	ND
18	DNA replication	*O*	30.6	31
12		*P*	50.1	46.5
23	Late-transcriptional control	*Q*	22.3	24
13 ⎫	Lysis	*S*	11.5	10.5
19 ⎭		*R + RZ*	16.0	15
3 ⎫		*Nu1*	18.9	17
2 ⎬	DNA encapsulation	*A*	(59)[d]	67
1 ⎭		*B*	(80)	100
8	Prohead assembly; scaffolding	*Nu3*	(33.4)	39
5	Capsomere	*E + D*	ND	45.5
4 ⎫			ND	19
10 ⎬	Head stabilization	*W + FII*	ND	45.5
26 ⎭			ND	28.5
14	Unknown step in head assembly		ND	15.5
7 ⎫			ND	22
20 ⎬	DNA injection		ND	43.5
16 ⎭			ND	69
sieA	Superinfection exclusion		ND	ND
mnt	Maintenance of lysogeny	None	9.7	ND
arc	Early-transcriptional control	None	6.2	ND
ant	Antirepressor	None	34.7	33
9	Baseplate or tail	*ZUVGTHMLKIJ*	71.8	76
a1	Antigen conversion		ND	ND

[a]Molecular weights calculated from gene sequences; references as indicated in the text.
[b]Molecular weights estimated from electrophoretic mobilities in SDS polyacrylamide gels, as reported by Youderian and Susskind (1980a).
[c]Not determined.
[d]Figures in parentheses are estimates derived from incomplete DNA sequence determinations (S. Casjens, personal communication).

given in Table I. One general feature of P22 genetic structure is immediately apparent: the genes are arranged in functional clusters (lysis, heads, etc.). A second feature is that the map order of functionally analogous genes in P22 and λ is almost perfectly conserved.

The structure represented in Fig. 1 is the P22 prophage. The prophage is convenient to picture, because it is linear and has unique ends (or junctions), unlike replicating or packaged P22 DNA. The P22 integration site is designated *ata*A by *Salmonella* geneticists. It is located near minute 7 in the standard map, between *pro*A and *pro*C (Sanderson and Roth, 1983). The orientation of the prophage is such that *int* (the left end of the conventional map) is nearer *pro*A, and *a*1 (the right end) is nearer *pro*C, so left-to-right in the prophage map corresponds to clockwise in the *Salmonella* map.

The prophage map shown in Fig. 1 can be converted, in two steps, to the P22 linkage map determined by phage crosses. The first is circularization by joining *att*L and *att*R, as happens in excisive recombination. The second is a distortion introduced by a gradient of recombination frequency. Recombination frequencies per base pair are elevated in the sequence segments that are most often represented in the terminal repeats of mature phage chromosomes. Thus, genes *3*, *2*, and *1* occupy a disproportionate share of a map in which distances are proportional to recombination frequencies.

The circularity of P22's vegetative linkage map is readily understood as a consequence of its replication and packaging mechanisms. Following infection, the linear phage chromosome becomes a circle. Later, replication in the rolling-circle mode generates concatemers, in which all of the linkages between sequence elements in the circular template are conserved. Finally, because the packaging apparatus cuts the concatemer at many different sites, not just at *pac*, no two sequence elements are invariably separated by packaging. If cutting occurred exclusively at *pac*, then the map would presumably be linear, like that of phage λ, with *pac* at the ends.

In what follows, genes and sites in the P22 chromosome are discussed in the order in which they occur in the prophage map. The functional clustering of P22 genetic elements makes this approach less arbitrary than it might seem.

A. Site-Specific Recombination System

Leong *et al.* (1985) have determined the DNA sequences of *att*P and *ata*A (*att*B). The two sequences share a 46-bp common core. Restriction maps of the two prophage sites *att*L and *att*R determined by these investigators are consistent with the idea that integrative and excisive recombination involve reciprocal crossing over in the common core sequence. By analogy with λ, these investigators proposed that the crossover site is located in the center of an imperfectly symmetric sequence segment in the common core that might be an Int binding site.

In further studies of the P22 site-specific recombination system, Leong *et al.* (1986) sequenced and identified the *int* and *xis* genes. Both are transcribed leftward in the prophage map. The sequence implies that

Int is a basic polypeptide of 387 residues; Xis is a basic polypeptide of 116 residues. A phage bearing an insertion in *int* is defective in both integration and excision; an insertion in *xis* leads to a defect in excision only.

The site-specific recombination system of λ has been the subject of extensive structural and mechanistic studies (for review, see Weisberg and Landy, 1983). Comparison of λ and P22 sequences reveals very little homology but conservation of a number of structural features, including the locations of *att*P, *int*, and *xis*. Lambda Int and Xis proteins are slightly smaller than their P22 counterparts but, like them, are basic and encoded by overlapping genes. The Int proteins of λ, P22, and coliphage φ80 have statistically significant amino acid sequence homology in a short segment near the carboxyl terminus; the Xis proteins are related by similarly limited homology at the amino terminus (Leong *et al.*, 1986). Another conserved structural feature of the site-specific recombination systems is binding by *E. coli* integrative host factor (IHF) to sites in *att*. IHF binds to three sites in λ *att*P, to two in P22 *att*P, and to one in P22 *att*B; the locations of two of the λ IHF-binding sites relative to the crossover site are conserved in P22 (Leong *et al.*, 1985). This conservation of structural features encourages speculation that site-specific recombination works by similar mechanisms in P22 and λ.

B. Homologous Recombination System

Three known P22 genes are involved, directly and indirectly, in homologous recombination. The *abc* (anti-recBCD) genes modulate the activities of the host cell RecBCD protein. The *erf* (essential recombination function) gene promotes recA-independent homologous recombination.

The *abc2* gene was first detected as the locus of mutations, designated X, that confer on P22 an inability to grow in a *polA*⁻ host (Yamamoto *et al.*, 1977). In subsequent studies (Murphy *et al.*, 1987b), the *abc* genes were sequenced and further characterized. The *abc2* gene probably encodes a small polypeptide. Although Abc2 protein has not been identified, the sequence of the minimum segment of the P22 chromosome that can supply *abc2* function in *trans* from a plasmid contains an open reading frame of 97 codons with a canonical translational initiation sequence and normal codon usage. P22 lacking *abc2* is grossly defective for replication in a *polA*⁻ host and mildly defective in a wild-type host, but it produces a normal burst size in a *recB*⁻ host. The *abc1* gene encodes a polypeptide of 94 amino acid residues. Its initiation codon overlaps the termination codon of *erf*. Unlike *abc2*, *abc1* is not required for replication in a *polA*⁻ host. However, the phenotype of P22 *abc1*⁻ is qualitatively similar to that of *abc2*⁻ in a wild-type host, although its growth defect there is minimal; it can be detected as a slightly reduced plaque size. P22 lacking both *abc* genes is fully replication-proficient in a *recB*⁻ host, suggesting that the *abc* genes both function in counteracting a deleterious effect of the host RecBCD protein. However, the two *abc* genes function independently, as shown by the observation that expression of either one alone from a plasmid partially complements the double mutant phage.

The *abc* genes are functional analogues of the λ *gam* gene (for review of the λ homologous recombination functions see Smith, 1983). A plasmid that expresses λ *gam* fully complements P22 *abc1⁻ abc2⁻* (Poteete and Fenton, 1984). Most of what is known about *abc* gene functions comes from comparing the effects of plasmid-borne *gam* and *abc* expression in *E. coli* (Poteete and Fenton, 1984, and unpublished results). Gam allows λ *red⁻ gam⁻* to grow in a *recA⁻* host; Abc1 and Abc2 do not. Gam allows phage T4 bearing an amber mutation in gene *2* to form plaques on a wild-type, nonsuppressing host (Friedman and Hays, 1986); Abc1 and Abc2 together (but neither separately) partially rescue T4 *2⁻*, allowing it to form pinpoint plaques. Gam induces rolling-circle replication by ColE1-related plasmids (Cohen and Clark, 1986); the induction of similar plasmid replication by P22 requires Erf function in addition to Abc. Finally, Gam partially inhibits host-cell-dependent homologous recombination between λ phages; Abc2 inhibits the same event more strongly. In both cases, only crossovers in a chi-containing interval are inhibited. In all of these tests, Gam behaves as if it made the cell phenotypically recBCD⁻. The activity of Abc is more subtle: it seems to inhibit the RecBCD recombinase strongly, but only to moderate the RecBCD nuclease activity. The differences between *gam* and *abc* are further indicated by an apparently complete lack of sequence homology and by an inversion of map order. In λ, *gam* is located to the right of the recombination-promoting *red* genes; in P22, the *abc* genes are to the left of the recombination-promoting *erf* gene. This is the only known case of nonconservation of map order among analogous functions in the two phages.

One question raised by the foregoing observations is why P22 would have two *abc* genes to do only part of what the *gam* gene does for λ. The answer may have to do with host range. Expression of *gam* is lethal for λ in *E. coli* that is lysogenic for phage P2 (Spi phenotype—see Smith, 1983), whereas a λ hybrid bearing P22 homologous recombination genes is able to grow in such a host (Hilliker and Botstein, 1976). Modulation, rather than inactivation, of RecBCD may be advantageous in some settings.

The product of the *erf* gene is a single-strand specific DNA-binding protein that can promote annealing of homologous single strands *in vitro* (Poteete and Fenton, 1983). It shares these properties with a number of proteins involved in replication and recombination, such as the RecA and Ssb proteins of *E. coli*, the gene *32* protein of phage T4, and the β protein of phage λ. The Erf protein differs from these others, though, in having a structure that is readily visualized by electron microscopy (Poteete *et al.*, 1983). A schematic drawing of the molecule is shown in Fig. 4. It is a ring with radially projecting structures like the teeth of a gear. It appears to consist of 12 of the 204-amino acid residue Erf monomers. The Erf mono-

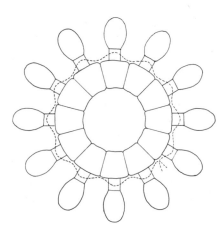

FIGURE 4. Schematic representation of Erf
protein bound to single-stranded DNA (dotted
line).

mer has two distinct domains: the aminoterminal portion of the molecule joins with others to form the ring; the carboxyterminal portion appears to be the "tooth." Amino acid sequence determinants of a number
of structural and functional elements of the Erf protein have been deduced from the properties of fragments of the molecule (Poteete *et al.*,
1983; Murphy *et al.*, 1987a). Digestion of Erf with elastase generates a
stable oligomeric aminoterminal fragment of approximately 136 residues
and a quasistable carboxyterminal fragment. The aminoterminal fragment oligomer retains the ringlike quaternary structure and single-
stranded DNA-binding specificity of the intact molecule, but it lacks the
prominent radially projecting structures.

Aminoterminal fragments of 95, 130, 149, and 190 residues generated
by amber mutant alleles of *erf* have been characterized. The 190-residue
fragment is stable *in vivo* but hypersensitive to proteases *in vitro*, where
it is rapidly degraded to a remnant that is slightly longer than the 149-
residue fragment. The 149- and 130-residue fragments are stable *in vitro*;
both form ringlike oligomers that resemble the elastase-generated aminoterminal fragment morphologically. The 149-residue fragment has the
same affinity for single-stranded DNA as intact Erf, whereas that of the
130-residue fragment is greatly decreased. The 95-residue fragment is
unstable *in vivo*. These observations have been interpreted as suggesting
that the Erf molecule consists of two distinct domains, joined by an
interdomain DNA-binding segment, as suggested in Fig. 4. According to
this view, residues between 130 and 149 are not integral parts of either
domain: not the aminoterminal domain because, unlike certain residues
between 95 and 130, they are dispensable for formation of the ring
oligomer; and not the carboxyterminal domain because, unlike residues
beyond 149, they are not made hyperlabile by disruption of the end of the
molecule. No function has yet been assigned to the carboxyterminal domain. It clearly has one, though, as the amber mutation that generates

the 190-residue fragment has a conditional lethal phenotype in a $recA^-$ nonsuppressing host.

The λ analogue of *erf* is *bet* (originally *red*β); plasmids that express *bet* complement P22 *erf*⁻ (Poteete and Fenton, 1984). Purified beta protein has DNA-binding properties similar to those of Erf but lacks Erf's distinctive gearlike morphology (Murphy and Hendrix, unpublished observations). The two genes have no obvious homology at the DNA or amino acid level. No P22 analogue of the λ *exo* gene has been identified to date.

There may be an additional P22 homologous recombination gene to the right of *erf*. Its existence is suggested by the properties of two deletion mutants, P22 Δ438 and P22 Δ439 (Semerjian and Poteete, unpublished results). Both deletions have the same right end point, in *sie*B. The longer deletion, Δ439, confers a growth defect; the other does not (both leave *erf* intact). A λ *bet* and *exo*-expressing plasmid complements the growth defect, suggesting that the problem is a recombination defect. An open reading frame of only 47 codons, whose termination codon overlaps the initiation codon of *erf*, is the most likely candidate for a gene that is removed by Δ439 but left intact by Δ438. A plasmid that contains this open reading frame and little else from P22 complements P22 Δ439, showing that the key missing locus encodes something that can work in trans.

C. Other P_L Operon Genes

1. *kil*

Expression of the P22 P_L operon kills the host. The key determinant of this killing appears to be a small open reading frame located to the right of *erf* and the possible recombination gene described above. This open reading frame has been tentatively named *kil*, by analogy with its λ analogue, which is nonhomologous but similar in size and map location (Greer, 1975; Ineichen *et al.*, 1981; Semerjian and Poteete, unpublished observations). The role of the *kil* gene in the life cycles of λ and P22 has yet to be determined.

2. *c3*

The *c3* gene is one of three discovered by Levine (1957) as complementation groups of clear-plaque mutants. Its action is necessary for establishment, but not maintenance, of lysogeny. There has been little characterization of its mechanism of action, but it is highly homologous to its λ counterpart, *c*III (Semerjian and Poteete, unpublished results). By analogy, it is possible to speculate that it works by inhibiting host cell-mediated degradation of the $c1$ protein. (For review of this issue in λ, see Wulff and Rosenberg, 1983.)

3. *17*

Gene *17* allows P22 to escape exclusion mediated by Fels-2 prophage, which is present in most of the *Salmonella* strains that are employed in genetic studies (D. Botstein and M. Susskind, personal communication). Its mechanism of action is unknown. Its sequence has not revealed much other than the sequence of the protein it encodes; no λ analogue is known, and it is not homologous to any λ sequences (Semerjian and Poteete, unpublished results).

4. *ral*

An open reading frame that is highly homologous to the *ral* gene of λ has been found in a corresponding position in the P22 genome (Semerjian and Poteete, unpublished observations). The products of the λ and P22 *ral* genes enhance modification by the *E. coli hsd* restriction-modification system (Loenen and Murray, 1986; Semerjian and Poteete, unpublished observations).

5. *sie*B

A number of *Salmonella* phages are sensitive to *sie*B-mediated super-infection exclusion. The mechanism of this exclusion involves an arrest of phage replication and gene expression midway through the lytic cycle. P22 itself bears a gene, *esc,* that makes it insensitive to *sie*B (Susskind *et al.*, 1974). Franklin (1985) has identified an open reading frame that overlaps the left (promoter-distal) half of gene *24;* unlike all the identified genes in this region, it is translated rightward. This property suggests that it might be the *sie*B gene, because *sie*B is the only gene in this region known to be expressed in a lysogen; all the others are repressed by the action of $c2$ protein at P_L. The results of deletion mapping experiments are consistent with the hypothesis that this open reading frame is the *sie*B gene; they also identify two candidates for *esc,* both of which are small leftward-translated open reading frames to the left of *sie*B (Semerjian and Poteete, unpublished results).

By examining the properties of λ lysogens of *Salmonella,* Susskind and Botstein (1980) found that λ has a *sie*B gene. The λ gene maps in the same place in its chromosome and excludes the same *Salmonella* phages as the P22 gene. The DNA sequence of this region of the λ genome (Ineichen *et al.*, 1981) reveals a rightward-oriented open reading frame between *ral* and *N* that is a likely candidate for *sie*B.

6. Others

Youderian and Susskind (1980b) identified eight proteins encoded by genes in the P_L operon between *int* and *erf*. These were designated EaA, EaC, EaD, EaE, EaF, EaG, and EaH (EaB, another member of this group, is encoded by a gene located between 9 and *att*). None of these proteins has a known function, with the possible exception of EaG, which may be the product of the *xis* gene.

D. Early Transcriptional Regulation

In the absence of gene 24 protein, few of the P22 genes involved in lytic growth are expressed, probably because of premature transcription termination. A substantial body of information indicates that gene 24 protein works by essentially the same mechanism as its λ analogue, the gene N protein, forming a complex with RNA polymerase and various other host proteins that ignores most transcription stop signals (Hilliker *et al.*, 1978; Chapter 4, this volume). The sequence of gene 24 reveals little homology with N, but a conservation of such features as map location and the size and charge of the encoded proteins (Franklin, 1985b). There is also significant homology in P22 with the sites near the beginnings of the P_L and P_R transcripts in λ where N protein is thought to act (Franklin, 1985a). The N and 24 proteins are not fully interchangeable; N protein seems to require its own sites, but 24 protein apparently can antiterminate λ P_R transcription (Friedman and Ponce-Campos, 1975; Hilliker and Botstein, 1976).

E. Repressor and Its Control

The c_2 repressor of P22 is a positive and negative transcriptional regulator and the key component of a regulatory mechanism that switches efficiently from lysogeny to lytic growth in response to inducing signals. Its action is almost exactly like that of λ repressor. This conservation of mechanism is interesting, because it occurs in systems with completely distinct specificities; neither repressor recognizes the operators of the other. Extensive studies of λ repressor and comparative studies of the repressors of P22 and coliphage 434 have produced a unified description of how they work, outlined below. It probably applies to all three repressors, although some features of the λ repressor have not been examined in the other two. (For a more detailed review, with specific λ references, see Johnson *et al.*, 1981.)

The active form of the repressor is an unstable dimer, which dissociates readily into monomers. The equilibrium between monomers and dimers is such that, in a lysogen, about 90% of the repressor is in the dimer form. Each monomer consists of two distinct domains: an aminoterminal domain that contains the DNA-binding site and determinants responsible for activation of transcription, and a carboxyterminal domain that mediates dimerization. The two domains retain these functions when separated from each other by proteolysis; the carboxyterminal fragment dimerizes normally, and the aminoterminal fragment binds to DNA. However, the affinity of the isolated aminoterminal domain for operator sequences is about 1000-fold lower than that of intact, dimeric repressor. (This lower affinity is readily understood as a consequence of reduced binding energy. The energy released by binding of a monomer is roughly half that released by binding of a dimer.) Proteolytic separation of repressor's amino- and carboxyterminal domains is the key event in lysogenic induction; activated RecA promotes cleavage of a specific peptide bond in the "hinge" region between the two domains.

Repressor exerts control over transcription by binding to two operators, O_L and O_R, on either side of its gene. The arrangement of repressor genes and operators exhibits some variability among the three phages. Lambda has two superinfection exclusion genes, rexA and rexB, between its repressor gene and O_L (Landsmann et al., 1982). Phage 434 has an analogous single gene, called hex (R. Yocum and M. Susskind, personal communication), in the same location. In P22, there are only 40 base pairs between c_2 and O_L, including a sequence with features that suggest that it might be a termination signal for the P_{RM} transcript (unpublished observations).

Repressor-binding sites are imperfectly symmetric sequences of 14–18 bp (the P22 sites are 18 bp). The available evidence indicates that the interaction between repressor and its binding site is based primarily on recognition of half-sites by symmetrically arrayed aminoterminal domains in the repressor dimer. Studies of repressor-DNA contacts indicate that the repressor sits on one "face" of the double helix, making base-specific contacts in the major groove at two successive intersections of the major groove with this face. Some of these aspects of repressor-DNA binding have been confirmed directly by X-ray crystallographic studies of a 434 repressor-DNA complex (Anderson et al., 1985).

Each operator consists of three repressor-binding sites. All six sites of any one phage have homology to each other, from which it is possible to abstract a symmetric consensus sequence. The consensus sequences of different phages are nonhomologous, reflecting the specificity of repressor-operator recognition and consequently of prophage immunity. The specific functions of the three O_L sites are not well understood; the only known activity of repressor at O_L is negative regulation of the overlapping promoter P_L. On the other hand, the three repressor-binding sites of O_R (in order, from left to right, O_R3, O_R2, and O_R1) have distinct, well-defined functional roles in the regulation of the divergent promoters P_R and P_{RM}. The P22 versions of these sequence elements are shown in Fig. 5.

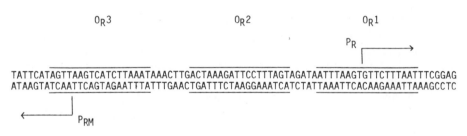

FIGURE 5. Structure of the O_R regulatory region. Repressor binding sites are indicated by horizontal lines immediately above and below the sequence; transcription start points are labeled P_{RM} and P_R.

The transcriptional effects of repressor binding to O_R sites can be summarized as follows: Repressor bound to O_R3 turns off P_{RM}; repressor bound to O_R2 stimulates P_{RM} and turns off P_R; and repressor bound to O_R1 turns off P_R. The transcriptional state of the system is determined by occupancy of the three sites. Site occupancy by repressor depends on the concentration of repressor, the different intrinsic affinities of the sites for repressor, and cooperative interactions between bound repressor molecules. O_R1 has the highest intrinsic affinity for repressor; the intrinsic affinities of the other two sites are lower and roughly equal. (Intrinsic affinity is defined here as the repressor-binding affinity of a site in the absence of functional adjacent sites.) Repressor exhibits a particular form of cooperative binding to operator sequences, called alternate pairwise. It appears that repressor bound to O_R2 can interact cooperatively with repressor bound to O_R3 or to O_R1, but not with both at once. These properties ensure that, over a certain range of repressor concentrations, the predominant configuration of the system is one in which O_R1 and O_R2 are occupied, whereas O_R3 is vacant. In this configuration, repressor stimulates its own transcription and turns off transcription of the lytic genes.

The complexity of repressor's action is puzzling at first sight, as it is apparent that qualitatively similar gene regulation could be achieved by much simpler systems. On the other hand, the conservation of most of the elements of this complexity—unstable dimeric repressors, tripartite operators, alternate pairwise cooperative binding, and an intrinsically weak P_{RM} under positive control by repressor—suggests that they must have an important function. Johnson et al. (1981) have pointed out that these complex features all have the effect of creating a system that efficiently switches between two transcriptional states, lytic and lysogenic, in an all-or-nothing fashion. The advantage of such a system to the phage is obvious: partial induction of a prophage, enough perhaps to kill the lysogen but not enough to produce a burst of phage, would be disadvantageous.

As an illustration of the working of the repressor O_R switch, consider a lysogen in which activated RecA has promoted cleavage of 90% of the repressor polypeptide chains. In principle, if the resulting mixture of repressor subunits and fragments came to equilibrium, the 10% remaining intact subunits would mostly associate with free carboxyterminal fragments; only 1% of the repressor would be in the form of dimers consisting of two intact subunits. Thus, destruction of 90% of the repressor in the cell could effectively reduce repressor activity by as much as 99%. Cooperative binding of repressor to O_R1 and O_R2 further amplifies the effect of reduced repressor activity. Over a certain concentration range, a small reduction in repressor level leads to a large reduction in the number of sites occupied. (The best-known example of this effect is seen in the case of cooperative oxygen binding by hemoglobin in the lung. In other tissues, in response to a small reduction in oxygen pressure, the protein efficiently sheds its bound oxygen.) Finally, positive control of the weak promoter P_{RM} works in reverse to destabilize the lysogenic state even further. Once O_R2 is vacated, the rate of transcription from P_{RM}, and hence of repressor synthesis, drops to an ineffectual level.

Repressor action at O_R3 could, in principle, serve to stabilize the lysogenic state and, at the same time, preserve inducibility. If O_R3 were partially occupied in a lysogen, it would be sensitive to minute changes in repressor concentration, in particular, possibly, to a decrease too small to cause significant shedding of repressor by O_R1 and O_R2. The effect of such a decrease would then be a small decrease in O_R3 occupancy, with a corresponding increase in the rate of transcription from P_{RM}. An increase in repressor concentration would have the opposite effect, increasing occupancy of O_R3 and decreasing transcription from P_{RM}. Negative autoregulation of this kind is homeostatic; it opposes change in either direction away from a programmed optimal repressor concentration. However, its significance in the overall regulation of lysogeny has not been established. The well-defined role of O_R3 is to serve as a binding site for Cro protein (see below).

Ballivet and Eisen (1978) reported the initial purification of the P22 repressor and characterization of its binding to DNA. They found that it binds specifically to the operators of both P22 and coliphage 21, as anticipated by the observation that λ hybrids bearing c2 have the same immunity specificity as phage 21, as well as gross homology in the repressor genes (Botstein and Herskowitz, 1974). Phage 21 repressor similarly binds to the operators of both phages (Ballivet et al., 1977). The sequences of the P22 and phage 21 operators are nearly identical (Poteete et al., 1980), as are the two repressors (Sauer et al., 1981; N. Franklin, personal communication). The actions of P22 repressor at O_R described above were documented by Poteete and Ptashne (1982). P22 repressor's domain structure was characterized by De Anda et al. (1983). RecA-mediated cleavage of repressor was characterized by Phizicky and Roberts (1980) and Sauer et al. (1982b).

Comparative studies of lambdoid phage repressors have contributed a number of insights into the molecular details of gene regulation. Two examples involving P22 repressor are particularly noteworthy.

The crystal structures of three site-specific DNA-binding proteins, λ repressor aminoterminal fragment, λ Cro, and *E. coli* CAP protein, reveal a conserved structural element consisting of two tandem α helices in a particular angular relationship, and connecting residues. This "helix-turn-helix" unit has been implicated as the structural determinant of site-specific DNA binding by a variety of physical and genetic studies. A large number of site-specific DNA-binding proteins, including P22 and 434 repressors, have amino acid sequence homologies that suggest that they use similar structures to bind to DNA (Sauer *et al.*, 1982c; Hecht *et al.*, 1983). A low-resolution X-ray crystallographic structure of 434 repressor bound to its operator revealed the predicted α helix lying in the major groove of the DNA (Anderson *et al.*, 1985). P22 and 434 repressors are more closely related in sequence to each other than either is to λ repressor. Wharton and Ptashne (1985) showed that changing five amino acid residues of 434 repressor in and adjacent to the "recognition helix" to the corresponding residues found in P22 repressor produced a functional repressor with the binding specificity of P22.

The second example involves the mechanism of positive control of P_{RM} by repressor. Hypothetical mechanisms can be sorted into two classes: those that invoke direct contact between repressor bound to O_R2 and RNA polymerase bound to P_{RM}, and those that invoke an indirect effect of repressor, mediated by an alteration of DNA structure consequent to repressor binding. Support for the direct contact hypothesis was obtained by isolation of a mutant λ repressor with a single amino acid substitution conferring a specific defect in positive control of P_{RM}; its DNA-binding properties were the same as wild type (Guarente *et al.*, 1982).

The similarities of P22 and λ repressors in structure, DNA binding, and regulatory action lead to the expectation that they would be found to employ the same mechanism of positive control. In particular, if the mechanism involves direct contact between RNA polymerase, then we would expect the spatial arrangement of P22 repressor bound to O_R2 and RNA polymerase bound to P_{RM} to resemble that of the λ system. In fact, the two arrangements differ substantially. The patterns of RNA polymerase and repressor contacts with DNA and the helix-turn-helix model of DNA binding that is thought to apply to both repressors suggest that direct contact could be made with the same site on RNA polymerase by both repressors. However, such contact would have to be made by noncorresponding structural elements in the two repressors (Poteete and Ptashne, 1982; Sauer *et al.*, 1982c; Hochschild *et al.*, 1983). This idea was borne out by the isolation of additional positive control mutants (Hochschild *et al.*, 1983). Mutants in λ repressor were found to have altered residues aminoterminal to the second α helix of the helix-turn-helix unit; the single P22 mutant characterized was found to have an altered residue at the carboxyterminal end of its corresponding helix. According to the

DNA-binding model, these noncorresponding loci in the two repressors would both be positioned very close to the same RNA polymerase-DNA contact on their respective DNAs.

F. Cro

The *cro* gene encodes a small protein (61 amino acid residues) that binds to the same sites in O_R as repressor. The affinity order of the sites for Cro is different, though; O_R3 is bound most tightly, followed by $O_R 1$ and O_R2 (Poteete *et al.*, 1986). P22 *cro*$^-$ mutants overproduce repressor and fail to turn down synthesis of early lytic proteins late in infection. Following infection of a wild-type host, the mutant phage is efficiently channeled into lysogeny and cannot form plaques, unless it also bears a mutation inactivating *c1* or *c2* (Winston and Botstein, 1981a). In these respects, P22 Cro closely resembles λ Cro, although the two proteins have very limited amino acid sequence homology and, like the phage repressors, recognize entirely different DNA sites. In light of the extraordinary conservation of structural organization and regulatory mechanisms in this region of the phage genome, it is reasonable to guess that P22 Cro works just like λ Cro.

Lambda Cro is a negative regulator of transcription (for a more detailed review, see Johnson *et al.*, 1981). It binds noncooperatively to the repressor binding sites, most tightly to O_R3. By binding to O_R3, Cro represses transcription from P_{RM}, an activity that is thought to be significant in prophage induction. According to this view, binding of Cro to O_R3 is the final step in switching from lysogeny to lytic growth; once Cro is present, no further transcription of repressor from P_{RM} can take place, and the system is committed to lytic growth. By binding to the other operator sites, Cro turns down transcription of all the early lytic genes, including its own.

Cro and repressor impose mutually exclusive transcriptional states. Each turns off transcription of the other's gene, and permits or promotes transcription of its own gene. This antagonism is illustrated by the phenomenon of antiimmunity, which is exhibited by certain mutant prophages. These prophages are unable to express lytic genes involved in DNA replication and host cell killing, and they have a temperature-labile repressor. When the lysogen is exposed to high temperature to inactivate repressor and then returned to low temperature, its recovery of immunity is impeded by the action of Cro. The heat-treated lysogens are not just nonimmune; they channel infecting wild-type phages into lytic growth. In this antiimmune state, O_R3 is presumably fully occupied by Cro, whereas O_R1 and O_R2 are partially occupied; the Cro produced by the mutant prophage can occupy the sites of a superinfecting phage in the same way. (The rate of P_R transcription permitted by Cro in this autoregulatory mode must be too low for effective expression of λ *cII* or P22 *c*1; see below). The observation that mutant P22 prophages can exhibit *cro*-dependent antiimmunity (Winston and Botstein, 1981a) strengthens the analogy between the λ and P22 regulatory systems.

G. *c*1

The *c*1 gene encodes a polypeptide of 92 amino acid residues that is about 50% homologous to its λ counterpart, the *c*II protein (Backhaus and Petri, 1984) and appears to work in the same way (Winston and Botstein, 1981b; M. Rosenberg, personal communication). A detailed account of λ *c*II function, including some comparisons with *c*1, is given by Ho *et al.* (1986). Briefly, *c*II protein activates transcription of three leftward λ promoters by binding to sequences overlapping their "−35" regions. The three promoters, P_{RE}, P_I, and P_{aQ}, are homologous but not identical; all are inactive in the absence of *c*II protein. P_{RE} overlaps the amino terminus–encoding end of *c*II; its transcript extends through the *cro* gene (in the antisense direction) and the repressor gene. A high level of repressor synthesis programmed by the P_{RE} transcript is essential to the establishment of lysogeny. P_I is located in the *xis* gene; its transcript encodes Int protein. Selective synthesis of Int—in particular, without concomitant synthesis of Xis—programmed by the P_I transcript, promotes integrative, but not excisive, recombination. P_{aQ} is located in gene *Q*; its transcript is thought to function as an antisense translational inhibitor of gene *Q* expression. Inhibition of gene *Q* expression delays expression of all the late lytic genes of the phage.

P22 appears to have analogues of all three *c*II-activated λ promoters. It contains a sequence that is highly homologous to λ P_{RE}, at the corresponding location (Backhaus and Petri, 1984). P22 *c*1 protein and λ *c*II protein are each able to stimulate transcription from both phages' P_{RE} promoters *in vitro*, but each exhibits a preference for its own; stimulation of transcription from the other phage's P_{RE} requires a higher concentration of the activator protein (Ho *et al.*, 1986; M. Rosenberg, personal communication). This specificity is also seen *in vivo* (Wulff and Mahoney, 1987). In addition, P22 has a promoter in its *xis* gene that is activated by *c*1 protein; unlike λ P_I it promotes rightward transcription (M. Rosenberg, personal communication). This property suggests that its transcript may function as an antisense translational inhibitor of *xis* expression. Finally, λ P_{aQ} is located in a segment of sequence that is identical in the two phages (M. Kroger and G. Hobom, personal communication).

The segment of DNA between *c*1 and *18* contains the start point for a small leftward transcript, called RNA b, that is produced from a promoter that is active in the absence of any phage-encoded regulatory proteins (Roberts *et al.*, 1976; Rosenberg and Court, 1979; Backhaus and Petri, 1984). The 3′ end of RNA b overlaps the carboxy terminus-encoding end of gene *c*1. It is analogous to the OOP RNA of λ, whose function has been obscure. Recent evidence suggests that OOP RNA may function as a negative regulator of *c*II expression (D. Wulff, personal communication).

H. DNA Replication Genes

The DNA replication genes of P22, *18* and *12*, can substitute as a block for their λ counterparts, *O* and *P*, in hybrid phages. However, λ phages bearing P22 replication functions do not complement the growth defects of λ phages bearing mutations in their own replication genes; similarly, λ *O* and *P* proteins are unable to help *18*$^-$ or *12*$^-$ mutants in *trans* (Hilliker and Botstein, 1976). These observations, viewed in light of what is known about λ DNA replication (see Chapter 3, this volume), suggest that the λ and P22 replication proteins are specific for their own replication origins.

Backhaus and Petri (1984) determined the sequences of *18* and *12*. They found that the aminoterminal halves of genes *18* and *O* are homologous. Gene *18* is still more homologous to the corresponding gene in the lambdoid phage 82; the homology in this case extends into the *ori* sequences that comprise the central part of the gene (Petri and Backhaus, 1984). Gene *12* protein is not homologous to λ *P* protein, but it is quite homologous to the *E. coli dna*B protein. This relationship between the *12* and *dna*B proteins is borne out by two other observations. First, P22 DNA replication, unlike that of λ, does not require a functional *dna*B gene (Botstein and Herskowitz, 1974; Schanda-Mulfinger and Schmieger, 1980). Second, purified gene *12* protein can substitute for *dna*B protein in an *in vitro* φX174 DNA replication assay (Wickner, 1984a). Wickner (1984a,b) has further characterized the activities of *12* protein, finding that it has an ATPase activity that is stimulated by single-stranded DNA and that it binds single-stranded DNA in the presence of ATP. In a purified system, substitution of *12* protein for *dna*B allows φX174 replication to bypass its normal requirement for *dna*C protein, thus mimicking P22 replication, which is *dna*C-independent *in vivo* (Schanda-Mulfinger and Schmieger, 1980). Formation of a complex containing *12* protein and single-stranded DNA depends on ATP but not on any specific replication origin; *dna*G primase recognizes this complex as a "promoter" for initiation of oligonucleotide synthesis. Wickner (1984a,b) speculates that *12* protein functions cooperatively with *18* protein, which, by analogy with λ, is probably an origin-specific DNA-binding protein. Transfer of *12* protein to the P22 replication origin mediated by *18* then triggers priming and DNA synthesis.

In λ, the DNA sequences between the DNA replication genes and the late-transcriptional regulator gene *Q* include one gene of known function, *ren*, and several other open reading frames of unknown function, all of which are dispensable for normal lytic growth and lysogeny (Toothman and Herskowitz, 1980; Kroger and Hobom, 1982). Although P22 lacks a *ren* gene (and is phenotypically *ren⁻*), the other sequences in this region are highly conserved (Toothman and Herskowitz, 1980; Backhaus and Petri, 1984; M. Kroger and G. Hobom, personal communication).

I. Late-Transcriptional Regulation

The P22 late-transcriptional regulatory gene, *23*, is homologous to λ gene *Q*; the encoded proteins are almost identical in amino acid sequence (M. Kroger and G. Hobom, personal communication). *Q* and *23* are functionally equivalent (Herskowitz, Toothman, and Hilliker, cited by Hilliker and Botstein, 1976). The gene *Q* protein works by antitermination of a short transcript, called 6S RNA, which is made from a promoter located about 50 bp to the right of *Q* (see Chapter 4, this volume). The sequences of P22 and λ diverge in this area; the -35 and -10 sequences of P22 P_{LATE} and its λ counterpart are the same, but sequences flanking them differ, as do the sequences of the small transcripts they direct in the absence of antitermination activity (Roberts *et al.*, 1976; M. Kroger and G. Hobom, personal communication).

A study by Weinstock *et al.* (1980) produced evidence that all of the P22 genes responsible for virion assembly are part of a single operon. Some, but not all, insertions of Tn1 in head genes, as well as in *ant*, were found to decrease expression of the tail gene (9). This polarity depended only on the orientation of the inserted Tn1, not on the locus of the insertion. Moreover, residual tail gene expression by phages containing both polar and nonpolar Tn1 insertions was found to depend on gene *23* function. The simplest explanation of these observations is that expression of the tail gene is dependent on transcription initiated far upstream, presumably at P_{LATE}. These results also show that *23* protein-potentiated transcription goes through at least one strong terminator, t_{ant} (see below), but can be stopped by another, in Tn1. Measurements of the kinetics of transcription of head and tail genes are consistent with the single-operon hypothesis (Casjens and Adams, 1985).

J. Lysis Genes

The DNA sequence of gene *13* reveals that it potentially encodes a polypeptide of 108 amino acid residues whose sequence suggests that it is an intrinsic membrane protein (Rennell and Poteete, 1985). Gene *13* protein is 90% homologous to λ gene *S* protein and so presumably functions in the same way. Lambda *S* protein works by insertion into the host cell's cytoplasmic membrane, where it causes a gross change in membrane permeability that is most readily explained by postulating that it creates channels through which any metabolite or small protein can diffuse

(Wilson, 1982). This nonspecific action of *S* and *13* proteins is illustrated by the observation that either protein can promote lysis in combination with P22 lysozyme, T4 lysozyme, or λ endolysin (Rennell and Poteete, 1985). The *13* and *S* proteins are the key regulators of the timing of lysis. In cells infected with mutant phages specifically lacking these functions, macromolecular synthesis and phage assembly continue long past the normal time of lysis.

Gene *19* protein is a lysozyme (Rao and Burma, 1971; Rennell and Poteete, 1985). It resembles phage T4 lysozyme in its substrate specificities and in amino acid sequence. The amino acid homology between T4 and P22 lysozymes is limited, but shared residues (26% of the total) are concentrated among those known to constitute the "core" of T4 lysozyme, including the active-site cleft. Alignment of the sequences further suggests that P22 lysozyme lacks two surface loops present in T4 lysozyme. These observations prompted Weaver *et al.* (1985) to propose that the two molecules have fundamentally similar structures. P22 lysozyme differs notably from its λ analogue, called endolysin, which apparently consists of the products of genes *R* (transglycosylase) and *RZ* (endopeptidase), in both sequence and enzymatic activity (Young *et al.*, 1979; Bienkowska-Szewczyk and Taylor, 1980).

About 2600 base pairs of DNA lie between genes *19* and *3*. This interval contains no known genes. In addition, almost all of it can be deleted without major effects on the ability of the phage to grow lytically or to form lysogens (A. R. Poteete and K. Chapin, unpublished results).

K. DNA Packaging Initiation Site (*pac*)

The results of a number of studies suggest that the P22 DNA packaging apparatus binds to concatemeric DNA at a site in gene *3*, called *pac*, and initiates packaging by cutting the DNA at any of a number of sites within a 100-bp sequence segment roughly centered around *pac* (Casjens *et al.*, 1987; Backhaus, 1985). The packaging apparatus component responsible for *pac* recognition is the gene *3* protein. Mutant alleles of gene *3*, called HT, confer altered site specificity on the packaging apparatus; they appear to exert their effects via an alteration of *3* protein rather than an alteration of the *pac* site (Schmieger, 1972; Raj *et al.*, 1974; Jackson *et al.*, 1982). One such allele, HT12/4, was found to differ from the wild-type gene by a sequence alteration resulting in a single amino acid substitution in *3* protein, and to direct the packaging apparatus to two new sites in the P22 genome (Casjens *et al.*, 1987). Comparison of the sequences in the vicinity of cuts made by wild-type and mutant *3* protein-directed packaging revealed a segment of 10 base pairs, seven of which were conserved among all three sites; the other three were conserved between the two sites recognized by the mutant. This 10-bp segment is thus likely to be a key determinant of *pac* function.

L. Head Genes

The activities of the P22 head genes are described in the chapters in this volume on bacteriophage assembly (Casjens and Hendrix) and DNA packaging (Black). In addition, regulation of head gene expression is discussed in the former. These topics will not be discussed here.

The cluster of head genes in the P22 genome includes one, gene *14*, whose function is not clearly defined. Youderian and Susskind (1980a) found that phages bearing amber mutations in this gene have a temperature-sensitive growth defect in nonsuppressing hosts, suggesting that the function of the *14* protein is more nearly essential at high temperature than at low temperature. Even a phage bearing two amber mutations in gene *14*, though, is only mildly defective at the nonpermissive temperature. Bazinet and King (1985) found that phages produced in the absence of *14* protein plate with reduced efficiency (relative to wild-type phages) on permissive host cells, although they adsorb with normal efficiency. This result suggests that P22 heads assembled in the absence of *14* protein are defective, even though *14* protein does not appear to be a component of the wild-type virion.

M. *imm*I Genes

The *ant* gene and others that control its expression are located in a part of the P22 genome that is sometimes called *imm*I. Historically, prophage immunity in P22 was found to consist of two determinants, *imm*C and *imm*I, which contain the *c2* and *mnt* genes, respectively. *imm*I is located between the head and tail genes. It has no λ counterpart, but hybrid λ phages bearing *imm*I can be formed by recombination between P22 and λ (Yamamoto *et al.*, 1978). *Salmonella* phage L, which is otherwise very closely related to P22, has no *ant* operon (Susskind and Botstein, 1978b). As outlined above, the lysis, head, and tail genes of P22 constitute a single operon. The *ant* operon is thus located within another operon but nevertheless is regulated nearly independently (see below).

The *mnt* gene encodes an 82 amino acid residue polypeptide that forms tetramers, which bind to a single site, called O_{mnt}, located between *mnt* and *arc* (see Fig. 6). Binding of Mnt turns down P_{ant} transcription and stimulates P_{mnt} transcription (Sauer *et al.*, 1983; Vershon *et al.*, 1985, 1987a). The action of Mnt repressor is thus formally similar to that of *c2* repressor; both stimulate transcription of their own genes, while repressing transcription of genes that promote lytic growth. Recent work (Liao and McClure, unpublished) suggests that Mnt stimulates transcription indirectly. RNA polymerase cannot bind to P_{mnt} and P_{ant} at the same time; the promoters thus compete. By selectively blocking RNA polymerase P_{ant} binding, Mnt passively stimulates transcription from P_{mnt}.

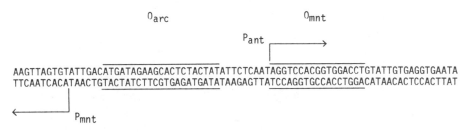

FIGURE 6. Structure of the $O_{arc}-O_{mnt}$ regulatory region. Repressor binding sites are indicated by horizontal lines immediately above and below the sequence; transcription start points are labeled P_{mnt} and P_{ant}.

Youderian *et al.* (1983) were able to identify a specific amino acid residue that contributes to the site specificity of Mnt binding, probably by contacting two symmetrically positioned bases in O_{mnt}. O_{mnt} is a 17-bp sequence with perfect symmetry around the central base pair. These investigators constructed a mutant O_{mnt}, bearing two symmetric base pair substitutions, to which wild-type Mnt binds poorly. They then selected mutant variants of *mnt* on the basis of their ability to repress transcripton from P_{ant} by binding to the mutant O_{mnt}. The mutant alleles of *mnt*, called bs (binding specificity), were found to differ from wild type by base substitutions resulting in the replacement of His_6 by Pro in Mnt. Studies of operator binding by Mnt and Mnt-bs revealed a nearly perfect specificity switch. The two repressors bind with approximately equal affinities to their preferred sites; each binds with 1000-fold lower affinity to the other repressor's preferred site. The techniques used to select bs mutants have been generalized to allow selection for any gene whose product can bind specifically to any given DNA sequence (Benson *et al.*, 1986).

The *arc* gene encodes a polypeptide of 53 amino acid residues that forms dimers, which bind to a 22-bp sequence, called O_{arc}, located in the region of overlap between the promoters P_{ant} and P_{mnt} (see Fig. 6). Binding of Arc turns down transcription from P_{ant}, thus repressing *arc* and *ant*, and from P_{mnt} (Susskind, 1980; Susskind and Youderian, 1982; Youderian *et al.*, 1982; Vershon *et al.*, 1985, 1987b). Arc is thus formally similar to Cro in its action.

The Arc and Mnt proteins share substantial amino acid sequence homology, yet they recognize operators that are not apparently related (Sauer *et al.*, 1983). Genetic studies (Youderian *et al.*, 1983; Vershon, 1986) suggest that some or all of the key determinants of site-specific DNA-binding in Mnt and Arc reside in the aminoterminal portions of the polypeptides. This suggestion is supported by an experiment in which the first 13 amino acid residues of Mnt were replaced with the first 10 of Arc. The resulting hybrid protein binds specifically to O_{arc} (Knight and Sauer, unpublished results).

Susskind and Botstein (1975) showed that antirepressor can reversibly inhibit operator binding by λ repressor. The reversibility of the inhibition implies that antirepressor action is mechanistically different from that of RecA, which promotes irreversible inactivation of repressor via proteolysis. Further studies have shown that antirepressor binds specifically to carboxyterminal fragments of P22 and λ repressors (De Anda, 1985).

The amino terminus-encoding end of the *ant* gene contains a leftward promoter that directs the synthesis of a 68 or 69 base transcript called *sar* RNA (small antisense RNA). The 5′ end of *sar* RNA is complementary to the *ant* ribosome-binding site; transcripts from P_{ant} and P_{sar} rapidly form complexes *in vitro* (Liao *et al.*, 1987). Experiments by Wu *et al.* (1987) have shown that *sar* RNA can repress synthesis of antirepressor from the P_{LATE} and P_{ant} transcripts *in vivo*. Mutations that inactivate P_{sar} (without altering the amino acid sequence of antirepressor) allow expression of *ant* from the P_{LATE} transcript and confer a clear-plaque phenotype on P22.

From the foregoing description, it is clear that expression of *ant* is regulated by three repressors: *mnt*, *arc*, and *sar*. Wu *et al.* (1987) propose that the sequence of events in *imm*I following infection by P22 is as follows.

1. At the beginning of the infectious cycle, none of the repressors is present, and transcription from P_{ant} ensues at a high rate. P_{sar} is a weaker promoter than P_{ant}; moreover, transcription from P_{ant} inhibits P_{sar} activity. Likewise, P_{mnt} is weak in the absence of regulatory proteins and is inhibited by P_{ant} activity. For these reasons, transcription from P_{sar} and P_{mnt} probably exerts little regulatory effect in the first few minutes of infection.
2. The burst of P_{ant} transcription produces a transiently high rate of Arc and antirepressor synthesis. As Arc accumulates, it turns down P_{ant} transcription to a low steady state.
3. Inhibition of P_{ant} transcription by Arc stimulates P_{sar}, leading to an accumulation of *sar* RNA, which acts as a translational inhibitor of antirepressor synthesis from residual P_{ant} transcripts.
4. Accumulated *sar* RNA also prevents antirepressor synthesis from P_{LATE} in infections that progress through the lytic pathway and from any transcripts resulting from residual P_{ant} activity under *mnt* repression in the lysogenic pathway. One aspect of *imm*I regulation that remains to be elucidated is the mechanism by which *mnt* repression is established in the lysogenic pathway.

A strong transcriptional terminator located between *ant* and 9, called t_{ant}, stops transcription from P_{ant} (Susskind and Youderian, 1982; Berget *et al.*, 1983). As discussed above, t_{ant} apparently does not stop 23 protein-potentiated transcription from P_{LATE}.

N. Tail Gene

The tail gene (9) encodes a polypeptide of 666 amino acid residues (Sauer *et al.*, 1982a). An experiment by Goldberg *et al.* (1982) suggests that the native tail protein is a trimer. These investigators identified mutant tail proteins with altered electrophoretic mobility in the native state. Mixed infection of mutant and wild type leads to the production of four species of tail protein: mutant, wild type, and two hybrid species of intermediate mobility. Preliminary x-ray crystallographic results also indicate that the native tail protein is a trimer (T. Alber, personal communication).

The mature tail protein is extraordinarily resistant to heat, protease, and SDS. Studies of its maturation have revealed the existence of two intermediates: a protease-sensitive monomer, and a protease-sensitive trimer, called a "protrimer" (Goldenberg and King, 1982). Assembly of the mature tail protein from monomers is naturally temperature-sensitive; its efficiency is 90% at 27°C, but only 15% at 42°C (Goldenberg *et al.*, 1982). Mutant tail proteins with increased temperature-sensitivity generally accumulate as monomers at the nonpermissive temperature (Yu and King, 1984). Like the wild-type protein, though, once matured at the permissive temperature, they are thermally stable (Goldenberg and King, 1981).

The tail protein, free or attached to heads, is an enzyme. It hydrolyzes rhamnosyl-1,3-galactose linkages in the O antigen part of the lipopolysaccharides of *Salmonella* serotypes A, B, and D (Iwashita and Kanegasaki, 1973). This endorhamnosidase activity is apparently not necessary for adsorption *per se*, but rather for progression of the phage particle from the O antigen to a secondary, more internal receptor (Berget and Poteete, 1980).

REFERENCES

Anderson, J. E., Ptashne, M., and Harrison, S. C., 1985, A phage repressor-operator complex at 7 A resolution, *Nature* 316:596.

Backhaus, H., 1985, DNA packaging initiation of *Salmonella* bacteriophage P22: Determination of cut sites within the DNA sequence coding for gene 3, *J. Virol.* **55**:458.

Backhaus, H., and Petri, J. B., 1984, Sequence analysis of a region from the early right operon in phage P22 including the replication genes 18 and 12, *Gene* 32:289.

Ballivet, M., and Eisen, H., 1978, Purification and properties of phage P22 c2 repressor, *Eur. J. Biochem.* **82**:175.

Ballivet, M., Reichardt, L. F., and Eisen, H., 1977, Purification and properties of coliphage 21 repressor, *Eur. J. Biochem.* **73**:601.

Bazinet, C. W., and King, J., 1985, A late gene product of phage P22 affecting virus infectivity, *Virology* 143:368.

Benson, N., Sugiono, P., Bass, S., Mendelman, L. V., and Youderian, P., 1986, General selection for specific DNA-binding activities, *Genetics* **114**:1.

Berget, P. B., and Poteete, A. R., 1980, Structure and functions of the bacteriophage P22 tail protein, *J. Virol.* **34:**234.

Berget, P. B., Poteete, A. R., and Sauer, R. T., 1983, Control of phage P22 tail protein expression by transcription termination. *J. Mol. Biol.* **164:**561.

Bienkowska-Szewczyk, K., and Taylor, A., 1980, Murein transglycosylase from phage λ lysate: Purification and properties, *Biochim. Biophys. Acta* 615:489.

Botstein, D., and Herskowitz, I., 1974, Properties of hybrids between *Salmonella* phage P22 and coliphage λ, *Nature* **251:**584.

Casjens, S., and Adams, M. B., 1985, Posttranscriptional modulation of bacteriophage P22 scaffolding protein gene expression, *J. Virol.* **53:**185.

Casjens, S., Hayden, M., Jackson, E., and Deans, R., 1983, Additional restriction endonuclease cleavage sites on the bacteriophage P22 genome, *J. Virol.* **45:**864.

Casjens, S., Huang, W. M., Hayden, M., and Parr, R., 1987, Initiation of bacteriophage P22 DNA packaging series: Analysis of a mutant that alters the DNA target specificity of the packaging apparatus, *J. Mol. Biol.* **194:**411.

Cohen, A., and Clark, A. J., 1986, Synthesis of linear plasmid multimers in *Escherichia coli* K-12, *J. Bacteriol.* **167:**327.

Davis, R. W., Botstein, D., and Roth, J. R., 1980, *Advanced Bacterial Genetics*, Cold Spring Harbor Laboratory, Cold Spring Harbor, NY.

De Anda, J. L., 1985, P22 antirepressor: Interactions with phage repressors, Ph.D. Dissertation, Massachusetts Institute of Technology, Cambridge, MA.

De Anda, J., Poteete, A. R., and Sauer, R. T., 1983, P22 c2 repressor: Domain structure and function, *J. Biol. Chem.* **258:**10536.

Fenton, A. C., and Poteete, A. R., 1984, Genetic analysis of the erf region of the bacteriophage P22 chromosome, *Virology* **134:**148.

Franklin, N. C., 1985a, Conservation of genome form but not sequence in the transcriptional antitermination determinants of bacteriophages λ, φ21, and P22, *J. Mol. Biol.* **181:**75.

Franklin, N. C., 1985b, "N" transcription antitermination proteins of bacteriophages λ, φ21, and P22, *J. Mol. Biol.* **181:**85.

Friedman, D. I., and Ponce-Campos, R., 1975, Differential effect of phage regulator functions on transcription from various promoters: Evidence that the P22 gene *24* and the λ gene *N* products distinguish three classes of promoters, *J. Mol. Biol.* **98:**537.

Friedman, S. A., and Hays, J. B., 1986, Selective inhibition of *Escherichia coli* RecBC activities by plasmid-encoded GamS function of phage lambda, *Gene* 43:255.

Goldenberg, D. P., and King, J., 1981, Temperature-sensitive mutants blocked in the folding or subunit assembly of the bacteriophage P22 tail spike protein. II. Active mutant proteins matured at 30 degrees C, *J. Mol. Biol.* **145:**633.

Goldenberg, D., and King, J., 1982, Trimeric intermediate in the *in vivo* folding and subunit assembly of the tail spike endorhamnosidase of bacteriophage P22, *Proc. Natl. Acad. Sci. USA* **79:**3403.

Goldenberg, D. P., Berget, P. B., and King, J., 1982, Maturation of the tail spike endorhamnosidase of *Salmonella* phage P22, *J. Biol. Chem.* **257:**7864.

Greer, H., 1975, The *kil* gene of bacteriophage lambda, *Virology* **66:**589.

Guarente, L., Nye, J. S., Hochschild, A., and Ptashne, M., 1982, Mutant λ phage repressor with a specific defect in its positive control function, *Proc. Natl. Acad. Sci. USA* **79:**2236.

Hecht, M. H., Nelson, H. C. M., and Sauer, R. T., 1983, Mutations in λ repressor's aminoterminal domain: Implications for protein stability and DNA binding, *Proc. Natl. Acad. Sci. U.S.A.* **80:**2676.

Hilliker, S., and Botstein, D., 1976, Specificity of genetic elements controlling regulation of early functions in temperate bacteriophages, *J. Mol. Biol.* **106:**537.

Hilliker, S., Gottesman, M., and Adhya, S., 1978, The activity of *Salmonella* phage P22 gene 24 product in *Escherichia coli*, *Virology* **86:**37.

Ho, Y.-S., Wulff, D., and Rosenberg, M., 1986, Protein–nucleic acid interactions involved in transcription activation by the phage lambda regulatory protein cII, in *Regulation of Gene Expression* (I. Booth and C. Higgins, eds.), pp. 79–103, Cambridge University Press, Cambridge, U.K.

Hochschild, A., Irwin, N. and Ptashne, M., 1983, Repressor structure and the mechanism of positive control, *Cell* **32**:319.

Ineichen, K., Shepherd, J. C. W., and Bickle, T. A., 1981, The DNA sequence of the phage lambda genome between P_L and the gene bet, *Nucleic Acids Res.* **9**:4639.

Iwashita, S., and Kanegasaki, S., 1973, Smooth specific phage adsorption: Endorhamnosidase activity of tail parts of P22, *Biochem. Biophys. Res. Commun.* **55**:403.

Jackson, E. N., Laski, F., and Andres, C., 1982, Bacteriophage P22 mutants that alter the specificity of DNA packaging, *J. Mol. Biol.* **154**:551.

Johnson, A. D., Poteete, A. R., Lauer, G., Sauer, R. T., Ackers, G. K., and Ptashne, M., 1981, λ Repressor and cro—components of an efficient molecular switch, *Nature* **294**:217.

Knight, J. A., Hardy, L. W., Rennell, D., Herrick, D., and Poteete, A. R., 1987, Mutations in an upstream regulatory sequence that increase expression of the bacteriophage T4 lysozyme gene, *J. Bacteriol.* **169**:4630–4636.

Kroger, M., and Hobom, G., 1982, A chain of interlinked genes in the *ninR* region of bacteriophage lambda, *Gene* **20**:25.

Landsmann, J., Kroger, M., and Hobom, G., 1982, the *rex* region of bacteriophage lambda: Two genes under three-way control, *Gene* **20**:11.

Leong, J. M., Nunes-Duby, S., Lesser, C. F., Youderian, P., Susskind, M. M., and Landy, A., 1985, The φ80 and P22 attachment sites: Primary structure and interaction with *Escherichia coli* integration host factor, *J. Biol. Chem.* **260**:4468.

Leong, J. M., Nunes-Duby, S. E., Oser, A. B., Lesser, C. F., Youderian, P., Susskind, M. M., and Landy, A., 1986, Structural and regulatory divergence among site-specific recombination genes of lambdoid phage, *J. Mol. Biol.* **189**:603.

Levine, M., 1957, Mutations in the temperate phage P22 and lysogeny in *Salmonella*, *Virology* **3**:22.

Levine, M., 1972, Replication and lysogeny with phage P22 in *Salmonella typhimurium*, *Curr. Top. Microbiol. Immunol.* **58**:135.

Liao, S.-M., Wu, T., Chiang, C. H., Susskind, M. M., and McClure, W. R., 1987, Control of gene expression in bacteriophage P22 by a small antisense RNA. I. Characterization *in vitro* of the P_{sar} promoter and the *sar* RNA transcript, *Genes Dev.* **1**:197.

Loenen, W. A. M., and Murray, N. E., 1986, Modification enhancement by the restriction alleviation protein (ral) of bacteriophage λ, *J. Mol. Biol.* **190**:11.

Murphy, K. C., Casey, L., Yannoutsos, N., Poteete, A. R., and Hendrix, R. W., 1987, Localization of a DNA-binding determinant in the bacteriophage P22 Erf protein, *J. Mol. Biol.* **194**:105.

Murphy, K. C., Fenton, A. C., and Poteete, A. R. 1987, Sequence of the bacteriophage P22 anti-RecBCD (abc) genes and properties of P22 abc region deletion mutants, *Virology* **160**:456.

Petri, J. B., and Backhaus, H., 1984, Structural organization of the *ori* site of phage P22; comparison with other lambdoid *ori* sites, *Gene* **32**:304.

Phizicky, E. M., and Roberts, J. W., 1980, Kinetics of RecA protein-directed inactivation of repressors of phage λ and phage P22, *J. Mol. Biol.* **139**:319.

Poteete, A. R., and Fenton, A. C., 1983, DNA-binding properties of the Erf protein of bacteriophage P22, *J. Mol. Biol.* **163**:257.

Poteete, A. R., and Fenton, A. C., 1984, Lambda *red*-dependent growth and recombination of phage P22, *Virology* **134**:161.

Poteete, A. R., and Ptashne, M., 1982, Control of transcription by the bacteriophage P22 repressor, *J. Mol. Biol.* **157**:21.

Poteete, A. R., Ptashne, M., Ballivet, M., and Eisen, H., 1980, Operator sequences of bacteriophages P22 and 21, *J. Mol. Biol.* **137**:81.

Poteete, A. R., Sauer, R. T., and Hendrix, R. W., 1983, Domain structure and quaternary organization of the bacteriophage P22 Erf protein, *J. Mol. Biol.* **171**:401.

Poteete, A. R., Hehir, K., and Sauer, R. T., 1986, Bacteriophage P22 Cro protein: Sequence, purification, and properties, *Biochemistry* **25:**251.

Raj, A. S., Raj, A. Y., and Schmieger, H., 1974, Phage genes involved in the formation of generalized transducing particles in *Salmonella*–phage P22, *Mol. Gen. Genet.* **135:**175.

Rao, G. R. K., and Burma, D. P., 1971, Purification and properties of phage P22-induced lysozyme, *J. Biol. Chem.* **246:**6474.

Rennell, D., and Poteete, A. R., 1985, Phage P22 lysis genes: Nucleotide sequences and functional relationships with T4 and lambda genes, *Virology* **143:**280.

Roberts, J. W., Roberts, C. W., Hilliker, S., and Botstein, D., 1976, Transcription termination and regulation in bacteriophages P22 and lambda, in: *RNA Polymerase* (R. Losick and M. Chamberlin, eds.), pp. 707–718, Cold Spring Harbor Laboratory, Cold Spring Harbor, NY.

Rosenberg, M., and Court, D., 1979, Regulatory sequences involved in the promotion and termination of RNA transcription, *Annu. Rev. Genet.* **13:**319.

Sanderson, K. E., and Roth, J. R., 1983, Linkage map of *Salmonella typhimurium*, edition VI, *Microbiol. Rev.* **47:**410.

Sauer, R. T., Pan, J., Hopper, P., Hehir, K., Brown, J., and Poteete, A. R., 1981, Primary structure of the phage P22 repressor and its gene *c2*, *Biochemistry* **20:**3591.

Sauer, R. T., Krovatin, W., Poteete, A. R., and Berget, P. B., 1982a, Phage P22 tail protein: Gene and amino acid sequence, *Biochemistry* **21:**5811.

Sauer, R. T., Ross, M. J., and Ptashne, M., 1982b, Cleavage of the λ and P22 repressors by *recA* protein, *J. Biol. Chem.* **257:**4458.

Sauer, R. T., Yocum, R. R., Doolittle, R. F., Lewis, M., and Pabo, C. O., 1982c, Homology among DNA-binding proteins suggests use of a conserved super-secondary structure, *Nature* **298:**447.

Sauer, R. T., Krovatin, W., DeAnda, J., Youderian, P., and Susskind, M. M., 1983, Primary structure of the *imm*I immunity region of bacteriophage P22, *J. Mol. Biol.* **168:**699.

Schanda-Mulfinger, U. E. M., and Schmieger, H., 1980, Growth of *Salmonella* bacteriophage P22 in *Escherichia coli dna*(Ts) mutants, *J. Bacteriol.* **143:**1042.

Schmieger, H., 1972, Phage P22-mutants with increased or decreased transduction abilities, *Mol. Gen. Genet.* **119:**75.

Schmieger, H., 1982, Packaging signals for phage P22 on the chromosome of *Salmonella typhimurium*, *Mol. Gen. Genet.* **187:**516.

Smith, G. R., 1983, General recombination, in: *Lambda II* (R. W. Hendrix, J. W. Roberts, F. W. Stahl, and R. A. Weisberg, eds.), pp. 175–210, Cold Spring Harbor Laboratory, Cold Spring Harbor, NY.

Susskind, M. M., 1980, A new gene of bacteriophage P22 which regulates synthesis of antirepressor, *J. Mol. Biol.* **138:**685.

Susskind, M. M., and Botstein, D., 1975, Mechanism of action of *Salmonella* phage P22 antirepressor, *J. Mol. Biol.* **98:**413.

Susskind, M. M., and Botstein, D., 1978a, Molecular genetics of bacteriophage P22, *Microbiol. Rev.* **42:**385.

Susskind, M. M., and Botstein, D., 1978b, Repression and immunity in *Salmonella* phages P22 and L: Phage L lacks a functional secondary immunity system, *Virology* **89:**618.

Susskind, M. M., and Botstein, D., 1980, Superinfection exclusion by λ prophage in lysogens of *Salmonella typhimurium*, *Virology* **100:**212.

Susskind, M. M., and Youderian, P., 1982, Transcription *in vitro* of the bacteriophage P22 antirepressor gene, *J. Mol. Biol.* **154:**427.

Susskind, M. M., Wright, A., and Botstein, D., 1974, Superinfection exclusion by P22 prophage in lysogens of *Salmonella typhimurium*. IV. Genetics and physiology of *sie*B exclusion, *Virology* **62:**367.

Toothman, P., and Herskowitz, I., 1980, Rex-dependent exclusion of lambdoid phages. II. Determinants of sensitivity to exclusion, *Virology* **102:**147.

Vershon, A. K., 1986, The Arc and Mnt repressors of bacteriophage P22, Ph.D. Dissertation, Massachusetts Institute of Technology, Cambridge, MA.

Vershon, A. K., Youderian, P., Susskind, M. M., and Sauer, R. T., 1985, The bacteriophage P22 Arc and Mnt repressors: Overproduction, purification, and properties, *J. Biol. Chem.* **260**:12124.

Vershon, A. K., Liao, S.-M., McClure, W. R., and Sauer, R. T., 1987a, Bacteriophage P22 Mnt repressor: DNA binding and effects on transcription *in vitro*, *J. Mol. Biol.* **195**:311–322.

Vershon, A. K., Liao, S.-M., McClure, W. R., and Sauer, R. T., 1987b, Interaction of the bacteriophage P22 Arc repressor with operator DNA, *J. Mol. Biol.* **195**:323–331.

Weaver, L. H., Rennell, D., Poteete, A. R., and Matthews, B. W., 1985, Structure of phage P22 gene 19 lysozyme inferred from its homology with phage T4 lysozyme: Implications for lysozyme evolution, *J. Mol. Biol.* **184**:739.

Weinstock, G. M., Susskind, M. M., and Botstein, D., 1979, Regional specificity of illegitimate recombination by the translocatable ampicillin-resistance element Tn1 in the genome of phage P22, *Genetics* **92**:685.

Weinstock, G. M., Riggs, P. D., and Botstein, D., 1980, Genetics of bacteriophage P22. III. The late operon, *Virology* **106**:82.

Weisberg, R. A., and Landy, A., 1983, Site-specific recombination in phage lambda, in: *Lambda II* (R. W. Hendrix, J. W. Roberts, F. W. Stahl, and R. A. Weisberg, eds.), pp. 211–250, Cold Spring Harbor Laboratory, Cold Spring Harbor, NY.

Wharton, R. P., and Ptashne, M., 1985, Changing the binding specificity of a repressor by redesigning an α-helix, *Nature* **316**:601.

Wickner, S., 1984a, DNA-dependent ATPase activity associated with phage P22 gene 12 protein, *J. Biol. Chem.* **259**:14038.

Wickner, S., 1984b, Oligonucleotide synthesis by *Escherichia coli* dnaG primase in conjunction with phage P22 gene 12 protein, *J. Biol. Chem.* **259**:14044.

Wilson, D. B., 1982, Effect of the lambda *S* gene product on properties of the *Escherichia coli* inner membrane, *J. Bacteriol.* **151**:1403.

Winston, F., and Botstein, D., 1981a, Control of lysogenization by phage P22. I. The P22 cro gene, *J. Mol. Biol.* **152**:209.

Winston, F., and Botstein, D., 1981b, Control of lysogenization by phage P22. II. Mutations (clyA) in the *c1* gene that cause increased lysogenization, *J. Mol. Biol.* **152**:233.

Wu, T., Liao, S.-M., McClure, W. R., and Susskind, M. M., 1987, Control of gene expression in bacteriophage P22 by a small antisense RNA. II. Characterization of mutants defective in repression, *Genes Dev.* **1**:204.

Wulff, D. L., and Mahoney, M. E., 1987, Cross-specificities between *cII*-like proteins and p_{RE}-like promoters of lambdoid bacteriophages, *Genetics* **115**:597.

Wulff, D. L., and Rosenberg, M., 1983, Establishment of repressor synthesis, in: *Lambda II* (R. W. Hendrix, J. W. Roberts, F. W. Stahl, and R. A. Weisberg, eds.), pp. 53–74, Cold Spring Harbor Laboratory, Cold Spring Harbor, NY.

Yamamoto, N., Ushijima, N., Gemski, P., and Baron, L. S., 1977, Genetic studies of hybrids between coliphage λ and *Salmonella* phage P22: Genetic analysis of the P22-λ class, *Mol. Gen. Genet.* **155**:117.

Yamamoto, N., Wohlhieter, J. A., Gemski, P., and Baron, L. S., 1978, λimmP22dis: A hybrid of coliphage λ with both immunity regions of *Salmonella* phage P22, *Mol. Gen. Genet.* **166**:233.

Youderian, P., and Susskind, M. M., 1980a, Identification of the products of bacteriophage P22 genes, including a new late gene, *Virology* **107**:258.

Youderian, P., and Susskind, M. M., 1980b, Bacteriophage P22 proteins specified by the region between genes 9 and erf, *Virology* **107**:270.

Youderian, P., Chadwick, S. J., and Susskind, M. M., 1982, Autogenous regulation by the bacteriophage P22 arc gene product, *J. Mol. Biol.* **154**:449.

Youderian, P., Vershon, A., Bouvier, S., Sauer, R. T., and Susskind, M. M., 1983, Changing the DNA-binding specificity of repressor, *Cell* **35**:777.

Youderian, P., Sugiono, P., Brewer, K. L., Higgins, N. P., and Elliott, T., 1988, Packaging the *Salmonella* chromosome with locked-in P22 prophages, *Genetics* (in press).

Young, R., Way, J., Way, S., Yin, J., and Syvanen, M., 1979, Transposition mutagenesis of bacteriophage Lambda: A new gene affecting cell lysis, *J. Mol. Biol.* **132**:307.

Yu, M.-H., and King, J., 1984, Single amino acid substitutions influencing the folding pathway of the phage P22 tail spike endorhamnosidase, *Proc. Natl. Acad. Sci. USA* **81**:6584.

Zinder, N. D., and Lederberg, J., 1952, Genetic exchange in *Salmonella, J. Bacteriol.* **64**:679.

CHAPTER 12

Bacteriophage Gene Products That Cause Human Disease

WILLIAM R. BISHAI AND JOHN R. MURPHY

I. INTRODUCTION

Bacteriophages are ubiquitous in nature. Indeed, bacteria for which no phages have been identified are exceptional cases, and this holds true among the pathogenic bacteria as well as the nonpathogenic. However, there are only a handful of pathogenic bacteria for which a virulence factor has been shown to be a phage-encoded gene: *Corynebacterium diphtheriae* (diphtheria), *Clostridium botulinum* (botulism), *Streptococcus pyogenes* (scarlet fever), *Staphylococcus aureus* (food poisoning), and *Escherichia coli* (noninvasive, hemorrhagic colitis). In each of these five cases, at least one of the virulence factors is an exotoxin, and in four of the five cases, the toxin's structural gene has been shown to be carried by a bacteriophage (this has not been rigorously proved for botulinum toxin).

Since the full list of virulence factors associated with an given pathogen is usually difficult to establish and often comprises complex multigene functions such as adherence factors, surface capsules, antigenic switching mechanisms, or enzyme secretion, it is little surprise that only the simplest of virulence factors, exotoxin production, has been demonstrated to be phage-encoded. With the application of molecular biological

WILLIAM R. BISHAI • Evans Department of Medicine and Clinical Research, Boston University Medical Center, and Department of Microbiology and Molecular Genetics, Harvard Medical School, Boston, Massachusetts 02115.   JOHN R. MURPHY • Evans Department of Medicine and Clinical Research, Boston University Medical Center, Boston, Massachusetts 02118.

techniques to the study of bacterial exotoxins, a common theme has been that many of the genes for these proteins have been found on mobile genetic elements (for review see Betley *et al.*, 1986) such as plasmids, transposons, or, as we shall discuss, phages. There seems to be a premium in microbial evolution on keeping these genes mobile. One can only speculate that harboring an exotoxin gene on a mobile element in only a few carrier organisms serves both to shelter the toxin from premature exposure to the host's immune system and to facilitate rapid *in situ* conversion of nontoxinogenic bacteria when a nonimmune host is encountered. As other, more complex mechanisms of pathogenesis beyond exotoxin production are unraveled, it will be of interest to see if they too are linked to mobile genetic elements.

II. DIPHTHERIA TOXIN

A. Diphtheria

Diphtheria is a paradigm among the infectious diseases, for it was one of the earliest bacterial diseases to be studied in detail. Indeed, early investigations into the nature of diphtheria were rapidly rewarded by the development of both an effective therapy for acute infection (antitoxin) and a highly successful vaccine (diphtheria toxoid) by the 1920s.

Diphtheria is most commonly an infection of the upper respiratory tract causing fever, sore throat, fatigue, and malaise. The thick, adherent gray-green membrane that forms on the tonsils and pharyngeal walls in many cases is what gives the disease its name (Greek: *diph*, leather, and *therios*, pouch). The combined effects of bacterial growth, toxin production, tissue necrosis, and the host's immune response give rise to this diphtheritic membrane. Although the throat is typically the only site from which the diphtheria bacillus, *Corynebacterium diphtheriae*, can be cultivated, tissue damage is widespread owing to the elaboration of diphtheria toxin. Neuritis and myocarditis are the most common clinical manifestations of intoxication, and fatalities are usually due to conduction disturbances in the heart or to myocardial failure. Antibiotics are of little use, but antitoxin if administered promptly can be life-saving.

The effects of immunization have made diphtheria a rare disease in industrialized nations. In the United States the annual incidence of respiratory diphtheria has dropped from more than 200,000 cases in 1921 (5–10% of which were fatal) to zero cases reported in 1986 (Immunization Practices Advisory Committee, 1985; Centers for Disease Control, 1987). And in a massive immunization campaign in Romania between 1958 and 1972, in which over 30 million vaccine doses were administered, the annual incidence of diphtheria has dropped from 600 per 100,000 to less than 1 per 100,000 (Saragea *et al.*, 1979).

B. Bacterial Host

The causative organism of diphtheria is the gram-positive bacillus *Corynebacterium diphtheriae* first observed by Klebs (1883) and later cultivated by Loeffler (1884). Based on his observation that *C. diphtheriae* could only be cultivated from the site of infection and not from the damaged internal organs, Loeffler postulated the existence of a soluble toxin, and 4 years later, Roux and Yersin (1888) succeeded in producing diphtherialike disease in animals injected with sterile filtrates from *C. diphtheriae* cultures.

The spread of diphtheria is by exposure to infected individuals—usually by droplet transmission or intimate contact. Toxinogenic *C. diphtheriae* may be identified by the production of immunoprecipitin lines when grown in a streak across a strip of filter paper containing antidiphtheria toxin serum (Elek test; Elek, 1948). Epidemiological studies have traditionally distinguished three subtypes of *C. diphtheriae: mitis, intermedius,* and *gravis;* these are identified by biochemical tests and colony morphology (Anderson *et al.,* 1931). Moreover, 33 phage types have been identified (Saragea *et al.,* 1979), and these have also been useful in epidemiological studies of the disease.

C. Corynephage β

Phages that infect *C. diphtheriae* (for reviews see Barksdale, 1970; Barksdale and Arden, 1974) have been known since d'Herelle (1918) isolated the first specimen from the manure of horses that had been immunized with extracts from diphtheria cultures. He demonstrated that these corynephages only formed plaques on nontoxinogenic strains of *C. diphtheriae,* but he did not establish a link between the pathogenicity of the diphtheria bacillus and lysogeny by a corynephage. The first suggestion that toxin production and phage infection were related came 33 years later, from Freeman (1951) and Freeman and Morse (1952). In an attempt to increase toxin yields by using lytic phages to prepare cell-free extracts, these investigators noted that on old plates, nontoxinogenic bacterial strains had converted to toxinogenicity after exposure to certain phages. They subsequently identified a temperate phage, now known as corynebacteriophage β, as the converting phage. This observation was confirmed by Groman (1953) and Barksdale and Pappenheimer (1954).

Corynephage β is structurally similar to many of the coliphages; it has an icosahedral head and a non-contractile tail as observed by electron microscopy (Fig. 1) (Toshach, 1950; Mathews *et al.,* 1966). Electron microscopy has also revealed that its genome consists of linear and circular double-stranded DNA molecules 2.3×10^7 daltons or 35 kilobases (kb) in length (Wolfson and Dressler as cited in Singer, 1973a). The lysogenic

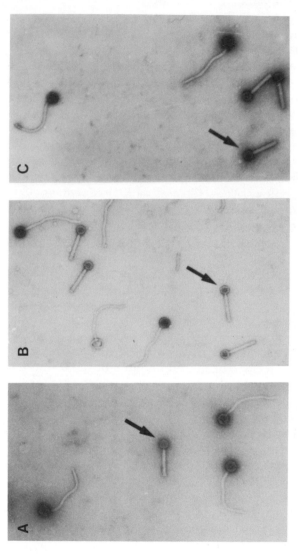

FIGURE 1. Transmission electron micrographs of corynephages (A) β, (B) γ, and (C) ω using negative staining with 1% uranyl acetate. Coliphage P4 (indicated by arrows) is used as a size standard. From Michel (1982).

phage is inducible by ultraviolet light or mitomycin C with a burst size of 30–60 plaque-forming units per cell after a 1-h latency period (Barksdale and Pappenheimer, 1954). Though β is a temperate phage, clear plaque-forming mutants can be readily isolated. Some of these lytic mutants (β_{clear} or β_c) fail to infect homoimmune lysogens, whereas others (β_{vir}) can superinfect homoimmune lysogens.

Although it was widely suspected in the 20 years following Freeman's discovery, there was no direct proof that the Tox character carried by the corynephages was indeed the diphtheria toxin structural gene. The Tox$^+$ phenotype could have been due to phage-borne regulatory gene whose expression correlated with toxin expression. Proof that corynephages carried the diphtheria toxin structural gene came when Uchida et al. (1971) isolated nitrosoguanidine-induced phage mutants that produced nontoxic, premature polypeptide chain termination mutants of diphtheria toxin that cross-reacted serologically with antitoxin. While helping to unravel the genetics of toxin production, these cross-reacting materials (CRMs) of diphtheria toxin have also proved invaluable in assigning the structure-activity relationships within the toxin polypeptide. Murphy et al. (1974) provided further proof that corynephages carry the toxin structural gene by showing that when added to an in vitro protein-synthesizing extract from E. coli, β-phage DNA directed the synthesis of authentic diphtheria toxin.

Mapping studies of the corynephage genome were begun by Holmes and Barksdale (1969), who studied the vegetatively (extrachromosomally) replicating phages. They were able to map the Tox character on the vegetative β genome relative to the extended host range markers h and h' and the immunity marker imm. The gene order was found to be h-tox-imm-h'. Matsuda et al. (1971) isolated 79 temperature-sensitive (ts) mutants of β_{vir} and used them to construct another map of the vegetative genome. Since toxin production is not essential for phage replication, none of their ts mutants mapped to the tox gene; however, they were able to identify 10 cistrons and to specify functions for some of them. Shortly thereafter, Singer (1973a,b) correlated the vegetative map of Holmes and Barksdale (1969) with that of Matsuda et al. (1971) and also mapped 10 new ts mutations. Singer was able to identify head-specific and tail-specific morphologic factors and show that the cistrons coding for each group were clustered at different ends of the phage genome. Singer's genetic map of the vegetative β genome is shown in Fig. 2.

Laird and Groman (1976a) studied the prophage form of corynephage β by inducing heteroimmune double lysogens and isolating mono-lysogenic recombinants. Their results showed that the prophage map is a circular permutation of the vegetative map. This led to the hypothesis that like coliphage λ, β-phage DNA has cohesive ends (cos) that circularize within the bacterial host, allowing for either vegetative replication or integration into the bacterial chromosome (Campbell, 1971). The prophage map of Laird and Groman (1976a) is also shown in Fig. 2. The

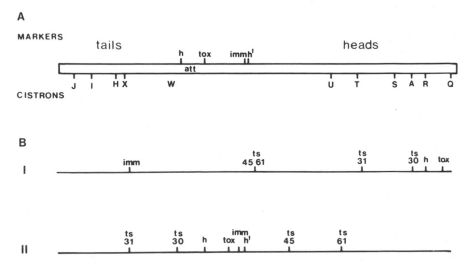

FIGURE 2. (A) Composite genetic map of the vegetative form of corynephage β based on the data of Singer (1973a) and Holmes and Barksdale (1969). Capital letters refer to cistrons. (B-I) Genetic map of the prophage form of corynephage β based on the data of Laird and Groman (1976a). (B-II) The vegetative map of Singer (1973a) with the ts markers of Laird and Groman (1976a) drawn in. From Michel (1982).

tox gene in this map is at one extreme end of the phage genome, directly adjacent to the phage attachment site attP. This observation has led to speculation that the tox gene originated from the bacterial chromosome by an aberrant excision event (Laird and Groman, 1976a; Pappenheimer, 1977).

More recently, the genetic maps of phage β have been complemented by the physical mapping of restriction endonuclease sites (Fig. 3). Costa et al. (1981) and Buck and Groman (1981) have shown that the β_c genome is 35 kb in length and has cos ends that can be dissociated by heating to 65°C or sealed by treatment with DNA ligase. The cos sites map to the ends of the linear vegetative map of Singer (1973a), and the tox gene was localized to a 1.7-kb segment of the genome that is directly adjacent to the attP site. β_{vir}, a lytic mutant of phage β, contains a 1-kb deletion about 5 kb to the left of the attP site in the region encoding tail morphologic genes (Costa et al., 1981). There is no evidence to suggest that this deletion is responsible for the lytic phenotype of β_{vir}, and it is more likely that β_{vir} contains small changes at an operator site controlling lysogeny that have escaped detection by restriction and heteroduplex analysis. The β_c and β_{vir} restriction map for several enzymes is shown in Fig. 4.

On the basis of these restriction maps, segments of the diphtheria toxin gene have been cloned and used to elucidate the DNA sequence of the tox gene (Kaczorek et al., 1983; Greenfield et al., 1983; Ratti et al.

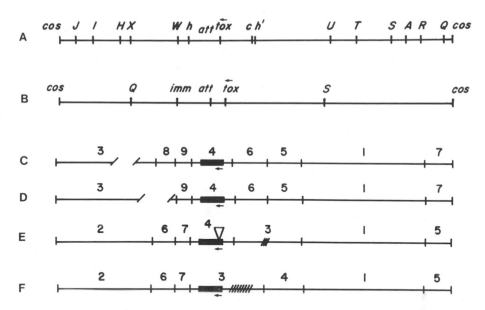

FIGURE 3. Comparison of the genetic maps corynephage β with the physical maps of β_c, β_{vir}, γ_c, and ω. Genetic maps: (A) the vegetative map of Singer (1973a) drawn as a prophage; (B) the prophage map of Laird and Groman (1976a). Physical maps: (C) β_c; (D) β_{vir}; (E) γ_c; (F) ω. The orientation of the *tox* gene is shown in all maps by a horizontal arrow. In the physical maps, vertical lines indicate the location of *Bam*HI restriction sites, and the numbers give the approximate length in kilobases of some of the fragments. The *tox* gene is indicated by the bold horizontal lines. Nonhomologous regions are shown as slashed areas, and the position of one of the insertions in γ_c is shown by a triangle. From Leong (1985).

1983). As suggested by the work of Holmes (1976) and Laird and Groman (1976b), the direction of transcription of the *tox* gene is toward the *attP* and *imm* loci. The sequencing data also confirmed the presence of a 25–amino acid leader peptide which directs the secretion of toxin into the extracellular space. Transcription is initiated 40 or 41 bases upstream from the CTG initiation codon at a sequence similar to the consensus sequence for *E. coli* promoters (Leong and Murphy, 1985).

D. Other Corynephages

Many different corynebacteriophages are known. In a comparative study, Holmes and Barksdale (1970) identified six different toxin-converting corynephages (α, β, δ, L, P, and π) and three nonconverting phages (γ, K, and ρ) on the basis of morphological, serological, and genetic characteristics. None of the criteria used to group the phages correlated with toxinogenicity; that is, many dissimilar phages were all toxinogenic. Groman (1984) has shown that toxinogenic corynephages can also be isolated from *Corynebacterium ulcerans*, a close relative of *C. diphthe-*

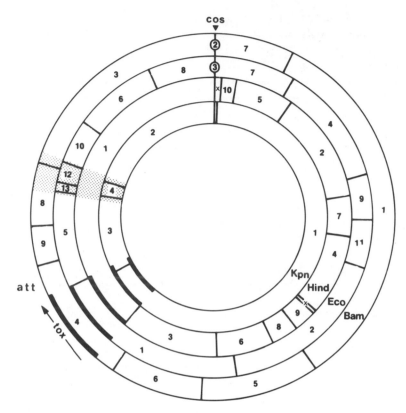

FIGURE 4. Composite phsycial map of corynephages β_c and β_{vir} for restriction endo-nucleases *Kpn*I, *Hind*III, *Eco*RI, and *Bam*HI. The stippled area shows DNA that is deleted in β_{vir}. The fragments are numbered by size for a given enzyme, with 1 designating the longest fragment. Adapted from Costa *et al.* (1981), and from Michel (1982).

riae, and that there are phages capable of infecting both *C. diphtheriae* and *C. ulcerans*.

Restriction endonuclease maps of some of these different cor-ynephages have now been compiled, and they show remarkable sim-ilarity, even though some have been maintained in laboratories for over 90 years. Corynephage γ was originally isolated as a nontoxinogenic phage from *C. diphtheriae* strain C7 (Groman and Eaton, 1955); it has a different host range from β, and its lysogens are not immune from β superinfection. Hybridization studies with ^{32}P-labeled *tox* mRNA showed that γ carries a cryptic *tox* gene that is not transcribed, and restriction mapping has revealed two DNA insertions in phage γ as com-pared to phage β, one of which is 1.5 kb in length and occurs at the 5' end of the *tox* gene (Michel *et al.*, 1982). Using DNA sequencing, Leong and Murphy (1985) have demonstrated that this is an insertionlike element with ends that are inverted repeats. It disrupts the signal sequence of the *tox* gene in phage γ and prevents *tox* translation. Other differences between β and γ are a 1.7-kb DNA insertion in γ in a region that specifies tail genes, and a substitution bubble seen in β/γ heteroduplexes at or near the *imm* locus. This substitution bubble may account for the heteroimmunity between these two phages.

Corynephage ω^{tox+} was isolated from the Park-Williams No. 8 (PW8) strain of *C. diphtheriae* (Park and Williams, 1896). Under optimal conditions, this bacterial strain will produce as much as 500 mg of diphtheria toxin per liter of culture (Righelato and Van Hemert, 1969)—about five times more than strain C7(ω^{tox+}), and for this reason it has been used commercially to make diphtheria toxin and toxoid. Morphologically, phage ω is identical to β. Restriction analysis of its genome shows three insertions relative to β, one of which is at the 5' end of the *tox* gene. This insertion near the *tox* gene does not, however, have any positive or negative regulatory effects on diphtheria toxin production (Rappuoli *et al.*, 1983a). Although host factors play a large role in the hypertoxinogenicity of PW8 (Pappenheimer, 1977), Rappuoli *et al.* (1983a,b) showed that phage ω, as well as phages β and γ, is capable of forming polylysogens by inserting a two different bacterial attachment sites, *attB1* and *attB2* (Rappuoli and Ratti, 1984). Both tandem and nontandem lysogens, which carry up to three prophage genomes, were characterized, and double lysogens were shown to produce twice as much diphtheria toxin under optimal conditions as single lysogens. Thus the *tox* gene dose also has an influence on toxin production.

Using molecular biological techniques, Buck *et al.* (1985) have reexamined the different corynephages first identified by Holmes and Barksdale (1970). They found that although the phages differed morphologically and serologically, restriction enzyme profiles of their genomes showed they were all similar with the exception of phage δ. They have argued that toxinogenic phages α, β, L, P, and π as well as nontoxinogenic phages γ, K, and ρ are all part of a highly related β-family of corynephages. Phage δ is most likely a representative of another family of corynephages.

Several studies have addressed the question of whether the *tox* gene is always phage-associated. Although strains can be isolated that are *tox*$^+$ but fail to produce phage (Rappuoli *et al.*, 1985), Southern blotting consistently reveals phage DNA in association with the *tox* gene. These strains are thus defective lysogens. Moreover, nontoxinogenic strains that carry cryptic *tox* genes (e.g., lysogens of phage γ) can be isolated by blotting techniques, but these also carry β-phage-like DNA (Groman *et al.*, 1983). Thus far no *C. diphtheriae* isolates have been found where the *tox* gene is not phage-associated (Groman *et al.*, 1983). There is one report of *C. ulcerans* carrying the *tox* gene without β-phage-like DNA, but it could be associated with a corynephage unrelated to β (Groman *et al.*, 1984).

E. Regulation of *tox* Expression

An important observation from the study of phage γ^{tox-} and nitrosoguanidine-induced *tox⁻* mutants of phage β is that a functional *tox* gene is not required for phage proliferation. Moreover, *tox* expression seems unrelated to the phage life cycle; toxin can be produced by lysogens (Matsuda and Barksdale, 1967), vegetatively replicating phage genomes (Matsuda and Barksdale, 1966), and nonintegrated exogenotes with lysogenic immunity (Gill *et al.*, 1972).

Although the diphtheria toxin gene must come from a corynephage, the expression of the *tox* gene is controlled by the host bacteria. Different bacterial strains lysogenic for the same toxinogenic phage may vary widely in the levels of toxin produced, whereas a given bacterial strain lysogenic for different phages makes the same amounts of toxin (Rappuoli *et al.*, 1983b).

Locke and Main (1931) and Pope (1932) were the first to note that among the many variables in toxin production, high levels of iron were particularly inhibitory. Pappenheimer and Johnson (1936) showed that toxin expression was maximal during the late log and early stationary phase of growth when iron in the growth media had been depleted. Strains that were high producers of toxin were ones that could continue to grow even when iron was depleted. The PW8 strain is the best example of this, and the amounts of toxin it produces during iron starvation are impressive. Under optimal conditions, 35% of its total protein synthesis (and 100% of its secreted protein) is diphtheria toxin (Pappenheimer, 1977).

The iron regulation of *tox* expression remained largely unstudied until the mid-1970s. Murphy *et al.* (1974) showed that *in vitro* protein-synthesizing extracts from *E. coli* produced toxin from β phage DNA whereas a similar extract from nonlysogenic *C. diphtheriae* did not. Moreover, no toxin was produced when the *C. diphtheriae* extract was mixed with the *E. coli* extract, indicating that host factors from *C. diphtheriae* inhibit the expression of *tox*. Two years later, Murphy *et al.* (1976) isolated a phage mutant β_{ct1}, which is relatively insensitive to iron inhibition. Since the *ct1* mutation is *cis*-dominant and the N-terminal amino acid sequence of tox_{ct1} is identical to that of authentic toxin, the mutation probably lies in the 5′ regulatory region of the *tox* gene.

Based on these observations, Murphy *et al.* (1976) proposed that *tox* expression is regulated by a bacteria-encoded repressor that in the presence of iron binds to an operator locus near the *tox* gene. The *ct1* mutation fits into this scheme as an operator-constitutive mutant in which repressor binding is inhibited owing to an alteration in the DNA sequence at the putative operator site (for review see Murphy and Bacha, 1979).

Welkos and Holmes (1981a) isolated a similar iron-insensitive phage mutant $\beta^{tox-201}$, which makes 200 times more toxin than β^{tox+} in the presence of iron (this is 8 times more that β_{ct1}). This regulatory mutation is also *cis*-dominant, but differs from β_{ct1} in that it produces four times more toxin than β^{tox+} even under low iron conditions. The mutation has been mapped to the 5' end of the *tox* gene (Welkos and Holmes, 1981b). The DNA sequences of the 5' regulatory regions of these mutants has not been reported.

Murphy's model predicts the existence of repressor mutants; these would be host mutations that result in constitutive, iron-insensitive toxin synthesis. Kanei *et al.* (1977) isolated such a bacterial mutant from strain C7 and have called it C7hm732. This strain overexpresses toxin in the presence of iron when lysogenized by either β^{tox+} or β_c^{tox-45} and thus is *trans*-dominant.

Further evidence in support of the iron-binding repressor came when Murphy *et al.* (1978) demonstrated that both iron and rifampicin (a potent inhibitor of transcription) give similar kinetics in inhibiting toxin synthesis. This suggests that iron regulation occurs at the level of transcription as predicted by the model. The postulated iron-binding repressor has not been purified or further characterized.

F. Diphtheria Toxin Structure and Function

Diphtheria toxin is one of the most lethal substances known with an LD_{50} (dose required to kill 50% of the animals tested) of about 100 ng/kg body weight for humans, rabbits, and guinea pigs (Gill, 1982). The toxin (for review see Collier, 1975; Murphy, 1976, 1985; Pappenheimer, 1977; Ward, 1987) is a 535–amino acid, single-chain polypeptide with a deduced molecular weight of 58,342 daltons (Greenfield *et al.*, 1983) and an apparent molecular weight on SDS-polyacrylamide gels of 62,000–63,000 daltons (Gill and Dinius, 1971; Collier and Kandel, 1971).

The toxin contains two disulfide loops (see Fig. 5), the first from cys_{186} to cys_{201} and the second from cys_{461} to cys_{471}. Three arginine residues occur in the first disulfide loop forming a protease sensitive site; in many preparations, the toxin has already been "nicked" within this loop by bacterial proteases. The same nicking process can be reproduced *in vitro* by exposure to dilute trypsin (Gill and Pappenheimer, 1971; Drazin *et al.*, 1971). Treatment of nicked toxin with reducing agents allows the separation of two fragments: the N-terminal portion, fragment A, is 193 amino acids long (MW 21,000); and the C-terminal portion, fragment B, is 342 amino acids long (MW 37,000).

Diphtheria toxin kills eukaryotic cells by enzymatically inactivating protein synthesis (Straus and Hendee, 1959; Collier and Pappenheimer, 1964). Fragment A carries the enzymatic function, and fragment B is responsible for the delivery of fragment A into the cell's cytoplasm. Fragment B carries two functional domains: membrane translocation and receptor binding.

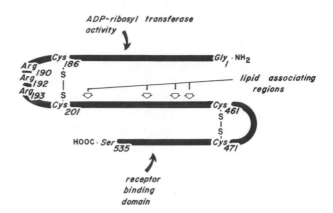

FIGURE 5. Schematic diagram of the structure-function relationships of diphtheria toxin. Fragment A is composed of residues 1 to 193, and fragment B stretches from 194 to 535.

Receptor binding is the first step in the intoxication process. The toxin binds to specific receptors on the surface of sensitive eukaryotic cells (Ittleson and Gill, 1973; Middlebrook et al., 1978). Binding of toxin to its receptor is saturable, and competition can be demonstrated using CRM197, a full-length, ADP-ribosyltransferase-negative, nontoxic, cross-reacting material of diphtheria toxin (Uchida et al., 1973; Ittleson and Gill, 1973). Although the exact nature of the diphtheria toxin receptor remains unclear, recent evidence suggests that the receptor in Vero cells is closely positioned to an anion transport channel (Olsnes and Sandvig, 1986; Sandvig and Olsnes, 1986).

Following receptor binding, the toxin is internalized by receptor-mediated endocytosis in coated pits (Moya et al., 1985), and fragment A is then translocated from the endocytic vesicle to the cytoplasm. The entry process is mediated by the N-terminal portion of fragment B or the portion of toxin from amino acid 194 to about 386. Eisenberg et al. (1984) have identified three hydrophobic stretches within this portion of the toxin that are capable of spanning a membrane, and Lambotte et al. (1980) have found regions of homology in this part of the toxin to both membrane-spanning domains and membrane surface-binding domains of other proteins. Others (Donovan et al., 1981; Kagan et al., 1981; Zalman and Wisnieski, 1984) have shown that fragments of toxin that contain this region are capable of forming channels in artificial membranes.

Membrane translocation is a triggered process that occurs at low pH (Sandvig and Olsnes, 1981). Lysosomotropic agents such as NH_4Cl and chloroquine, which interfere with acidification of lysosomes, also block the entry of diphtheria toxin (Draper and Simon, 1980). Sandvig and Olsnes (1982) and Marnell et al. (1984) have provided evidence suggesting that diphtheria toxin enters cells through endocytic vesicles in a pH-dependent fashion. The toxin denatures rapidly in vitro at low pH, and it is thought that a similar process at the membrane surface might lead to the exposure and insertion into the membrane of the fragment B hydrophobic domains.

The current model for toxin entry is that after binding, the toxin-receptor complex is internalized into endocytic vesicles, which are subsequently acidified. The acidification process triggers a conformational change within fragment B, enabling it to form channels across the endosomal membrane. Following proteolytic cleavage and disulfide bond reduction between the A and B fragments, fragment A passes through the channel and is liberated into the cytosol (for a review of membrane translocation see Neville and Hudson, 1986).

The third step in the intoxication process is the enzymatic inhibition of protein synthesis. Fragment A is an ADP-ribosylating enzyme that catalytically inactivates eukaryotic elongation factor 2 (EF-2) (Collier, 1967; Goor and Pappenheimer, 1967; for review of ADP-ribosylating enzymes see Ueda and Hayaishi, 1985). EF-2 is essential for transferring the nascent peptidyl-tRNA molecule from the aminoacyl site to the polypeptidyl site of the eukaryotic ribosome, and it is completely inactive when ADP-ribosylated. The reaction catalyzed by fragment A is shown below:

$$NAD^+ + EF\text{-}2_{active} \rightleftarrows ADP\text{-}ribose\text{-}EF\text{-}2_{inactive} + nicotinamide + H^+$$

At physiologic pH, the equilibrium for this reaction is far to the right, and the reaction is essentially quantitative. Yamaizumi et al. (1978) have shown that, owing to its catalytic nature, one molecule of fragment A is sufficient to kill a cell if introduced into the cytoplasm.

Van Ness et al. (1980) have identified the site of ADP ribosylation on EF-2 as being a posttranslationally modified histidine residue that has been named diphthamide (Fig. 6). All eukaryotic cells that have been characterized, as well as several archebacteria, have been shown to have diphthamide in their EF-2 (Gehrmann et al., 1985). Since mutant cell lines that fail to make diphthamide show normal growth properties (Moehring et al., 1980), the function of the diphthamide residue remains unclear. It has been suggested that diphthamide is a regulatory site on EF-2 that is modified during different phases of the cell cycle in order to

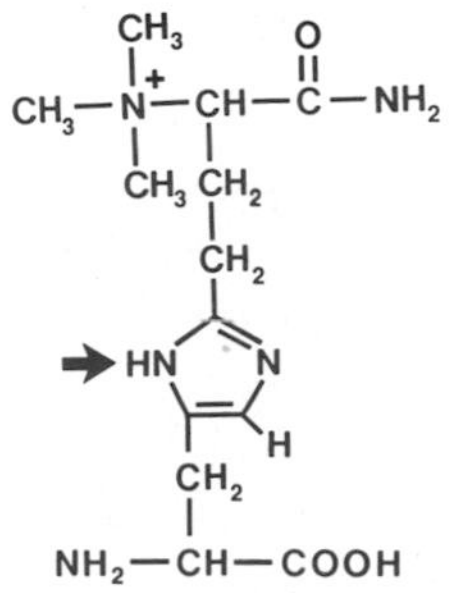

FIGURE 6. The structure of diphthamide, the modified histidine residue found on eukaryotic elongation factor 2. Diphtheria toxin fragment A catalyzes the transfer of ADP-ribose to the nitrogen indicated by the arrow. Modified from Van Ness et al. (1980).

modulate the level of protein synthesis (Lee and Iglewski, 1984). The discovery of an endogenous cytosolic ADP-ribosyltransferase activity in baby hamster kidney cells and beef liver supports this notion (Lee and Iglewski, 1984). As yet, however, the enzyme(s) responsible for this activity has not been purified.

The third and only other enzyme known that can ADP-ribosylate the diphthamide residue of EF-2 is *Pseudomonas aeruginosa* exotoxin A (Iglewski and Kabat, 1975). Functionally, it is very similar to diphtheria toxin, since it has an enzymatic domain and a binding/membrane translocation domain. However, diphtheria toxin and pseudomonas exotoxin A show little immunological cross-reactivity (Sadoff *et al.*, 1982), and the DNA and amino acid sequences are not homologous (Gray *et al.*, 1984). The three-dimensional structure of exotoxin A has been determined at the 3.0 Å level (Allured *et al.*, 1986), and it will be interesting to compare it to the crystal structure for diphtheria toxin once the latter has been solved.

G. Targeting Diphtheria Toxin-Related Hybrid Proteins to Cancer Cells

As an understanding of the structure-activity relationships of diphtheria toxin developed, it became increasingly attractive to target the toxin to specific cell types. The field of immunotoxin research (for review see Collier and Kaplan, 1984; Vitetta and Uhr, 1985) has for some years employed fragments of diphtheria toxin or the plant toxin, ricin, linked to antibodies, as experimental targeted cytotoxins. A more recent alternative approach is to use genetic engineering to construct hybrid toxins composed of a toxin fragment and targeting domain in a single polypeptide chain. Here a hybrid gene encodes the hybrid toxin protein. The advantages of this system are that the linkage between toxic fragment and the new binding domain is a peptide bond, the protein product is homogeneous, and the location of the fusion junction can be exactly specified.

Murphy *et al.* (1986, 1988) have constructed two diphtheria toxin-hormone gene fusions and used them to produce hybrid toxin proteins. In both cases they have truncated the diphtheria toxin portion at amino acid 485; this is 50 amino acids short of the C terminus of whole toxin. Thus the hybrid toxins are composed of all of fragment A (193 amino acids) and 292 amino acids of fragment B. The fusion junction was selected to leave much of the membrane translocation domains behind while deleting the diphtheria toxin receptor-binding domain.

The targeting portions of these toxins are the polypeptide hormones α-melanocyte-stimulating hormone (αMSH, 13 amino acids) and interleukin-2 (IL-2, 133 amino acids). In each instance, the polypeptide hormone has been shown to bind to surface receptors that are internalized and processed through acidified endocytic vesicles just like diphtheria toxin. These fusion proteins are envisioned as prototypes in the development of agents that may be useful in the treatment of malignant melanoma (αMSH toxin) and adult T-cell leukemia (IL-2 toxin). Since only activated and proliferating T cells express the IL-2 receptor, IL-2 toxin might also be useful as an immunosuppresive agent.

At present, the αMSH toxin produced by recombinant E. coli carrying an engineered hybrid toxin gene has been partially purified. The extracts are toxic for human malignant melanoma cells which bear the αMSH receptor and are nontoxic for other cell lines which are devoid of the αMSH receptor (Murphy et al., 1986).

The IL-2 toxin has been purified to apparent homogeneity and is selectively toxic for high-affinity IL-2 receptor-positive cell lines in vitro (Williams et al., 1987; Bacha et al., 1988). On the human C91/P1 T-cell line, the IC_{50} for inhibition of protein synthesis is 10^{-11} M with IL-2 toxin and 10^{-8} M with diphtheria toxin. Thus with this cell line the IL-2 toxin is approximately 1000 times more toxic than diphtheria toxin itself. Cells devoid of IL-2 receptors are resistant to inhibition of protein synthesis by IL-2 toxin. The toxicity of the hybrid toxin against receptor positive cells is inhibited by the addition of free IL-2, 33.B3 (an anti-IL-2 receptor monoclonal antibody), and chloroquine (an inhibitor of endosome acidification). These experiments clearly demonstrate that IL-2 toxin action is mediated throught the IL-2 receptor, and further that passage through and acidic vesicle is a required step in the intoxication process. Additional experiments have shown that IL-2 toxin catalyzes the ADP-ribosylation of EF-2 in target cells. Thus, IL-2 toxin is a new toxin that combines the potency of diphtheria toxin with the target cell specificity of IL-2.

III. BOTULINUM TOXIN

A. Botulism

Until recently, botulism was not considered a true infectious disease but rather an intoxication brought about by ingesting preformed botulinum toxin made by *Clostridium botulinum*. In addition to food-poisoning botulism, two infectious forms of the disease are now recognized: Infant botulism and wound botulism (Sugiyama, 1980). In infant botulism, *C. botulinum* has been shown to colonize the gastrointestinal tract of babies less than 6 months old and slowly elaborate toxin. Similarly, in wound botulism, which is exceedingly rare (6 cases in 1983–86), the bacteria colonize a break in the skin and intoxicate the host. All types of botulism result in flaccid paralysis.

On a molar basis, botulinum toxin is the most potent poison known to mankind, with the lethal dose being about 1 pmole for a human adult (20 ng/kg). The disease was first recognized over 200 years ago by German physicians who noted that the fatal syndrome sometimes resulted from eating spoiled sausage (*botulinum* is Latin for sausage). Studies in the 1920s, which defined the foods most often contaminated by *C. botulinum* and the conditions required to kill the bacterial spores, have greatly reduced the incidence of botulism from commercially canned foods. Although there have been occasional large outbreaks (30–60 cases) resulting from contaminated food being served in public places, most outbreaks in the United States now result from improperly cooked, home-canned foods and strike fewer than three individuals (Smith, 1977).

Depending on the amount of toxin ingested, botulism intoxication can be rapidly progressive and cause death within 24 h or be so mild that the patient may not seek medical advice. Symptoms usually appear about 24 h after ingesting toxin and typically consist of blurred or double vision, photophobia, slurred speech, and a flaccid, symmetric paralysis of the extremities. Constipation, urinary retention, and reduced salivation and tears also occur, but there is never any impairment of the sensory nervous system. All of these symptoms are a direct result of botulinum toxin's neurotoxicity—a blockade of cholinergic transmission outside the central nervous system. Death results from paralysis of the respiratory muscles or from respiratory complications such as pneumonia. With the availability of antitoxin and sophisticated means of supportive care, the mortality rate is now about 10% in the United States.

B. Bacterial Host

The genus *Clostridium* comprises gram-positive, spore-forming bacilli that are strictly anaerobic. The organisms are widely disseminated in soil, lakes, and ocean environments and are sometimes found in the intestinal flora of animals. Clostridial spores are resistant to extremes of temperature (including boiling for several hours) and can only be effectively eliminated by heating to 120°C for 30 min. *Clostridium botulinum* is defined as any clostridial isolate that produces botulinum toxin.

There are at least two different methods for classifying different *C. botulinum* strains. The first and most prevalent is based on the serotype of botulinum toxin the strain produces (Smith, 1977). Eight different serotypes (A, B, C_1, C_2, D, E, F, and G) are currently recognized. Types A, B, and E are most commonly associated with disease in humans. Types C and D cause botulism in animals, with type C best known for producing limberneck in waterfowl and type D for cattle botulism. Types F and G are natural isolates that have only rarely caused disease. Serological typing of *C. botulinum* on the basis of the toxin produced has proved problematic in several instances. Some *C. botulinum* strains have lost their toxinogenicity either spontaneously or by experimental manipulation. Other strains can be shown to produce more than one type of toxin (Giminez and Ciccarelli, 1970; Sugiyama *et al.*, 1972; Jansen, 1971).

A second method for classifying *C. botulinum* strains is based on their biochemical properties as well as their toxin serotype. Group I organisms (types A, B, and F) are proteolytic, group II (types B, E, and F) are nonproteolytic, group III (types C_1, C_2, and D) are weakly proteolytic or nonproteolytic, and group IV (type G) is proteolytic but nonsaccharolytic. Strains in the same group show cross-reactivity of surface and spore antigens, homology of chromosomal DNA and ribosomal RNA, and similarities in susceptibility to bacteriophages (Sugiyama, 1980).

C. Converting Bacteriophages of *C. botulinum*

Many features of *C. botulinum* growth suggested that the bacteria might carry phages. These hints included premature clearance of culture supernatants, intermittent failure to grow after transfer, and small foci of clearance within colonies (Dolman and Chang, 1972). Electron micrograph studies proved that although the yields of phage were often low, virtually every strain carried one or more temperate phages that could be induced by UV light or mitomycin C (Vinet and Fredette, 1968; Inoue and Iida, 1968; Eklund *et al.*, 1969; Dolman and Chang, 1972). Several different phage morphologies have been observed including icosahedral heads with contractile tails, bullrushy heads with contractile tails, and icosahedral heads with flexible tails (Dolman and Chang, 1972).

Inoue and Iida (1970) were the first to show a relationship between lysogeny and toxinogenicity. Since *C. botulinum* strains are all, by definition, toxinogenic, these investigators first converted a type C_1 strain to nontoxinogenicity by growth in the presence of acridine orange. It is noteworthy that the nontoxinogenic phenotype was stable for many passages, indicating that botulinum toxin type C_1 is not an essential protein for these *Clostridia*. They then converted the nontoxinogenic strain back to type C_1 toxinogenicity by adding a mitomycin-induced, cell-free lysate of the parent culture. Eklund *et al.* (1971) confirmed this finding; they also observed that two different phages could be isolated from their parent type C culture, but only one was toxin-converting.

The same experiment proved successful with *C. botulinum* type D (Inoue and Iida, 1971; Eklund *et al.*, 1972) but not for type C_2. Moreover, Inoue and Iida (1971) showed that with some strains a type C_1 phage could convert a cured type D bacterial strain to type C_1 toxin production. The phage-host relationship here appears to be that of pseudolysogeny, because growth in antiphage serum (Inoue and Iida, 1971) or induction of sporulation (Eklund *et al.*, 1972) removes toxinogenicity. Eklund and Poysky (1974) carried the analysis further by converting type C_1 bacteria to type D and then back to type C_1 with toxin-converting bacteriophages.

The demonstration of inter-*type* phage conversion in *C. botulinum* was followed by one of inter-*species* phage conversion. By curing both *C. botulinum* type C and *C. novyi* type A (a clostridial species producing a toxin involved in gas gangrene) of their respective phages, Eklund *et al.* (1974) found that the cured strains could subsequently be converted to produce the opposite toxin; that is, nontoxinogenic *C. botulinum* type C became indistinguishable from *C. novyi* type A when infected with phage NA1^{tox+} from *C. novyi*. These analyses showed that although there is biochemical and physiological heterogeneity among the clostridial species, a few parental strains may exist that, following infection with different converting phages, give rise to some of the different serotypic types of *C. botulinum* as well as some different clostridial species.

However, Oguma *et al.* (1976a) showed that the clostridial phages may not be as promiscuous as previously suggested. They demonstrated three different antigenic types of tox$^+$ phages for types C_1 and D toxin and showed that, although the phages were morphologically similar, they had specific host ranges. Moreover, some phages absorb to the bacterial surface but do not convert (Oguma and Sugiyama, 1978), although this may be an immunity phenomenon resulting from previous lysogenization by tox$^-$ phages (Oguma, 1976). Phages have also been shown to convert *C. botulinum* types C and D to hemagglutinin production (Oguma *et al.*, 1976b).

Virtually nothing is known of the genetics of these clostridial phages, and, as yet, no attempt has been made to determine whether the type C_1 and D converting phages carry structural genes for botulinum toxin types C_1 and D or are merely a genetic factor involved in the expression of the toxins. The role of bacteriophages in the toxinogenicity of *C. botulinum* types A, B, and E, which cause the majority of human disease, is still an open question.

D. Botulinum Toxin Structure and Function

In contrast to the genetics of *Clostridium botulinum* and its phages, much is known about the toxin the bacteria produce (for review see Sugiyama, 1980; Simpson, 1981). Although the eight serotypes of botulinum toxin are immunologically distinct, biochemically they appear to be quite homogeneous. They all have molecular weights between 140,000 and 170,000 daltons. They are synthesized as single polypeptide chains and are not secreted but rather released into the extracellular space by autolysis (Bonventre and Kempe, 1960a). All the toxins except type G have been purified, and type A has been crystallized (Abrams *et al.*, 1946). The botulinum toxins have disulfide bonds that are essential for toxicity (Sugiyama *et al.*, 1973).

Botulinum toxin requires proteolytic nicking for activation. Even after a culture has stopped growing and autolysis is complete, the toxicity of the culture supernatant continues to increase because of the action of endogenous clostridial proteases on the existing unnicked botulinum toxin (Bonventre and Kempe, 1960b). Types A and B toxins (which are produced by proteolytic strains of *C. botulinum*) are 10–100 times more potent than type E (which is produced by nonproteolytic strains). When type E toxin is nicked with trypsin, its specific toxicity approaches that of types A and B toxin (Duff *et al.*, 1956). Trypsin nicking, as well as the action of endogenous proteases, cleaves the botulinum toxins within their respective disulfide loops. Subsequent reduction liberates an N-terminal light chain (MW 50,000) and a C-terminal heavy chain (MW 100,000) (DasGupta and Sugiyama, 1972).

Botulinum toxins block the release of acetylcholine (ACh) from the presynaptic terminal at the neuromuscular junction, causing a flaccid paralysis of the motor nervous system (Burgen *et al.*, 1949). They also act at sites within the autonomic nervous system wherever ACh is the synaptic transmitter. The synthesis, storage, and metabolism of ACh are not affected in intoxicated nerve endings, but the production of end plate potentials (believed to be the result of vesicular release of ACh by the presynaptic neuron) is drastically reduced in response to nerve stimulation (Dreyer *et al.*, 1984).

A three-step model for intoxication has been proposed (Simpson, 1980). The first is binding to a specific receptor. At least one element of the receptor is a sialic acid-containing ganglioside of the G_{1b} series, which is only found on neural tissue (Kitamura *et al.*, 1980; Montecucco, 1986). Antibodies against botulinum toxin interfere with the intoxication process even after binding has occurred (Simpson, 1974), suggesting that binding is extracellular and that binding alone does not directly intoxicate the nerve terminal. Next, the toxin is thought to be internalized, possibly by receptor-mediated endocytosis. A study showing that NH_4Cl and methylamine-HCl antagonize botulinum toxin's action supports the endocytic vesicle internalization hypothesis (Simpson, 1983). Recent work has also shown that the heavy chains of botulinum toxin type B and tetanus toxin form channels in lipid bilayers in a pH-dependent fashion (Hoch *et al.*, 1985) and points to a membrane translocation function by the heavy chain of botulinum toxin. The third step is termed the "lytic" phase, where botulinum toxin interrupts the nerve terminal's capacity for evoked ACh release. Calculations show that between 1000 and 10,000 botulinum toxin molecules are capable of inactivating a single terminal (Hanig and Lamanna, 1979; Simpson, 1981), and the inactivation can last as long as months. These observations have led to the suggestion that the toxin's lytic function is enzymatic, although as yet no substrates have been identified. Some of the proposals for the lytic action of botulinum toxin are that it blocks ACh vesicle refilling (Boroff *et al.*, 1974), that it blocks calcium channels (Hirokawa and Heuser, 1980), and that it blocks the response of the end plate to increased intracellular calcium (Cull-Candy *et al.*, 1976).

The similarities between diphtheria toxin and botulinum toxin are striking. Both are lethal in nanogram quantities for mammals, and both accomplish this with a single polypeptide chain carrying at least three biochemical activities. Both have a trypsin-sensitive disulfide loop which divides the polypeptide into heavy and light chains with molecular weight ratios of about 2:1. The heavy chain in both instances mediates binding to a specific eukaryotic receptor and later is responsible for translocating the light chain into the cytosol. The light chain of diphtheria toxin, and perhaps botulinum toxin enzymatically inactivates a cytosolic target protein thereby causing cell intoxication.

IV. STREPTOCOCCAL PYROGENIC EXOTOXINS

A. Scarlet Fever

Scarlet fever is caused by group A streptococci, which elaborate streptococcal pyrogenic exotoxins (SPEs; also known as erythrogenic toxins or pyrogenic toxins). Streptococcal pharyngitis is one of the most common infections in humans, particularly among children aged 5–15 years. Scarlet fever results when strains of group A streptococci capable of making SPEs infect a host who is not immune to the toxin.

Scarlet fever is usually a self-limiting disease of about a week's duration. It is characterized by a diffuse rash which occurs about 2 days after the onset of sore throat. The rash starts on the neck and upper chest and spreads to the rest of the trunk and extremities; the erythema blanches on pressure. Other characteristic features include a white coating on the tongue with red, hypertrophied papillae protruding through (strawberry tongue) early in the disease, which converts to a uniformly beefy red appearance (raspberry tongue) later in the illness. The rash subsides in 4–5 days and is followed by extensive peeling of the damaged skin layers. The disease is usually contracted by direct (droplet) transmission from an infected individual. Since the organism can persist in the nasopharynx for weeks or months after symptoms have subsided, carrier rates for group A streptococci as high as 15% have been reported. Although streptococcal pharyngitis and scarlet fever are rarely life-threatening, antibiotic treatment is important to prevent the possible complications of group A streptococcal infection—abscess formation, acute rheumatic fever, and acute glomerulonephritis.

B. *Streptococcus pyogenes* and Its Toxins

Group A streptococci or *Streptococcus pyogenes* is responsible for most of the human pathogenicity among the beta-hemolytic streptococci. *Groups* are determined by serotyping acid extracts of the bacteria that contain the group-specific cell wall carbohydrate. Within group A, more than 60 *types* (determined by the cell wall M protein) exist. Human immunity to streptococcal infection is *type*-specific.

In addition to this serotypic variation, group A streptococci secrete over 20 extracellular proteins, many of which are antigenic and some of which have human toxicity. These proteins include streptokinase, streptodornase, hyaluronidase, diphosphopyridine nucleotidase, proteinases, amylases, and two hemolysins (streptolysins O and S) as well as the SPEs. Only the SPEs, of which there are three serotypes, have been linked to lysogeny by a streptococcal phage.

C. SPE-Converting Bacteriophages

SPE (erythrogenic toxin) was first identified as the cause of scarlet fever by Dick and Dick (1924). Shortly thereafter, Cantacuzene and Boncieu (1926) and Frobisher and Brown (1927) reported that an agent in sterile filtrates of scarlet fever-producing streptococci could impart toxinogenicity to nontoxic strains. Although this was later confirmed (Bingel, 1949), a bacteriophage was not identified as the converting agent until Zabriskie (1964) showed that streptococcal bacteriophage T12 forms lysogens in *S. pyogenes* T25$_3$ and causes a specific conversion to SPE production.

Lysogeny is prevalent among the group A streptococci, and Colon-Whitt *et al.* (1979) have shown that 90% of group A isolates are lysogenic for a phage, although many of these are not toxin-converting. All streptococcal bacteriophages studied thus far are morphologically similar to the Bradley class B1 phages (Bradley, 1967) with isometric polyhedral heads and long, unsheathed, noncontractile tails (Nida and Ferreti, 1982); they all carry double-stranded DNA.

Three serological types of SPEs (types A, B, and C) have been identified (Watson, 1960). With the development of antisera specific for each type of SPE, it has been possible to show that not only SPE type A toxin (Zabriskie, 1964) but also type C (Colon-Whitt *et al.*, 1979; Johnson *et al.*, 1980) and type B toxins (Nida and Ferretti, 1982) are phage-associated.

Nida and Ferretti (1982) isolated 10 different converting phages from cases of scarlet fever and showed that although each was serologically distinct and had a unique host range, all could convert nontoxinogenic streptococci to SPE production. Thus many different converting phages exist. As with toxinogenic corynebacteriophages, SPE-converting phages can produce toxin in either the lysogenic state (Johnson *et al.*, 1980), the pseudolysogenic state, where replication is extrachromosomal and a carrier state exists (Nida and Ferretti, 1982), or the virulent state (obligate lytic growth; McKane and Ferretti, 1981).

Although there were preliminary reports that phage mutants produced cross-reacting SPEs of altered toxicity (Johnson *et al.*, 1980), proof that converting phages actually carry the SPE structural genes was provided by molecular genetic techniques. Unlike corynephage research, in which the isolation of CRMs and the genetic mapping of phages preceded the application of molecular biological techniques, a physical (restriction) map of a streptococcal converting phage was determined (Johnson and Schlievert, 1983) in the absence of a genetic map or any confirmation that the phage genome carried the toxin structural gene. Johnson and Schlievert (1984) and Weeks and Ferretti (1984) demonstrated that phage T12 (Zabriskie's original converting phage) carries the structural gene for SPE type A by showing that cloned T12 DNA fragments direct the synthesis of SPE type A immunoreactivity in recombinant strains of *E. coli.*

The identification of the SPE type A structural gene (called *speA*) has made it possible to characterize toxinogenic streptococcal strains by hybridization techniques. Of particular interest are SPE type A-producing strains that do not yield phages. Is the *speA* gene sometimes bacterial and sometimes phage-borne? Johnson *et al.* (1986) examined the Southern hybridization of a *speA*-specific probe and a converting phage-specific probe to the chromosomal DNA of several SPE type A-producing but phage-negative streptococcal strains. They found that in all cases both phage sequences and *speA* sequences were present in the bacterial chromosome. This suggests that the strains contain defective prophages that have somehow lost their ability to excise and replicate. Their results also showed that the phage attachment site, *attP*, is adjacent to the *speA* gene on the phage genome, indicating that the toxin gene may have originated from the bacterial chromosome.

The *speA* gene has recently been sequenced (Weeks and Ferretti, 1986) and shown to encode a 221-amino acid polypeptide with a 30-amino acid leader peptide (total length, 251 amino acids). Bal-31 deletions of the 3' end of the gene (encoding the carboxy terminus) destroy the SPE type A immunoreactivity produced by recombinant *E. coli* carrying the gene. This implies that the major immunological epitopes of the toxin reside at the C terminus. The deduced amino acid sequence of SPE type A has extensive homology to staphylococcal enterotoxins type B and C_1, especially at the C terminus. A subsequent study has demonstrated immunological cross-reactivity between SPE type A and these two staphylococcal enterotoxins (Hynes *et al.*, 1987). The genes for staphylococcal enterotoxins B and C_1 are located on the bacterial chromosome, although they may be associated with a mobile element (Ranelli *et al.*, 1985).

The location of the structural genes for SPE types B and C has not been determined. At this time, nothing is known about the regulation of SPE type A expression in streptococci except that some lysogens produce far more toxin than others, and there is an A-T-rich region with several palindromes in the untranscribed sequences 5' to the *speA* gene which may serve a regulatory role.

D. Structure and Function of the SPEs

Genes for SPE production are widespread among the group A streptococci; about 90% of group A isolates make one or more of the three SPEs (Wannamaker, 1983). Although all three toxins are resistant to extremes of pH, there appear to be differences in heat stability and protease sensitivity. Aside from the immunological distinctions by which SPE types A, B, and C are defined, the three toxins can also be separated by differential solubility in various solvents (Cunningham et al., 1976). Purification schemes for each type have been reported (for review see Wannamaker, 1983). From the purification studies, SPE type B is reported to have a molecular weight of 21,900 (Barsumian et al., 1978a), and for type C it is 13,200 (Schlievert et al., 1977). The deduced molecular weight for mature SPE type A is 25,787 (Weeks and Ferretti, 1986).

Many different functions have been associated with the SPEs (for review see Alouf, 1980). These include pyrogenicity, enhanced susceptibility to endotoxic shock, increased permeability of the blood-brain barrier, T-cell mitogenicity, reduced clearance by the reticuloendothelial system, and cardiotoxicity (Barsumian et al., 1978b; Cunningham and Watson, 1978; Schlievert and Watson, 1978; Watson, 1960). The erythematous skin reaction, from which scarlet fever derives its name, is now believed to be a secondary result of the toxin's enhancement of the delayed type hypersensitivity response. The skin rash results from the combined presence of the SPEs and other streptococcal antigens to which the individual was previously sensitized (Schlievert et al., 1979).

Whether any of these tissue responses have a common basis at the cellular level is not known. Likewise, almost nothing is known of the mechanism of action of the three SPEs at the molecular level.

V. STAPHYLOCOCCAL ENTEROTOXINS

A. Staphylococcal Food Poisoning

Staphylococcal enterotoxins (SEs) cause an acute food poisoning syndrome that is second only to *Salmonella* infection as the leading cause of food-borne disease in the United States (MacDonald and Griffin, 1986). Like botulism, the illness results from ingesting preformed bacterial toxins and is not normally associated with infection by staphylococci.

Staphylococcal food poisoning follows a short incubation period (1–6 h) and usually only lasts about 10 h. It is typically associated with institutional outbreaks, striking many individuals who have dined together; as many as 75% of those exposed to the contaminated food develop symptoms. The toxin causes cramps and a secretory diarrhea (no blood or inflammatory cells are found in the stool), and unlike other noninvasive bacterial diarrheas, it is nearly always associated with vomiting. Although relatively short-lived, the diarrhea and vomiting can lead to severe fluid depletion, and 10–20% of patients require intravenous fluid to prevent hypovolemic shock, acidosis, or acute renal failure.

Staphylococcal food poisoning occurs when the bacteria are given the opportunity to multiply in contaminated food. Because staphylococci are normal inhabitants of the skin and can multiply at temperatures ranging from 4°C to 46°C, prevention of food poisoning rests largely on keeping potentially contaminated items, especially protein- or carbohydrate-rich foods, well refrigerated.

Seven separate SEs have been implicated in the pathogenesis of this disease. The toxins are distinguished serologically and are called types A, B, C_1, C_2, C_3, D, and E (Bergdoll, 1979). Only staphylococcal enterotoxin A (SEA), which is responsible for about 70% of staphylococcal food poisoning (Casman et al., 1967), has been shown to be phage-associated.

B. Staphylococcus aureus and Its Toxins

Staphylococcus aureus is a gram-positive, nonmotile, nonsporulating, aerobic bacterium that is coagulase-positive and ferments mannitol. Different strains elaborate several antigenic exotoxins in addition to the seven known enterotoxins. These include four hemolysins, leukocidin, coagulase, and hyaluronidase. S. aureus is responsible for numerous other forms of human pathology in addition to food poisoning, including purulent superficial infections, osteomyelitis, pneumonia, bacteremia, endocarditis, meningitis, abscesses, and genitourinary infections.

C. SE-Converting Bacteriophages

Bacteriophages that infect S. aureus have been known for many years and are the basis of a phage-typing system for this organism. Blair and Carr (1961) were the first to suggest a connection between lysogeny and toxinogenicity in the staphylococci when they used a phage to convert two of three nontoxic strains to the ability to produce alpha hemolysin (also known as lethal toxin). Read and Pritchard (1963) were the first to study lysogeny among the enterotoxic staphylococci. They found each of the 20 enterotoxic strains they studied to be lysogenic, but did not demonstrate phage conversion. However, they did show that defective lysogens could be isolated at high frequency that were immune to superinfection and continued to make SE, but failed to produce phage. Casman (1965) isolated phages from three enterotoxic staphylococcal strains and showed that only one of them (that from strain PS42D) could convert nontoxic strains to SEA production. Jarvis and Lawrence (1971) confirmed the conversion to the EntA phenotype (enterotoxin A or SEA production) by infection with this same phage. Thus lysogeny was linked with enterotoxinogenicity, but only with certain strains of *S. aureus*.

In a study of *S. aureus* strains that did not include the PS42D strain, Shafer and Iandolo (1978) showed that the EntA phenotype did not reside on a plasmid, although they did not rule out a prophage. The chromosomal location of the EntA phenotype mapped to the space between the *pur* (purine biosynthesis) and *ilv* (isoleucine and valine biosynthesis) markers (Pattee and Glatz, 1980). However, in four out of 27 strains studied by Mallonee *et al.* (1982), the EntA marker was chromosomal but was not located in the *pur-ilv* region. Thus a phenotypic marker associated with SEA production (not yet proved to be a structural gene for SEA) had been shown to be carried by a phage in one strain and chromosomally located but at variable locations in other strains.

Betley *et al.* (1984) have applied molecular cloning techniques to the study of SEA genetics. By cloning the gene for the EntA marker from the *pur-ilv* region and expressing it in *E. coli* to produce immunoreactive SEA, they proved that the phenotypic EntA marker was indeed the SEA structural gene, *entA*. Moreover, they found that the 8–12 kb of DNA surrounding the *entA* gene was conserved whether *entA* was in the *pur-ilv* region or elsewhere in the chromosome. Only strains that were EntA⁻ lacked the surrounding DNA sequences. This observation prompted speculation that *entA* might be part of a mobile genetic element.

Betley and Mekalanos (1985) used the cloned *entA* gene to reexamine the PS42D strain of *S. aureus* from which Casman (1965) had isolated the original EntA-converting phage. They confirmed the existence of the temperate phage and showed by hybridization techniques that it carries *entA*. Mapping and hybridization experiments showed that the PS42D phage integrates by the Campbell model of circularization and reciprocal crossover (Campbell, 1971) which is also employed by coliphage λ and corynephage β. Moreover, the *entA* gene is adjacent to the phage attachment site, *attP*, in the converting phage. All 10 SEA-producing strains examined by Betley and Mekalanos (1985) carried sequences homologous to the converting phage, and three of eight SEA-negative strains also carried converting phage sequences. Some of the lysogens carried converting phage DNA in the *pur-ilv* region, some in other locations, and some in both the *pur-ilv* region and elsewhere. At least one EntA⁺ strain that was positive for converting phage DNA in its chromosome failed to produce plaque-forming units upon induction and thus represents a defective lysogen.

The picture that emerges for SEA production is that the *entA* gene is carried by a temperate phage adjacent the the phage *attP* site. There are probably several *attB* sites within the *S. aureus* chromosome, the strongest of which lies between the *pur* and *ilv* genetic markers. The phage has a tendency to form defective lysogens, and thus many SEA-producing strains can be isolated that do not produce converting phages but that carry phage DNA in their chromosomes.

The genes for two other SE genes (types B and C_1) have been extensively studied and shown in at least one strain to be carried by a large penicillinase-encoding plasmid (56.2 kb; Altboum et al., 1985). In other strains, the entB gene appears to be chromosomal, although temperate phages or transposons have not been ruled out (Ranelli et al., 1985). SEB and SEC_1 have been sequenced (Huang and Bergdoll, 1970; Schmidt and Spero, 1983), as has the gene for SEA (Betley and Mekalanos, unpublished results reported in Betley et al., 1986). SEB and SEC_1 have 63% amino acid homology to one another and about 23% amino acid homology to SEA. SEB and SEC_1 have also been shown to have extensive amino acid homology to streptococcal pyrogenic exotoxin type A (SPE type A), whose gene is phage-borne.

Another staphylococcal toxin, toxic shock syndrome exotoxin (TSSE), has been associated with lysogenic strains (Schutzer et al., 1983), but a study of 17 phages isolated from TSSE-producing strains failed to show lysogenic conversion (Kreiswirth et al., 1983). The TSSE gene, however, does appear to be part of a larger DNA element (Kreiswirth et al., 1983), although whether it is a mobile element is not known. The alpha hemolysin-converting phage identified by Blair and Carr (1961) has received little attention since its original discovery.

D. Structure and Function of the SEs

The SEs are a structurally homogeneous but antigenically heterogeneous family of proteins. The seven serotypes currently recognized have been purified and have molecular weights from 27,000 to 30,000 daltons. Although they are defined serologically, antibody preparations exist that recognize multiple serotypes (Meyers et al., 1979; Thompson et al., 1984). The toxins are heat-stable, single-chain polypeptides. SEB and SEC_1 have disulfide loops that can be nicked by trypsin without a large loss of toxicity (Spero et al., 1973, 1976). However, unlike diphtheria and botulinum toxins, nicking is probably not a requirement for activity, since SEA is completely resistant to trypsin nicking (Spero et al., 1973).

The SEs cause vomiting and diarrhea, which can be reproduced in primates. The toxins are believed to act locally within the GI tract to produce these effects (Sugiyama and Hayama, 1965). Vomiting probably results from stimulation within the GI tract of autonomic afferents which ascend to the brainstem vomiting centers (Elwell et al., 1975). Recent evidence demonstrates that the emetic action of the SEs can be attenuated by treatment with cimetidine, an antagonist of the H2 histamine receptor (Scheuber et al., 1985), and suggests that the SEs may stimulate histamine receptors in the GI tract.

The diarrhea that accompanies staphylococcal food poisoning is thought to result from a toxin-mediated inhibitory effect on water absorption by epithelial cells (Elias and Shields, 1976; Liu and DuFault,

1977). The inhibition of water absorption is distinct from the mechanism of action of other diarrheagenic toxins like cholera toxin and the *E. coli* heat-labile and heat-stable toxins, which cause a secretion of electrolytes from the intestinal epithelial cells. The cellular and molecular mechanisms by which the SEs produce these pathogenic effects are not well understood at present.

VI. SHIGALIKE TOXINS OF *ESCHERICHIA COLI*

A. *E. coli*-Induced Enteric Diseases

Pathogenic *E. coli* strains fall into three categories: (1) noninvasive, enterotoxinogenic strains, which cause a secretory, nonhemorrhagic diarrhea similar to that seen in cholera; (2) enteroinvasive strains, which destroy the intestinal epithelium and cause a hemorrhagic diarrhea similar to that seen in shigellosis; and (3) "enteropathogenic *E. coli*" (EPEC), which are noninvasive but cause hemorrhagic diarrhea.

Enterotoxinogenic *E. coli* produce two well-characterized toxins: heat-labile toxin (LT) and heat-stable toxin (ST). LT is a high-molecular-weight (70,000 daltons), two-subunit, diarrheagenic toxin that is similar to cholera toxin in its mode of action (stimulation of adenylate cyclase in intestinal epithelial cells, resulting in fluid secretion). ST is smaller (MW 5000) and is a single-chain polypeptide that probably stimulates epithelial cell guanylate cyclase to produce a similar secretory diarrhea. Both of these toxins are encoded by *E. coli* plasmids (for review see Betley *et al.*, 1986).

Enteroinvasive strains of *E. coli* penetrate the epithelium of the large intestine and cause hemorrhagic diarrhea as well as systemic symptoms such as headache, fever, muscle pains, and chills. These *E. coli* strains are serologically related to the shigellae (Formal *et al.*, 1978) and can be identified by their ability to cause keratoconjunctivitis in guinea pigs (Séreny test; Séreny, 1955). The genetic basis of pathogenicity of these enteroinvasive organisms is not well understood.

Enteropathogenic *E. coli* strains do not invade (Séreny test negative), do not make LT or ST, but do produce a cytotoxin. These *E. coli* strains cause diarrhea (Williams Smith *et al.*, 1983) and hemorrhagic colitis (Johnson *et al.*, 1983) and have been associated with the hemolytic uremic syndrome (Karmali *et al.*, 1983). The cytotoxin of these strains was originally identified as an *E. coli* toxin distinct form LT and ST that was lethal for cultured Vero cells (Vero cell cytotoxin, VT; Konowalchuk *et al.*, 1977). O'Brien *et al.* (1983) showed that the Vero cell cytotoxicity could be neutralized by antibodies against shiga toxin (the major exotoxin produced by *Shigella dysenteriae* 1) and proposed the name shigalike toxin (SLT). The production of SLT in *E. coli* is phage-associated (for review, see O'Brien and Holmes, 1987).

B. SLT-Converting Coliphages

In 1971, before the Vero cell cytotoxin in *E. coli* extracts had even been described, Williams Smith and Linggood (1971) reported that lysates of *E. coli* strain H19 (of the 026:H11 serotype) transferred enterotoxinogenicity to *E. coli* K-12. Although they were unable to identify a phage from strain H19, they did note that the enterotoxin was distinct from that of the classical enterotoxic *E. coli* strains (LT-producing), because it caused dilation in ligated pig intestines. Similar results were reported by Scotland *et al.* (1980), who showed that Vero cell cytotoxin and enterotoxin from strain H19 were identical.

Williams Smith *et al.* (1983) were the first to isolate bacteriophages that transmitted the Vero cell cytotoxicity. Scotland *et al.* (1983) purified the toxin-converting phage from strain H19 and showed it to be a DNA phage with a genome about 45 kb in length. By electron microscopy it had a hexagonal head and a flexible, noncontractile tail. Although the *E. coli* H19 strain (serotype 026:H11) came from an outbreak of infantile diarrhea in Great Britain, O'Brien *et al.* (1984b) found SLT-converting phages from *E. coli* strain 933 (serotype O157:H7) isolated from a hemorrhagic colitis case in the United States. The H19 and 933 phages are morphologically similar but show differences in lysogenic immunity and host range. These differences indicate that a family of SLT-converting phages probably exists.

Newland *et al.* (1985) and Willshaw *et al.* (1985) cloned the SLT-converting genes from the 933 and H19 phages, respectively, into *E. coli* plasmids. By showing that cloned gene fragments produced immunoreactive polypeptide fragments, they established that these phages carry the SLT structural genes. Extensive restriction mapping showed that the 933 phage has a 53-kb DNA genome and that a 3-kb fragment carries sequences that encode both the A (31.5 kD) and the B (7 kD) subunits of the toxin. Southern blotting experiments showed that cloned DNA from the *E. coli* SLT gene is homologous to discrete DNA fragments from *Shigella dysenteriae* and *Shigella flexneri*. Huang *et al.* (1986) have shown that the cloned H19 SLT gene produces immunoreactive proteins of 31 and 5.5 kD and that part of the H19-converting phage is homologous to coliphage lambda. At this time, the level of homology between the 933 phage and the H19 phage has not been reported, nor have the nucleotide sequences of the various cloned SLT genes been published.

Strockbine *et al.* (1986) have reported a second cytotoxin from *E. coli* strain 933 (serotype 0157:H7), which they call shigalike toxin II (SLT-II). Its gene is more than 74% homologous to that of SLT-I, and it has the same biologic activities; however, it is not neutralized by antisera to shiga toxin. The gene for SLT-II is also carried by a coliphage.

SLTs have also been found in *Vibrio parahemolyticus* and *Vibrio cholerae* (O'Brien *et al.*, 1984a) and have been proposed as a cause for the residual pathogenicity of *V. cholerae* strains that have been deleted of cholera toxin genes. It is not clear whether the SLT produced by these vibrios are phage-associated. Mekalanos (unpublished results cited in Betley *et al.*, 1986) reports that phage DNA from *E. coli* SLT-converting phages is not homologous to DNA from *V. cholerae* 569B. These results suggest that if the SLT gene in *V. cholera* is phage-borne, the phage is not related to the SLT-converting coliphages.

C. Regulation of Toxin Expression

Like the expression of shiga toxin itself (Van Heyningen and Gladstone, 1953), the expression of SLT from *E. coli* is repressed by the presence of iron (O'Brien *et al.*, 1982). The toxin is not secreted into the extracellular space but must be liberated by cell lysis (O'Brien and LaVeck, 1983). Preliminary sequencing data (Calderwood and Mekalanos, cited in Betley *et al.*, 1986) suggests that the SLT A and B subunit genes are transcribed as a single operon with a 12-bp intergene spacer. Each has a hydrophobic leader peptide, indicating that the proteins are probably exported to the periplasmic space. These authors also report that SLT expression is under the negative control of an iron-responsive element encoded by the *fur* locus of *E. coli*.

D. Structure and Function of the SLTs

Considerably more is known about the structure and function of authentic shiga toxin than is known about the shigalike toxins. However, because the toxins have the same biological effects and are serologically and structurally related, they are likely to have similar mechanisms of action. O'Brien and LaVeck (1983) have purified SLT from *E. coli* strain H30 (serotype 026:H11) and compared its properties to authentic shiga toxin from *Shigella dysenteriae 1* strain 60S. Both toxins have the same isoelectric point (7.03) and the same heat stability profile (active after heating to 65°C for up to 30 min). Newland *et al.* (1985) showed that *E. coli* SLT is composed of two subunits, A (MW 31,500) and B (MW 7000), which is similar to the data of Olsnes *et al.* (1981) showing authentic shiga toxin to have an A_1B_n structure (A = 30,500 and B = 5000) where n was 6 or 7. The A chain of authentic shiga toxin is easily nicked within a trypsin-sensitive disulfide loop to give fragments A_1 (MW 27,500) and A_2 (MW 3000); the A or B chains alone are nontoxic (Olsnes *et al.*, 1981).

Functionally, both shiga toxin and SLT are cytotoxic *in vitro* and enterotoxic *in vivo*; they are also paralytic and lethal when injected into mice. Shiga toxin inhibits protein synthesis in cell-free systems (Brown *et al.*, 1981) by inactivating the eukaryotic 60S ribosome (Reisbig *et al.*, 1981). Trypsin-nicking of shiga toxin is a prerequisite for this cell-free activity. Recently, Obrig *et al.* (1985) have demonstrated that shiga toxin is, in fact, a ribonuclease that is specific for the 5S and 5.8S rRNA components of the 60S eukaryotic ribosomal subunit.

E. coli strains expressing SLT produce a hemorrhagic colitis because, unlike the other *E. coli* exotoxins (LT and ST), SLT is cytotoxic and destroys part of the intestinal epithelium. However, SLT-producing *E. coli* strains fail to penetrate the damaged colonic wall (in contrast to *S. dysenteriae*, which is enteroinvasive and expresses authentic shiga toxin) and thus do not produce the systemic symptoms associated with shigellosis.

VII. CONCLUDING REMARKS

Two intriguing questions arise from the discussion of bacteriophage-borne toxin genes: Where did they originate? And why have they persisted as phage genes?

With respect to the question of origin, several lines of evidence point to the bacterial chromosome as the source of the toxin genes. First, in the three cases where the phage attachment site (*attP*) has been mapped (corynebacteriophage β, streptococcal SPE-converting phage T12, and staphylococcal SEA-converting phage from PS42D), the respective toxin genes have been located adjacent to *attP*. This observation raises the possibility that an imprecise excision event from the bacterial chromosome accidently included the toxin gene. Second, none of the toxins discussed in this chapter have been shown to play an essential role in the life cycle of the respective phages. In fact, in most cases nontoxinogenic phages have been isolated, and toxinogenic phages have been mutated to nontoxinogenicity without a loss of phage viability or burst size. A third factor is that at least in the cases of diphtheria toxin and SLT, toxin expression appears to be regulated by elements whose genes are associated with the bacterial host. This is consistent with the idea that in these instances, phages picked up what were originally chromosomal genes but left behind the chromosomal regulatory systems. And finally, in the case of the staphylococcal enterotoxins and botulinum toxins where multiple serotypes exist, only staphylococcal enterotoxin type A (out of 7 serotypes) and botulinum toxins types C_1 and D (out of 8 serotypes) have been proved to be phage-associated. Indeed, SE types B and C_1 have been shown to be chromosomal, although there may be an association with a transposon. One can thus argue that perhaps all of the SE or botulinum toxin serotypes were originally chromosomal but only some have been picked up by phages.

In spite of these arguments, the theory that exotoxin genes originated in the bacterial chromosomes leaves several questions unanswered. In several cases, the toxin gene serves no obvious role in bacterial physiology, and it is difficult to imagine a selective advantage to the bacteria in having the toxin gene. Consider the botulinum toxins and staphylococcal enterotoxins where the ingested toxin causes disease, and there is little or no bacterial colonization of the host. What selective advantage do these proteins impart? Moreover, if the phage-associated toxin genes evolved from the bacterial chromosome, why have no examples of such chromosomal genes been found? In every example studied of toxinogenic, apparently nonlysogenic bacterial isolates of *C. diphtheriae*, SPE-producing *S. pyogenes*, and SEA-producing *S. aureus*, phage-homologous sequences have been found associated with the toxin gene. These toxinogenic strains that fail to yield phages are merely defective lysogens.

Perhaps the more puzzling question is the teleological one, which asks how the bacterial chromosome evolved such sophisticated, enzymatic proteins whose only substrates are eukaryotic, cytosolic macromolecules. The only known substrate for diphtheria toxin, for example, is eukaryotic elongation factor 2 (EF-2); shigalike toxins selectively cleave the 60S eukaryotic ribosomal subunit, and the botulinum toxins seem to enzymatically inhibit vesicular release at cholinergic nerve terminals. The recent discovery of a eukaryotic, ADP-ribosylating enzyme that carries out the same reaction on EF-2 as diphtheria toxin and that may be a regulatory enzyme for protein synthesis (Lee and Iglewski, 1984) poses an intriguing question. Are diphtheria toxin and the cellular ADP-ribosylating enzyme examples of convergent or divergent evolution?

If the diphtheria toxin gene originated from the *C. diphtheriae* chromosome, the cellular ADP-ribosyltransferase and diphtheria toxin are most likely examples of convergent evolution; that is, they are genes that evolved completely separately to perform the same function. The alternative hypothesis to the bacterial origin of bacteriophage-associated exotoxin genes is that the bacterial toxin genes *diverged* from ancestral genes that have also gone on to function as physiologic enzymes in eukaryotic systems. A highly speculative extension of this idea is that the bacteriophages that carry the modern-day exotoxin genes are vestigial remnants of ancient mobile genetic elements that transferred the genes between primordial eukaryotes and prokaryotes.

Regardless of where these exotoxin genes originated, the second question remains. Why do these exotoxin genes persist within phage genomes? All of the toxins presented here are highly antigenic, and in at least one case (diphtheria), immunity to the toxin alone is fully protective against large-scale colonization by toxinogenic bacteria. In an immune host, then, toxin expression is a liability to a bacterium. To persist in a partially immune population, toxin gene expression must be prevented in carriers who are immune to the toxin. When a nonimmune host is colonized, rapid growth and high-level toxin expression—before the immune system can respond—are the best way to proliferate.

Phage conversion is a highly efficient means of rapidly disseminating the toxin gene within a nonimmune host. In the case of *C. diphtheriae*, the bacteria double every hour *in vitro*, but in that same hour a lytic corynephage can produce 30–60 converting phages. Nontoxinogenic *C. diphtheriae*, *S. pyogenes*, *S. aureus*, and *E. coli* are all frequent if not constant members of the normal human flora. For these autochthonous organisms, *in situ* phage conversion represents a means of rapid spread of the toxin gene once a susceptible host has been infected with just a few toxinogenic organisms.

The current epidemiology of diphtheria illustrates that *in situ* phage conversion is an effective means of spread for an infectious disease in a largely immune population. While the carrier rate for *C. diphtheriae* in immunized populations has remained stable, the incidence of toxinogenic *C. diphtheriae* has dropped to near zero, because most isolates are now nontoxinogenic. At present, toxinogenic *C. diphtheriae* can only be isolated at high frequency in developing nations without adequate immunization programs, and most cases of diphtheria in developed nations can usually be traced to a traveler who has recently returned from an area where diphtheria is still endemic (Pappenheimer, 1984).

In situ phage conversion of *C. diphtheriae* was demonstrated in the case of a healthy woman from Toronto who was carrying three different strains of *C. diphtheriae*: A^{tox+}, B^{tox-}, and C^{tox+}. Except for their *tox* phenotype, strains A and B were identical morphologically and lysotypically. Restriction endonuclease fingerprints of chromosomal DNA from the three strains confirmed that A and B were an identical strain distinct from strain C. Southern blotting experiments, on the other hand, showed that A and C carried an identical prophage related to corynephage β (strain B was prophage negative). The most likely interpretation of these data is that corynephage from strain C^{tox+} converted strain B^{tox-} to toxinogenicity in this woman's upper respiratory tract (Pappenheimer and Murphy, 1983).

A second selective advantage that the phage location might confer upon the exotoxin genes is genetic variability. A common theme among the exotoxins discussed in this chapter is serotypic variation. Toxins produced by the same bacterial species that have identical mechanisms of action and similar molecular weights fail to cross-react with immune serum. There are eight serotypes of botulinum toxin, three serotypes of streptococcal pyrogenic exotoxin, and seven serotypes of staphylococcal enterotoxin. The shigalike toxins of *E. coli* show structural variations but do cross-react with polyclonal antibodies. Only diphtheria toxin appears to be structurally and antigenically homogeneous. Since a temperate phage undergoes many rounds of replication per burst in addition to the chromosomal replication it receives as a prophage on every mitotic division, phage genes have greater opportunity for mutation than chromosomal genes. The need for antigenic variation is probably one of the evolutionary forces that keep the genes for these exotoxins located on bacteriophages.

The existence of exotoxin protein genes on bacteriophages, and the more general association of toxins with other mobile genetic elements, still has much to teach us about both the evolution and epidemiology of bacterial pathogens. In addition to the clues these phages provide, further study of the toxins they encode is sure to illuminate the eukaryotic processes that the toxins disrupt.

REFERENCES

Abrams, A., Kegeles, G., and Hottle, G. A., 1946, The purification of toxin from *Clostridium botulinum* type A, *J. Biol. Chem.* **164:**63–79.

Allured, V. S., Collier, R. J., Carroll, S. F., and McKay, D. B., 1986, Structure of exotoxin A of *Pseudomonas aeruginosa* at 3.0-Ångstrom resolution, *Proc. Natl. Acad. Sci. USA* **83:**1320–1324.

Alouf, J. E., 1980, Streptococcal toxins (streptolysin O, streptolysin S, erythrogenic toxin), *Pharmacol. Ther.* **11:**661–717.

Altboum, Z., Hertman, I., and Sarid, S., 1985, Penicillinase plasmid-linked genetic determinants for enterotoxins B and C_1 production in *Staphylococcus aureus, Infect. Immun.* **47:**514–521.

Anderson, J. S., Happold, F. C., McLeod, J. W., and Thomson, J. G., 1931, The existence of two forms of diphtheria bacillus—*B. diphtheriae gravis* and *B. diphtheriae mitis*—and a new medium for their differentiation and for the bacteriological diagnosis of diphtheria, *J. Pathol. Bacteriol.* **34:**667–681.

Bacha, P., Williams, D. P., Waters, C., Williams, J. M., Murphy, J. R., and Strom, T. B., 1988, Interleukin-2 receptor targeted cytotoxicity. Interleukin-2 receptor-mediated action of a diphtheria toxin-related interleukin-2 fusion protein, *J. Exp. Med.* (in press).

Barksdale, L., 1970, *Corynebacterium diphtheriae* and its relatives, *Bacteriol. Rev.* **34:**378–422.

Barksdale, L., and Arden, S. B., 1974, Persisting bacteriophage infections, lysogeny, and phage conversions, *Annu. Rev. Microbiol.* **28:**265–299.

Barksdale, W. L., and Pappenheimer, A. M. Jr., 1954, Phage-host relationships in nontoxinogenic and toxinogenic diphtheria bacilli, *J. Bacteriol.* **67:**220–232.

Barsumian, E. L., Cunningham, C. M., and Schlievert, P. M., 1978a, Heterogeneity of group A streptococcal pyrogenic exotoxin type B, *Infect. Immun.* **20:**512–518.

Barsumian, E. L., Schlievert, P. M., and Watson, D. W., 1978b, Nonspecific and specific immunological mitogenicity by group A streptococcal pyrogenic exotoxins, *Infect. Immun.* **22:**681–688.

Bergdoll, M. S., 1979, Staphylococcal intoxications, In: *Foodborn Infections and Intoxications* (H. Riemann and F. L. Bryan, eds.), Academic Press, New York.

Betley, M. J., and Mekalanos, J. J., 1985, Staphylococcal enterotoxin A is encoded by phage. *Science* **229:**185–187.

Betley, M. J., Lofdahl, S., Kreiswirth, B. N., Bergdoll, M. S., and Novick, R. P, 1984, Staphylococcal enterotoxin A gene is associated with a variable genetic element, *Proc. Natl. Acad. Sci. USA* **81:**5179–5183.

Betley, M. J., Miller, V. L., and Mekalanos, J. J., 1986, Genetics of bacterial enterotoxins, *Annu. Rev. Microbiol.* **40:**577–605.

Bingel, K. F., 1949, Heue untersuchunen zur scharlachatiologie, *Dtsch. Med. Wochenschr.* **74:**703–706.

Blair, J. E., and Carr, M., 1961, Lysogeny in staphylococci, *J. Bacteriol.* **82:**984–993.

Bonventre, P. F., and Kempe, L. L., 1960a, Physiology of toxin production by *Clostridium botulinum* types A and B. I. Growth, autolysis, and toxin production, *J. Bacteriol.* **79:**18–23.

Bonventre, P. F., and Kempe, L. L., 1960b, Physiology of toxin production by *Clostridium botulinum* types A and B. IV. Activation of the toxin, *J. Bacteriol.* **79:**24–32.

Boroff, D. A., Del Castillo, J., Evoy, W. H., and Steinhardt, R. A., 1974, Observations on the action of type A botulinum toxin on frog neuromuscular junction, *J. Physiol. (Lond.)* **240:**227–253.

Bradley, D. E., 1967, Ultrastructure of bacteriophages and bacteriocins, *Bacteriol. Rev.* **31**:230–314.

Brown, J. E., Ussery, M. A., Leppla, S. H., and Rothman, S. W., 1981, Inhibition of protein synthesis by Shiga toxin. Activation of toxin and inhibition of peptide elongation, *FEBS Lett.* **117**:84–88.

Buck, G. A., and Groman, N. B., 1981, Physical mapping of β-converting and γ-nonconverting corynebacteriophage genomes, *J. Bacteriol.* **148**:131–142.

Buck, G. A., Cross, R. E., Wong, T. P., Loera, J., and Groman, N., 1985, DNA relationships among some *tox*-bearing corynebacteriophages, *Infect. Immun.* **49**:679–684.

Burgen, A. S. V., Dickens, F., and Zatman, L. J., 1949, The action of botulinum toxin on the neuromuscular junction, *J. Physiol. (Lond.)* **109**:10–24.

Campbell, A. M., 1971, Introduction to lambda, in: *The Bacteriophage Lambda* (A. D. Hershey, ed.), pp. 3–44, Cold Spring Harbor Laboratory, Cold Spring Harbor, NY.

Cantacuzene, J., and Boncieu, O., 1926, Modifications subies par des streptococques d'origine non-scarlatineuse qui contact des produits scarlatineux filtres, *C. R. Acad. Sci.* **182**:1185.

Casman, E. P., 1965, Staphylococcal enterotoxin, *Ann. N.Y. Acad. Sci.* **128**:124–131.

Casman, E. P., Bennett, R. W., Dorsey, A. E., and Issa, J. A., 1967, Identification of a fourth staphylococcal enterotoxin, enterotoxin D, *J. Bacteriol.* **94**:1875–1882.

Centers for Disease Control, 1987, Cases of notifiable diseases, United States, *Morb. Mort. Weekly Rep.* **35**:810.

Collier, R. J., 1967, Effect of diphtheria toxin on protein synthesis: Inactivation of one of the transfer factors, *J. Mol. Biol.* **25**:83–98.

Collier, R. J., 1975, Diphtheria toxin: Mode of action and structure, *Bacteriol Rev.* **39**:54–85.

Collier, R. J., and Kandel, J., 1971, Structure and activity of diphtheria toxin. I. Thiol-dependent disassociation of a fraction of toxin into enzymatically active and inactive fragments, *J. Biol. Chem.* **246**:1496–1503.

Collier, R. J., and Kaplan, D. A., 1984, Immunotoxins, *Sci. Am.* **253**:56–64.

Collier, R. J., and Pappenheimer, A. M. Jr., 1964, Studies on the mode of action of diphtheria toxin. II. Effect of toxin on amino acid incorporation in cell-free systems, *J. Exp. Med.* **120**:1019–1039.

Colon-Whitt, A., Whitt, R. S., and Cole, R. M., 1979, Production of an erythrogenic toxin (streptococcal pyrogenic exotoxin) by a nonlysogenized group-A streptococcus, in: *Pathogenic Streptococci* (M. T. Parker, ed.), pp. 64–65, Reedbooks Ltd., Chertsey, Surrey, U.K.

Costa, J. J., Michel, J. L., Rappuoli, R., and Murphy, J. R., 1981, Restriction map of corynebacteriophages β_c and β_vir and physical localization of the diphtheria *tox* operon, *J. Bacteriol.* **148**:124–130.

Cull-Candy, S. G., Lundh, H., and Thesleff, S., 1976, Effects of botulinum toxin on neuromuscular transmission in the rat, *J. Physiol. (Lond.)* **260**:177–203.

Cunningham, C. M., and Watson, D. W., 1978, Alteration of clearance function by group A streptococci and its relation to suppression of the antibody response, *Infect. Immun.* **19**:51–57.

Cunningham, C. M., Barsumian, E. L., and Watson, D. W., 1976, Further purification of group A streptococcal pyrogenic exotoxin and characterization of the purified toxin, *Infect. Immun.* **14**:767–775.

DasGupta, B. R., and Sugiyama, H., 1972, Role of a protease in natural activation of *Clostridium botulinum* neurotoxin, *Infect. Immun.* **6**:587–590.

d'Herelle, F., 1918, Technique de la recherche du microbe filtrant bacteriophage, *C. R. Soc. Biol.* **81**:1160.

Dick, G. F., and Dick, G. H., 1924, The etiology of scarlet fever, *JAMA* **82**:301–302.

Dolman, C. E., and Chang, E., 1972, Bacteriophages of *Clostridium botulinum*, *Can. J. Microbiol.* **18**:67–76.

Donovan, J. J., Simon, M. I., Draper, R. K., and Montal, M., 1981, Diphtheria toxin forms transmembrane channels in planar lipid bilayers, *Proc. Natl. Acad. Sci. USA* **78:**172–176.

Draper, R. K., and Simon, M. I., 1980, The entry of diphtheria toxin into the mammalian cell cytoplasm: Evidence for lysosomal involvement, *J. Cell Biol.* **87:**849–854.

Drazin, R., Kandel, J., and Collier, R. J., 1971, Structure and activity of diphtheria toxin. II. Attack by trypsin at a specific site within the intact toxin molecule, *J. Biol. Chem.* **246:**1504–1510.

Dreyer, F., Becker, C., Bigalke, H., Funk, J., Penner, R., Rosenberg, F., and Ziegler, M., 1984, Action of botulinum A toxin and tetanus toxin on synaptic transmission, *J. Physiol. (Paris)* **79:**252–258.

Duff, J. T., Wright, G. G., and Yarinsky, A., 1956, Activation of *Clostridium botulinum* type E toxin by trypsin, *J. Bacteriol.* **72:**455–460.

Eisenberg, D., Schwarz, E., Komaromy, M., and Wall, R., 1984, Analysis of membrane and surface protein sequences with the hydrophobic moment plot, *J. Mol. Biol.* **179:**125–142.

Eklund, M. W., and Poysky, F. T., 1974, Interconversion of type C and D strains of *Clostridium botulinum* by specific bacteriophages, *Appl. Microbiol.* **27:**251–258.

Eklund, M. W., Poysky, F. T., and Boatman, E. S., 1969, Bacteriophages of *Clostridium botulinum* types A, B, E, and F and nontoxinogenic strains resembling type E, *J. Virol.* **3:**270–274.

Eklund, M. W., Poysky, F. T., Reed, S. M., and Smith, C. A., 1971, Bacteriophage and the toxinogenicity of *Clostridium botulinum* type C, *Science* **172:**480–482.

Eklund, M. W., Poysky, F. T., and Reed, S. M., 1972, Bacteriophage and the toxinogenicity of *Clostridium botulinum* type D, *Nature New Biol.* **235:**16–17.

Eklund, M. W., Poysky, F. T., Meyers, J. A., and Pelroy, G. A., 1974, Interspecies conversion of *Clostridium botulinum* type C to *Clostridium novyi* type A by bacteriophage, *Science* **186:**456–458.

Elek, S. D., 1948, Recognition of toxicogenic bacterial strains *in vitro, Br. Med. J.* **1:**493–496.

Elias, J., and Shields, R., 1976, Influence of staphylococcal enterotoxin on water and electrolyte transport in the small intestine, *Gut* **17:**527–535.

Elwell, M. R., Liu, C. T., Spertzel, R. O., and Beisel, W. R., 1975, Mechanisms of oral staphylococcal enterotoxin B-induced emesis in monkey, *Proc. Soc. Exp. Biol. Med.* **148:**424–427.

Formal, S. B., O'Brien, A. D., Gemski, P., and Doctor, B. P., 1978, Invasive *Escherichia coli, J. Am. Vet. Med. Assoc.* **173:**596–598.

Freeman, V. J., 1951, Studies on the virulence of bacteriophage-infected strains of *Corynebacterium diphtheriae, J. Bacteriol.* **61:**675–688.

Freeman, V. J., and Morse, I. U., 1952, Further observations on the change to virulence of bacteriophage-infected avirulent strains of *Corynebacterium diphtheriae, J. Bacteriol.* **63:**407–414.

Frobisher, M., and Brown, J. H., 1927, Transmissible toxinogenicity of streptococci, *Bull. Johns Hopkins Hosp.* **41:**167–173.

Gehrmann, R., Henschen, A., and Klink, F., 1985, Primary structure of elongation factor 2 around the site of ADP-ribosylation is highly conserved from archaebacteria to eukaryotes, *FEBS Lett.* **185:**37–42.

Gill, D. M., 1982, Bacterial toxins: A table of lethal amounts, *Microbiol. Rev.* **46:**86–94.

Gill, D. M., and Dinius, L. L., 1971, Observations on the structure of diphtheria toxin, *J. Biol. Chem.* **246:**1485–1491.

Gill, D. M., and Pappenheimer, A. M. Jr., 1971, Structure-activity relationships in diphtheria toxin, *J. Biol. Chem.* **246:**1492–1495.

Gill, D. M., Uchida, T., and Singer, R. A., 1972, Expression of diphtheria toxin genes carried by integrated and nonintegrated phage beta, *Virology* **50:**664–668.

Giminez, D. F., and Ciccarelli, A. S., 1970, Another type of *Clostridium botulinum, Zentralbl. Bakteriol. Parasitnkd. Infektionskr. Hyg. Abt. 1 Orig.* **215:**221–224.

Goor, R. S., and Pappenheimer, A. M. Jr., 1967, Studies on the mode of action of diphtheria toxin. III. Site of toxin action in cell-free extracts, *J. Exp. Med.* **126**:899–912.

Gray, G. L., Smith, D. H., Baldridge, J. S., Harkins, R. N., Vasil, M. L., Chen, E. Y., and Heyneker, H. L., 1984, Cloning, nucleotide sequence, and expression in *Escherichia coli* of the exotoxin A structural gene of *Pseudomonas aeruginosa*, *Proc. Natl. Acad. Sci. USA* **81**:2645–2649.

Greenfield, L., Bjorn, M. J., Horn, G., Fong, D., Buck, G. A., Collier, R. J., and Kaplan, D. A., 1983, Nucleotide sequence of the structural gene for diphtheria toxin carried by corynebacteriophage β, *Proc. Natl. Acad. Sci. USA* **80**:6853–6857.

Groman, N. B., 1953, The relation of bacteriophage to the change of *Corynebacterium diphtheriae* from avirulence to virulence, *Science* **117**:297–299.

Groman, N. B., 1984, Conversion by corynephages and its role in the natural history of diphtheria, *J. Hyg. (Lond.)* **93**:405–417.

Groman, N. B., and Eaton, M., 1955, Genetic factors in *Corynbacterium diphtheriae* conversion, *J. Bacteriol.* **70**:637–640.

Groman, N., Cianciotto, N., Bjorn, M., and Rabin, M., 1983, Detection and expression of DNA homologous to the *tox* gene in nontoxinogenic isolates of *Corynebacterium diphtheriae*, *Infect. Immun.* **42**:48–56.

Groman, N., Schiller, J., and Russell, J., 1984, *Corynebacterium ulcerans* and *Corynebacterium pseudotuberculosis* responses to DNA probes derived from corynephage β and *Corynebacterium diphtheriae*, *Infect. Immun.* **45**:511–517.

Hanig, J. P., and Lamanna, C., 1979, Toxicity of botulinum toxin: A stoichiometric model for the locus of its extraordinary potency and persistence at the neuromuscular junction, *J. Theor. Biol.* **77**:107–113.

Hirokawa, N., and Heuser, J. E., 1980, Structural evidence that botulinum toxin blocks neuromuscular transmission by impairing the calcium influx that normally accompanies nerve depolarization, *J. Cell. Biol.* **88**:160–171.

Hoch, D. H., Romero-Mira, M., Ehrlich, B. E., Finkelstein, A., DasGupta, B. R., and Simpson, L. L., 1985, Channels formed by botulinum, tetanus, and diphtheria toxins in planar lipid bilayer: Relevance to translocation of proteins across membranes, *Proc. Natl. Acad. Sci. USA* **82**:1692–1696.

Holmes, R. K., 1976, Characterization and genetic mapping of nontoxinogenic (*tox*) mutants of corynebacteriophage beta, *J. Virol.* **19**:195–207.

Holmes, R. K., and Barksdale, L., 1969, Genetic analysis of *tox*+ and *tox*− bacteriophages of *Corynebacterium diphtheriae*, *J. Virol.* **3**:586–598.

Holmes, R. K., and Barksdale, L., 1970, Comparative studies with *tox*+ and *tox*− corynebacteriophages, *J. Virol.* **5**:783–794.

Huang, A., DeGrandis, S., Friesen, J., Karmali, M., Petric, M., Congi, R., and Brunton, J. L., 1986, Cloning and expression of the genes specifying shiga-like toxin production in *Escherichia coli* H19, *J. Bacteriol.* **166**:375–379.

Huang, I. Y., and Bergdoll, M. S., 1970, The primary structure of staphylococcal enterotoxin B. III. The cyanogen bromide peptides of reduced and amino-ethylated enterotoxin B and the complete amino acid sequence, *J. Biol. Chem.* **245**:3518–3525.

Hynes, W. L., Weeks, C. R., Iandolo, J. J., and Ferretti, J. J., 1987, Immunologic cross-reactivity of type A streptococcal exotoxin (erythrogenic toxin) and staphylococcal enterotoxins B and C1, *Infect. Immun.* **55**:837–838.

Iglewski, B. H., and Kabat, D., 1975, NAD-dependent inhibition of protein synthesis by *Pseudomonas aeruginosa* toxin, *Proc. Natl. Acad. Sci. USA* **72**:2284–2288.

Immunization Practices Advisory Committee, 1985, Diphtheria, tetanus, and pertussis: Guidelines for vaccine prophylaxis and other preventive measures, *Morb. Mort. Weekly Rep.* **34**:405–426.

Inoue, K., and Iida, H., 1968, Bacteriophages of *Clostridium botulinum*, *J. Virol.* **2**:537–540.

Inoue, K., and Iida, H., 1970, Conversion of toxinogenicity in *Clostridium botulinum* type C, *Jpn. J. Microbiol.* **14**:87–89.

Inoue, K., and Iida, H., 1971, Phage-conversion of toxinogenicity in *Clostridium botulinum* types C and D, *Jpn. J. Med. Sci. Biol.* **24**:53–56.

Ittelson, T. R., and Gill, D. M., 1973, Diphtheria toxin: Specific competition for cell receptors, *Nature* **242**:330–332.

Jansen, B. C., 1971, The toxic antigenic factors produced by *Clostridium botulinum* types C and D, *Onderstepoort J. Vet. Res.* **38**:93–98.

Jarvis, A. W., and Lawrence, R. C., 1971, Production of extracellular enzymes and enterotoxins A, B, and C by *Staphylococcus aureus, Infect. Immun.* **4**:110–115.

Johnson, L. P., and Schlievert, P. M., 1983, A physical map of the group A streptococcal pyrogenic exotoxin bacteriophage T12 genome, *Mol. Gen. Genet.* **189**:251–255.

Johnson, L. P., and Schlievert, P. M., 1984, Group A streptococcal phage T12 carries the structural gene for pyrogenic exotoxin type A, *Mol. Gen. Genet.* **194**:52–56.

Johnson, L. P., Schlievert, P. M., and Watson, D. W., 1980, Transfer of group A streptococcal pyrogenic exotoxin production to nontoxinogenic strains by lysogenic conversion, *Infect. Immun.* **28**:254–257.

Johnson, L. P., Tomai, M. A., and Schlievert, P. M., 1986, Bacteriophage involvement in group A streptococcal pyrogenic exotoxin A production, *J. Bacteriol.* **166**:623–627.

Johnson, W. M., Lior, H., and Bezanson, G. S., 1983, Cytotoxic *Escherichia coli* O157:H7 associated with haemorrhagic colitis in Canada, *Lancet* **1**:76.

Kaczorek, M., Delpeyroux, F., Chenciner, N., Streeck, R. E., Murphy, J. R., Boquet, P., and Tiollais, P., 1983, Nucleotide sequence and expression of the diphtheria tox228 gene in *Escherichia coli, Science* **221**:855–858.

Kagan, B. L., Finkelstein, A., and Colombini, M., 1981, Diphtheria toxin fragment forms large pores in phospholipid bilayer membranes, *Proc. Natl. Acad. Sci. USA* **78**:4950–4954.

Kanei, C., Uchida, T., and Yoneda, M., 1977, Isolation from *Corynebacterium diphtheriae* C7(β) of bacterial mutants that produce toxin in medium containing excess iron, *Infect. Immun.* **18**:203–209.

Karmali, M. A., Steele, B. T., Petric, M., and Lim, C., 1983, Sporadic cases of haemolytic-uremic syndrome associated with faecal cytotoxin and cytotoxin-producing *Escherichia coli* in stools, *Lancet* **1**:619–620.

Kitamura, M., Iwamori, M., and Nagai, Y., 1980, Interaction between *Clostridium botulinum* neurotoxin and gangliosides, *Biochim. Biophys. Acta* **628**:328–335.

Klebs, E., 1883, Ueber diphtheriae, *Verh. Cong. Inn. Med.* **2**:139–154.

Konowalchuk, J., Speirs, J. I., and Stavric, S., 1977, Vero response to a cytotoxin of *Escherichia coli, Infect. Immun.* **18**:775–779.

Kreiswirth, B. N., Lofdahl, S., Betley, M. J., O'Reilly, M., Schlievert, P. M., Bergdoll, M. S., and Novick, R. P., 1983, The toxic shock syndrome exotoxin structural gene is not detectably transmitted by a prophage, *Nature* **305**:709–712.

Laird, W., and Groman, N., 1976a, Prophage map of converting corynebacteriophage beta, *J. Virol.* **19**:208–219.

Laird, W., and Groman, N., 1976b, Orientation of the *tox* gene in the prophage of corynebacteriophage beta, *J. Virol.* **19**:228–231.

Lambotte, P., Falmagne, P., Capiau, C., Zanen, J., Ruysschaert, J.-M., and Dirkx, J., 1980, Primary structure of diphtheria toxin fragment B: Structural similarities with lipid-binding domains, *J. Cell Biol.* **87**:837–840.

Lee, H., and Iglewski, W. J., 1984, Cellular ADP-ribosyltransferase with the same mechanism of action as diphtheria toxin and *Pseudomonas* toxin A, *Proc. Natl. Acad. Sci. USA* **81**:2703–2707.

Leong, D., 1985, Characterization of the expression of the diphtheria tox gene in *Corynebacterium diphtheriae* and in *Escherichia coli*, Doctoral Thesis, Harvard University, Cambridge, MA.

Leong, D., and Murphy, J. R., 1985, Characterization of the diphtheria tox transcript in *Corynebacterium diphtheriae* and *Escherichia coli, J. Bacteriol.* **163**:1114–1119.

Liu, C. T., and DuFault, B. R., 1977, Effects of intestinal infusion of staphylococcal entero-toxin B (SEB) on water and electrolyte fluxes: Possible mechanisms of diarrhea, *Physiologist* **20**:57.

Locke, A., and Main, E. R., 1931, The relation of copper and iron to production of toxin and enzyme action, *J. Infect. Dis.* **48**:419–435.

Loeffler, F., 1884, Untersuchungen über die bedeutung der mikroörganismen für die enstehung der diphtherie beim menschen bei der taube und beim kalbe, *Mitt. Klin. Gesundh. Berlin* **2**:421–499.

MacDonald, K. L., and Griffin, P. M., 1986, Foodborne disease outbreaks, annual summary, 1982, *Morbid Mortal. Weekly Rep. Surveil. Summ.* **35**:7ss–16ss.

Mallonee, D. H., Glatz, B. A., and Pattee, P. A., 1982, Chromosomal mapping of a gene affecting enterotoxin A production in *Staphylococcus aureus, Appl. Environ. Microbiol.* **43**:397–402.

Marnell, M. H., Shia, S.-P., Stookey, M., and Draper, R. K., 1984, Evidence for penetration of diphtheria toxin to the cytosol through a prelysosomal membrane, *Infect. Immun.* **44**:145–150.

Mathews, M. M., Miller, P. A., and Pappenheimer, A. M. Jr., 1966, Morphological observations on some diphtherial phages, *Virology* **29**:402–409.

Matsuda, M., and Barksdale, L., 1966, Phage-directed synthesis of diphtherial toxin in non-toxinogenic *Corynebacterium diphtheriae, Nature* **210**:911–913.

Matsuda, M., and Barksdale, L., 1967, System for the investigation of the bacteriophage-directed synthesis of diphtherial toxin, *J. Bacteriol.* **93**:722–730.

Matsuda, M., Kanei, C., and Yoneda, M., 1971, Temperature sensitive mutants of non-lysogenizing corynebacteriophage βhv: Their isolation, characterization and relation to toxinogenesis, *Biken J.* **14**:119–130.

McKane, L., and Ferretti, J. J., 1981, Phage-host interactions and the production of type A streptococcal exotoxin in group A streptococci, *Infect. Immun.* **34**:915–919.

Meyers, R. F., Miller, L., Bennett, R. W., and MacMillan, J. D., 1979, Development of a monoclonal antibody capable of interacting with five serotypes of *Staphylococcus aureus* enterotoxin, *Appl. Environ. Microbiol.* **47**:283–287.

Michel, J. L., 1982, Restriction endonuclease mapping and characterization of corynephages beta, gamma and omega. Doctoral Thesis, Harvard University, Cambridge, MA.

Michel, J. L., Rappuoli, R., Murphy, J. R., and Pappenheimer, A. M. Jr., 1982, Restriction endonuclease map of the nontoxinogenic corynephage γ_c and its relationship to the toxinogenic corynephage β_c, *J. Virol.* **42**:510–518.

Middlebrook, J. L., Dorland, R. B., and Leppla, S. H., 1978, Association of diphtheria toxin with Vero cells: Demonstration of a receptor, *J. Biol. Chem.* **253**:7325–7330.

Moehring, J. M., Moehring, T. J., and Danley, D. E., 1980, Posttranslational modification of elongation factor 2 in diphtheria-toxin-resistant mutants of CHO-K1 cells, *Proc. Natl. Acad. Sci. USA* **77**:1010–1014.

Montecucco, C., 1986, How do tetanus and botulinum toxins bind to neuronal membranes? *Trends Biochem. Sci.* **11**:314–317.

Moya, M., Dautry-Varsat, A., Goud, B., Louvard, D., and Bouquet, P., 1985, Inhibition of coated pit formation in Hep_2 cells blocks the cytotoxicity of diphtheria toxin but not that of ricin toxin, *J. Cell. Biol.* **101**:548–559.

Murphy, J. R., 1976, Structure activity relationships of diphtheria toxin, in: *Mechanisms in Bacterial Toxicology* (A. W. Bernheimer, ed.), pp. 31–51, John Wiley, New York.

Murphy, J. R., 1985, The diphtheria toxin structural gene, *Curr. Top. Microbiol. Immunol.* **118**:235–251.

Murphy, J. R., and Bacha, P., 1979, Regulation of diphtheria toxin production, in: *Microbiology—1979* (D. Schlessinger, ed.), pp. 181–186, American Society for Microbiology, Washington.

Murphy, J. R., Pappenheimer, A. M. Jr., and Tayart de Borms, S., 1974, Synthesis of diphtheria *tox*-gene products in *Escherichia coli* extracts, *Proc. Natl. Acad. Sci. USA* **71**:11–15.

Murphy, J. R., Skiver, J., and McBride, G., 1976, Isolation and partial characterization of a corynebacteriophage β, *tox* operator constitutive-like mutant lysogen of *Corynebacterium diphtheriae, J. Virol.* **18:**235–244.

Murphy, J. R., Michel, J. L., and Teng, M., 1978, Evidence that the regulation of diphtheria toxin production is directed at the level of transcription, *J. Bacteriol.* **35:**511–516.

Murphy, J. R., Bishai, W., Borowski, M., Miyanohara, A., Boyd, J., and Nagle, S., 1986, Genetic construction, expression, and melanoma-selective cytotoxicity of a diphtheria toxin-related α-melanocyte stimulating hormone fusion protein, *Proc. Natl. Acad. Sci. USA* **83:**8258–8262.

Murphy, J. R., Williams, D. P., Bacha, P., Bishai, W., Waters, C., and Strom, T. B., 1988, Cell receptor specific targeted toxins: Genetic construction and characterization of an interleukin-2 diphtheria toxin-related fusion protein, *J. Receptor Res.* **8** (in press).

Neville, D. M. Jr., and Hudson, T. H., 1986, Transmembrane transport of diphtheria toxin, related toxins, and colicins, *Annu. Rev. Biochem.* **55:**195–224.

Newland, J. W., Strockbine, N. A., Miller, S. F., O'Brien, A. D., and Holmes, R. K., 1985, Cloning of shiga-like toxin structural genes from a toxin converting phage of *Escherichia coli, Science* **230:**179–181.

Nida, S. K., and Ferretti, J. J., 1982, Phage influence on the synthesis of extracellular toxins in group A streptococci, *Infect. Immun.* **36:**745–750.

O'Brien, A. D., and Holmes, R. K., 1987, Shiga and shiga-like toxins, *Microbiol. Rev.* **51:**206–220.

O'Brien, A. D., and LaVeck, G. D., 1983, Purification and characterization of a *Shigella dysenteriae* 1-like toxin produced by *Escherichia coli, Infect. Immun.* **40:**675–683.

O'Brien, A. D., LaVeck, G. D., Thompson, M. R., and Formal, S. B., 1982, Production of *Shigella dysenteriae* type 1-like cytotoxin by *Escherichia coli, J. Infect. Dis.* **146:**763–769.

O'Brien, A. D., Lively, T. A., Chen, M. E., Rothman, S. W., and Formal, S. B., 1983, *Escherichia coli* 0157:H7 strains associated with haemorrhagic colitis in the United States produce a *Shigella dysenteriae* 1 (shiga)-like cytotoxin, *Lancet* **1:**702.

O'Brien, A. D., Chen, M. E., Holmes, R. K., Kaper, J., and Levine, M. M., 1984a, Environmental and human isolates of *Vibrio cholerae* and *Vibrio parahaemolyticus* produce a *Shigella dysenteriae* 1 (shiga)-like cytotoxin, *Lancet* **1:**77–78.

O'Brien, A. D., Newland, J. W., Miller, S. F., Holmes, R. K., Williams Smith, H., and Formal, S. B., 1984b, Shiga-like toxin-converting phages from *Escherichia coli* strains that cause hemorrhagic colitis or infantile diarrhea, *Science* **226:**694–696.

Obrig, T. G., Moran, T. P., and Colinas, R. J., 1985, Ribonuclease activity associated with the 60S ribosome-inactivating proteins ricin A, phytolaccin and shiga toxin, *Biochem. Biophys. Res. Commun.* **130:**879–884.

Oguma, K., 1976, The stability of toxinogenicity in *Clostridium botulinum* types C and D, *J. Gen. Microbiol.* **92:**67–75.

Oguma, K., and Sugiyama, H., 1978, Adsorption to *Clostridium botulinum* cultures of phage controlling type C botulinum toxin production (40284), *Proc. Soc. Exp. Biol. Med.* **159:**61–64.

Oguma, K., Iida, H., Shiozaki, M., and Inoue, K., 1976a, Antigenicity of converting phages obtained from *Clostridium botulinum* types C and D, *Infect. Immun.* **13:**855–860.

Oguma, K., Iida, H., and Shiozaki, M., 1976b, Phage conversion to hemagglutinin production in *Clostridium botulinum* types C and D, *Infect. Immun.* **14:**597–602.

Olsnes, S., and Sandvig, K., 1986, Interactions between diphtheria toxin entry and anion transport in Vero cells. II. Inhibition of anion antiport by diphtheria toxin, *J. Biol. Chem.* **261:**1553–1561.

Olsnes, S., Reisbig, R., and Eiklid, K., 1981, Subunit structure of *Shigella* cytotoxin, *J. Biol. Chem.* **256:**8732–8738.

Pappenheimer, A. M. Jr., 1977, Diphtheria toxin, *Annu. Rev. Biochem.* **46:**69–94.

Pappenheimer, A. M. Jr., 1984, Diphtheria, in: *Bacterial Vaccines* (R. Germanier, ed.), pp. 1–36, Academic Press, Orlando, FL.

Pappenheimer, A. J. Jr., and Johnson, S. J., 1936, Studies in diphtheria toxin production. I. The effects of iron and copper, Br. J. Exp. Pathol. **17**:335–341.

Pappenheimer, A. M. Jr., and Murphy, J. R., 1983, Studies on the molecular epidemiology of diphtheria, Lancet **2**:923–926.

Park, W. H., and Williams, A. W., 1896, The production of diphtheria toxin, J. Exp. Med. **1**:164–185.

Pattee, P. A., and Glatz, B. A. 1980, Identification of a chromosomal determinant of enterotoxin A production in Staphylococcus aureus, Appl. Environ. Microbiol. **39**:186–193.

Pope, C., 1932, The production of toxin by C. diphtheriae. II. Effects produced by additions of iron and copper to the medium, Br. J. Exp. Pathol. **36**:373–380.

Ranelli, D. M., Jones, C. L., Johns, M. B., Mussey, G. J., and Khan, S. A., 1985, Molecular cloning of staphylococcal enterotoxin B gene in Escherichia coli and Staphylococcus aureus, Proc. Natl. Acad. Sci. USA **82**:5850–5854.

Rappuoli, R., and Ratti, G., 1984, Physical map of the chromosomal region of Corynebacterium diphtheriae containing corynephage attachment sites attB1 and attB2, J. Bacteriol. **158**:325–330.

Rappuoli, R., Michel, J. L., and Murphy, J. R., 1983a, Restriction endonucleas map of corynebacteriophage ω_c^{tox+} isolated from the Park-Williams No. 8 strain of Corynebacterium diphtheriae, J. Virol. **45**:524–530.

Rappuoli, R., Michel, J. L., and Murphy, J. R., 1983b, Integration of corynebacteriophages β^{tox+}, ω^{tox+}, and γ^{tox-} into two attachment sites on the Corynebacterium diphtheriae chromosome, J. Bacteriol. **153**:1202–1210.

Rappuoli, R., Ratti, G., Perugini, M., and Murphy, J. R., 1985, Detection and physical map of a ω^{tox+}-related defective prophage in Corynebacterium diphtheriae Belfanti 1030(–)$^{tox-}$, J. Virol. **54**:194–198.

Ratti, G., Rappuoli, R., and Giannini, G., 1983, The complete nucleotide sequence of the gene coding for diphtheria toxin in the corynephage omega (tox+) genome, Nucleic Acids Res. **11**:6589–6595.

Read, R. B. Jr., and Pritchard, W. L., 1963, Lysogeny among the enterotoxinogenic staphylococci, Can. J. Microbiol. **9**:879–889.

Reisbig, R., Olsnes, S., and Eiklid, K., 1981, The cytotoxic activity of Shigella toxin. Evidence for catalytic inactivation of the 60S ribosomal subunit, J. Biol. Chem. **256**:8739–8744.

Righelato, R. C., and Van Hemert, P. A., 1969, Growth and toxin synthesis in batch and chemostat cultures of Corynebacterium diphtheriae, J. Gen. Microbiol. **58**:403–410.

Roux, E., and Yersin, A., 1888, Contribution à l'étude de la diphthérie, Ann. Inst. Pasteur **2**:629–662.

Sadoff, J. C., Buck, G. A., Iglewski, B. H., Bjorn, M. J., and Groman, N. B., 1982, Immunological cross-reactivity in the absence of DNA homology between Pseudomonas toxin A and diphtheria toxin, Infect. Immun. **37**:250–254.

Sandvig, K., and Olsnes, S., 1981, Rapid entry of nicked diphtheria toxin into cells at low pH: Characterization of the entry process and effects of low pH on the toxin molecule, J. Biol. Chem. **256**:9068–9074.

Sandvig, K., and Olsnes, S., 1982, Entry of the toxic proteins abrin, modeccin, ricin, and diphtheria toxin into cells. II. Effect of pH, metabolic inhibitors, and ionophores and evidence for toxin penetration from endocytic vesicles, J. Biol. Chem. **257**:7504–7513.

Sandvig, K., and Olsnes, S., 1986, Interactions between diphtheria toxin entry and anion transport in Vero cells. IV. Evidence that entry of diphtheria toxin is dependent on efficient anion transport, J. Biol. Chem. **261**:1570–1575.

Saragea, A., Maximescu, P., and Meitert, E., 1979, Corynebacterium diphtheriae: Microbiological methods used in clinical and epidemiological investigations, Methods Microbiol. **13**:62–176.

Scheuber, P. H., Golecki, J. R., Kickhofen, B., Scheel, D., Beck, G., and Hammer, D., 1985, Skin reactivity of unsensitized monkeys upon challenge with staphylococcal enterotoxin B: A new approach for investigating the site of toxin action, *Infect. Immun.* **50:**869–876.

Schlievert, P. M., and Watson, D. W., 1978, Group A streptococcal pyrogenic exotoxin: Pyrogenicity, alteration of blood-brain barrier, separation of sites for pyrogenicity and enhancement of lethal endotoxin shock, *Infect. Immun.* **21:**753–763.

Schlievert, P. M., Bettin, K. M., and Watson, D. W., 1977, Purification and characterization of group A streptococcal pyrogenic extoxin type C, *Infect. Immun.* **16:**673–679.

Schlievert, P. M., Bettin, K. M., and Watson, D. W., 1979, Reinterpretation of the Dick test: Role of group A streptococcal pyrogenic exotoxin, *Infect. Immun.* **26:**467–472.

Schmidt, J. J., and Spero, L., 1983, The complete amino acid sequence of staphylococcal enterotoxin C_1, *J. Biol. Chem.* **258:**6300–6306.

Schutzer, S. E., Fischetti, V. A., and Zabriskie, J. B., 1983, Toxic shock syndrome and lysogeny in *Staphylococcus aureus*, *Science* **220:**316–318.

Scotland, S. M., May, N. P., Willshaw, G. A., and Rowe, B., 1980, Cytotoxic enteropathogenic *Escherichia coli*, *Lancet* **1:**90.

Scotland, S. M., Smith, H. R., Willshaw, G. A., and Rowe, B., 1983, Vero cytotoxin production in strain of *Escherichia coli* is determined by genes carried on bacteriophage, *Lancet* **2:**216.

Séreny, B., 1955, Experimental *Shigella* keratoconjunctivitis: A preliminary report, *Acta Microbiol. Acad. Sci. Hung.* **2:**293–296.

Shafer, W. M., and Iandolo, J. J., 1978, Staphylococcal enterotoxin A: A chromosomal gene product, *Appl. Environ. Microbiol.* **36:**389–391.

Simpson, L. L., 1974, Studies on the binding of botulinum toxin type A to the rat phrenic nerve-hemidiaphragm preparation, *Neuropharmacology* **13:**683–691.

Simpson, L. L., 1980, Kinetic studies on the interaction between botulinum toxin type A and the cholinergic neuromuscular junction, *J. Pharmacol. Exp. Ther.* **212:**16–21.

Simpson, L. L., 1981, The origin, structure, and pharmacological activity of botulinum toxin, *Pharmacol. Rev.* **33:**155–188.

Simpson, L. L., 1983, Ammonium chloride and methylamine hydrochloride antagonize clostridial neurotoxins, *J. Pharmacol. Exp. Ther.* **225:**546–552.

Singer, R. A., 1973a, Temperature-sensitive mutants of toxinogenic corynebacteriophage beta. I. Genetics, *Virology* **55:**347–356.

Singer, R. A., 1973b, Temperature-sensitive mutants of toxinogenic corynebacteriophage beta. II. Properties of mutant phages, *Virology* **55:**357–362.

Smith, L. D., 1977, *Botulism: The Organism, Its Toxins, the Disease.* Charles C. Thomas, Springfield, IL.

Spero, L., Warren, J. R., and Metzger, J. F., 1973, Effect of single peptide bond scission by trypsin on the structure and activity of staphylococcal enterotoxin B, *J. Biol. Chem.* **248:**7289–7294.

Spero, L., Griffin, B. Y., Middlebrook, J. L., and Metzger, J. F., 1976, Effect of single and double peptide bond scission by trypsin on the structure and activity of staphylococcal enterotoxin C, *J. Biol. Chem.* **251:**5580–5588.

Straus, N., and Hendee, E., 1959, The effect of diphtheria toxin on the metabolism of HeLa cells, *J. Exp. Med.* **109:**145–163.

Strockbine, N. A., Marques, L. R. M., Newland, J. W., Williams Smith, H., Holmes, R. K., and O'Brien, A. D., 1986, Two toxin-converting phages from *Escherichia coli* 0157:H7 strain 933 encode antigenically distinct toxins with similar biologic activities, *Infect. Immun.* **53:**135–140.

Sugiyama, H., 1980, *Clostridium botulinum* neurotoxin, *Microbiol. Rev.* **44:**419–448.

Sugiyama, H., and Hayama, T., 1965, Abdominal viscera as site of emetic action for staphylococcal enterotoxin in the monkey, *J. Infect. Dis.* **115:**330–336.

Sugiyama, H., Mizutani, K., and Yang, K. H., 1972, Basis of type A and F toxicities of *Clostridium botulinum* strain 84, *Proc. Soc. Exp. Biol. Med.* **141:**1063–1067.

Sugiyama, H., DasGupta, B. R., and Yang, K. H., 1973, Disulfide-toxicity relationship of botulinal toxin types A, E, and F, *Proc. Soc. Exp. Biol. Med.* **143:**589–591.

Thompson, N. E., Ketterhagen, M. J., and Bergdoll, M. S., 1984, Monoclonal antibodies to staphylococcal enterotoxins B and C: Cross-reactivity and localization of epitopes on tryptic fragments, *Infect. Immun.* **45**:281–285.

Toshach, S., 1950, Bacteriophages for *Corynebacterium diphtheriae, Can. J. Publ. Health* **41**:332–336.

Uchida, T., Gill, D. M., and Pappenheimer, A. M. Jr., 1971, Mutation in the structural gene for diphtheria toxin carried by temperate phage β, *Nature New Biol.* **233**:8–11.

Uchida, T., Pappenheimer, A. M. Jr., and Harper, A. A., 1973, Diphtheria toxin and related proteins. II. Kinetic studies on intoxication of HeLa cells by diphtheria toxin and related proteins, *J. Biol. Chem.* **248**:3845–3850.

Ueda, K., and Hayaishi, O., 1985, ADP-ribosylation, *Annu. Rev. Biochem.* **54**:73–100.

Van Heyningen, W. E., and Gladstone, G. P., 1953, The neurotoxin of *Shigellae shigae.* 3. The effect of iron on production of toxin, *Br. J. Exp. Pathol.* **34**:221–229.

Van Ness, B. G., Howard, J. B., and Bodley, J. W., 1980, ADP-ribosylation of elongation factor by diphtheria toxin: NMR spectra and proposed structures of ribosyl diphthamide and its hydrolysis products, *J. Biol. Chem.* **255**:10710–10716.

Vinet, G., and Fredette, V., 1968, Un bactériophage dans une culture de *Clostridium botulinum* C, *Rev. Can. Biol.* **27**:73–74.

Vitetta, E. S., and Uhr, J. W., 1985, Immunotoxins: Redirecting nature's poisons, *Cell* **41**:653–654.

Wannamaker, L. W., 1983, Streptococcal toxins, *Rev. Infect. Dis.* **5** (Suppl.):S723–S732.

Ward, W. H. J., 1987, Diphtheria toxin: A novel cytocidal enzyme, *Trends Biochem. Sci.* **12**:28–31.

Watson, D. W., 1960, Host-parasite factors in group A streptococcal infection. Pyrogenic and other effects of immunologic distinct exotoxins related to scarlet fever toxins, *J. Exp. Med.* **111**:255–284.

Weeks, C. R., and Ferretti, J. J., 1984, The gene for type A streptococcal exotoxin (erythrogenic toxin) is located in bacteriophage T12, *Infect. Immun.* **46**:531–536.

Weeks, C. R., and Ferretti, J. J., 1986, Nucleotide sequence of the type A streptococcal exotoxin (erythrogenic toxin) gene from *Streptococcus pyogenes* bacteriophage T12, *Infect. Immun.* **52**:144–150.

Welkos, S. L., and Holmes, R. K., 1981a, Regulation of toxinogenesis in *Corynebacterium diphtheriae.* I. Mutations in bacteriophage β that alter the effects of iron on toxin production, *J. Virol.* **37**:936–945.

Welkos, S. L., and Holmes, R. K., 1981b, Regulation of toxinogenesis in *Corynebacterium diphtheriae.* II. Genetic mapping of a *tox* regulatory mutation in bacteriophage β, *J. Virol.* **37**:946–954.

Williams, D., Parker, K., Bacha, P., Bishai, W., Borowski, M., Genbauffe, F., Strom, T. B., and Murphy, J. R., 1987, Diphtheria toxin receptor binding domain substitution with interleukin-2: Genetic construction and properties of a diphtheria toxin-related interleukin-2 fusion protein, *Protein Eng.* **1**:493–498.

Williams Smith, H., and Linggood, M. A., 1971, The transmissible nature of enterotoxin production in a human enteropathogenic strain of *Escherichia coli, J. Med. Microbiol.* **4**:301–305.

Williams Smith, H., Green, P., and Parsell, Z., 1983, Vero cell toxins in *Escherichia coli* and related bacteria: Transfer by phage and conjugation and toxic action in laboratory animals, chickens and pigs, *J. Gen. Microbiol.* **129**:3121–3137.

Willshaw, G. A., Smith, H. R., Scotland, S. M., and Rowe, B., 1985, Cloning of genes determining the production of Vero cytotoxin by *Escherichia coli, J. Gen. Microbiol.* **131**:3047–3053.

Yamaizumi, M., Mekada, E., Uchida, T., and Okada, Y., 1978, One molecule of diphtheria toxin fragment A introduced into a cell can kill the cell, *Cell* **15**:245–250.

Zabriskie, J. B., 1964, The role of temperate bacteriophage in the production of erythrogenic toxin by group A streptococci, *J. Exp. Med.* **119**:761–780.

Zalman, L. S., and Wisnieski, B. J., 1984, Mechanism of insertion of diphtheria toxin: Peptide entry and pore size determinations, *Proc. Natl. Acd. Sci. USA* **81**:3341–3345.

CHAPTER 13

Structure and Function of the Transcription Activator Protein cII and Its Regulatory Signals

YEN SEN HO AND MARTIN ROSENBERG

I. INTRODUCTION

When bacteriophage λ infects *E. coli* cells, the phage can develop along either of two pathways: a lytic pathway leading to the multiplication of progeny virus and lysis of the host cells, or a lysogenic pathway leading to the integration of phage DNA into the host genome and maintenance in a dormant state. The cII protein of phage λ is a transcriptional activator of gene expression; it plays a pivotal role in the lytic versus lysogenic developmental decision made by the phage after infection. The cII protein coordinately regulates transcription from three separate transcription units, each controlled by a cII-dependent promoter signal—P_{RE}, P_I, and P_{aQ} (Fig. 1). Two of the cII-dependent promoters, P_{RE} and P_I, control the expression of the two phage gene products, repressor (cI) and integrase (*int*), the first of which inhibits transcription of lytic functions, and the second which catalyzes the integrative recombination of the viral DNA into the host genome (Herskowitz and Hagen, 1980; Wulff and Rosenberg, 1983). The third promoter, P_{aQ}, is thought to direct the synthesis of an antisense RNA, the function of which is to reduce the expression of

YEN SEN HO AND MARTIN ROSENBERG • Department of Molecular Genetics, Research and Development Division, Smith Kline and French Laboratories, King of Prussia, Pennsylvania 19406-0939.

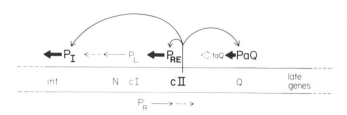

FIGURE 1. Schematic diagram showing the coordinately controlled cII-dependent transcription units on phage λ. Thick horizontal arrows indicate origin and direction of transcription from the three cII activated promoters, P_I, P_{RE}, and P_{aQ}. Also indicated is the proposed transcription terminator of the P_{aQ} transcription unit, t_{aQ}. Thin arrows indicate the origin and direction of transcription from the promoters, P_I and P_R, which control the major leftward and rightward operons of phage. The approximate position of the genes encoding integrase (int), N protein, repressor (cI), cII protein, and Q protein are also shown.

the λ Q gene product (Fig. 1) (Ho and Rosenberg, 1985; Hoopes and McClure, 1985). Q protein is an antiterminator for the gene expression of all phage late genes during lytic growth. The down-regulation of the Q gene favors lysogenic development.

It has been demonstrated that cII alone is both necessary and sufficient to activate P_{RE}, P_I, and P_{aQ} transcription (Shimatake and Rosenberg, 1981; Ho and Rosenberg, 1982, 1985; Ho et al., 1983). cII binding and transcription activation at these three promoters occur at essentially the same cII levels in vitro (Ho et al., 1983; Ho and Rosenberg, 1985). In addition, the three promoters also respond to cII at the same time following phage infection in vivo (Schmeissner et al., 1980, 1981; Ho and Rosenberg, 1985). These results clearly demonstrate that all three promoters function in concert to achieve the lysogenic growth response of the phage.

One of the most significant differences of cII protein is that it recognizes a direct repeat DNA sequence instead of a DNA sequence with twofold rotational symmetry, as is the case with the λ repressors cI and Cro, and the E. coli CRP protein, Trp repressor, and Lac repressor (Maniatis et al., 1975; Pabo and Lewis, 1982; Johnson et al., 1978; Anderson et al., 1981; Majors, 1978; Aiba and Krakow, 1981; McKay et al., 1982; Bennett et al., 1977; Dickson et al., 1975; Gilbert et al., 1976). It is of fundamental interest to understand how a regulatory protein that exists in tetrameric form recognizes and interacts with a direct-repeat DNA sequence.

In this chapter we will discuss the physical and chemical properties of the cII protein, the promoter signals it controls, and the specific DNA-protein interactions involved in transcription activation. We will review the experimental approaches and analyses that have led to our present understanding of the structure and function of cII and the DNA signals with which it interacts.

II. cII-REGULATED PROMOTER SIGNALS

The structure and transcription initiation sites of all three of the cII-dependent promoters on phage λ (P_{RE}, p_I, and P_{aQ}) have been well defined (Fig. 2) (Abraham et al., 1980; Davies, 1980; Hoess et al., 1980; Schmeissner et al., 1980, 1981; Ho and Rosenberg, 1985; Hoopes and McClure, 1985). These promoters exhibit little homology with the highly conserved −10 and −35 region hexamer consensus sequences for prokaryotic promoters. Yet they do share significant structural similarity to each other. This is not surprising, since none of these promoters function in an *in vitro* transcription system containing only RNA polymerase. Their function is completely dependent on the cII activator protein. Most notably, all three promoters contain the same tetranucleotide repeat sequence (TTGC) separated by six base pairs (N_6) positioned identically in their −35 regions with respect to their transcription start sites (Fig. 2). The occurrence of this $TTGCN_6TTGC$ repeat structure in all three signals led to the proposal that this sequence might define a site involved in the positive regulation mechanism common to these promoters (Ho and Rosenberg, 1982). As will be described below, it was demonstrated by both genetic and biochemical analysis that this tetranucleotide direct repeat is the core recognition structure for the sequence-specific cII-DNA interaction at these sites. These promoters also contain other structural homologies surrounding the −10 region. For example, the P_{aQ} and P_{RE} promoters contain an extensive homology within their −10 regions (12 of 13 identical consecutive residues), and the P_{aQ} and P_I promoters exhibit an exact 6-bp homology in the −15 to −20 region (Fig. 2). At present, there is no evidence suggesting that these sequences play a role in the cII activation mechanism. However, they are important determinants of overall promoter function and efficiency. There are two other $TTGCN_6TTGC$ sequences on the phage λ genome, which do not share these −10 region homologies. cII protein binds to these sequences as demonstrated by DNase footprinting analysis, but they do not exhibit any promoter function (Ho and Rosenberg, 1985).

Finally, it is of interest to mention that two of the cII-dependent

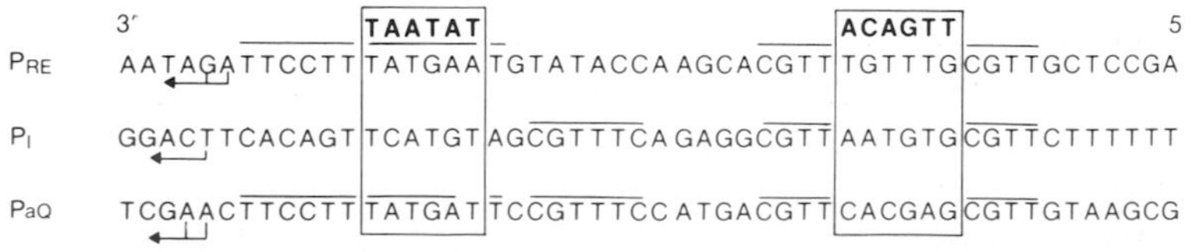

FIGURE 2. DNA sequences of the nontemplate strands of the three cII-dependent phage λ promoters, P_I, P_{RE}, and P_{aQ}. The transcription start sites are indicated by arrows. The boxed regions correspond to and are compared with the −10 and −35 region consensus sequences for promoters recognized by *Escherichia coli* RNA polymerase (Rosenberg and Court, 1979). The overscored areas represent regions of homology shared by these sequences.

728   YEN SEN HO and MARTIN ROSENBERG

```
                                          T
                                          A
                                          |
G          GC ACCA     C A A     G               TG  AT
C          CG TGGT      GTT      C               AC  TA
|          | | | |  ┘    ┘       |               | |  | |
S.D.       F-MET VAL  ARG  ALA  ASN  LYS  ARG  ASN  GLU  ALA

5'---ATCTAAGGAAATACTTACATATGGTTCGT GC AAACAAACGCAACGAGGCT---3'


        TAATAT                               ACAGTT


3'---TAGATTCCTTTATGAATGTATACCAAGCA CGTTTGTTTGCGTTGCTCCGA---5'
   ←─PRE
             G   ACG  T                    TTG   GTTAAGG
             C   TGC  A                    AAC   CAATTCC
                                            |      |  |
                                            T      T  C
                                            A      A  G
```

FIGURE 3. Nucleotide sequence in the region of structural overlap between the P_{RE} promoter and the NH_2-terminal end of the cII gene. The 6-bp consensus sequences for the -10 and -35 regions of prokaryotic promoters are indicated and aligned as in Fig. 2. The transcription initiation site of P_{RE} is indicated by the arrow. The TTGC tetranucleotide repeat sequence and the Shine–Delgarno region important for ribosome recognition of the cII gene are underscored. The F-met initiation codon and the first 10 amino acid residues of the cII protein are also indicated. Nucleotide changes shown below the sequence are promoter "down" mutations selected in P_{RE}, and nucleotide changes shown above the sequence are those selected as cII mutations.

promoters, P_{RE} and P_{aQ}, overlap with DNA sequences that encode other functions. In the case of P_{aQ}, the promoter sequence is positioned in the middle of the Q gene and has an anti-Q orientation (Fig. 1) (Ho and Rosenberg, 1985). In the case of P_{RE}, the promoter overlaps the NH_2-terminal coding region of the cII activator gene itself (Fig. 3) (Schmeissner et al., 1980; Wulff et al., 1980; Rosenberg et al., 1978a). It has been proposed that this overlap plays a role in the autoregulation of the synthesis of cII protein in vivo; however, at present there is little direct evidence for its support.

III. PHYSICAL, CHEMICAL, AND FUNCTIONAL CHARACTERIZATION OF PURIFIED cII PROTEIN

The important role of cII protein in the lysis-lysogeny decision of λ phage has been known for years, yet the detailed biochemical and functional studies of cII protein were hampered by its limited availability. To circumvent this limitation, the cII gene was cloned and overproduced by using an expression vector, pKC30, carrying the strong, regulatable λ phage promoter P_L (Shimatake and Rosenberg, 1981). The expression of cII protein from this vector was selectively induced by either temperature or chemical reagents (Mott et al., 1985). Using this vector system, cII protein was produced routinely at levels approaching 5% of total E. coli cellular protein. A relatively simple purification procedure was developed for the isolation of homogeneous cII protein at a final yield of 1–1.5 mg/g wet weight of cell culture (Ho *et al.*, 1982). This strategy has also been used to overexpress a variety of other potentially lethal gene products with great success (Rosenberg *et al.*, 1983).

Extensive physical and chemical characterization of pure cII protein has been carried out. To date, the amino acid composition, NH_2-terminal sequence, molar extinction coefficient, subunit and native molecular weight, oligomeric structure, isoelectric point, alpha helical content, and antigenic capability of cII protein have all been examined (Table I) (Ho *et al.*, 1982). Analysis of cII by both analytical ultracentrifugation and velocity sedimentation demonstrated that in solution at concentrations above 4×10^{-7} M, cII is a 44,000-MW tetramer. NH_2-terminal amino acid analysis indicated that the mature cII protein started from the third encoded amino acid, arginine (Ho *et al.*, 1982). Apparently, both the F-met and the second amino acid, valine, are removed to form the mature cII protein. The large quantities of protein available have allowed X-ray crystallographic studies to be initiated.

The regulatory function of cII protein on gene transcription has been demonstrated *in vitro* on all three promoter signals: P_{RE}, P_I, and P_{aQ} (Shimatake and Rosenberg, 1981; Ho and Rosenberg, 1982, 1985; Ho *et al.*, 1982, 1983). cII was both necessary and, most importantly, sufficient to activate transcription from these promoter signals in the reconstituted *in vitro* system (Fig. 4). Moreover, transcription *in vitro* initiated at precisely the same start sites as *in vivo*. Titration experiments with cII protein showed that activation on these three promoters occurred at the same cII concentration but reached rather different levels. For example, the P_{RE} promoter was at least four times more efficient than P_I (Ho *et al.*, 1983), whereas P_{aQ} and P_{RE} exhibited similar efficiencies (Ho and Rosenberg, 1985).

The differences in promoter efficiency might have resulted either from differences in cII interaction or from differences in RNA polymerase interaction at these signals. Since cII exhibited identical binding affinities

TABLE I. Physical and Chemical Properties
of cII Protein

Molecular weight	
Velocity sedimentation	43,600
Sedimentation equilibrium	44,000
SDS-PAGE	11,300
$S_{20,\omega}^{o}$	3.4S
ϵ_{280}	7.2×10^4
Subunit structure	Tetramer
Aminoterminal sequence	(fMet-Val)-Arg-Ala-Asn
Isoelectric point	8.8
α-Helix content	50–60%

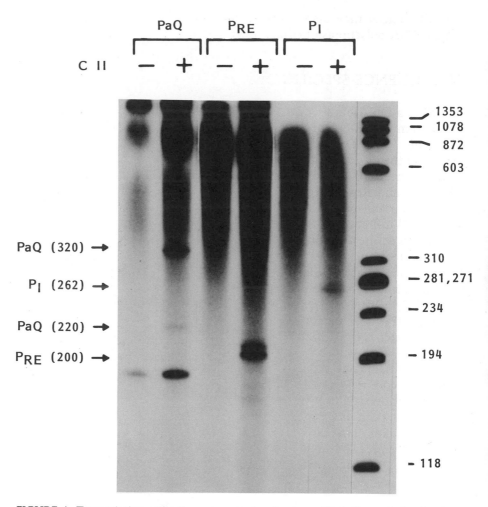

FIGURE 4. Transcription activation responses *in vitro* to purified *c*II protein for the three different phage λ promoters shown in Fig. 2. The autoradiogram shows a polyacrylamide gel electrophoretic analysis of ^{32}P-labeled RNA transcripts synthesized *in vitro* either in the presence (+) or absence (−) of purified *c*II protein. The various *c*II-induced transcripts are indicated, and their estimated sizes are given in parentheses. DNA fragments of the sizes indicated were used as markers.

for all three sites (see below), it appeared that the differences in promoter strength were due to RNA polymerase recognition and initiation. As has been mentioned previously, the −10 region sequences of P_{RE} and P_{aQ} were very similar, whereas the P_I sequence was quite different (Fig. 2). Presumably, the −10 region sequences of P_{RE} and P_{aQ} are more favorable for RNA polymerase recognition than that of P_I. Moreover, P_{RE} and P_{aQ} transcription both initiated with purine nucleotides (ATP), whereas P_I transcription initiated with a pyrimidine nucleotide (UTP). These start-site differences may also contribute to the different efficiencies with which RNA polymerase utilized these signals.

IV. SEQUENCE-SPECIFIC DNA BINDING

cII is a DNA-binding protein. This was first suggested by its strong interaction with DNA-agarose, which has been utilized in its purification (Ho et al., 1982). The sequence-specific interaction of cII and RNA polymerase at the P_{RE}, P_I, and P_{aQ} promoter signals was demonstrated later by using a variety of chemical and enzymatic probe techniques (Ho et al., 1983; Ho and Rosenberg, 1985). Promoter function studies on a large number of point mutations mapped in the P_{RE} region (Brachet and Thomas, 1969; Wulff et al., 1980, 1984; Rosenberg et al., 1978b) provide strong support to define the core sequence for cII recognition (Ho et al., 1983). DNA protection studies using either DNase and/or neocarcinostatin demonstrated that cII binds selectively in the homologous −35 regions of all three promoters. The protected regions encompassed some 20–25 bp and always centered on the common $TTGCN_6TTGT$ repeat sequence (Fig. 5). Titration experiments showed that cII exhibited essentially identical affinities, approximately 3×10^{-7} M, for all three sites. That these three cII binding sites have little in common other than the tetranucleotide repeat sequence strongly suggests that this repeat sequence is the important core recognition element for cII protein.

Protection studies were also used to examine the interaction of RNA polymerase, both alone and in the presence of cII, at all three promoters (Ho et al., 1983; Ho and Rosenberg, 1985). In the absence of cII, only at very high concentrations RNA polymerase did show a weak but reproducible protection pattern around the −10 regions of these three pro-

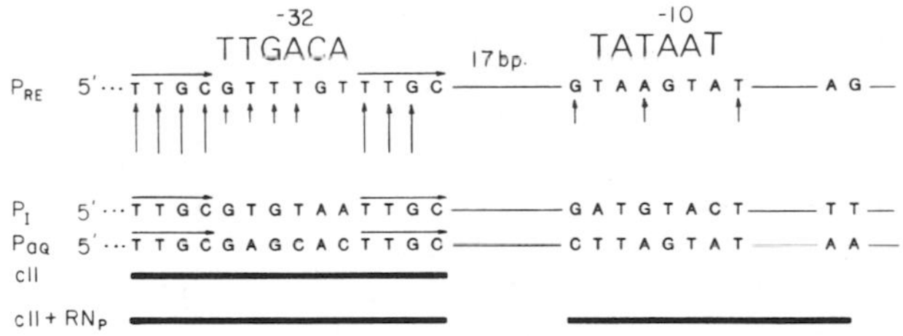

FIGURE 5. Comparison of the −10 and −35 region sequences of the P_{RE}, P_I, and P_{aQ} promoters aligned with respect to their cII-dependent transcription start sites (+1). Only the nontemplate strands are shown. The consensus −10 and −35 region sequences recognized by RNA polymerase are also shown for comparison, as is the consensus 17-bp separation between them. The regions of the promoter protected from nuclease digestion by cII and cII plus RNA polymerase are indicated by thick solid bars. The tetranucleotide repeat sequence is indicated by horizontal arrows. The long vertical arrows indicate residues that, when mutated, affect cII binding. Short arrows indicate positions that, when mutated, have no effect on cII binding.

moters. Although this kind of interaction did not give rise to any productive transcription, RNA polymerase might be capable of weak interaction (i.e., perhaps closed-complex formation) at these promoters in the absence of cII protein. In contrast to these results, when RNA polymerase interaction was examined in the presence of cII protein, the entire promoter region extending over some 45 bp was protected (Fig. 5). Clearly, cII caused RNA polymerase to bind and form a stable complex at each promoter signal. In addition, it was noted that the amount of cII required to achieve protection in the presence of RNA polymerase was approximately 10-fold lower than that needed alone to protect the promoter. That is, in the presence of RNA polymerase, half-maximal protection of the promoters occurred at a cII concentration of 3×10^{-8} M, instead of the 3×10^{-7} M for cII alone. Apparently, cII and RNA polymerase interact in a cooperative way at all three cII-dependent promoter signals. This cooperativity was also demonstrated in the transcription reaction, wherein the amount of cII utilized to achieve full activation was 10-fold lower than that required alone for DNA binding. Since the extent of cooperativity is similar for all three promoters, they respond to essentially identical levels of cII protein *in vitro*; this result is consistent with the coordinate function required of these signals during phage development.

In an effort to define more precisely the DNA sequences required for cII interaction, DNase-protection studies were also carried out on 18 different promoter mutations in the P_{RE} site (Ho and Rosenberg, 1982; Ho et al., 1983). Single-base-pair changes in both the -10 and -35 regions of P_{RE} were examined for their effects on cII binding. The results (summarized in Fig. 5) show that mutations in the -10 region have no effect on cII binding. Presumably, these mutations inactivate promoter function by affecting RNA polymerase interaction rather than cII interaction. In contrast, mutations in the -35 region of P_{RE} do affect cII binding. The mutations that abolish cII binding fall into the two tetranucleotide repeat sequences. Alterations in seven of the eight base pairs of the tetranucleotide repeat were shown to affect cII binding (Fig. 5). Only one mutation occurring in the repeat sequence (TTGCN$_6$TTGT) was found to be acceptable for both cII binding and promoter function.

Four other mutations, which occur within the 6-bp separation between the tetranucleotide repeats, had little if any effect on cII binding, but all eliminated promoter function. Strikingly, this 6-bp region is positioned exactly 17 bp upstream of the P_{RE} -10 region sequence. Thus, it is analogous in both size and position to the -35 region hexamer sequence found in other promoter signals (Rosenberg and Court, 1979). Although this sequence at P_{RE} bears little resemblance to the consensus -35 region hexamer (TTGACA), it must carry out a similar function, because single-base-pair changes in this region eliminate the promoter function. Apparently, cII binding in some way makes the poor -35 region recognizable by RNA polymerase for promoter function, either through altering the local conformation of the −35 region DNA sequence or through protein-protein interaction with RNA polymerase.

There are a large number of mutations positioned between the −10 and −35 regions of the promoter (Rosenberg and Court, 1979; Wulff and Rosenberg, 1983). None of these mutations affect P_{RE} function, which supports the general contention that this region of the promoter does not play a role in the sequence-specific protein-DNA interaction. Instead, it serves to properly position the −10 and −35 regions. The importance of this spacing for P_{RE} has now been domonstrated directly (Keilty and Rosenberg, 1987). A 2-bp insertion and a 2-bp deletion mutation were created in the P_{RE} spacer region at position −17 of the promoter. DNA-binding studies showed that cII still interacted with both of these mutant P_{RE} signals, but the transcription activation was eliminated completely both *in vitro* and *in vivo*.

The DNase protection studies on native and mutated P_{RE} promoters strongly indicate that the TTGC tetranucleotide repeat forms the core of the cII recognition site. Since the corresponding positions in each of the tetranucleotide repeats are separated by 10 bp (i.e., exactly one turn of the DNA helix), the two TTGC sequences are aligned on one side of the DNA. Thus, it was suggested that cII might bind primarily on one side of the DNA helix. Since the six-nucleotide sequence between the two TTGC repeat sequences might comprise the RNA polymerase interact sites at P_{RE}, it was proposed that the contact sites of RNA polymerase occur on the other side of the DNA helix.

Strong evidence supporting the conclusions drawn above was obtained by examining the close apposition of cII and DNA using methylation protection techniques (Ho *et al.*, 1983). The results indicated that all four G residues that occurred within the TTGC repeat sequence were protected by cII protein (Fig. 6A). No other purine residues outside or between the repeat sequences were strongly protected. The two pairs of protected G residues are closely juxtaposed in each of the repeat units and are aligned perfectly on one face of the DNA. Since methylation occurs at the N7 position of the G base, which occupies the DNA major groove, cII protein must bind at this major groove. In contrast to the G methylation pattern, the A residues showed dramatically enhanced methylation in the presence of cII protein (Fig. 6A). No other purines within or outside this region were affected. It is known that methylation of A residues occurs at the N3 position in the minor groove of duplex DNA (Siebenlist *et al.*, 1980; Singer, 1975; Lawley and Brookes, 1963). Thus, the methylation enhancement at these positions suggests that cII binding, rather than protecting the minor groove, makes this groove more accessible to DMS attack. This conformational change encompasses the −35 region nonconsensus hexamer sequences that may be responsible for RNA polymerase recognition, thereby leading to promoter function.

Methylation protection studies were also carried out in the presence of both cII and RNA polymerase (Ho *et al.*, 1983). The same four G

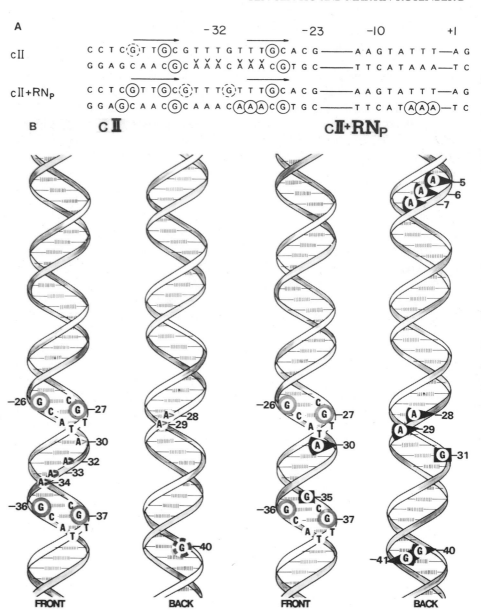

FIGURE 6. (A) Summary of the methylation protection studies carried out with cII alone and cII plus RNA polymerse (RN_P) at the P_RE promoter. Sequence alignment and all designations are the same as those used in Fig. 5. O, Strongly protected residue; ⊙, weakly protected residue; >, methylation enhanced residue. (B) Diagrammatic summary of the methylation-production studies carried out with cII alone and cII plus RNA polymerase at the P_RE promoter. Residues protected by cII alone: solid circle, strongly protected residue; dashed circle, weakly protected residue; >, methylation-enhanced residue. Residues protected by cII and RNA polymerase; wedge, strongly protected residue; box, weakly protected residue. Numbers indicate nucleotide position in the promoter relative to the transcription start site.

residues protected by cII alone remained protected. Apparently, cII remains bound to the same region after RNA polymerase binding. RNA polymerase binding results in strong protection of other purine residues positioned both outside and between the tetranucleotide repeat sequence, as well as in the -10 region. Most important, these binding sites are located on the side of the DNA opposite that which cII binds. Thus, all the evidence indicates that cII and RNA polymerase interact with DNA in the -35 region of the promoter by making contacts with different sides of the DNA helix, thereby sandwiching the DNA between them. These data are presented in schematic form in Fig. 6B.

V. DOMAIN ANALYSIS OF cII PROTEIN

The cII gene encodes a 97-amino acid polypeptide (Fig. 7) (Schwarz *et al.*, 1978). A variety of mutations have been characterized that map within the cII gene coding region of phage λ (Brachet and Thomas, 1969; Wulff *et al.*, 1980, 1984; Rosenberg *et al.*, 1978b). These mutants were characterized genetically, and more than 80 different single amino acid substitutions were defined by DNA sequence analysis (Table II). A representative set of more than 20 different single amino acid substitutions in cII, spanning the entire gene, were selected for more detailed biochemical study. Each mutant was cloned and overproduced in the *E. coli* expression vector system, pKC30, under the transcriptional control of the inducible phage λ P_L promoter. The various cII mutant proteins chosen for analysis were then characterized with respect to their ability to form tetramers, interact with DNA, and activate transcription (Ho *et al.*, 1987). The results of these experiments indicated that cII could be subdivided into several distinct domains (Fig. 7).

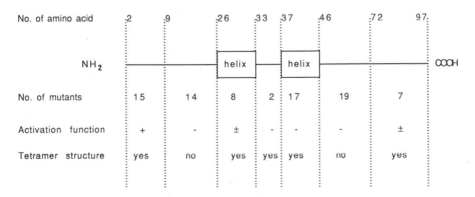

FIGURE 7. Domain structure of the cII protein; see text for details.

TABLE II. Amino Acid Substitutions in the cII Gene[a]

Codon	Wild type	Mutant[b]				
2	val	leu*	ALA*	asp*		
3	arg	CYS[d]				
4	ala	THR*[d]	VAL[c]			
5	asn	ASP[c]				
6	lys	glu	ARG[c]	ASN[c,g]		
7	arg	CYS*[c]	HIS[c]	CYS		
8	asn	ASP[c]	HIS[c]	SER[c]		
9	glu	gly*	ASP[d]			
10	ala	thr	val			
11	leu	pro				
13	ile	phe				
14	glu	lys				
15	ser	asn				
17	leu	ser				
19	asn	asp				
20	lys					
33	val	ala				
34	gly	ser*				
37	lys	arg*	glu*[e]			
38	ser	pro	leu*			
40	ile	asn*	thr	met	leu	
41	ser	gly*	asn	ile		
42	arg	gly*	trp*	lys	met	ser
44	lys	glu				
46	asp	gly*	SER[f]			
47	trp	arg				
51	phe	tyr	ser			
52	ser	leu	pro			
53	met	LYS*				
55	leu	phe*				
58	leu	phe				
59	glu	lys*				

Position				
21	ile	thr	asn	
24	leu	pro*		
25	gly	glu		
26	thr	ile		
27	glu	LYS*		
28	lys	glu˟		
29	thr	*ile*		
30	ala	thr		
31	glu	LYS*		
32	ala	*ser**	*val*	

Position				
52	val	*ala*		
57	met	*thr**		
58	ala	*thr*		
70	leu	*ser**	phe*	trp
71	ala	thr	val	
74	val	*ile*	ala	
75	ala	*thr*		
78	leu	*phe*		
92	gln	*arg**		
95	glu	*val*		

[a] Nonsense and frame shift mutations are not shown.

[b] Mutant key: aaa = cI⁻ phenotype; *aaa* = cII partial activity; AAA = cII⁺ phenotype.

[c] cy P_RE mutants (Wulff et al., 1983).

[d] Revertants of Leu2 or Asp2.

[e] Site-directed mutagenesis was carried out for changing the codon AAG (Lys37) to GAG. A short oligonucleotide 3'-CAAC-TACTCAGCGTC-5' was synthesized by Dr. Sathe, G. for directing the mutagenesis. The desired mutation was verified by M13 sequencing (data not shown).

[f] A revertant of Gly46.

[g] Bracket indicates double mutation.

* These cII mutants cloned for gene expression. The structural genes of the mutant cII proteins were cloned into the E. coli expression vector pKC30 under the control of the inducible phage lambda P_L promoter as described previously [Shimatake and Rosenberg, 1981]. One major change in the cloning strategy is to eliminate the lambda O protein coding sequence from the DNA fragment. Since O protein is always highly expressed in the pKC30 system, this change greatly facilitates the protein purification procedure.

A. The Amino-Terminal Domain: Amino Acid Residues 2–8

Nineteen different single amino acid mutations have been characterized in the seven amino acid codons positioned between residues 2 and 8 of the cII protein (Fig. 7). All of the mutants in this region, with the exception of a Lys to Glu alteration at position 6, exhibit cII$^+$ phenotype and cannot be distinguished either biochemically or genetically from wild-type cII. Examination of several representative mutants from this region indicates that these variant proteins form normal tetramers, bind selectively to DNA, and activate transcription. Clearly, the amino acid structure of the NH$_2$-terminal region is quite flexible. This finding contrasts sharply with that found for λ repressor. The NH$_2$-terminal region of the repressor is known to be important for DNA binding. Removal (or selective mutation) of this region dramatically reduces the binding affinity of the repressor for DNA (Eliason et al., 1985). The NH$_2$-terminal of λ repressor is thought to function as an arm, wrapping around the DNA helix and making contact with the phosphate backbone of the DNA, thereby stabilizing the interaction. The mutational flexibility exhibited by the corresponding NH$_2$-terminal region of cII indicates that it does not have a similar function. Since the sequence-specific DNA-binding affinity of cII is several orders of magnitude lower than that of the λ repressor, we assume a major reason for this difference resides in their NH$_2$-terminal regions.

B. The Oligomerization Domains: Amino Acid Residues 9–25 and 46–71

The oligomerization domains of cII are characterized by nine different substitutions between positions 9 and 25, and 15 different substitutions between positions 46 and 71. It is known the wild-type cII protein is a 44-kD tetramer in solutions composed of four identical subunits (Ho et al., 1983). The native molecular forms of the various cII mutant proteins were determined by a relatively simple procedure developed in our laboratory, which does not require extensive protein purification. The results indicate that there is a group of mutants representing amino acid alterations that affect protein oligomerization. These mutants clustered within two distinct regions of the protein, extending between amino acid residues 9 and 25 and between amino acid residues 46 and 71. Since all these variants exhibit a cII$^-$ phenotype, we conclude that the defectiveness of these proteins may result directly from their inability to form tetramers. In other words, these mutants define two regions of the cII protein which serve primarily a structural role in the formation of the active tetrameric form of cII protein.

During the analysis of the protein stability of various cII mutants, we found that many of the variants were far less stable in the E. coli host than wild-type cII. The results shown in Table III and Fig. 8 indicate that these mutants exhibit half-lives of less than 3 min (some as low as 36 sec), as compared to the 15-min half-life for wild-type cII. Most remarkably, these highly unstable variants are those that are unable to form tetramers. Apparently, there exists a strong correlation between tetramer formation and protein stability.

Recently, we have found an E. coli host strain that stabilizes this particular class of highly unstable cII mutant. In this host strain (HtpR$^-$, high-temperature production regulator), all the highly unstable cII mutants exhibit stabilities comparable to or greater than wild-type cII. For example, the highly unstable cII mutant, cII 3085(Glu^9 → Gly), which exhibits a half-life of <1 min in a normal host, exhibits a half-life of ≥ 20 min in the HtpR$^-$ host (Fig. 9). Although this protein now accumulates in the HtpR$^-$ background, it still does not form tetramers. Clearly, this

TABLE III. Native Molecular Forms and Stabilities
of cII and cII Mutants

Name	Codon of amino acid substitutions	Native molecular form[a]	Half-life (min)
cII		Tetramer (1, 2, 3)	15
Can1 cII	2	Tetramer (1, 2, 3)	49
3059ctrl	2, 4	Tetramer (3)	
3073	2	Tetramer (3)	
3107	7	Tetramer (3)	10
3085	9	Monomer (3)	0.8
2002	24	Monomer (3)	2.5
3606	28	Tetramer (3)	7
DYA-1	31	Tetramer (3)	10
3641	32	Tetramer (3)	3
3612	34	Tetramer (3)	3
3563	37	Tetramer (3)	15
SDM-1	37	Tetramer (3)	15
3062	38	Tetramer (1)	15
3283	39, 40	Tetramer (3)	14
3378	41	Tetramer (3)	15
3151	42	Tetramer (3)	15
3133	46	Tetramer and monomer (3)	
3600	55	Monomer (3)	0.7
3500	67	Monomer (3)	4
3331	70	Monomer (3)	0.6
3192	70	Monomer, and a small amount of tetramer (3)	1
3639	92	Tetramer (3)	4.5
3638	95	Tetramer (3)	5

[a]Determination methods are indicated in parenthesis: (1) velocity sedimentation with purified protein (Ho et al., 1982); (2) sedimentation equilibrium with purified protein (Ho et al., 1982); (3) velocity sedimentation with ^{35}S-methionine-labeled crude extract (Ho et al., 1987).

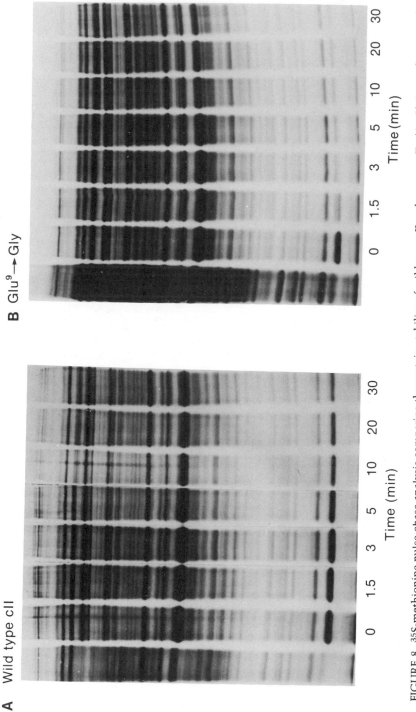

FIGURE 8. ^{35}S-methionine pulse-chase analysis comparing the protein stability of wild-type cII and mutant cIIs. (A–C) Autoradiograms of pulse-chase experiments of (A) wild-type cII, (B) cII mutants Glu^9 → Gly, and (C) Arg^{42} → Gly. The first lane of each autoradiogram is the control. The chasing times are given at the bottom of each lane. The migration positions of cII proteins are indicated by arrows. All of the pulse-chase experiments were done in the lysogen UC5822: N99 (λ int 6 red 3 CI^{857} cII 3067 Pam 3). (D) Half-log plot of representative examples of the half-life determination of cII and various cII mutants. All the mutants in the second α-helical DNA-binding region, including

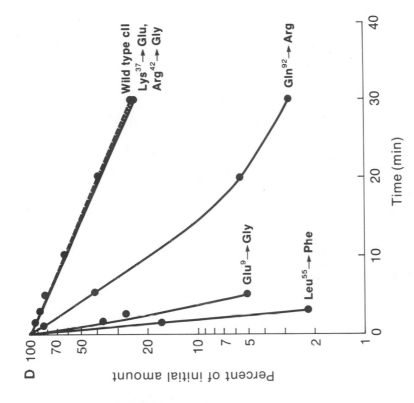

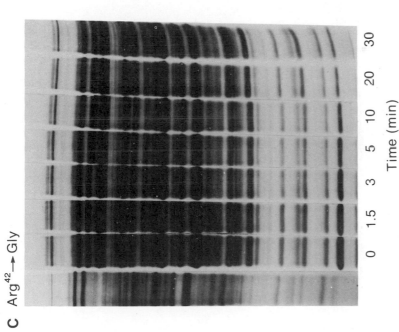

Lys[37] → Glu, Lys[37] → Arg, Ser[38] → Leu, Ile[40] → Asn, Ser[41] → Gly, and Arg[42] → Gly, have the same half-lives as wild-type cII protein. The mutants in the region of amino acid residues 9–25 and 46–71, including Glu[9] → Gly, Leu[24] → Pro, Leu[55] → Phe, Met[67] → Thr, Leu[70] → Ser, and Leu[70] → Phe, are very unstable. Their half-lives fall in the same category as Glu[9] → Gly and Leu[55] → phe, which are shown on this figure as two representative mutants of these two regions.

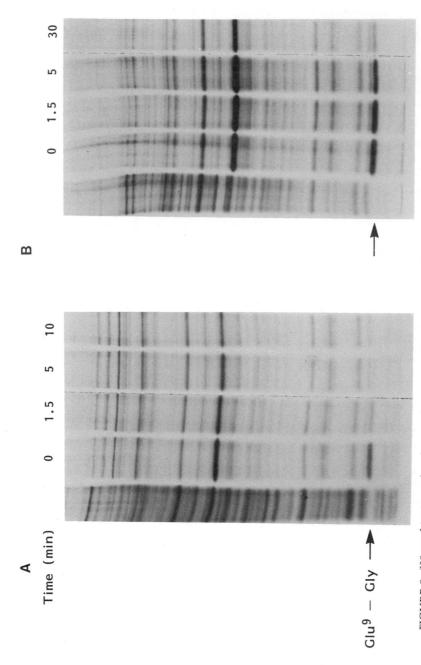

FIGURE 9. ³⁵S-methionine pulse-chase analysis comparing the protein stability of a highly unstable cII mutant, Glu⁹ → Gly, with wild-type cII in the HtpR⁻ and HtpR⁺ E. coli host strains (AR67 and AR65, respectively). The autoradiograms of pulse-chase experiments are shown as follows: (A) cII Glu⁹ → Gly in HtpR⁺ (AR65); (B) cII Glu⁹ → Gly in HtpR⁻

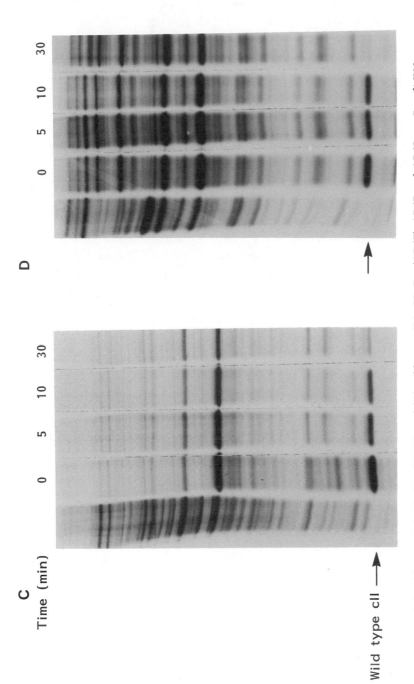

C

Time (min)

Wild type cII ⟶

D

Wild type cII ⟶

(AR67); (C) wild-type cI in HtpR⁺ (AR65); and (D) wild-type cII in HtpR⁻ (AR67). AR67 and AR65 are *E. coli* K12 derivatives designated as follows: AR67; CAG456(cI^{857} kil^- H1)galE::Tn10 (patent 14252); AR65: SC122(cI^{857} kil^- H1)galE::Tn10 (patent 14252).

additional independent correlation between this class of mutants and protein stability strengthens our previous conclusion that the two distinct regions defined by these mutants comprise structural domains crucial for stable tetramer formation. Interestingly, these two domains, which comprise 40% of the molecule, contain more than 60% of the hydrophobic residues of cII, implying that hydrophobic interaction might be directly involved in the subunit-subunit interaction in the tetrameric conformation.

C. The DNA-Binding Domain: Amino Acid Residues 26–45

We have characterized about 20 different amino acid substitutions in a region flanked by the two oligomerization domains. Genetic analysis indicates that most of these mutants are defective in positive regulation (Wulff et al., 1984). Yet, in contrast to the mutants located in the oligomerization domains, mutant proteins in this region retained their ability to form tetramers (Table III). This region of cII protein extends from amino acid position 26 to 45 and exhibits structural homology to the helix-turn-helix motif shown by a variety of other DNA binding proteins, such as λ repressor cI and λ cro (Fig. 10). Crystallographic study of several different DNA-binding regulatory proteins has indicated that this is the common structural motif used by these proteins to recognize their specific DNA-binding sites (Anderson et al., 1981; McKay and Steitz, 1981; Ohlendorf et al., 1982; Pabo and Lewis, 1982). This motif consists of two α-helical regions in the protein. They are 7 and 9 amino acid residues

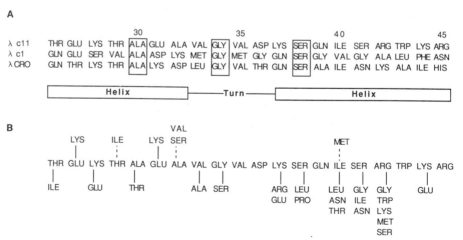

FIGURE 10. Amino acid sequences of the DNA binding domain. (A) Alignment of cII amino acid sequences in the region (from amino acid positions 26–45) corresponding to α-helices 2 and 3 of λ repressor and λ cro protein. Regions of amino acid identity are boxed. (B) Amino acid sequence and single amino acid substitutions in the proposed helix-turn-helix region of cII protein. The amino acid alterations shown below the sequence are defective in cII function. The amino acid changes shown above the sequence indicate mutations that maintain full (solid lines) or partial (dotted lines) cII function.

long, respectively, and separated by a short, 4-amino-acid-long "turn" region. This "turn" region permits the two helices to be juxtapositioned at an appropriate angle for their interactions with DNA.

Twelve different amino acid substitutions were defined in the postulated second α-helical DNA-binding region of the cII protein (Figs. 7, 10). We have overexpressed and purified five of these mutants: cII 3563 (Lys[37] to Arg), cII SDM-1 (Lys[37] to Glu), cII 3062 (Ser[38] to Leu), cII 3378 (Ser[41] to Gly), and cII 3151 (Arg[42] to Gly). Sedimentation analysis indicated that all these mutant proteins retained their ability to form tetramers (see Table III). Apparently, mutations in this region have little effect on overall cII structure. Moreover, most of these mutants retain their ability to bind DNA nonspecifically. However, DNase protection experiments (Fig. 11A) demonstrated that they have lost their ability to bind the specific cII recognition sequence. In addition, these mutants showed no activation function in *in vitro* transcription, even at greater than 10-fold higher concentrations of protein than those used for the wild-type protein (Fig. 11B). Clearly, the mutations in this region define a domain of cII protein important for DNA interaction (Figs. 7, 10). That many of these second helix mutations are conservative amino acid changes (e.g., Lys[37] to Arg, Ser[46] to Gly, Arg[42] to Lys) suggests that the specific side chains of these amino acid residues, rather than their general acidic/basic/polar/nonpolar properties, are important for DNA interaction. This biochemical evidence clearly indicates that the second helical region plays a key role in the sequence-specific DNA-protein recognition. This finding is also consistent with the predication made from the helix-turn-helix model which suggests that this region penetrates into the major groove of the DNA and makes highly specific contacts with the nucleotide bases exhibited in this groove.

We have also characterized several different amino acid substitutions in the proposed first α-helical DNA-binding region of the cII protein (Fig. 10). Analogous to the mutants discussed above, all these variant proteins form tetramers. Functionally, some of these are "up" mutations and some are "down" mutations. Genetic experiments indicate that the Lys[28] to Glu and the Ala[32] to Ser or Val alteration in this region results in a cII "down" effect. We have expressed and purified the severely defective Lys[28] to Glu protein. DNAase protection experiments demonstrated that in contrast to the mutations in the second α-helix described above, this mutant retains its ability to bind selectively to the appropriate DNA recognition site in the presence of RNA polymerase, albeit at greatly reduced affinity (Fig. 11A). When supplied in high concentration, this protein also activated *in vitro* transcription (Fig. 11). Two "up" mutations have been characterized in this same proposed first α-helical region, designated dya-8 (Glu[27] to Lys) and dya-1 (Glu[31] to Lys). These two cII mutants were obtained by selecting for cII-dependent promoter function at a defective P_{RE} signal containing an altered cII recognition element (Wulff *et al.*, 1984). Both mutants not only functioned at the detective promoter but also retained their ability to activate the wild-type signal.

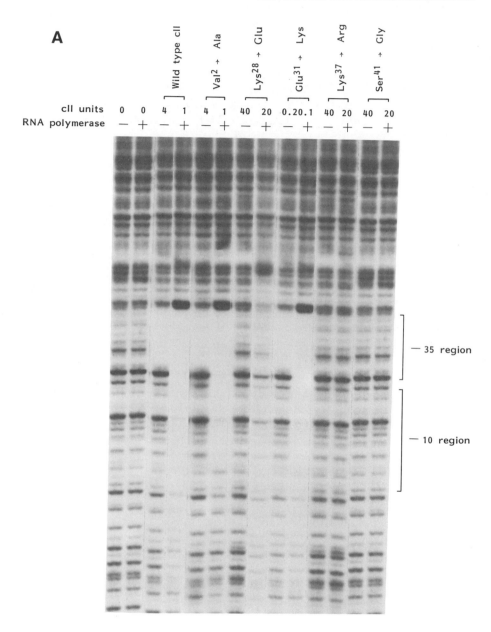

FIGURE 11. DNase protection and transcription activation analysis comparing the wild-type cII with cII mutants. (A) DNase I protection experiments were carried out essentially as described previously (Ho et al., 1983). Purified cII and cII mutant proteins were added as indicated. The relative units of protein are given at the top of each lane. One unit corresponds to a concentration of 0.35 µM tetramer. Where indicated, 0.6 units of RNA polymerase (sp. act. 320 µ/mg, Molecular Biology Division, Pharmacia) were added to the reaction. The purification of the mutant cII proteins was carried out as described by Ho et al.

B

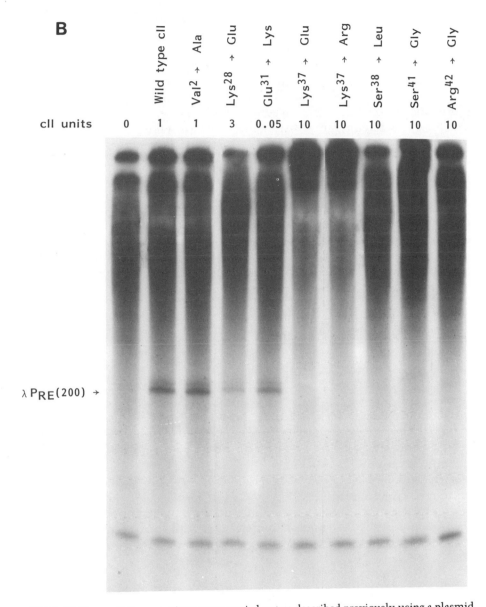

λ P$_{RE}$(200) →

(1987). (B) Transcription reactions were carried out as described previously using a plasmid that carries P$_{RE}$ promoter signal as DNA template (Ho et al., 1982). An autoradiogram is shown of a PAGE analysis of ^{32}P-labeled RNA transcripts synthesized in vitro in the presence of purified cII proteins. The relative units of protein are given at the top of each lane. One unit corresponds to a concentration of 45-nM tetramer. From left to right: No cII protein; wild-type cII; cII Val^2 → Ala; cII Lys^{28} → Glu; cII Glu^{31} → Lys; cII Lys^{37} → Glu; cII Lys^{37} → Arg; cII Ser^{38} → Leu; cII Ser^{41} → Gly; cII Arg^{42} → Gly.

We have over-produced and purified the dya-1 protein for bio-chemical studies. In the process of protein purification, this protein showed a very strong nonspecific DNA-binding affinity. Examination of the chromatographic behavior of this protein on DNA agarose columns also demonstrated that it had a very strong nonspecific interaction with calf thymus DNA. Moreover, high salt concentrations were required to elute this protein during phosphocellulose chromatography (0.68 M of salt for dya-1 as compared with 0.46 M salt for wild-type cII). In both *in vitro* transcription reactions and DNA footprinting experiments, this protein exhibited a dramatically enhanced (approximately 8-fold) ability to bind and function at P_{RE} promoter (Fig. 11). These results indicate that the mutant protein has dramatically increased nonspecific affinity for DNA which allows it to recognize and function with enhanced activity at the wild-type signal and also recognize and function at altered signals that would normally be defective.

The results on both "up" and "down" mutations strongly suggest that the first α-helical region plays a major role in determining the general affinity for DNA rather than the sequence-specific DNA interaction. The nature of the amino acid substitutions in these cII variants is most consistent with this contention. The lysine residue at these positions would be expected to favor ionic interaction between cII and DNA, whereas the acidic glutamate substitution would oppose this interaction. Clearly, the results from these mutational analyses not only support the contention that cII utilizes the helix-turn-helix motif for DNA interaction, but help to define further the more specialized and distinct functions of the two α-helical DNA-binding structures. They strongly implicate that the second helical region, which is the only region of the cII protein in which substitutions result in the selective loss of sequence-specific DNA binding while maintaining the ability to form tetramers and to bind DNA nonspecifically, plays a key role in highly specific protein-DNA recognition. On the other hand, the first α-helical region performs a primary function in stabilizing the nonspecific interactions of the protein with DNA via ionic interactions with the phosphate residues along the backbone of DNA.

D. The Carboxyterminal Domain: Amino Acid Residues 72–97

The last domain of the cII protein encompasses the carboxyterminal 25–amino acid residues (positions 72–97, Fig. 7). This region is characterized by seven amino acid substitutions, most of which exhibit a partial defective phenotype. These variant proteins appear to retain their ability to form tetramers; however, this ability may be somewhat impaired. Pulse-chase experiments demonstrated that although these mutants are more stable in *E. coli* than the highly unstable mutants described above, they are significantly less stable than is wild-type (Table III and Fig. 8).

In addition, we found that these carboxyterminal mutants were stabilized in the HtpR⁻ host just the same as the highly unstable mutants. These mutants are thus recognized by the same proteolytic system that degrades the highly unstable class of cII mutants, but they are less susceptible to this system, presumably because they still form tetramers. Apparently, the carboxyterminal domain of the protein is not essential for DNA interaction, but rather plays a structural role in helping to stabilize the formation of the tetrameric structure.

VI. CROSS-REACTIVITY OF λ cII AND P22 C1 PROTEINS ON PROMOTER SIGNALS FROM λ, P22, AND i21 PHAGES

There exist several other λ-related bactiophages that carry cII-like transcription activators, such as *Salmonella* phage P22 C1 and λ phage i21 cII. Amino acid sequence comparison shows that these two molecules share 50% and 32% homology with cII protein, respectively (Fig. 12A). Examination of the promoter signals activated by these proteins indicates that all of these signals share the common TTGCN₆TTGC/T repeat sequence identically positioned in each site (Fig. 12B). This remarkable conservation of both the activator proteins and the activator-dependent promoter signals reflects a common origin of evolution. Moreover, it predicts that each activator protein might recognize and cross-react with the homologous regions of these heterogeneous promoter signals.

To verify this prediction, the C1 gene of *Salmonella* phage P22, an analogue of λ cII gene, was cloned, overproduced, and purified to homogeniety (Ho, Pfarr, and Rosenberg, unpublished results). The activation function of pure λ cII and P22 C1 proteins at the P_RE promoter of phages λ, P22, and i21 was examined. The results shown in Fig. 13 indicate that both λ cII and P22 C1 protein activate transcription from all of these three promoters in the presence of excess RNA polymerase, although different amounts of activator are required for function at different sites (Ho and Rosenberg, unpublished results). DNase protection analysis demonstrated that, λ cII, and P22 C1 not only bind selectively to the −35 region sequence of their own P_RE promoter, they bind selectively to each others' P_RE promoter as well. Again, different levels of protein are required to achieve the complete protection (Ho and Rosenberg, unpublished results). These data not only support the contention that the TTGC repeat sequence is the core recognition element for λ cII protein, they strongly suggest that this contention is also valid for P22 C1. Figure 12B shows that the last base of the TTGC repeat sequence in P22 P_RE promoter is T instead of the C found in the λ P_RE promoter. The cross-reactivity of λ cII protein on P22 P_RE promoter indicates that this change is acceptable for cII function. As mentioned previously, there is a λ P_RE point mutation designated ctr 1 (Wulff *et al.*, 1984) which has the same base-pair substitution at this position as in P22 P_RE—that is, TTGCN₆TTG*T*. Transcription *in vitro* demonstrated that

A

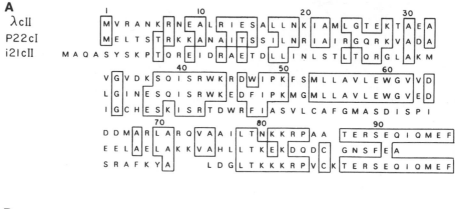

B

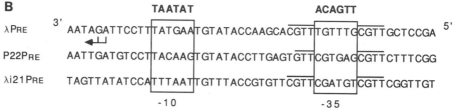

FIGURE 12. (A) Comparison of the amino acid sequence of the λ cII protein with the analogous transcrition activators, P22 Cl and i21 cII. The amino acid sequences are given in standard single-letter code. Regions of amino acid identity between these three proteins are boxed. (B) DNA sequences of the nontemplate strands of the three P$_{RE}$ promoters from phage λ, P22, and λ i21. The transcription start sites are indicated by arrows. The boxed regions correspond to and are compared with the −10 and −35 region consensus sequences for promoters recognized by E. coli RNA polymerase (Rosenberg and Court, 1979). The tetranucleotide repeat sequences are overscored.

the activation efficiency of cII protein for ctr 1 P$_{RE}$ was similar to that for wild-type P$_{RE}$ (Ho and Rosenberg, unpublished results). These data support our definition of the core recognition sequence and identify this single position in the TTGC repeat sequence where either of the two pyrimidines are acceptable for the specific protein-DNA interaction.

To our surprise, examination of cross-reactivity in vivo indicated that each of the activator systems exhibits specificity. That is, no cross-reactivity is observed between these different phage systems when examined by standard genetic trans-complementation tests or by supplying activator to heterologous P$_{RE}$–galK fusion. One possible explanation is that although the λ cII and P22 Cl recognize the same core TTGCN$_6$TTGC/T repeat sequence, the efficiency of these interactions is influenced by the particular sequence context surrounding the repeat unit. These quantitative differences in recognition efficiency could be responsible for the major physiological consequences observed. Moreover, there are clear

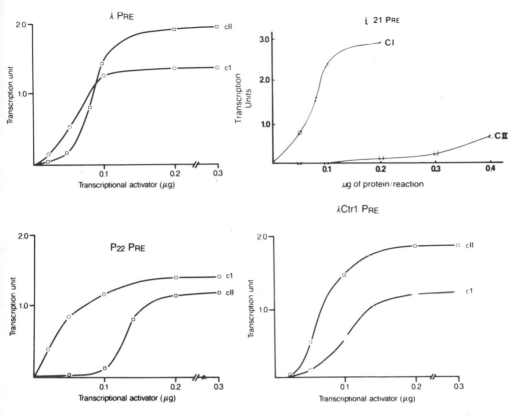

FIGURE 13. Comparison of transcription activation responses to cII protein for the four different P$_{RE}$ promoters of phage λ, P22, i21, and λ ctrl. Transcription reactions were carried out as described previously (Ho *et al.*, 1983). The transcription unit is arbitrary, and it is defined as follows: The intensity of each transcript induced by different amounts of cII proteins was first quantitated by using a Beckman DU-8 spectrophotometer with a gel scanning accessory, then normalized with the intensity of the transcript from ori as an internal control.

biochemical distinctions between the way the P22 C1 and λ cII proteins interact with DNA. For example, DNA-binding and competition experiments have demonstrated that P22 C1 forms more stable complexes with DNA than does λ cII, even at the phage λ recognition sites (Keilty and Rosenberg, unpublished results). Thus, it may be an inherent difference in the formation and kinetics of the activator-DNA complex and its recognition by RNA polymerase that results in the observed phage system specificity. Efforts are currently being directed toward altering the particular amino acids in the DNA-binding regions of P22 C1 and λ cII as well as changing the sequences in and around the tetranucleotide elements in various promoters. We expect that the detailed comparative study of two (or more) positive regulatory analogues should help discern the molecular details of the protein-DNA interactions and especially provide insight into the signal-recognition specificity and efficiency observed.

VII. CONTROL OF cII DEGRADATION

The level of cII protein in an infected cell has been proposed to be the crucial determinant in the lysis-lysogeny decision of phage λ (Herskowitz and Hagen, 1980). This level depends on the balance of the rate of synthesis (transcription, translation, processing, and oligomerization) and degradation of cII. cII is known to be relatively unstable in infected cells and can be detected only in the early stage of infection (Reichardt, 1975; Hoyt et al., 1982). The rate of degradation plays a key role in determining the levels of cII present in infected cells.

The importance of the host factor, hfl, and the λ cIII protein in cII degradation has been reviewed by Herskowitz and Hagen (1980) and Wulff and Rosenberg (1983). The general understanding is that the host HflA protein is partially responsible for controlling the degradation of cII protein. The λ cIII protein, which is necessary for high efficiency of lysogeny, was thought to be an antagonist of hflA. It enhances lysogenization by opposing the proteolytic consequences of this host factor (Gautsch and Wulff, 1974).

Recently, more detailed biochemical studies give new insight on the correlation of the host factor hfl and λ cIII protein with cII stability. By using ^{35}S-methionine pulse-chase analysis, the turnover rate of cII protein in different hfl$^-$ and cIII$^-$ backgrounds was examined. The results demonstrated that cIII not only protects cII against hfl-mediated degradation, it also enhances the stability of cII protein in hfl$^-$ host cells. This is true for cII made after infection (Hoyt et al., 1982) and for cII overproduced from expression vectors in both hflA$^-$ (Ho and Rosenberg, unpublished results) and hflB$^-$ host strains (Banuett et al., 1986). Figure 14A summarizes our results. The half-life (in minutes) of cII protein in lysogens carrying different combinations of hflA and λ cIII mutations varies as follows: 8 min in cIII$^-$ hflA$^+$, 14 min in cIII$^+$ hglA$^+$, 20 min in cIII$^-$ hflA$^-$, and 25 min in cIII$^+$ hflA$^-$. These results demonstrate that cIII protein has a protective effect on cII protein in the absence of hfl and thus cannot simply be an antagonist of host hfl factors. Perhaps cIII protein exerts its protective function by more than one mechanism. Clearly, a combination of cIII$^+$ and hfl$^-$ results in the highest stabilizing effect for cII, increasing its half-life up to 25 min.

We tested whether hflA$^-$ host strains can stabilize certain unstable cII mutant proteins and whether cIII protein can act as a general protease inhibitor. Several cII mutants were transformed into different cIII$^+$ versus cIII$^-$ and hflA$^-$ versus hflA$^+$ background host strains. A representative example is given in Fig. 14B. cII 3085, a Glu to Gly mutant at amino

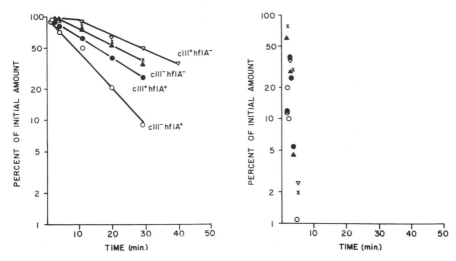

FIGURE 14. Comparison of the protein stability of wild-type and Glu^9 → Gly mutant cII in different hfl and λ cIII mutant lysogens. (A) Half-log plot of the half-life determination of wild-type cII. cIII$^-$ hflA$^+$ (UC5876):N99(λ int. 6 red. 3 cIII$_{co2}$ cI^{857} cII3067 Pam 3); cIII$^-$ hflA$^-$, the following two lysogens have been used; they are UC5882, N99 hflA-150 (λ int. 6 red. 3 cIII$_{co2}$ cI^{857} cII3067 Pam 3) and UC 5881, N99hfl-1 (λ int. 6 red. 3 cIII$_{co2}$ cI^{857} cII3067 pAM 3). cIII$^+$ hflA$^-$ (UC5835):N99hfl-1 (λ int. 6 red. 3 cI^{857} cII3067 Pam 3). (B) Half-log plot of the half-life determination of cII3085 (Glu^9 → Gly). The different lysogens used are the same as described above.

acid position 9, shows no change of its extremely short half-life in any of these host strains. These results suggest that the proteolytic mechanism involved in the normal turnover of cII protein is probably very different from that responsible for degrading the mutant protein. A second set of experiments supports this contention. As was mentioned previously, a HtpR$^-$ E. coli strain showed remarkable stabilizing effects on a whole class of highly unstable cII mutants that were incapable of properly forming oligomers. The half-lives of these mutants were extended from less than 3 min to 15 min or longer. Surprisingly, the half-life of wild-type cII in this strain remained totally unchanged (Fig. 9). Apparently, different degradation mechanisms are able to differentiate the nonfunctional monomer form of this protein from the functional tetramer. We expect that this is probably a general mechanism operative in bacteria and other organisms that can discriminate mutated defective, foreign, or otherwise altered forms of proteins from their normal counterparts.

ACKNOWLEDGMENTS. We thank Daniel Wulff for kindly providing us with certain E. coli and λ phage strains used in this work, and Ruth Hatton for editing and typing the manuscript.

REFERENCES

Abraham, J., Mascarenhas, D., Fischer, R., Benedik, M., Campbell, A., and Echols, H., 1980, DNA sequence of the regulatory region for the integration gene of bacteriophage, *Proc. Natl. Acad. Sci. USA* **77**:2477.

Aiba, H., and Krakow, J. S., 1981, Isolation and characterization of the amino and carboxyl proximal fragments of the adenosine cyclic 3',5'-phosphate receptor protein of *Escherichia coli*+, *Biochemistry* **20**:4774–4780.

Anderson, W. F., Ohlendorf, D. H., Takeda, Y., and Matthews, B. W., 1981, Structure of the cro repressor from bacteriophage and its interaction with DNA, *Nature* **290**:754–758.

Banuett, F., Hoyt, M. A., McFarlane, L., Echols, H., and Herskowitz, I., 1986, hflB, a new *Escherichia coli* locus regulating lysogeny and the level of bacteriophage lambda cII protein, *J. Mol. Biol.* **187**:213–224.

Belfort, M., and Wulff, D. L., 1973a, Genetic and biochemical investigation of the *Escherichia coli* mutant hfl-1 which is lysogenized at high frequency by bacteriophage lambda, *J. Bacteriol.* **115**:299.

Belfort, M., and Wulff, D. L., 1973b, An analysis of the processes of infection and induction of *E. coli* hfl-1 by bacteriophage lambda, *Virology* **55**:183.

Bennett, G. N., Brown, K. D., and Yanofsky, C., 1977, Nucleotide sequence of the promoter-operator region of the tryptophan operon for *E. coli* and *S. typhimurium*, *Fed. Proc.* **36**(3199):878.

Brachet, P., and Thomas, R., 1969, Mapping and functional analysis of y and cII mutants, *Mutat. Res.* **7**:257–264.

Davies, R. W., 1980, DNA sequence of the int-xis-P_I region of the bacteriophage lambda: Overlap of the int and xis genes, *Nucleic Acids Res.* **8**:1765–1782.

Dickson, R. C., Abelson, J., Barnes, W. M., and Reznikoff, W. S., 1975, Genetic regulation: The lac control region, *Science* **187**:27–35.

Eliason, J., Weiss, M., and Ptashne, M., 1985, NH_2-terminal arm of phage repressor contributes energy and specificity to repressor binding, *Proc. Natl. Acad. Sci. USA* **82**:2339–2343.

Gautsch, J. W., and Wulff, D. L., 1974, Fine structure mapping, complementation, and physiology of *Escherichia coli* hfl mutants, *Genetics* **77**:435.

Gilbert, W., Maxam, A., and Mirzabekov, A., 1976, Contacts between the lac repressor and DNA revealed by methylation, in: *Control of Ribosome Synthesis*, Alfred Benson Symposium IX (N. O. Kjeldgaard and O. Maaloe, eds.), p. 139, Academic Press, New York.

Herskowitz, I., and Hagen, D. A., 1980, The lysis-lysogeny decision of phage λ: Explicit programming and responsiveness, *Annu. Rev. Genet.* **14**:399–445.

Ho, Y. S., and Rosenberg, M., 1982, Characterization of the phage λ regulatory protein cII, *Ann. Microbiol. (Paris)* **133A**:215–218.

Ho, Y. S., and Rosenberg, M., 1985, Characterization of a third, cII-dependent, coordinately activated promoter on phage involved in lysogenic development, *J. Biol. Chem.* **260**:11838–11844.

Ho, Y. S., Lewis, M., and Rosenberg, M., 1982, Purification and properties of a transcriptional activator, *J. Biol. Chem.* **257**:9128–9134.

Ho, Y. S., Wulff, D., and Rosenberg, M., 1983, Bacteriophage protein cII binds promoters on the opposite face of the DNA helix from RNA polymerase, *Nature* **304**:703–708.

Ho, Y. S., Mahoney, M. E., Wulff, D. L., and Rosenberg, M., 1988, Identification of the DNA binding domain of the phage lambda cII transcriptional activator, and the direct correlation of cII protein stability with its oligomeric forms, *Genes Dev.* **2**:184–195.

Hoess, R. H., Foeller, C., Bidwell, K., and Landy, A., 1980, Site-specific recombination functions of bacteriophage λ: DNA sequence of the regulatory regions and overlapping structural genes for Int and Xis, *Proc. Natl. Acad. Sci. USA* **77**:2482–2487.

Hoopes, B., and McClure, W., 1985, A cII-dependent promoter is located within the Q gene of bacteriophage λ, *Proc. Natl. Acad. Sci. USA* **82**:3134–3138.

Hoyt, M. A., Knight, D. M., Das, A., Miller, H. I., and Echols, H., 1982, Control of phage λ development by stability and synthesis of cII protein: Role of the viral cIII and host hflA, himA, and himD genes, *Cell* **31**:565.

Johnson, A. D., Meyer, B. J., and Ptashne, M., 1978, Mechanism of action of the cro protein of bacteriophage, *Proc. Natl. Acad. Sci. USA* **75**:1783–1787.

Keilty, S., and Rosenberg, M., 1987, Constitutive function of a positively regulated promoter reveals new sequences essential for activity, *J. Biol. Chem.* **262**:6389–6395.

Lawley, P. D., and Brookes, P., 1963, Further studies on the alkylation of nucleic acids and their constituent nucleotides, *Biochem. J.* **89**:127–135.

Majors, J., 1978, Ph.D. Thesis, Harvard University, Cambridge, MA.

Maniatis, T., Ptashne, M., Backman, K., Kleid, D., Flashman, S., Jeffrey, A., and Mauer, R., 1975, Recognition sequences of repressor and polymerase in the operators of bacteriophage lambda, *Cell* **5**:109–113.

McKay, D. B., and Steitz, T. A., 1981, Structure of catabolite gene activator protein at 2.9 A resolution suggests binding to left-handed B-DNA, *Nature* **290**:744–749.

McKay, D. B., Weber, I. T., and Steitz, T. A., 1982, Structure of catabolite gene activator protein at 2.9-A resulution, *J. Biol. Chem.* **257**:9518–9524.

Mott, J. E., Grant, R. A., Ho, Y. S., and Platt, T., 1985, Maximizing gene expression from plasmid vectors containing the λ P_L promoter: Strategies for overproducing transcription termination factor p, *Proc. Natl. Acad. Sci. USA* **82**:88–92.

Ohlendorf, D. H., Anderson, W. F., Fisher, R. G., Takeda, Y., and Matthews, B. W., 1982, The molecular basis of DNA-protein recognition inferred from the structure of cro repressor, *Nature* **298**:718–723.

Pabo, C. O., and Lewis, M., 1982, The operator-binding domain of λ repressor-structure and DNA recognition, *Nature* **298**:443.

Reichardt, L., 1975, Control of bacteriophage lambda repressor synthesis after phage infection: The role of the N, cII, cIII and cro products, *J. Mol. Biol.* **93**:267.

Rosenberg, M., and Court, D., 1979, Regulatory sequences involved in the promotion and termination of RNA transcription, *Annu. Rev. Genet.* **13**:319–353.

Rosenberg, M., Court, D., Shimatake, H., Brady, C., and Wulff, D. L., 1978a, Structure and function of an intercistronic regulatory region in bacteriophage lambda, in: *The Operon* (J. H. Miller and W. S. Reznikoff, eds.), pp. 304–324, Cold Spring Harbor Laboratory, Cold Spring Harbor, NY.

Rosenberg, M., Court, D., Shimatake, H., Brady, C., and Wulff, D. L., 1978b, The relationship between function and DNA sequence in an intercistronic regulatory region in phage λ, *Nature* **272**:414 423.

Rosenberg, M., Ho, Y. S., and Shatzman, A., 1983, The use of pKC30 and its derivatives for controlled expression of genes, in: *Methods in Enzymology*, Vol. 101 (R. Wu, L. Grossman, and K. Moldave, eds.), pp. 123–138, Academic Press, New York.

Schmeissner, U., Court, D., Shimatake, H., and Rosenberg, M., 1980, Promoter for the establishment of repressor synthesis in bacteriophage λ, *Proc. Natl. Acad. Sci. USA* **77**:3191–3196.

Schmeissner, U., Court, D., Shimatake, H., and Rosenberg, M., 1981, Positively activated transcription of λ integrase gene initiates with Utp *in vivo*, *Nature* **292**:173–175.

Schwarz, E., Scherer, G., Hobom, G., and Kossel, H., 1978, Nucleotide sequence of cro, cII and part of the O gene in phage λ DNA, *Nature* **272**:410.

Shimatake, H., and Rosenberg, M., 1981, Purified regulatory protein cII positively activates promoters for lysogenic development, *Nature* **292**:128–132.

Siebenlist, U., Simpson, R. B., and Gilbert, W., 1980, E. coli RNA polymerase interacts homologously with two different promoters, *Cell* **20**:269–281.

Singer, B., 1975, The chemical effects of nucleic acid alkylation and their relation to mutagenesis and carcinogenesis, *Prog. Nucleic Acids Res. Mol. Biol.* **15**:219–284.

Wulff, D. L., and Rosenberg, M., 1983, Establishment of repressor synthesis, in: *The Bacteriophage Lambda*, Vol. 2 (J. Hendrix, J. Roberts, F. Stahl, and R. Weisberg, eds.), pp. 53–73, Cold Spring Harbor Laboratory, Cold Spring Harbor, NY.

Wulff, D. L., Beher, M., Isumi, S., Beck, J., Mahoney, M., Shimatake, H., Brady, C., Court, D., and Rosenberg, M., 1980, Structure and function of the cy control region of bacteriophage lambda, *J. Mol. Biol.* **138:**209–230.
Wulff, D. L., Mahoney, M., Shatzman, A., and Rosenberg, M., 1984, Mutational analysis of a regulatory region in bacteriophage λ that has overlapping signals for the initiation of transcription and translation, *Proc. Natl. Acad. Sci. USA* **81:**555–559.

Index